ALIMENTARY TRACT RADIOLOGY

Volume 2

ALIMENTARY TRACT RADIOLOGY

Fourth Edition

Edited by

Alexander R. Margulis, M.D.

Professor and Chairman,
Department of Radiology,
University of California,
San Francisco,
School of Medicine,
San Francisco, California

H. Joachim Burhenne, M.D., F.R.C.P. (C)

Professor and Head,
Department of Radiology,
University of British Columbia,
Vancouver, British Columbia, Canada

With 4454 illustrations, including 44 in color

The C. V. Mosby Company

ST. LOUIS · BALTIMORE · TORONTO   1989

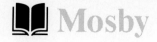 Mosby

Editor: George Stamathis
Developmental Editor: Kathryn H. Falk
Production Editor: Stephen Dierkes
Designer: Rey Umali

Fourth edition

The C. V. Mosby Company
11830 Westline Industrial Drive, St. Louis, Missouri 63146

Library of Congress Cataloging-in-Publication Data

Alimentary tract radiology.

    Includes bibliographies and index.
     1. Alimentary canal—Radiography. I. Margulis,
Alexander R. II. Burhenne, H. Joachim (Hans Joachim),
1925-   . [DNLM: 1 .Digestive System—radiography.
WI 141 A411]
RC804.R6A 1989   616.3′30757   88-8345
ISBN 0-8016-3191-2 (set)

CONTRIBUTORS

SERGIO A. AJZEN, M.D.

Fellow, Department of Radiology, University of British Columbia, Vancouver, British Columbia, Canada

GREGORY J. ALLEN, M.D.

Fellow, Department of Radiology, University of British Columbia, Vancouver, British Columbia

JOE ARIYAMA, M.D.

Associate Professor, Department of Gastroenterology, Jutendo University School of Medicine, Tokyo, Japan

THOMAS J. BECK, Sc.D.

Instructor in Radiology, The Russell H. Morgan Department of Radiology and Radiological Science, The Johns Hopkins University School of Medicine, Baltimore, Maryland

CHRISTOPH D. BECKER, M.D.

Fellow, Department of Radiology, University of British Columbia, Vancouver, British Columbia

ROBERT N. BERK, M.D.

Professor, Department of Radiology, University of California, San Diego, School of Medicine; Editor-in-Chief, American Journal of Roentgenology, San Diego, California

PIERRE BODART, M.D.

Professor and Chairman, Department of Diagnostic Radiology, Universite Catholique de Louvain, Cliniques Universitaires St. Luc, Brussels, Belgium

DOUGLAS P. BOYD, Ph.D.

Professor of Radiology (Physics), Department of Radiology, University of California, San Francisco, School of Medicine, San Francisco, California

ROBERT C. BRASCH, M.D.

Professor, Department of Radiology and Pediatrics, and Director, Contrast Media Laboratory, University of California, San Francisco, School of Medicine, San Francisco, California

THOMAS F. BUDINGER, M.D., Ph.D.

Professor of Radiology, Department of Radiology, University of California, San Francisco, School of Medicine, San Francisco, California; Henry Miller Professor of Bioinstrumentation, Department of Electrical Engineering and Computer Science, University of California at Berkeley; Division Head, Research and Radiology Biophysics, Lawrence Berkeley Laboratory, Berkeley, California

H. JOACHIM BURHENNE, M.D., F.R.C.P.(C)

Professor and Head, Department of Radiology, University of British Columbia, Head, Department of Radiology, Vancouver General Hospital, Vancouver, British Columbia, Canada

M. PAUL CAPP, M.D.

Professor and Chairman, Department of Radiology, University of Arizona, School of Medicine, Tucson, Arizona

DAVID C. CARTER, M.D.

Regius Professor of Clinical Surgery, University of Edinburgh Royal Infirmary, Edinburgh, Scotland

RONALD A. CASTELLINO, M.D.

Professor of Radiology, Director of Diagnostic Radiology, and Acting Chairman, Department of Diagnostic Radiology and Nuclear Medicine, Stanford University School of Medicine, Stanford, California

ARTHUR R. CLEMETT, M.D.

Professor of Radiology, New York Medical College; Clinical Professor of Radiology, New York University, New York, New York

RONALD A. COHEN, M.D.

Radiologist, Department of Radiology, Children's Hospital Medical Center of Northern California, Oakland, California

MICHAEL COLLIER, Ph.D.

Chief of Clinical Physics, Radiotherapy Service, Lawrence Berkeley Laboratories, Berkeley, California

PETER L. COOPERBERG, M.D.

Professor, Department of Diagnostic Radiology, University of British Columbia; Director, Department of Radiology, St. Paul's Hospital, Vancouver, British Columbia, Canada

v

PETER B. COTTON, M.D.

Professor of Medicine, Chief of Endoscopy, Division of Gastroenterology, Duke University Medical Center, Durham, North Carolina

LAWRENCE E. CROOKS, Ph.D.

Professor of Electrical Engineering, Department of Radiology, University of California, San Francisco, School of Medicine, San Francisco, California

PETER DAWSON, M.R.C.P., F.R.C.R.

Senior Lecturer, Department of Diagnostic Radiology, University of London, Royal Postgraduate Medical School, London, England

BARBARA E. DEMAS, M.D.

Assistant Professor of Radiology, Department of Radiology, University of California, San Francisco, School of Medicine, San Francisco, California

GERALD D. DODD, M.D.

Olga Keith and Harry Carothers Weiss Professor and Head, Division of Diagnostic Imaging, The University of Texas, M.D. Anderson Cancer Center, Houston, Texas

WYLIE J. DODDS, M.D.

Professor of Radiology and Medicine, The Medical College of Wisconsin, Milwaukee, Wisconsin

MARTIN W. DONNER, M.D.

Professor, The Russell H. Morgan Department of Radiology and Radiological Science, The Johns Hopkins University School of Medicine, Baltimore, Maryland

J. SCOTT DUNBAR, M.D.

Clinical Professor of Radiology, University of California, San Francisco, School of Medicine, San Francisco, California

J. STEPHEN FACHE, M.D.

Assistant Professor, Department of Radiology, University of British Columbia, Vancouver, British Columbia

MICHAEL P. FEDERLE, M.D.

Professor of Radiology, University of California, San Francisco, School of Medicine; Chief, Department of Radiology, San Francisco General Hospital, San Francisco, California

ROY A. FILLY, M.D.

Professor of Radiology and of Obstetrics, Gynecology, and Reproductive Medicine; Chief, Section of Diagnostic Ultrasonography, Department of Radiology, University of California, San Francisco, School of Medicine, San Francisco, California

HARVEY V. FINEBERG, M.D., Ph.D.

Dean, Harvard School of Public Health, Harvard University, Boston, Massachusetts

ISAAC R. FRANCIS, M.D.

Associate Professor of Radiology, Department of Radiology, University of Michigan School of Medicine, Ann Arbor, Michigan

PATRICK C. FREENY, M.D.

Clinical Professor of Radiology, Department of Radiology, The Virginia Mason Clinic, University of Washington School of Medicine, Seattle, Washington

BOB W. GAYLER, M.D.

Associate Professor, The Russell H. Morgan Department of Radiology and Radiological Science, The Johns Hopkins University School of Medicine, Baltimore, Maryland

DAVID W. GELFAND, M.D.

Professor and Chief of Gastrointestinal Radiology, Bowman Gray School of Medicine, Winston-Salem, North Carolina

GARY M. GLAZER, M.D.

Professor of Radiology, Department of Radiology; Director, Division of Magnetic Resonance Imaging, University of Michigan Hospitals, Ann Arbor, Michigan

BARRY B. GOLDBERG, M.D.

Professor of Radiology and Director, Division of Ultrasound, Thomas Jefferson University Hospital, Philadelphia, Pennsylvania

HENRY I. GOLDBERG, M.D.

Professor, Department of Radiology, University of California, San Francisco, School of Medicine, San Francisco, California

CHARLES A. GOODING, M.D.

Professor of Radiology and Pediatrics; Executive Vice Chairman, Department of Radiology, University of California, San Francisco, School of Medicine, San Francisco, California

GRETCHEN A. W. GOODING, M.D.

Professor, Department of Radiology, University of California, San Francisco, School of Medicine; Chief, Radiology Service, Veterans Administration Medical Center, San Francisco, California

PHILIP C. GOODMAN, M.D.

Associate Clinical Professor, Department of Radiology, University of California, San Francisco, General Hospital, San Francisco, California

PETER F. HAHN, M.D., Ph.D.

Assistant in Radiology, Department of Radiology, Massachusetts General Hospital, Boston, Massachusetts

ROBERT S. HATTNER, M.D.

Associate Professor, Department of Radiology, University of California, San Francisco, School of Medicine, San Francisco, California

HEDVIG HRICAK, M.D.

Professor of Radiology and Urology, University of California, San Francisco, School of Medicine, San Francisco, California

R. BROOKE JEFFREY, Jr., M.D.

Professor, Department of Radiology, University of California, San Francisco, School of Medicine, San Francisco, California

ELIAS KAZAM, M.D.

Professor of Radiology and Head, Division of Ultrasound and Computed Body Tomography, Department of Radiology, The New York Hospital–Cornell Medical Center, New York, New York

FREDERICK S. KELLER, M.D.

Professor of Radiology and Surgery; Chief, Angiography and Interventional Radiology, Department of Radiology, The University of Alabama at Birmingham, University of Alabama Hospital, Birmingham, Alabama

ROBERT KERLAN, M.D.

Assistant Clinical Professor of Radiology, University of California, San Francisco; Radiologist, Scripps Memorial Hospital, La Jolla, California

ROBERT E. KOEHLER, M.D.

Professor and Vice Chairman, Department of Radiology, The University of Alabama at Birmingham, University of Alabama Hospital, Birmingham, Alabama

GEORGE S. KOSSOFF, D.Sc.Eng.

Director, Ultrasonics Institute, Commonwealth Department of Health, Sydney, Australia

HERBERT Y. KRESSEL, M.D.

Professor, Department of Radiology, Hospital of the University of Pennsylvania, Philadelphia, Pennsylvania

IGNAZIO LaDELFA

Assistant Professor, Division of General Internal Medicine, Department of Medicine, St. Michael's Hospital, University of Toronto, Toronto, Ontario, Canada

FAYE C. LAING, M.D.

Professor, Department of Radiology, University of California, San Francisco, School of Medicine; Chief, Ultrasound Section, San Francisco General Hospital, San Francisco, California

IGOR LAUFER, M.D.

Professor, Department of Radiology and Chief, Gastrointestinal Radiology, Hospital of the University of Pennsylvania, Philadelphia, Pennsylvania

BRIAN C. LENTLE, M.D.

Professor and Head, Division of Nuclear Medicine, Department of Radiology, University of British Columbia and Vancouver General Hospital, Vancouver, British Columbia, Canada

GEORGE R. LEOPOLD, M.D.

Professor of Radiology and Chairman, Department of Radiology, University of California, San Diego, School of Medicine, San Diego, California

MARC S. LEVINE, M.D.

Associate Professor, Department of Radiology, Hospital of the University of Pennsylvania, Philadelphia, Pennsylvania

DAVID K.B. LI, M.D., F.R.C.P.(C)

Associate Professor, Department of Radiology, University of British Columbia, Vancouver, British Columbia, Canada

ARTHUR E. LINDNER, M.D.

Associate Professor of Medicine and Associate Dean, New York University School of Medicine, New York, New York

ANDERS LUNDERQUIST, M.D.

Professor, Department of Diagnostic Radiology; Head, Section for Gastrointestinal Radiology, University Hospital of Lund, Lund, Sweden

PIERRE H. G. MAHIEU

Chef de Clinique Associe, Universite Catholique de Louvain, Institut Chirurgical de Bruxelles and Cliniques Universitaires St. Luc, Brussels, Belgium

DANIEL MAKLANSKY, M.D.

Associate Clinical Professor, Department of Radiology, Mt. Sinai School of Medicine, The City University of New York, New York, New York

ALEXANDER R. MARGULIS, M.D.

Professor and Chairman, Department of Radiology, University of California, San Francisco, School of Medicine, San Francisco, California

JOHN A. MARKISZ, M.D., Ph.D.

Assistant Professor of Radiology, Head Division of Magnetic Resonance Imaging, The New York Hospital–Cornell Medical Center, New York, New York

MASAKAZU MARUYAMA, M.D.

Department of Internal Medicine, Cancer Institute Hospital, Tokyo, Japan; Emeritus Professor of Montendeo University; Visiting Professor of Korea University, and Visiting Professor of Peruvian University

JAMES J. McCORT, M.D.

Clinical Professor Emeritus, Department of Radiology, Stanford University School of Medicine, Stanford, California; Chairman, Department of Radiology, Santa Clara Valley Medical Center, San Jose, California

KENNETH L. MELMON, M.D.

Professor of Medicine and Pharmacology, Division of Clinical Pharmacology, Department of Medicine, Stanford University School of Medicine, Stanford, California

DIETER J. MEYERHOFF, Ph.D.

Research Specialist, Magnetic Resonance Unit, San Francisco VA Medical Center, University of California, San Francisco, San Francisco, California

MORTON A. MEYERS, M.D.

Professor and Chairman, Department of Radiology, State University of New York, Stony Brook, Health Sciences Center, Stony Brook, New York

ROBERT E. MINDELZUN, M.D.

Clinical Associate Professor of Radiology, Stanford University School of Medicine, Stanford, California; Chief, Division of Diagnostic Radiology, Santa Clara Valley Medical Center, Santa Clara, California

IAN W. MONIE, M.B., Ch.B., M.D. (Glas.)

Professor Emeritus of Anatomy and Embryology, Department of Anatomy, University of California, San Francisco, School of Medicine, San Francisco, California

ALBERT A. MOSS, M.D.

Professor and Chairman, Department of Radiology, University of Washington, School of Medicine, Seattle, Washington

J. ODO OP DEN ORTH, M.D.

Consultant Radiologist, Department of Radiology, St. Elizabeth's of Groote Gasthuis, Haarlem, The Netherlands.

GARY M. ONIK, M.D.

Senior Scientist, Allegheny-Singer Research Institute, Pittsburgh, Pennsylvania

THERON W. OVITT, M.D.

Department of Radiology, University of Arizona, Health Sciences Center, Tucson, Arizona

PHILIP E. S. PALMER, M.D., F.R.C.P., F.R.C.R.

Professor and Chairman, Department of Radiology, University of California, Davis, School of Medicine, Davis, California

THEODORE L. PHILLIPS, M.D.

Professor and Chairman, Department of Radiation Oncology, University of California, San Francisco, School of Medicine, San Francisco, California

DAVID C. PRICE, M.D.

Professor of Radiology and Medicine, Section of Nuclear Medicine, University of California, San Francisco, School of Medicine, San Francisco, California

JACQUES PRINGOT, M.D.

Professor, Department of Diagnostic Radiology, Université Catholique de Louvain, Cliniques Universitaires St. Luc, Brussels, Belgium

LESLIE E. QUINT, M.D.

Assistant Professor of Radiology, Department of Radiology, University of Michigan, School of Medicine, Ann Arbor, Michigan

MAURICE M. REEDER, M.D.

Professor and Chairman, Department of Radiology, University of Hawaii School of Medicine, Honolulu, Hawaii

ERNEST J. RING, M.D.

Professor and Head, Interventional Radiology, University of California, San Francisco, School of Medicine, San Francisco, California

JOSEF RÖSCH, M.D.

Professor and Head of Interventional Radiology, The Oregon Health Sciences University, Portland, Oregon

CHARLES A. ROHRMANN, Jr., M.D.

Professor and Vice-Chairman, Department of Radiology, University of Washington School of Medicine, Seattle, Washington

HENRIETTA KOTLUS ROSENBERG, M.D.

Senior Radiologist and Director, Division of Ultrasound, The Children's Hospital of Philadelphia, Professor of Radiology, University of Pennsylvania, School of Medicine, Philadelphia, Pennsylvnia

LEONARD ROSENTHALL, M.D.

Director, Division of Nuclear Medicine, and Professor, Department of Radiology, McGill University, Montreal, Quebec, Canada

WILLIAM A. RUBENSTEIN, M.D.

Associate Professor of Clinical Radiology, The New York Hospital–Cornell Medical Center, New York, New York

PIERRE SCHNYDER, M.D.

Privat Docent et Agrege, Department of Radiology, University of Lausanne, Lausanne, Switzerland

WILLIAM B. SEAMAN, M.D.

J. Picker Professor Emeritus, Department of Radiology, College of Physicians and Surgeons, Columbia University, New York, New York

HOWARD A. SHAPIRO, M.D.

Professor, Department of Medicine, University of California, San Francisco, School of Medicine, San Francisco, California

HIKOO SHIRAKABE, M.D.

Honorary Professor of Jutendo University School of Medicine, Chairman of Foundation for Detection of Early Gastric Carcinoma, and Directing Chief of Central Clinic, Tokyo, Japan

EDWARD B. SINGLETON, M.D.

Chief and Director of Radiology, St. Luke's Episcopal Hospital and Texas Children's Hospital; Professor of Radiology, Baylor College of Medicine; Clinical Professor of Radiology, University of Texas Medical School, Houston, Texas

JOVITAS SKUCAS, M.D.

Professor of Radiology, School of Medicine and Dentistry, University of Rochester, Rochester, New York

PREMYSL SLEZAK, M.D., Ph.D.

Associate Professor, Department of Diagnostic Radiology–Endoscopy Unit, Karolinska Hospital, Stockholm, Sweden

VERNON SMITH, M.S.C.

Associate Adjunct Professor, Department of Radiation Oncology, University of California, San Francisco, School of Medicine, San Francisco, California

†EDWARD A. SMUCKLER, M.D., Ph.D.

Former Professor and Chairman, Department of Pathology, University of California, San Francisco, School of Medicine, San Francisco, California

HARLAN J. SPJUT, M.D.

The Clarence and Irene Fulbright Professor, Department of Pathology, Baylor College of Medicine, Houston, Texas

DAVID D. STARK, M.D.

Associate Professor of Radiology, Harvard Medical School, Massachusetts General Hospital, Boston, Massachusetts

DAVID H. STEPHENS, M.D.

Professor of Radiology, Mayo Medical School; Department of Diagnostic Radiology, Mayo Clinic and Mayo Foundation, Rochester, Minnesota

GILES W. STEVENSON, M.D.

Professor and Chairman, Department of Diagnostic Radiology, McMaster University; Head of Section, Department of Radiology, Chedoke-McMaster Hospitals, Hamilton, Ontario, Canada

---

†Deceased

EDWARD T. STEWART, M.D.

Professor of Radiology and Chief of Gastrointestinal Radiology, Department of Radiology, Medical College of Wisconsin, Milwaukee, Wisconsin

IAN C. TALBOT, M.D.

Consultant Histo-Pathologist, St. Mark's Hospital, London, England

HOOSHANG TAYBI, M.D., M.Sc.

Clinical Professor of Radiology, University of California, San Francisco, School of Medicine, San Francisco, California; Radiologist, Department of Radiology, Children's Hospital Medical Center, Oakland, California

RUEDI F. THOENI, M.D.

Associate Professor, Department of Radiology and Chief of Computed Tomography/Gastrointestinal Radiology, University of California, San Francisco, School of Medicine, San Francisco, California

WILLIAM J. TUDDENHAM, M.D.

Professor, Department of Radiology, University of Pennsylvania, School of Medicine, Philadelphia, Pennsylvania

SUSAN D. WALL, M.D.

Assistant Professor, Department of Radiology, University of California, San Francisco, School of Medicine; Assistant Chief, Radiology, Veterans Administration Medical Center, San Francisco, California

MICHAEL W. WEINER, M.D.

Associate Professor of Medicine and Radiology, University of California, San Francisco, School of Medicine; Director of Magnetic Resonance Unit, San Francisco VA Medical Center, San Francisco, California

RALPH WEISSLEDER, M.D. Ph.D.

Department of Radiology, Massachusetts General Hospital, Boston, Massachusetts

WERNER WENZ, M.D.

Professor and Chairman, Department of Radiology, Klinikum der Albert-Ludwigs-Universität Freiburg, Freiburg, West Germany

JOSEPH P. WHALEN, M.D.

Professor and Chairman, Department of Radiology, Cornell University Medical College, Radiologist-in-Chief, The New York Hospital, New York, New York

JACK WITTENBERG, M.D.

Professor, Department of Radiology, Harvard Medical School, Boston, Massachusetts

KENNETH ZIRINSKY, M.D.

Assistant Professor of Radiology, The New York Hospital–Cornell Medical Center, New York, New York

PREFACE

The fourth edition of *Alimentary Tract Radiology* occurs at a time when radiology in general and gastrointestinal radiology in particular have been making significant advances. Ultrasonography has become much more sophisticated, and color Doppler has been introduced. Magnetic resonance imaging is advancing radiologic detection of multiple focal lesions in the liver and is showing great promise in the staging of carcinoma of the rectum and sigmoid. Enteroclysis is rapidly replacing conventional examination of the small bowel, and interventional radiology of the alimentary tract is becoming one of the most rapidly advancing areas in medicine, making a great impact on patient treatment. Gallstone lithotripsy in biliary ducts and the gallbladder is being investigated and promises revolutionary advances.

As before, this edition approaches the subject of alimentary radiology from the standpoint of pathology, technique, and imaging appearances and patterns.

Since the availability of equipment and talent varies so much from locale to locale, no attempt has been made for a fixed sequencing order of procedures for the diagnosis of various conditions. Approaches are presented, and their advantages and disadvantages are laid out.

We are presenting subjects that are controversial and therefore require some duplication to present different points of view. As before, we have been able to attract outstanding contributors from around the globe in an attempt to achieve completeness through diversity. We are grateful to our colleagues and hope that this edition of *Alimentary Tract Radiology* justifies their efforts.

Alexander R. Margulis
H. Joachim Burhenne

CONTENTS

ALIMENTARY TRACT RADIOLOGY

PART IX

PANCREAS

41 *Pathology*

HARLAN J. SPJUT

PANCREATITIS

MALFORMATIONS

CARCINOMAS

ENDOCRINE TUMORS

RARE TUMORS

Lesions of the pancreas and biliary tract are important not only in themselves but because of the involvement of adjacent organs. Pancreatic pseudocysts commonly impinge on nearby structures. A pseudocyst is most frequently associated with chronic alcohol abuse with related chronic pancreatitis. Biliary tract disease, trauma, hyperlipidemia, and the postoperative status are other background factors in the genesis of pseudocysts. Those occurring in adults usually follow acute or chronic pancreatitis, pseudocysts in children are usually related to trauma. The lesion is found in the head and body or both and is rarely confined to the tail of the pancreas. Because of its location a pseudocyst may displace the stomach anteriorly, displace the transverse colon, or extend into the pelvis and even into the mediastinum. Ordinarily pseudocysts are unicameral, and their wall is fibrous and devoid of an epithelial lining.[17]

Pseudocysts comprise approximately three fourths of the cysts of the pancreas, the remainder being true cysts. True cysts have an epithelial lining. They are generally classified as congenital or acquired cysts; the latter include retention cysts, parasitic cysts, and cysts that may accompany neoplasms.[9]

PANCREATITIS

Acute pancreatitis is associated commonly with alcoholism, but other factors—such as a pancreatic duct obstruction, reflux of bile, trauma, autoimmunization, and infection—are individually or in combination important as causes of pancreatitis. The pancreas is usually enlarged, firm, and edematous with chalky white areas of fat necrosis. If vessel necrosis occurs, there is a focal or extensive extravasation of blood (hemorrhagic pancreatitis).[7] Radiographically the abdominal films of the majority of patients are within normal limits; about one third show evidence of ileus, and a few show calcific densities in the pancreatic area.[4]

Suppurative pancreatitis may result from infection in a neighboring organ, such as appendicitis or a perforated peptic ulcer, but the most common cause of suppuration

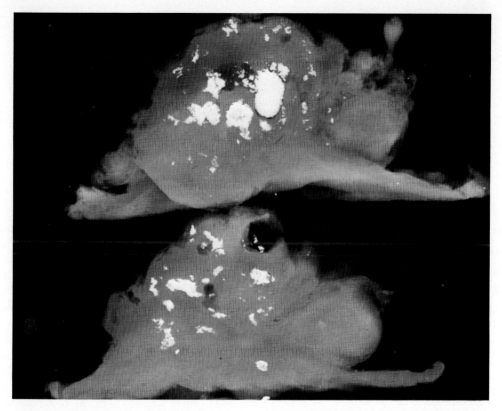

Fig. 41-1 Radiographs of pancreas involved by chronic pancreatitis. Multicalcific foci are evident.

(abscess) in the pancreas is preceding pancreatitis. Most abscesses are located in the left subphrenic or retroperitoneal spaces, having originated in the body or tail of the pancreas. Usually radiographs demonstrate the displacement of parapancreatic organs.[15]

In cases of chronic pancreatitis there is a progressive destruction of parenchyma along with a fibrous replacement of parenchyma, duct obliteration, or duct dilatation. More than half of these patients have radiographically detectable calcification in the pancreatic area. The small or large ducts contain calculi; interstitial calcification is uncommon[7] (Fig. 41-1).

MALFORMATIONS

An annular pancreas is a rare anomaly apparently caused by a failure of fusion between the ventral and dorsal buds of the developing pancreas. The ventral bud develops independently and surrounds the second portion of the duodenum. There may be sufficient constriction to produce symptoms, or the lesion may be found coincidentally. At times the constriction may be severe enough that the lesion is diagnosed during infancy. It is important to recall that an annular pancreas is commonly associated with other anomalies, including intestinal mal-

rotation, cardiac defects, imperforate anus, and duodenal bands. Many others as well have been found.[11]

Heterotopic pancreatic tissue has a reported incidence of 0.5% to 13.7%.[13] The common locations of aberrant pancreas are the stomach, duodenum, jejunum, Meckel's diverticulum, and ileum. Usually the nodule, which is yellowish, is located in the mucosa or submucosa of the bowel and occasionally is found in the serosa or the muscularis and may vary in size from less than a centimeter to 3 cm.

CARCINOMAS

Carcinomas of the pancreas cause more than 23,000 deaths per year in the United States. During the past four decades there has been an increase in the number of deaths caused by carcinomas of the pancreas. With rare exceptions a carcinoma of the pancreas is a disease of adulthood; 30 cases have been reported in children.[12]

Approximately two thirds of the carcinomas of the pancreas occur in the head; the remainder occur in the body or tail or involve the pancreas diffusely. Grossly, the lesion usually appears as a hard, ill-defined enlargement, commonly causing an obstruction of the duct of Wirsung and the common bile duct (Fig. 41-2). Much

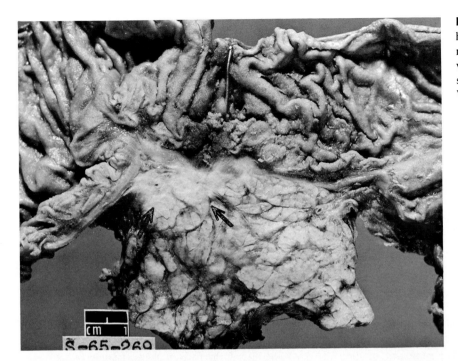

Fig. 41-2 Small carcinoma *(arrows)* of head of pancreas. Even though carcinoma is small, duodenal wall is invaded. Lymph nodes contained metastatic carcinoma. Probe is in ampulla of Vater.

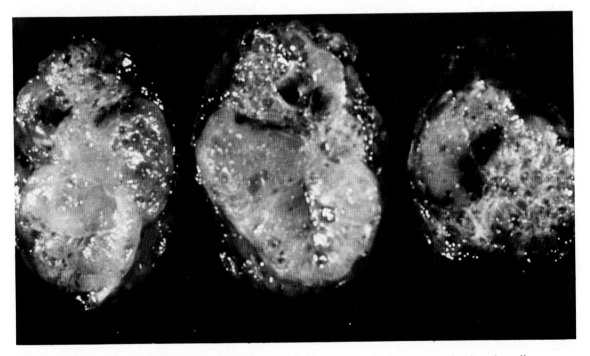

Fig. 41-3 Cross sections of microcystic adenoma of pancreas. It is well encapsulated, and small cysts are evident.

of the firmness of the cancer is caused by a commonly occurring fibrosis and chronic inflammation. Histologically, the majority of carcinomas of the pancreas are adenocarcinomas with varied degrees of differentiation and are probably ductal in origin. Occasional tumors have been reported that were thought to have been of acinar cell origin. A few of the reported carcinomas of the pancreas were squamous cell carcinomas, mixed squamous cell and adenocarcinomas, or pleomorphic carcinomas that might be mistaken for other lesions such as metastatic melanomas, rhabdomyosarcomas, and giant cell carcinomas.[21]

Cystadenocarcinomas of the pancreas are a variant of pancreatic carcinomas. Benign lesions designated as cystadenomas comprise approximately 10% of benign cystic lesions of the pancreas, and cystadenocarcinomas comprise approximately 1% of malignant neoplasms of the pancreas. These lesions are usually well encapsulated, lobulated, and multicystic and involve the body or tail. An interesting feature is that the majority of them occur in women. Histologically, these are often well-differentiated mucinous adenocarcinomas. In a few instances the capsule is calcified and may be identified as such radiographically. Approximately 80% of these lesions are present as a palpable upper abdominal mass that may reach 30 cm in size. In contrast to ordinary carcinomas of the pancreas, the cystadenocarcinoma is usually slow to metastasize and has a relatively good prognosis.[8] However, ReMine et al.[20] has observed that cystadenocarcinomas of a high grade are likely to have metastases at the time of abdominal exploration.

The solid and papillary epithelial neoplasm of the pancreas has a strong tendency to occur in women and is of low malignant potentential. It may reach 15 cm in size and is usually well circumscribed and at least partly cystic.[14]

Microcystic adenomas of the pancreas are benign multicystic tumors that tend to occur in persons beyond the age of 50 years, predominantly in women. It has distinctive gross (Fig. 41-3) and microscopic patterns. The tumor may vary in size from 2 cm to larger than 12 cm; it is a slowly growing lesion. Immunohistochemically and ultrastructurally microcystic adenomas apparently originate from the centroacinar cells.[1]

ENDOCRINE TUMORS

Endocrine tumors are capable of producing a variety of secretory products: insulin, pancreatic polypeptide, glucagon, gastrin, and vasoactive intestinal polypeptide. Symptoms are often related to the hormone secreted. Small tumors may be clinically silent, found incidentally at surgical exploration or at autopsy; malignant tumors are often large. It has been observed that most insulinomas are benign, whereas gastrinomas, glucagonomas and VIPomas are likely to be malignant.

Tumors of the islet cells may be associated with other endocrine neoplastic and hyperplastic lesions such as pheochromocytomas, medullary carcinomas of the thyroid, and adenomas of the pituitary. These have been divided into two groups: multiple endocrine neoplasia type 1 and multiple endocrine neoplasia type 2.[3] Histologically, pancreatic endocrine tumors are difficult to differentiate from those that are benign unless metastases

have occurred or there is an infiltration into the surrounding organs or tissues. Capsular invasion and blood vessel invasion have not in themselves been considered evidence of overt malignancy. These carcinomas are compatible with a long life even in the presence of metastases.[2,5,6,16,19]

RARE TUMORS

Pancreatoblastomas are usually found in children and rarely in adults. A pancreatoblastoma may form a pancreatic mass as large as 15 cm. Pulmonary and hepatic metastases may occur.[18] A leiomyosarcoma may present as a pancreatic mass larger than 15 cm and produce widespread metastases. Histologically and ultrastructurally the tumor is similar to leiomyosarcomas found elsewhere in the body.[10]

REFERENCES

1. Alpert, LC, et al: Microcystic adenoma (serous cystadenoma) of the pancreas, Am J Surg Pathol 12:251, 1988.
2. Bryant, LR, Moore, TC, and Carney, EK: Islet cell adenomas of the duodenum with recurrent peptic ulceration (Zollinger-Ellison), Ann Surg 160:104, 1964.
3. Carney, JS, et al: Familial pheochromocytoma and islet cell tumor of the pancreas, Am J Med 68:515, 1980.
4. Cogbill, CL, and Song, KT: Acute pancreatitis, Arch Surg 100:673, 1970.
5. Gould, VE, et al: The APUD cell system and its neoplasms, Surg Clin North Am 59:93, 1979.
6. Heitz, PU, et al: Pancreatic endocrine tumors: immunocytochemical analysis of 125 tumors, Hum Pathol 13:263, 1982.
7. Hermann, RE: Clinical aspects of pancreatitis, Postgrad Med 36:135, 1964.
8. Hodgkinson, DJ, ReMine, WH, and Weiland, LH: Pancreatic cystadenoma, Arch Surg 113:512, 1978.
9. Howard, JM, and Jordan, GL: Surgical diseases of the pancreas, Philadelphia, 1960, JB Lippincott.
10. Ishikawa, O, et al: Leiomyosarcoma of the pancreas, Am J Surg Pathol 5:597, 1981.
11. Kiernen, PD, et al: Annular pancreas, Arch Surg 115:46, 1980.
12. Lack, EE, et al: Tumors of the exocrine pancreas in children and adolescents, Am J Surg Pathol 7:319, 1983.
13. Lai, ECS, and Tompkins, RK: Heterotopic pancreas, Am J Surg 151:697, 1986.
14. Lieber, MR, et al: Solid and papillary epithelial neoplasm of the pancreas, Am J Surg Pathol 11:85, 1987.
15. Miller, TA, et al: Pancreatic abscess, Arch Surg 108:545, 1974.
16. Mukai, K, et al: Retrospective study of 77 pancreatic endocrine tumors using the immunoperoxidase method, Am J Surg Pathol 6:387, 1982.
17. O'Malley, VP, Cannon, JP, and Postier, RG: Pancreatic pseudocysts: cause, therapy and results, Am J Surg 150:680, 1985.
18. Palosaari, D, Clayton, F, and Seaman, J: Pancreatoblastoma in an adult, Arch Pathol Lab Med 110:650, 1986.
19. Peurifoy, JT, Gomez, LG, and Thompson, JC: Separate pancreatic gastrin cell and beta cell adenomas, Arch Surg 114:956, 1979.
20. ReMine, SG, et al: Cystic neoplasms of the pancreas, Arch Surg 122:443, 1987.
21. Tschang, TP, Garza-Garza, R, and Kissane, JM: Pleomorphic carcinoma of the pancreas, Cancer 39:2114, 1977.

42 *Ultrasonography*

GEORGE R. LEOPOLD

GENERAL CONSIDERATIONS

Since the previous edition of this text, new diagnostic approaches to patients with suspected pancreatic disease have appeared. Most clinicians and radiologists now agree that if the patient's symptoms are clearly related to the pancreas, computed tomography (CT) may be the test of choice. Possible exceptions are children and pregnant patients. The clear demonstration of the pancreas possible with CT, even in the presence of air-filled bowel and ascites, have earned this distinction. Excessive retroperitoneal fat, another deterrent to ultrasound, further enhances CT.

Ultrasonography still plays a vital role in the assessment of the pancreas, a once "hidden" organ. Many patients are referred with vague or unrelated symptoms. Now the preferred test for evaluating the gallbladder, ultrasonography often uncovers unsuspected pancreatic disease. In addition, the lower cost and ready availability of ultrasonography encourage clinicians to use it more often than CT (or for that matter, magnetic resonance imaging). Finally, the ability to bring the imaging equipment to the bedside of a critically ill patient is a major advantage in the minds of referring physicians. For these reasons, the utility of ultrasonography in evaluation of the pancreas has steadily increased.

No area of the abdomen is as complex to image with ultrasonography as the pancreas and bile ducts. To obtain a satisfactory study the examiner must possess thorough knowledge of both normal anatomy and the many common variants.[21,24] Differences in body habitus, excessive bowel gas, and overlying barium may necessitate a variety of scanning techniques, so a precise routine is not always possible. The wide spectrum of pathologic alterations produced by common pancreatic disorders must also be recognized.

Advances in technology have much improved pancreatic imaging. Articulated-arm static scanners have now almost completely given way to dynamic real-time units. In addition, phased array technology has markedly improved the resolution of such units. The analogy between x-ray fluoroscopy and static overhead films is entirely appropriate. Radiologists interested in gastrointestinal disease now wield real-time ultrasound machines with the same aplomb once accorded the fluoroscope. Yet, as before, instrumentation is far less important than the examiner's understanding of anatomy and pathology.

Given this set of circumstances, modern ultrasonography has emerged as an excellent noninvasive tool for evaluation of pancreatic and biliary disease.

PATIENT PREPARATION

No special preparation is required for pancreatic ultrasonography. The patient is requested to fast for at least 12 hours if possible (water is permitted) before the examination, so that the gallbladder is maximally distended. This also limits intake of gas-producing foods, which are potential examination problems. The ultrasonographic study should precede barium studies; in the usual suspensions given for radiography barium is impermeable to the beam.[29]

Supplemental regimes such as filling the stomach with water and administering antifoaming agents have been tried with varying degrees of success. Sommer et al.[48] have shown a slight improvement in scan quality following the administration of simethicone for several days before the examination. If water alone is used, some examiners recommend it to be allowed to sit for several hours to permit microbubbles of gas to escape. Others find that bubbles cause no significant interference and may actually aid in recognition of peristalsis during real-time observations. In an innovative approach, duCret, Jackson, and Rees have suggested the use of intravenous metoclopramide, an agent that stimulates gastric and duodenal peristalsis, before ultrasonography.[7] In their series, 44% of patients showed improved visualization on this protocol.

Despite these regimens, bowel gas remains the single most important obstacle to excellent ultrasound studies. Even with meticulous scanning technique, the pancreas cannot be visualized in 10% of patients.[52] Unfortunately, these patients often are seriously ill (inpatients, those receiving pain medications, those with ileus). CT is extremely beneficial in such patients.

CONDUCT OF THE EXAMINATION

This section provides guidelines for proper conduct of the examination. The approach described is not meant to be rigid; many laboratories use different approaches to obtain the essential information. The performance of the examination is much like that of an upper gastrointestinal series. Though methods may vary, certain key observations must be made at some time during the course of the study to assure maximum diagnostic results.

Real-time examination

Real-time study is now the accepted mode of imaging. This examination may be considered analogous to the fluoroscopic portion of an upper gastrointestinal series. The examiner quickly observes the orientation of the major upper abdominal viscera such as the liver and gallbladder. An assessment of the left hepatic lobe is important, because a large or prominent left lobe usually facilitates pancreatic scanning. The position of the splenic vein is noted and serves as a marker for the body and tail of the pancreas.[10,11,37] The inferior vena cava is identified to localize the pancreatic head. The axis of the portal vein is also identified, because the common hepatic bile duct—an important part of any pancreatic exam— lies just anterior to this structure.

This survey discloses any large, abnormal solid masses in the pancreatic region, and even small fluid-filled masses are readily apparent. The latter are carefully observed for peristalsis, characterized by either change of contour or jets of bubbles, which produce bright, moving echoes in the apparent mass. Fluid-filled bowel (usually gastric antrum or duodenum) may thus be eliminated as a source of diagnostic confusion.

In patients with gastric retention, the fluid-filled stomach may look remarkably like a pancreatic pseudocyst. When a left upper quadrant cystic mass is discovered, the patient is asked to drink ordinary tap water (which contains many small bubbles) under real-time observation. If the mass in question is stomach, it fills rapidly with bright echoes. This simple expedient greatly reduces the incidence of false positive diagnoses of pseudocyst.

If the pancreas is not satisfactorily identified, tap water or one of the fluids discussed previously is administered. Positional maneuvers are also helpful. When the patient assumes an upright or semiupright position, antral air rises to the fundus of the stomach, allowing better visualization of the body and tail of pancreas.[32] When the antrum is filled with fluid, it is often necessary to decrease overall system gain to prevent obscuring the pancreas. To study the pancreatic head, the patient is placed in right lateral decubitus position to fill the duodenum. This often allows differentiation between duodenum and pancreatic head, a potential pitfall for both ultrasound and CT.

Static gray scale examination

Once the mainstay of pancreatic sonography, static gray scale examination has been relegated to a secondary role. Such scans are helpful because of their wide-angle nature in convincing others of the observed real-time findings. The analogy between spot and overhead films in barium study of the gut is appropriate.

Some pseudocysts are so large that imaging with real-time instruments does not allow a complete assessment of the problem. Overall relationships are much clearer on static scans.

Endoscopic sonography

Combining ultrasonography with endoscopy has several compelling advantages. In addition to eliminating bowel gas problems, it permits higher-frequency transducers (7.5 MHz), which have much improved resolution. Although originally designed to evaluate esophageal and gastric wall invasion by tumor, early reports indicate success with endoscopic sonography in pancreatic diagnosis as well.[15,31] Its principal utility seems to be detecting very small masses, particularly insulinomas, that are not visualized by other imaging methods.

Operative sonography

Surgeons have recently begun to appreciate the value of sonography in the operating room. In the pancreas, potential uses include localization of small tumors, pancreatic calculi, and the pancreatic duct.[16] Visualization of these structures before dissection or ductography is often helpful in planning resection or decompression.[44,46] As with endoscopic sonography, high-frequency transducers can be used to provide images of extremely high resolution. As an intermediate step between endoscopic and intraoperative sonography, Okita has proposed its use during laparoscopy.[36] In his hands, the technique was useful in assessing the spread of pancreatic cancer and in directing biopsy of suspicious lesions.

NORMAL ANATOMY
Regional anatomy

The pancreatic head abuts the anterior (ventral) surface of the inferior vena cava and is usually apparent on both transverse and sagittal scans. The latter tend to be more useful, as the head is vertically oriented in most patients. The position of the head relative to the portal vein varies considerably. In some patients it is in contact with the portal vein, whereas in others a cephalocaudad separation of several centimeters is noted. Slight anterior indentation of the vena cava is seen in many normal subjects. The amount of indentation probably depends on distensibility of the inferior vena cava.

In the same plane the distal portion of the common bile duct passes over the portal vein and courses posteriorly into the pancreatic head (Fig. 42-1). This portion of the duct does not exceed 6 mm in diameter. A larger figure (up to 10 mm) may be accepted in patients with previous biliary surgery.[37]

If sagittal scanning is carried out slightly medial to the pancreatic head, the superior mesenteric vein is seen ventral and parallel to the inferior vena cava or abdominal aorta. A small amount of pancreatic tissue corresponding to the neck of the gland lies just anterior to this vessel. The uncinate process—a medial extension of the pancreatic head—may be seen just posterior to the vein. The uncinate is quite variable in size. It is significant because it is the only portion of the pancreas in which masses produce anterior displacement of the superior mesenteric vessels. Most masses causing anterior displacement are enlarged peripancreatic lymph nodes rather than primary pancreatic tumors.

Transverse scans of the pancreatic head (Fig. 42-2) also provide useful information. In these sections, the

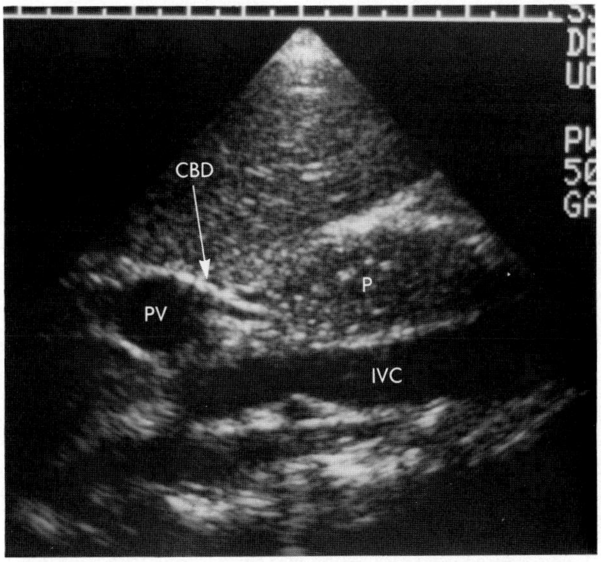

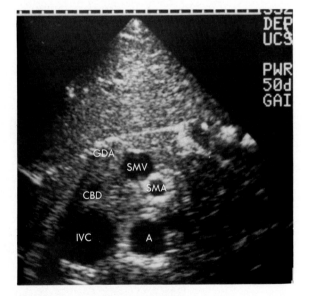

Fig. 42-1 Sagittal scan of pancreatic head, normal patient. *P,* pancreas; *IVC,* inferior vena cava; *PV,* portal vein; *CBD,* common bile duct.

Fig. 42-2 Transverse scan of pancreatic head, normal patient. Excellent definition of pancreas and surrounding vessels. *A,* aorta; *IVC,* inferior vena cava; *SMA,* superior mesenteric artery; *SMV,* superior mesenteric vein; *P,* pancreas; *CBD,* common bile duct; *GDA,* gastroduodenal artery.

intrapancreatic portion of the common bile duct can be identified in its short axis just anterior to the inferior vena cava. On the ventral surface of the gland, the gastroduodenal artery is also frequently seen.

The pancreatic body is easily identified by localization of the splenic vein. This is possible in either the sagittal or transverse plane. The splenic vein is closely related to the dorsal surface of the pancreatic body and tail, but its precise cephalocaudad relationship to the back of the pancreas is quite variable.

Because the body of the gland is oriented transversely, transverse scans are usually more informative (Fig. 42-3 and 42-4). The width of the body is noticeably less than that of the head. The pancreatic duct is easiest to visualize in the body of the gland, probably because its walls are perpendicular to the incident ultrasound beam.[26] In the head and tail, where this structure curves away from the transducer, demonstration of the duct is less common. In most individuals the duct appears as an echogenic line in the center of the gland; however, a

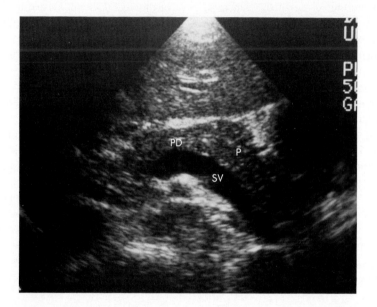

Fig. 42-3 Transverse scan of pancreatic body, normal patient. Contour defect shown is common normal varient. *P*, pancreas; *PD*, pancreatic duct; *SV*, splenic vein.

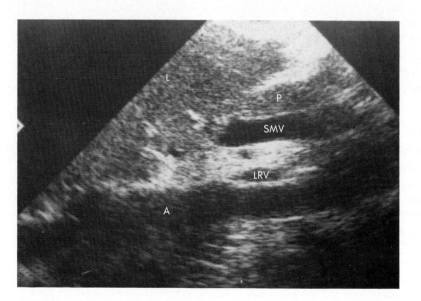

Fig. 42-4 Sagittal midline scan of normal patient, *P*, pancreas; *SMV*, superior mesenteric vein; *L*, liver; *A*, aorta; *LRV*, left renal vein.

small amount of fluid may be seen within its lumen.[6] Most authors agree that a width of more than 2 mm is abnormal.[52,55]

To identify the pancreatic duct with certainty, two other important structures must be visualized. These are the splenic vein and the posterior wall of the stomach. At times both have been mistaken for pancreatic duct. The distinction is made by observing sections immediately adjacent to the one in question. The splenic vein may be traced to its confluence with the superior mesenteric vein and into the liver. The posterior gastric wall can usually be traced to its junction with the anterior wall near the region of the pylorus. Finally, pancreatic parenchyma should appear both dorsal and ventral to the structure in question before it is referred to as being the pancreatic duct.

The tail of the pancreas is without question the most difficult portion of the gland to image ultrasonically. Excessive retroperitoneal fat and gaseous distention are the two primary causes of nonvisualization. Fortunately, these patients are the most amenable to examination by CT. As mentioned previously, filling of the stomach may render the tail visible in an anterior approach. It is also fortunate for ultrasonographers that disease in the pancreas tail is much less common than in the head and body.

Pancreatic size

Various authors have listed normal dimensions for the individual segments of the pancreas.[3,4,18] However, there has been no consensus about precisely where such measurements should be made. Because the pancreas is a curved organ, one must be wary of measurements obtained in a single plane. This is especially true of head measurements from longitudinal scans. Although most investigators conclude that 3.5 cm is the maximum normal diameter of the head and tail, with the body somewhat smaller, it is difficult to apply these figures in actual practice. As with liver and spleen, considerable anatomic variation of the pancreas defies simple uniplanar measurements.

Pancreatic texture

The fibrous pancreas is usually of greater echogenicity than the adjacent liver with its more homogeneous composition.[3,11,23] A comparison is commonly made between the body of the gland and the overlying left lobe of liver. In many normal patients, however, the texture of the two organs is nearly identical. It is likely that state of hydration, fasting, and numerous other factors influence pancreatic echogenicity. Furthermore, many patients have combined pancreatic and liver disease, making direct comparison of parenchymal echoes less reliable. In some patients ultrasonography visualizes the retroperitoneal vessels, but the contours of the gland itself cannot

be distinguished from surrounding retroperitoneal tissues. CT has been of assistance in clarifying these findings. In many older patients, small lobules of fat are interspersed with pancreatic parenchyma, presumably as a consequence of aging.[60] There is no associated pancreatic insufficiency.[33]

Some researchers have also noted that the texture of the pancreatic echogenicity differs in children.[13] Although overall the pancreas may appear less echogenic than in adults, the individual echoes from within it are of greater intensity. The mechanism responsible for this is obscure.

Though pancreatic textural changes are somewhat helpful, quantitative analytic methods may yield even more information in ultrasonic instruments of the next decade.

PANCREATIC PATHOLOGY
Pancreatitis

Inflammatory disease of the pancreas, regardless of cause (alcoholic, traumatic, viral, or biliary) often produces ultrasonographic changes. Even using the crude bistable equipment of nearly two decades ago, early researchers recognized morphologic changes believed to be characteristic.[3,10] Their description included visualization of the organ (not thought possible in the normal state) and textural change caused by pancreatic edema. Modern gray scale studies have both confirmed and extended these observations.[6,9,28]

Texture

It is now possible to demonstrate parenchyma in nearly all patients. The most consistent textural change in pancreatitis is loss of echogenicity (Fig. 42-5). This is presumably caused by interstitial edema of the gland.[6] No ultrasonic features clearly distinguish acute pancreatitis from more chronic forms of the disorder.[1,42] Not all cases of pancreatitis display this textural change, however. In some cases enlargement of the gland is the only telltale finding; in others, the gland appears perfectly normal.

Size

Diffuse enlargement remains one of the more helpful diagnostic features of both acute and chronic pancreatitis. In end-stage disease, the gland atrophies to a stringlike structure that cannot be visualized ultrasonographically.

One of the most disturbing features of this disorder is its occasional tendency to involve only a segment of the gland, usually the head. The result is masslike enlargement indistinguishable from carcinoma. Such swellings may cause an obstruction of the common bile duct and even clinical jaundice. Textural changes have not allowed differentiation between pancreatitis and carcinoma, as was previously hoped. Continued work with tissue char-

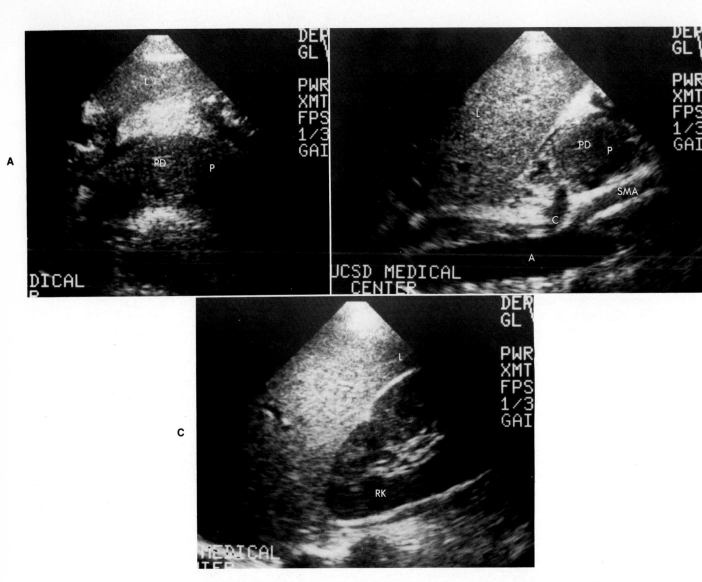

Fig. 42-5 A, Transverse scan showing markedly enlarged, sonolucent pancreas *(P)* as compared to the more echogenic left lobe of liver *(L); PD,* pancreatic duct. **B,** Sagittal scan of same patient demonstrates relationships of the enlarged pancreas to the celiac *(C)* and superior mesenteric arteries *(SMA). A,* Aorta. **C,** Right parasagittal scan shows that liver is abnormally dense when compared to kidney parenchyma *(RK),* invalidating the comparison made in **A.**

acterization and better endoscopic probes may alter the situation.

Other findings

Punctate, high-intensity echoes (Fig. 42-6), sometimes accompanied by acoustic shadowing, appear in the parenchyma in cases of long-standing pancreatitis.[54] These almost certainly represent calcifications but are more easily demonstrated with plain radiographs of the abdomen.

The two major complications of pancreatitis are pseudocyst formation (discussed in a later section) and retroperitoneal hemorrhage.[19] The latter is probably produced by the action of proteolytic enzymes on pancreatic vessels, sometimes resulting in massive hemorrhage. In such cases ultrasonography can often detect the hemorrhage and predict its extent. CT, however, does a better job of defining the total extent of hemorrhage or edematous change occurring in the peripancreatic area.[20] Repeat studies using both methods are very helpful in monitoring the progress of these patients.

Clinical utility

Patients who have all the classic signs and symptoms of acute pancreatitis do not need imaging studies to establish the diagnosis. Indeed, such patients commonly

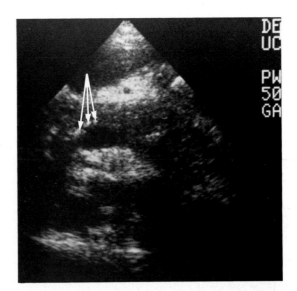

Fig. 42-6 Transverse scan in patient with chronic pancreatitis. Small, punctate echoes *(arrows)* represent calcifications.

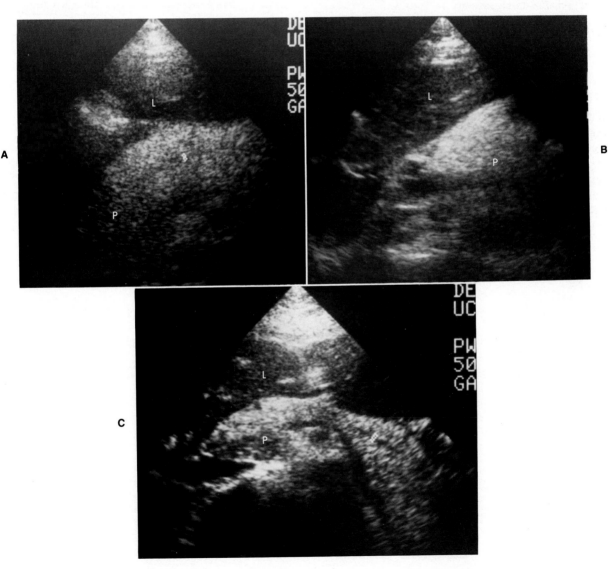

Fig. 42-7 A, Transverse scan in patient with chornic pancreatitis. Patient demonstrates both pancreatic enlargement and increased parenchymal echogenicity. *L,* Liver; *P,* pancrea. **B,** Sagittal scan in same patient. **C,** Another patient with chronic pancreatitis showing a normal-sized gland but marked textural changes.

have ileus of the bowel overlying the pancreas, making sonographic visualization difficult or impossible.

In patients with chronic pancreatitis, however, ultrasonography may have a more definitive role. There is usually a long history of unexplained epigastric or left upper quadrant pain. Serum and urinary enzyme studies are normal. Ultrasonography may show a diffuse (common) or focal (uncommon) enlargement of the gland and thus provide a presumptive diagnosis. In most cases, the gland has increased echogenicity—sometimes this is the only finding (Fig. 42-7). The technique is of greater use in detecting serial changes or complications of pancreatitis than in making the primary diagnosis.[8,9,53] If pancreatitis progresses to form an abscess, CT is much more reliable in making the diagnosis. Small gas bubbles in the inflammatory mass are easily identified with CT but often invisible on ultrasound.

If the inflammatory process has produced peripancreatic phlegmon, the extent of this process also is more easily determined with CT.[22,51,52]

Cysts

One of the valuable features of pancreatic ultrasonography has been its contribution to the diagnosis of cystic disease. The vast majority of cystic lesions are pseudocysts occurring as a consequence of pancreatitis or, more rarely, trauma. Because ultrasonography can be performed serially without risk or discomfort to the patient, important information is emerging about the evolution and resolution of pseudocysts.[27]

Ordinary pseudocysts

The usual pseudocyst is a well-circumscribed, fluid-filled mass lying within or immediately adjacent to the head, body, or tail of the gland. With the high-resolution capabilities of present equipment pseudocysts as small as 1.5 cm are easily demonstrable. They may be either unilocular or multilocular. Echoes often appear in the dependent portion of the pseudocyst (Fig. 42-8), and there may be a fluid-solid interface that changes position in decubitus scans. The solid material represents debris (partially autolyzed pancreas) or in some cases organized blood. If hemorrhage into a pseudocyst has been extensive, thick fibrous synechiae form throughout the lesion. These dense bands are quite different from the delicate septations multilocular lesions. Septated pseudocysts are of particular concern because it is technically more difficult to create adequate drainage for each individual compartment. Detection of a pseudocyst should not preclude careful examination of the remainder of the gland. If pseudocyst is found in the body or tail, a more proximally located carcinoma may be the cause. Unfortunately, masses detected in these circumstances stand a chance of being either focal pancreatitis or cancer, and the diagnosis is still usually in doubt.

Considerable enthusiasm has developed for percutaneous drainage of pseudocysts.[25] Sonography is helpful both in placement of drainage tubes and in follow-up of such patients. If drainage procedures are planned, CT is often used to assure that all locules of the lesion have been visualized.

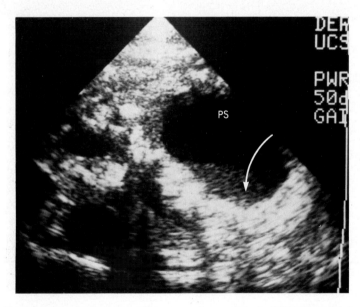

Fig. 42-8 Transverse scan of patient with pancreatic pseudocyst *(PS)*. Note debris *(arrow)* in dependent portion of cyst.

Ectopic pseudocysts

Pseudocysts may appear at locations in the body remote from the pancreatic bed (Fig. 42-9). In addition to spread along fascial planes of the retroperitoneal space, the digestive nature of pancreatic fluid also enables it to penetrate them.

The lesser sac is one of the common ectopic sites (Fig. 42-10). Others pass through the diaphragm and present as a mediastinal mass. If spread is lateral, the cyst may form medial or lateral to the spleen.

Pseudocysts may also occur in the pelvis, the scrotum, and even the groin. In addition to these peculiar extraorgan sites, direct extension into the solid organs of the abdomen (liver, spleen, and kidneys) also occurs.

When pseudocysts are ectopically located and the clinical history does not suggest pancreatic disease, diagnosis is difficult. Correct interpretation of the findings requires a high index of suspicion. If the diagnosis of ectopic pseudocyst is considered, percutaneous needle aspiration of fluid for amylase content confirms the diagnosis. No significant complications from this procedure have been reported.

Temporal relationships

A fascinating aspect of pancreatic pseudocysts uncovered by ultrasonography is their evanescent nature.[2,39] Commonly, 1 to 3 cm fluid-filled collections are found within or adjacent to the pancreas only to disappear on subsequent examination. There is usually no change in symptoms. Presumably some of these lesions are capable of reestablishing communication with the pancreatic duct and decompressing themselves.[30]

Larger pseudocysts also occasionally disappear. In such cases, the mechanism is often rupture with escape of fluid into the free peritoneal space (Fig. 42-10, *C*). This is usually referred to as pancreatic ascites.[38] Although rupture was previously considered lethal, more recent experience teaches otherwise.

It is now clear that pseudocyst formation and resolution are far more common and dynamic than previously suspected. Continued close observation should provide even more information regarding the natural history of these lesions.

False-positive pseudocysts

Several pitfalls complicate the diagnosis of pseudocyst.[47] Probably the most important of these complicating pitfalls is fluid-filled gut. Although the stomach is the most troublesome viscus, the duodenum and other loops of small bowel and colon also occasionally cause confusion.

This problem is much less common now that real time is the primary method of evaluation. Still, absence of peristalsis does not exclude fluid-filled bowel as a source of misdiagnosis, and provocative maneuvers should be used. If a nasogastric tube is in place, injection of air or tap water during the real-time examination usually solves the problem. If no tube is in place, having the patient drink tap water during the period of observation is also effective.

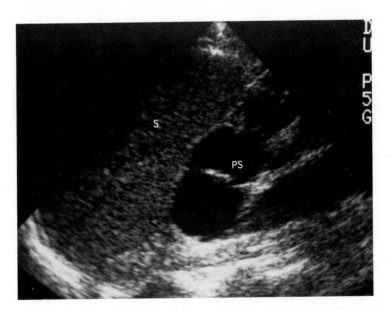

Fig. 42-9 Coronal scan of patient with multilocular pseudocyst in hilus of spleen *(S)*. *PS*, Pseudocyst.

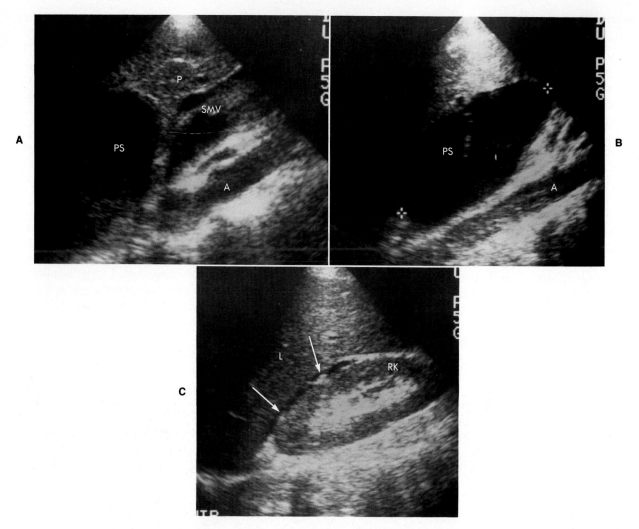

Fig. 42-10 A, Sagittal midline scan showing pancreatic pseudocyst in lesser sac. Pancreatic body is totally separate from lesion. *P,* Pancreas; *PS,* pseudocyst; *A,* aorta; *SMV,* superior mesenteric vein. **B,** Sagittal scan centered slightly higher than in **A,** demonstrating cephalad extent of pseudocyst. **C,** Right parasagittal scan in same patient shows small collection of pancreatic ascites *(arrows)* in Morrison's pouch. *L,* Liver; *RK,* right kidney.

Generalized ascites passes freely through the foramen of Winslow into the lesser peritoneal sac. Although this fluid collection may superficially resemble a pancreatic pseudocyst, no real mass effect is evident. Surrounding liver and loops of bowel project into the collection rather than being displaced by it.

Other cystic lesions

Though far less common than pseudocysts, other cysts of the pancreas do occur. True congenital cysts are quite rare, but in the presence of autosomal dominant polycystic renal disease the pancreas is occasionally involved.[43] These cysts are usually quite small and of no apparent clinical significance. Though they are ordinarily devoid of internal echoes, trauma and internal hemorrhage can produce a more complex appearance, as is the case with pseudocysts.

Cystadenomas and cystadenocarcinomas of the pancreas present ultrasonographically as fluid-filled lesions with multiple internal septations.[58,59] These cysts may be difficult to differentiate from a trabeculated pseudocyst. The clinical history is often helpful, because cystadenomas have a predilection for young women and the tail of the pancreas. There are no reliable ultrasound criteria for distinguishing benign from malignant forms.

Microcystic cystadenoma of the pancreas deserves special mention. In these patients, cysts are present but are not demonstrable by ultrasonography. They appear as large solid masses, occasionally containing calcification, that produce acoustic shadowing.

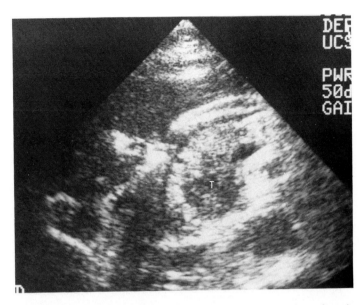

Fig. 42-11 Transverse scan demonstrates sonolucent mass *(T)* in region of uncinate—proven pancreatic cancer. Focal pancreatitis could have identical appearance.

Carcinomas

As the incidence of gastric malignancy has declined, pancreatic carcinoma has shown a distressing increase. Because symptoms from this tumor occur relatively late, its cure rate has been low. Only an occasional patient with a small tumor causing early obstructive jaundice is likely to be cured by surgery.

Because pancreatic cancer has become a major health problem, it is logical to expect that new diagnostic methods such as ultrasonography and CT would be applied with the hope of an earlier diagnosis. Unfortunately, there is no convincing evidence that either method has improved the long-term survival of these patients.

By the time pancreatic cancers can be detected by ultrasonography, they are usually extensive. Although lesions smaller than 3 cm have occasionally been described, these are usually found when the tumor markedly distorts the gland's external contour. If smaller tumors are entirely intrapancreatic in location, they usually pass unnoticed.[49,50]

Fig. 42-11 is typical of pancreatic carcinomas discovered by ultrasonography. These are usually large lesions and totally unresectable. Although some authors state that carcinomas are less echogenic than normal pancreatic parenchyma, textural features are quite variable and often confusing.[41] Ultrasonography, like CT, must therefore rely on contour abnormality or the presence of a sizable mass to suggest the diagnosis of pancreatic cancer. In their present state of development, such tools are not effective screening methods for pancreatic cancer.

Many authors believe that screening will be done with a biochemical marker, or perhaps some combination of marker and imaging study.

In some cancers a dilated pancreatic duct may be imaged (Fig. 42-12). At times this is the only clue to the presence of a tumor.[17] Unfortunately, this finding is also seen in chronic pancreatitis and is therefore nonspecific.

The most valuable role played by ultrasonography is demonstration of metastatic disease and secondary effects on the common bile duct. Unfortunately, regional metastases to peripancreatic nodes and hematogenous dissemination to liver are common. Even when the primary tumor is small, extensive metastases are frequent.

Although adenocarcinoma is by far the commonest solid tumor of the pancreas, ultrasonographers need to be aware of other neoplasms that may have a similar appearance. Pleomorphic carcinoma,[58] epithelial neoplasm,[14] islet cell tumors,[40] and metastases[56] (Fig. 42-13) have all been reported.

Pancreatic biopsy

Attention has recently focused on ultrasonography and CT as localizing methods to guide percutaneous puncture of pancreatic masses.[12,13,34,45] If such localizing methods are properly used, many patients with incurable disease will be spared the risk and expense of laparotomy to confirm the diagnosis of inoperable pancreatic carcinoma. This procedure is a fine-needle aspiration rather than an actual biopsy. It is therefore necessary that the cellular aspirate be properly prepared and the services of

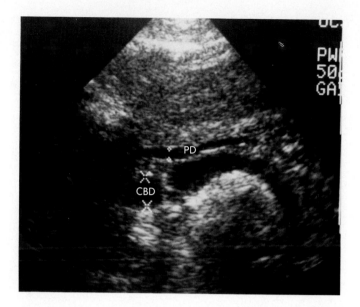

Fig. 42-12 Transverse scan shows both dilated pancreatic duct *(PD)* and intrapancreatic common bile duct *(CBD)*. Cause was tiny lesion of pancreatic head that could not be imaged by either CT or ultrasound.

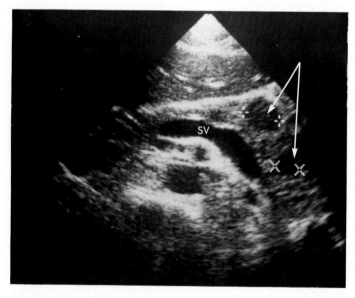

Fig. 42-13 Transverse scan in patient with diffuse histiocytic lymphoma. Nodular masses of tumor *(arrows)* are evident in pancreatic parenchyma. *SV,* splenic vein.

pathologist skilled in interpreting such specimens be available.

Ohto has reported the use of real-time ultrasonography in guiding puncture of the duct of Wirsung for evaluation of both inflammatory and neoplastic conditions of the pancreas.[35]

REFERENCES

1. Alpern, M, Sandler, M, and Kellman, G: Chronic pancreatitis: ultrasonic features, Radiology 155:215, 1985.
2. Bradley, E, and Clements, J: Spontaneous resolution of pancreatic pseudocysts: implications of timing of operative intervention, Am J Surg 129:23, 1975.
3. Burger, J, and Blauenstein, V: Current aspects of ultrasound scanning of the pancreas, AJR 112:405, 1974.

4. de Graaff, C, et al: Gray scale echography of the pancreas: re-evaluation of normal size, Radiology 129:157, 1978.

5. Didier, D, Deschamps, J, and Rohmer, P: Evaluation of the pancreatic duct: a reappraisal based on a retrospective correlative study by sonography and pancreatography in 117 normal and pathologic subjects, Ultrasound Med Biol 9:509, 1983.

6. Doust, B, and Pearce, J: Gray scale ultrasonic properties of the normal and inflamed pancreas, Radiology 120:653, 1976.

7. duCret, R, Jackson, V, and Rees, C: Pancreatic sonography: enhancement by metoclopramide, AJR 146:341, 1986.

8. Duncan, J, Imire, C, and Blumgart, L: Ultrasound in the management of acute pancreatitis, Br J Radiol 49:858, 1976.

9. Ferrucci, J: Radiology of the pancreas, 1976: Sonography and ductography, Radiol Clin North Am 14:543, 1976.

10. Filly, R, and Freimanis, A: Echographic diagnosis of pancreatic lesions, Radiology 96:575, 1970.

11. Ghorashi, B, and Rector, W: Gray scale sonographic anatomy of the pancreas, J Clin Ultrasound 5:25, 1977.

12. Goldstein, H, et al: Percutaneous fine needle biopsy of the pancreas and other abdominal masses, Radiology 123:319, 1977.

13. Fleischer, A, Parker, P, and Kirchner S: Sonographic findings of pancreatitis in children, Radiology 146:151, 1983.

14. Friedman, A, Lichtenstein, J, and Fishman, E: Solid and papillary epithelial neoplasm of the pancreas, Radiology 154:333, 1985.

15. Fukuda, M, Nakano, Y, and Saito, K: Endoscopic ultrasonography in the diagnosis of pancreatic carcinoma, Scand J Gastroenterol 19(suppl 94):65, 1984.

16. Gorman, B, Charboneau, W, and James, E: Benign pancreatic insulinoma: preoperative and intraoperative sonographic localization, AJR 147:929, 1986.

17. Gosink, B, and Leopold, G: The dilated pancreatic duct: Ultrasonic evaluation, Radiology 126:475, 1978.

18. Haber, K, Freimanis, A, and Asher, W: Demonstration and dimensional analysis of the normal pancreas with gray scale echography, AJR 126:624, 1976.

19. Hancke, S, Holm, HH, and Koch, F: Ultrasonically guided percutaneous fine needle biopsy of the pancreas, Surg Gynecol Obstet 140:361, 1975.

20. Hashimoto, B, Laing, F, and Jeffrey, R: Hemorrhagic pancreatic fluid collections examined by ultrasound, Radiology 150:803, 1984.

21. Hatchette, J, Shuler, S, and Mursion, P: Scintiphotos of the pancreas: analysis of 134 studies, J Nucl Med 13:51, 1972.

22. Jeffrey, R, Laing, F, and Wing, V: Extrapancreatic spread of acute pancreatitis: new observations with real time ultrasound, Radiology 159:707, 1986.

23. Johnson, M, and Mack, L: Ultrasonic evaluation of the pancreas, Gastrointest Radiol 3:257, 1978.

24. Kreel, L, Sandin, B, and Slvain, G: Pancreatic morphology: A combined radiological and pathological study. Clin Radiol 24:154, 1973.

25. Kuligowska, E, and Olsen, W: Pancreatic pseudocysts drained through a percutaneous transgastric approach, Radiology 154:79, 1985.

26. Lawson, T, Berland, L, and Foley, W: Ultrasonic visualization of the pancreatic duct, Radiology 144:865, 1982.

27. Leopold, G: Pancreatic echography: a new dimension in the diagnosis of pseudocyst, Radiology 104:365, 1972.

28. Leopold, G: Echographic study of the pancreas, JAMA 232:287, 1975.

29. Leopold, G, and Asher, W: Deleterious effects of gastrointestinal contrast material on abdominal echography, Radiology 98:637, 1971.

30. Leopold, G, Berk, R, and Reinke, R: Echographic-radiological documentation of spontaneous rupture of a pancreatic pseudocyst into the duodenum, Radiology 102:699, 1972.

31. Lutz, H, and Heyder, N: Transgastric ultrasonography of the pancreas, Ultrasound Med Biol 9:503, 1983.

32. MacMahon, H, Bowie, J, and Beezhold, C: Erect scanning of pancreas using a gastric window, AJR 132:587, 1979.

33. Marks, W, Filly, R, and Callen, P: Ultrasonic evaluation of normal pancreatic echogenicity and its relationship to fat deposition, Radiology 137:475, 1980.

34. Ohto, M, et al: Ultrasonically guided percutaneous contrast medium injection and aspiration biopsy using a real time puncture transducer, Radiology 136:171, 1980.

35. Ohto, M, et al: Real time sonography of the pancreatic duct: Application to percutaneous pancreatic ductography, AJR 134:647, 1980.

36. Okita, K, Kodama, M, and Takemoto, T: Laparoscopic ultrasonography, Scand J Gastroenterol 19(suppl 94):91, 1984.

37. Sample, W, et al: Gray scale ultrasonography: techniques in pancreatic scanning, Appl Radiol 4:63, 1975.

38. Sankaran, S, and Walt, A: Pancreatic ascites, Arch Surg 111:430, 1976.

39. Sarti, D: Rapid development and spontaneous regression of pancreatic pseudocysts documented by ultrasound, Radiology 125:789, 1977.

40. Shawker, T, Doppman, J, and Dunnick, N: Ultrasonic investigation of pancreatic islet cell tumors, J Ultrasound Med 1:193, 1982.

41. Shawker, T, Garra, B, and Hill, M: The spectrum of sonographic findings in pancreatic carcinoma, J Ultrasound Med 5:169, 1986.

42. Shawker, T, Linzer, M, and Hubbard, V: Chronic pancreatitis: size and echo amplitude, J Ultrasound Med 3:267, 1984.

43. Shirkoda, A, and Mittelstaedt, C: Demonstration of pancreatic cysts in adult polycystic disease by computed tomography and ultrasound, AJR 131:1074, 1978.

44. Sigel, B, Machi, J, and Ramos, J: The role of imaging ultrasound during pancreatic surgery, Ann Surg 200:486, 1984.

45. Smith, E, et al: Percutaneous aspiration biopsy of the pancreas under ultrasonic guidance, N Engl J Med 292:825, 1975.

46. Smith, S, Vogelzang, R, and Donovan, J: Intraoperative sonography of the pancreas, AJR 144:557, 1985.

47. Sokoloff, J, et al: Pitfalls in the echographic evaluation of pancreatic disease, J Clin Ultrasound 2:321, 1975.

48. Sommer, G, Filly, R, and Laing, F: Simethicone as a patient preparation for abdominal ultrasonography, Radiology 125:219, 1977.

49. Walls, W, and Templeton, A: Ultrasonic demonstration of inferior vena caval compression: guide to pancreatic head enlargement with emphasis on neoplasm, Radiology 123:165, 1977.

50. Walls, W, et al: B-scan ultrasound evaluation of the pancreas, Radiology 114:127, 1975.

51. Warshaw, A: Inflammatory masses following acute pancreatitis, Surg Clin North Am 54:621, 1974.

52. Weill, F, Brun, P, and Rohmer, P: Migrations of fluid of pancreatic origin, Ultrasound Med Biol 9:485, 1983.

53. Weill, F, et al: Ultrasonography of the normal pancreas: success rate and criteria for normality, Radiology 123:417, 1977.

54. Weinstein, B, Weinstein, D, and Brodmerkl, G: Ultrasonography of pancreatic lithiasis, Radiology 134:185, 1980.

55. Weinstein, D, and Weinstein, B: Ultrasonic demonstration of the pancreatic duct: an analysis of 41 cases, Radiology 130:729, 1979.

56. Wernecke, K, Peters, P, Galanski, M: Pancreatic metatases: US evaluation, Radiology 160:399, 1986.

57. Wolfman, N, Karstaedt, N, and Kawamoto, E: Pleomorphic carcinoma of the pancreas: computed tomographic, sonographic, and pathologic findings, Radiology 154:329, 1985.

58. Wolfman, N, Ramquist, N, and Karstaedt, N: Cystic neoplasms of the pancreas: CT and sonography, AJR 138:37, 1982.

59. Wolson, A, and Walls, W: Ultrasonic characteristics of cystadenomas of the pancreas, Radiology 119:205, 1976.

60. Worthen, N, and Beabeau, D: Normal pancreatic echogenicity: relations to age and body fat, AJR 139:1095, 1982.

43 Radiology of the Pancreas: Diagnostic and Interventional Techniques

PATRICK C. FREENY

A variety of radiologic and fluoroscopically assisted endoscopic techniques are available for evaluation and management of patients with suspected pancreatic disease. The techniques of performing these examinations are crucial for accurate diagnosis and successful patient management.

DIAGNOSTIC EXAMINATIONS

Pancreatic diseases produce a variety of morphologic changes in the gland that can be detected by different imaging modalities. Each modality images different anatomic parts of the pancreas.

Plain radiographs depict changes in the chest or abdomen that result from pancreatic disease. However, with the exception of showing pancreatic ductal calcifications or a soft tissue mass in the region of the pancreas, they do not image the gland directly. Similarly, though barium studies depict changes in the gastrointestinal tract that are caused by pancreatic pathology, they do not image the gland directly.

The cross-sectional modalities of sonography, computed tomography (CT) and magnetic resonance imaging (MRI), visualize the pancreatic parenchyma, main pancreatic duct and biliary tract, major peripancreatic blood vessels, and the organs and structures surrounding the pancreas. Endoscopic retrograde cholangiopancreatography (ERCP), percutaneous pancreatography, and percutaneous transhepatic cholangiography (PTC) image only the pancreatic or biliary ducts. Angiography images the pancreatic and peripancreatic arteries and veins, but also shows the parenchyma if high-dose contrast infusion is used.

The techniques of transhepatic pancreatic venography, fine-needle aspiration biopsy (FNAB), and percutaneous needle aspiration are employed to obtain blood, tissue, or fluid samples for laboratory evaluation.

The initial diagnostic procedure and subsequent sequence of examinations for evaluation of patients with potential pancreatic disease thus depend on the disease suspected and the structures of the gland (parenchyma, blood vessels, ducts) most likely to be involved by the pathologic process or most likely to show diagnostic morphologic changes.

INTERVENTIONAL PROCEDURES

The techniques of ERCP and PTC have been extended to encompass interventional procedures. Endoscopic placement of biliary and pancreatic duct stents and endoscopic papillotomy can be used for treatment of ductal obstruction caused by both neoplastic and inflammatory diseases. Biliary duct obstruction also can be relieved by percutaneous transhepatic catheter or endoprosthesis placement.

Angiographic techniques of transcatheter embolization can be used to control bleeding caused by inflammatory or neoplastic pancreatic diseases and to control symptoms resulting from hepatic metastases from functioning islet cell neoplasms.

Catheters also can be placed percutaneously within pancreatic or peripancreatic fluid collections, pseudocysts, or abscesses for drainage.

DIAGNOSTIC EXAMINATIONS: TECHNIQUES AND NORMAL ANATOMY
Sonography

The development of high-resolution real-time sonographic scanners has facilitated evaluation of the pancreas and, equally important, the biliary tract. Sonography can be performed both transcutaneously and directly on the surface of the pancreas during surgery (intraoperative sonography).[13]

Techniques

Current real-time scanners usually employ transducers that operate at a frequency of 3 to 7.5 MHz. Most transducers are sector scanners that encompass an arc of 30 to 120 degrees. The transducers can be oriented in virtually any plane, so that the pancreatic gland parenchyma, pancreatic and biliary ducts, and major peripancreatic arteries and veins can be displayed on multiple images. Because intestinal gas interferes with sonographic imaging, the liver, spleen, and kidneys often are used as acoustic windows. Alternatively, the stomach and duodenum can be filled with orally ingested fluid, yielding a temporary window.

Intraoperative sonography is now often employed to evaluate the pancreas for the presence of small tumors, usually islet cell neoplasms.[9] Because the transducer is applied directly to the surface of the surgically exposed gland, high-frequency (7.5 to 10 MHz) transducers can be used to produce high-resolution images.[9]

Normal anatomy

The pancreatic features assessable by sonography include gland size and parenchymal texture pattern, pancreatic duct caliber, wall thickness, regularity, the presence of intraductal filling defects (calculi or neoplasms), peripancreatic blood vessels, and intrapancreatic and extrapancreatic bile duct anatomy.[13]

The echogenicity of the normal pancreatic parenchyma is homogeneous, equivalent to or slightly greater than that of the normal liver and slightly less than that

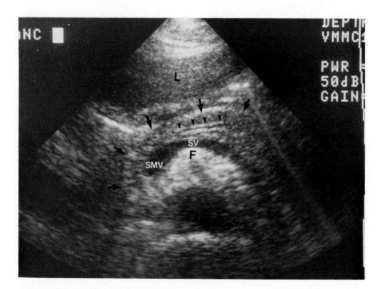

Fig. 43-1 Pancreatic sonography. Real-time sonogram of a normal pancreas *(arrows)* shows echo texture pattern equal to liver *(L)*) and less than retropancreatic fat *(F)*. Splenic *(SV)* and superior mesenteric *(SMV)* veins and segment of normal pancreatic duct *(arrowheads)* are seen.

of the retroperitoneal fat. The pancreatic duct is a thin, tubular structure with smooth, parallel walls (Fig. 43-1). The internal diameter usually measures only 2 to 3 mm.[6] High-resolution transducers usually can display the celiac, superior mesenteric, hepatic, splenic, and occasionally gastroduodenal arteries and the splenic, superior mesenteric, and portal veins. The intrapancreatic segment of the common bile duct, the common hepatic duct, and the gall bladder are seen routinely.

Computed tomography

CT is currently the most important technique for imaging the pancreas. It has a high diagnostic accuracy rate for both neoplastic and inflammatory disease.[6]

Technique

Current CT scanners operate at scan speeds of less than 2 seconds and use automatic table incrementation. Examinations are performed following oral contrast administration and during injection of a bolus of intravenous contrast. Thus the pancreatic parenchyma, pancreatic and biliary ducts, peripancreatic arteries and veins, and surrounding solid and hollow organs are imaged with precise anatomic detail.

The best anatomic detail is obtained using 5 or 10 mm collimation and contiguous scans. Intravenous contrast is administered as a bolus of 150 to 180 ml of 60% iodinated agent via a peripheral vein.[5,6] The bolus is given over 60 to 90 seconds, with the scan sequence initiated after the first 50 ml has been given. This produces an increase in pancreatic parenchymal attenuation of about 50 to 60 HU (Hounsfield units) over a noncontrast baseline, thus aiding in detection of small, hypervascular or hypovascular intrapancreatic masses (Fig. 43-2). In addition, contrast enhancement of the peripancreatic blood vessels aids in diagnosis, particularly in assessing the resectability of neoplasms.

CT of the pancreas should also include evaluation of the liver and the rest of the abdomen. This is important for detection of metastases from primary pancreatic neoplasms, for evaluation of the extent of involvement in pancreatic inflammatory disease (pancreatitis), and for detection of incidental pathology or other abnormalities that can mimic pancreatic disease.[7]

Normal anatomy

Bolus-enhanced CT of the pancreas displays the pancreatic parenchyma, pancreatic and biliary ducts, peri-

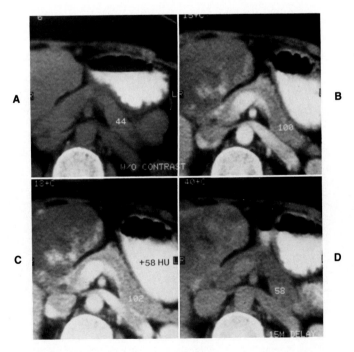

Fig. 43-2 Pancreatic CT. **A,** Single level bolus-dynamic scan shows attenuation of normal pancreatic parenchyma of 44 HU. **B** and **C,** Scans during bolus-dynamic phase show increase parenchymal attenuation to maximum of 102 HU, 58 HU above baseline. Note excellent contrast enhancement of peripancreatic vessels. **D,** Fifteen-minute delayed scan shows decrease of attenuation to 58 HU, only 14 HU above baseline.

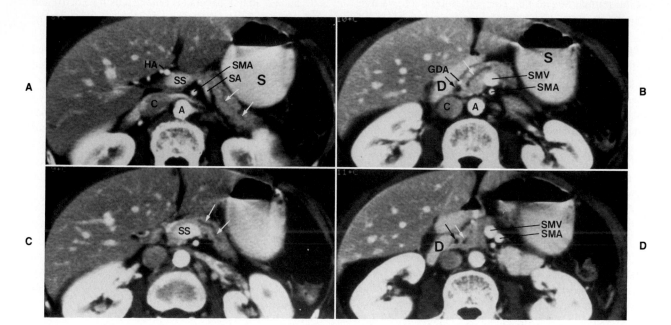

Fig. 43-3 Pancreatic CT. **A** and **B,** Contiguous 10 mm bolus-dynamic scans show normal pancreatic duct (white arrows) in body and tail of gland. **C** and **D,** Scans at level of head show pancreatic duct *(white arrows)* and common bile duct *(black arrows)* on cross section. Contrast opacifies stomach *(S)* and duodenum *(D)*. *HA,* hepatic artery; *GDA,* gastroduodenal artery; *SA,* splenic artery; *SMA,* superior mesenteric artery; *SMV,* superior mesenteric vein; *A,* aorta; *C,* inferior vena cava. *SS,* junction of splenic vein-superior mesenteric vein.

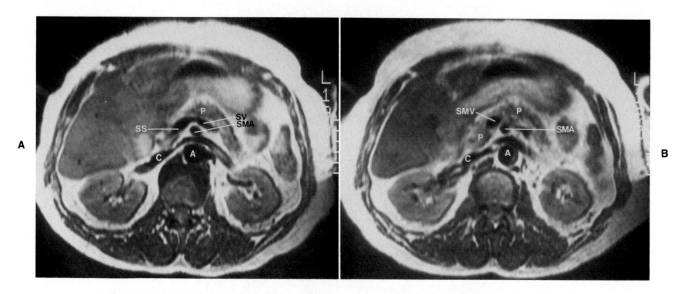

Fig. 43-4 Pancreatic MRI. **A** and **B,** Normal pancreas MRI (1.5 T; SE, TR 2000/TE 25) shows gland parenchyma *(P)* as area of low signal intensity. Gland is surrounded by peripancreatic fat of high signal intensity. Peripancreatic vessels have no signal (flow void), indicating vessel patency. *A,* aorta; *C,* inferior vena cava; *SMA,* superior mesenteric artery; *SMV,* superior mesenteric vein; *SV,* splenic vein; *SS,* junction of superior mesenteric-splenic veins.

pancreatic vessels, normal peripancreatic fascia, and surrounding solid and hollow organs (Fig. 43-3).

The normal pancreatic parenchyma shows homogeneous contrast enhancement.[5] The texture may be smooth or may show a lobulated pattern caused by normal amounts of fat within and along the lobular septae of the gland. Segments of the normal pancreatic duct and intrapancreatic segment of the common bile duct are usually seen.[1,6] The pancreatic duct diameter is about 2 to 4 mm, and the intrapancreatic common bile duct diameter is usually less than 6 to 7 mm. The contrast sensitivity of CT makes detection of pancreatic and biliary duct calculi highly accurate.

The peripancreatic arteries and veins are displayed precisely by bolus-enhanced CT (Fig. 43-4). However, because these structures run obliquely through the standard axial CT planes, only short segments usually are seen on each scan. Thus the sequence of scan images of the vessels must be visually collated. This is also true of the pancreas and pancreatic duct, as well as the surrounding solid and hollow organs.

Magnetic resonance imaging

MRI is the newest imaging technique to be applied to the pancreas. Though it has not yet significantly improved diagnosis of pancreatic disease, the future holds much promise.[11,23]

Technique

Techniques of MRI of the pancreas have not been well defined. The morphologic appearance of the pancreas varies, depending on the magnetic field strength of the scanner and the pulse sequences that are selected.

MRI scanners operating at low field strength (0.35 to 0.5 T) probably yield the best image of the pancreas when using averaging of multiple short-TR/short-TE spin-echo pulse sequences. Units operating at high field strength (1.5 T) probably yield the best image when using T_2-weighted spin-echo sequences (TR, 2000; TE, 35, 70).[21]

Normal anatomy

MRI displays the normal pancreatic parenchyma, peripancreatic blood vessels, and upper abdominal solid organs but does not reliably show the pancreatic duct or surrounding hollow organs as well as CT does (Fig. 43-4). In addition, detection of intraductal calculi or tumoral calcification is inherently less than with CT.[11,21] Thus MR is less precise than CT for evaluation of patients with suspected chronic pancreatitis.[11]

A major advantage of MRI is its ability to image the peripancreatic blood vessels without the use of intravenous contrast. Flowing blood produces a signal void; thus

tumor invasion or thrombosis of arteries or veins are clearly depicted by MRI as vessels with increased signal.[21]

Endoscopic retrograde cholangiopancreatography

The pancreatic duct can be altered by both inflammatory and neoplastic disease. Thus ERCP is highly sensitive for diagnosis of ductal carcinoma and pancreatitis.[6]

Interventional ERCP techniques applicable to the pancreas include endoscopic papillotomy and endoscopic placement of biliary and pancreatic duct stents for treatment of benign and malignant ductal obstruction.[16,19]

Technique

ERCP is performed using a side-viewing endoscope and a variety of cannulas with both tapered and nontapered tips or tiny needlelike tips.[6] Using needle cannulas, the accessory or minor papilla can be cannulated with a relatively high degree of reliability.

The cannula is manipulated under direct vision by the endoscopist, while the radiologist fluoroscopically monitors the procedure during injections of contrast agent and records the ductal anatomy on film. Careful fluoroscopic monitoring is also essential during endoscopic papillotomy and placement of pancreatic or biliary duct stents.

Normal anatomy

The normal pancreatic duct has smooth, parallel walls that gradually taper from the papilla to the tail of the gland[6,22] (Fig. 43-5). The normal diameter of the main duct is about 3 to 5 mm in the head, 2 to 3 mm in the body, and 1 to 2 mm in the tail of the gland.[6] The small lateral side branches are evenly distributed along the course of the main duct, and several prominent ducts are often seen draining the head and uncinate portion of the gland (Fig. 43-5, A). The accessory duct extends from the minor papilla, which is about 1.5 to 2.0 cm proximal to the main papilla, to join the main pancreatic duct in the neck of the gland (junction of head and body) (Fig. 43-5, B). The minor papilla is patent in 30% to 60% of patients and thus may act as an accessory route of drainage if the main duct is blocked between the major papilla and the accessory duct junction.[6]

The major (duct of Wirsung) and minor (duct of Santorini) ducts fail to fuse in about 5% to 7% of patients, producing a pancreas divisum.[6] In this case, both the major and minor papillae must be cannulated to display the anatomy of the entire pancreatic ductal system. A small duct of Wirsung should not be misinterpreted as an obstructed main duct.[3]

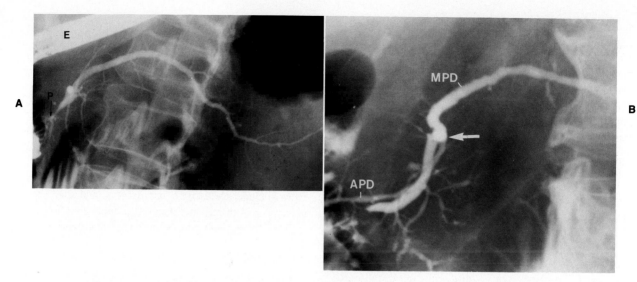

Fig. 43-5 Normal ERCP. **A,** Main pancreatic duct shows smooth, tapering walls from papilla *(P)* to tail. Lateral side branches are evenly spaced. Larger branches from uncinate are seen *(arrowheads)*. *E,* endoscope. **B,** Close-up of normal ERCP of head of pancreas shows junction *(arrow)* of accessory (APD) and main (MPD) pancreatic ducts.

Percutaneous transhepatic cholangiography

The intrapancreatic segment of the common bile duct often is altered by carcinoma or pancreatitis.[6,22] PTC can be used for diagnostic evaluation of the biliary ducts if obstructive jaundice is present, or the techniques can be extended for percutaneous placement of transhepatic or endoprosthetic biliary drainage catheters.[12,18]

Technique

PTC is performed from a right lateral intercostal or left subcostal approach with local anesthetic and mild intravenous sedation.[4,20] The standard PTC needle is a thin, flexible 22- or 23-gauge needle.[4] It is advanced into the liver under fluoroscopic control, avoiding the pleural space, and small amounts of contrast are injected as the needle is withdrawn. When a bile duct is entered, contrast is injected, opacifying the biliary tract.

Patients with bile duct obstruction can undergo drainage via the percutaneous tract used for the PTC. Several needle-catheter sets are available commercially, including a .018-inch guidewire that passes through a 21-gauge PTC needle. A standard PTC is performed, opacifying the bile ducts and identifying the obstruction. The wire can then be advanced through the needle into the punctured bile duct and manipulated across the obstruction. A permanent transhepatic catheter or endoprosthesis can then be advanced over the wire.[4,18,20]

Angiography

CT and ERCP have replaced angiography for diagnosis of most pancreatic diseases.[7] However, angiography continues to play an important role in evaluating patients with equivocal CT or ERCP findings, assessing vascular anatomy before pancreatic surgery, and diagnosing and controlling pancreatic hemorrhage, usually caused by severe pancreatic inflammatory disease.[6]

Technique

Pancreatic angiography usually is performed via a femoral artery approach. Selective and superselective visceral catheters are then used to catheterize the celiac and superior mesenteric arteries and their major branches (hepatic, gastroduodenal, splenic, dorsal pancreatic, and inferior pancreaticoduodenal). Accurate angiographic diagnosis depends on complete opacification of the intrapancreatic and peripancreatic vascular network. This is best achieved with superselective, high-volume injections.[6]

Normal anatomy

The blood supply to the pancreas arises from branches of the splenic artery (dorsal pancreatic artery, pancreatica magna artery), the gastroduodenal artery (anterior and posterior superior pancreaticoduodenal artery, transverse pancreatic artery), and the superior mesenteric artery (anterior and posterior inferior pancreaticoduodenal arteries).[6] Selective injection of these main vessels, or superselective injection of the major branches, produces excellent filling of the pancreatic vasculature (Fig. 43-6).

Transhepatic pancreatic venography

In some patients with functioning islet cell tumors, the primary tumor cannot be localized preoperatively by

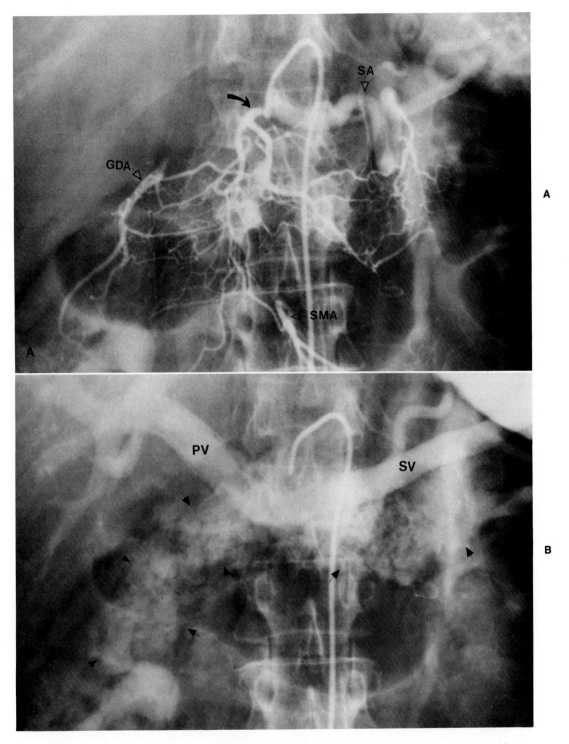

Fig. 43-6 Pancreatic angiogram. **A** and **B,** High-volume selective dorsal pancreatic artery *(curved arrow)* injection (**A,** arterial phase) shows filling of intrapancreatic vessels and retrograde filling of splenic *(SA)*, gastroduodenal *(GDA)*, and superior mesenteric *(SMA)* arteries *(arrows)*. Parenchymal phase (**B**) shows normal lobular pattern of pancreatic parenchyma (arrows) and filling of splenic vein *(SV)* and portal vein *(PV)*.

CT, MRI, sonography, or angiography. In these patients, transhepatic pancreatic venography (TPV) with selective venous sampling is a useful method for tumor localization.[2,6]

Technique

TPV is performed in a fashion similar to PTC: a 21-gauge needle is placed into the hepatic parenchyma via a right lateral intercostal approach using local anesthesia and mild intravenous sedation. Contrast is injected as the needle is withdrawn. When a portal vein branch is entered, a .018-inch guidewire is passed through the needle and manipulated into the portal vein. A No. 5 or 6.5 French catheter is passed over the wire and into the main pancreatic vein branches of the splenic and superior mesenteric veins.[6] Venous blood samples are then collected and sent for laboratory assay for the appropriate pancreatic hormone (for example, gastrin or insulin). A map of the sampled pancreatic veins and their hormone levels is then constructed to locate the tumor for the surgeon.[2]

Normal anatomy

The pancreatic veins are paired with the corresponding pancreatic arteries and have the same names (dorsal pancreatic vein, transverse pancreatic vein, and so on). The posterosuperior pancreatic vein usually is a branch of the main portal vein, and the anterosuperior vein is a branch of the gastrocolic trunk, which enters at the lateral confluence of the superior mesenteric and main portal veins.[6]

Fine-needle aspiration biopsy

Pancreatic masses often have a nonspecific appearance and may be caused by inflammatory disease or by different types of neoplasm. Though ductal adenocarcinoma is usually incurable, other neoplasms such as islet cell carcinoma and lymphoma may respond to chemotherapy or radiation therapy or be curable by surgical resection. Thus a specific pathologic diagnosis must be made to assure proper patient management.[6] This can be accomplished safely and effectively with radiologically-guided FNAB.

Technique

Most pancreatic biopsies are performed with a 22- or 23-gauge needle.[10] Precise guidance that permits visualization of the needle tip will result in a positive biopsy in about 80% to 85% of cases[10] (Fig. 43-7). Examples of guidance techniques are fluoroscopic guidance with ERCP, angiography, PTC, bile duct drainage catheter, or endoprosthesis for targeting; CT; or sonography with transducer biopsy guide. The needle is introduced percutaneously using sterile technique, local anesthesia, and intravenous sedation. Suction is applied with a 10 ml syringe as the needle is rotated and oscillated. The as-

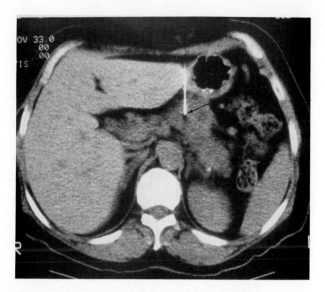

Fig. 43-7 FNAB. CT-guided FNAB shows 23-gauge needle *(arrow)* in focal mass (adenocarcinoma) in pancreatic body.

pirate is placed on glass slides and stained with a quick-stain technique. This material is examined immediately for cytologic diagnosis. Additional material can be obtained for a cell block, which can be evaluated with both light and electron microscopy.[6]

Recent reports indicate improved results with similar safety using an 18-gauge cutting biopsy needle.[15] The biopsy needle design is commercially available as Tru Cut and is operated with a spring-driven biopsy gun. Lees and Rode reported that biopsies performed with this technique were better tolerated by the patient than conventional fine-needle aspiration biopsies.[15]

Fine-needle fluid aspiration and percutaneous pancreatography

Using the same techniques as described for aspiration biopsy, 22- and 23-gauge needles can be placed in pancreatic fluid collections in patients with pancreatitis to determine the presence of infection.[8,24] The needles are inserted under CT or sonographic guidance into various locations within the fluid collections to assure that appropriate sampling of the fluid is achieved (Fig. 43-8). The material is then sent for Gram stain and culture. This technique has assumed increasing importance in management of patients with severe pancreatitis.[8,24]

The primary uses of percutaneous pancreatography are to guide FNAB and to define ductal anatomy before pancreatic surgery for patients in whom ERCP is unsuccessful in obtaining ductal opacification.[14,17] The procedure is performed under combined sonographic and fluoroscopic guidance. A puncture site is usually chosen in the midbody of the pancreas, close to the skin surface. The needle is inserted under mild intravenous sedation

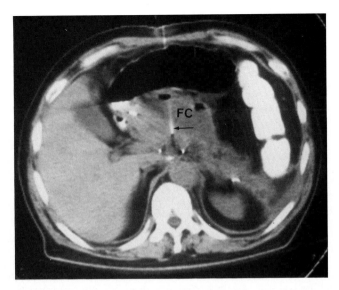

Fig. 43-8 Fine-needle fluid aspiration. CT-guided fluid collection *(FC)* aspiration showed bacterial infection, leading to successful percutaneous catheter drainage.

and a local anesthetic. When the needle tip echo is noted within the duct, the stylet is removed and pancreatic juice aspirated. Contrast is then injected to opacify the ductal system. It is best to limit the amount of contrast to an amount equal to or less than the amount of aspirated pancreatic juice.[17] This will reduce or virtually eliminate overdistention and subsequent pancreatitis.

Percutaneous catheter drainage

Percutaneous catheter drainage is a nonsurgical alternative for treatment of infected and noninfected pancreatic fluid collections or pseudocysts. The indications, techniques, and results are discussed in Chapter 46.

REFERENCES

1. Berland, LL, et al: Computed tomography of the normal and abnormal pancreatic duct: correlation with pancreatic ductography, Radiology 141:715-724, 1981.
2. Cho, KJ, et al: Localization of the source of hyperinsulinism: percutaneous transhepatic portal and pancreatic vein catheterization with hormone assay, AJR 139:237, 1982.
3. Classen, M, and Phillip, J: Endoscopic retrograde cholangiopancreatography (ERCP) and endoscopic therapy in pancreatic disease, Clin Gastroenterol 13:819, 1984.
4. Ferrucci, JT, Jr, Mueller, PR, and Harbin, WP: Percutaneous transhepatic biliary drainage: technique, results, and applications, Radiology 135:1, 1980.
5. Freeny, PC: Computed tomography of the pancreas, Clin Gastroenterol 13:791, 1984.
6. Freeny, PC, and Lawson, TL: Radiology of the pancreas, New York, 1982, Springer-Verlag.
7. Freeny, PC, Marks, WM, and Ball, TJ: Impact of high-resolution computed tomography on utilization of ERCP and angiography, Radiology 142:35, 1982.
8. Gerzof, SG, et al: Role of guided percutaneous aspiration in early diagnosis of sepsis, Dig Dis Sci 29:950, 1984.
9. Gorman, B, et al: Benign pancreatic insulinoma: preoperative and intraoperative sonographic localization, AJR 147:929, 1986.
10. Hall-Craggs, MA, and Lees, WR: Fine-needle aspiration biopsy: pancreatic and biliary tumors, AJR 147:399, 1986.
11. Jenkins, JPR, et al: Quantitative tissue characterization in pancreatic disease using magnetic resonance imaging, Br J Radiol 60:333, 1987.
12. Lammer, J, and Neumayer, K: Biliary drainage endoprostheses: experience with 201 placements, Radiology 159:625, 1986.
13. Lees, WR: Pancreatic ultrasonography, Clin Gastroenterol 13:763, 1984.
14. Lees, WR, and Heron, CW: US-guided percutaneous pancreatography: experience in 75 patients, Radiology 165:809, 1987.
15. Lees, WR, and Rode, J: 18 swg cutting biopsy of the pancreas: feasibility, results, and safety. Presented at the Seventy-second Scientific Session and Annual Meeting of the Radiologic Society of North America, Chicago, November 30, 1986.
16. Marks, WM, et al: Endoscopic retrograde biliary drainage, Radiology 152:357, 1984.
17. Matter, D, et al: Pancreatic duct: US-guided percutaneous opacification, Radiology 163:635, 1987.
18. May, GR, et al: Diagnosis and treatment of jaundice, RadioGraphics 6:847, 1986.
19. McCarthy, J, Greenen, JE, and Hogan, WJ: Preliminary experience with endoscopic stent placement in benign pancreatic diseases, Gastrointest Endosc 34:16, 1988.
20. Mueller, PR, et al: Obstruction of the left hepatic duct: diagnosis and treatment by selective fine-needle cholangiography and percutaneous biliary drainage, Radiology 145:297, 1982.
21. Stark, DD, and Bradley, WG, Jr: Magnetic resonance imaging, St. Louis, 1988, The C.V. Mosby Co.
22. Stewart, ET, Vennes, JA, and Geenen, JE; Atlas of endoscopic retrograde cholangiopancreatography, St. Louis, 1977, The C.V. Mosby Co.
23. Tscholakoff, D, et al: MR imaging in the diagnosis of pancreatic disease, AJR 148:703, 1987.
24. vanSonnenberg, E, et al: Complicated pancreatic inflammatory disease: diagnostic and therapeutic role of interventional radiology, Radiology 155:335, 1985.

44 *Radionuclide Examinations*

BRIAN C. LENTLE

The pancreas, situated retroperitoneally high in the epigastrium, was a particularly difficult organ to image noninvasively before ultrasonography and computed tomography (CT) became available. Indeed the organ still remains difficult to examine in some patients, a fact reflected in the variety of methods available to evaluate pancreatic morphology.

It is something of a paradox that the pancreas is metabolically active and physiologically important but that its examination by radionuclide methods has virtually ceased to have any role in day-to-day clinical practice. To some extent this is caused by the tendency of the pancreas's commonest gross diseases—carcinoma and pancreatitis, for example—to result in nonfunction of the entire organ.[2] Disorders of pancreatic endocrine function have generally not required imaging methods for diagnosis, although an understanding of diabetes mellitus and its nosology has been advanced by radioimmunoassay of plasma insulin concentrations.[35]

RADIOPHARMACEUTICALS

After some unsuccessful approaches to imaging of the pancreas with radionuclides[24] a method was developed that reflected the considerable rate of protein synthesis in normal pancreatic tissue. Blau had reported the incorporation of selenium-75 (^{75}Se) methionine into proteins when the selenium was substituted for the atom of sulfur normally present in the essential amino acid methionine.[3] ^{75}Se-selenomethionine can be produced either by chemical or biologic synthesis; it has also been used for tumor scintigraphy[25] and localization of parathyroid adenomas.[23]

Of an injected dose of ^{75}Se-methionine 6% to 7% is taken up within the pancreas in the first hour.[17] Uptake per gram is greatest in small bowel mucosa, and liver extraction is only 15% that of the pancreas—but the mass of the liver and its position relative to the pancreas contribute to the difficulties in pancreatic imaging by radionuclide methods.

Although methionine, of the essential amino acids, has one of the lowest pancreas-to-liver ratios,[29] the use of other labeled amino acids for single photon imaging has been no more successful.[7,29,32] Positron tomography has prompted the examination of ^{11}C-labeled (C is carbon) compounds such as ^{11}C–DL-tryptophan,[5,13,27] but no consistent role for such techniques either in elucidating disease processes or in clinical practice has yet emerged. Syrota et al. believe that such a role will emerge in the future.[28]

There have been attempts made to image, scintigraphically, islet cells in animals and in patients with insulinomas, but up to the present they have not been consistently successful.[1,4]

Perhaps the methods that have proved most valuable in radionuclide examinations of the pancreas are those that are not directed at the pancreas at all. Scintigraphy with gallium-67 (^{67}Ga) citrate and radiolabeled granulocytes is usually undertaken to search for otherwise occult infection. These methods are valuable in that they capitalize on the fact that such whole-body searches do not cause incremental radiation exposure (with radionuclide investigations the dose commitment is defined when the radiotracer is injected rather than with each image obtained). The localization of ^{67}Ga-citrate at inflamed sites is well recognized if poorly understood,[30] whereas the localization of radiolabeled granulocytes at sites of inflammation is conceptually simple, although the actual labeling is demanding in terms of the support services necessary.

CLINICAL METHODS

Imaging of the pancreas with ^{75}Se-selenomethionine was performed with a dose of 250 μCi (microcuries) (9.25 mBq) and, until single photon emission computed tomography because available, the gamma-camera head was positioned with a small degree of cephalad tilt. This, with occasional use of left anterior oblique positioning, helped to minimize the impact on the images of liver activity; nevertheless it became usual to attempt subtractive imaging using liver scintigraphy performed with technetium-99m (^{99}Tc) sulfide colloid.[9] Clearance of ^{75}Se-selenomethionine into the pancreas is very rapid, and images can be obtained within minutes of intravenous injection. The poor photon flux made it desirable to obtain serial 10-minute images for up to 1 hour. Because disease usually resulted in nonvisualization of the pancreas, it proved ineffective to define exposure in terms of count density, at least in respect to the pancreas.

DISEASES OF THE PANCREAS
Carcinoma

Pancreatic scintigraphy, using ^{75}Se-selenomethionine, was used for a brief time to examine the pancreas when carcinoma was suspected. Resolution was poor, and, despite careful positioning of the gamma-camera head and dual nuclide subtractive techniques, the method was limited in its usefulness. With the development of such alternative methods of examining the pancreas as ultra-

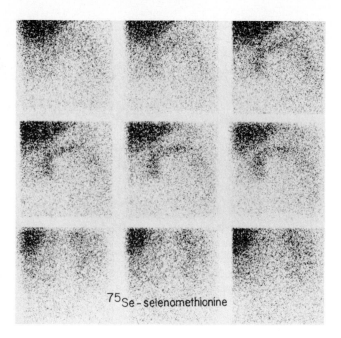

Fig. 44-1 Coronal sectional images of a normal pancreas made with ^{75}Se-selenomethionine. Note uptake of tracer in liver.

sonography, CT, and endoscopic retrograde pancreatography, this technique for examining the pancreas is rarely, if ever, used.

Although the normal pancreas is relatively easily defined as such, particularly using single-photon tomography (Fig. 44-1), disease of any kind results in limited or absent uptake of ^{75}Se-selenomethionine, with the additional complication that there is sometimes slight localization of this tracer in the tumor, reflecting its anabolic metabolism (Fig. 44-2). In one of the larger studies the method had a sensitivity and a specificity of only 0.65 and 0.64, respectively, for all disease.[11] (Higher sensitivities had been reported earlier,[26] presumably in more highly selected groups of patients.)

Pancreatitis

Pancreatitis has been identified as a cause of nonvisualization of the pancreas on imaging with ^{75}Se-selenomethionine, and of course pancreatitis may complicate carcinoma, particularly of the pancreatic head. These facts probably contribute to the nonspecificity of the method just described.

Pancreatitis can also be visualized directly using either ^{67}Ga-citrate or the patient's own radiolabeled granulocytes. The former technique potentially reveals either a tumor or inflammatory process, but in practice pancreatic carcinoma is rarely imaged in a satisfactory way with ^{67}Ga because of limitations on resolution. In an appropriate clinical context ^{67}Ga localization in the region of the pancreas suggests a diagnosis of pancreatitis.[20]

Granulocytes have been labeled with indium-111

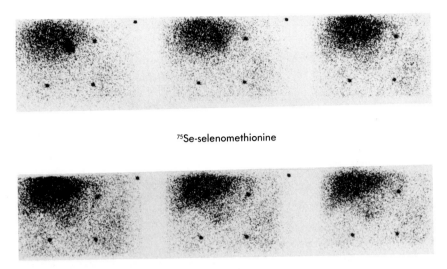

⁷⁵Se-selenomethionine

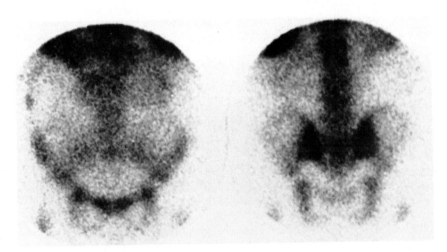

Fig. 44-2 Coronal sectional images of patient with adenocarcinoma of pancreatic head. Disrupted pancreatic morphology is evident in comparison with Fig. 44-1.

Fig. 44-3 Anterior and posterior views of lower trunk. Localization of ^{111}In-labeled granulocytes in epigastrium of patient subsequently shown to have pancreatitis. There is normal visualization, in addition, of liver, spleen, and bone marrow.

(^{111}In) oxine and tropolone, ^{99}Tc colloids, and more recently with ^{99m}Tc–hexamethyl propylene amine oxine.[19] Such radiolabeled granulocytes provide an elegant and more specific method of disclosing focal sepsis (Fig. 44-3). Although no study limited to patients suspected of having pancreatitis has been reported in this context, a sensitivity and a specificity of the order of 0.85 and 0.95, respectively, have been reported in localizing occult intraabdominal infection with ^{111}In-labeled leukocytes.[10] In general this technique is most effectively used in the absence of localizing symptoms and signs. When the clinical findings point to a pancreatitis, other imaging methods are usually more appropriate.[16]

Pancreatic pseudocyst

In a patient with a pseudocyst complicating pancreatitis or other diseases, such a lesion is best identified and characterized by techniques that are directed to morphologic display, such as CT and ultrasonography. Nevertheless, since a pseudocyst represents a fluid collection that is not in rapidly dynamic equilibrium with the extravascular-extracellular (interstitial) space, any technique displaying these spaces more than very transiently will permit recognition of a pseudocyst as a photon-deficient lesion in the region of the pancreas.[14] Such photon-deficient areas may even be recognized when relatively low photon fluxes are available, for example with

^{67}Ga-citrate scintigraphy[21] (although this tracer has been reported to localize in an infected pseudocyst[15]).

There is an additional report of a pseudocyst being imaged by virtue of how much ^{75}Se-selenomethionine (used to image the pancreas) it contains,[18] an observation that will probably hold true for the more recently developed labeled amino acids already described.

Finally, it is known that intrasplenic dissection by pancreatic pseudocysts may occur.[18] This phenomenon has been observed on appropriate images made with ^{99m}Tc-sulfide colloid.[12,22,33,34]

Disordered pancreatic exocrine function

The pancreatic ductal system has been explored using a retrograde injection of ^{99m}Tc-labeled compounds in dogs.[32] No application of this technique to human disease has emerged.[31]

Measurement of ^{75}Se-selenomethionine in the duodenal aspirate[6] and ^{14}C in the breath after administration of ^{14}C-palmitin[36] have been suggested as tests of pancreatic exocrine function. The ^{75}Se-selenomethionine scan itself has been used to assess improved pancreatic function after surgery for pancreatitis.[8]

REFERENCES

1. Balachandran, S, et al: Tissue distribution of C-14-, I-125- and I-131-diphenylhydantoin in the toadfish, rat and human with insulinomas, J Nucl Med 16:775, 1975.
2. Barkin, J, et al: Computerized tomography, diagnostic ultrasound, and radionuclide scanning: comparison of efficacy in diagnosis of pancreatic carcinoma, JAMA 238:2040, 1977.
3. Blau, M: Biosynthesis of [^{75}Se]-selenomethionine and [^{75}Se]-selenocystine, Biochem Biophys Acta 49:389, 1961.
4. Boyd, CM: Studies on the tissue distribution of I-125 iodopropamide in the dog, J Nucl Med 12:117, 1971.
5. Buonocore, E, and Huber, KF: Positron-emission computed tomography of the pancreas: a preliminary study, Radiology 133:195, 1979.
6. Chen, I-W, et al: C-14 tripalmitin breath test as a diagnostic aid for fat malabsorption due to pancreatic insufficiency, J Nucl Med 15:1125, 1974.
7. Cottrell, MF, Taylor, DM, and McElwain, TJ: Investigations of F-18-p-fluorophenylalamine for pancreas scanning, Br J Radiol 46:277, 1973.
8. Eaton, SB, et al: Evaluation of corrective surgery for pancreatitis by Se-75 selenomethionine pancreatic imaging, AJR 112:678, 1971.
9. Eaton, SB, et al: Radioisotopic "subtraction" scanning for pancreatic lesions, AJR 89:1033, 1967.
10. Froelich, JW, and Swanson, D: Imaging of inflammatory processes with labeled cells, Semin Med 14:128, 1984.
11. Hall, FJ, Cooper, M, and Hughes, RG: Pancreatic cancer screening: analysis of the problem and the role of radionuclide imaging, Am J Surg 134:544, 1977.
12. Hanelin, J, and Carlson, DH: A case of pancreatic pseudocyst extending into the spleen with associated subcapsular hemorrhage, Clin Nucl Med 3:232, 1978.
13. Hayes, RL, et al: Synthesis and purification of C-11-carboxy-labeled amino acids, Int J Appl Radiat Isotop 29:186, 1978.
14. Jackson, FI, and Lentle, BC: Scintigraphic recognition of pancreatic pseudocysts, Clin Nucl Med 1:145, 1976.
15. Kennedy, TD, et al: Identification of an infected psuedocyst of the pancreas with ^{67}Ga-citrate, J Nucl Med 16:1132, 1975.
16. Knochel, JQ, et al: Diagnosis of abdominal abscesses with computed tomography, ultrasound, and In-111 leukocyte scans, Radiology 137:425, 1980.
17. Lathrop, KA, Honston, RE, and Blau, M: Radiation dose to humans from Se-75 selenomethionine, J Nucl Med (MIRD suppl 6, pamphlet 9) p 10, 1972.
18. Mattar, AG, and Prezio, JA: Visualization of pancreatic pseudocyst, J Nucl Med 16:326, 1975.
19. McAfee, JG, Subramanian, G, and Gagne, G: Technique of leukocyte harvesting and labeling: problems and perspectives, Semin Nucl Med 14:83, 1984.
20. Myerson, PJ, et al: Gallium-67 spread into the anterior pararenal space in pancreatitis: case report, J Nucl Med 18:893, 1977.
21. Park, HM: Pancreatic pseudocyst: photopenic abdominal lesion on gallium-67 imaging, Clin Nucl Med 1:269, 1976.
22. Parker, JA, Popky, GL, and Younis, MT: Use of the spleen scan in evaluation of pancreatic pseudocyst, Clin Nucl Med 1:132, 1976.
23. Potchen, EJ, Watts, HG, and Awwad, HK: Parathyroid scintiscanning, Radiol Clin N Am 5:267, 1967.
24. Shapiro, R: Radioopacification of the pancreas: a review of experimental efforts, Semin Roentgenol 3:318, 1968.
25. Spencer, RP, et al: Uptake of selenomethionine by mouse and in human lymphomas, with observations on selenite and selenate, J Nucl Med 8:197, 1967.
26. Staab, EV, et al: Pancreatic radionuclide imaging using electronic subtraction technique, Radiology 99:633, 1971.
27. Syrota, A, et al: [C-11] methionine pancreatic scanning with positron emission computed tomography, J Nucl Med 20:778, 1979.
28. Syrota, A, et al: The role of positron emission tomography in the detection of pancreatic disease, Radiology 143:249, 1982.
29. Taylor, DM, and Cottrall, MT: Evaluation of amino-acids labeled with F-18 for pancreas scanning in radiopharmaceuticals and labeled compounds, vol 1, Vienna 1973, International Atomic Energy Agency.
30. Tsan, MF: Mechanism of gallium 67 accumulation in inflammatory lesions, J Nucl Med 26:88, 1985.
31. Varley, PF, Silvis, SE, and Shafer, RB: Pancreatic scanning using retrograde injection of technetium-99m-labeled compounds, J Nucl Med 18:676, 1977.
32. Varma, VM: Pancreatic concentration of I-125-labeled phenylalamine in mice, J Nucl Med 10:219, 1969.
33. Warshaw, AL, et al: Intrasplenic dissection by pancreatic pseudocysts, N Engl J Med 287:72, 1972.
34. Wellisch, M, and Holmquest, D: Diagnosis of a pancreatic pseudocyst from the liver-spleen scan, J Nucl Med 14:107, 1973.
35. Yalow, RS, and Berson, SA: Immunoassay of endogenous plasma insulin in man, J Clin Invest 39:1157, 1960.
36. Youngs, GR, et al: Radioselenium in duodenal aspirate as an assessment of pancreatic exocrine function, Br Med J 2:252, 1971.

45 *Nonneoplastic Lesions*

PATRICK C. FREENY
CHARLES A. ROHRMANN, JR.

PANCREATITIS: GENERAL CONSIDERATIONS

Two international symposia have recently been held to evaluate the current understanding of pancreatitis, to correlate new data regarding function and morphology, and to offer an improved classification system. The first was held in Cambridge in 1983, and the second in Marseille in 1984.[73,134]

Cambridge and Marseille classifications
Acute pancreatitis

The 1983 Cambridge Symposium defined acute pancreatitis as an acute inflammatory disease of the pancreas typically presenting with abdominal pain, and usually associated with raised pancreatic enzymes in blood or urine.[134] Although acute pancreatitis can recur, the original 1963 Marseille subdivision of relapsing acute pancreatitis was eliminated.[133]

The 1984 Marseille Symposium defined acute pancreatitis essentially in the same terms as the Cambridge group, but included morphologic changes in the definition.[73] The Marseille classification emphasized the gradation of morphologic changes seen in acute pancreatitis. In the mild form, peripancreatic fat necrosis and interstitial edema are present, but pancreatic necrosis is absent. The mild form can develop into severe disease with extensive peripancreatic and intrapancreatic fat necrosis, parencymal necrosis, and hemorrhage. These changes may be focal or diffuse. Both exocrine and endocrine function of the pancreas may be impaired to a variable extent and for a variable duration. However, occasionally there is little correlation between the severity of the clinical features and the morphologic findings.

The Marseille Symposium noted that if the primary cause or complications of the acute inflammatory process (such as biliary tract stones or pseudocysts) are corrected, normal restitution of clinical, morphologic, and functional changes occurs. Only rarely does acute pancreatitis lead to chronic pancreatitis. In some cases, scarring, parenchymal fibrosis, or pseudocysts can persist and lead to obstructive pancreatitis. However, this is a different disease process than typical chronic pancreatitis.[73]

Chronic pancreatitis

Chronic pancreatitis was defined at the 1983 Cambridge Symposium as a continuing inflammatory disease of the pancreas, characterized by irreversible morphologic change, and typically causing pain and/or permanent loss of exocrine and endocrine function.[134] Patients with chronic pancreatitis also may have acute clinical exacerbations of pain—but the condition can be painless, and the only evidence of an inflammatory process may be fibrosis due to previous inflammation.

The Marseille and Cambridge clinical definitions of chronic pancreatitis also were similar, but the Marseille classification again included morphology.[73] Chronic pancreatitis is characterized by irregular sclerosis with destruction and permanent loss of exocrine parenchyma. All types of inflammatory cells can be present in varying degrees, as well as edema and focal necrosis. Cysts and pseudocysts—with or without infection and communicating or not communicating with ducts—are not uncommon. Compared to the degree of acinar destruction, the islets of Langerhans are relatively well preserved.

The changes of chronic pancreatitis may be focal, segmental, or diffuse, and they may be associated with varying degrees of pancreatic duct dilatation. Duct dilatation is usually associated with strictures or intraductal protein plugs and calculi (calcification), although occasionally no apparent cause of dilatation is seen.

The following descriptive terms, based predominately on structural features, can be used: (1) chronic pancreatitis with focal necrosis; (2) chronic pancreatitis with segmental or diffuse fibrosis; and (3) chronic pancreatitis with or without calculi.

The Marseille classification also included a distinctive morphologic form of chronic pancreatitis, termed *obstructive chronic pancreatitis*. It is characterized by dilatation of the pancreatic duct proximal to an occlusion (due, for example, to a tumor or scar), diffuse atrophy of the acinar parenchyma, and uniform diffuse fibrosis. Calculi are uncommon in obstructive chronic pancreatitis. In obstructive chronic pancreatitis, both structural and functional changes tend to improve if the obstruction is corrected; if the obstruction persists, functional and morphologic changes usually progress. Chronic pancreatitis that is caused by acute pancreatitis is believed to be secondary to an inflammatory stricture and consequent pancreatic duct obstruction.

The Cambridge sections on imaging and function recognized that there may be major discrepancies between the clinical severity of the inflammatory process, the degree of functional exocrine and endocrine impairment of the gland, and the morphologic changes depicted by ultrasound (US), computed tomography (CT), and endoscopic retrograde cholangiopancreatography (ERCP). It

was also apparent that diagnosis of mild to moderately severe chronic pancreatitis often requires a combination of modalities, including clinical evaluation, laboratory studies and function testing, and one or more imaging procedures. Accordingly, a classification of the severity of the morphologic changes in chronic pancreatitis was proposed (Table 45-1).[13]

☐ **TABLE 45-1**

Cambridge classification of pancreatic morphology in chronic pancreatitis

Changes	Endoscopic retrograde cholangiopancreatography‡	Computed tomography and ultrasound‡
Normal	MPD* normal No abnormal LSB†	MPD not more than 2 mm in diameter Normal gland size and shape Homogeneous parenchyma
Equivocal	MPD normal Less than 3 abnormal LSB	Only one of the following signs MPD 2-4 mm in diameter Gland enlarged (less than 2 times normal) Heterogeneous parenchyma
Mild	MPD normal Greater than 3 abnormal LSB	Two or more signs for diagnosis MPD 2-4 mm in diameter Slight gland enlargement Heterogeneous parenchyma Small cavities (less than 10 mm)
Moderate	MPD changes Positive LSB changes	MPD irregularity Focal acute pancreatitis* Increased echogenicity of MPD walls Gland contour irregularity

Marked
Any of the above changes plus one or more of the following:
Cavity greater than 10 mm in diameter
Intraductal filling defects
Calculi
MPD obstruction, stricture
Severe MPD irregularity
Contiguous organ invasion

(From Axon, ATR, et al: Gut 25:1107, 1984.)
MPD, Main pancreatic duct. LSB-lateral side branch ducts.
†*LSB*, Lateral side branch ducts.
‡Focal change: less than one-third of gland involved.

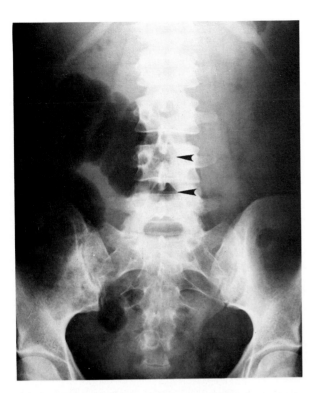

Fig. 45-1. Acute pancreatitis (colon cutoff sign). Conventional radiograph of abdomen shows dilatation of proximal transverse colon and abrupt termination of gas shadow *(arrowheads)*.

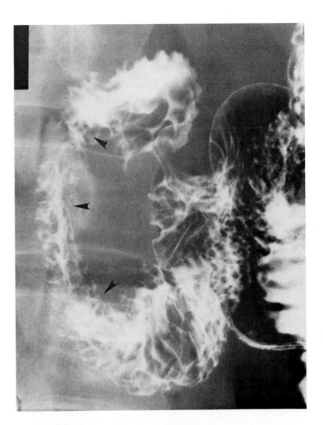

Fig. 45-2. Acute pancreatitis. Double contrast examination of duodenum shows persistent spasm, effacement of medial wall, and spiculation of folds *(arrowheads)*.

RADIOLOGIC DIAGNOSIS OF PANCREATITIS
Acute pancreatitis

The role of radiology is determined by the type of pancreatitis. The diagnosis of acute pancreatitis is based on clinical and laboratory findings; thus radiology has very little application during the acute stage of the disease. In rare instances when the clinical diagnosis is in doubt, radiologic evaluation may provide valuable information. The primary abnormalities that may be included in the differential diagnosis of acute pancreatitis are gastric or duodenal ulcers, primary biliary tract disease, mesenteric vascular insufficiency or infarction, abdominal aortic aneurysm, gynecologic or renal disease, and some rare hematologic dyscrasias.

Conventional radiographs of the chest and abdomen are often abnormal during acute pancreatitis but rarely yield a specific diagnosis.[10,38,121] The most common findings include pleural effusion, basilar atelectasis, and a focal or generalized ileus. Two findings that are quite suggestive of primary pancreatic disease include a focal duodenal ileus and the colon cutoff sign (Fig. 45-1). In both cases the ileus is caused by inflammation by pancreatic enzymes that reach the duodenum by direct spread from the head of the pancreas or that reach the colon by migration through the transverse mesocolon and the phrenicocolic ligament.[107]

Barium examinations of the upper gastrointestinal tract or colon may either demonstrate findings that are indicative of pancreatitis or, more important, indicate the presence of other abnormalities that are mimicking the symptoms of acute pancreatitis, such as gastroduodenal ulcerations. The most characteristic findings of acute pancreatitis are found in the duodenum. These include widening of the C-loop due to enlargement of the head of the pancreas, mucosal edema, and spiculation of the folds (Fig. 45-2). These findings may be demonstrated by conventional barium examination, hypotonic duodenography, or double contrast gastroduodenography. Also, pancreatic enzymes may spread along the small bowel mesentery, producing a paralytic ileus, compression, or stenosis of the distal duodenum, small bowel, or cecum. Barium examination of the colon may demonstrate effacement of the inferior haustra of the transverse colon or focal spasm at the level of the splenic flexure along with narrowing of the lumen or spiculation of the folds (Fig. 45-3). If severe, this process may result in colonic necrosis, abscess, fistula, or stenosis.[35,46,156]

A radiologic diagnosis of acute pancreatitis can be

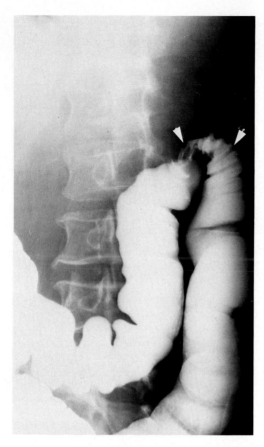

Fig. 45-3. Acute pancreatitis. Barium examination of colon shows focal, irregular stenosis of splenic flexure *(arrowheads)* due to contiguous pancreatic inflammation.
(Courtesy Dr. Howard Ansel.)

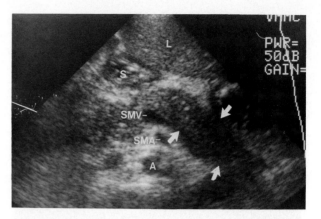

Fig. 45-4. Acute pancreatitis. Axial real-time ultrasonogram of pancreas *(arrows)* shows gland to be slightly enlarged and hypoechoic relative to liver *(L)*. *S*, Gastric antrum; *SMV*, superior mesenteric vein; *SMA*, superior mesenteric artery; *A*, aorta.
(From Freeny PC: Acute and chronic pancreatitis: current concepts of diagnosis. In Margulis, AR, and Gooding, CA, editors: Diagnostic radiology 1987. San Francisco, 1987, University of California in San Francisco.)

edematous pancreatitis is characterized by gland enlargement and decreased parenchymal echogenicity[54,92] (Fig. 45-4). Hemorrhagic and necrotic pancreatitis also produces gland enlargement, but hemorrhage and necrosis are seen as areas of inhomogeneous, increased parenchymal echogenicity.

The complications of acute pancreatitis, such as intrapancreatic or peripancreatic fluid collections, pseudocysts, phlegmons, and abscesses, often can be recognized by carefully performed US.[54,82,83,92]

Computed tomography

Patients with mild or edematous pancreatitis may not have any detectable change in size or appearance of the gland. In the absence of morphologic changes, some have suggested that this mild form of the disease be classified as hyperamylasemia. These patients represent about 29% of cases with mild or edematous acute pancreatitis.[143] In the remainder of patients, a spectrum of morphologic changes is seen, depending on the severity of the inflammatory process.[54]

The morphologic changes of acute edematous pancreatitis include enlargement and indistinctness of the gland margins, parenchymal inhomogeneity, thickening of the anterior pararenal fascia, and occasionally small fluid collections within or adjacent to the pancreas[40,52,54] (Fig. 45-5).

Acute hemorrhagic pancreatitis usually results in more marked gland enlargement. Parenchymal hemorrhage can be seen as an area of increased attenuation, and parenchymal necrosis can be identified as an area of non–contrast-enhancing parenchyma during bolus-dynamic contrast-enhanced CT[14,52,87] (Figs. 45-6 and 45-7). The morphologic evolution of pancreatic necrosis may follow

made by identifying characteristic morphologic changes of the pancreas, usually by US or CT, or by identifying one of the complications associated with the inflammatory process, such as fluid collections or pseudocyst formation.* Although US can be used for evaluation of acute pancreatitis, there is a high frequency of indeterminate examinations in critically ill patients caused by inability to image the entire gland and peripancreatic spaces. Even in expert hands, using meticulous technique and high-resolution real-time scanners, US can identify only 78% of the abnormalities, which are easily detected by CT.[83] CT is thus the preferred method for initial evaluation of patients with acute pancreatitis, whereas US often can be used efficaciously to follow the temporal changes of abnormalities recognized by CT.[92]

Ultrasonography

The ultrasonographic findings of acute pancreatitis depend on the severity of the inflammatory process. Acute

---

*References 52, 54, 82, 83, 92, 143.

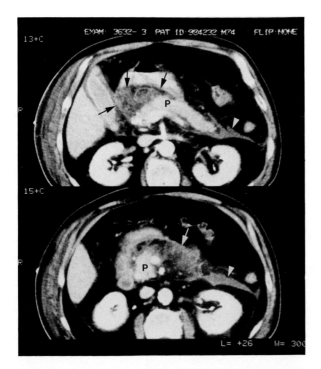

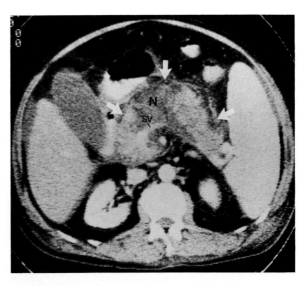

Fig. 45-6. Acute necrotizing pancreatitis. Bolus-dynamic CT scan of pancreas *(arrows)* shows gland enlargement. Areas of decreased attenuation are zones of necrosis *(N)*. Spleen is enlarged because of compression of splenic vein *(SV)* (congestive splenomegaly).
(From Freeny PC: Acute and chronic pancreatitis: current concepts of diagnosis. In Margulis, AR, and Gooding, CA, editors: Diagnostic radiology 1987. San Francisco, 1987, University of California in San Francisco.)

Fig. 45-5. Acute pancreatitis. **A** and **B,** Bolus-enhanced CT scan of pancreas shows peripancreatic fluid collection *(arrows)* and fluid ventral to anterior pararenal fascia *(arrowheads)*. Pancreatic parenchyma *(P)* shows normal, homogeneous contrast enhancement.

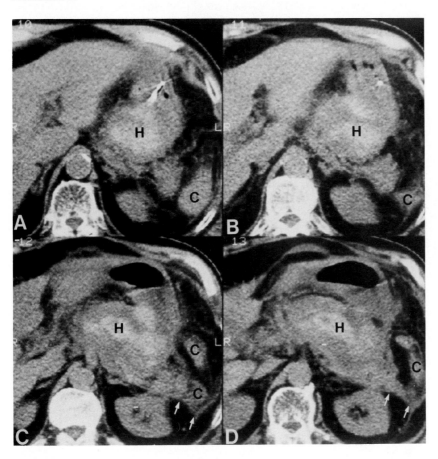

Fig. 45-7. Acute hemorrhagic pancreatitis. **A** to **D,** CT scans of pancreas without contrast show central area of increased attenuation due to hemorrhage *(H)*. **C** and **D,** Arrows show extension of the inflammatory process laterally along the left anterior pararenal fascia and adjacent to the splenic flexure of the colon *(C)*.
(From Freeny PC: Acute and chronic pancreatitis: current concepts of diagnosis. In Margulis, AR, and Gooding, CA, editors: Diagnostic radiology 1987. San Francisco, 1987, University of California in San Francisco.)

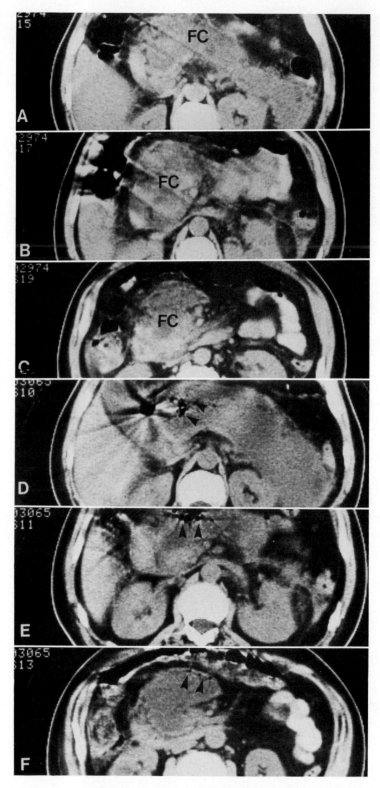

Fig. 45-8. Evolution of infected pancreatic fluid collection. **A** to **C,** CT scans of pancreas without contrast show large fluid collection *(FC)* in pancreatic bed caused by pancreatic necrosis. **D** to **F,** Scans 6 days later show gas within fluid collection *(arrowheads)*. Note development of convex margins of *FC* (**A** to **D**). Infection confirmed by needle aspiration.

(From Freeny PC: Acute and chronic pancreatitis: current concepts of diagnosis. In Margulis, AR, and Gooding, CA, editors: Diagnostic radiology 1987. San Francisco, 1987, University of California in San Francisco.)

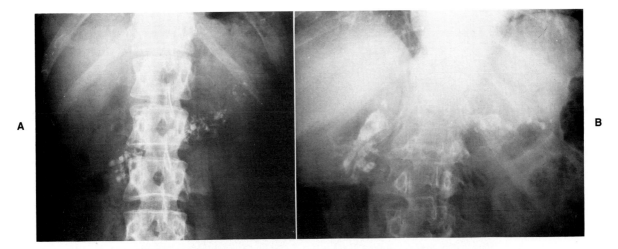

Fig. 45-9. A, Chronic pancreatitis. Conventional radiograph of abdomen shows small calcifications distributed throughout pancreas. **B,** Hereditary pancreatitis. Multiple large calcifications with peripheral density and central lucency are distributed throughout pancreas.

a relatively typical course. White et al. have demonstrated a pattern consisting of gland enlargement with convex margins and progressively diminished parenchymal attenuation values[172] (Fig. 45-8). The area of necrosis often involves the entire gland and assumes a saclike configuration with a contrast-enhancing capsule. The development of infected necrosis results in extremely high morbidity and mortality, and is discussed in more detail in the section about staging of severity of pancreatitis.

The CT diagnosis of acute pancreatitis, as with US, is aided by identification of the complications of the inflammatory process, such as intrapancreatic and peripancreatic fluid collections, pancreatic ascites, pseudocyst, phlegmon, and abscess.[52,54,142]

Chronic pancreatitis

The diagnosis of chronic pancreatitis, like that of acute pancreatitis, is based chiefly on clinical and laboratory findings. However, the clinical features frequently are more diverse and nonspecific, and hence the diagnosis may be more difficult to establish, particularly during the early course of the disease. Thus radiologic evaluation often plays a crucial role in the initial diagnosis.

Conventional radiographs of the abdomen show pancreatic calcifications in 27% to 65% of patients[74] (Fig. 45-9). The great majority of pancreatic calcifications seen radiologically are caused by chronic alcoholic pancreatitis. Although they are virtually pathognomonic of this disease, they tend to occur relatively late and may not be detectable until about 8 years following the onset of the disease. They are intraductal in location and may vary in size. In the rare hereditary form of pancreatitis, the calculi are large, often greater than 2 cm in diameter, with a peripheral density and central lucency (Fig. 45-

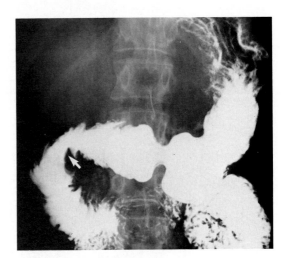

Fig. 45-10. Chronic pancreatitis. Upper GI series shows mucosal irregularity and spiculation of duodenum along with proximal narrowing *(arrow)*. Small calcifications are seen in pancreatic bed.

9, *B*). In addition, calcifications may also occur in patients with cystic fibrosis, kwashiorkor, hyperparathyroidism, pancreatic carcinoma, and cystic pancreatic neoplasms.

Barium examinations of the upper gastrointestinal tract and colon may reveal a variety of changes.[54] The most common abnormalities are found in the stomach and duodenum and include extrinsic displacement or compression by an enlarged pancreas and mucosal irregularities caused by the chronic inflammatory reaction produced by pancreatic enzymes* (Fig. 45-10). Although

---

*References 4, 8, 13, 18, 49, 68.

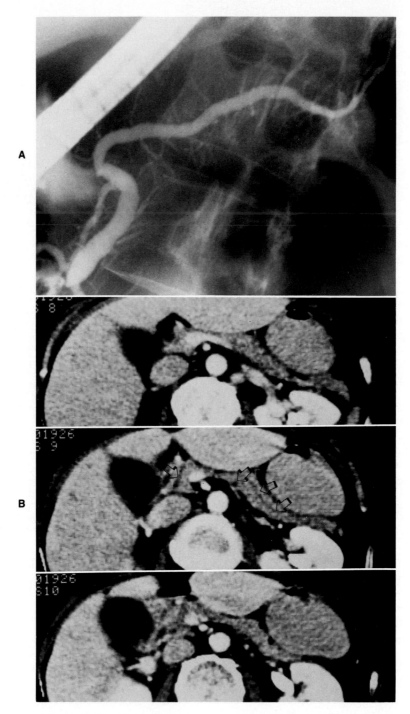

Fig. 45-11. Chronic pancreatitis: mild changes. **A,** ERCP shows normal main pancreatic duct and minimal ectasia and "nipping" of origins of multiple lateral side branches. **B,** Sequential bolus-dynamic CT scans of pancreas show normal gland contour and parenchyma. Main pancreatic duct *(arrow)* is of normal caliber.

(From Freeny PC: Acute and chronic pancreatitis: current concepts of diagnosis. In Margulis, AR, and Gooding, CA, editors: Diagnostic radiology 1987. San Francisco, 1987, University of California in San Francisco.)

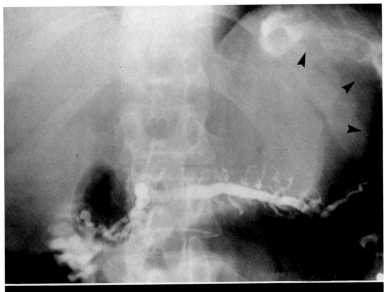

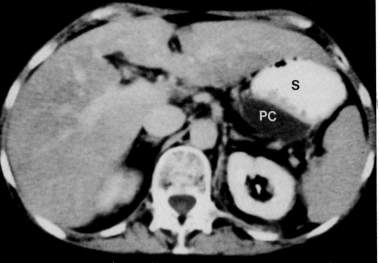

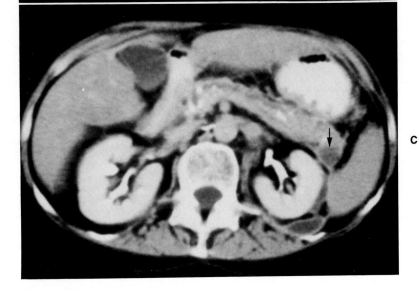

Fig. 45-12. Chronic pancreatitis: marked changes. **A,** ERCP shows marked main pancreatic duct dilatation, ectasia of lateral side branches, and small calculi. Note evidence of displacement of stomach *(arrowheads);* contrast is from duodenal gastric reflux during ERCP. **B,** Bolus-dynamic CT scan shows pseudocyst *(PC)* displacing stomach *(S).* **C,** Scan at level of pancreas shows marked changes of chronic pancreatitis: main pancreatic duct dilatation, intraductal calculi, and mild atrophy of gland parenchyma. Second pseudocyst *(arrow)* exists in tail of gland, and fluid is in left posterior pararenal space.

(From Freeny PC: Acute and chronic pancreatitis: current concepts of diagnosis. In Margulis, AR, and Gooding, CA, editors: Diagnostic radiology 1987. San Francisco, 1987, University of California in San Francisco.)

these examinations are useful when positive, 50% of conventional barium examinations and 20% of hypotonic duodenograms may be negative in patients with proved pancreatic enlargement. Even with severe steatorrhea, pancreatic exocrine insufficiency rarely produces radiographically demonstrable small bowel abnormalities. Occasionally, severe atrophy or loss of the normal jejunal mucosal pattern is visible. The colon is less frequently involved by chronic than by acute pancreatitis. This is caused by the relative lack of exudation of pancreatic enzymes as exocrine function is destroyed by the progression of chronic pancreatitis.

The radiologic diagnosis of chronic pancreatitis has been improved by the use of the imaging modalities of US, CT, and ERCP. The role of magnetic resonance imaging (MRI) is unknown, but perhaps it will become a valuable modality.

Ultrasonography

The US findings of chronic pancreatitis include a focal or diffuse increase in gland size or, in cases of advanced disease and atrophy, a small, diminutive gland; irregular or lobulated contour, or loss of gland margins due to pancreatic fibrosis; hyperechoic and inhomogeneous parenchymal echo texture pattern; intraductal calculi; and pancreatic duct dilatation (the duct may also be small or not identifiable if there is diffuse sclerosis)* (Fig. 45-11).

Computed tomography

The CT findings of chronic pancreatitis include alterations in gland size (focal or diffuse enlargement, or gland atrophy), irregular margins, pancreatic duct dila-

*References 1, 15, 16, 54, 92, 112, 138, 140.

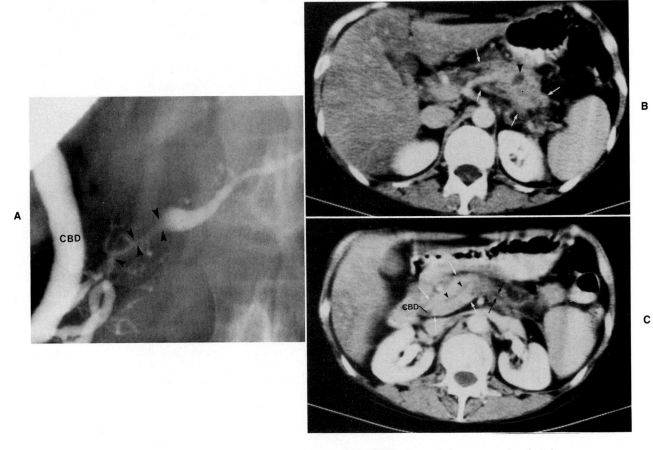

Fig. 45-13. Chronic pancreatitis: marked changes. **A,** ERCP shows 3.5 cm stenosis of main pancreatic duct at junction of head-body *(arrowheads)*, irregularity of upstream main duct, and ectatic and partially amputated lateral side branches. *CBD,* Common bile duct. **B,** Bolus-dynamic CT scan shows enlargement of tail of gland *(arrows)*, parenchymal inhomogeneity, and small cyst *(arrowhead)*. Inflammatory process extends into peripancreatic fat. **C,** Scan at level of head of pancreas shows normal-appearing parenchyma *(white arrows)* and main pancreatic duct *(arrowheads)*. Dilated upstream duct is visible *(black arrows)*. *CBD,* Common bile duct.
(From Freeny PC: Acute and chronic pancreatitis: current concepts of diagnosis. In Margulis, AR, and Gooding, CA, editors: Diagnostic radiology 1987. San Francisco, 1987, University of California in San Francisco.)

tation, and intraductal calculi[52,54,97] (Figs. 45-11 to 45-13). Secondary findings include intrapancreatic or peripancreatic cysts or fluid collections, thickening of peripancreatic fascia, and evidence of vascular involvement (arterial pseudoaneurysm formation or venous occlusion and varices)[52,54] (Fig. 45-12).

Endoscopic retrograde cholangiopancreatography

ERCP is the most sensitive modality for detection of chronic pancreatitis. The ERCP findings have been described in multiple reports and include clubbing and dilatation of the lateral side branches, narrowing ("nipping") of the origins of the side branches from the main duct, main duct marginal irregularities, strictures, focal or diffuse dilatation, or multifocal strictures and intervening areas of dilatation ("chain of lakes"), and intraductal protein plugs or calculi* (Figs. 45-11 to 45-13). These findings may be diffuse (Figs. 45-11 and 45-12) or focal (Fig. 45-14). Communicating cysts may be small or large and can be filled during contrast injection. The intrapancreatic segment of the common bile duct also may be narrowed[144,153] (Fig. 45-15).

Rarely, the main pancreatic duct is completely obstructed. This may be caused by an intraductal calculus or ductal fibrosis. In the latter case, differentiation from a pancreatic neoplasm may be difficult, and angiography may be required[88,124] (Fig. 45-16).

---

*References 28, 85, 127, 129, 144, 153.

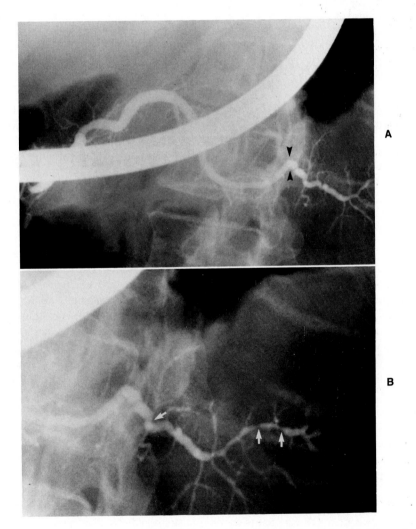

Fig. 45-14. Focal chronic pancreatitis. **A,** ERCP shows abrupt onset *(arrowheads)* of irregularity of main pancreatic duct in tail of gland. Lateral side branches also are ectatic. **B,** Magnified view of tail shows irregularity of main duct, multifocal stenoses *(arrows)*, and ectasia of lateral side branches.
(From Freeny PC: Acute and chronic pancreatitis: current concepts of diagnosis. In Margulis, AR, and Gooding, CA, editors: Diagnostic radiology 1987. San Francisco, 1987, University of California in San Francisco.)

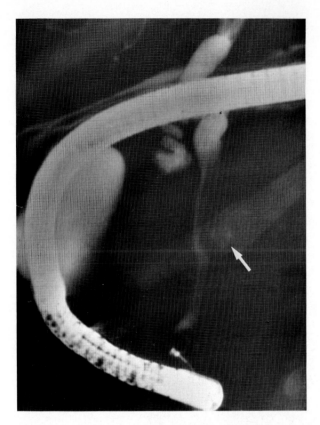

Fig. 45-15. Chronic pancreatitis. ERCP shows long, smooth narrowing of common bile duct. Pancreatic calcification *(arrow)* is seen adjacent to duct.

Angiography

Before the development and use of US, CT, and ERCP, pancreatic angiography frequently was used as one of the initial procedures for the diagnosis of suspected chronic pancreatitis. Angiography is now only rarely used for diagnosis; most often it is employed as a preoperative procedure to define upper abdominal vascular anatomy for the surgeon or to identify vascular complications, such as pseudoaneurysms, in patients with severe pancreatitis or pseudocyst formation.[53,80,94] In some cases, however, the findings of chronic pancreatitis and pancreatic carcinoma may overlap, and a specific diagnosis may not be possible on the basis of either US, CT, or ERCP. In this situation, angiography may be useful for further evaluation[53] (Fig. 45-16).

Correlation of CT and ERCP

ERCP is more sensitive than CT for detection of changes of chronic pancreatitis because mild to moderate changes are limited to the main duct and side branches and are very difficult to detect with CT.[152] In some cases, however, CT may provide additional information about

---

the gland parenchyma and about associated findings not depicted by ERCP, such as noncommunicating cysts and vascular involvement (Fig. 45-14). Thus a combination of both studies provides the best overall morphologic assessment of chronic pancreatitis.

CLINICAL AND RADIOLOGIC STAGING OF PANCREATITIS
Acute pancreatitis

Acute pancreatitis represents a spectrum of inflammatory disease ranging from mild, self-limiting edematous pancreatitis to severe and often fatal hemorrhagic and necrotic pancreatitis. The prognosis or mortality of the disease reflects this continuum. Patients with edematous pancreatitis have a mortality rate of about 4% (usually due to a serious complication or to exacerbations and evolution into a more severe form), whereas the rate may increase as high as 80% to 90% in patients with hemorrhagic pancreatitis.[117]

Clinical staging

It is important to attempt to identify early those patients in a high-risk category to ensure appropriate clinical and surgical management decisions. The objective criteria of Ranson are the most widely used[117] (see box). A relationship exists between the number of prognostic signs and the incidence of death or complications requiring at least 7 days in intensive care units. "Mild" pancreatitis is defined as two or less signs, and most of these patients have self-limited disease; three to five signs represents "moderate" pancreatitis, and more than six

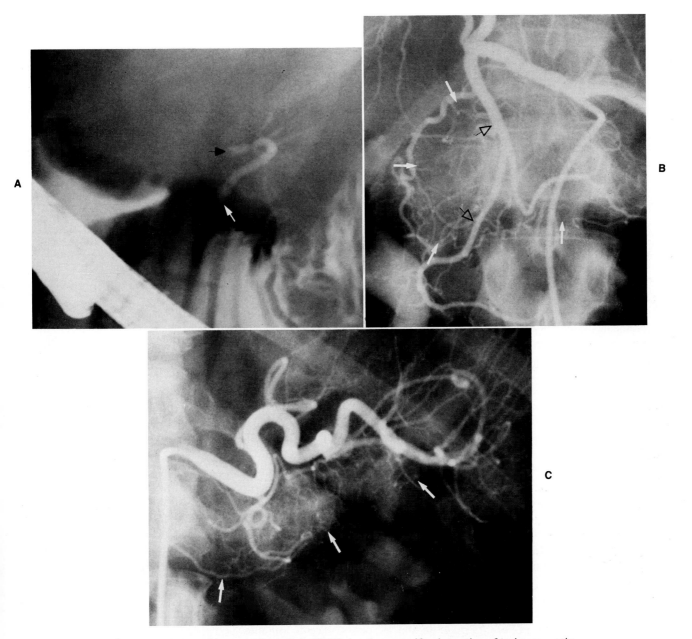

Fig. 45-16. Pancreatitis or carcinoma? **A,** ERCP shows nonspecific obstruction of main pancreatic duct *(arrow)*. Papilla is in transverse duodenum *(white arrow)*. Selective hepatic, **B,** and splenic, **C,** arteriograms show typical changes of pancreatitis: gland is moderately enlarged and hypervascular, and small intrapancreatic vessels *(white arrows)* are minimally deformed and tortuous. Gastroduodenal artery *(open arrows)* is displaced anteromedially. Venous phases (not shown) were normal. Inflammatory ductal stricture and chronic pancreatitis were found at surgery.

signs indicates "severe" disease. Unfortunately, some patients with so-called mild pancreatitis develop severe, sometimes fatal complications, whereas those with three to five signs may have only mild, uncomplicated disease.[5,78,118]

Recent work by Buchler et al. has shown that the use of serum determinations of antiproteases (α-1, α-2), complement factors (C3, C4), and C-reactive protein during the initial clinical episode of acute pancreatitis can reliably distinguish edematous pancreatitis from necrotizing pancreatitis.[23] The antiproteases and complement factors have a detection rate for pancreatic necrosis of 74% to 85%, and C-reactive protein of 95%. The combined use of these serum parameters may soon prove to be invaluable in the staging of acute pancreatitis.

Radiologic (morphologic) staging

Only recently have attempts been made to correlate the clinical severity of pancreatitis with morphologic changes as depicted by US or CT.*

Initial comparative studies of US and CT in detecting complications of pancreatitis (fluid collections, pseudocysts, abscesses, and phlegmon formation; vascular involvement was not considered) showed a high incidence of nondiagnostic US studies (up to 38%), indicating that CT is preferable for evaluation of patients with acute pancreatitis.[14,143] More recently, Jeffrey and co-workers, using meticulous US scanning techniques and high-resolution real-time scanners, were able to reduce the number of inadequate examinations.[83] However, this study involved only determination of extrapancreatic fluid collections, with no consideration given to identifying other complications. In this setting they were still able to identify only 78% of the abnormalities identified by CT.[83]

The consequences of missing or misinterpreting major complications of acute pancreatitis are increased patient morbidity and mortality. Thus the limitations inherent in high-resolution real-time ultrasound, even in expert hands, are too great to obviate CT as the initial imaging modality.

The most important morphologic CT features for staging the severity of the inflammatory process are the presence of parenchymal necrosis (Fig. 45-6) and the development and persistence of intrapancreatic or peripancreatic fluid collections, pancreatic ascites, and pancreatic abscess. Secondary findings that may indicate a more severe clinical course are extension of a fluid collection into the mediastinum, vascular involvement (venous occlusion or pseudoaneurysm formation), bile duct obstruction, extension of the extrapancreatic inflamma-

---

*References 5, 7, 14, 22, 78, 117.

□ **TABLE 45-2**

Morphologic factors of mortality in necrotizing pancreatitis (in 205 patients)

		Patients (%)	Mortality (%)
Extent of pancreatic necrosis:			
30%		38.5	7.6
50%		36.6	24.0
Subtotal or total gland necrosis		24.9	51.0
Extrapancreatic necrosis	Positive	46.8	34.4
	Negative	53.2	15.6
Pancreatogenic ascites	Positive	56.1	36.5
	Negative	43.9	8.9
Bacterial contamination (in 138 patients)	Positive	40.6	32.1
	Negative	59.4	9.8

(From Beger, HG, and Buchler, M: Outcome of necrotizing pancreatitis in relation to morphological parameters. In Malfertheiner, P, Ditschuneit, H, editors: Diagnostic procedures in pancreatic disease, Berlin, 1986, Springer-Verlag.)

tory reaction to involve contiguous organs (for example, the stomach, duodenum, colon, spleen, or liver), and pulmonary involvement ("pancreatitis" lung). This latter complication is not a CT diagnosis, but a clinical diagnosis, aided by a chest roentgenogram.[54]

PARENCHYMAL NECROSIS

Parenchymal necrosis is the most important prognostic CT finding, short of frank pancreatic abscess (Table 45-2).[7] Necrosis is identified by CT as areas of non–contrast-enhancing pancreatic parenchyma[14,87,171] (Fig. 45-6). The approximate percentage of gland necrosis correlates with patient mortality.

The presence of bacterial contamination of necrotic pancreas substantially increases patient mortality, irrespective of the percentage of gland necrosis (Table 45-3).[8] Early diagnosis and surgical debridement can lower morbidity and mortality. However, the only reliable method of diagnosing the presence of bacterial contamination, short of surgery, is guided percutaneous fine-needle aspiration.[60,161] The liberal use of fine-needle aspiration is important for early detection of bacterial contamination, indicating need for surgical debridement.

FLUID COLLECTIONS

Fluid collections are common sequelae of acute pancreatitis. Many of the collections are small and resolve spontaneously, whereas others may enlarge, become infected, or persist.[19] In the latter case, an inflammatory fibrous capsule usually forms, and the collections are properly termed *pseudocysts*.[141]

□ **TABLE 45-3**

Morphologic alterations and associated mortality rates in patients with bacterially contaminated and sterile pancreatic necrosis

Morphologic alteration	No.	Bacteriologically positive		Bacteriologically negative	
		No. (%)	Mortality (%)	No. (%)	Mortality (%)
Minor necrosis (30%)	36	12 (26.7%)	0	24 (34.8%)	0
Extended necrosis (50%)	49	18 (40%)	38.9	31 (44.9%)	12.9
Subtotal/total necrosis	29	15 (33.3%)	66.7	14 (20.3%)	14.3
Extrapancreatic necrosis	55	27 (60%)	59.3	28 (40.6%)	10.7
Ascites	67	32 (71.1%)	53.1	35 (50.7%)	17.1

(From Beger, HG, and Buchler, M: In Malfertheiner, P, and Ditschuneit, H, editors: Diagnostic procedures in pancreatic disease, Berlin, 1986, Springer-Verlag.)

Fluid collections have a spontaneous resolution rate of about 40% to 50% within the first 6 weeks.[18,19] After this time, the chance of spontaneous resolution is small, and the incidence of complications increases to almost 60%, compared with an incidence of about 20% during the initial 6 weeks.[19] In recent reports by Ranson and Balthazar et al., 35 (45.7%) of 83 patients with acute pancreatitis had fluid collections demonstrated on initial CT scans.[5,117] Spontaneous resolution occurred in 19 (54.3%). The remaining 16 (45.7%) persisted, and all became infected. In the entire group, 18 patients developed pancreatic abscess, and all but two of these occurred in preexisting fluid collections. Thus, early detection (usually by CT) and careful serial observation (which can be performed with CT or US) are essential (Fig. 45-8). Percutaneous fine-needle aspiration should be performed if clinical or morphologic findings indicate possible sepsis or infection.[60,160]

PANCREATIC ASCITES

Pancreatic ascites is caused by disruption of the pancreatic duct with leakage of pancreatic juice into the peritoneal cavity. Ductal rupture probably is caused by necrosis of the duct and adjacent parenchyma. Mortality rates are as high as 15% to 20% for untreated cases, and may increase to almost 60% if the fluid becomes infected[7,21] (Table 45-3).

The presence of free fluid within the peritoneal cavity can be detected with US or CT, the diagnosis of pancreatic ascites confirmed by percutaneous aspiration of the fluid and amylase determination, and the site of duct rupture documented by ERCP.[54] Bacterial contamination should always be suspected, and a culture and Gram's stain should be obtained from the percutaneous aspirate.

PANCREATIC ABSCESS

Pancreatic abscess is a focal collection of liquid pus, usually with a fairly well-defined wall or capsule. It may develop within a preexisting fluid collection or pseudocyst, or within an area of parenchymal gland necrosis (Fig. 45-8). Most abscesses associated with acute pancreas exist within the pancreatic bed, but they may develop in areas of the abdomen or pelvis remote from the pancreas, essentially in the same locations as pancreatic fluid collections or pseudocysts.[54] Diagnosis of infection can be suspected if gas is present within the collection, but percutaneous aspiration is the only reliable method for confirmation of the diagnosis[54,60,162] (Fig. 45-8).

Morphologic versus clinical staging

Several recent series have correlated CT morphology and clinical or operative findings in patients with acute pancreatitis.[5,14,23,118] The results of these studies indicate that CT is very accurate in staging the severity of acute pancreatitis—that is, in detecting parenchymal necrosis and fluid collections and abscesses—and may show evidence of necrosis or abscess formation before clinical suspicion of the complication. The presence of these CT findings correlates more closely with final clinical outcome and mortality (the number of patients needing surgical pancreatic necrosectomy or drainage and debridement of pancreatic abscess) than simple Ranson scoring (discussed earlier in chapter). This is to be expected, since the Ranson criteria are designed to identify statistically groups of patients with acute pancreatitis who are at high risk for development of complications, rather than to identify specific patients, as CT is able to do.[118]

The findings of these studies indicate that it is important to obtain baseline CT scans of patients with a clinical diagnosis of acute pancreatitis. If the Ranson score is low, and CT shows only mild changes, then further studies are not necessary unless the patient's clinical condition deteriorates. The use of laboratory parameters as recommended by Buchler et al. (antiproteases, complement factors, and C-reactive protein) may also prove to be valuable for early detection of pancreatic necrosis.[22]

Chronic pancreatitis

The severity of chronic pancreatitis can be staged by assessing the degree of exocrine or endocrine dysfunction of the pancreas, the morphologic findings depicted by US, CT, or ERCP, or by the clinical syndrome manifested by the patient (for example, pain or complications related to exocrine or endocrine dysfunction, such as malabsorption and diabetes). The most important goal in overall assessment of the individual patient (that is, in the diagnosis and therapeutic decision) is to be able to correlate morphology and function with the clinical status of the patient.

The imaging section of the Cambridge Symposium developed an international classification of the morphologic changes of chronic pancreatitis[3,133] (Table 45-1). Subsequently, several reports have been published that correlate morphology, function, and clinical status of patients with chronic pancreatitis.*

Morphology and function

These reports can be summarized by saying that in mild or eary chronic pancreatitis, the most accurate diagnosis is achieved by the use of both function tests and imaging modalities, primarily CT and ERCP. The correlation is excellent in most cases; still, there are a few patients with minimal morphologic changes but marked functional abnormalities, and a few with marked morphologic changes but minimal functional alteration.

An important new observation concerns the relationship of pancreatic ductal calculi and exocrine function. In the past, duct calculi were believed to indicate advanced disease and severe exocrine dysfunction. In Lankisch et al.'s recent series, however, it was shown that 50% of patients with calculi had only mild to moderate exocrine dysfunction.[90]

Morphology, function, and clinical course

If all stages of chronic pancreatitis—mild to severe—are considered, the severity of the patient's clinical course (the amount of pain, presence of diabetes mellitus, malabsorption, and complications such as acute pancreatitis, acute pancreatic necrosis, and extrapancreatic manifestations) cannot be predicted directly from the morphologic changes and vice versa. There is also no significant correlation between the degree of exocrine gland dysfunction and the severity of clinical symptoms.[101]

---

*References 20, 21, 61, 84, 90, 99, 101.

However, if patients with only advanced stages of chronic pancreatitis are considered (defined as having more than 75% reduction of enzyme and/or bicarbonate secretion in the SEC-C test), there is a significant correlation between the clinical and morphologic severity of the disease in 80% of patients.[101] Similarly, there is poor correlation of morphology and function in patients with mild to moderate disease (less than 50% to 75% reduction of enzymes and/or bicarbonate). Advanced morphologic changes in ERCP or CT are found in 65% of these patients. As noted by Malfertheiner, these findings raise the question of whether the morphologic grading of ERCP and CT is incorrect or whether the morphologic changes might precede the clinical course. Additional studies need to be performed to evaluate these questions.

ETIOLOGY OF PANCREATITIS: RADIOLOGIC EVALUATION

Radiology plays a crucial role in identifying correctable causes of pancreatitis. This is particularly true for patients with acute or acute relapsing pancreatitis, who are often found to have biliary tract disease or a structural abnormality of the upper gastrointestinal tract or pancreatic duct.

Biliary tract disease

Biliary tract disease is the most common cause of acute pancreatitis in the United States. In most patients calculi are found within the gallbladder or common bile duct. The development of US has revolutionized the approach to these patients by permitting immediate and accurate evaluation of the gallbladder, biliary ducts, and pancreas.[30,31,65,108,109] In many patients a diagnosis of cholelithiasis or choledocholithiasis and associated acute edematous pancreatitis can be made by US and ERCP soon after hospital admission.

The current use of ^{99m}Tc-HIDA, a radiopharmaceutical capable of opacifying the biliary ducts and gallbladder has been shown to be efficacious in evaluating patients with pancreatitis and suspected biliary tract disease, and in differentiating acute pancreatitis from acute cholecystitis.[51,140,145,146,170]

A variety of inflammatory, neoplastic, and congenital abnormalities of the common bile duct have been associated with pancreatitis. These include choledochal cysts, parasitic infestations, sclerosing cholangitis, stenosis of the sphincter of Oddi, and bile duct tumors.[6,63,111,114,164] Stenosis of the sphincter of Oddi is being recognized with increasing frequency and may be a more common cause of acute relapsing pancreatitis than heretofore realized. Each of these abnormalities can be evaluated by ERCP or PTC.

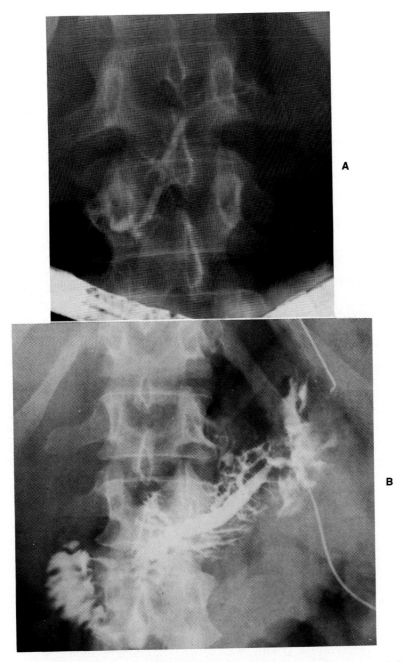

Fig. 45-17. Pancreas divisum. **A,** ERCP shows large ventral pancreas with changes of chronic pancreatitis. **B,** Operative pancreatogram shows more severe inflammatory changes in dorsal duct system.

Stomach and duodenum

Primary abnormalities of the stomach and duodenum have also been associated with pancreatitis. These may be diagnosed by barium studies and include penetrating ulcers and tumors of the stomach and duodenum, intraluminal and conventional duodenal diverticula, afferent loop obstruction, and regional enteritis involving the stomach and duodenum.[91,93,174]

Pancreas divisum

Considerable controversy exists about the significance of pancreas divisum (failure of the dorsal and ventral ducts of Wirsung and Santorini to fuse—with an incidence of about 9%) relative to pancreatitis (Fig. 49-19). Initial reports by Gregg[70] and Rösch et al.[128] described an incidence of pancreatitis of 21% to 45% in patients with pancreas divisum. The cause of the pancreatitis was believed to be due to stenosis of the minor papilla, which serves as the main excretory pathway in patients with pancreas divisum.[32]

Recent reports by Delhaye et al.[39] and Sugawa et al.,[151] however, showed that the frequency of pancreas divisum was the same in patients with pancreatitis (acute and chronic) and in a series of patients investigated by ERCP for other reasons. These authors concluded that pancreatitis did not occur with increased frequency in patients with pancreas divisum.

It is nevertheless clear that if minor papillary stenosis occurs in a patient with pancreas divisum, recurrent attacks of pancreatitis are likely to result, caused by obstruction (Fig. 45-17). In these patients, ERCP of the minor papilla may show pancreatic duct dilatation, and

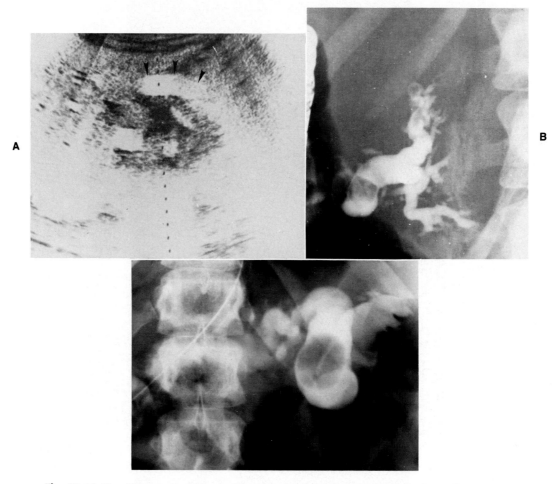

Fig. 45-18. Hereditary pancreatitis. **A,** Transverse ultrasonogram demonstrates 2-cm dilatation of main pancreatic duct *(arrowheads)*. **B,** Endoscopic retrograde injection of ventral pancreatic duct demonstrates marked ectasia of side branches and main duct. Multiple calculi are evident, most notably within portion of duct adjacent to papilla. **C,** Intraoperative injection of dorsal portion of pancreatic ductal system likewise shows marked dilatation and intraductal concretions. These were not calcified and were not visible on plain film radiographs.

ultrasonography of the pancreatic duct during secretin stimulation may show abnormally prolonged ductal dilatation.[170] It has been shown by Bolondi et al.[15] that the normal pancreatic duct dilates from 1.2 mm normal basal value to 2.9 mm after secretin stimulation. Thus, to use the criteria of Warshaw and colleagues for identification of patients with minor papilla stenosis, the duct must dilate for a prolonged time.[170] In these patients, minor duct papillotomy produces good results in most patients.[167]

Hereditary pancreatitis

Hereditary pancreatitis is a rare disorder of unknown pathophysiology that is transmitted as an autosomal dominant with variable penetrance.[71,86,96] The onset of symptoms is often during childhood, but the diagnosis is frequently delayed because of the nonspecificity of the clinical picture.[136] Plain films reveal large, round, peripherally dense pancreatic calculi in 60% of patients* (Fig. 45-9, *B*). Pancreatography characteristically demonstrates a markedly increased caliber and length of the main pancreatic duct and dilatation of the lateral side branches[98,116,126,136] (Fig. 45-18). These radiologic findings can assist in establishing the diagnosis earlier in the course of the patient's disease and in planning surgical treatment.[98,102,116,126]

Traumatic pancreatitis

Traumatic pancreatitis follows blunt or penetrating abdominal trauma in about 3% to 12% of cases.[68,156] The

---

*References 62, 68, 71, 86, 95, 136.

injury may vary from a simple contusion to complete transsection of the gland, resulting in either acute or chronic pancreatitis.[158] In many cases the pancreatic injury may be masked by multiple injuries to other abdominal organs or to the central nervous system. A delay in diagnosis and treatment may result in the formation of a pancreatic fistula, pseudocyst, or abscess, each of which is associated with a high morbidity and mortality. ERCP, CT, US, and angiography may be used for diagnosis during the acute or chronic phase.[67,147,154,161] The findings depend on the severity of the injury and usually are similar to the changes of pancreatitis produced by other causes. One exception is complete transsection of the gland with disruption of the main pancreatic duct.[161]

COMPLICATIONS OF PANCREATITIS: RADIOLOGIC DETECTION AND TREATMENT

One of the most important roles of radiology is the diagnosis and evaluation of complications of acute and chronic pancreatitis. These complications are responsible for a significant proportion of the morbidity and mortality of inflammatory disease of the pancreas. However, if detected early, they often can be treated appropriately without sequelae.

Pancreatic and extrapancreatic fluid collections

An intrapancreatic or extrapancreatic fluid collection is a potential complication of either acute or chronic pancreatitis and occurs in up to 50% of patients.[44,106,131,175] These fluid collections are composed of blood, pancreatic enzymes, fluid, and debris. They result from intrapan-

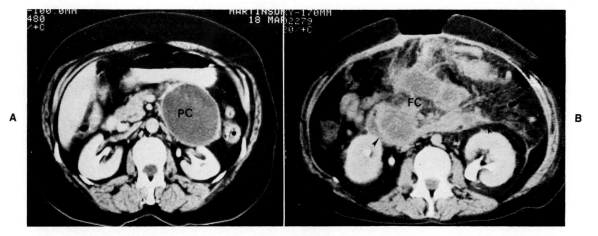

Fig. 45-19. Pancreatic extrapancreatic fluid collections. **A,** CT scan at level of pancreas shows well-marginated, intrapancreatic fluid collection typical of pseudocyst *(PC)*. **B,** CT scan of another patient slightly below level of pancreas shows poorly marginated, multiloculated extrapancreatic fluid collection *(FC)* along with bilateral thickening of anterior pararenal fascia *(arrowheads)*. Defect in anterior abdominal wall is postoperative.

creatic activation of enzymatic precursors with damage to the acinar cells and subsequent autodigestion and propagation of tissue necrosis.[175] Although the term "pseudocyst" implies the presence of a wall or containing structure, the fluid collections are often uncontained and poorly circumscribed (Fig. 45-19).[42] They are most frequently found in the lesser sac and anterior pararenal space, and about 20% are multiple.[106,131,142] Less common sites include the perihepatic and perisplenic spaces, the mediastinum, the mesentery and the pelvis.[54] Continuity with the pancreatic ductal system is common and can be demonstrated by pancreatography in 50% to 80% of cases.[54,125]

Conventional radiographs

Pancreatic or extrapancreatic fluid collections may produce findings on the chest radiograph that include elevation of the left diaphragm, pleural effusion, atelectasis or consolidation, and, rarely, a mediastinal mass.[54] Abdominal films may show displacement of the gastric air bubble or bowel gas shadows, a soft tissue mass, or pancreatic calcifications, possibly of a curvilinear type in a cyst wall (Fig. 45-20).

Barium studies

Pancreatic fluid collections displace some part of the upper gastrointestinal tract in 75% of cases.[130] The degree and vector of displacement depend on the size and location of the fluid collection (Fig. 45-21). The adjacent wall of the displaced viscera may be smooth or irregular,

depending on the amount of contiguous inflammation. If the fluid collection ruptures into the adjacent stomach or bowel, it may fill with gas or interstitial fluid and debris. Rarely, the communication may be demonstrated during contrast radiography[18,72] (Fig. 45-22).

Ultrasonography and computed tomography

Fluid collections associated with pancreatitis are evanescent lesions that may develop and spontaneously resolve within a few weeks.[18,29,135] Many can be demonstrated by US. Initially they are seen as irregularly marginated, sonolucent structures. As they mature, a fibrous capsule develops, their periphery becomes more sharply defined, and strong posterior wall acoustic enhancement is seen. This mature fluid collection is properly termed a pseudocyst. Pseudocysts may be entirely sonolucent, or they may contain numerous echoes because of septations or necrotic debris.[64] Spontaneous resolution has been observed in about 20% of cases followed by serial ultrasonograms.[64] Those that resolve usually do so within 6 weeks of initial detection.[19]

Although US is quite sensitive in detecting fluid collections, the ability of CT to provide detailed anatomic definition of the pancreas and surrounding structures has made it the single best imaging modality for evaluation of suspected fluid collections. Current-generation high-resolution scanners can detect fluid collections as small as 5 mm in diameter, define their relationship to adjacent structures, and demonstrate their full extent and location, particularly those located in unusual locations, such as

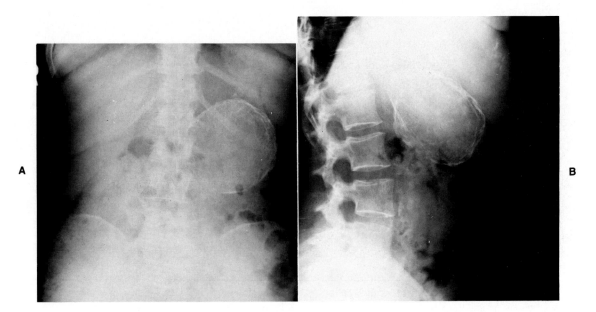

Fig. 45-20. Pancreatic cyst. Anterior, **A,** and lateral, **B,** conventional radiographs show densely calcified rim of true pancreatic cyst. (Courtesy Dr. S.H. Tsai.)

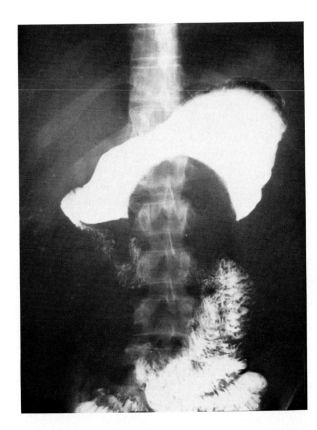

Fig. 45-21. Pancreatic pseudocyst. Barium upper GI series shows marked impression on greater curvature of stomach.

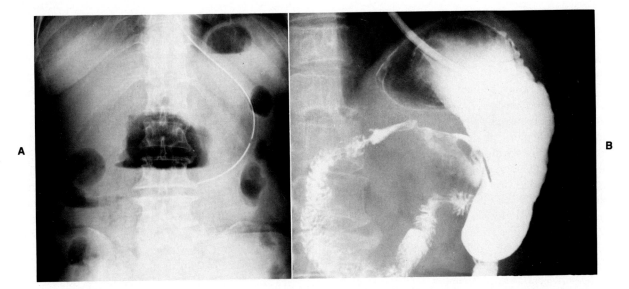

Fig. 45-22. Pancreatic pseudocyst rupturing into stomach. **A,** Upright conventional radiograph shows air-fluid level in pseudocyst following rupture into stomach. **B,** This communication is confirmed by iodinated contrast upper GI series.

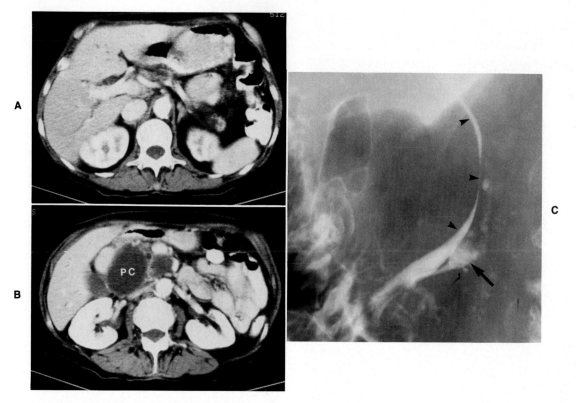

Fig. 45-23. Chronic pancreatitis: bile duct obstruction caused by pseudocyst. **A,** CT scan shows dilated intrahepatic bile ducts. **B,** Scan at lower level shows loculated pseudocyst *(PC)* in head of pancreas. **C,** ERCP shows obstruction of main pancreatic duct by calculus *(arrow)* and displacement and partial obstruction of common bile duct *(arrowheads)* caused by pseudocyst.
(From Freeny, PC: Complications of pancreatitis: diagnosis and management. Gastrointestinal radiology, categorical course syllabus, Miami, 1987, American Roentgen Ray Society.)

within the spleen or liver, the mediastinum, or the lower abdomen.[54]

The CT appearance of fluid collections depends on their stage of development.[54,142] Acute or early collections are seen as poorly marginated areas of diminished attenuation surrounding or even remote from the pancreas, or as focal collections within the pancreatic parenchyma (Fig. 45-19). As they mature, they appear as well-marginated round or oval collections of fluid with a discernible wall or capsule. In the latter instance, the collections are properly referred to as pseudocysts[142] (Fig. 45-23).

CT also is an excellent modality for detection of secondary complications of fluid collections, such as infection, hemorrhage, or involvement of adjacent structures (gastrointestinal tract, spleen or liver, blood vessels, urinary tract or kidney).[54]

Secondary infection of pancreatic pseudocysts can be suspected by CT if gas bubbles or increased attenuation of the fluid contents is seen.[54,105] However, some fluid collections do not manifest any changes indicating in-

fection, and a definite diagnosis is possible only if cultures of the fluid are positive (Fig. 45-24). Therefore an important function of CT is to provide guidance for fine-needle aspiration of the fluid collection so that material can be obtained for bacteriologic examination.[60,162]

Percutaneous catheter drainage

Infected fluid collections can be treated effectively by percutaneous catheter drainage.[55,59] The initial fine-needle aspiration should be used to determine the presence of infection and the quality of the fluid—that is, whether there is sufficient liquid to be drained via catheter).

We have treated 20 patients with 32 localized, infected pancreatic fluid collections.[55] Five of the patients were critically ill with respiratory and renal failure requiring ventilatory support, dialysis, or both. The collections were intrapancreatic or peripancreatic in 24 cases, but 8 were located at sites remote from the pancreas. In these latter cases, CT was essential for detection and planning of percutaneous access routes for catheter drainage.

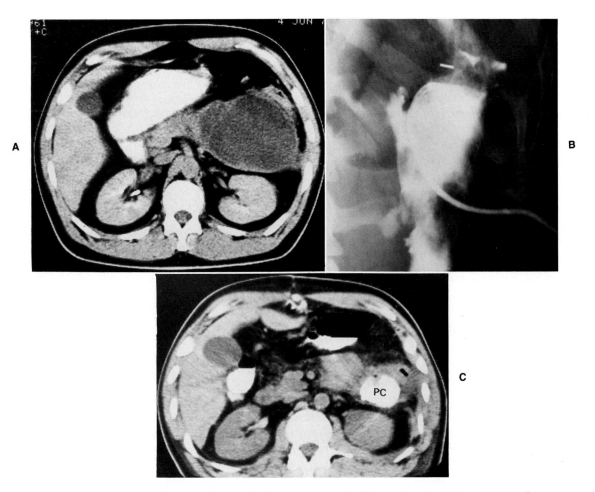

Fig. 45-24. Infected pseudocyst: percutaneous drainage. **A,** CT scan shows pseudocyst in tail of pancreas. Fine-needle aspiration showed infection. **B,** Percutaneous catheter drainage has been performed. Contrast study shows filling of cyst. **C,** CT scan following drainage and injection of dilute contrast shows decompression of entire cyst *(PC)*.

(From Freeny, PC: Complications of pancreatitis: diagnosis and management. Gastrointestinal radiology, categorical course syllabus, Miami, 1987, American Roentgen Ray Society.)

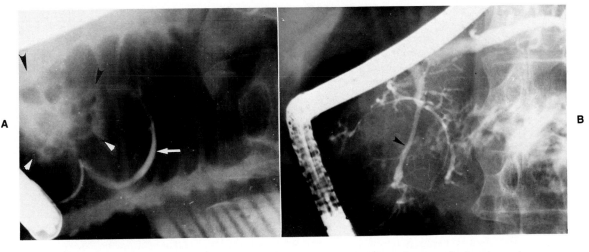

Fig. 45-25. Pancreatic pseudocysts. **A,** ERCP shows communication of pancreatic duct *(arrow)* with pseudocyst *(arrowheads)* in pancreatic head. **B,** Noncommunicating pseudocyst narrows main pancreatic duct *(arrowhead)* and displaces branch ducts. Inflammatory changes are evident in all segments of ductal system.

Patients with infected pancreatic pseudocysts also should have an ERCP before catheter drainage to determine if a pancreatic duct fistula is present and to assess the status of the duct[145] (Fig. 45-25). If the main pancreatic duct between the communicating fluid collection and the papilla is obstructed by a calculus or stricture (Fig. 45-23), percutaneous catheter drainage is likely to result in a pancreatic-cutaneous fistula, and drainage should be performed only if the patient is a prohibitive operative risk, or if a transgastric approach is technically feasible. In the latter case the potential for a pancreatic-cutaneous fistula is virtually eliminated by placing the catheter through the stomach.[110]

Percutaneous catheter drainage was successful in 19 of the 20 patients with infected fluid collections (Fig. 45-24). Only one patient required surgical drainage because of recurrence of the collection. There were three complications: two patients had episodes of hemorrhage from the catheters (both stopped spontaneously and required no treatment), and one patient required surgical placement of a left chest tube to drain an empyema caused by catheter transgression of the pleural space.

Catheter drainage of pancreatic fluid collections may be prolonged. In our series, drainage averaged 60 days.[55] Patients with isolated collections required an average of 29 days of drainage, whereas those with pancreatic duct fistulas required 99 days, and those with gastrointestinal fistulas required 104 days. Frequent contrast studies and

catheter manipulations and changes are necessary to maintain adequate drainage.

Pancreatic phlegmon

Pancreatic phlegmon is characterized by marked enlargement of the pancreas and peripancreatic soft tissues caused by inflammation, edema, and tissue necrosis. Patients with phlegmons usually have had a severe episode of pancreatitis and have a longer duration of abdominal pain, fever, and leukocytosis than patients with no phlegmon formation.[148] It is important to differentiate a phlegmon from an abscess or pseudocyst, since they usually resolve spontaneously and surgical intervention is unnecessary and carries a significant morbidity and mortality.[166]

Phlegmons cause significant displacement of the stomach and duodenum. In the past they were confused with pseudocysts on the basis of findings seen on barium examination[139] (Fig. 45-26). Currently they can be diagnosed accurately in most patients by either US or CT. The typical US findings consist of marked enlargement of the pancreas by a solid mass of highly echogenic tissue (Fig. 45-26). Serial scans can be used to follow the regression of the mass and often show evanescent areas of sonolucency that probably represent areas of liquefaction necrosis.[50] These areas must not be mistaken for abscess formation, and their appearance should be correlated with the clinical condition of the patient, which,

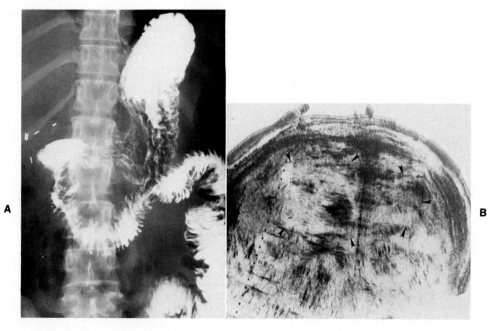

Fig. 45-26. Pancreatic phelgmon. **A,** Upper GI series shows widening of duodenal C-loop, mucosal edema, and spiculation of folds. **B,** Transverse ultrasonogram shows marked enlargement of pancreas along with numerous irregular echoes *(arrowheads)*.

unlike the septic course caused by abscesses, should be one of progressive improvement.

The CT appearance of a pancreatic phlegmon is characterized by enlargement of the pancreas, obliteration of its margins, thickening of peripancreatic soft tissue planes, and extrapancreatic inflammatory mass(es) with no evidence of a wall or capsule[52,148] (Fig. 45-27). The attenuation values of the phlegmonous tissues are varied, usually averaging more than 20 HU (Hounsfield units). CT may show focal areas of necrosis or collections of fluid within the phlegmonous masses. Secondary complications—such as biliary duct obstruction, gastrointestinal, renal or ureteral involvement, or splenic vein obstruction—also can be demonstrated by CT[52] (Fig. 45-27). The usually long duration of fever and leukocytosis makes exclusion of superimposed bacterial infection essential. This can be accomplished by using CT- or US-guided fine-needle aspiration.[148]

Pancreatic abscess

Abscess formation has an overall incidence of about 4% in patients with pancreatitis but may be as high as 50% to 75% in patients with severe hemorrhagic or necrotizing pancreatitis.[54,115,166] It may arise de novo within the pancreas by communication with viscera or as a complication of a preexisting phlegmon or pancreatic fluid collection (Fig. 45-22). Patients with an untreated pancreatic abscess have a mortality of about 100%; if the abscess is recognized early and treated adequately, the mortality is about 65%.[115]

Although abnormal fluid collections can be detected by a variety of techniques, including plain radiographs, contrast studies, US, and CT, there is only one specific finding indicative of an abscess: an *extraluminal collection of gas*.[54,160] This finding is best detected by a plain radiograph of the abdomen or a CT scan[54,58,105] (Fig. 45-28). Although contrast studies may aid in differentiating intraluminal from extraluminal gas, they may also delay

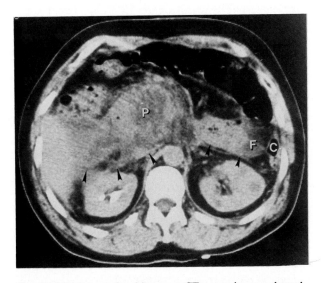

Fig. 45-27. Pancreatic phlegmon. CT scan shows enlarged, unhomogeneous pancreas *(P)* with areas of low parenchymal attenuation. Note loss of tissue planes and bilateral thickening of anterior pararenal fascia *(arrowheads)*. Low-density fluid collection is present in left anterior pararenal space *(F)*, and involves the colon *(C)*.

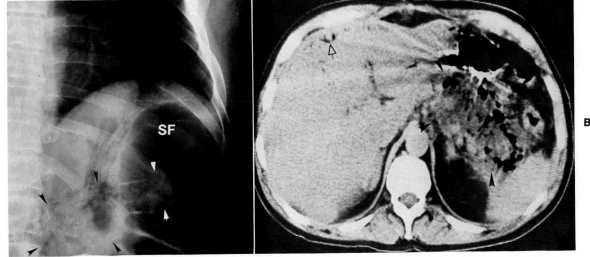

Fig. 45-28. Pancreatic abscess. **A,** Radiograph of abdomen shows abnormal gas bubbles in left upper quadrant *(arrowheads)* and dilatation of splenic flexure of colon *(SF)*. **B,** CT scan shows gas-containing abscess of pancreas *(arrowheads)*. Also note gas in periphery of liver in portal veins *(arrow)*.

the opportunity to perform a CT scan, which is the most specific imaging modality, for both detection and definition of the extent or boundaries of an abscess.

Plain films should be obtained in a routine serial fashion in patients with hemorrhagic or necrotizing pancreatitis. The presence of an abnormal gas collection, which may present in the form of a collection of small bubbles or a single large bubble, or the presence of clinical findings suggesting sepsis should be followed by a CT scan.

The CT features of pancreatic abscesses are varied.[48,54] During the acute phase of abscess formation, the findings are usually nonspecific and may be similar to those associated with acute pancreatitis and phlegmon formation. The pancreas is usually enlarged and has indistinct margins, the surrounding soft tissue planes are obliterated, and a distinct fluid collection usually is not seen. The subacute or chronic stage of abscess development is manifested by a focal or multifocal low-attenuation fluid collection with thick, irregular walls. Gas bubbles often can be seen within the fluid, usually indicating the presence of gas-forming bacteria[48] (Fig. 45-28). However, a fistula to the GI tract can produce a similar appearance without the presence of infection[104] (Fig. 45-22). Thus, regardless of the CT findings, if an abscess is suspected clinically, a guided fine-needle aspiration should be performed to obtain material for culture.[79]

Percutaneous catheter drainage

Percutaneous catheter drainage can be used to treat pancreatic abscesses that are composed of focal, homogeneous collections of infected fluid, or pus.[55] Thus the CT morphology of the abscess is crucial for appropriate patient selection: abscesses that are poorly defined, that are composed of extensive necrotic, inhomogeneous tissue, or that are not accessible by a safe percutaneous route should not be drained by percutaneous catheter placement (Fig. 45-29). Initial fine-needle aspiration also should be performed to confirm the presence of infection and to determine that the fluid is drainable by catheters. Follow-up CT scans and contrast studies of the catheters are important to confirm that the abscess has been evacuated completely and that it is responding (that is, decreasing in size) to treatment (Fig. 45-24).

Pancreatic necrosis

The acute inflammatory process of pancreatitis may progress and result in areas of parenchymal necrosis, probably caused by ischemia. It is essential to detect the presence of necrosis, since it is usually associated with a more fulminant clinical course and a high mortality due to pulmonary, renal, and cardiovascular complications. Septic complications also dominate in the later

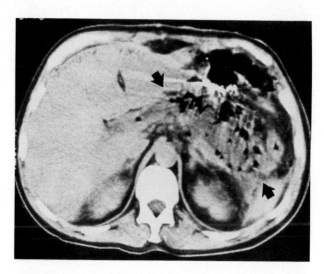

Fig. 45-29. Pancreatic necrosis and abscess. CT scan shows pancreatic abscess containing gas and necrotic debris *(arrows)*. CT morphology indicates need for surgical debridement.
(From Freeny, PC: Complications of pancreatitis: diagnosis and management. Gastrointestinal radiology, categorical course syllabus, Miami, 1987, American Roentgen Ray Society.)

stages, when areas of devitalized, necrotic tissue become infected; this results in higher rates of mortality.

Early surgical debridement and drainage of necrotic parenchyma and infected fluid are crucial for preventing a high mortality, which is often more than 60% if superimposed bacterial infection occurs.[8] Early diagnosis of pancreatic necrosis is therefore essential. This can be accomplished by combining bolus-dynamic CT scanning with clinical monitoring of the patient, especially daily determinations of C-reactive protein levels. The C-reactive protein levels rise early with the onset of necrosis. When 100 mg/100 ml is used as the discriminating point, an overall detection rate of 95% is usual.[23]

CT is useful to confirm the clinical and laboratory diagnosis, localize the areas of necrosis, and estimate the extent of necrosis.[9] The bolus-dynamic CT findings of pancreatic necrosis are characterized by zones of low-attenuation, non–contrast-enhancing parenchyma within the pancreas[87,88] (Fig. 45-6). As the areas of necrosis become subacute or chronic, they may assume a saclike configuration with a thick, smooth rim or capsule.[172] The attenuation values of the necrotic tissue average about 20 to 40 HU. CT-guided fine-needle aspiration can be performed to detect infection. This is essential since the combination of necrosis and infection have a mortality of 39% to 67%, compared with 13% to 14% with necrosis alone.[8] The consistency and quality of the necrotic debris prevent evacuation by even large-bore (24 to 30 F) cath-

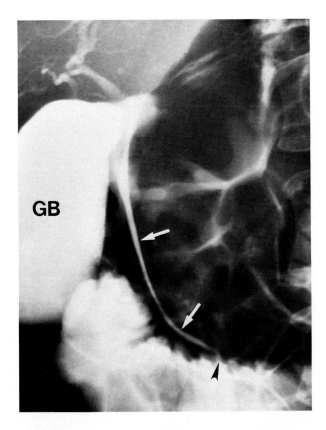

Fig. 45-30. Pancreatic pseudocyst. ERCP shows long, smooth narrowing and displacement of common bile duct *(arrows)*. Papilla is in transverse duodenum *(arrowhead)*. Gallbladder *(GB)* is filled with contrast material.

eters. Thus surgical debridement is necessary, and percutaneous catheter treatment should be avoided.

Biliary complications

Since the common bile duct traverses the pancreatic parenchyma in approximately 75% of individuals, any neoplastic or inflammatory process in the pancreatic head may cause common bile duct obstruction.[54] Although common bile duct deformity may be seen in up to two thirds of patients with pancreatitis, cholestasis occurs in less than half of these cases.[169] A pseudocyst may cause biliary obstruction in 10% of cases.

Common bile duct deformity in patients with pancreatic inflammatory disease results from acute inflammation with edema, from compression by a cystic mass, or from chronic inflammation with fibrosis. Although a spectrum of ductal deformity is possible, chronic pancreatitis (Fig. 45-14) and a pseudocyst (Fig. 45-30) typically produce a long, gently tapered narrowing. Since the effect of acute inflammation may be transient, prediction of the ultimate state of the bile duct by cholangiography must be made with care.

Nonoperative biliary drainage

Patients who are poor operative risks, or who are critically ill with cholangitis, can be temporarily or per-

manently treated with percutaneous or endoscopic biliary decompression[27] (Fig. 45-31).

Vascular complications

The vascular system can be involved by the inflammatory process of pancreatitis in several ways: pancreatic enzymes can cause direct erosion of pancreatic or peripancreatic arteries with resulting hemorrhage or formation of pseudoaneurysms, or the inflammatory process may cause thrombosis of the splenic or superior mesenteric veins, resulting in the development of varices.* Bolus-dynamic CT produces excellent opacification of the arteries and veins surrounding the pancreas and thus is an excellent modality for identifying these vascular complications.[52,54]

Acute pancreatic hemorrhage can be suspected by CT if one can identify a focal collection of fluid (blood) with increased attenuation, or recognize an interim increase in the attenuation values of the fluid within a previously demonstrated pseudocyst or fluid collection.[54]

Arterial pseudoaneurysms can develop within the pancreatic parenchyma, adjacent to the gland, or within a pseudocyst. They can be diagnosed by angiography (Fig.

---

*References 54, 57, 76, 80, 122, 149, 165, 171.

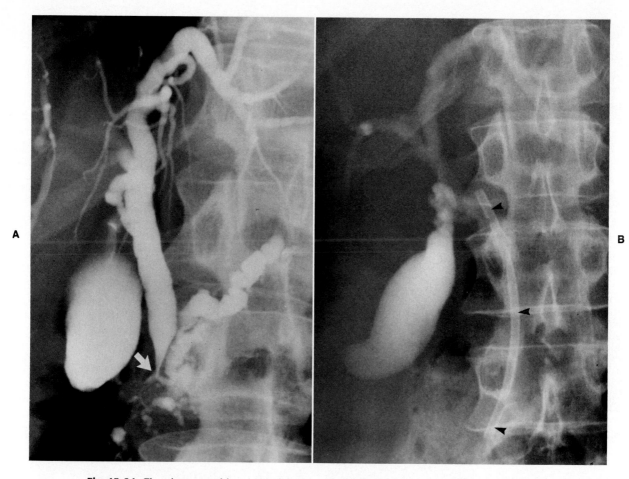

Fig. 45-31. Chronic pancreatitis: pancreatic and common bile duct stenosis. **A,** ERCP shows stenosis of pancreatic and common bile ducts *(arrow)* with upstream dilatation and pancreatic duct changes of chronic pancreatitis. **B,** Endoscopic stent *(arrowheads)*, placed in bile duct for decompression. (From Freeny, PC: Complications of pancreatitis: diagnosis and management. Gastrointestinal radiology, categorical course syllabus, Miami, 1987, American Roentgen Ray Society.)

45-32) or CT by demonstrating a contrast-enhancing mass[24,54,80] (Fig. 45-33).

Venous occlusion can be seen directly by angiography as an abrupt cutoff of the contrast-filled vein (Fig. 45-34), or indirectly by CT or angiography as collateral vessels enlarge and perigastric or mesenteric varices develop (Fig. 45-33).

Transcatheter embolization, which has been used for many years to treat gastrointestinal bleeding, also can be used to treat acute hemorrhage or pseudoaneurysms caused by pancreatitis.[54,150,163,165]

Pancreatic ascites

Pancreatic ascites is caused by extravasation of pancreatic enzymes from a ruptured pancreatic duct.[54,132] Although CT can detect the presence of ascites, the fluid

must be shown to have a high amylase for a specific diagnosis of pancreatic ascites to be made.[54] The exact site of ductal rupture usually is not evident on the CT scan and can best be determined by retrograde pancreatography.[37,38,130]

Gastrointestinal complications

The inflammatory reaction associated with acute pancreatitis can extend beyond the gland to involve virtually any portion of the GI tract from the esophagus to the colon.[54] CT can demonstrate the spread of the pancreatic inflammatory process to contiguous or remote segments of the GI tract. In addition, it may show communications or fistulas between a fluid collection or pseudocyst and a contiguous segment of the stomach or bowel, or it can identify potential sites of GI tract involvement[47] (Fig.

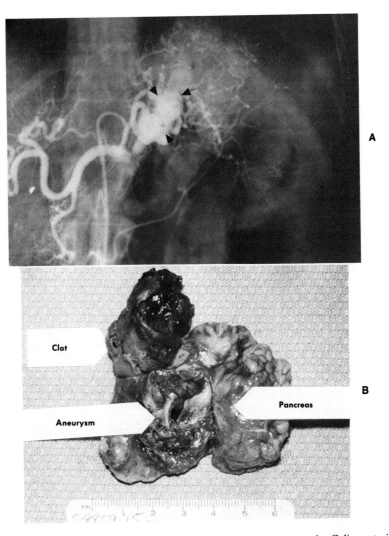

Fig. 45-32. Chronic relapsing pancreatitis and splenic artery aneurysm. **A,** Celiac arteriogram shows lobulated splenic artery aneurysm *(arrows)*. Venous phase (not shown) showed splenic vein occlusion. **B,** At surgery, pancreas showed chronic inflammation and aneurysm was embedded within tail, necessitating distal pancreatectomy and splenectomy.

45-27). Contrast studies (barium or water-soluble media) also may be useful to demonstrate a suspected fistula or stenosis[157] (Figs. 45-3, 45-10, and 45-24).

Ossseous complications

Pancreatitis has been implicated in the pathogenesis of several types of osseous lesions, including polyarthritis, aseptic necrosis of the femoral or humeral heads, mottled calcific metaphyseal lesions, and focal areas of cortical destruction in the long bones and in the small tubular bones of the hands and feet. In some cases the bone lesions are associated with skin lesions resembling erythema nodosum.[54] Both the osseous and cutaneous lesions are thought to be the result of fat necrosis due to high levels of circulating pancreatic lipase.[17]

Pulmonary complications

Respiratory failure is a recognized complication of acute pancreatitis and may be caused by injury of the alveolocapillary membrane by high levels of circulating triglycerides.[168] Sometimes referred to as "pancreatitis lung," it is characterized by a diffuse alveolar infiltrate and the frequent development of pleural and pericardial effusions.[26,104]

Unilateral or bilateral pancreatic-pleural fistulas may result from posterior leakage by dissection or pancreatic

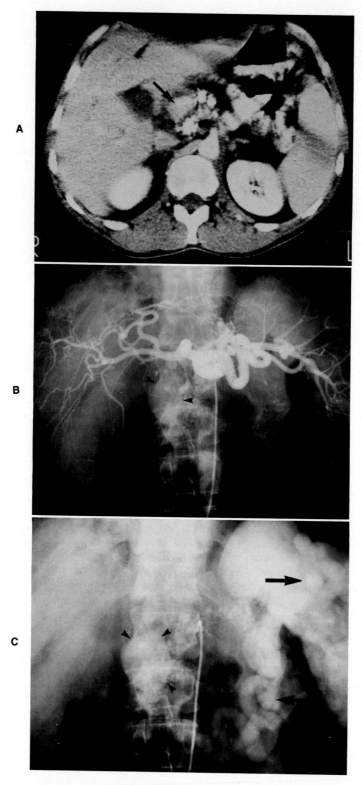

Fig. 45-33. Chronic calcific pancreatitis: arterial pseudoaneurysm and splenic vein obstruction. **A,** CT scan of head of pancreas shows a contrast-enhancing mass *(arrow)* within small pseudocyst. Note perigastric varices caused by splenic vein obstruction. **B,** Celiac arteriogram shows pseudoaneurysm arising from gastroduodenal artery *(arrowheads).* **C,** Venous phase shows contrast within pseudoaneurysm *(arrowheads)* and large perigastric varices *(arrows).*
(From Freeny, PC: Complications of pancreatitis: diagnosis and management. Gastrointestinal radiology, categorical course syllabus, Miami, 1987, American Roentgen Ray Society.)

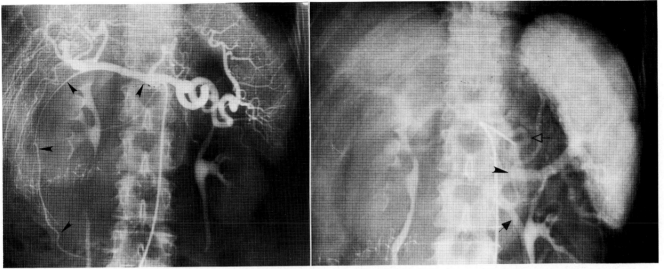

Fig. 45-34. Pancreatic pseudocyst. **A,** Celiac arteriogram shows displacement of hepatic and gastroduodenal arteries by large avascular mass *(arrowheads)* due to a pseudocyst. Spleen is enlarged, and intrasplenic vessels are separated and straightened, indicating congestive splenomegaly. **B,** Venous phase of selective splenic injection shows occlusion of splenic vein *(arrowhead)*, dilated gastric vein *(open arrow)*, and retrograde flow in inferior mesenteric vein *(closed arrow)*.

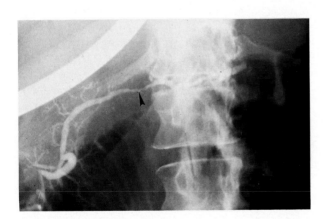

Fig. 45-35. Chronic pancreatitis. ERCP shows focal stenosis of pancreatic duct at head-body junction *(arrowhead)*. Prestenotic dilatation of main duct and side branches is evident. Patient underwent distal pancreatectomy.

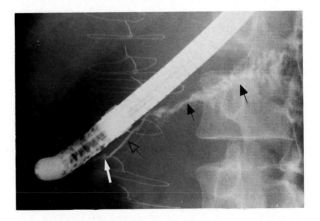

Fig. 45-36. Postoperative distal pancreatectomy. Patency of pancreaticojejunal anastomosis is confirmed by endoscopic retrograde pancreatography. Endoscopic cannula *(white arrow)*, pancreatic duct *(open arrow)*, and jejunum *(closed arrows)* are shown.

enzymes along the retroperitoneum, through the esophageal or aortic hiatus, and into the mediastinum or pleural space. Rarely, a transdiaphragmatic route is taken.

PREOPERATIVE AND POSTOPERATIVE RADIOLOGIC EVALUATION OF PANCREATITIS
Acute pancreatitis

The primary role of radiology in the preoperative evaluation of patients with acute or acute relapsing pancreatitis is the detection of a surgically correctable cause. These have been discussed previously and include biliary tract disease, lesions of the upper GI tract, and structural abnormalities of the pancreatic or biliary ducts.[81] The primary procedures used are US and CT, oral cholecystography, barium studies of the upper gastrointestinal tract, ERCP, and percutaneous transhepatic cholangiography (PTC).[34]

Chronic pancreatitis

Preoperative radiologic evaluation of patients with chronic pancreatitis has several purposes. First, pancreatic and biliary duct anatomy determine whether the patient is managed medically or surgically. In some cases surgery may be judged to be of no value, and an unnecessary laparotomy is thus avoided. In other cases the appropriate type of surgical resection or drainage procedure is based on the morphologic changes of the pancreatic and biliary ducts.[32] Such a case is illustrated by Fig. 45-35.

Second, preoperative definition of pancreatic and peripancreatic vascular anatomy is essential for the safe performance of major pancreatic surgery.[80] A lack of knowledge of the presence of one or more of the potential anomalous vascular patterns of the pancreas may result in inadvertent ligation of a major vessel with subsequent infarction of the liver, stomach, duodenum, or spleen.[66,118,120,177] In addition, knowledge of the presence of an arterial pseudoaneurysm or venous occlusion with associated varices may be crucial in planning the proper surgical procedure and in avoiding intraoperative and postoperative hemorrhage[56] (Figs. 45-32 to 45-34).

Finally, careful definition of the full extent of pancreatic or peripancreatic fluid collections or abscesses is essential in executing the complete drainage of these lesions. The presence of numerous loculations or the migration of fluid to remote areas may be overlooked without adequate preoperative studies (Fig. 45-19). Diagnostic imaging of the postoperative pancreas is useful in defining postoperative complications or in confirming the adequacy of pancreatic or biliary anastomoses with the intestinal tract.[103,173] Fig. 45-36 demonstrates the patency of a pancreaticojejunal anastomosis.

VASCULAR DISEASES

Primary vascular diseases of the pancreas are quite rare and usually are encountered unexpectedly during unrelated visceral angiography.

Hereditary hemorrhagic telangiectasia (Osler-Weber-Rendu disease) is transmitted as an autosomally dominant disease and is characterized by multiple telangiectases involving the skin, mucous membranes, lungs, liver, pancreas, and other sites.[12] Angiographic evaluation has demonstrated a spectrum of findings ranging from small telangiectases to large arteriovenous fistulas.[75,89] Although the pancreas may be involved, the most common manifestations are found in the liver and lungs.

Primary pancreatic *arteriovenous malformations* are rare. In most cases they are associated with hereditary hemorrhagic telangiectasia, but they may also be isolated lesions within the pancreas.[54] They are often discovered during angiographic evaluation for occult GI hemorrhage or are found incidentally at surgery or during unrelated visceral angiography.[69,113]

Pancreatic *hemangiomas* and *cavernous lymphangiomas* are extremely rare lesions.[113] In one case report, a lymphangioma was discovered by the presence of multiple phlebolith-like calcifications within a pancreatic mass.[41]

CONGENITAL ABNORMALITIES
Abnormalities of development

Although rarely of clinical consequence, congenital anomalies of the pancreas are well documented as representing radiographic abnormalities with varying symptoms.[11,43] Anomalies of pancreatic embryogenesis result mainly in the ectopic location of pancreatic tissue and in variations in ductal fusion or location.

The adult pancreas is the result of the embryologic fusion of two components. These arise as ventral or dorsal outpouchings from the foregut just distal to the stomach. The ventral portion arises as a component of the embryonic biliary duct system, which during maturation rotates posterior to the duodenum to fuse with the dorsal component (Fig. 45-37). In addition, nests of aberrant pancreatic tissue may be located in any position along the GI tract or within its accessory organs.

Aberrant (heterotopic) pancreas

Buds of anomalously placed pancreatic tissue are most commonly found in the stomach.[11,43] Other sites include the duodenum, small intestine, esophagus, gallbladder, spleen, and Meckel's diverticula.[155] Heterotopic tissue is found incidentally in 1 of 500 surgical cases and in 1 of 10 autopsies. It is usually identified as a smooth submucosal nodule with a central umbilication[123] (Fig. 45-

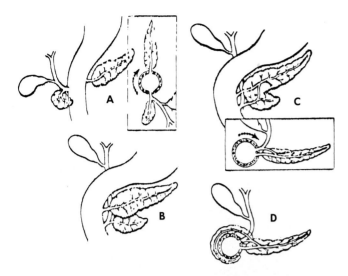

Fig. 45-37. Embryologic development of pancreas. Lecco's theory of embryonic development of normal pancreas, **A** to **C,** and annular pancreas, **D.**
(From Lloyd-Jones, W, Mountain, JC, and Warren, W: Ann Surg 176:163, 1972.)

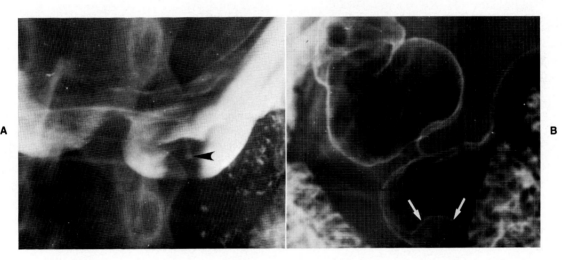

Fig. 45-38. Ectopic pancreas. Compression, **A,** and air contrast, **B,** views of gastric antrum demonstrate centrally umbilicated smooth mass *(arrows)* along greater curvature. Central umbilication *(arrowhead)* represents orifice of rudimentary duct system.

38). However, atypical presentations, such as large masses, prolapsing polyps, and annular configurations, are also possible.[155] Fig. 45-38 demonstrates a typical heterotopic pancreatic nodule in the gastric antrum. The diagnosis is infrequently made preoperatively and requires demonstration of the rudimentary duct system within the nodule.[11,43,123,155]

Annular pancreas

When the ventral component of the pancreas fails to rotate normally around the duodenum, the potential for an annular pancreas arises[62,94] (Fig. 45-37). This circumstance has been found in approximately 1 of 7000 au-topsies or in 1 of 22,000 laparotomies.[119] An annular pancreas can be symptomatic in adults as well as in the pediatric age group, with a peak adult incidence occurring between 40 and 50 years of age. The reason for this late onset of symptoms in a congenital abnormality is thought to relate to a higher incidence of inflammatory reaction in patients with an annular pancreas.[42,119] Because of the variability of the completeness of the ring of pancreatic tissue about the duodenum and the intensity of potential inflammatory disease, symptoms may be variable or nonexistent.

Radiographic diagnosis depends on the demonstration of an annular constriction in the proximal or mid–de-

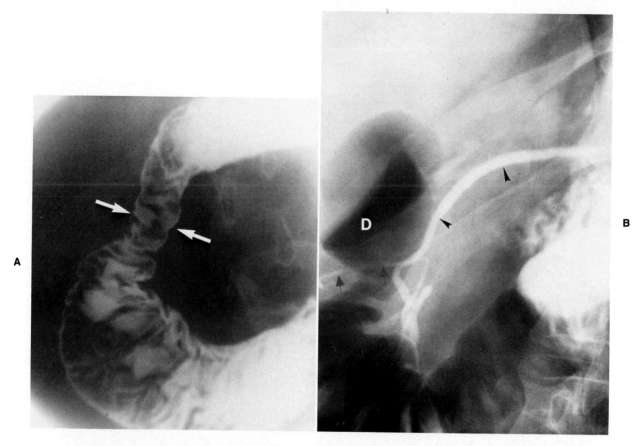

A

B

D

Fig. 45-39. Annular pancreas. **A,** Upper GI series shows smooth, extrinsic, circumferential narrowing of proximal duodenum *(arrows).* **B,** ERCP shows accessory pancreatic duct *(arrows)* encircling duodenum *(D).* Main duct *(arrowheads)* is normal. (See Fig. 49-19).

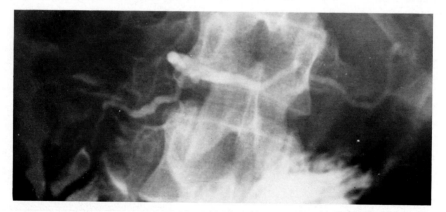

Fig. 45-40. Cystic fibrosis. ERCP shows irregular narrowing of main pancreatic duct. There is limited filling of branch ducts.

scending duodenum[208] (Fig. 45-39). The degree of obstructive dilatation of the duodenum bulb and stomach is variable. Demonstration of the annular duct by operative pancreatography or by ERCP confirms the diagnosis[62,77,137] (Fig. 45-39).

ABNORMALITY OF FUNCTION: CYSTIC FIBROSIS

Although cystic fibrosis (mucoviscidosis) is known to be transmitted as an autosomal recessive disorder, its pathophysiology remains undefined.[36,176] Both serous and mucous secretions are abnormally concentrated, producing inspissation, obstruction, and abnormal function in many organs.[2] In the GI tract both tubular and solid organs are affected. The manifestations that may be present in the newborn or neonatal period are considered in Chapter 78. In the adult, progressive pancreatic insufficiency caused by ductal obstruction, episodes of acute pancreatitis, and fibrosis are variable occurrences.[176] Cholecystitis, cholelithiasis, and biliary cirrhosis—along with potential portal hypertension and esophageal varices—are the principle effects within the hepatobiliary tract.[2,45,159] Deterioration of the pancreas may be associated with fine granular pancreatic calcifications. Although episodes of acute pancreatitis are rare, they generally are related to a superimposed factor and when present may be manifested radiographically by the typical signs of acute pancreatitis detailed earlier in this chapter. The pancreatic duct may be narrowed, irregular, or possibly obstructed (Fig. 45-40).

Intestinal maldigestion, although frequently severe, does not consistently produce radiographically detectable small bowel abnormalities.[36,175] When abnormalities are present, fold thickening and modest dilatation are notable features. Intestinal obstruction due to fecal impaction, volvulus related to colonic enlargement, and pneumatosis cystoides intestinalis have been reported. A barium enema may reveal multiple filling defects caused by difficulties in cleansing and resultant adherent mucus. Dilatation of the colonic glands may produce an abnormal, lacy mucosal pattern.[176]

REFERENCES

1. Alpern, MB, et al: Chronic pancreatitis: ultrasonic features, Radiology 155:215, 1985.
2. Anderson, CM, and Goodchild, MC: Cystic fibrosis: manual of diagnosis and management, Oxford, 1976, Blackwell Scientific Publications.
3. Axon, ATR, et al: Pancreatography in chronic pancreatitis: international definitions, Gut 25:1107, 1984.
4. Balthazar, EJ: Effects of acute and chronic pancreatitis on the stomach: patterns of radiographic involvement, Am J Gastroenterol 72:568, 1979.
5. Balthazar, EJ, et al: Acute pancreatitis: prognostic value of CT, Radiology 156:767, 1985.
6. Bar-Meir, S, et al: Biliary and pancreatic duct pressures measured by ERCP manometry in patients with suspected papillary stenosis, Dig Dis Sci 24:209, 1979.
7. Beger, HG, and Buchler, M: Outcome of necrotizing pancreatitis in relation to morphological parameters. In Malfertheiner, P, and Ditschuneit, H, editors: Diagnostic procedures in pancreatic disease, Berlin, 1986, Springer-Verlag.
8. Beger, HG, et al: Bacterial contamination of pancreatic necrosis: a prospective clinical study, Gastroenterology 91:433, 1986.
9. Beger, HG, et al: How do imaging methods influence the surgical strategy in acute pancreatitis? In Malfertheiner, P, and Ditschuneit, H, editors: Diagnostic procedures in pancreatic disease, Berlin, 1986, Springer-Verlag.
10. Berenson, JE, Spitz, HB, and Felson, D: The abdominal fat necrosis sign, Radiology 100:567, 1971.
11. Besemann, EF, Auerbach, SH, and Wolfe, WW: The importance of roentgenologic diagnosis of aberrant pancreatic tissue in the gastrointestinal tract, Am J Roentgenol 107:71, 1969.
12. Bird, RM, and Jaques, WE: Vascular lesions of hereditary hemorrhagic telangiectasia, N Engl J Med 260:597, 1959.
13. Blackstone, MO, and Mizuno, H: Reactive duodenal changes in chronic pancreatitis simulating the contiguous spread of pancreatic carcinoma, Am J Dig Dis 22:658, 1977.
14. Block, S, et al: Sensitivity of imaging procedures and clinical staging for necrotizing pancreatitis, Digestion 30:102, 1984.
15. Bolondi, L, et al: Secretin administration induces a dilatation of main pancreatic duct, Dig Dis Sci 29:802, 1984.
16. Bolondi, L, et al: Critical evaluation and controversial points of ultrasound findings in chronic pancreatitis. In Malfertheiner, P, and Ditschuneit, H, editors: Diagnostic procedures in pancreatic disease, Berlin, 1986, Springer-Verlag.
17. Boswell, SH, and Baylin, GJ: Metastatic fat necrosis and lytic bone lesions in a patient with painless acute pancreatic, Radiology 106:85, 1973.
18. Bradley, EL, and Clements, JL: Spontaneous resolution of pancreatic pseudocysts, Am J Surg 129:23, 1975.
19. Bradley, EL, Clements, JL, and Gonzales, AC: The natural history of pancreatic pseudocysts: a unified concept of management, Am J Surg 137:135, 1979.
20. Braganza, JM, Hunt, LP, and Warwick, F: Relationship between pancreatic exocrine function and ductal morphology in chronic pancreatitis, Gastroenterology 82:1341, 1982.
21. Broe, PJ, and Cameron, JL: Pancreatic ascites and pancreatic pleural effusions. In Bradley, EL, III, editor: Complications of pancreatitis: medical and surgical management, Philadelphia, 1982, WB Saunders.
22. Buchler, M, Malfertheiner, P, and Beger, HG: Correlation of imaging procedures, biochemical parameters, and clinical stage in acute pancreatitis. In Malfertheiner, P, and Ditschuneit, H, editors: Diagnostic procedures in pancreatic disease, Berlin, 1986, Springer-Verlag.
23. Buchler, M, et al: Sensitivity of antiproteases, complement factors and C-reactive protein in detecting pancreatic necrosis: results of a prospective clinical study, Int J Pancreatology 1:227, 1986.
24. Burbige, EJ, et al: Colonic varices: a complication of pancreatitis with splenic vein thrombosis, Am J Dig Dis 23:752, 1978.
25. Burke, JW, et al: Pseudoaneurysms complicating pancreatitis: detection by CT, Radiology 161:447, 1986.
26. Case records of the Massachusetts General Hospital: Case 40-1975, N Engl J Med 293:764, 1975.

27. Chuang, VP, et al: Angiography of pancreatic arteriovenous malformation, AJR 129:1015, 1977.

28. Classen, M, and Phillip, J: Endoscopic retrograde cholangiopancreatography (ERCP) and endoscopic therapy in pancreatic disease, Clin Gastroenterol 13:819, 1984.

29. Clements, JL, Jr, Bradley, EL, and Eaton, SB, Jr: Spontaneous internal drainage of pancreatic pseudocysts, Am J Roentgenol 126:985, 1976.

30. Cooperberg, PL, and Burhenne, HT: Real time ultrasonography, N Engl J Med 302:1277, 1980.

31. Cooperberg, PL, and Gibney, RG: Imaging of the gallbladder, 1987, Radiology 163:605, 1987.

32. Cooperman, AM, and Hoerr, SO: Surgery of the pancreas: a text and atlas, St Louis, 1977, The CV Mosby Co.

33. Cotton, PB: Congenital anomaly of pancreas divisum as a cause of obstructive pain and pancreatitis, Gut 21:105, 1980.

34. Cotton, PB, and Beales, JSM: Endoscopic pancreatography in management of relapsing acute pancreatitis, Br Med J 1:608, 1974.

35. Dallemand, S, et al: Colonic necrosis complicating pancreatitis, Gastrointest Radiol 2:27, 1977.

36. Danks, DM, Allan, J, and Anderson, CM: A genetic study of fibrocystic disease of the pancreas, Ann Hum Genet 28:323, 1965.

37. Davis, RE, and Graham, DY: Pancreatic ascites, the role of ERCP, Am J Dig Dis 20:977, 1975.

38. Davis, S, Probhoo, SP, and Gibson, MJ: The plain abdominal radiograph in acute pancreatitis, Clin Radiol 31:87, 1980.

39. Delhaye, M, Engelhome, L, and Cremer, M: Pancreas divisum: congenital anatomic variant or anomaly? contribution of endoscopic retrograde dorsal pancreatography, Gastroenterology 89:951, 1985.

40. Dembner, AG, et al: A new computed tomographic sign of pancreatitis, AJR 133:477, 1979.

41. Dodds, WJ, Margolin, FR, and Goldberg, HI: Cavernous lymphangioma of the pancreas, Radiol Clin Biol 38:267, 1969.

42. Doubilet, H, and Worth, MH: Pseudocyst of annular pancreas demonstrated by operative pancreatography, Surgery 58:824, 1965.

43. Eklof, O: Accessory pancreas in the stomach and duodenum, Acta Chir Scand 121:19, 1961.

44. Erb, WH, and Grimes, EL: Pseudocysts of the pancreas, Am J Surg 100:30, 1960.

45. Esterly, JR, and Openheimer, GH: Observations in cystic fibrosis of the pancreas. I. The gallbladder, Bull Johns Hopkins Hosp 110:247, 1962.

46. Farman, J: Colonic complications of pancreatitis. In Marshak, RH, Lindner, AE, and Maklansky, D, editors: Radiology of the colon, Philadelphia, 1980, WB Saunders.

47. Federle, MP, and Burke, VD: Pancreatitis and its complications: computed tomography and sonography, Sem US CT MR 5:414, 1984.

48. Federle, MP, et al: Computed tomography of pancreatic abscesses, AJR 136:879, 1981.

49. Feinberg, SB, and Tully, TE: Secondary gastric mural abnormalities simulating primary disease in isolated chronic left subphrenic abscess and isolated chronic pancreatitis, Am J Roentgenol 122:413, 1974.

50. Ferrucci, JT, Jr: Radiology of the pancreas, 1976: sonography and ductography, Radiol Clin North Am 14:543, 1976.

51. Fonseca, C, et al: 99m Tc-IDA imaging in the differential diagnosis of acute cholecystitis and acute pancreatitis, Radiology 130:525, 1979.

52. Freeny, PC: Computed tomography of the pancreas, Clin Gastroenterol 13:791, 1984.

53. Freeny, PC, Ball, TJ, and Ryan, J: Impact of the new diagnostic imaging methods of pancreatic angiography, AJR 133:619, 1979.

54. Freeny, PC, and Lawson, TL: Radiology of the pancreas, New York, 1982, Springer-Verlag.

55. Freeny, PC, et al: Infected pancreatic fluid collections: percutaneous catheter drainage, Radiology, 1988. (in press)

56. Frey, CF: Pancreatic pseudocysts—operative strategy, Ann Surg 188:652, 1978.

57. Gadaiz, TR, Trunkey, D, and Kieffer, RF, Jr: Visceral vessel erosion associated with pancreatitis: case reports and a review of the literature, Arch Surg 113:1438, 1978.

58. Gerzof, SG, Robbins, AH, and Birkett, DH: Computed tomography in the diagnosis and management of abdominal abscesses, Gastrointest Radiol 3:287, 1978.

59. Gerzof, SG, et al: Percutaneous drainage of infected pancreatic pseudocysts, Arch Surg 119:888, 1984.

60. Gerzof, SG, et al: Role of guided percutaneous aspiration in early diagnosis of pancreatic sepsis, Dig Dis Sci 29:950, 1984.

61. Girdwood, AH, et al: Structure and function in noncalcific pancreatitis, Dig Dis Sci 29:721, 1984.

62. Glazer, GM, and Margulis, AR: Annular pancreas: etiology and diagnosis using endoscopic retrograde cholangiopancreatography, Radiology 133:303, 1979.

63. Goldberg, PB, et al: Choledochocele as a cause of recurrent pancreatitis, Gastroenterology 78:1041, 1980.

64. Gonzalez, AC, Bradley, EL, and Clements, JL: Pseudocyst formation in acute pancreatitis: ultrasonographic evaluation of 99 cases, Am J Roentgenol 127:315, 1976.

65. Goodman, AJ, et al: Detection of gallstones after acute pancreatitis, Gut 26:125, 1985.

66. Gordon, DH, et al: Accessory blood supply to the liver from the dorsal pancreatic artery: an unusual anatomic variant, Cardiovasc Radiol 1:199, 1978.

67. Gougon, FW, et al: Pancreatic trauma: a new diagnostic approach, Am J Surg 132:400, 1976.

68. Graham, JM, Mattox, KL, and Jordan, GL, Jr: Traumatic injuries to the pancreas, Am J Surg 136:744, 1978.

69. Grannis, FW, et al: Diagnosis and management of an arteriovenous fistula of pancreas and duodenum, Mayo Clin Proc 48:780, 1973.

70. Gregg, JA: Pancreas divisum: its association with pancreatitis, Am J Surg 134:539, 1977.

71. Gross, JB, Gambill, EE, and Ulrich, JA: Hereditary pancreatitis, Am J Med 33:358, 1962.

72. Guyer, PB, and Amin, PH: Radiological demonstration of spontaneous rupture of pancreatic pseudocysts, Br J Radiol 43:342, 1970.

73. Gyr, KE, Singer, MV, and Sarles, H, editors: Pancreatitis: concepts and classification: proceedings of the Second International Symposium on the Classification of Pancreatitis, Marseille, March 28-30, 1984, Amsterdam, 1984, Excerpta Medica.

74. Hacken, JB, and Baer, JW: Calcifications within the duct of Wirsung in calcific pancreatitis, Gastrointest Radiol 3:173, 1978.

75. Halpern, M, Turner, AF, and Citron, BP: Hereditary hemorrhagic telangiectasia: an angiographic study of abdominal visceral angiodysplasias associated with gastrointestinal hemorrhage, Radiology 90:1143, 1968.

76. Harris, RD, Anderson, JE, and Coel, MN: Aneurysms of the small pancreatic arteries: a cause of upper abdominal pain and intestinal bleeding, Radiology 115:17, 1975.

77. Heyman, RL, and Whelan, TJ: Annular pancreas: demonstration of the annular duct on cholangiography, Ann Surg 165:470, 1967.

78. Hill, MC, et al: Acute pancreatitis: clinical vs. CT findings, AJR 139:263, 1982.

79. Hill, MC, et al: Role of percutaneous aspiration in diagnosis of pancreatic abscess, AJR 141:1035, 1983.

80. Hofer, BO, Ryan, JA, Jr, and Freeny, PC: Surgical significance of vascular changes in chronic pancreatitis, SGO 164:499, 1987.

81. Howard, JM, and Jordan, GL: Surgical diseases of the pancreas, Philadelphia, 1960, JB Lippincott.

82. Jeffrey, RB, Jr, Federle, MP, and Laing, FC: Computed tomography of mesenteric involvement in fulminant pancreatitis, Radiology 147:185, 1983.

83. Jeffrey, RB, Jr, Laing, FC, and Wing, VW: Extrapancreatic spread of acute pancreatitis: new observations with real-time US, Radiology 159:707, 1986.

84. Jensen, AR, et al: Pattern of pain, duct morphology, and pancreatic function in chronic pancreatitis, Scand J Gastroenterol 19:334, 1984.

85. Kasugai, T, Kuno, N, and Kizu, M: Manometric endoscopic retrograde pancreatocholangiography: technique, significance, and evaluation, Am J Dig Dis 19:485, 1974.

86. Kattwinkel, J, et al: Hereditary pancreatitis: three new kindreds and a critical review of the literature, Pediatrics 51:55, 1973.

87. Kivisaari, L, et al: Early detection of acute fulminant pancreatitis by contrast-enhanced computed tomography, Scand J Gastroenterol 18:39, 1983.

88. Kruse, A, Thommesen, P, and Frederiksen, P: Endoscopic retrograde cholangiopancreatography in pancreatic cancer and chronic pancreatitis: differences in morphologic changes in the pancreatitis duct and the bile duct, Scand J Gastroenterol 13:513, 1978.

89. Lande, A, Bedford, A, and Schechter, LS: The spectrum of arteriographic findings in Oster-Weber-Rendu disease, Angiology 27:223, 1976.

90. Lankisch, PG, et al: Pancreatic calcifications: no indicator of severe exocrine pancreatic insufficiency, Gastroenterology 90:617, 1986.

91. Lawson, TL: Intraluminal duodenal diverticulum, Am J Dig Dis 19:673, 1974.

92. Lees, WR: Pancreatic ultrasonography, Clin Gastroenterol 13:763, 1984.

93. Legge, DA, Hoffman, HN, II, and Carlson, HC: Pancreatitis as a complication of regional enteritis of the duodenum, Gastroenterology 61:834, 1971.

94. Levin, DC, Wilson, R, and Abrams, HL: The changing role of pancreatic arteriography in the era of computed tomography, Radiology 136:245, 1980.

95. Lloyd-Jones, W, Mountain, JC, and Warren, KW: Annular pancreas in the adult, Ann Surg 176:163, 1972.

96. Logan, A, Schlicke, CP, and Manning, GB: Familial pancreatitis, Am J Surg 112:142, 1966.

97. Maier, W: Computed tomography in chronic pancreatitis. In Malfertheiner, P, and Ditschuneit, H, editors: Diagnostic procedures in pancreatic disease, Berlin, 1986, Springer-Verlag.

98. Maier, W: Grading of acute pancreatitis by computed tomography morphology. In Malfertheiner, P, and Ditschuneit, H, editors: Diagnostic procedures in pancreatic disease, Berlin, 1986, Springer-Verlag.

99. Malfertheiner, P: Combined functional and morphological diagnostic approach in chronic pancreatitis. In Malfertheiner, P, and Ditschuneit, H, editors: Diagnostic procedures in pancreatic disease, Berlin, 1986, Springer-Verlag.

100. Malfertheiner, P, et al: Exocrine pancreatic function in correlation to morphologic findings (assessed by different imaging parameters) in chronic pancreatitis. In Gyr, KE, Singer, MV, and Sarles, H, editors: Pancreatitis: concepts and classification, Amsterdam, 1984, Excerpta Medica.

101. Malfertheiner, P, et al: Correlation of morphological lesions, functional changes, and clinical stages in chronic pancreatitis. In Malfertheiner, P, and Ditschuneit, H, editors: Diagnostic procedures in pancreatic disease, Berlin, 1986, Springer-Verlag.

102. Malik, SA, Van Kley, H, and Knight, WA: Inherited defect hereditary pancreatitis, Am J Dig Dis 22:999, 1977.

103. Manegold, BC: Endoscopic retrograde pancreatography (ERP) in pre- and post-operative pancreatic disease. In Anacker, H, editor: Efficiency and limits of radiologic examination of the pancreas, Stuttgart, 1975, Georg Thieme Verlag.

104. McKenna, JM, et al: The pleuropulmonary complications of pancreatitis, Chest 71:197, 1977.

105. Mendez, G, Jr, and Isikoff, MB: Significance of intrapancreatic gas demonstrated by CT: a review of nine cases, AJR 132:59, 1979.

106. Mendez, G, Jr, Isikoff, MB, and Hill, MC: CT of acute pancreatitis: interim assessment, AJR 135:463, 1980.

107. Meyers, MA, and Evans, JA: Effects of pancreatitis on the small bowel and colon: spread along mesenteric planes, Am J Roentgenol 119:151, 1973.

108. Mullin, GT, et al: Arthritis and skin lesions resembling erythema nodosum in pancreatic disease, Ann Intern Med 68:75, 1968.

109. Neoptolemos, JP, et al: The urgent diagnosis of gallstones in acute pancreatitis: a prospective study of three methods, Br J Surg 71:230, 1984.

110. Nunez, D, Jr, et al: Transgastric drainage of pancreatic fluid collections, AJR 145:815, 1985.

111. Ohmori, K, et al: Pancreatic duct obstruction by a benign polypoid adenoma of the ampulla of Vater, Am J Surg 132:662, 1976.

112. Otte, M: Ultrasound in chronic pancreatitis. In Malfertheiner, P, and Ditschuneit, H, editors: Diagnostic procedures in pancreatic disease, Berlin, 1986, Springer-Verlag.

113. Pack, GT, Trinidad, SS, and Lisa, JR: Rare primary somatic tumors of the pancreas, Arch Surg 77:1000, 1958.

114. Pellegrini, CA, et al: Acute pancreatitis of rare causation, Surg Gynecol Obstet 144:899, 1977.

115. Pemberton, JH, Nagorny, DM, and Dozois, RR: Pancreatic abscess. In Go, VLW, editor: The exocrine pancreas, New York, 1986, Raven Press.

116. Perrault, J, Gross, JB, and King, JE: Endoscopic retrograde cholangiopancreatography in familial pancreatitis, Gastroenterology 71:138, 1976.

117. Ranson, JHC: Etiological and prognostic factors in human acute pancreatitis: a review, Am J Gastroenterol 77:633, 1982.

118. Ranson, JHC, et al: Computed tomography and the prediction of pancreatic abscess in acute pancreatitis, Ann Surg 201:656, 1985.

119. Ravitch, MM: The pancreas in infants and children, Surg Clin North Am 55:377, 1975.

120. Redman, HC, and Reuter, SR: Angiographic demonstration of surgically important vascular variations, Surg Gynecol Obstet 129:33, 1969.

121. Renert, WA, Kit, MG, and Capp, MP: Acute pancreatitis, Sem Roentgenol 8:405, 1973.

122. Reuter, SR, Redmond, HC, and Joseph, RR: Angiographic findings in pancreatitis, Am J Roentgenol 107:56, 1969.

123. Rohrmann, CA, Delaney, JH, and Protell, RL: Heterotopic pancreas diagnosed by cannulation and duct study, AJR 128:1044, 1977.

124. Rohrmann, CA, Jr, Silvis, SE, and Vennes, JA: The significance of pancreatic ductal obstruction in differential diagnosis of the abnormal endoscopic retrograde pancreatogram, Radiology 121:311, 1976.

125. Rohrmann, CA, Vennes, JA, and Silvis, SE: Evaluation of the endoscopic pancreatogram, Radiology 113:297, 1974.

126. Rohrmann, CA, et al: The diagnosis of hereditary pancreatitis by pancreatography, Gastrointest Endosc 27:168, 1981.

127. Rösch, W: Report on a symposium "10 years of ERCP": diagnostic and therapeutic aspects, European Society of Gastrointestinal Endoscopy, Newsletter 15:7, 1981.

128. Rösch, W, et al: The clinical significance of the pancreas divisum, Gastrointest Endosc 22:206, 1976.

129. Sahel, J: Endoscopic retrograde pancreatography findings and their grading in chronic pancreatitis. In Malfertheiner, P, and Ditschuneit, H, editors: Diagnostic procedures in pancreatic disease, Berlin, 1986, Springer-Verlag.

130. Sankaran, S, Sagawa, C, and Walt, AJ: Value of endoscopic retrograde cholangiography in pancreatic ascites, Surg Gynecol Obstet 148:185, 1979.

131. Sankaran, S, and Walt, AJ: The natural and unnatural history of pancreatic pseudocysts, Br J Surg 62:37, 1975.

132. Sankaran, S, and Walt, AJ: Pancreatic ascites: recognition and management, Arch Surg 111:430, 1976.

133. Sarles, H, editor: Pancreatitis: symposium of Marseille, April 25-26, 1963, Basel, 1963, S. Karger.

134. Sarner, M, and Cotton, PB: Definitions of acute and chronic pancreatitis, Clin Gastroenterol 13:865, 1984.

135. Sarti, DA: Rapid development and spontaneous regression of pancreatic pseudocysts documented by ultrasound, Radiology 125:789, 1977.

136. Sato, T, and Saitoh, Y: Familial chronic pancreatitis associated with pancreatic lithiasis, Am J Surg 127:511, 1974.

137. Scherer, K, Soehendra, N, and Dahm, K: Diagnosis of annular pancreas, Rofo 129:70, 1978.

138. Shawker, TH, Linzer, M, and Hubbard, VS: Chronic pancreatitis: the diagnostic significance of pancreatic size and echo amplitude, Radiology 154:568, 1985.

139. Shafer, RB, and Silvis, SE: Pancreatic pseudo-pseudocysts, Am J Surg 127:320, 1974.

140. Shuman, WP, et al: Radionuclide hepatobiliary imaging and real-time ultrasound in the detection of acute cholecystitis [letter], Radiology 152:238, 1984.

141. Shwachman, H, Lebenthal, E, and Khaw, KT: Recurrent acute pancreatitis in patients with cystic fibrosis with normal pancreatic enzymes, J Pediatr Surg 55:86, 1975.

142. Siegelman, SS, et al: CT of fluid collections associated with pancreatitis, AJR 134:1121, 1980.

143. Silverstein, W, et al: Diagnostic imaging of acute pancreatitis: a prospective study in 102 patients utilizing CT and sonography, AJR 137:497, 1981.

144. Silvis, SE, and Schuman, BM: Benign conditions of the pancreas. In Stewart, ET, Vennes, JA, and Geenen, JE, editors: Atlas of endoscopic retrograde cholangiopancreatography, St Louis, 1977, The CV Mosby Co.

145. Silvis, SE, Vennes, JA, and Rohrmann, CA: Endoscopic pancreatography in the evaluation of patients with suspected pancreatic pseudocysts, Am J Gastroenterol 61:452, 1974.

146. Smith, R, Rosen, JM, and Alderson, PO: Gallbladder perforation: diagnostic utility of cholescintigraphy in suggested subacute or chronic cases, Radiology 158:63, 1986.

147. Soroudi, M, and Bookstein, JJ: Angiography in acute pancreatic transection, Radiology 115:309, 1975.

148. Sostre, CF, et al: Pancreatic phlegmon: clinical features and course, Dig Dis Sci 30:918, 1985.

149. Stanley, JC, et al: Major arterial hemorrhage: a complication of pancreatic pseudocysts and chronic pancreatitis, Arch Surg 111:435, 1976.

150. Stuckman, ML, et al: Major gastrointestinal hemorrhage from peripancreatic vessels in pancreatitis: treatment by embolotherapy, Radiology 154:559, 1985.

151. Sugawa, C, et al: Pancreas divisum: is it a normal anatomic variant? Am J Surg 153:62, 1987.

152. Swobodnik, W, et al: Ultrasound, computed tomography and endoscopic retrograde cholangiopancreatography in the morphologic diagnosis of pancreatic disease, Klin Wochenschr 61:291, 1983.

153. Takemoto, T, and Kasugai, T: Endoscopic retrograde cholangiopancreatography, New York, 1979, Igaku-Shoin Medical Publishers.

154. Taxier, M, et al: Endoscopic retrograde pancreatography in the evaluation of trauma to the pancreas, Surg Gynecol Obstet 150:65, 1980.

155. Thoeni, RF, and Gedgaudas, RK: Ectopic pancreas: usual and unusual features, Gastrointest Radiol 5:37, 1980.

156. Thompson, RJ, Jr, and Hinshaw, DB: Pancreatic trauma, Ann Surg 163:153, 1966.

157. Thompson, WM, Kelvin, FM, and Rice, RP: Inflammation and necrosis of the transverse colon secondary to pancreatitis, AJR 128:943, 1977.

158. Torrance, B: Traumatic lesions of the pancreas. In Howat, HT, and Sarles, H, editors: The exocrine pancreas, Philadelphia, 1979, WB Saunders.

159. Tucker, AS, Mathews, LW, and Doershuk, CF: Roentgen diagnosis of complications of cystic fibrosis, Am J Roentgenol 89:1048, 1963.

160. Tylen, U, and Dencker, H: Roentgenologic diagnosis of pancreatic abscess, Acta Radiol 14:9, 1973.

161. Vallon, AG, Lees, WR, and Cotton, PB: Grey-scale ultrasonography and endoscopic pancreatography after pancreatic trauma, Br J Surg 66:169, 1979.

162. vanSonnenberg, E, et al: Complicated pancreatic inflammatory disease: diagnostic and therapeutic role of interventional radiology, Radiology 155:335, 1985.

163. Vujic, I, et al: Pancreatic and peripancreatic vessels: embolization for control of bleeding in pancreatitis, Radiology 150:51, 1984.

164. Waldram, R, et al: Chronic pancreatitis, sclerosing cholangitis and sicca complex in two siblings, Lancet 1:550, 1975.

165. Walter, JR, et al: Angiography of massive hemorrhage secondary to pancreatic disease, Radiology 124:337, 1977.

166. Warshaw, AL: Inflammatory masses following acute pancreatitis: phlegmon, pseudocyst, abscess, Surg Clin North Am 54:621, 1974.

167. Warshaw, AL: Reply to selected summary: more doubts about the clinical significance of pancreas divisum, Gastroenterology 93:1140, 1987.

168. Warshaw, AL, et al: The pathogenesis of pulmonary edema in acute pancreatitis, Ann Surg 182:505, 1975.

169. Warshaw, AL, et al: Persistent obstructive jaundice, cholangitis, and biliary cirrhosis due to common bile duct stenosis in chronic pancreatitis, Gastroenterology 70:562, 1976.

170. Warshaw, AL, et al: Objective evaluation of ampullary stenosis with ultrasonography and pancreatic stimulation, Am J Surg 149:65, 1985.

170a. Weissmann, HS, et al: Rapid and accurate diagnosis of acute cholecystitis with 99m Tc-HIDA cholescintigraphy, AJR 132:523, 1979.

171. White, AF, Baum, S, and Buranasiri, S: Aneurysms secondary to pancreatitis, Am J Roentgenol 127:393, 1976.

172. White, EM, et al: Pancreatic necrosis: CT manifestations, Radiology 158:343, 1986.

173. White, TT: Reoperative gastrointestinal surgery, Boston, 1979, Little Brown & Co.

174. Wilk, PJ, Mollura, J, and Danese, CA: Jaundice and pancreatitis caused by a duodenal diverticulum, Am J Gastroenterol 60:273, 1973.

175. Winship, D: Pancreatitis: pancreatic pseudocysts and their complications, Gastroenterology 73:593, 1977.

176. Wood, RE, Boat, TF, and Doershuk, CF: Cystic fibrosis, Am Rev Respir Dis 113:833, 1976.

177. Yeo, R, and Powell, K: Avascular gastric necrosis: a complication of partial gastrectomy following interruption of the splenic artery or its branches, Br J Surg 54:707, 1967.

46 *Neoplastic Lesions*

DAVID H. STEPHENS

Developments of the past several years have greatly advanced our ability to diagnose pancreatic neoplasms. After decades of reliance on indirect manifestations, the radiologic diagnosis of pancreatic tumors at last can be based primarily on the altered composition and morbid anatomy of the pancreas itself. There exists a choice of ways to depict the form and substance of the gland as well as its ducts and vessels. Meanwhile, radiologic participation in the diagnosis and management of patients with pancreatic neoplasms has been expanded to include percutaneous biopsy and certain palliative procedures.

ADENOCARCINOMA (DUCTAL CARCINOMA)

"Cancer of the pancreas" usually refers to the common form of pancreatic malignancy, adenocarcinoma that arises from ductal epithelium of the gland. One of the most formidable diseases of our time, this neoplasm is now the fourth leading cause of death from cancer in the United States.[90] No more than 1% to 2% of its victims live 5 years beyond the time of diagnosis.[1,2] For reasons not fully explained, the disease has become increasingly prevalent in the latter half of this century. Pancreatic carcinoma is known to occur more often in men than in women and to affect most commonly the elderly and middle aged. Otherwise, extensive epidemiologic study has identified no clearly defined segment of the population to be at particularly high risk. For practical purposes, therefore, diagnostic investigation is currently limited to individuals who are symptomatic.

Clinical presentation

Presenting signs and symptoms vary among patients who are referred for radiologic investigation because of suspected pancreatic carcinoma.[58,61] Pain, weight loss, and jaundice are the common complaints. Regardless of the part of the gland involved, most patients with pancreatic cancer have experienced pain by the time they consult a physician. The pain is usually felt deep in the upper abdomen, but it may penetrate to the back or be localized there. Early in the illness the discomfort is usually vague, but as the disease progresses, the pain often becomes intense and unremitting. The degree of weight loss varies from slight to profound and is not necessarily related to the size or extent of the tumor.

Although jaundice may be the initial complaint, it is usually preceded or accompanied by discomfort.[61] When patients with cancer of the pancreatic head seek attention before they become jaundiced, the symptoms are not very different from those caused by tumors elsewhere in the organ or, for that matter, from symptoms of a variety of other conditions. Less common indications for a radiologic search for pancreatic carcinoma include metastatic carcinoma of unknown primary source and certain disorders, such as unexplained venous thrombosis, that suggest the presence of an occult malignancy. Steatorrhea, pancreatitis, and diabetes are other conditions that may be associated with pancreatic cancer.

Morbid anatomy

An understanding of the gross pathologic anatomy of pancreatic carcinoma provides the soundest foundation for radiologic diagnosis of the disease. Ductal-type pancreatic carcinomas are predominantly solid scirrhous lesions. However, because they are generally hypovascular, these tumors are subject to ischemia and may undergo internal necrosis. Some pancreatic carcinomas are well defined, but others are exceedingly infiltrative. Although most of these tumors will have grown large enough to cause a conspicuous alteration in the form of the gland by the time they come to attention, this is not always the case. Occasional pancreatic carcinomas become symptomatic before they produce gross distortion of the organ's contours.[37] On the other hand, carcinomas of the pancreas often incite a desmoplastic response in the surrounding parenchyma,[20] a process that can add volume to the mass.

As it grows, the tumor surrounds, constricts, and eventually obliterates the ducts and vessels within its path. The common bile duct, lying within or adjacent to the head of the pancreas, is especially vulnerable to obstruction by tumors arising in the pancreatic head. The main pancreatic duct seldom escapes constriction or occlusion from tumors arising anywhere in the organ. The ductal system above an obstruction becomes dilated. Pancreatic parenchyma upstream from an obstructing tumor may become inflamed or undergo atrophy. Thus, a tumor in the head or neck of the pancreas is frequently accompanied by ductal distention and parenchymal thinning in the body and tail of the gland.

By the time they are diagnosed, most pancreatic carcinomas have extended beyond the confines of the gland, which, unlike other organs, has no strong capsular barrier. There is a predilection for perivascular and perineural extension along the course of neighboring splanchnic vessels. Regional lymph nodes, the liver, and peritoneal surfaces are common sites of metastasis.

Sectional imaging: general considerations

Almost entirely as a result of recent advances in sectional imaging, radiologists have the ability to diagnose or exclude cancer of the pancreas with unprecedented accuracy in ways that barely jeopardize the patient's safety or comfort. The diagnostic process begins with activation of the machinery that produces graphic images. An examination of the pancreas by whatever method must be conducted in a manner that is suitable to the problem at hand, and the meaning of the resulting images must be interpreted with skill. With so much attention directed toward the technology of imaging, the interpretative aspects have received perhaps less emphasis than they deserve.

Anyone who has had more than a little experience interpreting abdominal images of patients suspected to have pancreatic carcinoma knows that the task can be a substantial challenge. Contrary to what is sometimes taught, cancers of the pancreas, even those in the gland's body or tail, are not always massive tumefactions by the time they cause symptoms. The interpreter should therefore be familiar with and alert for the subtle manifestations of the disease. Excluding pancreatic carcinoma can be even more difficult than making a positive diagnosis, since variations in pancreatic morphology and an assortment of pathologic processes other than pancreatic carcinoma can mimic the appearance of a pancreatic cancer.

Despite these potential difficulties, an accurate diagnosis or confident exclusion of pancreatic carcinoma is possible by noninvasive imaging in all but exceptional cases. Sometimes more than one imaging method is required, and often it is appropriate to confirm the radiologic diagnosis with percutaneous biopsy. A more invasive procedure may be needed as a guide to treatment or to evaluate a specific effect of the tumor, but when noninvasive examinations are carefully performed and skillfully interpreted, invasive procedures are not often needed for radiologic diagnosis.

The sequence in which imaging procedures should be employed in the diagnosis of pancreatic cancer does not easily lend itself to a universally applicable algorithmic scheme. Many patients are sent for evaluation because of vague complaints, in which case cancer of the pancreas is only one of many conditions to be excluded. In those circumstances computed tomography (CT) is likely to be the procedure of choice, since it can provide a comprehensive examination of the abdomen as well as a detailed depiction of the pancreas. If a pancreatic tumor is revealed by CT, an accurate assessment for evidence of unresectability can be made,[34,51] and when appropriate, a percutaneous biopsy can be performed. Thus a precise radiologic diagnosis, an assessment of potential resectability, and a biopsy for microscopic confirmation can all be accomplished with a single radiologic procedure. For the same reasons, CT is also the current procedure of choice in the workup of most patients who are strongly suspected to have pancreatic cancer.

Ultrasonography may be the preferred initial procedure in a patient who is undergoing an investigation primarily to determine the cause of jaundice, or in a patient whose symptoms suggest biliary tract disease as a cause of abdominal pain. In those situations, as in most ultrasonographic survey examinations of the upper abdomen, a thorough depiction of the pancreas is usually attempted. A case can also be made for the routine use of ultrasonography as the first imaging procedure for patients who are suspected to have pancreatic cancer,[99] especially in practices where CT is not as readily accessible as ultrasonography. Ultrasonography is less expensive than CT, but as a rule it does not provide the breadth of potentially useful information that is available from a comprehensive CT study. Like CT, ultrasonography can be used for percutaneous pancreatic biopsy. The complementary roles of CT and sonography are discussed later.

Magnetic resonance imaging (MRI) of the pancreas is already capable of providing information comparable to that obtained from CT.[8,96,102] Like CT, MRI provides a comprehensive display of anatomy, including an evaluation of the blood vessels commonly affected by pancreatic cancer. Mainly because of the expense, time, and technical complexity currently involved in producing a diagnostically suitable MRI examination of the pancreas, the method has not yet supplanted CT or ultrasonography as an initial procedure to evaluate patients suspected to have pancreatic disease.[96] With further advances in this emerging modality, that situation could change.

Although their images are derived from entirely different physical properties, CT, ultrasonography, and MRI have much in common in diagnosing or excluding pancreatic carcinoma. For each of these methods, major keys to success are a commitment to excellent technique and a knowledge of relevant normal and pathologic anatomy. Because CT has become the principal imaging procedure to diagnose pancreatic cancer, the greatest amount of discussion in this section is devoted to CT. Most of the findings described and illustrated by CT, however, are no less applicable to sonography and MRI.

Computed tomography
Technical considerations

Since carcinoma of the pancreas is likely to be only one of the diagnostic possibilities under consideration in a patient sent for CT evaluation, it is often appropriate for the examination to include the entire abdomen and pelvis. An examination of most of the abdomen, at least from the dome of the diaphragm to below the level of the kidneys, is worthwhile even when a strong clinical suspicion of pancreatic cancer is the primary indication for the study. This permits an evaluation of the most common sites of metastasis. For most purposes, scanning the abdomen with contiguous slices of 10 mm thickness is sufficient.

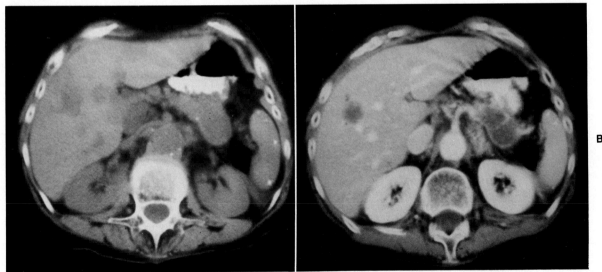

Fig. 46-1 Carcinoma of pancreatic tail with hepatic metastasis and encasement of splentic artery. Case illustrates advantages of intravenous contrast enhancement. **A,** Unenhanced CT scan shows a slightly hypodense oval mass arising from pancreatic tail. Within liver are several hypodense zones, at least some of which represent normal blood vessels. **B,** With contrast enhancement unenhanced pancreatic tumor is seen to encase opacified, irregularly narrowed splenic artery. Normal vessels in liver are enhanced, whereas metastatic lesion and slightly dilated bile ducts adjacent to it remain unenhanced.

Intravenous contrast enhancement serves a number of worthwhile purposes: to accentuate differences between enhancing normal tissue and unenhancing primary or metastatic tumor; to evaluate the effects of a tumor on neighboring vessels; and to define pancreatic and biliary ductal anatomy (Fig. 46-1). To achieve these goals, the delivery of contrast material should be coordinated with scanning in such a way that the entire liver and pancreas are depicted while there are adequate amounts of contrast material within the circulation, but before iodinated material has entered hypovascular tumor tissue. With current CT equipment this can be accomplished by scanning at contiguous anatomic levels, beginning shortly after bolus injection of contrast material and continuing the series during and after rapid infusion of additional material. The contrast material can be delivered manually or by automatic power injector.[64]

Whether an unenhanced series of scans should be made is a matter of individual considerations. Because ductal-type pancreatic carcinomas and their intrahepatic metastases are hypovascular, there is little diagnostic advantage to obtaining a preliminary series of unenhanced scans, although there may be a valid clinical reason to withhold contrast material. On the other hand, unenhanced scans may provide all the information that is required, thereby obviating the need to give the patient intravenous contrast material. Preliminary scans may also call attention to a localized region of the pancreas that appears likely to harbor a tumor. In that case, highly collimated scans made with dynamic contrast enhancement at the level of concern may provide exceptionally detailed images.[45] For most purposes, however, a technique of rapid incremental scanning during the vascular phase of contrast enhancement is effective and practical.

Primary signs

The primary features of pancreatic carcinoma displayed by CT are related to the presence of a tumor that enlarges the gland, distorts its contour, alters its density, or invades adjacent tissues.

MASS EFFECT

Typically, pancreatic cancer enlarges only part of the gland, changing the contour in a more or less abrupt fashion (Figs. 46-1 to 46-3). Uncommonly, the entire gland appears enlarged, but even then the configuration as well as the size of the organ is altered.[103,106] Although most pancreatic cancers are obvious as tumefactions, subtle masses may be difficult to appreciate. Because the dimensions of the normal pancreas are so variable, it is seldom worthwhile to measure the image of a pancreas in an attempt to determine whether or not the organ or a part of it is pathologically enlarged. A subjective interpretation, based on careful observation of a large number of normal and abnormal pancreatic images, is generally more reliable. It is especially important to evaluate

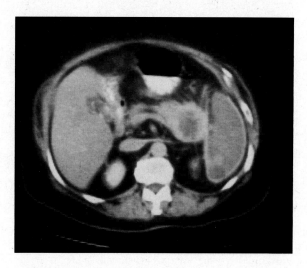

Fig. 46-2 Carcinoma of pancreatic tail with splenic infarction. Unenhancing spherical tumor in tail of pancreas has occluded splenic artery, causing splenic infarction. Interior of spleen is mostly unenhanced, indicating lack of perfusion, although there is enhancement of subcapsular rind of splenic tissue.

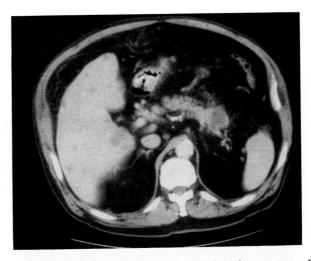

Fig. 46-3 Small carcinoma of pancreatic tail with multiple hepatic metastases. Primary tumor, 2 cm in diameter, is conspicuous as unenhancing mass that protrudes from otherwise lobulated anterior surface in pancreas. Liver contains many small metastatic lesions.

the entire configuration of the organ and to correlate the size and form of each part with the appearance of other parts. In that way, small tumors may be recognized as disproportionate enlargements. Changes in texture should also be noted. A solid tumor within a pancreas that is otherwise characterized by prominent surface lobularity may be apparent as a soft tissue mass that focally obliterates the normal lobular pattern.

Approximately two-thirds of pancreatic carcinomas occur in the head of the gland, which is normally the

thickest part of the organ as displayed in cross section. Focal enlargements in that location may not be as obvious as they would be in the thinner body or tail. Tumors of the pancreatic head that do not obstruct the common bile duct early in their growth are usually recognizable as masses by the time they cause symptoms. Tumors arising in the central portion of the pancreatic head tend to produce a spherical enlargement of the head (Fig. 46-4, *B*). When a tumor of the pancreatic head is associated with atrophy of the body and tail, the disproportionate en-

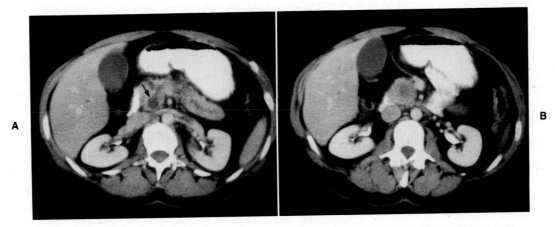

Fig. 46-4 Carcinoma of pancreatic head obstructing pancreatic duct and common bile duct. **A,** CT scan showing dilated main pancreatic duct in neck, body, and tail of pancreas. Common bile is also dilated *(arrow)* as it enters pancreatic head. **B,** At lower level, obstructing tumor (unenhancing mass within pancreatic head) causes rounded enlargement of head and leftward displacement of superior mesenteric vein.

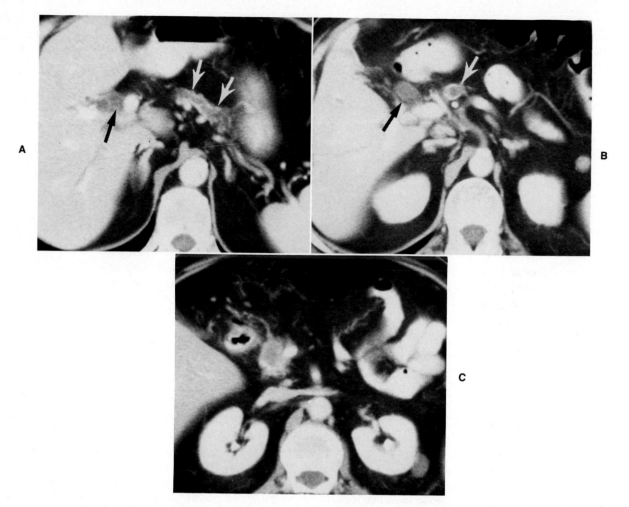

Fig. 46-5 Small carcinoma of head of pancreas with dilatation of main pancreatic duct and atrophy of pancreatic parenchyma above tumor. **A** and **B,** Main pancreatic duct is dilated throughout neck, body, and tail of pancreas *(white arrows),* and surrounding parenchyma is markedly thinned. Extrahepatic bile duct *(black arrows)* and intrahepatic ducts are slightly dilated. **C,** In pancreatic head, obstructing tumor is seen as small unenhancing mass. Tumor, which could not be separated surgically from portal vein, was unresectable.

largement of the head becomes more conspicuous (Fig. 46-5). Even the smaller tumors are usually apparent when the images are carefully analyzed. Particular attention should be paid to the uncinate process, which is usually wedge-shaped as it extends behind the superior mesenteric vein. Tumors of the uncinate process enlarge that structure and cause it to become rounded (Fig. 46-6).

ALTERATION OF DENSITY

On scans made without contrast enhancement, the radiographic density of a solid pancreatic carcinoma may be recognizably less than that of normal parenchyma, or there may be no perceptible difference.[103] Necrosis causes further diminution of density, and when there is

liquifaction, the density of the necrotic cavity approaches that of water (see Fig. 46-10).[53] Contrast enhancement accentuates the difference in density between carcinoma and normal pancreatic parenchyma by causing transient opacification of the parenchyma (or its vascular bed) while leaving the hypovascular tumor unenhanced (Figs. 46-1 to 46-5). This effect is best achieved when scans are made during the phase of relatively dense vascular enhancement. Demonstration of relative radiolucency in a pancreatic carcinoma is especially useful to detect a tumor when the mass effect is inconspicuous (Fig. 46-7). Rarely, it may be the only CT clue to the existence of a tumor. It should be noted, however, that not all pancreatic carcinomas exhibit this effect.

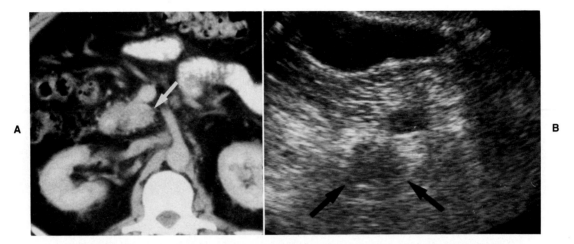

Fig. 46-6 Carcinoma of uncinate process; complementary use of ultrasound. **A,** CT scan showing subtle enlargement and rounding of uncinate process *(arrow)* as only positive CT finding in man with otherwise unexplained abdominal pain. **B,** Sonogram of pancreatic head, which shows uncinate process to contain small hypoechoic mass *(arrows). st,* Water-filled stomach. Workup also revealed pulmonary metastases. Carcinoma of pancreas was confirmed by CT-guided biopsy, and pulmonary metastases was confirmed by transthoracic needle aspiration.

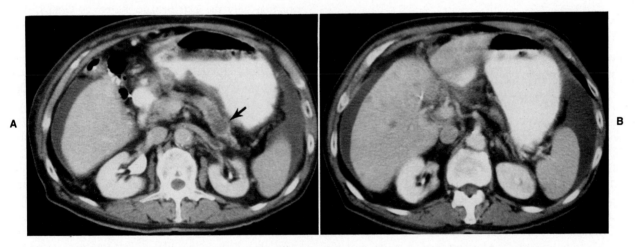

Fig. 46-7 Small pancreatic carcinoma with liver metastases and ascites. **A,** Within tail of pancreas is small unenhancing tumor *(arrow)* that does not cause obvious pancreatic enlargement, although tip of pancreatic tail beyond tumor is atrophic. **B,** Liver contains multiple tiny metastases. Hepatic lesions and primary tumor were isodense with adjacent parenchyma on unenhanced scans (not shown).

EXTRAPANCREATIC EXTENSION

Direct extension of pancreatic cancer is most often shown by CT to occur in a retropancreatic direction, toward the aorta along the courses of the celiac and superior mesenteric arteries. This form of extension causes an obliteration of the fat that normally surrounds and sharply defines these arterial trunks.[65,103] Either or both arteries may be involved. The tumor may completely encase the vessel, or it may only partially obscure a margin. The lumen of an encased artery may be identified when the bloodstream is opacified with intravenous contrast material (Fig. 46-8). Usually the pancreatic origin of such a tumor is obvious, but sometimes the extrapancreatic extension is more conspicuous than the intrapancreatic component. In that circumstance, perivascular retropancreatic extension is a particularly useful diagnostic sign. It is one of the most characteristic features of ductal-type pancreatic carcinoma.[103] Direct extension can also

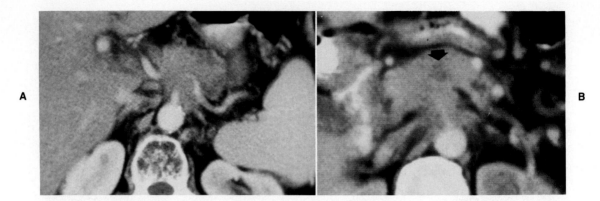

Fig. 46-8 Carcinoma of body of pancreas with retropancreatic extension. **A,** Celiac axis and its hepatic and splenic branches are encased by tumor that extends from body of pancreas to anterior margin of aorta. **B,** In another case, superior mesenteric artery, its lumen opacified with contrast material, is surrounded by abnormal tissue. Small intrapancreatic portion of tumor is seen only as an unenhancing zone *(arrow)* within body of pancreas.

occur in other directions, such as toward the porta hepatis, although cranial or caudal extention is not as easily recognized on cross sectionally–oriented CT scans.[51]

Secondary signs

Secondary effects of pancreatic cancer are sometimes the most prominent CT manifestations of the disease. Rarely, they are the only positive findings.

DUCTAL OBSTRUCTION

One of the most common secondary effects is ductal dilation resulting from obstruction. The pancreatic duct, biliary system, or both may be affected. As already mentioned, pancreatic and biliary ducts are displayed to best advantage when the surrounding parenchyma and adjacent vessels have been opacified with intravenous contrast material.[4]

Dilatation of the main pancreatic duct may occur upstream from an obstructing tumor located in any part of the pancreas, but it occurs most often as a result of obstruction in the head or neck of the gland. The dilated main duct in the tail or body of the pancreas appears as a smooth or beaded radiolucent column[5,53] (Fig. 46-4, *A*). In the vertically oriented head of the pancreas the duct is projected on end. Often the pancreatic parenchyma surrounding the dilated duct is thinned (Figs. 46-5 to 46-9). A less common consequence of pancreatic ductal obstruction is the formation of one or more retention cysts or pseudocysts upstream from the occlusion.[47]

Most carcinomas of the head of the pancreas, and some that originate elsewhere in the gland, eventually obstruct the common bile duct. Whether that occurs early or late depends mainly on the location of the tumor relative to the passage of the duct. In most cases of biliary obstruction from pancreatic cancer, intrahepatic ducts

and extrahepatic ducts are both dilated (Fig. 46-5). Often the extrahepatic ducts are dilated to a greater degree than the intrahepatic ducts, and in some cases of early obstruction only the extrahepatic system is dilated. The gallbladder may or may not be distended when the extrahepatic bile duct is obstructed.

As mentioned earlier, cancers of the pancreatic head not infrequently come to clinical attention before they obstruct the common bile duct. In fact, some of the larger tumors of the pancreatic head are encountered in anicteric patients. On the other hand, some of the smallest tumors detected are those that obstruct the duct and produce jaundice at an early stage of growth.

When either pancreatic or biliary ductal obstruction is caused by carcinoma, the obstructing tumor, although it may be subtle, is usually apparent (Fig. 46-5). Infrequently, the only positive CT finding is dilatation of one or both ductal systems. Even in these cases the series of scans should show the dilated duct to terminate within the pancreatic substance (Fig. 46-9, *A*), thus indicating the location of the obstruction (Fig. 46-9, *B*). In the absence of an intraductal stone or history of either pancreatitis or iatrogenic injury, the likely cause of this form of obstruction is tumor. In some cases direct opacification of the duct may be necessary to define the obstructing lesion,[31] but often a sonographic examination will confirm the neoplastic nature of the obstruction (Fig. 46-9).

VASCULAR INVOLVEMENT

The effects of a pancreatic carcinoma on neighboring vessels are among the most influential considerations in evaluating the feasibility of surgical resection, and involvement of splanchnic arteries is well shown by contrast-enhanced CT.[34,51] The appearance of neoplastic encasement of the superior mesenteric artery and celiac axis

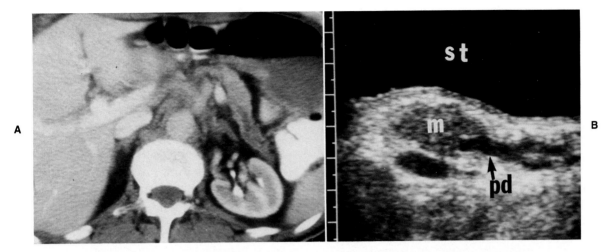

Fig. 46-9 Nonexpanding carcinoma of pancreas obstructing main pancreatic duct. **A,** CT scan showing dilatation of main pancreatic duct and parenchymal thinning in tail of pancreas. Dilated pancreatic duct terminates abruptly in solid tissue, isodense with normal parenchyma, at junction of body and tail. Fat adjacent to celiac axis appears infiltrated. Findings are highly indicative of pancreatic carcinoma, but definite tumor mass is not identified. **B,** Transverse sonogram shows oval hypoechoic mass *(m),* corresponding to solid tissue seen on CT, at termination of dilated duct *(pd)* in pancreatic tail. Fluid-filled stomach *(st)* provides effective acoustic window.

has already been described (Fig. 46-8). The splenic artery (Figs. 46-1 and 46-8, *A*) and hepatic artery (Fig. 46-8, *A*) are also subject to encasement. When occlusion of the splenic artery or one of its branches causes infarction in the portion of the spleen supplied by the affected vessel, the resulting abnormality of splenic perfusion may be seen on contrast-enhanced CT scans (Fig. 46-2).[14]

Venous involvement may be more difficult to recognize, in part because the terminal portions of the splenic

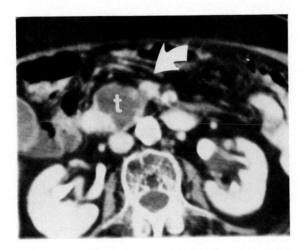

Fig. 46-10 Carcinoma of pancreatic head invading superior mesenteric vein. Small nubbin of tumor projects into contrast-enhanced lumen of superior mesenteric vein *(arrow)* from mostly necrotic tumor *(t)* in adjacent pancreatic head.

and superior mesenteric veins and the origin of the portal vein are not entirely separated from the pancreatic surface by intervening fat. Nevertheless, compression or invasion of a major vein can often be demonstrated by contrast enhancement (Fig. 46-10).[34] Evidence of venous occlusion may appear as distention of the affected vein and its tributaries proximal to the obstruction.

INVOLVEMENT OF ADJACENT ORGANS

Since the pancreas does not have an effective capsular covering, carcinomas arising from the organ have a tendency to involve neighboring structures by direct extension. On CT scans, involvement of the stomach or intestine is best appreciated when the lumen of the involved viscus is distended with contrast material. Other organs sometimes affected by direct extension are the spleen and either adrenal gland or kidney.

METASTASES

Metastases are very common CT findings in patients with pancreatic carcinoma. The biologic nature of this tumor is such that metastases are frequently present even when the primary tumor is relatively small and the clinical illness is of recent onset. Metastases are found by CT most often in the liver. As noted earlier, these are hypovascular lesions, best displayed on contrast-enhanced scans (Figs. 46-1 and 46-3). Hepatic metastases from a ductal pancreatic carcinoma tend to be smaller on the average than metastases from less common, slower growing types of pancreatic malignancy

(Figs. 46-24 and 46-25), probably because patients with the metastatic ductal type of pancreatic cancer do not survive long enough to develop large metastases. Lymph nodes are the next most frequent sites in which metastases are discovered. Usually they are located in the vicinity of the pancreas. Nodal enlargement in this disease tends to be moderate rather than massive. Peritoneal and serosal implants are usually small deposits, often invisible to current CT scanning. However, peritoneal carcinomatosis usually produces ascites, and the finding of ascites in the presence of a pancreatic carcinoma (Fig. 46-7) can be considered presumptive evidence of carcinomatosis.[34]

Ultrasonography

Most of the pathologic anatomy of pancreatic carcinoma that is displayed by CT is also demonstrable by ultrasonography, although the information is of a different nature because ultrasound images depict the acoustic properties of tissues rather than their attenuation of x-ray beams. Ultrasonographic images may be obtained in a variety of anatomic planes; with real-time instrumentation it can provide a continuous display of anatomy.

Technical considerations

Because of its versatility, real-time ultrasonography has become the preferred sonographic method to evaluate the pancreas and related abdominal structures. Regardless of the instrumentation used, a successful ultrasonographic examination of the pancreas requires considerable skill on the part of the sonographer to overcome a variety of natural obstacles. Meticulous attention to technical detail can produce highly accurate sonographic results in the assessment of most patients suspected to have pancreatic cancer.[99]

The limitations of ultrasonography in pancreatic imaging are related mostly to the inability of sound waves to penetrate certain biologic substances, i.e., bowel gas, bone, and excessive fat. The presence of gas in the gastrointestinal lumen is the most common deterrent to complete depiction of the pancreas, most often preventing adequate display of the organ's body or tail. In many cases this problem can be overcome by distending the stomach with fluid to provide a medium for transmission of sound[7,60,99] (Figs 46-6, *B* and 46-9, *B*). The left lobe of liver and the spleen are also used as acoustic windows. Scanning should be performed in supine and erect or semierect positions and in posterior oblique positions as required.

Primary signs

Neoplastic enlargements and distortions of pancreatic contour as displayed by ultrasound are similar to those demonstrated by CT. Most bulky pancreatic tumors are readily demonstrated as masses, but subtle changes in contour may not be shown as clearly as with CT scans.

A more important contribution of ultrasound is the demonstration of altered parenchymal texture. This capability permits detection of an intrapancreatic tumor even in the absence of obvious change in the contour of the organ. Most pancreatic adenocarcinomas are hypoechoic relative to normal parenchyma[99,105] (Figs. 46-6, *B*, 46-9, *B*, and 46-11, *B*). This pattern illustrates the generally featureless internal composition of typical

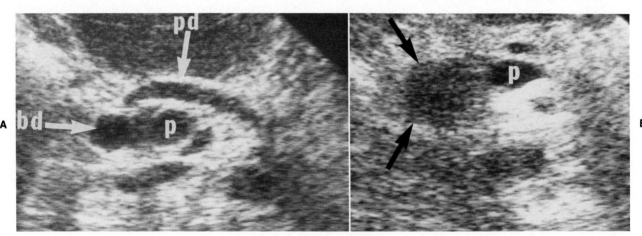

Fig. 46-11 Carcinoma of pancreatic head obstructing common bile duct and main pancreatic duct. **A,** Transverse sonogram showing dilated main pancreatic duct *(pd)* in body and tail of gland and dilated common bile duct *(bd)* just above pancreatic head. **B,** At lower level, hypoechoic mass *(arrows)* in head of pancreas is shown. *p*, Portal vein. Subsequently tumor was resected. (From Ormson, MJ, Charboneau, JW, and Stephens, DH: Sonography in patients with a possible pancreatic mass shown on CT, AJR 148:551-555, © by Am Roentgen Ray Soc 1987.)

pancreatic carcinomas. Tumors that have undergone internal necrosis have varied echo patterns, but those tumors are usually larger lesions that are also apparent as masses.[8] Attenuation of sound by solid pancreatic tumors is similar to that of other solid tissues. Sound is usually transmitted through the mass but becomes diminished in intensity so that structures beyond the tumor are visible but displayed with less pronounced density.[105]

Secondary signs

Real-time ultrasonography is especially well suited to demonstrate pancreatic and biliary ductal dilation.[57] The ultrasonographic appearance of normal and dilated ducts of both systems and the techniques to display them are described in the radiologic literature[57,104] and in other chapters of this text. It will suffice here to note again that considerable skill on the part of the operator is required for consistent delineation of relevant ductal anatomy. When obstruction is caused by pancreatic carcinoma, the dilated pancreatic or bile duct can usually be traced to its termination in the mass (Figs. 46-9, B, and 46-11), but occasionally the tumor itself cannot be shown, in which case ductal dilatation may be the only ultrasonographic evidence of the disease.

Many of the vascular alterations that occur as a result of pancreatic carcinoma are demonstrable by ultrasonography. Displacement of a neighboring vessel may be indirect evidence of an adjacent pancreatic mass. Involvement of the splenic vein is suggested when the vein cannot be seen despite adequate demonstration of the pancreatic bed and deeper structures.[105]

Hepatic metastases and ascites are other common secondary findings. Metastatic involvement of regional lymph nodes may also be seen, but not as often on sonograms as on CT scans.

Complementary roles of CT and ultrasonography

Although CT and ultrasonography both have high rates of success in detecting or excluding pancreatic cancer,[34,99] there are circumstances in which the results of either procedure may be less than conclusive. In a significant minority of cases, despite the best efforts of the sonographer, it may not be possible with ultrasound to depict the entirety of the pancreas or to display all pertinent extrapancreatic anatomy. There are also cases in which the significance of an ultrasonographic finding is indeterminate, even though the feature in question is well displayed. In these situations, CT, with its comprehensive display of anatomy, can usually overcome the inherent inadequacies of the ultrasonographic examination or provide enough additional information to solve the diagnostic problem.

It is perhaps not as well recognized that ultrasonography can be equally complementary to CT. Ultrasonography is especially useful to evaluate an inconclusive CT finding that raises the question of the presence of a pancreatic mass.[72] A limited real-time examination, directed toward solving a specifically defined problem, can be performed rapidly and economically and, more often than not, can add the decisive information. Ultrasonography is especially worthwhile to differentiate between a subtle pancreatic mass (Figs. 46-6 and 46-9) and a normal variation in pancreatic configuration (Fig. 46-12). This is

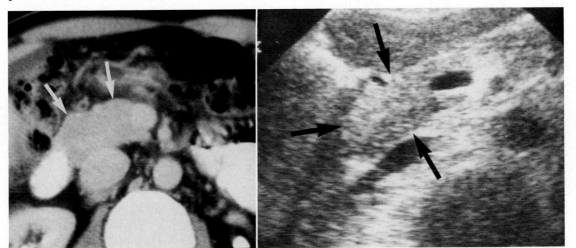

Fig. 46-12 Normal variant. **A,** On CT scan, pancreatic head *(arrows)* shown to be prominent and lobular but of uniform density. It does not have spherical shape typical of carcinoma in this location (see Fig. 46-4, *B*); scans above this level (not shown) showed no ductal dilatation. **B,** Transverse sonogram shows normal echotexture in pancreatic head *(arrows)*, identical to that in remainder of gland. (From Ormson, MJ, Charboneau JW, and Stephens, DH: Sonography in patients with a possible pancreatic mass shown on CT, AJR 148:551-555, © by Am Roentgen Ray Soc 1987.)

done by demonstrating whether or not the region of concern has a normal echo pattern relative to the adjacent pancreatic tissue. Only exceptionally is a directed real-time ultrasonographic examination unsuccessful in solving such a problem. In that case a more invasive procedure, such as endoscopic pancreatography, may be required.

Magnetic resonance imaging

Initially hampered by poor spatial resolution and less than optimal image contrast,[94] MRI of the pancreas has improved to the point that it can produce information in patients suspected to have pancreatic cancer comparable to that provided by CT[96,102] (Fig. 46-13). In a recently reported series of 10 pancreatic adenocarcinomas studied by MRI, the tumors had a variety of signal intensities. On T_1 or T_2-weighted images the signal intensities of the tumors ranged from higher than to the same as those of normal pancreatic tissue.[102]

Advantages of MRI include delineation of vessels without the need for contrast material and the production of images that are free of artifactual degradation from metal clips in postoperative patients. Abdominal MRI is still being refined, and the efficiency of various scanning techniques is still under investigation. Already a clinically applicable method of pancreatic imaging in selected cases,[102] MRI almost certainly will assume an increasingly prominent role in the evaluation of pancreatic disease.

Differential diagnosis
Normal variants

Occasional variations in the size or shape of the normal pancreas can resemble a pancreatic mass. Any part of the gland may be disproportionately thicker than usual. Anomalies of fusion of the dorsal and ventral pancreatic anlagen can simulate a mass in the pancreatic head.[12,92] A normal uncinate process may be more rounded than usual, giving an appearance similar to that caused by a small tumor in the location. On CT scans, homogeneous parenchymal contrast enhancement, isodense with that in the remainder of the gland, is an indication that the region in question is more likely to be normal tissue than a lesion (Fig. 46-12, A). With ultrasonography, a normal echo pattern (the same as that in adjacent pancreatic tissue) has like significance (Fig. 46-12, B). The complementary use of ultrasound and CT in indeterminate cases has been discussed. If the issue cannot be resolved by noninvasive imaging, endoscopic pancreatography may be indicated.[92] When the evidence of a mass is not compelling, however, a follow-up noninvasive imaging procedure may be a reasonable approach.

Extrapancreatic structures, especially neighboring parts of the GI tract, can simulate a pancreatic mass. This problem can be avoided on CT by making sure that the nearby gastrointestinal lumen is filled with either a radiopaque or radiolucent contrast material.[81] Adjacent loops of bowel encountered at ultrasonography may be seen to change configuration on serial images, or, if real-time scanning is used, peristalsis may be observed. The search continues for a practical gastrointestinal contrast material for MRI.

Extrapancreatic masses

Mass lesions originating from neighboring structures may simulate primary pancreatic tumors, but most extrapancreatic masses can be recognized as being separate from the pancreas on careful inspection of the images.

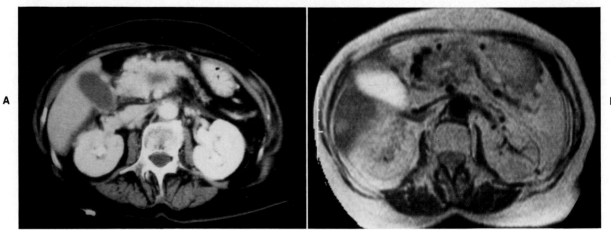

Fig. 46-13 Carcinoma of pancreatic head with liver metastases. **A,** Contrast-enhanced CT and, **B,** T_2-weighted magnetic resonance images, both showing large, centrally ischemic tumor arising from pancreatic head. Tail of pancreas is atrophic. Dilated veins on lateral surface of tumor are enhanced on CT scan and have low signal intensity on MRI. Metastatic lesion in right lobe of liver is better shown by MR, but hepatic metastases at other levels were shown equally well by both methods.

Often an interface can be identified between the mass and the pancreas. The abilities of ultrasound and MRI to display anatomy in a variety of orientations can be advantageous in that regard. Enlarged lymph nodes lying adjacent to the pancreas are a relatively common occurrence. In cases of lymphoma, however, the lymphadenopathy is not likely to be confined to the peripancreatic region. Sometimes the site of origin of a very large tumor is more difficult to determine than is the origin of a small tumor. Ductal adenocarcinomas of the pancreas, however, are seldom huge, although less common pancreatic neoplasms can be very large.

Other pancreatic neoplasms

Pancreatic neoplasms other than ductal adenocarcinomas often have radiologic and clinical characteristics that indicate that they are something other than the ductal type of pancreatic cancer. These tumors are discussed in subsequent sections of this chapter.

Carcinoma versus pancreatitis

Pancreatic carcinoma and pancreatitis have many gross pathologic features in common. Pancreatic enlargement, ductal obstruction and dilatation, cyst formation, infiltration of adjacent tissues, and ascites can occur with either condition. To complicate matters further, cancer of the pancreas may be accompanied by inflammation, and a pancreas already involved with chronic inflammation can develop a carcinoma.

Despite their similarities, carcinoma and pancreatitis can usually be distinguished from each other, especially when clinical and laboratory information is correlated with radiologic findings. Although phlegmonous swelling of the pancreas might sometimes resemble a neoplasm, the clinical picture in that condition is one of acute or recently acute pancreatitis. Extrapancreatic spread of acute inflammation usually occurs in the form of an effusion that extends into the anterior pararenal space or lesser sac, whereas neoplastic extension tends to be perivascular and retropancreatic.

Chronic pancreatitis is more difficult to distinguish from carcinoma, and even the previously established diagnosis of chronic pancreatitis does not exclude coexisting carcinoma. It is particularly difficult to determine the nature of a focal enlargement, although additional findings may be influential. The presence of hepatic or nodal metastases, for example, indicates malignancy, whereas intraductal pancreatic calcification indicates chronic pancreatitis. An inflammatory mass may contain dilated intrapancreatic ductal branches, with or without calculi, whereas ducts become obliterated when they are engulfed by neoplasm. A necrotic carcinoma may have a cavitary appearance similar to that of a pseudocyst, but the thickness and irregularity of its wall will frequently indicate the probability of a necrotic neoplasm rather than

an inflammatory pseudocyst. Although retropancreatic fat may become obliterated in advanced chronic pancreatitis, selective perivascular extension along the major mesenteric arteries (Fig. 46-8) is a feature of cancer rather than inflammation.

The most difficult diagnostic problem is presented by a focal solid mass with no ancillary features to indicate whether it is inflammatory or neoplastic. The tissue similarities of a mass of solid fibrinous pancreatitis and a desmoplastic adenocarcinoma can be such that they have identical appearances by CT, ultrasonography, ductography, angiography, and even gross inspection.[71,72] There is not yet any substantive indication that MRI will be able to resolve this problem.[102] Since a sample biopsy that is negative for carcinoma does not exclude the possibility of malignancy, there may be no immediate method to determine the nature of such a mass short of surgical resection and meticulous pathologic examination. Depending on the clinical circumstances, it may be more prudent in some cases to follow the appearance of the mass with serial noninvasive imaging.

Direct ductography: pancreatic and biliary
Endoscopic retrograde
cholangiopancreatography

In current practice endoscopic retrograde cholangiopancreatography (ERCP) usually plays a supplementary role in the evaluation of patients suspected to have pancreatic cancer. The method may be used to clarify ambiguous information from CT or ultrasonography.[17,31,32,70] Because it affords an endoscopic view of the duodenum, ERCP has advantages in differentiating duodenal or ampullary carcinomas from periampullary cancers of the pancreatic head. Endoscopy is also used for placement of endoprostheses to relieve biliary obstruction.

As performed by skilled endoscopists ERCP is a highly successful procedure with a low incidence of serious complications. Pancreatic ductography is accomplished in approximately 90% of cases and cholangiography in a smaller proportion.[18] In cancer of the pancreas the most frequent positive findings involving the main pancreatic duct are stenosis and complete obstruction.[6] Stenosis is usually focal (Fig. 46-14), but it may involve a considerable length of the duct. Ductal narrowing may be concentric or eccentric, smooth or irregular. Lateral branches at the site of the tumor are usually obliterated, and the main duct upstream from a stenotic lesion is often dilated. When the duct is completely obstructed, the column of contrast material terminates in either an abrupt (Fig. 46-15, A), or tapered fashion. If a tumor has undergone cystic necrosis, contrast material may enter the cavity. Rarely, the only positive finding is evidence of a space-occupying parenchymal lesion extrinsic to the main duct, causing displacement or obstruction of side branches.[91] Cancers of the head of the pancreas may

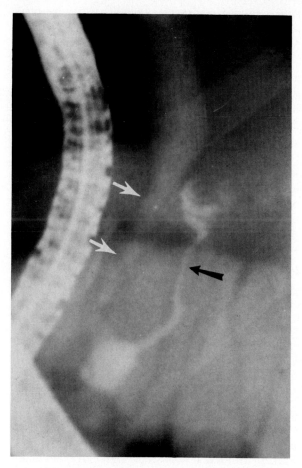

involve the common bile duct in similar manners, causing stenosis, obstruction, or extrinsic compression. When the common bile duct is affected, the nearby pancreatic duct is usually also involved[77] (Fig. 46-14).

Experienced observation is helpful to distinguish subtle abnormalities from variations of normal. It is necessary to recognize congenital anomalies, such as incomplete fusion of the dorsal and ventral pancreatic remnants (pancreas divisum). This anomaly can cause a pattern that resembles obstruction of the main pancreatic duct.[18] Differentiation between carcinoma and pancreatitis can be especially difficult because most alterations of ductal pattern caused by neoplasm can also result from inflammation.[18,80] As described elsewhere in this text, however, there are usually features that permit the distinction to be made,[85] especially when the ERCP is correlated with the findings of sectional imaging.

Percutaneous transhepatic cholangiography

The information provided by transhepatic cholangiography is limited to a depiction of the biliary system. Although the findings may be highly indicative of pancreatic carcinoma, they reveal neither the extent of the tumor nor the presence of metastasis. Delineation of the biliary tree above an obstruction is helpful to the surgeon contemplating a biliary bypass operation, but that information is usually obtainable by noninvasive means. Of perhaps more relevance, transhepatic cholangiography is an integral part of percutaneous biliary drainage procedures (Fig. 46-16).

Pancreatic carcinomas characteristically obstruct the common bile duct at the level of the pancreatic head and cause generalized dilatation of the biliary tree proximal to the obstruction. The ductal dilatation often ends in an

Fig. 46-14 Carcinoma of pancreatic head. ERCP showing high-grade stenosis of main pancreatic duct *(black arrow)* and tapered narrowing of adjacent common bile duct *(white arrows)*.

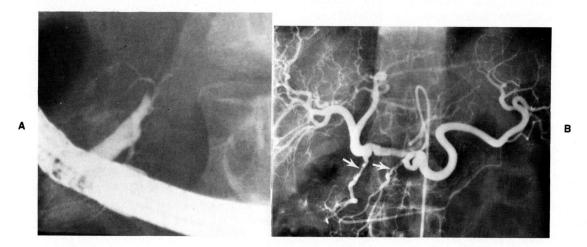

Fig. 46-15 Carcinoma of pancreatic head. **A,** ERCP showing abrupt obstruction of main pancreatic duct in head of pancreas. **B,** Celiac arteriogram showing irregular narrowing of gastroduodenal and dorsal pancreatic arteries *(arrows)* as result of neoplastic encasement.

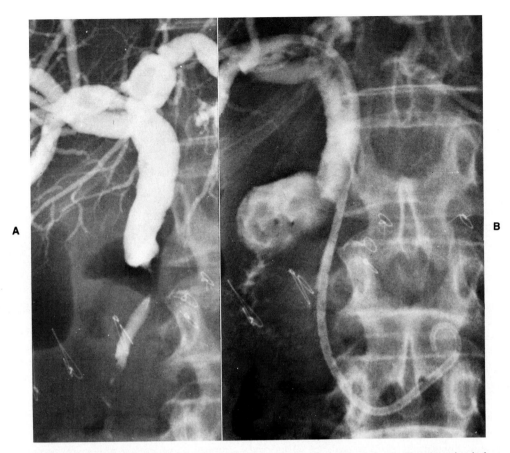

Fig. 46-16 Carcinoma of head of pancreas obstructing common bile duct. **A,** Transhepatic chol-angiogram showing focal constriction of bile duct at level of pancreatic head with dilatation of biliary tree above partial obstruction. **B,** Transhepatic internal biliary decompression established by passing drainage catheter beyond obstructing tumor and into duodenum.

abruptly tapered deformity with a nipplelike extension or an asymmetric rattail configuration.[28] The patterns of obstruction, however, are quite variable and not necessarily specific for pancreatic cancer. When the obstruction is incomplete, the stenotic segment may be either short (Fig. 46-16, *A*) or long, but it usually has a form that suggests extrinsic constriction. Sometimes, as a result of metastatic nodal involvement, pancreatic cancer causes obstruction near the porta hepatis.

Angiography

The role of angiography in the primary diagnosis of the ductal type of pancreatic cancer has almost disappeared with the widespread availability of noninvasive imaging and ERCP. Current angiography is most often a search for evidence of unresectability or an attempt to define vascular anatomy before surgical intervention.[32] The frequency with which angiography is used for these purposes varies among practices.

Most authorities employ selective catheterization of the celiac and superior mesenteric arteries, followed (when needed and as technically feasible) by selective injection of branches directly supplying the pancreas.[82,86] Rapid serial filming displays arterial, capillary, and venous phases of opacification. Ancillary techniques include magnification, subtraction, and pharmacologic vasoconstriction or vasodilatation.

Since the usual pancreatic carcinoma does not possess a prominent bed of intrinsic tumor vessels, angiographic features of the tumor are related to its effects on preexisting vessels. The sign generally regarded to be most characteristic of pancreatic cancer is arterial encasement, which appears as narrowing or irregularity of the affected artery (Fig. 46-15, *B*). Neoplastic encasement is sometimes smooth, but an irregular pattern is much more indicative of pancreatic carcinoma.[41,59]

Involvement of the major extrapancreatic arteries, such as the splenic, hepatic, celiac, superior mesenteric, or gastroduodenal artery, indicates that the tumor has spread beyond the confines of the pancreas. Major neighboring veins may also be affected. The splenic, superior mesenteric, or portal vein may become narrowed, compressed, or occluded.[10]

Although some angiographic abnormalities, such as irregular arterial narrowing, are characteristic of carcinoma, many of the vascular alterations are not specific. Atherosclerosis, for example, is a much more common cause of smooth arterial narrowing than is cancer. Pancreatitis can produce many of the same kinds of angiographic changes as those caused by carcinoma.

Gastrointestinal examinations

Barium examinations are no longer among the principal diagnostic procedures to search for evidence of pancreatic cancer in practices with more rewarding methods of imaging available. However, a barium study may be among the first procedures requested for a patient with pancreatic carcinoma whose symptoms are more suggestive of a primary disorder of the alimentary canal. In that situation a barium examination might afford the radiologist the opportunity to indicate that the abnormality is primarily pancreatic. By their nature, the effects of pancreatic cancer on the alimentary canal are indirect and generally nonspecific. Although some radiographic signs are more characteristic than others, almost any of them can also be caused by conditions other than pancreatic carcinoma. Moreover, barium examination of patients with pancreatic carcinoma often reveal no evidence whatsoever of the disease. Fortunately, it is no longer necessary to rely on results of these studies as the principal radiologic indicators of pancreatic cancer.

The secondary effects of pancreatic carcinoma on the hollow viscera of the alimentary canal have long been recognized. They are thoroughly reviewed, amply illustrated, and critically appraised in a number of publications, including the first two editions of this text.[13,24,62]

The likelihood that a pancreatic mass will involve a portion of the GI tract is related to the size of the mass and its proximity to the neighboring viscus. Masses that arise from the head of the pancreas tend to involve the inner curvature of the duodenal loop (Fig. 46-17) and the inferior surface of the gastric antrum. Tumors of the pancreatic body are likely to involve the posterior or inferior aspect of the gastric body or antrum, and tumors arising from the tail of the pancreas tend to involve the posterior aspect or lesser curvature of the gastric fundus. Tumors of the body or tail of the pancreas may also involve the distal portion of the duodenum or duodenojejunal junction. The transverse colon or splenic flexure may also be affected by pancreatic carcinoma. Gastrointestinal effects of pancreatic carcinoma include compression or indentation (Fig. 46-17), distortion of mucosal folds, ulceration (Fig. 46-17), and stenosis or obstruction.

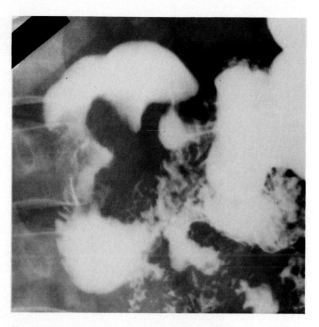

Fig. 46-17 Carcinoma of head of pancreas. Barium upper GI tract examination showing compression and invasion of second portion of duodenum with ulceration on inner wall. This configuration has been called reverse-3 sign of Frostberg.[36]

Percutaneous biopsy

Biopsy of pancreatic tumors by percutaneous needle aspiration has become a standard radiologic procedure. It offers the opportunity to establish histologic or cytologic diagnosis without exploratory laparotomy. Fluoroscopy, ERCP, and angiography have all been used to guide the placement of biopsy needles, but the obvious advantages of CT or ultrasonography have made these newer techniques the preferred methods of radiologic guidance in most situations.[67,73,98]

Biopsy techniques vary among practices, depending on personal preferences and available cytopathologic services. Technical details are described in another chapter. At one time most aspirates obtained from the thin (21- to 23-gauge) needles used to biopsy the pancreas were suitable only for cytologic study. However, fine needles with cutting tips currently make it possible to obtain tissue cores suitable for histologic diagnosis as well. Pathologists at my institution are usually able to make an immediate positive diagnosis, either from frozen section of a histologic specimen or from cytologic material. Thus microscopic confirmation is often established within minutes after a single puncture of the tumor is made. The availability of immediate pathologic interpretation enables the radiologist to limit the passes to no more than the number required to obtain adequate material.

The safety and efficacy of percutaneous fine-needle biopsy of pancreatic tumors is established. Complications are extremely rare, although at least one case of seeding of tumor cells along the needle path has been reported.[29] The likelihood of obtaining a positive microscopic diagnosis is quite high in pancreatic cancer, but failure to demonstrate malignancy does not exclude carcinoma. False-positive results, on the other hand, are practically nonexistent in the hands of pathologists experienced with the procedure.

Clinical benefits

Benefits that accrue to patients as a result of advances in the radiologic diagnosis of pancreatic cancer are not easy to measure in an objective manner, but there is no doubt that progress in radiology has altered very significantly the diagnostic evaluation and management of many patients with this disease. Compared to what was formerly required, current methods to establish the diagnosis are remarkably safe, swift, and economical. There is also little question that for many patients the disease is being diagnosed earlier than in the past. The availability of accurate noninvasive techniques has encouraged physicians to refer patients at a stage when symptoms are vague and nonspecific, and when pancreatic cancer is the cause of those symptoms, the tumor usually can be detected.

Unfortunately, the potential for earlier diagnosis of pancreatic carcinoma in symptomatic patients has not had a noticeably favorable effect on the extremely poor survival rates associated with this disease. It is true that resectable tumors are being found by noninvasive imaging,[34,49] and almost certainly there are individuals who owe their lives to the radiologic detection of their disease. However, a large proportion of resectable tumors become clinically evident because they obstruct the bile duct and cause jaundice early in their growth. It can be assumed that most jaundice-producing tumors would have been discovered and resected, if possible, whether or not there had been a preoperative radiologic diagnosis. Furthermore, only a relatively small proportion of patients whose primary pancreatic carcinomas are resected are then cured of their cancer.[25,34] At least among symptomatic patients, the major obstacle to discovery of the disease at a curable stage is not so much a deficiency in our diagnostic capabilities as the biologic nature of the disease. By the time a patient with ductal pancreatic carcinoma even suspects that he or she is ill, the disease in all but exceptional cases has already advanced beyond the stage of curability by any current method of treatment. This is true even though the primary tumor may be relatively small (Fig. 46-3 to 46-7).

Among the large majority of patients with symptomatic pancreatic cancer whose disease is incurable, there are still significant benefits to be derived from radiologic imaging. With nonvasive determination of unresectabily

many patients can be spared an operation or angiographic procedure. Although criteria for resectability vary among surgeons,[19,30,69] the demonstration of such findings as extrapancreatic tumor extension, metastasis, invasion of adjacent organs, involvement of extrapancreatic vessels, and ascites are generally considered to preclude successful extirpation.[34] Absence of these features on even the best of current imaging examinations does not guarantee that a tumor will be resectable, but imaging does serve to select those patients most likely to benefit from surgical intervention as opposed to those in whom an attempted curative resection would be futile. To obtain microscopic confirmation of pancreatic carcinoma, all that is required in most cases is percutaneous aspiration, which can often be accomplished in an outpatient setting in a matter of several minutes. Other radiologically guided interventional procedures that may offer palliation to some patients with pancreatic cancer are percutaneous biliary drainage to relieve jaundice or itching and celiac ganglion block to relieve pain.[44]

Among the patients who benefit most from modern pancreatic imaging are those who are suspected to have pancreatic cancer but do not. In these patients the demonstration of a pancreas that appears entirely normal in form and substance is an important finding that allows attention to be directed toward other possible explanations for the symptoms. The same examination that is used to display the pancreas can also be extended to evaluate other sites likely to harbor a lesion. The decline in the use of exploratory laparotomy to search for the cause of vague abdominal symptoms is a fairly accurate measure of the effectiveness of contemporary abdominal imaging to accomplish the same goal.

UNUSUAL CARCINOMAS OF THE EXOCRINE PANCREAS
Pleomorphic carcinoma

Pleomorphic, or sarcomatoid, carcinoma of the pancreas is a rare form of pancreatic cancer characterized histologically by anaplastic mononuclear cells, multinucleated giant cells, and spindle cells.[20,107] This aggressive malignancy is even more rapidly lethal than ductal adenocarcinoma of the pancreas, and widespread metastatic disease is invariably present at the time of initial evaluation.

The striking feature on abdominal imaging, in addition to the pancreatic mass, is massive lymphadenopathy — so extensive that the disease is likely to be mistaken for lymphoma.[107] However, the presence of a pancreatic mass similar in appearance to an ordinary pancreatic cancer, together with the fulminant clinical course, should indicate the possibility of a primary pancreatic cancer. Similarly, the presence of massive and extensive lymphadenopathy, which is not a usual feature of ductal carcinoma, should suggest the pleomorphic variety. Percutaneous biopsy may be indicated to exclude with certainty a more treatable disease, such as lymphoma.

Acinar cell carcinoma

Another uncommon cancer of the exocrine pancreas is acinar cell carcinoma.[20] A peculiar proclivity of this type of pancreatic carcinoma is the production of a clinical syndrome resulting from focal necrosis of subcutaneous and intraosseous fat.[79] This rare condition, attributed to the release of pancreatic lipase into the bloodstream, is not limited to acinar cell carcinoma, but also occurs in pancreatitis and, rarely, in association with ductal pancreatic carcinoma.

Awareness of the association between the syndrome of metastatic fat necrosis and an otherwise occult pancreatic neoplasm should lead to an imaging examination of the pancreas in patients afflicted with the syndrome. In one reported case of this association, CT scans revealed a large, well-defined tumor arising from the pancreatic tail.[79] The tumor, an acinar cell carcinoma, was subsequently resected.

Mucin-hypersecreting tumor of the pancreatic duct

Yet another rare carcinoma of the pancreas is this relatively well differentiated papillary tumor that arises from and is confined to the mucosal lining of the main pancreatic duct. Itai et al.,[50] who reported 5 cases, speculate that it is the same tumor that some pathologists designate as colloid carcinoma.[20] The tumor produces mucin in such quantity that it causes pronounced dilatation of the main pancreatic duct with consequent thinning of the pancreatic parenchyma. The markedly dilated duct, which is filled with radiolucent mucin, and the thinned parenchyma constitute the main findings on CT. On ERCP the orifice of the pancreatic duct is widely patent, and it is sometimes impossible to fill the entire duct with contrast material. Within the duct there are filling defects that may represent either excrescences of tumor or globs of mucin.[50]

Solid and papillary epithelial neoplasm

This uncommon pancreatic tumor is known by a variety of descriptive but somewhat cumbersome names: solid and papillary epithelial neoplasm, papillary and epithelial neoplasm, papillary and cystic neoplasm, and papillary carcinoma.[3,36,55] As its names imply, the tumor has a mixed composition. It apparently begins as a solid tumor but undergoes varying degrees of cystic degeneration due to necrosis and hemorrhage. Papillary excrescences are a unique histologic feature. Although they are of ductal origin and low-grade malignancy, these tumors grow slowly and seldom metastasize or extend

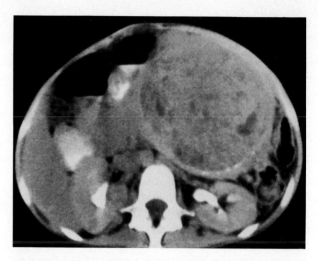

Fig. 46-18 Solid and papillary epithelial neoplasm. Huge, spherical, well-defined tumor arising from pancreatic tail contains both solid and cystic components. Calcification is present in peripheral capsule. Originally designated pathologically as cystadenocarcinoma, resected tumor was subsequently reclassified as solid and papillary epithelial neoplasm.

beyond their enveloping fibrous capsule. Most can be excised, and excision is usually curative. Unlike other malignant pancreatic neoplasms, these tumors have an excellent prognosis.

Solid and papillary epithelial neoplasms of the pancreas have a definite predilection for young women and adolescent girls, and a disproportionate number of the patients reported to date with this condition have been black or oriental.[3,36,55] Symptoms are usually related to local effects of the expanding mass; therefore most of the tumors are large by the time their presence is manifest.

Solid and papillary epithelial neoplasms examined by sectional imaging have consistently appeared as large, rounded, well-defined pancreatic masses.[3,36,55] The interior of the tumor may be either solid or cystic or, as in the majority of cases, of mixed solid and cystic composition (Fig. 46-18). Calcification is relatively uncommon, and when it occurs, it is usually peripheral (Fig. 46-18). These tumors can resemble serous or mucinous cystic neoplasms or islet cell carcinomas, and it is probable that many of them have been misclassified as such in the past. Conceivably, one of these tumors could also resemble a ductal adenocarcinoma, although in most cases the large size of the mass and its sharp definition, together with the clinical setting, should lead the interpreter away from that diagnosis. Needless to say, it is of considerable importance that this highly curable pancreatic neoplasm not be mistaken for a much more lethal form of cancer.

CYSTIC NEOPLASMS

Cystic neoplasms have been classified traditionally as either cystadenoma or cystadenocarcinoma. Recently these designations have been modified and to some extent replaced by a classification based on distinctive pathologic characteristics that correlate with the clinical behavior of the tumors.[15,16] Two types are recognized: microcystic adenoma, also called serous or glycogen-rich cystadenoma; and mucinous cystic, or macrocystic, neoplasms. Microcystic adenomas (serous cystadenomas) are invariable benign, whereas mucinous cystic (macrocystic) tumors may be either benign (mucinous cystadenoma) or malignant (cystadenocarcinoma). Unlike the microcystic adenoma, which has no reported malignant potential, the mucinous cystadenoma has a very considerable malignant potential.

Morphologic features of pancreatic cystic neoplasms usually make these tumors readily apparent on imaging examinations, and in most cases they can be distinguished from ordinary ductal carcinoma. Both types of cystic neoplasm are typically large at discovery, and both types are of mixed cystic and stromal composition. The solid elements tend to be well vascularized and occasionally contain calcification. Despite the characteristics that the two types of cystic neoplasm have in common, however, there are also radiologically demonstrable ar-chitectural features that can be used to differentiate them from each other. This exercise has practical significance because of the differences in clinical behavior between microcystic adenomas and mucinous cystic neoplasms.

Microcystic adenoma (serous cystadenoma)

As its name indicates, this tumor is made up of small cysts, varying in diameter from less than a millimeter to 2 cm. Occasionally one of these tumors has a few cysts with diameters greater than 2 cm. The numbers of cysts can vary from several to innumerable. In its classic form microcystic adenoma has a honeycomb appearance on cross-sectional display. Sometimes there is a central fibrotic scar that gives rise to radiating septations. When calcification is present, it is likely to be within the central scar.

Sectional imaging accurately depicts the morphology and internal architecture of most microcystic adenomas.[35,48,108] By CT, the features are best displayed on scans made with contrast enhancement, which exaggerates the difference in density between the enhancing stroma and unenhancing cystic spaces (Fig. 46-19, *A*). Occasionally the individual cysts are so small that the cystic composition of the mass may be difficult to perceive on a CT scan. Ultrasound is especially suited to display the cystic structure of these tumors (Fig. 46-19, *B*), even in masses that are not conspicuously cystic by CT. The central scar, if present, may be shown by either method. Stromal hypervascularity is a well-known an-

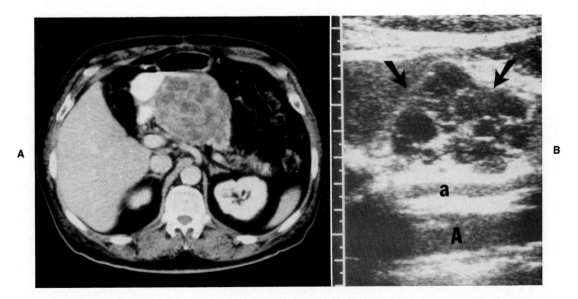

Fig. 46-19 Microcystic adenoma (serous cystadenoma). **A,** Contrast-enhanced CT showing large pancreatic mass composed of numerous small cysts with enhancing walls. **B,** Sagittal sonogram showing the multicystic appearance of another microcystic adenoma *(arrows)*. Note enhanced through-transmission of sound, which clearly defines aorta *(A)* and superior mesenteric artery *(a)* behind mass.

giographic feature of the tumors now called microcystic adenomas.[33]

Since microcystic adenomas are not regarded as susceptible to malignant transformation, the decision whether such a tumor should be surgically removed should not have to be based on that contingency, provided that the nature of the tumor can be established by nonoperative means. Thus far there has been an understandable reluctance on the part of surgeons to leave these large tumors alone, and in some cases resection is indicated because of problems associated with the mass itself. Whether features displayed by radiologic imaging will prove reliable enough to obviate an operation that is not otherwise indicated remains to be determined. Experience to date indicates that some microcystic adenomas have appearances characteristic enough to permit a confident diagnosis of that benign tumor, whereas others are not so easily classified. It will be of interest to learn whether MRI will provide more definitive information. In any case, even when a precise preoperative diagnosis of microcystic adenoma cannot be made with certainty, there are usually radiologic features that permit the possibility to be suggested, thereby alerting the surgeon and perhaps averting a more extensive operation than is necessary.

Mucinous cystic neoplasms (macrocystic cystadenoma and cystadenocarcinoma)

The cysts that occur in mucinous cystic neoplasms are usually larger than those in microcystic adenomas. In mucinous cystic tumors the cysts may be solitary or multiple, unilocular or multilocular (Fig. 46-20). Sometimes excrescences of tumor project into the cystic spaces from outer walls or septa (Fig. 46-21). Calcifications tend to be peripherally located. Signs of malignancy include invasion of contiguous organs and metastases involving the liver or regional lymph nodes. In the absence of such overt evidence of malignancy it is not possible to determine radiologically whether a mucinous cystic tumor is a cystadenoma or cystadenocarcinoma. Since malignant tissue frequently exists in only a portion of such a tumor, biopsy of a section may fail to indicate the malignant nature of a cystadenocarcinoma. For that reason—and because of the recognized tendency for mucinous cystadenomas to become malignant—there is a consensus that all mucinous cystic tumors should be removed if possible.[15,35]

CT (Figs. 46-20, A and 46-21), ultrasonography (Fig. 46-20, B), and MRI are capable of displaying much of the morphology and internal architecture that characterizes mucinous cystic neoplasms.[35,48,108] Sometimes it is difficult to distinguish one of these tumors from a microcystic adenoma having larger than usual cysts, from a ductal adenocarcinoma that has undergone cavitary necrosis, or from a large islet cell tumor with cystic degeneration. Cystic lymphangioma, a rare benign tumor, can have an identical CT appearance to mucinous cystic neoplasms.[63,74] Pseudocysts and congenital cysts are more common masses that can be difficult to distinguish from a mucinous cystic tumor, especially one that occurs

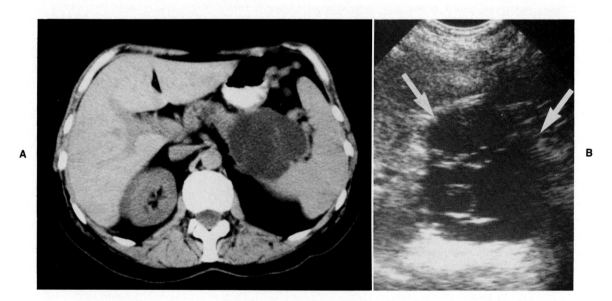

Fig. 46-20 Mucinous cystic (macrocystic) neoplasm. **A,** CT scan showing large cystic mass arising from pancreatic tail. Mass has internal septations, but individual cystic compartments are considerably larger than those of microcystic adenoma in Fig. 46-19. **B,** Sonogram of same tumor *(arrows).* At pathologic examination no malignant tissue was found.

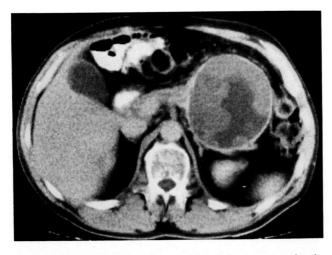

Fig. 46-21 Mucinous cystic neoplasm (cystadenocarcinoma). Large encapsulated mass arising from pancreatic tail contains solid tumor tissue as well as fluid. Hepatic metastases (not shown) were visible at other levels.

in the form of a solitary unilocular cyst with no conspicuous soft tissue component. The absence of a history of pancreatitis or of any other radiologic evidence of pancreatitis is a clue that such a cyst could be neoplastic rather than inflammatory. If the lesion is aspirated, an analysis of the fluid should be helpful to differentiate between a mucinous cystic neoplasm and a nonneoplastic cyst.

ISLET CELL NEOPLASMS (APUDOMAS)

Neoplasms that arise from the islets of Langerhans occur in both benign and malignant forms. Benign islet cell adenomas come to clinical attention only as a result of their endocrine activity, whereas islet cell carcinomas are important because of their malignancy, whether or not they are hormonally active. Many islet cell carcinomas, however, do secrete excessive hormone, in which case their presenting symptoms are usually related to the endocrinopathy rather than the tumor mass. Islet cell tumors are part of a group of endocrine neoplasms, collectively called apudomas, that arise from a widely dispersed system of polypeptide-secreting cells of neuroectodermal origin. The acronym *APUD* (amine precursor uptake and decarboxylation) is derived from the common chemical properties of these cells.[68,75]

Depending on the hormones they secrete, functioning islet cell tumors are responsible for a variety of syndromes.[52,68] The two best known conditions are (1) the complex of hypoglycemic symptoms that result from hy-

persecretion of insulin by the beta-cell tumor, insulinoma, and (2) the Zollinger-Ellison syndrome, caused by hypersecretion of gastrin by the non-beta tumor, gastrinoma. The pathophysiology and radiographic features of the Zollinger-Ellison syndrome are described elsewhere in this text. Syndromes caused by other non-beta islet cell tumors are less familiar. The watery diarrhea, hypokalemia, and hypochlorhydria (WDHH) syndrome, also known as pancreatic cholera, is attributed to hypersecretion of vasoactive intestinal peptide (VIP), and the responsible tumor is called a vipoma. Tumors that secrete glucagon (glucagonomas) cause a syndrome characterized by hyperglycemia and a migratory necrolytic erythematous rash. Other functioning tumors are so rare that clinical features are not well defined, although diarrhea and weight loss have been associated with most cases of somatostatinoma.[83]

Because pancreatic apudomas have the capacity to secrete hormones other than those indigenous to the pancreas, they may cause endocrinopathies, such as Cushing's syndrome (from hypersecretion of adrenocorticotropic hormone), which are more often attributable to hyperactivity of other glands. Conversely, hyperactivity of endocrine cells outside the pancreas can cause disorders that are usually associated with islet cell tumors.[68] Islet cell tumors, together with tumors of the parathyroid glands, pituitary gland, and sometimes the adrenal cortex, are common components of the multiple endocrine neoplasia type 1 (MEN-I) syndrome.[68]

Since the diagnosis of functioning islet cell tumors is usually established or suspected on the basis of clinical and laboratory information, the primary role of radiology is to provide preoperative assessment of the location and number of tumors. The extent of the lesion and the presence of metastasis is additional worthwhile information. Although the individual types of islet cell tumors vary in their size, distribution, number, and incidence of malignancy, there are characteristics of each type that influence the likelihood of successful radiologic demonstration.

Insulinoma

About 85% of insulinomas are benign adenomas.[95] They occur as discrete tumors, usually solitary but often multiple, with no particular predilection for any part of the pancreas. Although occasional insulinomas are greater than 5 cm in diameter, most are considerably smaller, ranging from a few millimeters to 2 cm.[26] Surgical removal of insulin-secreting adenomas is usually curative.

Accurate localization of insulinomas greatly facilitates surgical resection. A variety of radiologic techniques, varying in accuracy, invasiveness, and cost, have been employed for that purpose. With any technique the rate of success is related to the skill and dedication applied to the task. Angiography, CT, ultrasonography, and venous sampling have all been shown to be effective in the preoperative localization of insulinomas, and there is every reason to believe that MRI will also be of value.[102] Intraoperative ultrasonography adds yet another degree of accuracy to the radiologic localization of insulinomas within the pancreas.[42]

Ultrasonography

Ultrasonography is a noninvasive, relatively inexpensive, and, with real-time instrumentation, acceptably sensitive method for preoperative localization of insulinomas. With a success rate between 60% and 70%,[42,43] real-time ultrasonography has become the initial localizing procedure, and frequently the only one required, in my institution.[42] Meticulous technique, applied at least as skillfully as in the search for pancreatic carcinoma, is a prerequisite for demonstrating small insulinomas in any part of the gland.

Intraoperative high-frequency ultrasonography is more sensitive than preoperative ultrasonography. Frequently it can reveal intrapancreatic tumors so small that they cannot be detected by direct palpation of the gland. Intraoperative ultrasonography has been especially useful in patients whose pancreatic anatomy has been distorted by previous surgery and in patients, such as those with the MEN-I syndrome, who are likely to have multiple small islet cell tumors.[42] By displaying the relationship of an insulinoma to the pancreatic duct or bile duct, intraoperative ultrasonography can facilitate enucleation of the tumor (Fig. 46-22, *B*).

Most insulinomas are distinctly hypoechoic relative to normal pancreatic parenchyma (Fig. 46-22, *A* and *B*). A small proportion, however, are hyperechoic or isoechoic. Hyperechoic and isoechoic tumors are more common in younger patients, whose normal pancreatic parenchyma tends to be less echogenic than in later life.[42] Although isoechoic tumors are difficult to perceive, they are often surrounded by a visible echogenic halo.[42]

Computed tomography

Reported rates of success with CT scans in the localization of insulinomas range from 50%[56,93] to 80%.[87] Best results are achieved with a dynamic technique of scanning that produces high-resolution images in rapid succession while there is a high concentration of contrast material in the circulation. Rossi and co-workers[87] recommend multiple bolus injections, contiguous overlapping slices of 1 cm thickness, and 0.6 cm table incrementation.

Because of their hypervascularity, typical insulinomas become transiently hyperdense relative to normal parenchyma with dynamic contrast enhancement (Fig. 46-22, *C*). Some insulinomas are also evident as discrete masses that project beyond the normal pancreatic contour, but small tumors within the substance of the gland can be seen only if there is differential contrast enhancement.

Angiography

Angiography has been reported to localize insulinomas in up to 90% of cases,[38] although rates of success in most series are somewhat lower.[23,76] Greatest accuracy is achieved with selective—when necessary, superselective—arterial injections. Stereoscopy, magnification, and subtraction are helpful to detect smaller lesions and tumors otherwise obscured by superimposed structures. Angiography can be supplemented by a CT scan performed with contrast material injected directly into the celiac axis through the arterial catheter.[56] Angiographically, insulinomas appear as intensely vascular, sharply defined masses (Fig. 46-22, *D*). The homogeneous vascular blush persists into the venous phase. Although it is sensitive, angiography is associated with a significant number of false-positive results.[84] Other relative disadvantages include its costliness and invasiveness.

Other localizing techniques

Rates of success as high as 97% have been reported with pancreatic venous sampling,[11,22,84] but this invasive, technically difficult, and time-consuming procedure has not met with widespread acceptance. MRI has been used in only a few cases of insulinoma so far, but early results

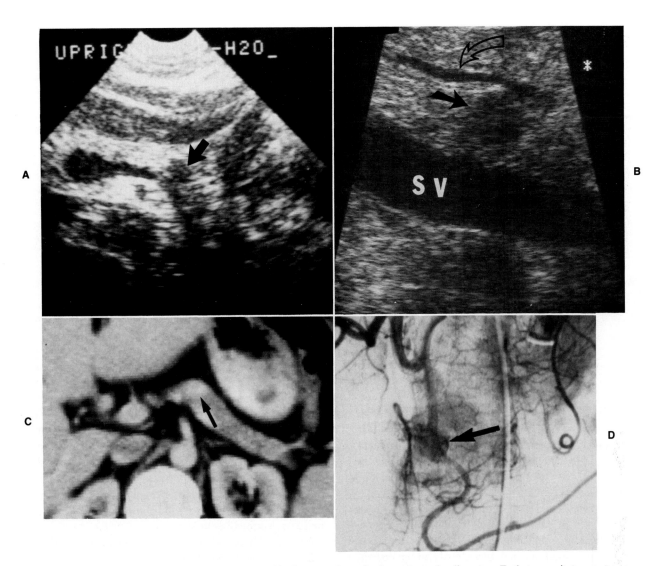

Fig. 46-22 Solitary insulinomas *(black arrows),* each about 1 cm in diameter. Each tumor is depicted by different modality. **A,** Preoperative sonogram showing hypoechoic lesion in pancreatic body. **B,** Intraoperative sonogram showing discrete hypoechoic lesion in substance of pancreas, between main pancreatic duct *(open arrow)* and splenic vein *(sv).* **C,** CT scan showing enhancing tumor in body of pancreas (same tumor as in **A**). **D,** Subtraction angiogram showing hypervascular tumor in pancreatic head. **A** and **B** (From Gorman, B, et al: Benign pancreatic insulinoma: preoperative and intraoperative sonographic localization, AJR 147:929-934, © by Am Roentgen Ray Soc, 1986.)

are promising.[102] Success was reported recently with scintigraphy in the case of an insulinoma that was demonstrable because of its increased uptake of ^{99m}Tc-methylene diphosphonate.[78]

Gastrinoma

Gastrin-secreting tumors occur in a variety of sizes, but often they are small and multiple.[84] As is the case with other islet cell tumors, gastrinomas that are part of the MEN-I syndrome are especially likely to be multiple. About half of all gastrinomas exhibit malignant behavior by the time they are discovered, although the malignancy

is usually of low grade. The radiologic diagnosis of malignancy depends on identification of metastatic tumor, which may be occult or direct extrapancreatic extension. Not all cases of Zollinger-Ellison syndrome are caused by a discrete pancreatic tumor, since excessive amounts of gastrin may also be elaborated by islet cell hyperplasia, diffuse microadenomatosis, metastases, or extrapancreatic gastrinoma.[52]

For these reasons the source of gastrin hypersecretion is likely to escape detection by any current method of imaging in a significant proportion of patients who have the Zollinger-Ellison syndrome. Nevertheless, a sizable

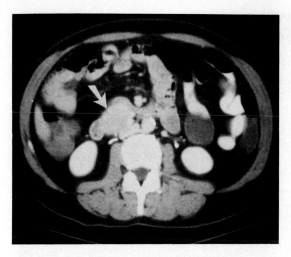

Fig. 46-23 Gastrinoma. CT scan shows enhancing mass *(arrow)* arising from inferior aspect of pancreatic head.

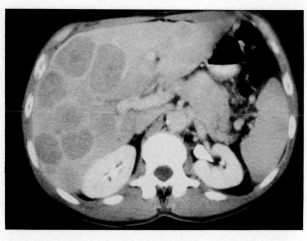

Fig. 46-24 Glucagon-secreting islet cell carcinoma with hepatic metastases. Mass arising from body and tail of pancreas undergoes enhancement, indicating that it is well vascularized.

proportion of gastrinomas can be detected. In each of three recently reported series dealing with CT in the evaluation of patients with these tumors, dynamic contrast-enhanced CT scans displayed the tumor in the majority of cases.[56,87,93] If the tumor is sufficiently vascular, it will become hyperdense with dynamic enhancement, and if it is sufficiently large or superficial, it may be obvious as a mass[65] (Fig. 46-23). Other methods of noninvasive sectional imaging have not been used as often as CT in the evaluation of patients with excessive gastrin secretion, but preliminary experience with MRI suggests that its capabilities and limitations may be similar to those of CT.[102] Sectional imaging also affords an opportunity to evaluate the liver and node-bearing regions for metastasis. Angiography has been only moderately successful in localizing the source of excessive gastrin production, mainly because of the same factors that often inhibit successful evaluation by sectional imaging.[66,84]

Other functioning tumors

Vipomas, glucagonomas, and somatostatinomas are generally large when discovered, and they are often malignant. Although few of any one type have been studied by contemporary imaging, sizable tumors of these uncommon types, as well as their metastases, have been readily displayed by CT scans[9,83] (Fig. 46-24) and by other modalities.[39,40,101]

Nonfunctioning islet cell carcinoma

Islet cell tumors that do not cause a recognizable syndrome related to overproduction of hormone are called "nonfunctioning," even though they may secrete one or more hormones in amounts too small to be measured or

to cause an endocrine disorder. Benign adenomas in this category remain clinically silent, but malignant nonfunctioning islet cell tumors are life-threatening neoplasms that do cause symptoms. Presenting signs and symptoms of nonfunctioning islet cell carcinomas are usually related to local effects of the tumor. They include pain, a sensation of pressure, and occasionally a palpable mass.[54]

Islet cell carcinomas differ enough from the ductal type of adenocarcinomas in prognosis and treatment to make it worthwhile to distinguish between these two types of pancreatic cancer.[54] Islet cell carcinomas grow relatively slowly and are not as rapidly fatal as ductal carcinomas. Even the presence of metastasis does not preclude extended survival. Moreover, islet cell carcinomas and their metastases often respond to systemic chemotherapy, whereas ordinary pancreatic cancer does not.

Although nonfunctioning islet cell carcinomas are sometimes radiographically indistinguishable from ductal carcinoma, they often have features that help to differentiate them from the more common form of cancer.[27] Functioning islet cell carcinomas, especially the uncommon types, have morphologic features identical to those of nonfunctioning islet cell carcinomas, but their islet cell origins are clinically evident because of the associated endocrine syndromes. As a general rule, islet cell carcinomas tend to be larger than ductal carcinomas at the time of discovery. Approximately 25% of them contain calcification[27,93] (Fig. 46-25), whereas calcification is rare in ordinary pancreatic carcinoma.

Calcification is best demonstrated by CT scans, but it can often be seen on plain radiographs.[46] Although ne-

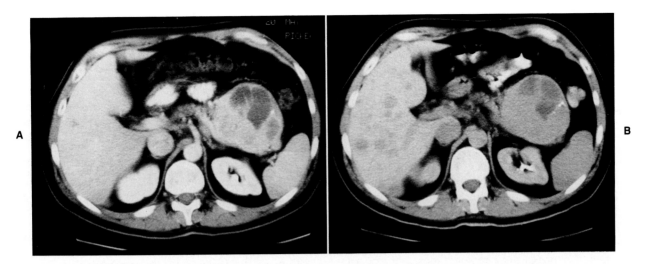

Fig. 46-25 Nonfunctioning islet cell carcinoma with hypervascular hepatic metastases. Advantage of delayed scanning. **A,** Contrast-enhanced CT scan showing large pancreatic tumor containing small calcification. Tumor has both solid enhancing tissue and necrotic unenhancing components. **B,** Delayed scan, taken about 4 hours after administration of intravenous contrast material, shows multiple hepatic metastases, most of which were invisible on earlier scan **(A).**

crotic cavitation is common in larger islet cell carcinomas, the solid portions of these tumors are often hypervascular and therefore subject to intravenous contrast enhancement on CT scans. One feature notably lacking among islet cell carcinomas is the type of retropancreatic periarterial extension that is a common CT feature of ductal carcinoma.[27] These more or less distinguishing characteristics of islet cell carcinoma have been documented most extensively by CT,[27,93] but many of the same

features can also be displayed by other imaging methods, notably MRI[94] (Fig. 46-26).

Radiologic imaging is also useful to demonstrate metastases from these tumors. They too may provide a clue as to the type of primary pancreatic carcinoma. Whereas hepatic metastases from ductal adenocarcinomas are usually relatively small, metastatic islet cell carcinoma in the liver is often in the form of relatively large tumor masses (Figs. 46-24 and 46-26). Also, solid metastatic tumor from islet cell carcinoma is likely to be hypervascular, which is not the case with ductal carcinoma. Because hepatic metastases of islet cell origin may undergo contrast enhancement on CT scans, these lesions sometimes become isodense with normal liver. For that reason, it may be worthwhile to obtain a series of scans of the liver, either before enhancement or at a later time, when most of the contrast material has been cleared from the circulation (Fig. 46-25).

NONEPITHELIAL NEOPLASMS
Lymphoma

Pancreatic lymphoma is usually of a non-Hodgkin's variety. Lymphomatous involvement of the pancreas is often associated with generalized disease, in which case the pancreatic tumor is likely to be accompanied by lymphadenopathy at other sites. In most cases the diagnosis of lymphoma will already have been established by the time the pancreatic involvement is discovered. In cases of widespread disease there is seldom any difficulty distinguishing lymphoma from a primary pancreatic carcinoma, but one type of pancreatic carcinoma that can

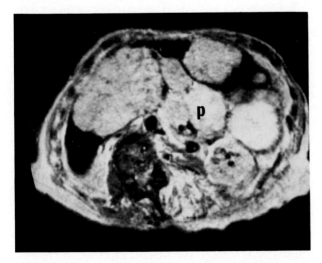

Fig. 46-26 Nonfunctioning islet cell carcinoma with large hepatic metastases. T_2-weighted magnetic resonance image shows primary pancreatic tumor *(p)* and large metastatic tumors in liver as sharply defined masses of high-signal intensity.

resemble extensive lymphoma is pleomorphic carcinoma, which typically produces massive metastatic lymphadenopathy. This highly aggressive tumor has already been discussed.

When the pancreas is the primary site of lymphoma, the tumor may appear on pancreatic images as a soft-tissue mass that cannot be distinguished from carcinoma.[100] Sometimes there are clinical or radiologic features to indicate the lymphomatous nature of the mass, or at least to indicate that it is something other than a ductal adenocarcinoma,[100] but even in those cases appropriate treatment usually requires accurate histologic classification. Occasionally this can be accomplished by needle biopsy, but often a precise classification of lymphoma requires more tissue than can be obtained by needle aspiration. For unexplained reasons, most primary pancreatic lymphomas arise within the head of the gland.[100] In that location they may obstruct the bile duct or pancreatic duct in the same manner as carcinoma.

Connective tissue tumors

Primary pancreatic neoplasms of connective tissue origin are rare. They occur in benign as well as malignant forms. Among the benign varieties are leiomyoma, fibroma, hemangioma, and lymphangioma. They are seldom of clinical significance, although some tumors, such as cystic lymphangioma, can grow to a large size. The corresponding sarcomas vary in the aggressiveness of their behavior, but they often become very large, and most are eventually lethal.

Radiologic experiences with these rare tumors is limited. Cyst lymphangiomas have been reported to resemble mucinous cystic neoplasms on CT scans.[63,74] Angiomatous tumors of the pancreas may contain radiographically visible phleboliths or other calcifications.[21,97] Leiomyosarcomas are likely to be large masses with prominent necrotic cavities.[89]

METASTATIC NEOPLASMS

Metastatic involvement of the pancreas is possible from almost any type of primary malignancy. Common primary sites include breast, lung, kidney, skin (melanoma), and GI tract.[20,88] Cancer that is metastatic to the pancreas may take the form of multiple nodules on the surface of the gland, or it may appear as a solitary localized mass.[88] In the latter case it can resemble a primary pancreatic neoplasm. However, a history of primary malignancy in another organ or an unusual radiologic feature of the pancreatic tumor may indicate the metastatic nature of the tumor. If histologic diagnosis of the pancreatic mass is of practical importance, percutaneous or surgical biopsy may be indicated.

REFERENCES

1. Aoki, K, and Ogawa, H: Cancer of the pancreas: international mortality trends, World Health Stat Rep 31:2, 1978.
2. Axtell, LM, Asire, AJ, and Myers, MH: Cancer patient survival, End Results in Cancer, Report No. 5, 1976, pp. 130.
3. Balthazar, EJ, et al: Solid and papillary epithelial neoplasm of the pancreas: radiographic, CT, sonographic, and angiographic features, Radiology 150:39, 1984.
4. Baron, RL, et al: Computed tomographic features of biliary obstruction, AJR 140:1173, 1983.
5. Berland, LL, et al: Computed tomography of the normal and abnormal pancreatic duct: correlation with pancreatic ductography, Radiology 141:715, 1981.
6. Bilbao, MK, and Katon, RM: Neoplasms of the pancreas. In Stewart, ET, et al, editors: Atlas of endoscopic retrograde cholangiopancreatography, St. Louis, 1977, The CV Mosby Co.
7. Bowie, JD, and MacMahon, H: Improved techniques in pancreatic sonography, Semin Ultrasound 1:170, 1980.
8. Bowie, JD, and Moosa, AR: Ultrasonography and computed tomography in the diagnosis of pancreatic tumors. In Moosa, AR, editor: Tumors of the pancreas, Baltimore, 1980, Williams & Wilkins.
9. Breatnach, ES, et al: CT of glucagonomas, J Comput Assist Tomogr 9:25, 1985.
10. Buranasiri, S, and Baum, S: The significance of the venous phase of celiac and superior mesenteric arteriography in evaluating pancreatic carcinoma, Radiology 102:11, 1972.
11. Cho, KJ, et al: Localization of the source of hyperinsulinism: percutaneous transhepatic portal and pancreatic vein catheterization with hormone assay, AJR 139:237, 1982.
12. Churchill, RJ, Reynes, CJ, and Love, L: Pancreatic pseudotumors: computed tomography, Gastrointest Radiol 3:251, 1978.
13. Clemett, AR: Examination of the pancreas. In Margulis, AR, and Burhenne, HJ, editors: Alimentary tract roentgenology, ed 2, vol 2, St. Louis, 1973, The CV Mosby Co.
14. Cohen, BA, Mitty, HA, and Mendelson, DS: Computed tomography of splenic infarction, J Comput Assist Tomogr 8:167, 1984.
15. Compagno, J, and Oertel, JE: Microcystic adenomas of the pancreas (glycogen-rich cystadenomas): a clinicopathologic study of 34 cases, Am J Clin Pathol 69:289, 1978.
16. Compagno, J, and Oertel, JE: Mucinous cystic neoplasms of the pancreas with overt and latent malignancy (cystadenocarcinoma and cystadenoma): a clinicopathologic study of 41 cases, Am J Clin Pathol 69:573, 1978.
17. Cotton, PB, et al: Gray-scale ultrasonography and endoscopic pancreatography in pancreatic diagnosis, Radiology 134:453, 1980.
18. Cotton, PB: Progress report: ERCP, Gut 18:316, 1977.
19. Crile, G, Jr: The advantages of bypass operations over pancreatoduodenectomy in the treatment of pancreatic carcinoma, Surg Gynecol Obstet 130:1049, 1970.
20. Cubilla, AL, and Fitzgerald, PJ: Surgical pathology of tumors of the exocrine pancreas. In Moosa, AR, editor: Tumors of the pancreas, Baltimore, 1980, Williams & Wilkins.
21. Dodds, WJ: Margolin, FR, and Goldberg, HI: Cavernous lymphangioma of the pancreas, Radiol Clin (Basel) 38:267, 1969.
22. Doppman, JL, et al: The role of pancreatic venous sampling in the localization of insulinomas, Radiology 138:557, 1981.
23. Dunnick, NR, et al: Localizing insulinomas with combined radiographic methods, AJR 135:747, 1980.
24. Eaton, SB, Jr, and Ferrucci, JT, Jr: Radiology of the pancreas and duodenum, Philadelphia, 1973, WB Saunders.
25. Edis, AJ, Kiernan, PD, and Taylor, WF: Attempted curative

resection of ductal carcinoma of the pancreas: review of Mayo Clinic experience, 1951-1975, Mayo Clin Proc 55:531, 1980.

26. Edis, AJ, et al: Insulinoma—current diagnosis and surgical management, Curr Probl Surg 13:1, 1976.

27. Eelkema, EA, et al: CT features of nonfunctioning islet cell carcinoma, AJR 143:943, 1984.

28. Evans, JA: Specialized roentgen diagnostic technics in investigation of abdominal disease, Radiology 82:579, 1964.

29. Ferrucci, JT, Jr, et al: Malignant seeding of the tract after thin-needle aspiration biopsy, Radiology 130:345, 1979.

30. Fortner, JG, et al: Regional pancreatectomy: en bloc pancreatic, portal vein and lymph node resection, Ann Surg 186:42, 1977.

31. Freeny, PC, Bilbao, MK, and Katon, RM: "Blind" evaluation of endoscopic retrograde cholangiopancreatography (ERCP) in the diagnosis of pancreatic carcinoma: the "double duct" and other signs, Radiology 119:271, 1976.

32. Freeny, PC, Marks, WM, and Ball, TJ: Impact of high-resolution computed tomography on utilization of ERCP and angiography, Radiology 142:35, 1982.

33. Freeny, PC, et al: Cystic neoplasms of the pancreas: new angiographic and ultrasonographic findings, AJR 131:795, 1978.

34. Freeny, PC, et al: Pancreatic ductal adenocarcinoma: diagnosis and staging with dynamic CT, Radiology 166:125, 1988.

35. Friedman, AC, Lichtenstein, JE, and Dachman, AH: Cystic neoplasms of the pancreas: radiological-pathological correlation, Radiology 149:45, 1983.

36. Friedman, AC, et al: Solid and papillary epithelial neoplasm of the pancreas, Radiology 154:333, 1985.

37. Frostberg, N: A characteristic duodenal deformity in cases of different kinds of perivaterial enlargement of the pancreas, Acta Radiol (Ther) (Stockh) 19:164, 1938.

38. Fulton, RE, et al: Preoperative localization of insulin-producing tumors of the pancreas, Am J Roentgenol 123:367, 1975.

39. Gerlock, AJ, Jr, et al: Pancreatic somatostatinoma: histologic, clinical, and angiographic features, AJR 133:939, 1979.

40. Gold, RP, et al: Radiologic and pathologic characteristics of the WDHA syndrome, AJR 127:397, 1978.

41. Goldstein, HM, Neiman, HL, and Bookstein, JJ: Angiographic evaluation of pancreatic disease: a further appraisal, Radiology 112:275, 1974.

42. Gorman, G, et al: Benign pancreatic insulinoma: preoperative and intraoperative sonographic localization, AJR 147:929, 1986.

43. Gunther, RW, et al: Islet-cell tumors: detection of small lesions with computed tomography and ultrasound, Radiology 148:485, 1983.

44. Haaga, JR, et al: Improved technique for CT-guided celiac ganglia block, AJR 142:1201, 1984.

45. Hosoki, T: Dynamic CT of pancreatic tumors, AJR 140:959, 1983.

46. Imhof, H, and Frank, P: Pancreatic calcification in malignant islet cell tumors, Radiology 122:333, 1977.

47. Itai, Y, Moss, AA, and Goldberg, HI: Pancreatic cysts caused by carcinoma of the pancreas: a pitfall in the diagnosis of pancreatic carcinoma, J Comput Assist Tomogr 6:772, 1982.

48. Itai, Y, Moss, AA, and Ohtomo, K: Computed tomography of cystadenoma and cystadenocarcinoma of the pancreas, Radiology 145:419, 1982.

49. Itai, Y, et al: Computed tomographic appearance of resectable pancreatic carcinoma, Radiology 143:719, 1982.

50. Itai, Y, et al: Mucin-hypersecreting carcinoma of the pancreas, Radiology 165:51, 1987.

51. Jafri, SZH, et al: Comparison of CT and angiography in assessing resectability of pancreatic carcinoma, AJR 142:525, 1984.

52. Jaspan, JB, et al: Clinical features and diagnosis of islet cell

tumors. In Moosa, AR, editor: Tumors of the pancreas, Baltimore, 1980, Williams & Wilkins.

53. Karasawa, E, et al: CT pancreatogram in carcinoma of the pancreas and chronic pancreatitis, Radiology 148:489, 1983.

54. Kent, RB, van Heerden, JA, and Weiland, LH: Nonfunctioning islet cell tumors, Ann Surg 193:185, 1985.

55. Kim, SY, Lim, JH, and Lee, JD: Papillary carcinoma of the pancreas: findings of US and CT, Radiology 154:338, 1985.

56. Krudy, AG, et al: Localization of islet cell tumors by dynamic CT: comparison with plain CT, arteriography, sonography, and venous sampling, AJR 143:585, 1984.

57. Laing, FC, et al: Biliary dilatation: defining the level and cause by real-time US, Radiology 160:39, 1986.

58. Mack, E: Clinical aspects of pancreatic disease, Semin Ultrasound 1:166, 1980.

59. Mackie, CR, et al: Prospective evaluation of angiography in the diagnosis of patients suspected of having pancreatic cancer, Ann Surg 189:11, 1979.

60. MacMahon, H, Bowie, JD, and Beezhold, C: Erect scanning of pancreas using a gastric window, AJR 132:587, 1979.

61. Malagelada, JR: Pancreatic cancer: an overview of epidemiology, clinical presentation, and diagnosis, Mayo Clin Proc 54:459, 1979.

62. Margulis, AR: Neoplasms of the pancreas. In Margulis, AR, and Burhenne, HJ, editors: Alimentary tract roentgenology, vol 2, ed 2, St. Louis, 1978, The CV Mosby Co.

63. Mathieu, D, et al: Correlation between imaging and pathologic study in cystic pancreatic neoplasms. Scientific exhibit presented at the 73rd Scientific Assemble and Annual Meeting of the Radiological Society of North America, Chicago, Nov 29 to Dec 4, 1987.

64. McCarthy, S, and Moss, AA: The use of a flow rate injector for contrast-enhanced computed tomography, Radiology 151:800, 1984.

65. Megibow, AJ, et al: Thickening of the celiac axis and/or superior mesenteric artery: a sign of pancreatic carcinoma on computed tomography, Radiology 141:449, 1981.

66. Mills, SR, et al: Evaluation of angiography in Zollinger-Ellison syndrome, Radiology 131:317, 1979.

67. Mitty, HA, Efemidis, SC, and Yeh, HS: Impact of fine-needle biopsy on management of patients with carcinoma of the pancreas, AJR 137:1119, 1981.

68. Modlin, IM: Collective reviews: endocrine tumors of the pancreas, Surg Gynecol Obstet 149:751, 1979.

69. Moosa, AR, Lewis, MH, and Mackie, CR: Surgical treatment of pancreatic cancer, Mayo Clin Proc 54:468, 1979.

70. Moss, AA, et al: The combined use of computed tomography and endoscopic retrograde cholangiopancreatography in the assessment of suspected pancreatic neoplasm: a blind clinical evaluation, Radiology 134:159, 1980.

71. Neff, CC, et al: Inflammatory pancreatic masses: problems in differentiating focal pancreatitis from carcinoma, Radiology 150:35, 1984.

72. Ormson, MJ, Charboneau, JW, and Stephens, DH: Sonography in patients with a possible pancreatic mass shown on CT, AJR 148:551, 1987.

73. Otto, R, and Deyhle, P: Guided puncture under real-time sonographic control, Radiology 134:784, 1980.

74. Pandolfo, I, et al: Cystic lymphangioma of the pancreas: CT demonstration, J Comput Assist Tomogr 9:209, 1985.

75. Pearse, AGE: Cytochemical and ultrastructure of polypeptide producing cells of the APUD series, and the embryologic, physiologic and pathologic implications of the concept, J Histochem Cystochem 17:303, 1969.

76. Pistolesi, GF, et al: Angiographic diagnosis of endocrine tumors of the pancreas, Radiol Clin (Basel) 46:401, 1977.

77. Plumley, TF, et al: Double duct sign: reassessed significance in ERCP, AJR 138:31, 1982.

78. Price, J, et al: Uptake of ^{99m}Tc-methylene diphosphonate by pancreatic insulinoma, AJR 149:69, 1987.

79. Radin, DR, et al: Pancreatic acinar cell carcinoma with subcutaneous and intraosseous fat necrosis, Radiology 158:67, 1986.

80. Rallis, PW, et al: Endoscopic retrograde cholangiopancreatography (ERCP) in pancreatic disease, Radiology 134:347, 1980.

81. Raptopoulos, V, et al: Fat-density oral contrast agent for abdominal CT, Radiology 164:653, 1987.

82. Reuter, SR: Superselective pancreatic angiography, Radiology 92:74, 1969.

83. Roberts, L, Jr, et al: Somatostatinoma of the endocrine pancreas: CT findings, J Comput Assist Tomgr 8:1015, 1984.

84. Roche, A, Raisonnier, A, and Gillon-Savouret, MC: Pancreatic venous sampling and arteriography in localizing insulinomas and gastrinomas: procedure and results in 55 cases, Radiology 145:621, 182.

85. Rohrmann, CA, Jr, Silvis, SE, and Vennes, JA: The significance of pancreatic ductal obstruction in differential diagnosis of the abnormal endoscopic retrograde pancreatogram, Radiology 121:311, 1976.

86. Rosch, J, and Grollman, JR: Superselective arteriography in the diagnosis of abdominal pathology: technical considerations, Radiology 92:1008, 1969.

87. Rossi, A, et al: CT of functioning tumors of the pancreas, AJR 144:57, 1985.

88. Rumancik, WM, et al: Metastatic disease to the pancreas: evaluation by computed tomography, J Assist Comput Tomogr 8:829, 1984.

89. Sheedy, PF, II, et al: Computed tomography of the body: initial clinical trial with the EMI prototype, Am J Roentgenol 127:23, 1976.

90. Silverberg, E, and Lubera, J: Cancer statistics, CA 37:2, 1987.

91. Silvis, SE, Rohrmann, CA, and Vennes, JA: Diagnostic criteria for evaluation of the endoscopic pancreatogram, Gastrointest Endosc 20:51, 1973.

92. Soulen, MC, et al: Pancreas divisum: CT scanning and ERCP correlation. Paper presented at the 72nd Scientific Assemble and Annual Meeting of the Radiological Society of North America, Chicago, Nov 30 to Dec 5, 1986.

93. Stark, DD, et al: CT of pancreatic islet cell tumors, Radiology 150:491, 1984.

94. Stark, DD, et al: Magnetic resonance and CT of the normal and diseased pancreas: a comparative study, Radiology 150:153, 1984.

95. Stefanini, P, et al: Beta-islet cell tumors of the pancreas: results of a study on 1067 cases, Surgery 75:597, 1974.

96. Steiner, E, et al: MR imaging of pancreatic carcinoma: comparison with CT. Paper presented at the 73rd Scientific Assembly and Annual Meeting of the Radiological Society of North America, Chicago, Nov 29 to Dec 4, 1987.

97. Stephens, DH, et al: Computed tomography of the liver, AJR 128:579, 1977.

98. Sundaram, M, et al: Utility of CT-guided abdominal aspiration procedures, AJR 139:1111, 1982.

99. Taylor, KJW, et al: Ultrasonographic scanning of the pancreas: prospective study of clinical results, Radiology 138:211, 1981.

100. Teefey, SA, Stephens, DH, and Sheedy, PF, II: CT appearance of primary pancreatic lymphoma, Gastrointest Radiol 11:41, 1986.

101. Thomas, ML, Lamb, GHR, and Barraclough, MA: Angiographic demonstration of a pancreatic "vipoma" in the WDHA syndrome, Am J Roentgenol 127:1037, 1976.

102. Tscholakoff, D, et al: MR imaging in the diagnosis of pancreatic disease, AJR 148:703, 1987.

103. Ward, EM, Stephens, DH, and Sheedy, PF, II: Computed tomographic characteristics of pancreatic carcinoma: an analysis of 100 cases, Radiographics 3:547, 1983.

104. Weinstein, DP, and Weinstein, BJ: Ultrasonic demonstration of the pancreatic duct: an analysis of 41 cases, Radiology 130:729, 1979.

105. Weinstein, DP, Wolfman, NT, and Weinstein, BJ: Ultrasonic characteristics of pancreatic tumors, Gastrointestinal Radiol 4:245, 1979.

106. Wittenberg, J, et al: Non-focal enlargement in pancreatic carcinoma, Radiology 144:131, 1982.

107. Wolfman, NT, Karstaedt, N, and Kawamoto, EH: Pleomorphic carcinoma of the pancreas: computed-tomographic, sonographic, and pathologic findings, Radiology 154:329, 1985.

108. Wolfman, NT, et al: Cystic neoplasms of the pancreas: CT and sonography, AJR 138:37, 1982.

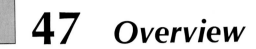

47 *Overview*

DAVID K.B. LI

In the past decade, unprecedented technologic innovations in imaging have changed the diagnostic approach to the pancreas, and in some instances altered the method of therapy.[8] Pancreatic imaging has advanced rapidly as indirect methods such as barium examination and angiography have been supplanted by direct methods such as computed tomography (CT) and ultrasound (US). These imaging methods, coupled with advances in catheter and needle techniques, have extended the radiologist's professional expertise into the area of biopsy and therapy. In the jaundiced patient with incurable pancreatic cancer, percutaneous methods of internal drainage can now be used as an alternative method to surgical bypass procedures. An exploratory laparotomy to document incurable carcinoma of the pancreatic body or tail can be replaced by radiologically guided percutaneous biopsy. Patients with pseudocysts or abscesses may undergo radiologically guided percutaneous drainage as a definitive therapeutic procedure.

IMAGING MODALITIES

A variety of methods to image the pancreas are now available and have been described in greater detail in the preceding chapters. US and CT are now the most widely used techniques because of their ability to directly visualize the pancreas in cross-sections noninvasively.[33,48,53] They permit assessment not only of the pancreas but also of contiguous organs and anatomic compartments. Though CT is now commonly available, US is undoubtedly more widespread in its distribution and more accessible than CT. US is also portable. No known risks are associated with US, whereas CT adds to a patient's radiation exposure and carries the small but additional risk attending the use of intravenous contrast. A major limitation of US is the ability of sound waves to penetrate bowel gas, bone, and excessive fat. Attention to technical details, such as distending the stomach and duodenum with fluid to provide a US window and scanning in multiple positions, can overcome some of these difficulties.[3] Nevertheless, a technically unsatisfactory examination occurs in between 10% and 15% of patients. Though CT is more expensive, of slightly greater risk, and more limited in the planes of examination available, it does overcome many of the drawbacks of US. The examinations are less operator dependent. With current CT scanners and careful attention to oral contrast administration and bolus injection of intravenous contrast, technically unsatisfactory examinations are very uncommon, even in thin patients.[41] The ability to examine all pancreatic segments with equal precision permits a high examiner confidence level, particularly with a normal examination. Most radiologists now agree that if the patient's symptoms are clearly related to the pancreas, CT is the imaging method of choice, with the exception of children and pregnant patients.[25] The complementary role of CT and US has been discussed in other chapters. Perhaps not as well recognized, and worth repeating, is the value of a limited real-time US examination to evaluate an inconclusive CT finding resulting from either a subtle pancreatic mass or a normal variation in pancreatic configuration. The demonstration of a normal echo pattern in the region of concern relative to the adjacent pancreatic tissue can be extremely helpful in excluding pathologic conditions.[39]

Magnetic resonance imaging (MRI) is the newest imaging technique to be applied to the pancreas. Initial image quality has been restricted by poor spatial resolution, suboptimal image contrast, motion artifacts, and lack of a satisfactory gastrointestinal contrast agent.[47] Neither has the potential for in vivo tissue characterization been realized. It is hoped, however, that recent improvements in technology including the use of fast imaging methods, motion artifact suppression techniques, intravenous contrast, and the development of an adequate gastrointestinal contrast agent may lead to advances in this area. A major advantage of MRI is its ability to image the peripancreatic blood vessels without the use of intravenous contrast and the potential to demonstrate tumor invasion.[50] Other advantages include the lack of ionizing radiation, the ability to produce images in multiple planes, and the production of images that are free of artifactual degradation from metallic clips in postoperative patients.

Pancreatic angiography, endoscopic retrograde cholangiopancreatography (ERCP),[10,36] percutaneous transhepatic cholangiography[37] (PTC) and percutaneous pancreatic ductography[31] (PPD) are all invasive procedures with low, but defined risks. These tests are more limited than the cross-sectional techniques because they are organ specific, restricted either to the blood vessels or biliary or pancreatic ducts.[18] These examinations require special equipment, which limits their availability, and they all require well-developed operator expertise.

Conventional examinations such as plain films, barium examinations, and intravenous cholangiography have all declined in importance in the primary evaluation of the pancreas. Radionuclide scanning with ^{75}Se-seleno

methionine now has little practical importance and is rarely if ever used.[32] Positron emission tomography (PET) offers the potential for assessing the biologic activity of the gland. It remains, however, in the investigational stage, and no consistent role either in elucidating disease processes or in clinical practice has yet emerged.[4]

CLINICAL PANCREATIC IMAGING

Advances in imaging make it difficult for referring physicians to appreciate fully the efficacy and limitations of the numerous radiologic procedures available. The use of algorithms or flow charts has recently been popularized. The suggested approach, however, may not be the most applicable one for every institution. It is subject to the limitations and availability of equipment and the experience and expertise of the physicians involved.[17] The radiologist has a role as a consultant to discuss the clinical problem with the referring physician and then to decide on the most expeditious and cost-effective method or combination of procedures to provide the most specific answers to the clinicians' questions.

Acute pancreatitis

The diagnosis of acute pancreatitis is based on the appropriate clinical history and findings, confirmed by simple laboratory tests. When the presentation is atypical or confusing, diagnostic imaging studies may be necessary. In the uncomplicated and mild cases, acute pancreatitis may not produce any contour alterations, and only subtle textural alterations may be appreciated on US. Though early pancreatitis may not be demonstrated by CT, it is still the preferred method for the initial evaluation of acute pancreatitis where the clinical presentation is atypical or confusing. This is because of the high frequency of indeterminate examinations in critically ill patients, caused by the inability to image the entire gland and peripancreatic spaces because of intestinal ileus.[26,45] More recently it has been recommended that CT be performed on all patients with moderate or severe clinical forms of pancreatitis to evaluate the presence and severity of the initial attack and as a prognostic indicator of morbidity and mortality.[1] One of the most important roles of radiology is the diagnosis and in some cases treatment[51] of the complications of acute pancreatitis, including pancreatic and extrapancreatic fluid collection,[44,49] pancreatic phlegmon,[54] abscess,[13] necrosis,[56] and hemorrhage.[5,52,55]

Jaundice

The purpose of imaging in patients with jaundice includes determining if biliary tract obstruction is present, the etiology of the biliary obstruction, the site and location of the obstructing lesion, and the choice of therapy, whether surgical, radiologic, or endoscopic.[16] The ability of ultrasound to delineate both intrahepatic and extrahepatic bile duct dilatation is well documented.[9] Though CT may have slightly better diagnostic specificity in determining the site and etiology of obstruction,[2] most agree that US is the primary procedure of choice in patients with jaundice because of its equal sensitivity, greater speed of performance, and lower cost.[21,29] CT is reserved only when the initial US is equivocal and more confidence is required before proceeding to direct cholangiography.

The next diagnostic procedure in the evaluation of jaundice patients after US is direct cholangiography. PTC is now widely used and has a low complication rate. In institutions where the expertise is available, ERCP is an alternative method for direct visualization of the bile ducts. It has the added advantage of evaluation of the pancreatic ducts. Both PTC and ERCP can provide a precise definition of the site and cause of the obstructing lesion.[35] PTC and ERCP are also essential preliminary procedures before any interventional procedure, whether surgical or radiologic.[15,30,34] Both methods also permit the diagnosis of conditions such as choledocholithiasis, papillary stenosis, and sclerosing cholangitis, which may produce obstruction in the presence of nondilated bile ducts.

ABDOMINAL PAIN

Patients with carcinoma of the pancreas and chronic pancreatitis may present with abdominal pain, which becomes unremitting as the disease progresses. Earlier symptoms such as fatigue, weakness, weight loss, and nausea may be sufficiently vague that the patient does not consult a physician until pain is experienced. Because of its lower cost and ready availability and because it is the preferred test for evaluating the gallbladder, US is commonly the first procedure performed and often uncovers unsuspected pancreatic disease.[6] CT, however, is considered the imaging method of choice for the pancreas because of its extremely low rate of technically unsatisfactory examination, higher confidence level in a negative examination, improved ability to stage tumor extension,[19] and sensitivity in detecting smaller areas of calcification in chronic pancreatitis.[14] However, masses discovered in the pancreas by CT and US are not sufficiently distinctive to allow definitive histologic diagnosis. Focal inflammatory masses are indistinguishable from tumor.[38] The diagnosis of malignancy may be suggested by the identification of liver metastasis and periaortic lymphadenopathy. Definitive diagnosis, however, commonly requires a fine-needle aspiration biopsy.[24]

When a dilated pancreatic duct is seen on either CT or US and a mass is not identified, direct delineation of duct morphology, either by ERCP or PPD,[31] may be helpful for diagnosis and therapy planning. Pancreatic ductography can also be combined with fine-needle aspiration biopsy.

Angiography has little to contribute in the diagnosis of adenocarcinoma. Occasionally, it has been used in the staging of small carcinomas and in the determination of resectability. Unfortunately, patients rarely present for diagnosis at a stage when the carcinoma is surgically curable. The new imaging techniques have not significantly changed the survival of a patient with carcinoma of the pancreas.[27] The principal reason for this poor prognosis is not any limitation of the imaging techniques but that patients present relatively late in the course of the disease.

Pancreatic insufficiency

The clinical diagnosis of pancreatic insufficiency may be difficult. Manifestations of exocrine pancreatic insufficiency include weight loss, diarrhea, steatorrhea, bloating, and abdominal pain. Diabetes, the result of endocrine pancreatic insufficiency, may be associated. Once the diagnosis has been suggested by laboratory tests and confirmed by a favorable response to oral pancreatic enzyme replacement therapy, a cause for pancreatic insufficiency should be sought. CT plays a key role in identifying causes such as obstruction of the pancreatic outflow resulting from tumor or stone, atrophy of the pancreas, or absence of pancreatic tissue.[43] ERCP may be helpful if CT is negative.

ENDOCRINOLOGIC SYNDROMES

Hormone-secreting islet cell tumors often cause symptoms when the primary tumor is small. Hormones that are hypersecreted include insulin, gastrin, vasoactive intestinal peptide, glucagon, and somatostatin. Because the diagnosis of functioning islet cell tumors is usually established on the basis of clinical and laboratory findings, the challenge for radiology is the preoperative assessment of the location, extent and number of tumors and the presence or absence of metastasis.[28] With a success rate between 60% and 70% for insulinoma, real-time US is the initial localizing procedure in some institutions.[22,23] Though the results with earlier CT scanners were discouraging,[11,12,46] detection rates have improved by use of current scanners, with rapid sequential scanning and multiple bolus injection of intravenous contrast.[41,42] Recent results approach the accuracy of angiography. The combination of superselective pancreatic arteriography and pancreatic venous sampling[7,40] remains the gold standard for preoperative localization: however, the procedure is invasive, technically difficult, and time consuming and therefore not widely available.[20] More recently, intraoperative high-frequency ultrasound has been used with success.[22] It is able to reveal intrapancreatic tumors so small that they cannot be detected even by direct palpation of the gland.

Epigastric mass

A clinically palpable epigastric mass may be explained by nonneoplastic causes such as an aortic aneurysm or a prominent but normal left lobe of the liver. These abnormalities, as well as other cystic solid masses, are easily imaged by US. CT, however, can be extremely useful in suggesting the organ from which the mass may have originated by virtue of its exquisite demonstration of anatomy.[33] This has some importance in prognosis because, for example, an adenocarcinoma arising from the pancreas has a different prognosis from one arising from the kidney or adrenal gland. In general, masses that lie anterior to the splenic vessels are pancreatic or gastric in origin. Masses posterior to the splenic vein are extrapancreatic and may arise from the kidney, adrenal gland, or other retroperitoneal structures. Exceptions to this rule have been reported but are rare. Often the pancreas may be clearly identified and seen to be displaced or separated distinctly by a fat plane from an extrapancreatic mass.

REFERENCES

1. Balthazar, EJ, et al: Acute pancreatitis: prognostic value of CT, Radiology 156:767, 1985.
2. Baron, RL, et al: Computed tomographic features of biliary obstruction, AJR 140:1173, 1983.
3. Bowie, JD, and MacMahon, H: Improved techniques in pancreatic sonography, Semin Ultrasound 1:170, 1980.
4. Buonocore, E, and Huber, KF: Positron-emission computed tomography of the pancreas: a preliminary study, Radiology 133:195, 1979.
5. Burke, JW, et al: Pseudoaneurysms complicating pancreatitis: detection by CT, Radiology 161:447, 1986.
6. Campbell, JP, and Wilson, SR: Pancreatic neoplasms: how useful is evaluation with US? Radiology 167:341, 1988.
7. Cho, KJ, et al: Localization of the source of hyperinsulinism: percutaneous transhepatic, portal and pancreatic vein catheterization with hormone assay, AJR 139:237, 1982.
8. Clark, LR, et al: Pancreatic imaging, Radiol Clin North Am 23:489, 1985.
9. Cooperberg, PL, et al: Accuracy of common hepatic duct size in the evaluation of extrahepatic biliary obstruction, Radiology 135:141, 1980.
10. Cotton, PB, et al: Gray-scale ultrasonography and endoscopic pancreatography in pancreatic diagnosis, Radiology 134:453, 1980.
11. Dunnick, NR, et al: Computed tomographic detection of nonbeta pancreatic islet cell tumors, Radiology 135:117, 1980.
12. Dunnick, NR, et al: Localizing insulinomas with combined radiographic methods, AJR 135:747, 1980.
13. Federle, MP, et al: Computed tomography of pancreatic abscess, AJR 136:179, 1981.
14. Ferrucci, J, Jr, et al: Computed body tomography in chronic pancreatitis, Radiology 130:175, 1979.
15. Ferrucci, JT, Jr, et al: Interventional radiology of the biliary tract, Gastroenterology 82:974, 1982.
16. Ferrucci, JT, Jr, et al: Advances in the radiology of jaundice: a symposium and review, AJR 141:1, 1983.
17. Foley, WD, et al: Computed tomography, ultrasonography, and endoscopic retrograde cholangiopancreatography in the diagnosis of pancreatic disease: a comparative study, Gastrointest Radiol 5:29, 1980.
18. Freeny, PC, et al: Impact of high-resolution computed tomography on utilization of ERCP and angiography, Radiology 142:35, 1982.
19. Freeny, PC, et al: Pancreatic ductal adenocarcinoma: diagnosis and staging with dynamic CT, Radiology 166:125, 1988.
20. Fulton, RE, et al: Preoperative localization of insulin producing tumors of the pancreas, AJR 123:367, 1975.
21. Gibson, RN, et al: Bile duct obstruction: radiologic evaluation of level, cause and tumor resectability, Radiology 160:43, 1986.
22. Gorman, B, et al: Benign pancreatic insulinoma: preoperative and intraoperative sonographic localization, AJR 147:929, 1986.
23. Gunther, RW, et al: Islet-cell tumors: detection of small lesions with computed tomography and ultrasound, Radiology 148:485, 1983.
24. Hall-Craggs, MA, and Lees, WR: Fine-needle aspiration biopsy: pancreatic and biliary tumors, AJR 147:399, 1986.
25. Hessel, SJ, et al: A prospective evaluation of computed tomography and ultrasound of the pancreas, Radiology 143:129, 1982.
26. Jeffrey, RB, Laing, FC, and Wing, VW: Extrapancreatic spread of acute pancreatitis: new observations with real-time US, Radiology 159:707, 1986.
27. Kairaluoma, MI, et al: Impact of new imaging techniques on survival in cancer of the head of the pancreas and the periampullary region, Acta Chir Scand 151:69, 1985.
28. Krudy, AG, et al: Localization of islet cell tumors by dynamic CT: comparison with plain CT, arteriography, sonography and venous sampling, AJR 143:585, 1984.
29. Laing, FC, et al: Biliary dilatation: defining the level and cause by real-time US, Radiology 160:39, 1986.
30. Lammer, J, and Neumayer, K: Biliary drainage endoprosthesis: experience with 201 placements, Radiology 159:625, 1986.
31. Lees, WR, and Heron, CW: US-guided percutaneous pancreatography: experience in 75 patients, Radiology 165:809, 1987.
32. Li, DKB: Pancreas: nuclear medicine. In Margulis, AR and Burhenne, HJ, editors: Alimentary tract radiology, ed 3, St. Louis, 1983, The CV Mosby Co.
33. Li, DKB: Pancreas: computed tomography. In Margulis, AR, and Burhenne, HJ, editors: Alimentary tract radiology, ed 3, St. Louis, 1983, The CV Mosby Co.
34. Marks, WM, et al: Endoscopic retrograde biliary drainage, Radiology 152:357, 1984.
35. Matzen, P, et al: Accuracy of direct cholangiography by endoscopic or transhepatic route in jaundice: a prospective study, Gastroenterology 81:237, 1981.
36. Moss, AA, et al: Combined use of computed tomography and endoscopic retrograde cholangiopancreatography in the assessment of suspected pancreatic neoplasm: a blind clinical evaluation, Radiology 134:159, 1980.
37. Mueller, PR, et al: Fine-needle transhepatic cholangiography: reflections after 450 cases, AJR 136:85, 1981.
38. Neff, CC, et al: Inflammatory pancreatic masses: problems in differentiating focal pancreatitis from carcinoma, Radiology 150:35, 1984.
39. Ormson, MJ, Charboneau, JW, and Stephens, DH: Sonography in patients with a possible pancreatic mass shown on CT, AJR 148:551, 1987.
40. Roche, A, et al: Pancreatic venous sampling and arteriography in localizing insulinomas and gastrinomas: procedure and results in 55 cases, Radiology 145:621, 1982.

41. Rossi, P, et al: Multiple bolus technique vs. single bolus or infusion of contrast medium to obtain prolonged contrast enhancement of the pancreas, Radiology 144:929, 1982.

42. Rossi, P, et al: CT of functioning tumors of the pancreas, AJR 144:57, 1985.

43. Shuman, WP, et al: Pancreatic insufficiency: role of CT evaluation, Radiology 158:625, 1986.

44. Siegelman, SS, et al: CT of fluid collections associated with pancreatitis, AJR 134:1121, 1980.

45. Silverstein, W, et al: Diagnostic imaging of acute pancreatitis: prospective diagnosis using CT and sonography, AJR 137:497, 1981.

46. Stark, DD, et al: CT of pancreatic islet cell tumors, Radiology 150:491, 1984.

47. Stark, DD, et al: Magnetic resonance and CT of the normal and diseased pancreas: a comparative study, Radiology 150:491, 1984.

48. Taylor, KJW, et al: Ultrasonographic scanning of the pancreas: prospective study of clinical results, Radiology 138:211, 1981.

49. Torres, WE, et al: Percutaneous aspiration and drainage of pancreatic pseudocysts, AJR 147:1007, 1986.

50. Tscholakoff, D, et al: MR imaging in the diagnosis of pancreatic disease, AJR 148:703, 1987.

51. vanSonnenberg, E, et al: Complicated pancreatic inflammatory disease: diagnostic and therapeutic role of interventional radiology, Radiology 155:335, 1985.

52. Walter, JF, Chuang, VP, and Bookstein, JJ: Angiography of massive hemorrhage secondary to pancreatic disease, Radiology 124:337, 1977.

53. Ward, EM, Stephens, DH, and Sheedy, PF: Computed tomographic characteristics of pancreatic carcinoma: an analysis of 100 cases, RadioGraphics 3:547, 1983.

54. Warshaw, AL: Inflammatory masses following acute pancreatitis, Surg Clin North Am 54:621, 1974.

55. White, AF, Barum, S, and Buranasiri, S: Aneurysms secondary to pancreatitis, AJR 127:393, 1976.

56. White, EM, et al: Pancreatic necrosis: CT manifestations, Radiology 158:343, 1986.

PART X

LIVER AND BILIARY TRACT

48 *Pathology*

EDWARD A. SMUCKLER
HARLAN J. SPJUT

DISEASES THAT AFFECT THE LIVER
  Newborn period
  Childhood and adolescence
  Adulthood

The liver is a complex organ noted for the diversity of its functions, the admixture of its cell types, and the dual vascular supply. The principal functions of the liver are carried out by the parenchymal cells, which in the adult constitute roughly 90% of the liver's volume but only 70% of its total number of cells. These cells form plasma proteins and clotting factors and participate in lipid and carbohydrate metabolism. Two other functions of these parenchymal cells are the secretion of specific bile salts to aid in digestion and the excretion of other molecules harmful to the organism. This particular function also includes a distinct secretory-excretory pathway formed initially by the walls of the hepatic cells (the bile canaliculi), then by parenchymal cells modified for duct function, and finally by a ductal system and a storage reservoir, the gallbladder. The liver is abundantly supplied by both the portal vein drawing blood from the intestinal tract and by the hepatic artery supplying as much as 20% of the total blood flow to the liver. The complex organ structure is supported by a fibrous network that contains both the major secretory-excretory ducts, the vasular supply, and the lymphatics.[12]

It is important to recall that there are changes in both structure and function of the liver that occur with age. The neonatal liver lacks many of the putative "luxury" functions seen in the adult; these are acquired in time during childhood and adolescence. Similarly, the liver changes in structure during the same period, enlarging and remodeling. The adult liver is subject to environmental and hormonal factors significantly altering its function and specific intracellular structure. Also, there is remarkable regenerating capacity of this organ.[7]

DISEASES THAT AFFECT THE LIVER

Diseases that affect the liver include inborn errors of metabolism, direct toxic effects, nutritional disorders, and infectious diseases. The expression of these diseases varies with the age of the individual and, to an extent, with the geographic origin of the patient. The particular disease must be taken in context with the regenerative capacity of the liver. Some injuries heal without scarring (for example, most acute hepatitis), and in some the pattern of the disease is really the result of the aberrant scarring regenerative pattern. The latter is best exemplified by cirrhosis. The abundant vascular supply to the liver also makes it a secondary catching site for both cellular and macromolecular complexes within the circulation; metastases to liver from the colon are common. The abundant cellular element lining the sinusoids provides one of the richest sources of the reticuloendothelial system within the body. Collections of debris, immune complexes, and macromolecules by these cells are readily identified and even mark this cell population, as in hemosiderosis.[38] The use of Thorotrast and the phagocytic activity of these cells have resulted in a number of radiation-induced liver diseases and cancer.[31]

The following discussion of diseases of the liver is divided into life periods of affected individuals.

Newborn period

Liver diseases that manifest most frequently during the newborn period include errors of development and inborn errors of metabolism. Infectious disease affecting the liver of the newborn should not be overlooked.

Errors of development

Embryologically the liver develops as an outgrowth of a bud of the primitive GI tract. The development of both the parenchyma and the excretory-secretory system from this bud takes place during early fetal life. It has been suggested that maldevelopment can occur with failures to maintain the continuity of the connection between the parenchymal aspect of the liver and the GI tract— the biliary duct system. These are referred to as biliary atresias and have been separated into intrahepatic biliary atresia, in which there is failure of formation of the biliary radicals within the liver, and extrahepatic biliary atresia, in which the duct connecting the liver to the gut fails to develop at all, or fails to develop normally.[39] The former is associated with an absence of bile ducts seen histologically, the latter with a distorted or absent extrahepatic duct system. Under these circumstances accumulation of excretory products including bilirubin occurs early in the newborn period. Significant interest in detection of this modification early during newborn life is prompted by the potential therapeutic modification of the disease.[16] Both surgical intervention and radiologic assay of the integrity of the duct system is of prime importance. It should be noted, however, that there is some disagreement concerning the development of this disease. One school of thought suggests that failure of the parenchymal cells to produce secretory products and therefore provide

the developmental stimulus for these ducts may underlie the disease. It remains, however, that in a large number of cases histologic evidence of malformation and maldevelopment of the extrahepatic ducts is apparent.

Inborn errors of metabolism

Inborn errors of metabolism, specifically storage diseases, appear in the newborn period, when the fetus can no longer depend on the maternal circulation for homeostasis. These are frequently associated with liver enlargement and with the deposition within hepatic parenchymal cells of the products of the abnormal intracellular enzymatic environment. Notable among these are the glycogen storage diseases and to a lesser extent mucolipidoses and mucopolysaccharidoses. Glycogen storage can accommodate within the cell sap or within specific organelles (lysosomes). The latter two diseases are most frequently associated with single membrane–limited body storage seen by electron microscopy. These livers enlarge, and some increased fibrosis may occur. These change the density of the liver cell to radiation. Radiodensity assays for assessment of the basis of liver enlargement have been made by computer-assisted tomography. A specific disease of alpha$_1$-antitrypsin deficiency is mentioned later.

Infection

The newborn liver is subject to infection most commonly by viral organisms. The compromised immunologic status of the newborn permits opportunistic viral pathogens, including the cytomegaloviruses and herpesviruses, to produce parenchymal disease. In these instances the target is the parenchymal cell. Disruption of the cells with the appearance of dead cells and a modification of function in other sublethally infected cells results in jaundice, in cell death, and in an inflammatory exudate consisting primarily of lymphocytes and plasma cells with a relative absence of polymorphonuclear leukocytes. This infection affects both the lobule and the portal areas.[19] One unique feature of the newborn liver is the appearance of cells with multiple nuclei. This specific response seems unique in the newborn period, and it is not clear whether this represents fusion of parenchymal cells or cytokinesis without mitosis. With recovery, complete healing can occur. Prenatal viral infections of the liver are recognized. With severe infection a disordered structure follows that may evolve to cirrhosis.

The fetal and newborn liver is the site of extramedullary hematopoiesis. In those specific diseases (associated with decreased or altered red blood cell formation, including erythroblastosis) the presence and increased quantities of hematopoietic elements within the liver can be noted.

Childhood and adolescence

The predominant modifications seen during childhood and adolescence include inborn errors of metabolism, infection, and neoplastic infiltrations.

The inborn errors of metabolism frequently become accentuated as development occurs. These include glycogen storage diseases, mucolipidosis, and mucopolysaccharide storage alterations mentioned above. In all instances hepatic enlargement is predominant, principally because of an enlargement of the individual parenchymal cells. Most marked histologic alterations occur primarily in parenchymal cells; however, in several of the mucolipidoses, the endothelial lining cells may also show significant deposition of these macromolecules. The predominant clinical feature of the disease is related to the defect in enzyme function, and although the liver is enlarged it frequently is functional.

A specific disease frequently noted in childhood and adolescence period is alpha$_1$-antitrypsin deficiency.[10] In this specific instance the failure to form an alpha$_1$-antitrypsin agent and secrete it into the circulation is believed to underlie the alteration. The particular modifications in the liver, however, are not explicable simply on this basis. Notably there is an increase in fibrosis from portal area to portal area, trapping groups of liver cells. Those parenchymal elements that are most adjacent to these fibrous septa and portal areas frequently show rounded bodies in the cytoplasm that are PAS positive—diastase resistant, as revealed by special staining techniques. Ultrastructural analysis reveals them to be dilated portions of the endoplasmic reticulum containing inspissated alpha$_1$-antitrypsin protein material. This is a progressive disease, expressed primarily in the homozygous individual. Many may develop cirrhosis in young adulthood and a few may become victims of hepatocellular carcinoma.

Another unique disease of childhood and adolescence is Reye's syndrome.[29] This particular illness affects multiple organ systems, but specifically in the liver is associated with a deposition of lipid throughout the lobules in fine vesicular form. This latter change is considered a diagnostic feature of the illness. The disease also presents altered blood chemistry, coma, and is frequently associated with death. The liver is frequently enlarged because of the infiltration of fat. The individual liver cells contain lipid droplets; the nucleus is maintained in a centrocellular position; and the droplets rarely coalesce to form cysts. Of particular significance is the fact that the radiodensity of the liver is modified, and computer-assisted tomography has made suggestive diagnosis of diffuse lipid deposition. The cause of Reye's syndrome is not known: a specific modification of mitochondria occurs in parenchymal cells, but it also occurs in sinusoidal lining cells as well as in other parts of the body.

Infectious hepatitis occurs during childhood and adolescence. In this period most infectious diseases still are viral, and the classical alterations of infectious hepatitis occur. These are discussed subsequently.

Childhood is also associated with toxic liver injury caused by accidental ingestion of a variety of poisonous materials. The specific modifications of the liver depend on the age and the time sequence following the ingestion. Classically, toxic hepatitis is associated with a zonal injury of cells and a degeneration of those generally in the central lobular area. Also, in large part single episodes of sublethal ingestion are associated with complete healing.

Adulthood

During the adult period the most frequent hepatic diseases are infections caused by viral agents and by toxic or nutritional injury. Parasitic diseases have become increasingly important as immigrants arrive from countries in which parasitic diseases are common. Most nutritional disease in Western cultures is associated with alcohol imbibition. Altered healing resulting from either infection or nutritional agents can be associated with cirrhosis. The development of cancer, both as secondary seeding from distant sites and as primary hepatomas, occurs with significant frequency.

Infection

Viral hepatitis is the most common infectious hepatitis disease seen in the adult. There are at least four and potentially five viral etiologic agents; the most common are hepatitis A, hepatitis B, and the hepatitis of the non-A, non-B viral agent. The morphologic changes associated with the infections are identical grossly, and microscopically are indistinguishable. More recently immunocytochemical and electron microscopic evidence suggests that hepatitis A and B infections may be separated. This can also be accomplished by immunologic means using serum samples. This is important because hepatitis A is not associated with chronic disease, whereas B and potentially non-A, non-B may persist and produce an ongoing smoldering infection, ultimately leading to cirrhosis.

The first modification that occurs in the liver following infection is located in the parenchymal cells. The hallmark of the disease is liver cell death. Lack of selective permeability results in a shrunken, eosinophilic cell designated as acidophilic necrosis. In addition there is a diffuse infiltration of lymphocytes and plasma cells, but no neutrophils. This involves both the portal areas as well as the parenchymal zone. The loss of parenchymal cells is a stimulus for cellular division, and regeneration begins to occur almost immediately. This is noted as binucleate cells and cells in mitosis. The deposition of lipid in this disease is notably absent. With resolution, both the number of cells undergoing necrosis and those cells in mitosis decrease, and the inflammatory exudate disappears. Complete resolution restores the liver to normal structure.

The course of these diseases is usually a matter of weeks, at times months. In some instances, however, a smoldering ongoing infection occurs, designated chronic hepatitis. In the liver a persistence of cell death occurs within the lobule, and an inflammatory exudate of greater or lesser degree occurs in the portal tracts, spreading from the portal tracts to the lobules. The intensity of the exudate and frequency of cell death separate the disease into a spectrum, at one end designated chronic persistent hepatitis associated with a prolonged survival and at the other end designated as chronic active hepatitis that may be associated with the development of cirrhosis and death.

In these latter instances, the sequence of degeneration, with continued loss of parenchymal cells, regeneration, and the development of fibrous (collagen) tissue within the lobule, takes place.[34] In the classic chronic active hepatitis increased degrees of fibrosis occur within the portal area stretching from portal area to portal area, isolating lobules with an intact central vein and maintaining the relationship of the central vein to the portal area. The disease is progressive; fibrosis increases when continued impairment of circulation and excretory function takes place. These latter circumstances lead to further cell loss, regeneration, and fibrosis, resulting in cirrhosis.

In this disease in the initial part of the infection, the liver may be enlarged because of the presence of edema and the inflammatory exudate. Later the enlargement is persistent because of the increased fibrosis and the regenerative nodules, but distorted in structure. Finally, as the fibrosis persists, the number of liver cells decreases, and the liver decreases in size and becomes shrunken and hard. The pattern of formation of fibrosis is similar to that seen in alcohol-based cirrhosis, discussed subsequently.

There are several results of cirrhosis. Liver cells are not perfused because of vascular shunts between the portal and systemic venous system, reducing the effective parenchymal mass. This decreases effective hepatic func-

tion, resulting in decreased plasma proteins and detoxification mechanism. The individual liver cells have decreased "luxury" function because of the stimulus for regeneration.[33] The fibrosis increases resistance to blood flow, increasing portal venous pressure and resulting in splenic enlargement and portal systemic venous anastomoses. The latter includes eosphageal varices, whose rupture constitutes a significant cause of death in these individuals.

There are two other modifications of parenchymal structure that may be infectious in origin and related to chronic hepatitis. These are designated primary biliary cirrhosis[27] and chronic sclerosing cholangitis.[37] In the former, an apparent destructive mechanism is established in which there is alteration in the ductal elements in the intralobular bile ducts. The cells swell, become vacuolated, and are associated with an intense lymphocytic infiltration, frequently with germinal centers in the lymphoid aggregates. This disease is then associated with fibrosis and the formation of cirrhosis. Characteristically it occurs in women at midlife and is ushered in by itching, but without defined jaundice. In contrast, chronic sclerosing cholangitis occurs during the same period and initially is associated with a relative paucity of intralobular bile ducts seen in histologic section. At a later time there is increased fibrosis in the portal areas and in and about the bile ducts. Radiologically, this disease is characterized by a "beaded" appearance in retrograde cholangiography.

Nutritional and alcohol-based liver disease

There is little question that the association of large alcohol intake with degenerative liver disease is established throughout the world.[4,11] The mechanism whereby the alcohol and its attendant dietary indiscretion produces this disease is not known. The characteristic features of nutritional or alcohol-based liver disease includes the presence of fat within the hepatic parenchymal cells, the presence of cell loss with single shrunken acidophilic cells, the appearance of specific intracellular proteins—alcoholic hyaline—and the presence of neutrophils within these cells (Fig. 48-1). In the most severe form, alcoholic hepatitis, the liver is frequently enlarged and tender.

A fatty liver can be produced in association with dietary indiscretion in which the cells are massively filled with lipid (Fig. 48-2). The liver is enlarged and tense and frequently shows that altered density revealed by computer-assisted tomography. These are reversible changes, however, and abstinence is associated with resolution. Continued alcoholic indiscretion is associated with increased fibrosis and degeneration in regeneration

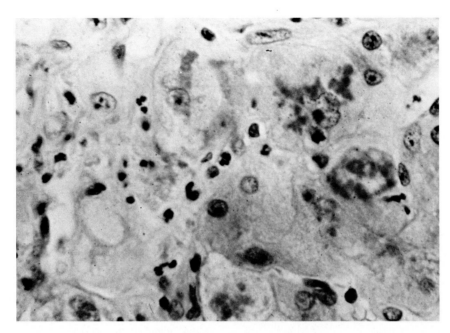

Fig. 48-1 Micrograph showing characteristic features of alcoholic hepatitis with both acute inflammation and intercellular, eosinophilic hyaline material, alcoholic hyaline. (×250.)

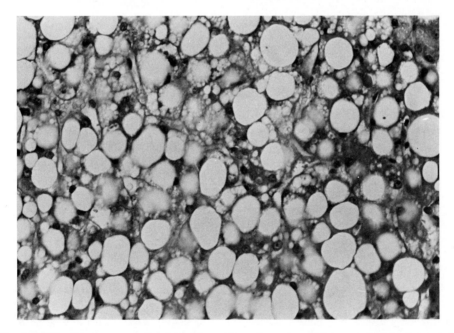

Fig. 48-2 Micrograph representing alcohol-based fatty change in which many cells have large cystic spaces filled with neutral lipid. (×100.)

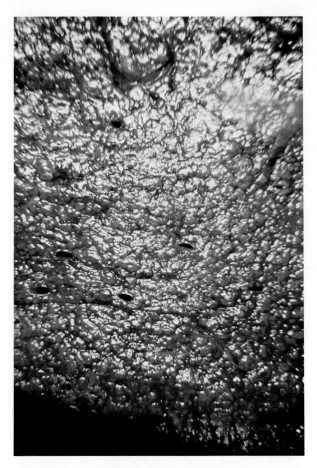

Fig. 48-3 Gross photograph showing finely nodular surface of cirrhotic liver, surface expression of fixed fibrous septa, and regenerative nodules.

associated with cirrhosis (Fig. 48-3). In these particular instances, however, the fibrosis affects the lobule itself, separating the structure into pseudolobules lacking the appropriate histologic relationship of the central vein in the portal area. This results in a marked distortion of vascular flow, with an increase in portal pressure and the development of venous collaterals within the esophagus, retroperitoneal space, hemorrhoidal plexus, and anterior abdominal wall.

Neoplastic disease

A number of benign tumors and tumorlike lesions occur in the liver. Among these are hemangiomas, bile duct adenomas, Meyenburg's complex, hepatic adenomas, diffuse nodular hyperplasia, and focal nodular hyperplasia. Hemangiomas are usually found incidentally during a laparotomy or autopsy. Rarely are they symptomatic, but intraabdominal bleeding may be seen. Likewise, bile duct adenomas are usually found incidentally and are small surface nodules, commonly solitary. Mey-

enburg's complex is a small conglomeration of dilated bile ducts, frequently in multiple areus.[8,15]

Nodular regenerative hyperplasia may or may not result in enlargement of the liver. There is diffuse fine nodularity of the liver, but the absence of associated fibrosis serves to distinguish it from cirrhosis. The lesion may be accompanied by splenomegaly, portal hypertension, and esophageal varices, among other things.[25] Adenomas in a number of patients are associated with steroid intake—often androgens or oral contraceptives.[22] Adenomas are most often solitary and may exceed 10 cm in diameter. There seems to be an increased incidence of hepatic adenomas related to the use of oral contraceptives. The women who take them are at risk of hemorrhage into or from the adenoma. Focal nodular hyperplasia (FNH) is grossly and histologically distinctive from hepatic adenoma (Fig. 48-4). The lesion is usually single but may present as multiple nodules; they are more common in women than in men and are not necessarily related to oral contraceptives.

FNH may vary in size from a few millimeters to more than 10 cm. Hepatic adenoma is distinguished from FNH in that adenoma is composed of parenchymal cells with little nuclear atypia, absence of bile ducts, and little or no fibrosis. FNH is a nodule in which bile ducts are found; fibrous septae that tend to radiate from a central scar are histologic highlights and separate FNH from hepatic adenoma with ease.[13,26]

Of primary malignant hepatic tumors hepatocellular carcinoma is the most common and receives considerable attention. In the United States, hepatocellular carcinoma arises in cirrhotic livers in about 75% of cases. Possible etiologic factors include hepatitis as related to HBsAg, aflatoxins, trypsonemia, alpha$_1$-antitrypsin deficiency, and hemochromatosis. Grossly hepatocellular carcinoma often presents as a single large mass but may be multinodular or even diffuse throughout the liver (Fig. 48-5). Several histologic types have been recognized: trabecular, clear cell, adenoid, syncytial, and fibrolamellar. The latter appears to have a better prognosis than do the other types.[5,9]

Cholangicellular carcinoma is a rare form of primary tumor that is often multinodular and by biopsy is difficult to distinguish from metastatic adenocarcinoma. A rare form of intrahepatic ductal carcinoma is bile duct cystadenocarcinoma. The tumor is demonstrable by ultrasonography and CT. It has a better prognosis than does cholangiocellular carcinoma.[35] Angiosarcomas occur in children as well as in adults. In the latter they have been associated with Thorotrast and exposure to vinyl chloride.[28]

Although hepatocellular carcinoma occurs occasionally in childhood, hepatoblastoma is for all practical pur-

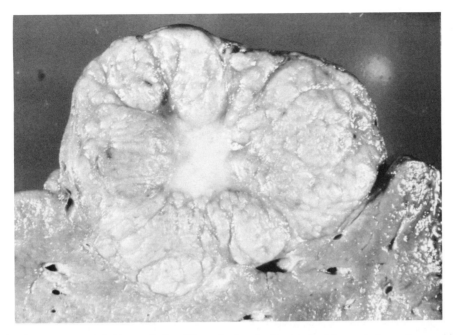

Fig. 48-4 Focal nodular hyperplasia of liver. Lesion is characterized by central scar (grey-white area) and tendency of fibrous bands to radiate from scar.

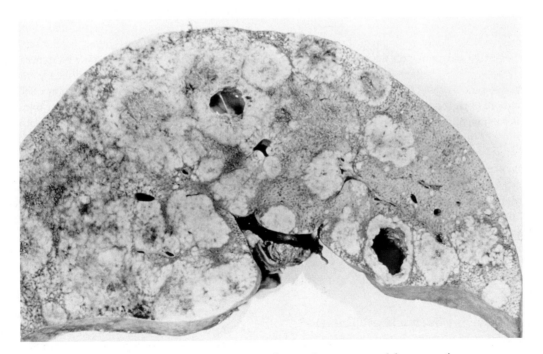

Fig. 48-5 Multifocal hepatocellular carcinoma. Some tumor nodules are cystic.

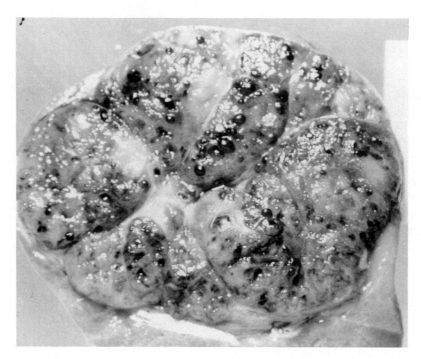

Fig. 48-6 Hepatoblastoma in child. Tumor was resected surgically and measured 5.5 cm in greatest dimension.

poses a tumor found exclusively in infants and children. It is a tumor composed dominantly of immature hepatocytes resembling embryonic or fetal liver. Mesenchymal components have been well characterized electron microscopically and immunohistochemically (Fig. 48-6).[1,14]

The liver is commonly involved with metastases; perhaps 50% or more of persons with metastatic tumors will have liver involvement. This is especially true of carcinomas arising in the large bowel, stomach, pancreas, and lung. Direct invasion also occurs from carcinomas of the gallbladder, stomach, and pancreas, for example.

Most benign and malignant neoplastic diseases are detectable by modern imaging techniques. Of equal importance is the anatomic delineation of the tumors and the detection of multiple tumors, since they relate to the chance of successful surgical resection. Even malignant tumors are resected with some expectancy of lengthy survival; this applies to selected metastases to the liver as well.[21,24]

Extrahepatic excretory ducts and gallbladder

Diseases of the duct system are not common; those of the gallbladder are more frequent. The storage of bile in the gallbladder and the modification of the relationship of water, salts, lipid, and proteins frequently are associated with a formation of a supersaturated solution in which crystallization occurs. This is especially frequent in instances in which there is increased pigment as a result of red blood cell lysis. The presence of this abnormal bile produces several changes within the wall of the gallbladder, including an acute and chronic inflammatory exudate, with a resultant resolution in fibrosis. Acute cholecystitis[32] is associated with hyperemia, thickening of the gallbladder wall due to acute inflammatory exudate and edema, at times ulceration of the mucosa, and serositis. The presence of abnormal bile is believed to be the precipitating factor, focally disrupting the wall and providing a nidus for stone formation. With repeated bouts of acute infection or even in the absence of clinically defined acute bouts, the gallbladder wall may thicken the lamina propria and part of the muscle area itself (Rokitansky-Aschoff space). The muscular wall enlarges in response to the presence of the epithelial structures. In such a circumstance gallstones are almost always found in the gallbladder. At this point one is usually dealing with chronic colecystitis.

Approximately 90% of gallstones are of the mixed variety: cholesterol, bile pigments, and calcium carbonate. About 20% of these mixed gallstones contain enough calcium to be radiopaque. The remainder of gallstones are pure cholesterol or pigment stones. Cholesterol stones are usually solitary, whereas the others are likely to be multiple. The formation of stones remain a point of discussion and experimental endeavor. It has been suggested that infectious or inflammatory changes in the composition of the bile lead to stone formation. Recently it has been shown that changes in the lipids of bile with pre-

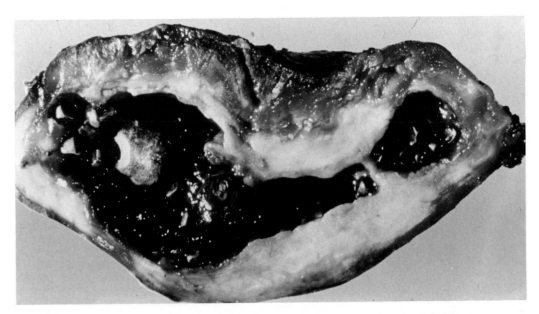

Fig. 48-7 Carcinoma of gallbladder. Thick grey-white areas are carcinoma. Several gallstones are seen in lumen.

cipitation of cholesterol and increased mucous secretion lead to stone formation in experimental animals.[23] Gallstones are an important source of disease, being associated with cholecystitis. Their passage through the biliary tract leads to obstruction, colic, or both, perforation of the gallbladder, and the common assertion that stones and carcinoma are causally related.

Neoplastic transformation does occur in the excretory system: 90% of the primary carcinomas of the gallbladder are associated with chronic cholecystitis and cholelithiasis.[30] Other factors that may be related to the genesis of carcinoma include adenomas. Histologically, Kozuka et al. demonstrated that adenomas of the gallbladder, particularly those of 1 cm or more in diameter, may evolve into carcinoma.[18] Also, carcinoma is situ (CIS) of the gallbladder as an only lesion and associated with invasive carcinoma has been described.[2] Dysplasia may accompany CIS. Thus there is a histologic chain that may link dysplasia to carcinoma. Grossly, CIS is difficult to see, although the gallbladder wall is usually thickened and the mucosal surface may be granular or have a slightly raised plaque.

Carcinomas of the gallbladder are usually advanced at the time of diagnosis, accounting for the poor prognosis (Fig. 48-7). The carcinomas average 3 cm or more in their greatest dimension. They may present as papillary tumors, ulcerated lesions, or diffuse thickening of a portion of or the whole gallbladder wall. Histologically, carcinomas may be subclassified as papillary carcinomas, adenocarcinomas, undifferentiated carcinomas, mucinous carcinomas, adenocarcinomas with a squamous component, or purely squamous cell carcinomas.

Carcinomas, adenomas, and villous tumors sometimes involve or arise in the papilla. The common duct and cystic duct are also sites of carcinomas, usually adenocarcinomas. Carcinomas at the bifurcation of the hepatic ducts are often poorly differentiated and provoke considerable fibrous reaction. Despite their location, surgical resection is possible in about half of the patients.[6,36] Rarely, other malignant tumors (such as rhabdomyosarcoma) arise in the biliary tract and only exceptionally in the gallbladder. The tumors are seen more frequently in children than in adults.[3]

Two important benign lesions that may mimic carcinoma clinically are choledochal cysts and sclerosing cholangitis. Both lesions have radiographic features that usually lead to a diagnosis.[17,20] Sclerosing cholangitis may occur alone or with chronic ulcerative colitis and involves extrahepatic and intrahepatic bile ducts.

REFERENCES

1. Abenoza, P, et al: Hepatoblastoma: an immunohistochemical and ultrastructural study, Hum Pathol 18:1025, 1987.
2. Albores-Saavedra, J, et al: Carcinoma in situ of the gallbladder, Am J Surg Pathol 8:323, 1984.
3. Aldabagh, SM, Shibata, CS, and Taxy, JB: Rhabdomyosarcoma of the common bile duct in an adult, Arch Pathol Lab Med 110:547, 1986.
4. Avogaro, P, Sirtori, CR, and Tremoli, E: Metabolic effects of alcohol, Amsterdam, 1979, Elsevier/North Holland Biomedical Press.
5. Berman, MM, Libbey, NP, and Foster, JH: Hepatocellular carcinoma, Cancer 46:1448, 1980.
6. Blackman, E, and Nash, SV: Diagnosis of duodenal and ampullary epithelial neoplasms by endoscopic biopsy: a clinicopathologic and immunohistochemical study, Hum Pathol 16:901, 1985.

7. Bucher, NLR, and Malt, RA: Regeneration of liver and kidney, New York, 1973, Little, Brown.

8. Chandra, RS, et al: Benign hepatocellular tumors in the young, Arch Pathol Lab Med 108:168, 1984.

9. Craig, JR, et al: Fibrolamellar carcinoma of the liver: a tumor of adolescents and young adults with distinctive clinico-pathologic features, Cancer 46:372, 1980.

10. Cutz, E, and Cox, DW: α-Antitrypsin deficiency: the spectrum of pathology and pathophysiology, Prog Pediatr Pathol 5:1, 1979.

11. Edmondson, HA: Pathology of alcoholism, Am J Clin Pathol 74:725, 1980.

12. Elias, H, Pauly, JE, and Burns, ER: Histology, ed 4, New York, 1978, John Wiley & Sons.

13. Fechner, RE: Benign hepatic lesions and orally administered contraceptives, Hum Pathol 8:255, 1977.

14. Gonzalez-Crussi, F, Upton, MP, and Maures, HS: Hepatoblastoma, Am J Surg Pathol 6:599, 1982.

15. Govindarajan, S, and Peters, RL: The bile duct adenoma, Arch Pathol Lab Med 108:922, 1984.

16. Kasai, M: Treatment of biliary atresia with special reference to hepatic porto-enterostomy and its modification, Prog Pediatr Surg 6:5, 1974.

17. Kimura, K, et al: Choledochal cyst, Arch Surg 113:159, 1978.

18. Kozuka, S, et al: Relation of adenoma to carcinoma in the gallbladder, Cancer 50:2226, 1982.

19. Krugman, S, and Gocke, DJ: Viral hepatitis, vol. 40. Major problems in internal medicine, Philadelphia, 1978, W.B. Saunders.

20. LaRusso, NF, et al: Primary sclerosing cholangitis, N Engl J Med 310:899, 1984.

21. Lim, RC, and Bongard, FS: Hepatocellular carcinoma, Arch Surg 119:637, 1984.

22. Lipstate, LK, Shomeyer, FW, and Welsh, RA: Benign hepatocellular tumors: a regional survey, South Med J 74:397, 1981.

23. MacPherson, BR, Pemsingh, RS, and Scott, GW: Experimental cholelithiasis in the ground squirrel, Lab Invest 56:138, 1987.

24. Malt, RA: Surgery for hepatic neoplasms, N Engl J Med 313:1591, 1985.

25. Miyai, K, and Bonin, ML: Nodular regenerative hyperplasia of the liver, Am J Clin Pathol 73:267, 1980.

26. Moesner, J, et al: Focal nodular hyperplasia of the liver, Acta Pathol Microbiol Scand 85:113, 1977.

27. Nakanuma, Y, and Olita, G: Histometric and serial section observation of the intrahepatic bile ducts in primary biliary cirrhosis, Gastroenterology 76:1326, 1979.

28. Noronka, R, and Gonzalez-Crussi, F: Hepatic angiosarcoma in childhood, Am J Surg Pathol 8:863, 1984.

29. Partin, JC, Schubert, WK, and Partin, JS: Mitochondrial ultrastructure in Reye's syndrome (encephalopathy and fatty degeneration of the viscera), N Engl J Med 285:1339, 1971.

30. Piehler, JM, and Crichlow, RW: Primary carcinoma of the gall bladder, Surg Gynecol Obstet 147:929, 1978.

31. Selinger, M, and Koff, RS: Thorotrast and the liver: a reminder, Gastroenterology 68:799, 1975.

32. Sjodahl, R, Taresson, C, and Wettetors, J: On the pathogenesis of acute cholecystitis, Surg Gynecol Obstet 146:199, 1976.

33. Smuckler, EA, Koplitz, RM, and Sell, S: α-Fetoprotein in toxic liver injury, Cancer Res 36:4558, 1976.

34. Stern, R: Experimental aspects of hepatic fibrosis, Prog Liver Dis 6:173, 1978.

35. Takayasu, K, et al: Imaging diagnosis of bile duct cystadenocarcinoma, Cancer 61:941, 1988.

36. Tsuzuki, T, et al: Carcinoma of the bifurcation of the hepatic ducts, Arch Surg 118:1147, 1983.

37. Wiesner, RH, and LaRusso, NF: Clinicopathologic features of the syndrome of primary sclerosing cholangitis, Gastroenterology 79:200, 1980.

38. Wisse, E, and Knook, DL: Kufer cells and other liver sinusoidal cells, Amsterdam, 1977, Elsevier/North Holland Biomedical Press.

39. Witzleben, CL: Extrahepatic biliary atresia: concepts of cause, diagnosis and management, Perspect Pediatr Pathol 5:41, 1979.

49 *Radiology of the Gallbladder*

ROBERT N. BERK
H. JOACHIM BURHENNE

PLAIN ABDOMINAL RADIOGRAPHY

The oldest radiologic imaging technique for detection of gallbladder disease is the plain radiograph of the abdomen. This simple and inexpensive examination is sometimes neglected in today's era of high-technology imaging. The plain film examination requires no special preparation of the patient, and the results are known immediately. It permits the diagnosis of several acute and chronic gallbladder diseases.

Cholelithiasis

Radiologic examination of the biliary tract began almost immediately after Roentgen's discovery of the x-ray. The first radiographs of gallstones were published in 1896.[195] Plain film detection of gallstones depends on their calcium content (Fig. 49-1). Gallstones can even be detected today by this radiographic technique in Egyptian mummies.[89] It is estimated that in the United States 10% of men and 20% of women between the ages of 55 and 65 have gallstones.[78]

The solubility of cholesterol in bile depends on the relative concentrations of cholesterol, bile salts, and lecithin in bile.[2] When these proportions are disturbed for any reason, the bile becomes lithogenic, and cholesterol precipitates, forming gallstones. Cholesterol is not radiopaque; consequently, most gallstones in the United States, at least, are not visible on plain abdominal radiography. Some gallstones are composed of calcium bilirubinate or have a mixed composition and contain sufficient calcium to be detectable. The concentration of calcium is sufficient to make calculi radiopaque on plain abdominal radiographs in only 10% to 15% of patients,[22,59] so the plain radiograph is of relatively little value in the detection of cholelithiasis, as compared with cholecystography. An analysis of 481 gallstones from eleven countries demonstrated that 13.1% of the stones consisted entirely of one or more calcium salts.[205]

Plain radiography of the abdomen may display gas-containing fissures within gallstones. This has been referred to as the "Mercedes-Benz" sign. Gas-containing calculi may be observed to float within bile when examined under real-time sonography.[17]

Computed tomography (CT) is often the first imaging

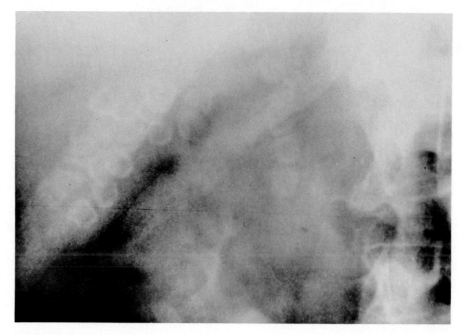

Fig. 49-1 Plain film demonstrates multiple calcified gallstones outlining gallbladder and common duct in asymptomatic patient.

modality used in the diagnosis of patients with suspected abdominal disease. This imaging modality is more sensitive to gallstone detection than plain film radiography. Eighty percent of gallstones found to be present by ultrasonography or surgical proof can be detected with CT. A recent report yielded an accuracy of 89.8% with a specificity of 100% and a sensitivity of 79.1% for CT in the determination of cholelithiasis.[15]

In diseases associated with an increased incidence of cholelithiasis, such as hemolytic anemias, Crohn's disease, cirrhosis, diabetes mellitus, and hyperparathyroidism,[48,74,192] it may be possible to establish the diagnosis of primary disease as well as to detect the gallstones on the plain radiograph. In patients with sickle cell anemia, the thickened trabecular architecture of the skeleton may be visible as well as the gallstones. Abnormal loops of intestine may be apparent in patient's with Crohn's disease, ascites may be visible in those with cirrhosis, severe vascular calcification may be present in diabetic patients, and pancreatic calcification may be identified in those with hyperparathyroidism.

Not all round or oval calcifications in the right upper quadrant are caused by gallstones.[59] An oral cholecystogram should be performed to confirm the diagnosis of cholelithiasis before surgery. Careful consideration must be given to calcification of the kidney from a wide variety of renal diseases, including tuberculosis, kidney stones, renal cysts and tumors, nephrocalcinosis, and calculi and

calyceal diverticula. A calculus in the appendix may resemble a gallstone when the appendix is in an abnormal location or when the appendix has perforated and the appendicolith is free in the peritoneal cavity. Calcifications in the liver, adrenal gland, costal cartilages, lymph nodes, arteries, and veins may have the appearance of gallstones.

Acute cholecystitis

Acute cholecystitis nearly always results from obstruction of the cystic duct by a gallstone.[215] Hyperemia and edema of the gallbladder wall follow and lead to an acute inflammatory infiltrate, hemorrhage, and necrosis. If the calculus disimpacts, as it does in 85% of patients, the acute inflammatory process rapidly subsides.[61] However, if the obstruction persists, the disease may progress to empyema and perforation of the gallbladder, along with a localized abscess in the right upper quadrant, or to generalized peritonitis.

The findings on the abdominal radiography depend on the stage and severity of the disease. If the inflammatory reaction is mild, the radiograph may be normal or reveal only the presence of gallstones. Progression of the disease in the gallbladder and extension of the inflammatory process to adjacent peritoneal surfaces cause a reflex inhibition of motility in adjacent segments of the intestine (sentinel ileus).[79,118,217] The abdominal radiograph shows a paralytic ileus along with distended, air-filled loops of

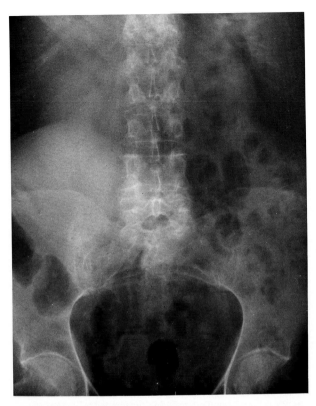

Fig. 49-2 Plain abdominal radiograph showing mass in right upper quadrant adjacent to liver caused by empyema of gallbladder.

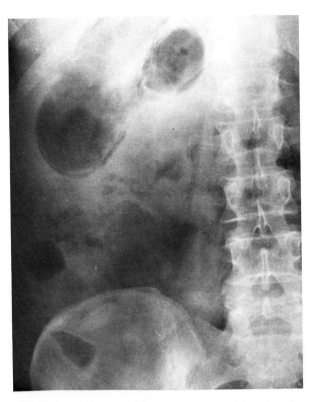

Fig. 49-3 Plain abdominal radiograph showing emphysematous cholecystitis. Intraluminal and intramural air are visible in body and neck of gallbladder.

bowel and multiple air-fluid levels localized in the right upper quadrant of the abdomen. The distended gallbladder may be visible as a mass adjacent to the liver. If the colon does not participate in the paralytic ileus, the radiographic findings may simulate a mechanical small bowel obstruction. When empyema of the gallbladder develops, a mass adjacent to the liver may be apparent on the abdominal radiograph (Fig. 49-2). Occasionally, the radiologic diagnosis of perforation of the gallbladder can be made if gallstones are identified free in the peritoneal cavity remote from the gallbladder.[112] If the inflammatory process subsides despite the persistence of cystic duct obstruction, the gallbladder may distend with mucus, producing hydrops.[215] In this circumstance the enlarged gallbladder is usually visible on the abdominal radiograph.[22]

Emphysematous cholecystitis is an uncommon variant of acute cholecystitis in which gas is present in the gallbladder wall and in the lumen.[106,157] The gas is caused by infection with gas-forming organisms of the genus *Clostridium*, though some cases are caused by anerobic streptococci, *Escherichia coli*, and staphylococci. Gangrene is a common pathologic feature.[145] In distinction

from ordinary acute cholecystitis, 20% of patients with emphysematous cholecystitis have diabetes. In addition, the incidence of emphysematous cholecystitis is three times greater in men than in women.[215] A substantial number of patients do not have associated cholelithiasis.[145] Hence emphysematous cholecystitis is quite distinct from typical acute cholecystitis. The pathogenesis of this form of emphysematous cholecystitis probably is occlusion of the cystic artery with subsequent ischemia, necrosis, and infection of the gallbladder.[14,44,145] Because of the high incidence of gangrene, it is not surprising that the diagnosis implies a risk of gallbladder perforation five times that expected from ordinary acute cholecystitis.[44]

Gas usually is not visible until at least 24 to 48 hours after the onset of cholecystitis.[142] Radiographs made after this interval show gas in the lumen of the gallbladder.[14] Radiographs made after this interval show gas in the lumen of the gallbladder,[14] in the gallbladder wall, and occasionally in the tissues adjacent to the gallbladder, indicating a pericholecystic abscess (Fig. 49-3). When the cystic duct is patent, gas may be seen in the biliary ducts.[94] The presence of free intraperitoneal gas as a

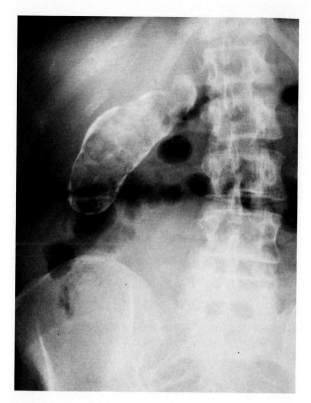

Fig. 49-4 Plain abdominal radiograph showing porcelain gallbladder. Large lower abdominal mass caused by uterine fibroid is also apparent.

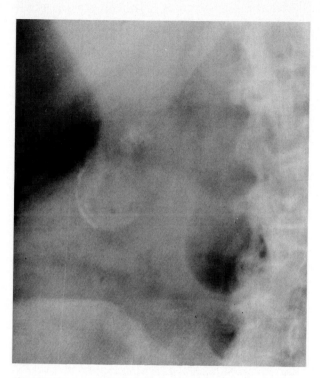

Fig. 49-5 Large calcified gallstone surrounded by calcified gallbladder wall and calcified impacted cystic duct stone seen on plain abdominal radiography.

complication of emphysematous cholecystitis has been reported.[173]

Porcelain gallbladder

Extensive calcification in the wall of the gallbladder has been named calcifying cholecystitis, cholecystopathia chronica calcarea, or simply calcified gallbladder.[40] The term *porcelain gallbladder* has been used to emphasize the blue discoloration and brittle consistency of the gallbladder wall.[164] Because most cases of gallbladder calcification are not reported, the incidence of the disease is difficult to determine; however, various studies of postoperative gallbladder specimens show a 0.06% to 0.8% occurrence of extensive mural calcification.[40] The disease is five times more frequent in women than in men. The mean age is 54 years, with a range of 38 to 70 years. A paucity of symptoms is characteristic, so that the diagnosis frequently is made by detection of a palpable mass in the right upper quadrant or by discovery of typical gallbladder calcification on abdominal radiographs.[51]

Pathologically the calcification occurs in two forms.[161] In one variety there is a broad continuous band of calcification in the muscularis; in the other form there are multiple, punctate calcifications that occur in the glandular spaces of the mucosa. Gallstones are present in nearly all instances of gallbladder calcification, and usually a stone obstructs the cystic duct with hydrops of the gallbladder.[166] The gallbladder wall is thickened by chronic inflammation, and the mucosa is often denuded. The contents usually are sterile.[122]

Most authors consider the calcification to be a sequela of a low-grade chronic inflammation, but others have emphasized the possibility that the calcification may be secondary to intramural hemorrhage or an imbalance in calcium metabolism.[51,65,164]

Plain abdominal radiographs show a characteristic ring of calcification that conforms to the shape and location of the gallbladder. The thickness of the calcification varies, and the distribution is often uneven and discontinuous. A porcelain gallbladder must be distinguished from a single, large, calcified gallstone (Fig. 49-4 and 49-5).

A review of the literature reveals 26 examples of carcinoma occurring in the presence of a porcelain gallbladder. The tumors are predominantly diffusely infiltrating adenocarcinoma, though cases of squamous cell carcinoma have been described.[168] It is clear that a porcelain gallbladder is uncommon in cases of carcinoma

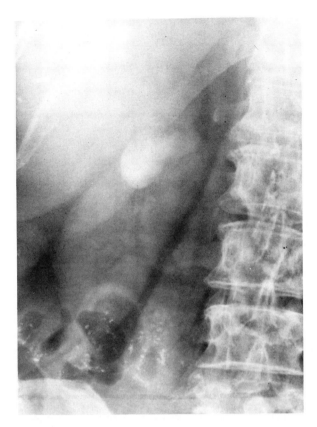

Fig. 49-6 Plain abdominal radiograph showing milk of calcium bile in gallbladder. Limy bile in gallbladder simulates normal oral cholecystogram.

of the gallbladder, but the frequency of carcinoma in cases of a porcelain gallbladder is striking. Polk estimated the frequency to be 22%.[168] Most authors agree that carcinoma occurs in cases of a porcelain gallbladder with sufficient frequency to warrant prophylactic cholecystectomy for patients with a porcelain gallbladder, even when the disease is asymptomatic.[2]

Milk of calcium bile

Milk of calcium bile, or the "limy bile syndrome," is characterized by the presence of radiopaque material in the gallbladder sufficient to produce opacification of the gallbladder on plain abdominal radiographs. The putty-like material in the gallbladder lumen is composed of calcium carbonate or, less often, calcium phosphate or calcium bilirubinate.[29] The cystic duct is obstructed by a gallstone, and the gallbladder is chronically inflamed. Holden and Turner[105] reported six cases in which passage of the limy bile and associated gallstones occurred spontaneously.

Milk of calcium bile may simulate the findings of a normally opacified gallbladder following oral cholecys-

tography (Fig. 49-6). Differentiation requires knowledge of whether the patient was given cholecystographic contrast material. In other cases the limy bile has a granular pattern that suggests the correct diagnosis.

Spontaneous biliary-enteric fistula

Spontaneous communication between the biliary tract and intestine is the result of erosion of a gallstone in 90% of cases, though 6% develop because of penetration of a peptic ulcer in the common duct, and the remaining 4% result from a tumor or trauma.[101] In 80% to 90%, the gallstone passes spontaneously without causing symptoms.[174] However, if the gallstone is larger than 2.5 cm, it may cause an obturation type of intestinal obstruction (gallstone ileus).[76]

Spontaneous biliary-enteric fistula caused by passage of a gallstone between the gallbladder and intestine is preceded by recurrent episodes of acute cholecystitis.[111] Wakefield and co-workers[214] reported a series of 176 fistulas in which 57% involved the duodenum, 18% were into the colon, and the remainder were multiple or involved the stomach. Gallstones may also erode into a bronchus or into the pleural cavity, portal vein, renal pelvis, urinary bladder, or aorta.[36,190,214]

Of all intestinal obstructions, gallstone ileus is the most insidious and difficult to diagnose clinically.[111] The mortality of the disease is five times that of any other small bowel obstruction. The average age of these patients is 69 years. Eighty-eight percent of instances of gallstone ileus occur in women.[37]

The intestinal obstruction may be constant or intermittent and usually occurs in the terminal ileum, where the stone is unable to pass through the ileocecal valve (60% of cases).[75,216] The next most common locations are the proximal ileum (24% of cases) and the distal jejunum (9% of cases), where spasm or a simple diameter disproportion is the cause of the obstruction.[111] Erosion into the colon occurs in less than 5% of cases. A cholecystocolonic fistula may cause diarrhea because of the effect of bile salts on the colonic mucosa (choleretic enteropathy).[93,104,198] Erosion of the gallstone into the stomach may cause pyloric obstruction.[176]

The radiologist is in a unique position to establish the diagnosis of gallstone ileus because of the classic features of the disease on the plain abdominal radiograph. First described by Rigler and co-workers[179] in 1941, the cardinal plain film radiographic findings are hoop-shaped, dilated loops of small bowel; air in the biliary tree; and a gallstone in an ectopic location in the abdomen. Barium studies are often useful in confirming the presence of intestinal obstruction, in identifying the obturating calculus, and in demonstrating the cholecystoenteric fistula.[210]

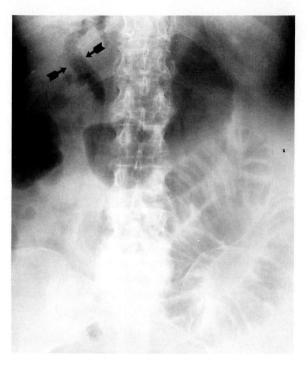

Fig. 49-7 Plain abdominal radiograph showing gallstone ileus. Loops of dilated small intestine and air in biliary tree *(arrows)* are evident.

Eisenman and co-workers[63] suggested that there is a characteristic appearance of the small bowel on supine plain abdominal radiographs in cases of gallstone ileus, which they termed *loop obturation pattern*. In this pattern there is minimal to moderate gaseous distention of the small bowel, prominent valvulae conniventes that do not show extreme degrees of effacement, clear delineation of the fluid-containing loops of bowel, and frequently a radial configuration of the loops of bowel.

Gas in the gallbladder or biliary tree is visible in nearly two thirds of patients with gallstone ileus[63] (Fig. 49-7). Balthazar and Schechter[14] identified air in the gallbladder exclusively in 25% of 16 cases of gallstone ileus. They emphasized that air in a shrunken gallbladder helps establish a prompt diagnosis. A suspicion of gallstone ileus or the finding of gas in the biliary tree is sufficient indication to perform a barium examination of the upper gastrointestinal tract if additional studies are necessary to establish the diagnosis. Gas in the biliary tree may result from previous surgery, including a choledochoduodenostomy, cholecystojejunostomy, or sphincterotomy. Rarely, gas may be caused by ascending cholangitis as a result of a gas-forming organism or by the reflux of air through a patulous sphincter of Oddi in aged patients.[191] Gas in the portal venous system usually collects toward the periphery of the liver, whereas gas in the bile duct is more prominent in the region of the porta hepatis.[79] Occasionally, fat surrounding the common bile duct may simulate gas within the duct.[194] However, the fat is not as radiolucent as gas in the bile duct and does not involve intrahepatic portions of the biliary tree.

The third radiographic finding in the classic triad associated with gallstone ileus is the presence of a gallstone in an ectopic location in the abdomen. This can be detected in between one fourth and one half of patients with the disease.[63,79,179]

Gallstone ileus should be treated by emergency surgery in which the obstructing stone is removed through a small enterotomy incision.[111,216] Surgical treatment of the cholecystoduodenal fistula is almost never indicated acutely. Recurrent gallstone ileus caused by a second stone that was located in the gallbladder or in the intestine during the first episode has been described.[210]

ORAL CHOLECYSTOGRAPHY

Oral cholecystography was developed in 1923 to become the principal diagnostic technique for gallbladder disease. As recently as 10 years ago, about 4 million oral cholecystograms were performed annually in the United States.[41] The use of oral cholecystography, however, has sharply decreased in medical institutions where ultrasonography is available. Cholecystosonography with real-time high-resolution sector scanners is less time consuming and has largely replaced oral cholecystography as the first technique in evaluation of the patient with suspected gallbladder disease.[50] The accuracy of both techniques is comparable for the diagnosis of cholecystolithiasis with a sensitivity and specificity of over 95%.[77] We must remember, however, when considering these high accuracy figures, that patients diagnosed as having no gallstones usually have poor follow up. Oral cholecystography has also been used recently for evaluation of chemolitholysis therapy and for targeting during gallstone fragmentation by extracorporeal shockwave lithotripsy.

Most physicians consider oral cholecystography to be an uncomplicated radiologic procedure that is simple to perform and easy to interpret; yet, in reality, few examinations in radiology require more expertise on the part of the radiologist.

The major use of oral cholecystography is for the diagnosis of cholelithiasis.[219] At present the examination is done only when clinical findings suggest the presence of cholelithiasis, and its use may increase with gallstone lithotripsy becoming a clinically accepted procedure. It is not customary to perform the study to detect gallstones in asymptomatic individuals, although this may be worthwhile in exceptionally high-risk groups such as diabetics, American Indians, and patients with hemolytic anemia, Crohn's disease, or cirrhosis.[5] Oral cholecystography should not be attempted in patients with impaired liver function or biliary obstruction in whom the serum bilirubin is 2 mg/100 ml or higher, because with this degree of cholestasis the possibility of opacification of the gallbladder is negligible.

Accuracy

The results of reports indicating an accuracy rate of oral cholecystography in the range of 97% to 99%* are misleading in that the studies involve only patients in whom a positive oral cholecystogram was correlated with the pathologic findings at surgery. These data indicate that the interpretation of an oral cholecystogram is nearly 100% correct when gallstones are visible in an opacified gallbladder or when there is nonvisualization of the gallbladder on two consecutive studies and extrabiliary causes of nonvisualization have been excluded. Hence the studies show that false-positive cholecystograms are exceedingly rare. However, these reports give no indication of the number of patients who have gallstones but in whom the cholecystogram is interpreted as being normal (false-negative findings). Before the introduction of ultrasonography, this information was impossible to obtain, because performing cholecystectomy indiscriminately in patients who have an apparently normal oral cholecystogram is not justified.

Consequently, reports of incidence of false-negative results of oral cholecystography have only recently become available. Studies correlating sonography, cholecystography, and surgical findings have established an 89% to 96% overall detection rate for cholelithiasis on oral cholecystography.* Thus it seems clear that even with ideal radiographic technique and good opacification of the gallbladder, gallstones that are 2 to 3 mm or less in diameter may occasionally be missed when only one or two are present in the gallbladder.[9,41] The accuracy of oral cholecystography in detecting gallstones is probably closer to 90% than to 98%.[41] Consequently, when a patient's symptoms are highly suggestive of gallbladder disease or when a patient has acute pancreatitis that might be caused by cholelithiasis, a normal oral cholecystogram should not be taken as conclusive evidence against the presence of gallstones.

Technique
Preparation of the patient

Recent experimental data in dogs and humans indicate that the active enterohepatic recirculation of bile salts plays a major role in facilitating both the intestinal ab-

sorption and hepatic excretion of Telepaque.[25,85,132,133] Consequently, it is important to ensure that fat is given in the diet at the same time that Telepaque is administered. Fat stimulates the release of cholecystokinin, which causes the gallbladder to contract and to empty bile salts stored in the gallbladder into the intestine. The fat content of the diet given with the other, more water-soluble, oral cholecystographic materials is less important in terms of absorption. However, these agents are rapidly absorbed from the intestine, and if they are excreted into bile when the gallbladder is still contracted as a result of a meal, they will be lost into the intestine. Thus water-soluble contrast agents should not be given with food.

The optimal dose of Telepaque and the other oral cholecystographic contrast agents has not been sufficiently studied. Some use 2 g rather than the usual 3 g dose to avoid dense opacification of the gallbladder in which gallstones could be obscured.[103] This is not a problem if compression spot films are made. Administering more than 3 g of Telepaque may be necessary in obese patients, but the routine use of larger doses should be avoided because of the likelihood that the degree of toxicity produced by the contrast agent is proportional to the amount of the compound given. The routine 1-day use of a double dose (6 g) is not warranted, because most of the reported cases of renal failure caused by oral cholecystographic contrast materials have been in patients who received high doses of the compounds.[26] More than two consecutive doses are not indicated, because such examinations are not associated with a higher incidence of improved gallbladder opacification.[153]

Care should be taken not to dehydrate the patient following the administration of the contrast agent because of the potent uricosuric effect of the compounds.[169] Water should be allowed as desired.

Because Telepaque frequently has a cathartic effect, it is not necessary to routinely administer a laxative to eliminate fecal material, which might interfere with optimal visualization of the gallbladder. Contrarily, it has been shown that castor oil does not interfere with opacification of the gallbladder when it is given with the Telepaque.[141,193] Indeed, because castor oil stimulates the gallbladder to contract, there is experimental evidence to suggest that castor oil could improve the absorption and excretion of Telepaque.[26]

Patients should be evaluated for a history of previous allergic reaction to any of the radiographic contrast materials before one proceeds with oral cholecystography. Cross-reactions with the urographic and angiographic contrast materials may occur. Adverse reactions in a patient with a known allergy to contrast materials can be avoided by treating the patient with corticosteroids and

---

*References 4, 11, 12, 70, 153, 160, 210, 220.
†References 16, 50, 54, 71, 81, 129, 140, 224.

antihistaminics before administering the cholecysto-graphic contrast agent.

Radiographic technique

Ideally, a preliminary plain abdominal radiograph of the abdomen should be made before the administration of contrast material. This is done to detect radiopaque gallstones that might be obscured by contrast material in the gallbladder and to recognize milk of calcium bile, which could be confused with a normally opacified gall-bladder. This is in keeping with the basic radiologic tenet that a preliminary radiograph should be made before any contrast agent is used. However, it is impractical in most cases to require patients to make an additional trip to the radiology department for the preliminary examination, and only 8% of 45 radiologists surveyed by Harned and LaVeen[95] required an initial radiograph. Consequently, one must weigh the inconvenience and expense of the preliminary radiograph against the number of times gall-bladder disease will be overlooked without it. If upright spot films of the gallbladder are made with graded compression, it is exceedingly rare that radiopaque gall-stones cannot be identified in the fundus of the opacified gallbladder. Indeed, this occurred in only 2% of Harned and LaVeen's cases. However, one must keep in mind that if the preliminary radiograph is omitted, rare false-negative cholecystograms might occur. In special cases such as patients with apparently normal cholecystograms who have characteristic symptoms of biliary colic and/or in whom significant symptoms persist, a plain ab-dominal radiograph should be made sometime in the ra-diologic workup.

Care must be taken to make the radiographs of the gallbladder at the appropriate time following the admin-istration of contrast material. Poor gallbladder opacifi-cation will occur if the radiographs are taken prematurely or if they are delayed. Whalen and co-workers[218] studied 50 patients having cholecystography with Telepaque and showed that peak opacification of the gallbladder oc-curred between 14 and 19 hours after ingestion of the contrast material. Using Bilopaque in 50 patients, Oli-phant and co-workers[162] determined that optimal gall-bladder opacification occurred at 10 hours. Conse-quently, timing of the radiographs depends on which contrast material is used.

The actual number and type of radiographs made as a part of a cholecystogram vary depending on the indi-vidual preference of the radiologist, but in all cases the following principles must be observed: (1) upright spot films made at fluoroscopy or right lateral decubitus ra-diographs should be included if gallstones are not evident on prone or supine radiographs; (2) at least one radiograph should include the entire abdomen; (3) the radiographs should be of excellent technical quality using low-kilovoltage technique; and (4) the radiographs should be viewed before the patient leaves the department so that additional films can be made as necessary.

Small gallstones are often invisible on supine and prone abdominal radiographs even when they are nu-merous. The accuracy of the cholecystogram is signifi-cantly impaired unless upright or decubitus projections of the gallbladder are obtained to allow the calculi to collect by gravity in the dependent portion of the gall-bladder or to form a layer in the bile.[67,91,137] Upright spot films made at fluoroscopy with graded compression of the gallbladder are indispensable unless gallstones are obvious on the supine or prone radiographs. Jensen and Kaude[116] showed that fluoroscopy with 70 mm film from the output screen of the image intensifier is an acceptable substitute for full-scale spot film radiography.

A right lateral decubitus projection of the abdomen is helpful when spot films are unsuccessful and has been recommended by some to replace fluoroscopy.[149] How-ever, decubitus views are usually not as good technically unless the radiographic table is equipped with a special attachment. A simple device for this purpose has been recommended by Miller.[148] With decubitus projections, visualization of the dependent portion of the gallbladder is left to chance, and compression under direct visual control is impossible. Amberg and co-workers[6] have rec-ommended elevating the patient's hips in the lateral de-cubitus position to improve visualization of the dependent portion of the gallbladder when it is obscured on the conventional decubitus projection.[6]

One radiograph should include the entire abdomen so that a gallbladder in an unusual position will not be over-looked and a mistaken diagnosis of nonvisualization will be avoided.[66]

The radiographs of every patient having cholecystog-raphy must be reviewed by a radiologist or a knowl-edgeable surrogate before the patient leaves the radiology department so that additional projections can be made if the first films are inadequate.[102] Hence the examination must be tailored to the special needs of each patient. If the fundus of the gallbladder still cannot be freed of overlying fecal material, an enema may eliminate the problem. In some cases a fatty meal is useful in con-tracting the gallbladder so that the fundus can be dem-onstrated adequately. When these maneuvers fail, to-mography,[47] stereoscopic radiographs, or ultrasound studies of the gallbladder may be necessary.

Fatty meal

The routine use of a fatty meal in oral cholecystog-raphy has been recommended by various authors.[97,149,185] It is generally agreed, however, that the response of the gallbladder to a fatty meal is too variable to permit valid conclusions regarding the ability of the gallbladder to empty normally.[40,100,132,223]

Miller and co-workers[149] emphasized the importance of giving a fatty meal routinely to visualize the neck of the gallbladder, where they believe stones are often missed. However, Laufer and Gledhill[128] compared the diagnoses before and after a fatty meal in 231 patients undergoing cholecystography and found only one patient in whom a stone was detected radiographically only after the fatty meal. In this case the stone was missed on the original film because of overlying gas, not because it was hidden in the neck of the gallbladder. Similar results were reported by Harvey and co-workers.[97]

Visualization of the cystic and common ducts is no justification for the routine use of a fatty meal. If the gallbladder is opacified on the oral cholecystogram, it is safe to assume that there are no calculi in the cystic duct. Furthermore, it can be assumed that there are no gallstones in the common duct if there are none in the gallbladder. Choledocholithiasis in the absence of gallstones in the gallbladder in patients without a cholecystectomy is exceedingly rare. If a patient has cholelithiasis, the common duct should be opacified by operative cholangiography performed routinely during cholecystectomy.[41] Consequently, there is no need to attempt to visualize the common duct preoperatively.

In view of the considerable inconvenience, expense, and additional radiation exposure involved in the use of a fatty meal, there is little objective data to justify its routine use in cholecystography. A fatty meal may be useful in specific circumstances, such as when the fundus of the gallbladder cannot otherwise be separated from fecal material in the colon or when the initial radiograph suggests the presence of adenomyomatosis or cholesterolosis.

Problem of impaired first-dose visualization

Repeat exmination in cases of impaired visualization of the gallbladder on a single-dose oral cholecystogram is required with disturbing regularity and represents an important practical problem.[21] The incidence varies depending on the degree of gallbladder opacification that individual radiologist are willing to accept as adequate for diagnosis on the first-dose examination. In both the series by Rosenbaum[183] and the series by Berk,[20] 15% of patients having cholecystography required a second examination because of impaired first-dose visualization. Mujahed and co-workers[153] found a second-dose examination necessary in 25% of their cases, and approximately one half of the patients in the study by Stanley and co-workers[202] required a second study.

The difficulty arises from the fact that gallbladder opacification is not always optimal on the first study and can sometimes be improved by a second dose of contrast material. As a result, initial nonvisualization of the gallbladder does not definitely indicate the presence of gallbladder disease, and a second study is required before a diagnosis can be made. Between 10% and 20% of patients with no visualization of the gallbladder after a single dose of contrast material have a normal cholecystogram on the second-dose examination. Equally troublesome is faint opacification at the first study. The initial visualization may be so poor, even in the absence of disease, that a second examination is necessary to obtain maximum opacification in an attempt to identify or exclude gallstones accurately. In this group 65% to 75% of cases are normal on the second examination.[21] In either case failure to repeat the cholecystogram significantly vitiates the diagnostic accuracy of the procdedure and invites unacceptable diagnostic error.

Poor visualization of the gallbladder after a single dose of contrast material not only occurs in a significant percentage of apparently normal patients, but it occurs regularly in patients with acute pancreatitis[120,172,199] or acute peritonitis[187]; after trauma,[110,210] surgery,[187] or fasting[226]; in patients with pernicious anemia[131]; in infants under 6 months of age[96]; and in women in the late months of pregnancy.[130] Kaden and co-workers[120] showed that approximately two thirds of 25 patients with acute pancreatitis had nonvisualization or poor visualization of the gallbladder when the examination was performed during the first week of an acute exacerbation of the disease. Subsequent cholecystograms performed after recovery showed that the gallbladders in these patients were normal. Similar results were obtained by Silvani and McCorkle[199] in their series of 28 patients with acute pancreatitis.

The cause of inadequate radiographic visualization of the gallbladder in the absence of gallbladder disease has not been clearly defined. Impaired first-dose opacification in apparently normal patients may be the result of impaired intestinal absorption and/or deficient hepatic excretion of Telepaque in the absence of circulating bile salts.[26,132,133] This occurs in patients who are fasting or are on a low-fat diet in whom bile salts are sequestered in the gallbladder. Poor absorption of the contrast material may also be related to diminished secretion of pancreatic juice along with an associated decrease in intestinal pH.[26,171] Stagnation of nonopaque bile in the gallbladder in fasting patients may prevent filling of the gallbladder with contrast material and prevent opacification.[226] Poor visualization in patients with acute pancreatitis may be related to the fact that the patients are usually fasting because of abdominal pain and as part of their therapy. This would not explain the persistent failure to visualize the gallbladder after a patient resumed a normal diet, as described by Sanchez-Ubeda and co-workers.[187] However, their data may be in error in view of the more recent report of Roller and co-workers,[182] who were able to obtain satisfactory gallbladder opacification in 89% of patients with acute pancreatitis before discharge from the hospital when the examination was performed after solid food was resumed.

Techniques to eliminate the need for second-dose cholecystogram

Burhenne and Obata[42] have recommended avoiding the problem of having to perform a second cholecystogram in patients with initial nonvisualization or poor visualization of the gallbladder by administering two consecutive 3 g doses of Telepaque each evening before the day that the radiographs are to be made. Their data from over 600 single-visit oral cholecystograms indicate that failure of the gallbladder to opacify under these circumstances is reliable evidence of gallbladder disease when extrabiliary causes of nonvisualization such as liver disease are excluded. Their simple technique is one solution to the problem of having to perform second-dose cholecystograms.

Koehler and Kyaw[127] were able to reduce the incidence of poor first-dose opacification of the gallbladder from 54% to 15% by giving the Telepaque tablets over a 6-hour period the day before the study rather than giving the total dose with the evening meal the evening before the examination in the conventional manner. Similar results were reported by Nelson.[156] Fischer and Burgener[72] showed in nine volunteers that a 3 g dose of Bilopaque given in four divided doses over 6 hours produced at least the same radiographic density of the gallbladder as a single 3 g dose. They have recommended the fractionated dose because the lower peak blood concentrations of the Bilopaque achieved with the divided dose should predispose patients to fewer toxic reactions than with the single-dose method. In distinction to the value of fractionating the dose with Telepaque, Michael and co-workers[147] demonstrated that fractionating the dose of Cholebrine was counterproductive, because gallbladder visualization was significantly better when Cholebrine was given in a single dose. The reason for this difference between Cholebrine and Telepaque is not known.

Administering Oragrafin to patients with first-dose nonvisualization or poor visualization of the gallbladder is a useful alternative to performing a second-day cholecystogram (reinforcement cholecystography).[28,56,167] This technique may save the patient a day of hospitalization by eliminating the need for a second-day examination. Radiographs made 4 hours after the administration of 6 g of Oragrafin showed sufficient improvement

in opacification to allow a diagnosis in 80% of the patients with initial poor visualization in Beseman's study.[28] If the original cholecystogram showed nonvisualization of the gallbladder, the chance of increased opacification with Oragrafin was only 13%. However, in a series of 115 patients with initial nonvisualization, Crummy[56] showed that persistent failure to visualize the gallbladder on radiographs made 5 hours after a second dose of 3 g of Oragrafin was conclusive evidence of gallbladder disease when extrabiliary causes of nonvisualization were excluded.[45]

Visualization of the common duct is accurate evidence that there has been adequate intestinal absorption and hepatic excretion of the contrast material to opacify the gallbladder. Nonvisualization of the gallbladder in this circumstance indicates the presence of cystic duct obstruction. Tomography of the right upper quadrant of the abdomen can reduce the need for a second cholecystogram by demonstrating opacification of the common bile duct in the absence of gallbladder visualization. This is the case in 70% to 80% of patients with nonvisualization of the gallbladder on cholecystography.* Tomography may reveal calcification in the obstructing cystic duct calculus that was not visible on the conventional cholecystogram or identify the stone as a crescentic filling defect in the cystic duct.[204] Routine tomography is not recommended because of the additional time, expense, and radiation exposure it requires.

Nathan and Newman[154] and Muhletalar and co-workers[151] have pointed out that the detection of conjugated Telepaque and conjugated Bilopaque in the intestine on radiographs of patients with nonvisualization of the gallbladder after a single dose of either contrast agent has the same significance as visualization of the common bile duct and indicates cystic duct obstruction. Conjugated contrast material may be identified on the radiograph as a homogeneous, uniform density that is easily distinguishable from the granular particulate appearance of unabsorbed, unconjugated contrast material. Its presence in the small bowel or colon indicates that the contrast material has been adequately absorbed from the intestine and properly excreted by the liver. Therefore failure of the gallbladder to opacifiy in these circumstances is the result of cystic duct obstruction.

Wherever ultrasonography is available, it is often used for final evaluation of the gallbladder in patients with impaired opacification of the gallbladder after single-dose oral cholecystography.[54,71,129] The accuracy of ultrasonography is the same as that of cholecystography, the results are known immediately, and direct evidence of the presence of cholelithiasis is provided, so ultrasound

---

*References 121, 138, 144, 170, 203, 204.

studies are well suited in this circumstance. Today, this technique is evolving as the primary technique for the detection of gallbladder disease.[50,224]

Causes and significance of nonvisualization of gallbladder after second-dose cholecystogram

Failure to visualize the gallbladder after the administration of two consecutive doses of cholecystographic contrast material is reliable evidence of gallbladder disease if other causes of nonvisualization can be excluded. In the series of 5000 patients having oral cholecystography reported by Mujahed and co-workers,[153] 14% of the group that had persistent nonvisualization of the gallbladder on consecutive studies had an extrabiliary cause for the nonvisualization. Two thirds of these patients had liver disease. The others had either had a previous cholecystectomy, had pyloric canal obstruction, or had received no contrast material. All the patients who had consecutive nonvisualization with no extrabiliary reason for nonvisualization had gallbladder disease at surgery—nearly always chronic cholecystitis and cholelithiasis. Hence failure of the gallbladder to opacify after a second dose of contrast material is highly reliable evidence of gallbladder disease. Further evaluation by intravenous cholangiography, tomography, or ultrasound is unnecessary.

There are a large number of extrabiliary causes of nonvisualization of the gallbladder (see box on right). Low-Beer and co-workers[135] presented evience that small bowel disease is rarely a cause of nonvisualization of the gallbladder on oral cholecystography with Oragrafin. They reported 84 patients with diseases that produce malabsorption (celiac disease, Crohn's disease, ileal resection, small intestine diverticulosis) in whom 95% had satisfactory gallbladder opacification. Goldberg[83] noted that in his experience patients with Crohn's disease or ileal resection may have nonvisualization of the gallbladder on oral cholecystography with Telepaque because of impaired intestinal absorption of the contrast materials, perhaps related to a deficiency of bile salts.

CHOLECYSTOKININ AND CHOLECYSTOGRAPHY

Fatty food intolerance, heartburn, flatulence, epigastric fullness, and upper abdominal discomfort are often considered to be classic symptoms of cholelithiasis. However, patients with a normal cholecystogram have these dyspeptic complaints as frequently as those with gallstones.[69]

In the United States the only universally accepted cause for recurrent biliary-type pain is gallstones. Patients with undiagnosed abdominal pain related to the ingestion of fatty foods who have a normal cholecysto-

---

□ EXTRABILIARY CAUSES OF NONVISUALIZATION OF THE GALLBLADDER □

1. Fasting
2. Failure to ingest contrast material
3. Vomiting
4. Nasogastric suction
5. Esophageal disease
   a. Zenker's diverticulum
   b. Epiphrenic diverticulum
   c. Esophageal obstruction
   d. Hiatus hernia
6. Gastric retention
7. Gastrocolic fistula
8. Acute pancreatitis
9. Acute peritonitis
10. Severe trauma
11. Postoperative ileus
12. Liver disease
13. Dubin-Johnson syndrome
14. Previous cholecystectomy
15. Cholestyramine
16. Infants under 6 months of age
17. Crohn's disease
18. Pregnancy
19. Pernicious anemia

---

gram and ultrasound examinations are sometimes diagnosed in Europe as having biliary dyskinesia. The clinical manifestations, pathologic changes, and results of surgery are so variable that most surgeons are reluctant to perform a cholecystectomy in these patients. A reliable radiographic procedure for the diagnosis of biliary dyskinesia is not available.

Diagnosis of biliary dyskinesia on oral cholecystography

The fatty meal has been used since the inception of oral cholecystography in an effort to recognize abnormalities in gallbladder evacuation in patients who have symptoms of biliary tract disease but a normal cholecystogram. Unfortunately, the degree that the normal gallbladder empties following a fatty meal varies widely and thus has little diagnostic significance.[41,82,100,134,223]

It has been suggested that persistent visualization of the gallbladder 36 hours after the administration of Telepaque is diagnostic of biliary dyskinesia.[1] However, despite preliminary data to the contrary, it is clear that normal patients have persistent opacification of the gallbladder at 36 hours. Visualization of the gallbladder at 36 hours is the result of enterohepatic recirculation of conjugated Telepaque.[166] Prolonged opacification is closely related to diet and to the degree of initial opacification. Patients should be expected not to empty their gallbladders if they had little or no fat in their diet following the cholecystogram.

Cholecystokinin

In 1928, Ivy and Oldberg[114] showed that fat in the small intestine stimulates the release of a substance that activates gallbladder contraction. This hormone, which they termed *cholecystokinin* (CCK), is a polypeptide with the active portion of the molecule residing in the C-terminal octapeptide fragment.[175] The octapeptide, synthesized by Ondetti and co-workers[163] in 1970, is more easily produced and promises to be an inexpensive alternative to the extracted preparation for use in place of a fatty meal during cholecystography. Hopman and co-workers[108] compared commercially available fatty meals and intravenous bolus injection of CCK and concluded that emptying rate or maximal gallbladder contraction were not significantly different. They concluded that the use of intravenous CCK does not offer any advantage over the ingestion of fatty meals in radiographic gallbladder studies.

Technique

CCK cholecystography is performed by giving 0.02 µg/kg of the octapeptide intravenously after first opacifying the gallbladder by oral cholecystography in the usual manner.[43,53,86-88,155,211] Four or five serial radiographs of the gallbladder are then made with the patient in the prone oblique position during the 15- to 20-minute interval after the injection. A positive examination is defined differently by various investigators but is one in which (1) the CCK induces the patient's symptoms (usually upper abdominal pain),[155,211] and/or (2) the radiographs show incomplete emptying and/or spasm of the gallbladder.[43,53,84,86] Incomplete emptying implies a reduction in volume of less than 20% to 50% in the 15- to 20-minute interval.[43,53,84,86-88]

Accuracy

Goldstein and co-workers[86-88] were enthusiastic about their experience with CCK cholecystography performed between 1959 and 1972, in which the diagnosis of the cystic duct syndrome was apparently made correctly on the basis of a positive test in 28 patients.[43,53] The response to CCK was considered abnormal when the gallbladder emptied less than 50%. In many of these cases the gallbladder assumed a globular configuration ("fighting gallbladder"), as if it were attempting to empty against increased resistance. All the patients with deficient gallbladder contraction developed upper abdominal pain after the CCK injection. Cholecystectomy was performed in 25 of the 28 patients. All but three of these were relieved of their symptoms during follow-up periods ranging from 6 months to 11 years. Histologic examination of the gallbladder showed varying degrees of chronic cholecystitis with kinks or narrowing of the cystic duct in 18 of the 25 patients. The gallbladder was normal in five, and histologic data were not available in two. CCK cholecystography was performed in 17 control subjects. In every instance the gallbladder contracted 50% or more, and no patients had upper abdominal pain (Table 49-1).

Valberg and co-workers[211] had an equally good experience with CCK in 13 patients with typical attacks of biliary-like pain who had normal conventional cholecystograms (Table 49-1).

In a third optimistic report, Nathan and co-workers[155] compared the results of CCK cholecystography in 141 patients with the results in 142 controls (35 physicians, 107 nonphysicians). Nathan and co-workers differed from Goldstein and co-workers[87] in that the former did not concern themselves with the degree of gallbladder emptying but considered only spasm of the gallbladder to be significant (Table 49-1).

Goldberg and co-workers[84] were equally sanguine about the value of CCK cholecystography in detecting patients with disease of the biliary tract in the presence of a normal conventional cholecystogram (Table 49-1).

Consequently, despite the fact that (1) different criteria were used to define a "positive" response to CCK, (2) the CCK was injected at different rates, (3) the control subjects were evaluated by varying standards according to the investigator, and (4) the patients were followed for different lengths of time postoperatively, all the authors mentioned were able to reach the same conclusion—that nearly all patients with biliary-type pain who have a cholecystectomy based on a "positive" response to CCK are cured even though they have a normal, conventional cholecystogram.

Despite these favorable reports,* CCK cholecystography has not been accepted enthusiastically as an accurate diagnostic modality in this enigmatic group of patients. Some radiologists are skeptical because of their own unsatisfactory experience with a fatty meal during cholecystography, in which the response of the gallbladder is variable and the production of symptoms is difficult to evaluate. In addition, there is a lack of confidence in CCK cholecystography because investigators do not agree on what constitutes a "positive" response to CCK.

Dunn and co-workers[60] emphasized that none of the previous reports on CCK cholecystography interpreted the results without knowledge of the patient's clinical

---

*References 43, 53, 84, 86-88, 155, 211.

☐ **TABLE 49-1**

Cholecystokinin cholecystography

	Goldstein et al.	Valberg et al.	Nathan et al.	Goldberg et al.	Dunn et al.
Rate of injection (minutes)	3	1	½	1 to 3	¾
Definition of a positive test	Failure to empty the gallbladder more than 50%	Pain	Spasm of the gallbladder and/or pain	Failure to empty the gallbladder more than 80% and pain	Spasm of the gallbladder and/or pain
Cure after cholecystectomy in patients with positive test	22 of 25 (88%)	12 of 13 (92%)	77 of 79 (97%)	14 of 15 (93%)	17 of 20 (85%)
Control studies					
Number	17	30	142	0	44
Result	0 failed to empty the gallbladder more than 50%	0 had pain	3% or less had spasm of the gallbladder; 9% or less had pain		28 had spasm of the gallbladder; 27% had pain

Data from Goldstein, F, Grunt, R, and Margulies, M: Am J Dig Dis 19:835, 1974; Valberg, LS, et al: Gastroenterology 60:1020, 1971; Nathan, MH, et al: AJR 110:240, 1970; Goldberg, HI, et al: Invest Radiol 7:447, 1972; and Dunn, FH, et al: JAMA 228:997, 1974.

condition. They performed CCK cholecystography in 44 control subjects and in 74 patients with a history suggestive of gallbladder disease but in whom routine cholecystography was normal. The radiographs were evaluated by three radiologists without knowledge of the patient's history. The authors concluded that CCK cholecystography as currently performed and interpreted is of little or no value in the diagnosis and management of patients with possible acalculous biliary tract disease. They gave four reasons for their assertion:

1. The incidence of "abnormal" gallbladder contraction in normal subjects is high (14% to 36%).
2. CCK cholecystography does not help predict which patients will be cured by cholecystectomy. Their results show that patients with both normal and abnormal responses to CCK usually are cured or improved by cholecystectomy.
3. CCK cholecystography does not help predict histologic findings in the gallbladder. Patients with normal and abnormal CCK responses who underwent cholecystectomy had similar histologic findings in their gallbladders.
4. There is a high degree of observer disagreement (approximately 28%) in the interpretation of the radiographs.

Davis and co-workers[58] showed no statistically sig-

nificant differences when observing gallbladder contraction with sonography, scintigraphy, and CCK cholecystography in the investigation of chronic acalculous cholecystitis. The results make it unlikely that the degree of contraction as observed by any of these techniques can be used to indicate the presence of chronic acalculous cholecystitis.

HYPERPLASTIC CHOLECYSTOSES

Hyperplastic cholecystosis is a general term introduced by Jutras[119] in 1960 for a group of abnormalities of the gallbladder that appear to be separate from inflammatory diseases.[27] Hyperplasia implies a benign proliferation of normal tissue elements, whereas cholecystosis indicates a pathologic process that is distinct from inflammation. The two main categories of hyperplastic cholecystoses are cholesterolosis and adenomyomatosis. According to Jutras, both types cause functional abnormalities of the gallbladder, including hyperconcentration, hypercontraction, and hyperexcretion. These can be detected on radiographs made during cholecystography and are clues to the diagnosis.

Cholesterolosis

Cholesterolosis, or "strawberry gallbladder," is characterized by abnormal deposits of cholesterol esters in

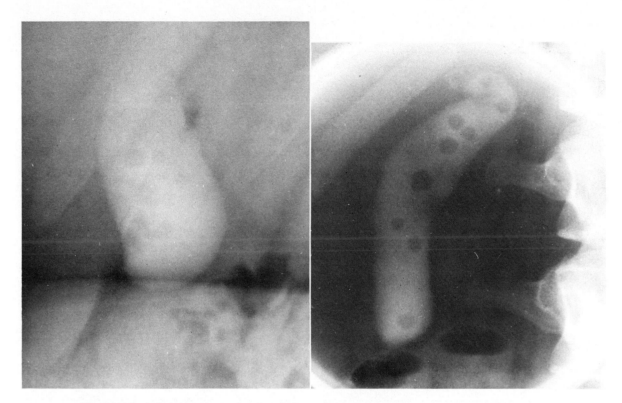

Fig. 49-8 Oral cholecystograms showing cholesterolosis of gallbladder in two patients. Numerous filling defects are visible in gallbladder. Defects maintained same location in gallbladder despite changes in patient's position, indicating that they are fixed to wall.

fat-laden macrophages in the lamina propria of the gall-bladder.[27] The lipid creates coarse, yellow, speckled excrescences on the surface of the reddened hyperemic gallbladder mucosa and gives the latter a strawberry appearance. The cause of the cholesterol deposition is unknown, although it has been attributed to excess cholesterol absorption across the gallbladder mucosa. Cholesterolosis is not related to the serum cholesterol concentration, but cholesterol stones develop in 50% to 70% of patients with the abnormality.[115]

When the cholesterol deposits are of sufficient size, the cholecystogram shows fixed radiolucencies, either localized or generalized, in the opacified gallbladder (Fig. 49-8). The lipid protrusions into the gallbladder lumen may be single or multiple, usually vary in size, are of uneven distribution, and may involve any portion of the gallbladder. The lesions often are best seen on radiographs made after partial evacuation of the gall-bladder and on radiographs made with compression. Indirect radiographic findings include hyperconcentration and hyperexcretion, which are general features of all the hyperplastic cholecystoses.[119] Cholesterolosis can be differentiated from cholelithiasis by determining that the radiolucent defects are fixed in position within the gall-bladder on radiographs made in different positions; gallstones usually are free to move about and to collect by gravity in the dependent portion of the gallbladder or to form a layer in the bile.

The management of patients with cholesterolosis is uncertain. Some surgeons reserve cholecystectomy in such patients for those who also have cholelithiasis and are symptomatic. However, in 269 cases of cholesterolosis without gallstones reported by Salmenkivi,[186] about 90% had complete or partial relief of symptoms following surgery.

Adenomyomatosis

Adenomyomatosis consists of proliferation of mucosa, increased thickness of the muscle coat, and the formation of outpouchings of mucosa into or through the muscularis.[27,119] These diverticula, which are termed *Rokitansky-Aschoff sinuses,* may be segmental or diffuse throughout the gallbladder (Fig. 49-9).

Radiographically the sinuses are seen as multiple or single oval collections of contrast material of varying size adjacent to the lumen of the gallbladder (Fig. 49-

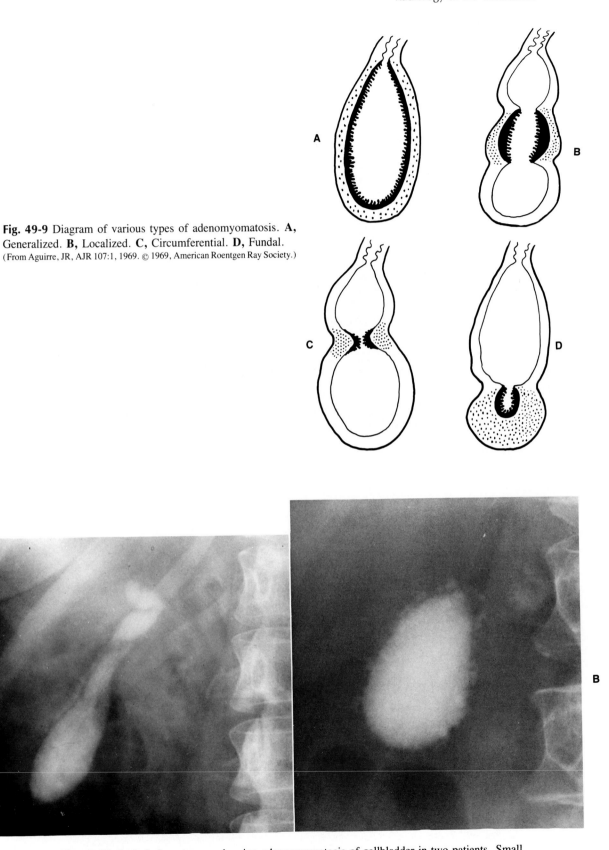

Fig. 49-9 Diagram of various types of adenomyomatosis. **A,** Generalized. **B,** Localized. **C,** Circumferential. **D,** Fundal. (From Aguirre, JR, AJR 107:1, 1969. © 1969, American Roentgen Ray Society.)

Fig. 49-10 Oral cholecystogram showing adenomyomatosis of gallbladder in two patients. Small outpouchings of gallbladder wall filled with contrast material are visible. **A,** Localized. **B,** Generalized.

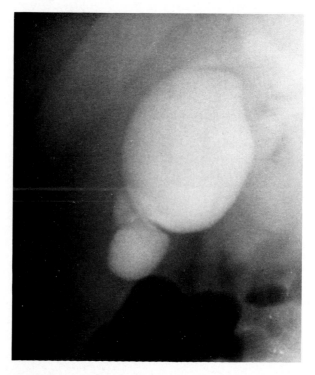

Fig. 49-11 Oral cholecystogram showing circumferential type of adenomyomatosis with compartmentalization of gallbladder.

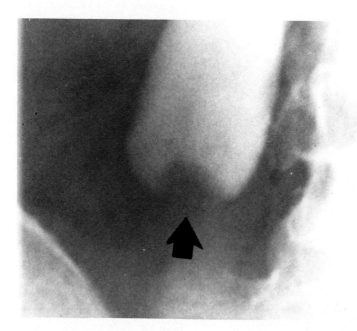

Fig. 49-12 Oral cholecystogram showing fundal adenomyoma of gallbladder *(arrow)*.

10). Any portion of the gallbladder may be involved. At times calcified concretions are present within the diverticula. Adenomyomatosis is often associated with compartmentalization of the gallbladder caused by septal folds or annular thickening of the gallbladder wall (Fig. 49-11). Whether compartmentalization is the cause or effect of adenomyomatosis is not certain. Compartmentalization may result from circumferential adenomyomatosis, a congenital septum, or adenomyomatosis superimposed on a congenital septum. Aguirre and coworkers[3] believe that the circumferential form of adenomyomatosis producing compartmentalization originates in a congenital septum. It is often difficult to determine by cholecystography whether the stenosis is a simple septum or whether the adenomyomatosis is already present.

The combination of adenomyomatosis and cholesterolosis is not unusual, and gallstones are often present. Like cholesterolosis, adenomyomatosis is often more easily identified and appears more marked on radiographs made after partial emptying of the gallbladder. Fundal adenomyomatosis has various radiologic patterns, ranging from a filling defect or mass in the fundus caused by focal hyperplsaia of the gallbladder wall to multiple diverticular outpouchings filled with contrast material or small calculi localized to the fundus (Fig. 49-12).

Adenomyomatosis is observed much more commonly pathologically than radiographically. In one series, 50% of patients having cholecystectomy for gallstones had associated adenomyomatosis that was not apparent on cholecystography.[136] Whether a cholecystectomy should be performed in a patient with adenomyomatosis depends on the severity and duration of the symptoms and the presence of cholelithiasis.

NORMAL VARIATIONS OF THE GALLBLADDER

The size, shape, and position of the gallbladder as seen on cholecystography vary considerably in normal patients, depending on the body habitus of the patient, the degree of filling of the gallbladder, the amount of distention of the adjacent transverse colon, the position in which the radiograph is made, and the type of contrast material used. Tall, slender individuals tend to have vertically oriented, long gallbladders that may lie in the right iliac fossa; in mesomorphic patients the gallbladder usually is horizontal, tortuous, oriented in a lateral plane, and high in the right upper quadrant of the abdomen. When the gallbladder has no mesentery and is closely applied to the undersurface of the liver, little change in shape and position occurs with differences in position of the patient, except for the fundus. The liver edge serves as a fulcrum for changes in the position of the fundus in relation to the body of the gallbladder. When the gallbladder is on a long mesentery, it can be quite mobile and change position and shape to a considerable extent, depending on gravity. Superimposition of the fundus on the body may simulate duplication of the gallbladder unless the gallbladder is visualized in profile using fluoroscopy to determine the optimal position.

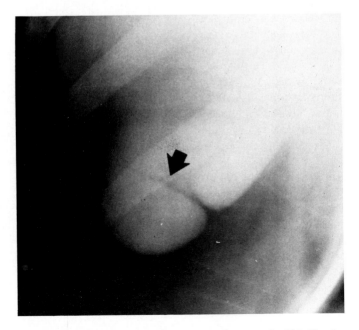

Fig. 49-13 Oral cholecystogram showing phrygian cap of gallbladder *(arrow)*.

Phrygian cap

A phrygian cap is a normal variation in the shape of the gallbladder in which the fundus appears to be folded on the body (Fig. 49-13). The name is taken from the similarly shaped headdress worn as a sign of liberation by slaves in ancient Greece. In 1935 Boyden[35] studied the morphology and pathogenesis of the phrygian cap and, contrary to the accepted view at that time, recognized it as having no clinical importance. He described two types, depending on whether the serosa of the gallbladder was included in the septum between the fundus and the body. Similar folding located more proximally in the body of the gallbladder is not unusual and has no significance except that it must be differentiated from compartmentalization of the gallbladder associated with adenomyomatosis. Indeed, such folds may predispose the patient to circumferential adenomyomatosis. When adenomyomatosis involves the septum, the fold or narrowing usually is thicker, and evacuation radiographs of the gallbladder show focal spasm and diverticular outpouchings in the region of the infolding.

Layering of contrast material

With the patient in the erect position, layers of bile are present in the gallbladder that increase in specific gravity from the neck to the fundus. Visual demonstration of this layering phenomenon occurs duuring cholecystography with the patient in the erect position whenever rapid filling of the gallbladder causes incomplete mixing of nonopaque and contrast-laden bile. When there is incomplete mixing, discrete bands of radiolucent bile can be identified separately from layers of bile containing contrast material on upright radiographs. The layer that has been in the gallbladder the longest has the highest specific gravity and therefore is dependent. Incomplete mixing detected on prone or supine radiographs may simulate cholelithiasis.

Layering of contrast material in the gallbladder is much more common during intravenous cholangiography than during oral cholecystography, because rapid filling of the gallbladder with contrast material during intravenous studies does not allow adequate time for uniform mixing.

Bryk and Moadel[39] showed that layering of contrast material occurred in only 6% of patients on upright radiographs made during oral cholecystography. However, when a fatty meal was given to these patients, layering was noted in most cases on upright radiographs made 2 hours later. In these cases the layering phenomenon appeared to be the result of rapid refilling of the gallbladder with nonopaque bile following partial emptying of the gallbladder.

Precipitation of contrast material

Because the glucuronide conjugate of Telepaque excreted by the liver is relatively water soluble, the contrast material is neither reabsorbed from the normal gallbladder nor precipitated in the gallbladder lumen.[26] Rarely, however, presumably because of the presence in the gallbladder of bacteria capable of producing glucuronidase, Telepaque glucuronide is deconjugated and Telepaque precipitates in the bile.[208] This action produces amorphous radiopaque densities in the gallbladder that collect in the fundus on radiographs made with the patient in the upright position (Fig. 49-14).

Differentiation from small radiopaque calculi depends on the fact that the precipitate does not persist on subsequent plain abdominal radiographs, whereas radiopaque calculi remain unchanged. In addition, for reasons that are obscure, Telepaque rarely precipitates a second time on a later cholecystogram.

CONGENITAL ANOMALIES
Anomalies of position

An abnormal position of the gallbladder occurs in association with situs inversus.[30] In other cases the gallbladder may be left sided in relation to the inferior aspect

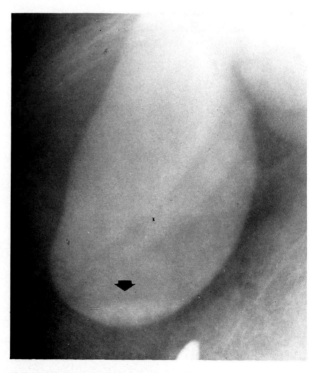

Fig. 49-14 Oral cholecystogram (upright projection) showing precipitation of Telepaque in fundus of gallbladder *(arrow)*.

of the left lobe of the liver, in which case the cystic duct may terminate in the right hepatic duct.[206] Rarely, the gallbladder may be on the left, associated with isolated transposition of the liver. In this case, the liver and the gallbladder usually are located directly anterior to the stomach.

When the gallbladder lies completely within the parenchyma of the liver, major diagnostic and therapeutic difficulties arise if acute cholecystitis occurs. A liver scan, ultrasound studies, and hepatic angiography suggest the presence of a hepatic abscess. Rarely, gallstones can be identified in the gallbladder within the liver on plain abdominal radiographs. The gallbladder may be located behind the liver (retrohepatic)[90] and may even be retroperitoneal or interposed between the liver and the diaphragm (suprahepatic).[212,225] Isolated cases have been reported of an ectopic gallbladder located in the falciform ligament in the abdominal wall.[98] An abnormally situated gallbladder in a retrorenal location may simulate a mass lesion.[62]

The gallbladder may be unusually mobile when it is on a long mesentery. In such cases herniation into the foramen of Winslow is possible. Vint[213] reported four surgically proved cases. The key radiologic finding is displacement of the gallbladder medial to the duodenal bulb, which is best seen on frontal projection with the gallbladder and the stomach opacified with barium. The gallbladder appears to drape over the apex of the bulb, and the adjacent walls of these structures conform closely to each other. The clinical significance of herniation of the gallbladder is unknown. It may be intermittent and asymptomatic in some patients, but in others it is believed to be the cause of vague abdominal discomfort. Hernia-tion and strangulation of the gallbladder through the foramen of Winslow, however, has been reported in one instance.[10]

Duplication

The appearance of a double gallbladder on cholecystography most often is proved to be a tortuous gallbladder with overlap of the fundus, body, and neck on one projection or a gallbladder with compartmentalization. To establish the diagnosis, two separate gallbladder lumina and two distinct cystic ducts must be demonstrated. Shehadi and Jacox[196] reported an incidence of 1 in 12,000 cholecystograms (Fig. 49-15).

Roedert and co-workers[180] reported a patient with triplication of the gallbladder in whom one gallbladder had acute cholecystitis and cholelithiasis and another had adenocarcinoma.

In these cases revacuolization of the primitive gallbladder is incomplete, resulting in a persistent longitudinal septum that divides the gallbladder lengthwise, creating a bifid gallbladder or a true duplication.[34]

Agenesis

Agenesis of the gallbladder is virtually impossible to distinguish radiographically from acute cholecystitis with obstruction of the cystic duct. However, two thirds of the patients with this anomaly have other malformations, such as congenital heart lesions, imperforate anus, or rectovaginal fistula.[99] Consequently, the diagnosis should be suspected in patients with multiple congenital anomalies who have opacification of the common bile duct without gallbladder visualization on oral cholecystography or intravenous cholangiography.

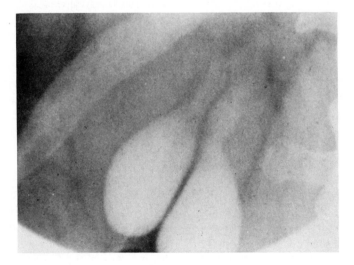

Fig. 49-15 Oral cholecystogram showing duplication of gallbladder. Two separate cystic ducts were identified at surgery.

Surgical exploration with operative cholangiography may be misleading.[206] A left-sided or intrahepatic gallbladder, an atrophic gallbladder, or one surrounded by adhesions may be mistaken for agenesis of the gallbladder.

More recent reports in the literature on agenesis of the gallbladder strongly suggest a familial hereditary trait.[222]

Multiseptate gallbladder

Croce[55] defined the multiseptate gallbladder as a solitary gallbladder, usually in normal position and size, characterized externally by a faintly bosselated surface and internally by the presence of multiple septa of variable size and number. The chambers thus formed communicate with each other by one or more orifices from the fundus to the cystic duct. Histologically the walls of the septa are characterized by a layer of muscle between the two epithelial surfaces, a finding that appears to exclude the hypothesis that the anomaly is the result of arrested vacuolization of the epithelial bud of the gallbladder or an extension of the valves of Heister from the cystic duct.[200]

Stasis of bile in the gallbladder predisposes the patient to infection and gallstone formation. The diagnosis can be made radiographically as long as complicating gallstones do not occlude the cystic duct and prevent opacification of the gallbladder. The multicystic honeycomb character of the gallbladder is apparent on oral cholecystography.[33]

The multiseptate gallbladder must be differentiated from the hypoplastic changes that occur in the gallbladder in patients with cystic fibrosis of the pancreas.

Heterotopic pancreatic and gastric tissue

Aberrant pancreatic tissue and gastric mucosa occur in a variety of locations throughout the gastrointestinal tract. Rarely, implants of these tissues have been reported in the gallbladder.[19,139,158] In such cases the cholecystogram may show a mural nodule in the gallbladder similar to cholesterolosis and various benign tumors. When the lesion is located at the neck of the gallbladder or cystic duct, partial or intermittent obstructions may cause nonvisualization of cholecystography and may result in cholecystitis.

CHOLELITHIASIS

An estimated 15 million Americans have gallstones, 85% of which are composed predominantly of cholesterol.[52] A prerequisite for the formation of cholesterol gallstones is bile containing insufficient bile salts and lecithin in proportion to cholesterol to maintain the cholesterol in solution by the detergent-like property of the

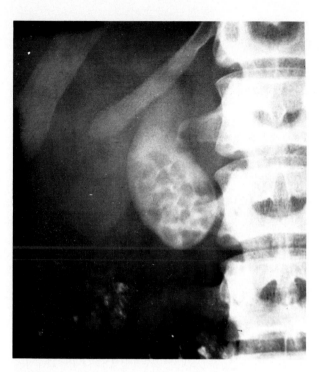

Fig. 49-16 Oral cholecystogram showing multiple gallstones in gallbladder.

bile salts.[177] Such lithogenic bile may result from a decrease in the size of the bile salt pool because of disease or resection of the terminal ileum or may result from increased hepatic cholesterol synthesis. Stones composed of bilirubin are less common and occur when there is excessive red blood cell destruction such as in patients with sickle cell anemia.

Kishk and co-workers[124] demonstrated that patients with gallstones exhibit a higher resting gallbladder volume with less fractional emptying after a fatty meal, and with a higher residual volume after the meal, when compared to normal control subjects. These authors suggest that in some patients decreased gallbladder contractility may contribute to gallstone development or proliferation.

Oral cholecystography is also being used as a method for observing the results of medical treatment of gallstones (Fig. 49-16). Thistle and Hofmann[209] have demonstrated that the oral administration of chenodoxycholic acid, one of the bile salts, decreases cholesterol saturation in bile and dissolves gallstones. By performing serial oral cholecystograms on patients with opacified gallbladders and cholelithiasis, these investigators observed the dissolution of gallstones over a period of 6 months in 12 of 19 patients receiving the compound.

Gallstones vary markedly in number, size, and shape, so that cholecystography may demonstrate gallstones as

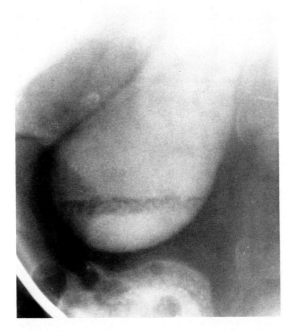

Fig. 49-17 Oral cholecystogram (upright projection) showing gallstones floating in gallbladder.

large as 4 or 5 cm, as well as some that are no more than 1 or 2 mm. A single stone may be present, or there may be as many as 100 or more. When tiny stones are numerous, they often have a sandlike or gravellike consistency and are visible only on upright or lateral decubitus projections of the gallbladder. Gallstones are nearly always freely movable in the gallbladder and readily change position on radiographs made in different positions. The stones usually fall by gravity to the dependent portion of the gallbladder. Not infrequently they form a layer in the bile, depending on their specific gravity in relation to that of the bile[57] (Fig. 49-17). Occasionally, a stone becomes adherent to the gallbladder wall and simulates a mural lesion such as a cholesterol polyp.

Reports of the spontaneous disappearance of gallstones are not rare, so that when there is a significant interval between the demonstration of calculi and surgery, a repeat cholecystogram should be performed.[8] This is especially important if the gallstones are small. In some cases, particularly after pregnancy, it may be that bile that was lithogenic returns to normal and the gallstones dissolve. In other cases the gallstones are passed into the duodenum via the cystic duct and common bile ducts with or without symptoms of biliary colic. Gas fissuring of gallstones may reduce the specific gravity of the stones, so that they float in bile and are more likely to enter the cystic duct and be passed spontaneously. Splitting of gallstones along the gas-filled faults causes spon-

---

☐ CAUSES OF FIXED FILLING DEFECT(S) IN OPACIFIED GALLBLADDER ☐

1. Cholesterolosis
2. Adenomyomatosis
3. Adherent gallstone
4. Adenoma
5. Papilloma
6. Carcinoid tumor
7. Carcinoma
8. Metastasis
9. Mucosal hyperplasia
10. Inflammatory polyp
11. Epithelial cyst
12. Mucous retention cyst
13. Spurious defect of infundibulum
14. Heterotopic pancreatic or gastric tissue
15. Parasitic granuloma
16. Varices
17. Arterial tortuosity and aneurysm

---

taneous fragmentation of the stones, which also predisposes them to spontaneous passage.[146]

NEOPLASMS
Benign tumors

True benign tumors of the gallbladder are exceedingly rare. Adenomas, the most common type, usually occur as flat elevations located in the body of the gallbladder.[45] Adenomas almost invariably occur in or near the fundus and must be distinguished pathologically from adenomyomatosis, which is a hyperplastic change in the gallbladder wall. Papillomas may occur singly or in groups and may be scattered over a large part of the mucosal surface of the gallbladder.[143]

When a benign tumor is present, the cholecystogram discloses one or more small round or oval radiolucent defects fixed to the wall of an opacified gallbladder.[92,159,207] Often the lesion is better delineated after partial contraction of the gallbladder. Radiographs made in various positions and with different degrees of compression confirm that the defect is not freely movable within the gallbladder.

In most patients with a fixed filling defect demonstrated on cholecystography, surgery proves that the defect is a pseudotumor rather than a true benign neoplasm. Of the many varieties of pseudotumors of the gallbladder that can be identified during cholecystography, a solitary cholesterol polyp is the most common. However, mucosal hyperplasia, inflammatory polyps, mucous cysts, and granulomas caused by parasitic infections also occur (see box above). Polypoid masses containing metachromatic sulfatides produce fixed defects in the wall of the gallbladder and occur in patients with metachromatic leukodystrophy.[126] Occasionally when gallstones are coated with tenacious mucus, they adhere to the gallbladder wall and present as fixed filling defects on oral cholecystography.

Cimmino[46] reported a case of noninvasive papillary adenocarcinoma in which the tumor was evident as a solitary fixed defect in a well-opacified gallbladder. Others have been reported,[83] but such cases are so unusual that cholecystectomy is not indicated to exclude carcinoma in patients in whom a solitary fixed defect is detected in the gallbladder at cholecystography.

Malignant tumors

Primary carcinoma of the gallbladder is nearly always a rapidly progressive disease, with a mortality approaching 100%.[18,107,123,125,178] Although it is associated with cholelithiasis in about 80% to 90% of cases, direct proof is lacking to implicate the gallstones as the carcinogenic agent.[150] Patients with a porcelain gallbladder also have an increased incidence of carcinoma of the gallbladder.[24] The latter is twice as common as carcinoma of the bile ducts and occurs most frequently in women 60 years of age or older.

Parker and Joffee[165] and Rogers and co-workers[181] reported patients who had calcification in mucinous adenocarcinoma of the gallbladder in which fine punctate calcifications were identified in the region of the gallbladder on plain abdominal radiographs. This type of calcification is distinct from that associated with a porcelain gallbladder and has also been described in primary and metastatic lesions in cases of mucinous adenocarcinoma of the colon.

When bloodborne metastases to the gallbladder occur, they are often caused by melanoma.[13,197] In a review by Willis[221] of 21 reported cases of metastases to the gallbladder, two thirds were caused by melanoma. Indeed, 15% of patients with metastatic melanoma have gallbladder involvement, indicating that the propensity for melanoma to metastasize to the gastrointestinal tract includes the gallbladder.[197] The metastases usually involve the mucosa of the gallbladder and are accompanied by liver metastases in most instances. According to Shimkin and co-workers,[197] the metastases first appear as small, flat, subepithelial nodules that become polypoid and even pedunculated as they grow into the gallbladder lumen.

ABNORMALITIES IN SIZE
Cholecystomegaly

Enlargement of the gallbladder in the absence of obstruction of the biliary tract has been reported by various investigators to be a sequela of both truncal and selective vagotomy.[7] In one of the earliest studies on the subject, Johnson and Boyden reported that the fasting gallbladder volume doubles in patients following a reduction of secretin-induced choleresis.[23] Gallbladder emptying probably remains normal, although this has been the subject of considerable debate.[32,68,109] Amberg and co-workers[7] showed that the response of the dog gallbladder to CCK is unchanged after truncal vagotomy. Despite theoretic reasons for expecting an increased tendency to form gallstones in patients with an enlarged gallbladder after vagotomy, there has been no clinical evidence that this is the case.[109,152]

Bloom and Stachenfeld[31] reported three patients with diabetes mellitus in whom the gallbladder was enlarged three to nine times normal size on cholecystography. In their series of 25 patients with diabetes, 16% had an enlarged gallbladder, whereas none was detected in 50 control patients. There was no correlation between cholecystomegaly and the clinical manifestations of diabetes, the severity of disease, or the mode of therapy. The gallbladder enlargement in these cases probably is related to an autonomic neuropathy. An analogy between postvagotomy and diabetic cholecystomegaly appears to be likely. However, enlargement of the gallbladder in diabetics may result from an abnormality of the gallbladder musculature, an alteration of the amount of character of bile, or a change in gallbladder function. Regardless of the pathogenesis, it appears appropriate to evaluate patients with a large gallbladder for diabetes.[80]

Microgallbladder in mucoviscidosis

A small, contracted, poorly functioning gallbladder with marginal irregularities and multiple weblike trabeculations may be present in patients with cystic fibrosis of the pancreas.[30,64,113,184,189] The pathologic changes in the gallbladder are presumed to be produced by the thick tenacious bile and mucus that are part of the disease. The findings are similar to those of a congenital multiseptate or hypoplastic gallbladder.

Displacement

Displacement and/or deformity of the gallbladder may result from dilatation of adjacent structures such as the duodenum and colon or may be produced by mass lesions in the right upper quadrant, particularly those arising in the liver or porta hepatis region.[117] Consequently, deformity of the gallbladder may be the first or only clue to the diagnosis of disease in a number of organs that are in proximity to the gallbladder.

It can be assumed that any mass adjacent to the gallbladder is capable of deforming its outline. Fisher[73] classified the origin of such masses as either hepatic or extrahepatic and described her own cases of multicentric

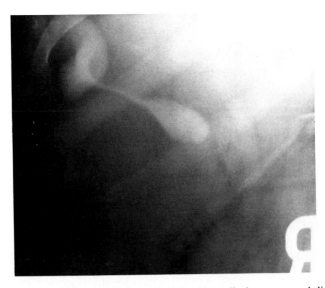

Fig. 49-18 Oral cholecystogram showing striking stretching, displacement, and distortion of gallbladder caused by adjacent large angiosarcoma of liver.

hepatoma, hepar lobatum caused by tertiary syphilis, and lymphadenopathy caused by histiocytic lymphoma in which there were extrinsic pressure defects on the gallbladder.

Other masses in the liver that can displace or deform the contour of the gallbladder include solitary hepatoma, hemangioma, metastases, regenerating nodules, hydatid cysts, polycystic disease and abscesses, and granulomas.[38,49,188] Joffe and Babenco[117] emphasized that mass lesions in the liver produce discrete localized defects in the gallbladder that are persistent and reproducible (Fig. 49-18). The deformity tends not to vary in relation to the patient's position. In cases of gallbladder displacement caused by distention of the colon or duodenum, the defect in the contour of the gallbladder is changeable and inconsistent. In these situations the cause of the abnormality usually is readily apparent.

Extrahepatic masses that may be evident by virtue of their effect on the gallbladder include retroperitoneal tumors, pancreatic pseudocysts, and lymphadenopathy, usually caused by one of the lymphomas.

Recognition of defects in the contour of the gallbladder may provide the first evidence that an abnormality is present and that additional studies with ultrasound, angiography, or CT are indicated to establish a definite diagnosis.

REFERENCES

1. Adams, TW, and Foxley, EG: A diagnostic technique for acalculous cholecystitis, Surg Gynecol Obstet 142:168, 1976.
2. Admirand, WH, and Small, DM: The physiochemical basis of cholesterol gallstone formation in man, J Clin Invest 47:1043, 1968.
3. Aguirre, JR, Boher, RO, and Guraieb, S: Hyperplastic cholecystoses: a new contribution to the unitarian theory, AJR 107:1, 1969.
4. Alderson, DA: The reliability of Telepaque cholecystography, Br J Surg 47:655, 1960.
5. Amberg, J: Radiology of the biliary tract. In Sleisenger, MH, and Fordtran, JS, editors: Gastrointestinal disease, Philadelphia, 1973, WB Saunders.
6. Amberg, JR, Zboralske, FF, and Johnson, ER: The inclined lateral decubitus position for cholecystography, AJR 92:1128, 1964.
7. Amberg, JR, et al: Effect of vagotomy on gallbladder size and contractility in the dog, Invest Radiol 8:371, 1973.
8. Arcomano, JP, Schwinger, HN, and DeAngelis, J: The spontaneous disappearance of gallstones, AJR 99:637, 1967.
9. Ashmore, JD, et al: Experimental evaluation of operative cholangiography in relation to calculus size, Surgery 40:191, 1956.
10. Bach, DB, et al: Herniation and strangulation of the gallbladder through the foramen of Winslow, AJR 142:541, 1984.
11. Baker, HI, and Hodgson, JR: Oral cholecystography: an evaluation of its accuracy, Gastroenterology 34:1137, 1958.
12. Baker, HL, and Hodgson, JR: Further studies on the accuracy of oral cholecystography, Radiology 74:239, 1960.
13. Balthazar, EJ, and Javors, B: Malignant melanoma of the gallbladder, Am J Gastroenterol 64:332, 1975.
14. Balthazar, EJ, and Schechter, LS: Air in the gallbladder: a frequent finding in gallstone ileus, AJR 131:219, 1978.
15. Barakos, JA, et al: Cholelithiasis: evaluation with CT, Radiology 162:415, 1987.
16. Bartrum, RJ, Crow, HC, and Foote, SR: Ultrasonic and radiographic cholecystography, N Engl J Med 296:538, 1977.
17. Becker, CD, and Vock, P: Appearance of gas-containing gallstones on sonography and computed tomography, Gastrointest Radiol 9:323, 1984.
18. Beltz, WR, and Condon, RE: Primary carcinoma of the gallbladder, Ann Surg 180:180, 1974.
19. Bentivegna, S, and Hirschl, S: Heterotopic gastric mucosa in the gallbladder presenting as a symptom-producing tumor, Am J Gastroenterol 57:423, 1972.

20. Berk, RN: The consecutive dose phenomenon in oral cholecystography, AJR 110:230, 1970.
21. Berk, RN: The problem of impaired first-dose visualization of the gallbladder, AJR 113:186, 1971.
22. Berk, RN: Radiology of thhe gallbladder and bile ducts, Surg Clin North Am 53:973, 1973.
23. Berk, RN: Oral cholecystography. In Berk, RN, and Clemett, AR, editors: Radiology of the gallbladder and bile ducts, Philadelphia, 1977, WB Saunders.
24. Berk, RN, Armbuster, TG, and Saltzstein, SL: Carcinoma of the porcelain gallbladder, Radiology 106:29, 1973.
25. Berk, RN, Goldberger, LE, and Loeb, PM: The role of bile salts in the hepatic excretion of iopanoic acid, Invest Radiol 9:7, 1974.
26. Berk, RN, and Loeb, PM: Pharmacology and physiology of the biliary radiographic contrast materials, Semin Roentgenol 11:147, 1976.
27. Berk, RN, van der Vegt, E, and Lictenstein, JE: Hyperplastic cholecystoses: cholesterolosis and adenomyomatosis, Radiology 146:593, 1983.
28. Beseman, EF: Can ipodate calcium save the patient one day in hospitalization? AJR 110:226, 1970.
29. Besic, LR, Krawzoff, G, and Tiesenga, MF: Limy bile syndrome, JAMA 193:145, 1965.
30. Blanton, DE, Bream, CA, and Mandel, SR: Gallbladder ectopia, AJR 121:396, 1974.
31. Bloom, AA, and Stachenfeld, R: Diabetic cholecystectomy, JAMA 208:357, 1969.
32. Bouchier, IAD: The vagus, the bile and gallstones, Gut 11:799, 1970.
33. Bova, JG: Gallstones simulated by gallbladder septation, AJR 140:287, 1983.
34. Boyden, EA: The accessory gallbladder, an embryological and comparative study of aberrant biliary vesicles occurring in man and domestic animals, Am J Anat 38:177, 1926.
35. Boyden, EA: The "phrygian cap" in cholecystography, AJR 33:589, 1935.
36. Broadbent, NRG, and Taylor, DEM: Gallstone erosion of the aorta, Aust NZ J Surg 45:207, 1975.
37. Brochis, JG, and Gilbert MC: Intestinal obstruction by gallstones, Br J Surg 44:461, 1956.
38. Brust, RW, and Conlon, PC: Roentgenologic manifestations of primary hepatoma with particular reference to some unusual cholecystographic findings, AJR 87:777, 1962.
39. Bryk, D, and Moadel, E: Layering of contrast material in oral cholecystography, Am J Dig Dis 20:727, 1975.
40. Buckstein, J: The digestive tract in roentgenology, ed 2, vol 2, Philadelphia, 1953, JB Lippincott.
41. Burhenne, HJ: Problem areas in the biliary tract, Curr Probl Radiol 5:1, 1975.
42. Burhenne, HJ, and Obata, WG: Single-visit oral cholecystography, N Engl J Med 292:627, 1975.
43. Camishion, RC, and Goldstein, F: Partial, non-calculous cystic duct obstruction (cystic duct syndrome), Surg Clin North Am 47:1107, 1967.
44. Campbell, EW, and Rogers, CL: Submucosal gallbladder emphysema, JAMA 227:790, 1974.
45. Christensen, AH, and Ishak, KG: Benign tumors and pseudotumors of the gallbladder, Arch Pathol 90:423, 1970.
46. Cimmino, CV: Carcinoma in a well-functioning gallbladder, Radiology 71:563, 1958.
47. Cockrell, CH, and Chio, SR: Upright tomographic oral cholecystography, Radiology 151:797, 1984.
48. Cohen, S, et al: Liver disease and gallstones in regional enteritis, Gastroenterology 60:237, 1971.
49. Conlon, PC, and Brust, RW: Cholecystography as an aid in the localization of upper abdominal masses, AJR 88:756, 1962.
50. Cooperberg, PL, and Burhenne, HJ: Real-time ultrasonography: diagnostic technique of choice in calculous gallbladder disease, N Engl J Med 302:1277, 1980.
51. Cornell, CM, and Clarke, R: Vicarious calcification involving the gallbladder, Ann Surg 149:267, 1959.
52. Coyne, MJ, et al: Treatment of gallstones with chenodeoxycholic acid and phenobarbital, N Engl J Med 292:604, 1975.
53. Cozzolino, HJ, et al: The cystic duct syndrome, JAMA 185:920, 1963.
54. Crade, M, et al: Surgical and pathologic correlation of cholecystosonography and cholecystography, AJR 131:227, 1978.
55. Croce, EJ: The multiseptate gallbladder, Arch Surg 107:104, 1973.
56. Crummy, AB: Five-hour reinforcement cholecystography, Gastrointest Radiol 1:91, 1976.
57. Culp, WL: Buoyancy of gallstones in varying concentrations of contrast media, AJR 143:79, 1984.
58. Davis, GB, et al: Cholecystokinin, cholecystography, and scintigraphy: detection of chronic acalculous cholecystitis, AJR 139:1117, 1982.
59. Donner, MW, and Weiner, S: Diagnostic evaluation of abdominal calcifications in acute abdominal disorders, Radiol Clin North Am 2:145, 1964.
60. Dunn, FH, et al: Cholecystokinin cholecystography, JAMA 228:997, 1974.
61. duPlessis, DJ, and Jersky, J: Management of acute cholecystitis, Surg Clin North Am 53:1071, 1973.
62. Ehman, RL, and Morrish, HF: Retrorenal gallbladder: a case report, J Can Assoc Radiol 34:321, 1983.
63. Eisenman, JI, Finck, EJ, and O'Loughlin, BJ: Gallstone ileus: a review of the roentgenographic findings and report of a new roentgen sign, AJR 101:361, 1967.
64. Esterly, JR, and Oppenheimer, EH: Observations in cystic fibrosis of the pancreas. I. The gallbladder, Bull Johns Hopkins Hosp 110:247, 1962.
65. Etala, E: Cancer de la vesicular bilar, Prensa Med Argent 49:2283, 1962.
66. Etter, LE: Left-sided gallbladder, AJR 70:987, 1953.
67. Ettinger, A: The value of the upright position in gallbladder examination, Radiology 34:481, 1940.
68. Fagerberg, S., et al: Vagotomy and gallbladder function, Gut 11:789, 1970.
69. Farrar, ZT: Underdiagnosis of biliary tract disorders, Gastroenterology 51:1074, 1966.
70. Ferguson, AN, and Palmer, WL: Cholecystography: its clinical evaluation, JAMA 100:809, 1933.
71. Ferrucci, JT: Body ultrasonography, part 2, N Engl J Med 300:590, 1979.
72. Fischer, HW, and Burgener, FA: Fractionated dose administration schedule for cholecystography, Invest Radiol 9:24, 1974.
73. Fisher, MS: Hepar lobatum and other less exotic causes of gallbladder deformity, Radiology 91:308, 1968.
74. Flye, MW, and Silver, D: Biliary tract disorders and sickle cell disease, Surgery 72:361, 1972.
75. Foss, HL, and Summers, JD: Intestinal obstruction from gallstones, Ann Surg 115:721, 1942.
76. Fox, PF: Planning the operation for cholecystenteric fistula with gallstone ileus, Surg Clin North Am 50:93, 1970.
77. Fried, L, et al: Oral cholecystography and cholecystosonography: a prospective trial, J Can Assoc Radiol 34:342, 1983.
78. Friedman, DK, Kannel WB, and Dawber, TR: Epidemiology of gallbladder disease: observations in Framingham study, J Chronic Dis 19:273, 1966.

79. Friman-Dahl, J: Roentgen examinations in acute abdominal diseases, ed 2, Springfield, Ill, 1960, Charles C Thomas.

80. Gitelson, S, Oppenheim, D, and Schwartz, A: Size of the gallbladder in patients with diabetes mellitus, Diabetes 18:493, 1969.

81. Goldberg, BB, Harris, K, and Broocker, W: Ultrasound and radiographic cholecystography: a comparison, Radiology 111:405, 1974.

82. Goldberg, HI: Cholecystokinin cholecystography, Semin Roentgenol 11:175, 1976.

83. Goldberg, HI: Small bowel disease and oral cholecystography, Gastroenterology 71:529, 1976.

84. Goldberg, HI, et al: Contractility of the inflamed gallbladder: an experimental study using the technique of cholecystokinin cholecystography, Invest Radiol 7:447, 1972.

85. Goldberger, LE, Berk, RN, and Loeb, PM: Biopharmaceutical factors influencing intestinal absorption of iopanoic acid, Invest Radiol 9:16, 1974.

86. Goldstein, F, Ginsberg, DK, and Johnson, RG: Biliary dyskinesia—report of two cases with physiologic studies, Am J Gastroenterol 36:268, 1961.

87. Goldstein, F, Grunt, R, and Margulies, M: Cholecystokinin cholecystography in differential diagnosis of acalculous gallbladder disease, Gastroenterology 62:756, 1972.

88. Goldstein, F, Grunt, R, and Margulies, M: Cholecystokinin cholecystography in the differential diagnosis of acalculous gallbladder disease, Am J Dig Dis 19:835, 1974.

89. Gray, PHK: Radiography of ancient Egyptian mummies, Medical Radiography and Photography, vol 43, Eastman Kodak, 1967.

90. Greaves, FW, Nguyen, KT, and Sauerbrei, EE: Retrohepatic gallbladder diagnosed by sonography and scintigraphy, J Can Assoc Radiol 34:319, 1983.

91. Greenwood, F, and Samuel, E: The pathological gallbladder, Br J Radiol 21:438, 1948.

92. Grieco, RV, Bartone, NF, and Vasiles, A: A study of fixed filling defects in the well opacified gallbladder and their evaluation, AJR 90:844, 1963.

93. Grossman, ET: Cholecystocolic fistula—an unusual cause of diarrhea, Am J Gastroenterol 55:277, 1971.

94. Harley, WD, Kirkpatrick, RH, and Ferrucci, JT: Gas in the bile ducts (pneumobilia) in emphysematous cholecystitis, AJR 131:661, 1978.

95. Harned, RK, and LaVeen, RF: Preliminary abdominal films in oral cholecystography: are they necessary? AJR 130:477, 1978.

96. Harris, RC, and Caffey, J: Cholecystography in infants, JAMA 153:1333, 1953.

97. Harvey, TC, Thwe, M, and Low-Beer, TS: The value of the fatty meal in oral cholecystography, Clin Radiol 27:117, 1976.

98. Hatfield, PM, and Wise, RE: Anatomic variation in the gallbladder and bile ducts, Semin Roentgenol 11:157, 1976.

99. Haughton, V, and Lewicki, AW: Agenesis of the gallbladder: is preoperative diagnosis possible? Radiology 106:305, 1973.

100. Heaton, KW, and Gibson, MJ: The use of fatty meals in oral cholecystography: report of a postal survey in England and Wales, Clin Radiol 24:90, 1973.

101. Hicken, NF, and Coray, QB: Spontaneous gastrointestinal biliary fistulas, Surg Gynecol Obstet 83:723, 1946.

102. Hodgson, JR: The technical aspects of cholecystography, Radiol Clin North Am 8:85, 1970.

103. Hodgson, JR, and Baker, HL: New concepts in cholecystography and cholangiography, Postgrad Med 26:283, 1959.

104. Hofman, AF: The syndrome of ileal disease and the broken enterohepatic circulation, Gastroenterology 52:752, 1967.

105. Holden, WS, and Turner, MJ: Disappearing limy bile, Clin Radiol 23:500, 1972.

106. Holgerson, LO, White, JL, and West, JP: Emphysematous cholecystitis: a report of five cases, Surgery 69:102, 1971.

107. Holmes, SL, and Mark, JBD: Carcinoma of the gallbladder, Surg Gynecol Obstet 135:561, 1971.

108. Hopman, WPM, et al: Gallbladder contraction: effects of fatty meals and cholecystokinin, Radiology 157:37, 1985.

109. Hopton, DS: The influence of the vagus nerves on the biliary system, Br J Surg 60:216, 1973.

110. Howard, JM: Gallbladder function (cholecystographic studies) following non-specific trauma, Surgery 36:1051, 1954.

111. Hudspeth, AS, and McGuirt, WF: Gallstone ileus, a continuing surgical problem, Arch Surg 100:668, 1970.

112. Isch, JH, Finneran, JC, and Nahrwold, DL: Perforation of the gallbladder, Am J Gastroenterol 55:451, 1971.

113. Isenberg, JN, et al: Clinical observations on the biliary system in cystic fibrosis, Gastroenterology 65:134, 1976.

114. Ivy, AC, and Oldberg, E: A hormone mechanism for gallbladder contraction and evacuation, Am J Physiol 86:559, 1928.

115. Jacobs, LA, et al: Hyperplastic cholecystoses, Arch Surg 104:193, 1972.

116. Jensen, R, and Kaude, J: Oral cholecystography, Acta Radiol 10:499, 1970.

117. Joffe, N, and Babenco, GO: Localized deformity of the gallbladder secondary to hepatic mass lesions, AJR 121:412, 1974.

118. Johnson, CD, and Rice, RP: Acute abdomen: plain radiographic evaluation, RadioGraphics 5:259, 1985.

119. Jutras, JA: Hyperplastic cholecystoses, AJR 83:795, 1960.

120. Kaden, VG, Howard, JM, and Doubleday, LC: Cholecystographic studies during and immediately following acute pancreatitis, Surgery 38:1082, 1955.

121. Kalisher, L, Sternhill, V, and Ferrucci, JT: Tomographic demonstration of the common bile duct following nonvisualization at oral cholecystography, Am J Gastroenterol 60:632, 1973.

122. Kazmierski, RH: Primary adenocarcinoma of gallbladder with intramural calcification, Am J Surg 82:248, 1951.

123. Keill, RH, and DeWeese, MS: Primary carcinoma of the gallbladder, Am J Surg 125:726, 1973.

124. Kishk, SMA, et al: Sonographic evaluation of resting gallbladder volume and postprandial emptying in patients with gallstones, AJR 148:875, 1987.

125. Klein, JB, and Finck, FM: Primary carcinoma of the gallbladder, Arch Surg 104:769, 1972.

126. Kleinman, P, Winchester, P, and Volberg, F: Sulfatide cholecystosis, Gastointest Radiol 1:99, 1976.

127. Koehler, PR, and Kyaw, MM: Effect of fractionated administration of Telepaque on gallbladder visualization, Radiology 108:517, 1973.

128. Laufer, I, and Gledhill, L: The value of the fatty meal in oral cholecystography, Radiology 114:525, 1975.

129. Leopold, GR, et al: Gray scale ultrasonic cholecystography, a comparison with conventional radiographic techniques, Radiology 121:445, 1976.

130. Levyn, L, Beck, EC, and Aaron, AH: Further cholecystographic studies in the late months of pregnancy, AJR 30:774, 1933.

131. Lindquist, T, and Sohrne, G: X-ray investigation of the gallbladder in pernicious anemia, Acta Med Scand 116:117, 1944.

132. Loeb, PM, Berk, RN, and Barnhart, JL: The dependence of the biliary excretion of iopanoic acid on bile salts, Gastroenterology 74:174, 1978.

133. Loeb, PM, et al: The effect of fasting on gallbladder opacification: a controlled study in normal volunteers, Radiology 126:395, 1978.

134. Lorman, HG, and Rosenbaum, HD: How to do an oral cholecystogram, Semin Roentgenol 11:165, 1976.

135. Low-Beer, TS, Heaton, KW, and Roylance, J: Oral cholecystography in patients with small bowel disease, Br J Radiol 45:427, 1972.

136. Lubera, RJ, Clinie, ARW, and Kling, GE: Cholecystitis and the hyperplastic cholecystoses: a clinical, radiologic and pathologic study, Am J Dig Dis 12:696, 1967.

137. Lubert, M, and Krause, GR: Upright cholecystography using the fluoroscopic spotfilmer with graded compression, Radiology 61:879, 1953.

138. Margulies, M, and Wohl, GT: Routine tomography in gallbladder nonvisualization: a method for extended positive diagnosis, AJR 117:400, 1973.

139. Martinez, LO, and Gregg, M: Aberrant pancreas in the gallbladder, J Can Assoc Radiol 24:234, 1973.

140. McCluskey, PL, et al: Use of ultrasound to demonstrate gallstones in symptomatic patients with normal oral cholecystogram, Am J Surg 138:655, 1979.

141. McConnell, RW, and Rice, RP: Effect of Neoloid on Telepaque cholecystography, AJR 101:617, 1967.

142. McCorkle, H, and Fong, EE: Clinical significance of gas in the gallbladder, Surgery 11:851, 1942.

143. McGregor, JC, and Cordiner, JW: Papilloma of the gallbladder, Br J Surg 61:356, 1974.

144. Melnick, GS, and LoCurcio, SB: The "non-visualized" gallbladder, Radiology 108:513, 1973.

145. Mentzer, RM, et al: A comparative appraisal of emphysematous cholecystitis, Am J Surg 129:10, 1975.

146. Meyers, MA, and O'Donohue, N: The Mercedes-Benz sign: an insight into the dynamics of formation and disappearance of gallstones, AJR 119:63, 1973.

147. Michael, JA, Nelson, JA, and Koehler, PR: The effect of fractionated administration of iocetamic acid (Cholebrine) on gallbladder visualization, Radiology 119:537, 1976.

148. Miller, RE: Simple apparatus for decubitus films with horizontal beam, Radiology 97:682, 1970.

149. Miller, RE, Chernish, SM, and Rodda, BE: Cholecystography: a cost reduction study, Radiology 110:61, 1974.

150. Milner, LR: Cancer of the gallbladder, its relationship to gallstones, Am J Gastroenterol 39:480, 1963.

151. Muhletalar, CA, Gerlock, AJ, and Avant, GR: Conjugated sodium tyropanoate (Bilopaque) in the bowel: significance of its presence or absence after first dose oral cholecystography, Radiology 141:311, 1981.

152. Mujahed, Z, and Evans, JA: The relationship of cholelithiasis to vagotomy, Surg Gynecol Obstet 133:656, 1971.

153. Mujahed, Z, Evans, JA, and Whalen, JP: The nonopacified gallbladder on oral cholecystography, Radiology 112:1, 1974.

154. Nathan, MH, and Newman, A: Conjugated iopanoic acid (Telepaque) in the small bowel, Radiology 109:545, 1973.

155. Nathan, MH, et al: Cholecystokinin cholecystography, AJR 110:240, 1970.

156. Nelson, HL: Fractional cholecystography: surgical significance, J Am Osteopath Assoc 73:440, 1974.

157. Nelson, SW: Extraluminal gas collections due to diseases of the gastrointestinal tract, AJR 115:225, 1972.

158. Nickerson, WR, and Boschetti, AE: Heterotopic gastric mucosa of gallbladder, Am J Surg 125:345, 1973.

159. Ochsner, SF: Solitary polypoid lesions of the gallbladder, Radiol Clin North Am 14:501, 1966.

160. Ochsner, SF: Performance and reliability of cholecystography, South Med J 63:1268, 1970.

161. Ochsner, SF, and Carrera, GM: Calcification of the gallbladder (porcelain gallbladder), AJR 89:847, 1963.

162. Oliphant, M, Whalen, HP, and Evans, JA: Time of optimal gallbladder opacification with Bilopaque (tyropanoate sodium), Radiology 112:531, 1974.

163. Ondetti, MA, et al: Cholecystokinin-pancreaozymin: recent developments, Am J Dig Dis 15:149, 1970.

164. Osler, W: The principles and practice of medicine, ed 10, New York, 1925, Appleton-Century-Crofts.

165. Parker, GW, and Joffee, N: Calcifying primary mucus-producing adenocarcinoma of the gallbladder, Br J Radiol 45:468, 1972.

166. Phemister, DB, Rewbridge, AG, and Rusisill, H: Calcium carbonate gallstones and calcification of the gallbladder following cystic duct obstruction, Ann Surg 94:493, 1931.

167. Pogonowska, MJ, and Collins, LC: Immediate repeat cholecystography with Oragrafin calcium after initial nonvisualization of the gallbladder, Radiology 93:179, 1969.

168. Polk, HC: Carcinoma and the calcified gallbladder, Gastroenterology 50:582, 1966.

169. Postlehwaite, AE, and Kelley, WN: Radiocontrast agents and aspirin, JAMA 219:1479, 1972.

170. Price, WH: Gallbladder dyspepsia, Br Med J 2:138, 1963.

171. Radakovich, M, Greenlaw, RH, and Strain, WH: Iodinated organic compounds as contrast media for radiographic diagnoses. X. Interrelationship of gallbladder and pancreas, Soc Exp Biol Med 77:156, 1951.

172. Radakovich, M, et al: Iodinated organic compounds as contrast media for radiographic diagnoses, XIV. The influence of pancreatic function on cholecystography, NY State J Med 51:2880, 1951.

173. Radin, DR, and Halls, JM: Emphysematous cholecystitis presenting with pneumoperitoneum, AJR 149:1175, 1987.

174. Railford, TS: Intestinal obstruction due to gallstones (gallstone ileus), Ann Surg 153:830, 1961.

175. Rayford, PL, Miller, TA, and Thompson, JC: Secretin, cholecystokinin and newer gastrointestinal hormones, N Engl J Med 294:1093, 1976.

176. Redding, ME, Anagnostopoulous, CE, and Wright, HK: Cholecystopyloric fistula with gastric outlet obstruction, Ann Surg 176:210, 1972.

177. Redinger, RN, and Small, DM: Bile composition, bile acid metabolism and gallstones, Arch Intern Med 130:618, 1972.

178. Richard, PF, and Cantin, J: Primary carcinoma of the gallbladder: study of 108 cases, Can J Surg 19:27, 1976.

179. Rigler, LG, Bormen, CN, and Noble, JF: Gallstone obstruction: pathogenesis and roentgen manifestations, JAMA 77:1753, 1941.

180. Roedert, WJ, Mersheimer, WL, and Kazarian, KK: Triplication of the gallbladder with cholecystitis, cholelithiasis and papillary adenocarcinoma, Am J Surg 121:746, 1971.

181. Rogers, LF, et al: Calcifying mucinous adenocarcinoma of the gallbladder, Am J Gastroenterol 59:441, 1973.

182. Roller, J, et al: Oral cholecystography (OCG) in patients with acute alcoholic pancreatitis, Gastroenterology 73:218, 1977.

183. Rosenbaum, HD: The value of re-examination in patients with inadequate visualization of the gallbladder following a single dose of Telepaque, AJR 82:1011, 1959.

184. Rovsing, H, and Sloth, K: Microgallbladder and biliary calculi in mucoviscidosis, Acta Radiol 14:588, 1973.

185. Sachs, MD, and Partington, PF: The distended gallbladder, AJR 83:835, 1960.

186. Salmenkivi, K: Cholesterolosis of the gallbladder: a clinical study based on 269 cholecystectomies, Acta Chir Scand Suppl 324:1, 1964.

187. Sanchez-Ubeda, R, Ruzicka, FF, and Rousselot, LM: Effect of peritonitis of nonbiliary origin on the function of the gallbladder

as measured by cholecystography: its frequency and its duration, N Engl J Med 257:389, 1957.

188. Sandy, RE: Cholecystography in the presence of polycystic disease of the liver, Radiology 85:895, 1965.

189. Sauvegrain, J, and Feigelson, J: Cholecsytography in mucoviscidosis, Ann Radiol 13:311, 1970.

190. Schwegler, N, and Endrei, E: Gallstone in the lung, Radiology 115:541, 1975.

191. Scott, MG, Pygott, F, and Murphy, L: Significance of gas or barium in the biliary tract, Br J Radiol 27:253, 1954.

192. Selle, JG, et al: Cholelithiasis in hyperparathyroidism, a neglected manifestation, Arch Surg 105:369, 1972.

193. Sengpiel, GW: The compatibility of castor oil and Priodax in concurrent examination of the colon and gallbladder, Radiology 53:75, 1947.

194. Shaub, MS, Birnbaum, WW, and Meyer, HL: Peribiliary fat, a new roentgenographic finding, AJR 123:330, 1975.

195. Shehadi, WH: History of radiology of the biliary tract, Appl Radiol 6:141, 1977.

196. Shehadi, WH, and Jacox, HW: Clinical radiology of the biliary tract, New York, 1963, McGraw-Hill.

197. Shimkim, PM, Soloway, MS, and Jaffe, E: Metastatic melanoma of the gallbladder, AJR 116:393, 1972.

198. Shocket, E, Evans, J, and Jonas, S: Cholecystoduodenocolic fistula, Arch Surg 101:523, 1970.

199. Silvani, HL, and McCorkle, HJ: Temporary failure of gallbladder visualization by cholecystography in acute pancreatitis, Ann Surg 127:1207, 1948.

200. Simon, M, and Tandon, BN: Multiseptate gallbladder: a case report, Radiology 80:84, 1963.

201. Sparkman, RS, and Jernigan, R: Visualization of the gallbladder and bile ducts following trauma, Surgery 41:595, 1957.

202. Stanley, RJ, et al: A comparison of three cholecystographic agents: a double blind study with and without a fatty meal, Radiology 112:513, 1974.

203. Stephens, DH, Carlson, HC, and Gisvold, JJ: Tomography in problem cholecystograms, Radiol Clin North Am 14:15, 1976.

204. Stephens, DH, Gisvold, JJ, and Carlson, HC: Tomography of the gallbladder in oral cholecystography, Gastrointest Radiol 1:93, 1976.

205. Sutor, DJ, and Wooley, SE: The nature and incidence of gallstones containing calcium, Gut 14:215, 1973.

206. Taybi, H: The biliary tract in children. In Margulis, AR, and Burhenne, HJ, editors: Alimentary tract roentgenology, ed 2, vol 2, St Louis, 1973, The CV Mosby Co.

207. Ten Eyck, EA: Fixed defects in the gallbladder wall, Radiology 71, 840, 1958.

208. Theander, G: Pseudoconcretions in precipitate of contrast medium in the gallbladder, AJR 86:828, 1969.

209. Thistle, JL, and Hofmann, AF: Efficacy and specificity of chenodeoxycholic acid therapy for dissolving gallstones, N Engl J Med 289:655, 1973.

210. Ulreich, S, and Massi, J: Recurrent gallstone ileus, AJR 133:921, 1979.

211. Valberg, LS, et al: Biliary pain in young women in the absence of gallstones, Gastroenterology 60:1020, 1971.

212. Van Gansbeke, D, et al: Suprahepatic gallbladder: a rare congenital anomaly, Gastrointest Radiol 9:341, 1984.

213. Vint, WA: Herniation of the gallbladder through the epiloic foramen into the lesser sac: radiologic diagnosis, Radiology 86:1035, 1966.

214. Wakefield, EG, Vicker PM, and Walter, W: Cholecystoenteric fistulas, Surgery 5:674, 1939.

215. Way, LW, and Sleisenger, MH: Acute cholecystitis. In Sleisenger, MH, and Fordtran, JH, editors: Gastrointestinal diseases, Philadelphia, 1973, WB Saunders.

216. Way, LW, and Sleisenger, MH: Gallstone ileus. In Sleisenger, MH, and Fordtran, JH, editors: Gastrointestinal diseases, ed 2, Philadelphia, 1978, WB Saunders.

217. Weens, HS, and Walker, LA: The radiologic diagnosis of acute cholecystitis and pancreatitis, Radiol Clin North Am 2:89, 1964.

218. Whelan, JP, Rizzutti, RJ, and Evans, JA: Time of optimal gallbladder opacification with Telepaque (iopanoic acid), Radiology 105:523, 1972.

219. Whitehouse, WM: Correlation of surgical pathology with Telepaque cholecystography in doses of two grams, Surg Gynecol Obstet 100:211, 1955.

220. Wickbom, IG, and Rentzhog, U: The reliability of cholecystography, Acta Radiol 44:185, 1955.

221. Willis, RA: The spread of tumors in the human body. ed 2, London, 1952, Butterworth.

222. Wilson, JE, and Deitrick, JE: Agenesis of the gallbladder: case report and familial investigation, Surgery 99:106, 1986.

223. Wise, RE: Pitfalls in roentgenographic diagnosis of gallbladder disease, Lahey Clin Found Bull 15:109, 1966.

224. Wolson, A, and Goldberg, BB: Gray-scale ultrasonic cholecystography, a primary scanning procedure, JAMA 240:2073, 1978.

225. Youngwirth, LD, Peters, JC, and Perry, MC: The suprahepatic gallbladder: an unusual anatomical variant, Radiology 149:57, 1983.

226. Zboralski, FF, and Amberg, JR: Cholecystocholestasis: a cause of cholecystographic error, Am J Dig Dis 7:339, 1962.

50 *Radiology of the Liver and Biliary Tract*

ARTHUR R. CLEMETT

GENERAL CONSIDERATIONS

Advances in imaging modalities of the liver and biliary tract in recent years have resulted in radical changes in the ability of the radiologist to make precise diagnoses of diseases of the liver. Ultrasound, computed tomography (CT), magnetic resonance imaging (MRI), and the development of new radionuclides and new nuclear medicine imaging techniques have played a major role in our ability to evaluate liver diseases. With progress, however, have come the problems of application of multiple imaging techniques and the need to reduce the incidence of false-positive studies.[72,84,156,197,216]

These newer modalities provide useful and diagnostic information about lesions of the biliary tract. Direct cholangiography, however, remains the most efficient and efficacious modality for biliary tract imaging. Recent years have seen an increasing use of direct cholangiography, such as percutaneous cholangiography. In centers where requisite endoscopic skills are available, endoscopic retrograde cholangiopancreatography (ERCP), is the primary method of direct cholangiography. In some institutions percutaneous cholangiography is the primary choice for lesions suspected in the liver or at the porta hepatis, whereas ERCP is the preferred technique for direct cholangiography of lesions below the hilum in the extrahepatic ducts and at the junction of common duct, pancreatic duct, and duodenum (Figs. 50-1 and 50-2).

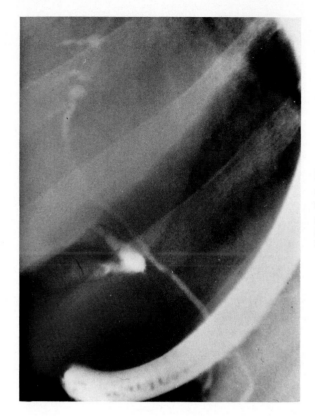

Fig. 50-1 ERCP in jaundiced patient. Marked narrowing (duodenoscope, which is 10 mm in diameter, is guide) of entire extrahepatic duct system is characteristic of primary sclerosing cholangitis.
(From Berk, RN, and Clemett, AR: Radiology of the gallbladder and bile ducts, Philadelphia, 1977, WB Saunders.)

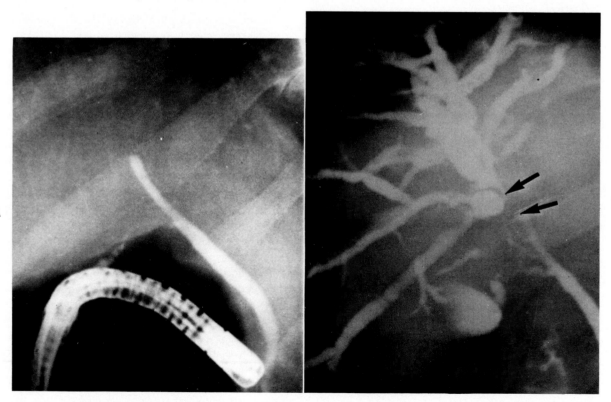

Fig 50-2 A, ERCP in jaundiced patient. There is complete obstruction of common hepatic duct.
B, Percutaneous transhepatic cholangiogram done a few minutes later identifies lesion (*arrows*) as short stricture characteristic of scirrhous carcinoma of common hepatic duct.
(From Berk, RN, and Clemett, AR: Radiology of the gallbladder and bile ducts, Philadelphia, 1977, WB Saunders.)

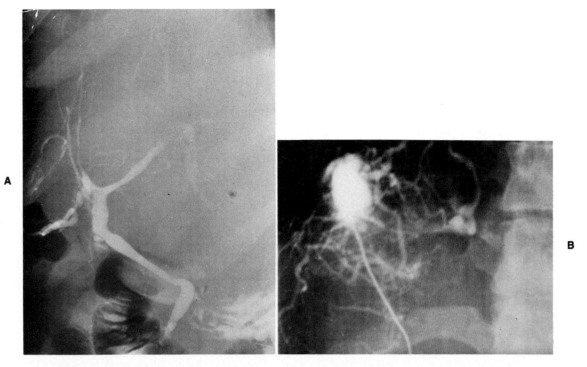

Fig. 50-3 A, ERCP in jaundiced patient with known chronic active hepatitis. Obstructive jaundice caused by bile duct lesion is excluded. Elongation and narrowing of intrahepatic ducts is consistent with diffuse hepatomegaly, and there is mass effect with displacement of intrahepatic ducts and common hepatic duct. **B,** Percutaneous transhepatic cholangiogram shows spider-web configuration of hepatic veins in Budd-Chiari syndrome, which confirms speculation that changes noted are due to hypertrophy of caudate lobe, a characteristic finding in Budd-Chiari syndrome.
(From Berk, RN, and Clemett, AR: Radiology of the gallbladder and bile ducts, Philadelphia, 1977, WB Saunders.)

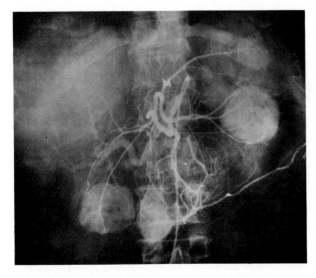

Fig. 50-4 Selective angiography in patient with known carcinoid tumor demonstrates four metastases in periphery of left lobe of liver.

Additional studies, such as angiography, ultrasound, CT, MRI, and nuclear medicine scans, are then done as indicated in a given case (Fig. 50-3).

This chapter on the diagnosis of liver diseases and diseases of the biliary tract will focus primarily on plain film studies, angiography,, and direct cholangiography. In some cases the clinical situation clearly dictates the diagnostic procedure of choice (Fig. 50-4). In other cases a combination of procedures is necessary for proper diagnostic interpretation.[31,83,208]

Knowledge of the internal architecture of the liver is important and sometimes essential for the proper interpretation of liver angiograms, particularly cholangiograms. The hepatic arteries, portal vein branches, and bile ducts follow the internal segmental anatomy of the liver[174] (Fig. 50-5), but the hepatic veins have an arrangement unrelated to the segmental distribution. The major hepatic veins are the right, middle, and left, but numerous variations and supplemental veins may be encountered.[60]

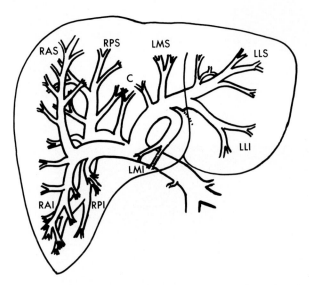

Fig. 50-5 Diagram of segmental anatomy of intrahepatic portal veins. Right and left lobes are divided by plane extending from gallbladder fossa to inferior vena cava. *RAS*, Right anterior superior; *RAI*, right anterior inferior; *RPS*, right posterior superior; *RPI*, right posterior inferior; *LMS*, left medial superior; *LMI*, left medial inferior (quadrate lobe in classical anatomy); *LLS*, left lateral superior; *LLI*, left lateral inferior; *C*, caudate lobe.

CONGENITAL LESIONS

Anomalies of the liver and biliary atresia are described in Chapter 71. Most diseases considered here are clearly congenital, but classification of some is arbitrary, since the cause is uncertain.

Biliary hypoplasia

Biliary hypoplasia, a poorly understood condition, is probably related to so-called intrahepatic biliary atresia.[19] The cause is unknown. Destruction of the duct system by inflammation and bile stasis has been suggested as the cause, along with primary dysplasia.[105] This entity raises the question of a real difference between what is termed *neonatal hepatitis* and *intrahepatic biliary atresia*.

In its severe form the extrahepatic duct system may be hypoplastic, but the characteristic anatomic finding is a hypoplastic intrahepatic duct system. The ducts are diminutive and sometimes fibrotic.[152] The pathologic anatomy is evident on the operative cholangiogram (Fig. 50-6). Intralobular bile ducts are diminished in number on liver biopsy[222] or even absent.[196] Cholestasis is frequent, and inflammation and fibrosis may vary from none[196] to severe.[88] The clinical course is quite variable. Jaundice is often intermittent but may be absent in some patients and severe in others. The prognosis is generally

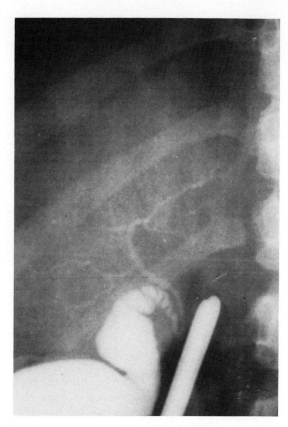

Fig. 50-6 Biliary hypoplasia in 7-year-old child. Operative cholangiogram with clamp on common bile duct shows reflux into diminutive intrahepatic ducts.

more favorable than in biliary atresia. Long survival with good health is possible if the complications of secondary biliary cirrhosis and portal hypertension do not occur.

Bile duct variations

The segmental anatomy of the bile ducts is schematically illustrated in Fig. 50-7. A number of variations may occur in the junctional arrangement of the segmental or divisional ducts[108] (Fig. 50-8). Knowledge of the segmental anatomy of the bile ducts and these variations is vital to both surgeon and radiologist[226] to avoid the biliary fistula that occurs with accidental transection of aberrant ducts.[239]

Congenital diaphragm of the common hepatic duct

Very few cases of a congenital diaphragm of the common hepatic duct have been reported. Histologically these thin webs or diaphragms may have a structure similar in all respects to the common hepatic duct wall[170] or may be fibrous with isolated areas of cartilage, large nerves,

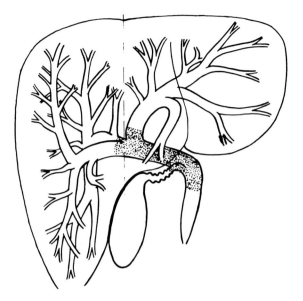

Fig. 50-7 Segmental anatomy of bile ducts. Shaded portion indicates area in which numerous variations in junctional arrangement occur.

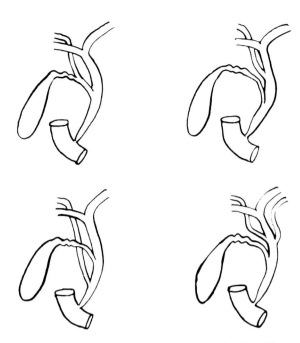

Fig. 50-8 Some bile duct variations as determined in 400 consecutive biliary operations.[108]

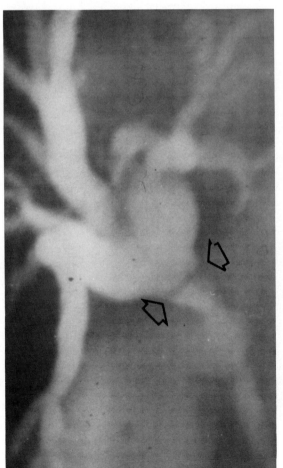

Fig. 50-9 Congenital diaphragm of common hepatic duct in 41-year-old patient (*arrows*).
(Courtesy Dr. Jack Wittenberg.)

and vascular channels.[75] There is no doubt about the congenital nature of this lesion, but, curiously, clinical manifestations appear late, from the second to the fifth decade of life in reported cases. Partial obstruction and a weblike defect in the common hepatic duct are the characteristic radiologic features (Fig. 50-9). Bile stasis, stone formation, and secondary biliary cirrhosis are the complications that eventually cause clinical symptoms. Surgical excision of these congenital diaphragms is curative.[58]

Congenital bronchobiliary fistula

Congenital bronchobiliary fistula is probably the result of the union of an anomalous bronchial bud with an anomalous bile duct in the 5- to 6-week-old embryo or a foregut duplication extending from the laryngotracheal outgrowth to the hepatic diverticulum of the 6- to 7-week-old embryo. The condition is very rare.[211] The fistulas originate at or near the carina and usually terminate at the level of left hepatic duct. In addition to respiratory and bile duct epithelium, the fistula may contain esophageal mucosa.[234]

Clinically cough productive of yellow or green sputum is present from the first days of life, and signs of atelectasis or pneumonia appear. The diagnosis is made by endoscopy, bronchography, or cholecystocholangiography.[70] Successful surgical excision of the fistula is curative.

Choledochal cyst

A choledochal cyst is a segmental dilatation of the extrahepatic bile duct that at times also involves the adjacent cystic duct or contiguous intrahepatic bile ducts. These lesions may be demonstrated by CT scanning,[11] ultrasound,[205] or cholescintigraphy.[104] Direct cholangiography, however, best defines the anatomic extent of the choledochal cyst (Fig. 50-10).

Choledochal cysts are not uncommon; more than 1000 cases have been reported.[76,100,110] The lesion is four times as common in females as in males. The incidence is high in Japan. More than one third of the reported cases have been Japanese. More than half of the cases are discovered

before the age of 10 years, but many cases first become evident in young adult life, and approximately 8% are first discovered in patients over 40 years of age. Symptoms have been present for months or years in most of the patients. The major clinical findings are jaundice, right upper quadrant pain, and a right upper quadrant mass. However, this classic triad exists only in a minority of the patients.

Histologically the cyst wall is usually fibrous without an epithelial lining,[110,131] even in the newborn with a choledochal cyst.[255] The origin of the choledochal cyst has been disputed in the past, but there is a growing body of evidence suggesting that most cases represent an acquired lesion that is due to an anomalous junction of the common duct and the main pancreatic duct that permits free reflux of pancreatic juice into the common duct with resultant injury to the common duct.[17,18,138,163]

The usual complications of choledochal cysts are stone formation and recurrent cholangitis, both the likely result of bile stasis and mucosal destruction. These progress to biliary cirrhosis and portal hypertension in some cases.[78] Perforation and bile peritonitis may occur.[91,122,125] There is a significant incidence of bile duct carcinoma in patients with a choledochal cyst.[153,240] Some tumors are

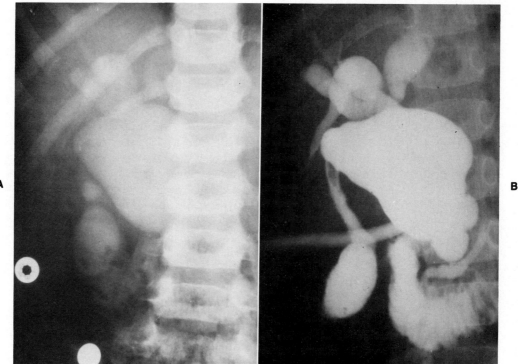

Fig. 50-10 Choledochal cyst in 7-year-old child. **A,** Intravenous cholangiogram. **B,** Operative cholangiogram. Note that distal common duct enters lateral aspect of main pancreatic duct about 2 cm proximal to duodenal papilla.

present at the time that the cyst is first recognized,[14] although others develop months or years after surgical treatment.[245] In contrast to the usual bile duct tumor, these carcinomas tend to be quite aggressive and metastasize early and widely.

Choledochocele

A choledochocele is a benign cystlike dilatation of the intramural segment of the distal common bile duct protruding into the duodenal lumen. It is controversial whether this entity represents an intramural variation of choledochal cyst or an acquired lesion (for example, from papillitis).[214] The choledochocele may remain asymptomatic or cause symptoms similar to those of choledocholithiasis, such as intermittent right upper quadrant pain, obstructive jaundice, and pancreatitis. The diagnosis is difficult and has usually been missed even at cholecystectomy. Choledochocele may be complicated by choledocholithiasis and can be treated by endoscopic retrograde sphincterotomy (Fig. 50-11).[24]

Caroli's disease

The cardinal features of Caroli's disease, or communicating cavernous ectasia, are segmental saccular dilatation of intrahepatic bile ducts, a predisposition to biliary calculus formation and cholangitis, and absence of cirrhosis or portal hypertension.[180] The disease is familial and may be evident at birth, but most cases of this rare entity are recognized in young adults. The symptoms of abdominal pain and fever are caused by stone formation and cholangitis. The course remains relatively benign until recurrent cholangitis results in liver abscesses, the most common cause of death in these patients.[181] Secondary biliary cirrhosis may also occur.[107]

Plain films may show hepatomegaly. The diagnosis can be made or suspected by CT scanning,[133] ultrasound,[23,178] or hepatic scintigraphy.[236] Direct cholangiography should be done in all cases, however, to confirm the diagnosis and to evaluate the possible formation of stasis calculi (Fig. 50-12).

Intrahepatic cystic dilatation of bile ducts has been associated with the (extrahepatic) choledochal cyst,[92] and some authors regard it as a variant of the choledochal cyst. Caroli's disease, however, is probably a distinctly

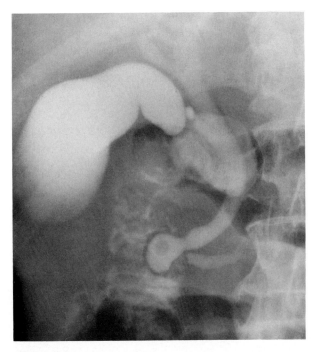

Fig. 50-11 Direct cholangiogram shows clublike configuration of distal common duct caused by choledochocele. Also stone within it.

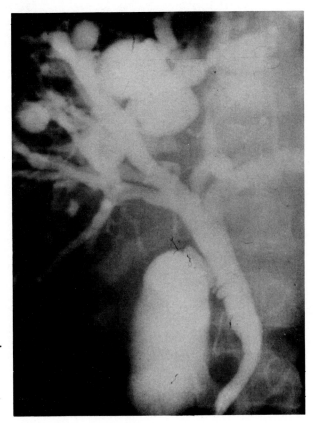

Fig. 50-12 Percutaneous cholangiogram demonstrating Caroli's disease in 10-year-old child with recurrent fever and right upper quadrant pain.
(Courtesy Plinio, Rossi, MD; from Berk, RN, and Clemett, AR: Radiology of the gallbladder and bile ducts, Philadelphia, 1977, WB Saunders.)

separate entity. Some reported cases have shown features of congenital hepatic fibrosis;[119] these diseases may be related. In most instances, however, Caroli's disease is readily distinguished on clinical and pathologic grounds. In congenital hepatic fibrosis the communicating cystic malformations involve smaller intrahepatic bile ducts and fibrosis predominates, causing portal hypertension, which is the essential clinical feature of the disease.[95,111]

DIFFUSE LIVER DISEASES
Hepatomegaly

Gross hepatomegaly is readily recognized on plain films supplemented by gastrointestinal studies and may be caused by a large number of diffuse diseases or by a single or multiple focal lesions, such as abscesses, cysts,

or tumors. The diffuse lesions seldom have characteristic appearances on special studies. Scans reveal hepatomegaly with either homogeneous distribution of the radioactivity or irregular, patchy uptake. Exceptionally, diffuse infiltrative lesions, such as Gaucher's disease, may simulate metastatic tumor on liver scans (Fig. 50-13).

With liver enlargement caused by diffuse disease, arteries are stretched and elongated, and irregular distribution of contrast may occur in the sinusoidal phase in such diverse conditions as cirrhosis and fatty liver, collagen disease,[5] and chronic active hepatitis. These appearances may be quite indistinguishable from multiple small metastases or multiple abscesses.[5] Diffuse infiltrative lesions often cause elongation and narrowing of intrahepatic bile ducts. In some instances associated ab-

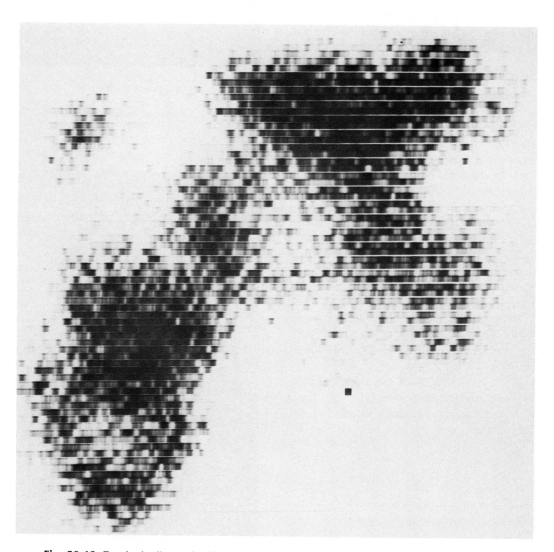

Fig. 50-13 Gaucher's disease in 36-year-old patient. Defects on liver scan simulate metastatic carcinoma.

normalities in other organs, such as bone (Fig. 50-14), spleen, lungs, heart, or gastrointestinal (GI) tract, may provide clues to the nature of the liver disease.

Cirrhosis

Radiologic findings in cirrhosis vary with the stage of the disease. The liver may be large, with features of diffuse hepatomegaly. When collapse, contraction, and scarring become prominent, the hepatic artery branches of the affected area become tortuous or like a corkscrew in appearance. Regenerating nodules cause stretching of hepatic artery branches. Contraction of the right lobe along with extensive regeneration of the left is a common pattern in cirrhosis (Fig. 50-15), but a dominant regenerating nodule may be found in any location.

Hepatic veins are relatively delicate structures with meager supporting elements. Cirrhosis causes severe alterations in hepatic vein structure before significantly affecting portal vein branches. These changes, which

may be demonstrated by free and wedged hepatic venography, consist of loss of branching, loss of tapering, and deformity of the veins (Fig. 50-16). These findings have a positive correlation with the severity of progressive cirrhosis.[229] Hepatic venous bed distortion by regenerating nodules is the source of the outflow obstruction in cirrhosis, but the venographic deformities do not necessarily correlate with portal hypertension.[229]

In biliary cirrhosis diffuse narrowing and diminished branching of intrahepatic bile ducts are frequent.[148] Similar changes occur in Laennec's cirrhosis, in which there is diffuse liver enlargement. The extrahepatic ducts are normal or may be slightly dilated. With atrophy of a part of the liver in cirrhosis, crowding and distortion of ducts occur, and with hypertrophy there is elongation and stretching of ducts (Fig. 50-17). With extensive fibrosis and regenerating nodules, the distortion of intrahepatic ducts may be severe and indistinguishable from the changes caused by diffuse metastatic tumor (Fig. 50-18).

Radioisotope scans reveal the size and shape of the cirrhotic liver. Uptake may be homogeneous but is usually irregular or patchy in character. This is caused by scarring, variations in uptake by regenerating nodules, and the contrast between hepatic parenchyma and vascular spaces. ^{99m}Tc-sulfur colloid scans show increased uptake in the spleen and bone marrow as compared with that in the liver,[208] and the relative difference reflects the severity of the liver disease.

Hepatic outflow obstruction in cirrhosis causes a rise in hepatic interstitial pressure, which in turn induces an increase in bile flow[149] and hepatic lymph formation. A two- to 100-fold increase in thoracic duct flow may be

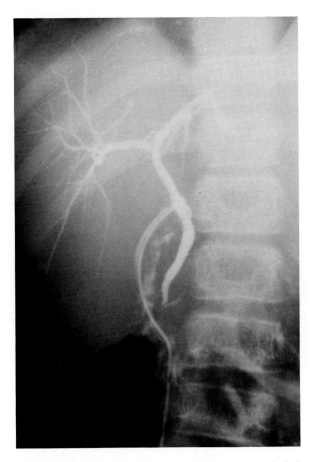

Fig. 50-14 Thalassemia with extramedullary hematopoiesis in liver. Intrahepatic ducts are elongated and narrowed. Note changes in lumbar spine.

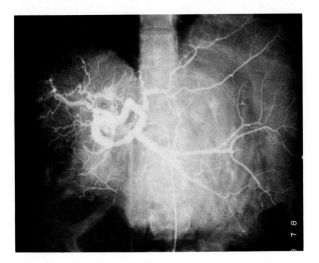

Fig. 50-15 Cirrhosis. Arteries in right lobe are tortuous and distorted because of contraction, whereas those on left are elongated and narrowed because of regenerating nodules.

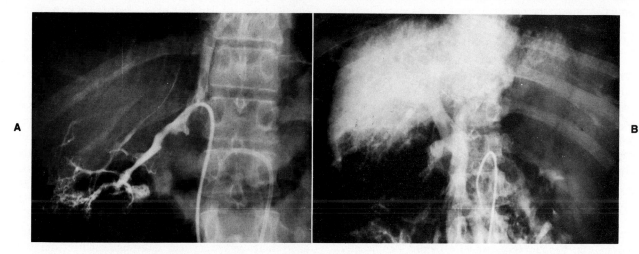

Fig. 50-16 A, Marked deformity and distortion of hepatic veins caused by macronodular regeneration in cirrhosis. **B,** Although venous phase of this superior mesenteric arteriogram shows shunting because of portal hypertension, intrahepatic portal branches appear normal. Separation of liver parenchyma from lateral abdominal wall is due to ascites.

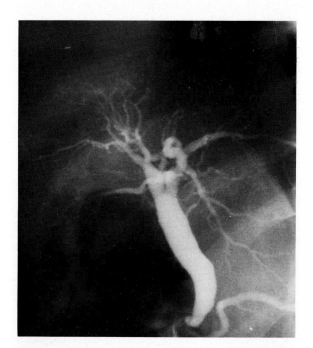

Fig. 50-17 ERCP in cirrhotic patient shows crowded and distorted ducts in shrunken right lobe and elongation and stretching of ducts in left lobe.
(From Berk, RN, and Clemett, AR: Radiology of the gallbladder and bile ducts, Philadelphia, 1977, WB Saunders.)

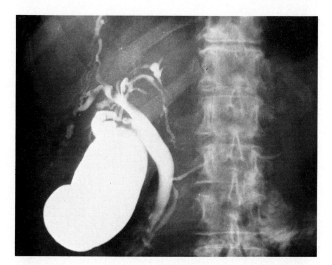

Fig. 50-18 ERCP in cirrhotic patient reveals marked distortion and encasement of intrahepatic ducts by regenerating nodules and fibrosis. Findings are indistinguishable from diffuse metastatic tumor.

found in cirrhosis. Lymphangiography reveals the thoracic duct diameter, normally 1 to 5 mm, to be increased, and the duct is tortuous.[59,225] Intrahepatic injection of contrast media results in a high incidence of lymphatic visualization in cirrhosis.[43] Lymphatic visualization also occurs frequently in a variety of other primary liver diseases and in extrahepatic bile duct obstruction. In fact, with an injection-withdrawal technique for percutaneous cholangiography, there is lymphatic visualization in more than 10% of cases.[46] With intrahepatic injection of contrast media, gross enlargement of hepatic lymphatics as well as increased lymphatic flow may be demonstrated in cirrhotic patients (Fig. 50-19).

VASCULAR DISEASES
Portal hypertension

Cirrhosis is the major cause of portal hypertension in North America. Several other entities must be considered in any given case, especially when liver function is relatively normal. These include schistosomiasis,[25,50] portal vein thrombosis, splenic vein thrombosis, hepatic vein obstruction, sarcoidosis,[176] hepatoportal sclerosis, congenital hepatic fibrosis, partial nodular transformation of the liver,[224] hepatic artery-portal vein shunts,[97] cystic fibrosis,[94] and portal vein aneurysm.[112,246]

Budd-Chiari syndrome

The majority of hepatic vein occlusions or obstructions go unnoticed because of the rapid development of collateral circulation. This is often so effective that significant hepatic congestion or hemodynamic alterations do not occur. The clinical features of the less frequent *symptomatic* hepatic vein obstruction, the Budd-Chiari syndrome, depend on the rapidity and extent of the venous obstruction. Hepatomegaly and ascites are the major manifestations. Jaundice is relatively infrequent and often mild when it occurs. In some cases portal hypertension and its consequences are prominent clinical features.

The Budd-Chiari syndrome may be caused by thrombosis of hepatic veins or the intrahepatic vena cava; webs or membranes in this part of the cava; venous obstruction by tumors, cysts, or abscesses; and even mechanical derangement caused by torsion of the liver by a diaphragmatic hernia.[44] The cause of hepatic vein thrombosis is unknown in a majority of cases. Specific causes include polycythemia vera,[187] chronic leukemia,[192] hepatic vein invasion by *Aspergillus* species in patients with leukemia,[272] poisoning by *Senecio* alkaloids,[154] oral contraceptives,[67,233] and trauma. Hepatocarcinoma and metastatic carcinoma are the usual tumors causing the syndrome, but any mass obstructing hepatic venous return, such as renal carcinoma invading the cava, leiomyosar-

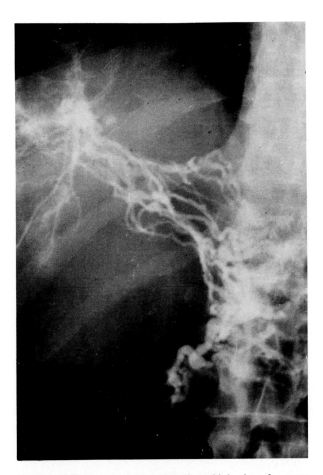

Fig. 50-19 Percutaneous intraparenchymal injection of contrast media in cirrhotic patient demonstrates gross enlargement of hepatic lymphatics and increased hepatic lymph flow.

coma of the inferior vena cava,[129,231] or right atrial myxoma,[73] can produce this.

Webs or diaphragms of the intrahepatic vena cava as causes of the Budd-Chiari syndrome are important because they are amenable to surgical cure. They are relatively infrequent in the western world but have been reported to cause one third of the cases of Budd-Chiari syndrome in Japan. The pathogenesis of these lesions is sometimes obscure. Many seem to be congenital, with gradual fibrosis and constriction of the lumen finally leading to symptoms,[114,212] whereas others are clearly caused by venous thrombosis.[256]

Arterial portography and splenoportography are usually inconclusive in establishing the diagnosis of Budd-Chiari syndrome. Inferior vena cavography followed by catheter exploration of the hepatic vein orifices should be done in all cases. Hepatic vein injections may reveal distortion of the veins, strictures, webs, or thrombi. Col-

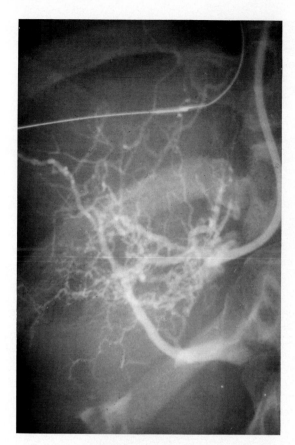

Fig. 50-20 Budd-Chiari syndrome. Injection into portal vein reveals spider-web pattern and filling of another hepatic vein through collaterals.

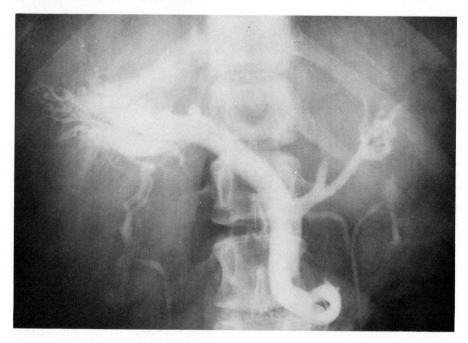

Fig. 50-21 Hepatoportal sclerosis. Operative portogram shows patent extrahepatic portal vein. Splenectomy several years previously accounts for small splenic vein. Normal segmental anatomy of intrahepatic portal veins is replaced by cluster of collateral vessels.

lateral hepatic venous pathways may be demonstrated. In the spider-web network pattern (Fig. 50-20) the vessels do not correspond to any normal hepatic venous pattern, a fact that is considered pathognomonic of the Budd-Chiari syndrome.[142] Intraparenchymal angiography can demonstrate thrombotic, neoplastic, and membranous obstructions of hepatic veins and vena cava.[201]

Hepatoportal sclerosis

Intrahepatic portal vein obstruction in the absence of cirrhosis or other specific causes of portal vein obstruction has been designated by many terms, including *hepatoportal sclerosis,*[175] *idiopathic portal hypertension,*[34] *primary portal hypertension,*[242] *noncirrhotic intrahepatic portal hypertension,*[273] *noncirrhotic portal fibrosis,*[34] *intrahepatic portal vein occlusion,*[244] and *obliterative portal venopathy.*[186] The disease is not rare. It accounts for up to 16% of cases in some series of patients with portal hypertension,[273] and it seems to be particularly prevalent in India.[34,184]

Careful evaluation of the intrahepatic portal vein branches on a technically good splenoportogram should differentiate hepatoportal sclerosis from cirrhosis in most cases, except those in which very small peripheral veins are occluded by thrombi.[242] There is gross irregularity of the intrahepatic portal venous pattern, and large segmental branches may show abrupt truncation by thrombi. In some cases portal vein to portal vein collaterals are prominent (Fig. 50-21). Similar or identical radiologic findings have been noted in schistosomiasis[50] and partial nodular transformation of the liver,[224] and theoretically they might also be present in congenital hepatic fibrosis and sarcoidosis.

Hepatic artery aneurysm

Hepatic artery aneurysms are classified as true or false aneurysms. Etiologic factors, listed here in order of frequency,[98] are infection[5]; atherosclerosis[165]; external[47,99] or operative[32] trauma; and specific vascular diseases, such as periarteritis nodosa[35,134] or necrotizing angitis associated with drug abuse.[102] The lesions may also be congenital.

As in any other aneurysm, calcification does not occur but is quite rare.[125] Large aneurysms may reveal themselves by extrinsic pressure on adjacent structures.[37] Accurate diagnosis, of course, depends on angiography.

Periarteritis nodosa

Hepatic artery involvement in periarteritis nodosa results in changes identical to those in other visceral arteries, namely, the formation of multiple small aneurysms of medium-size arteries. Similar changes may occur in

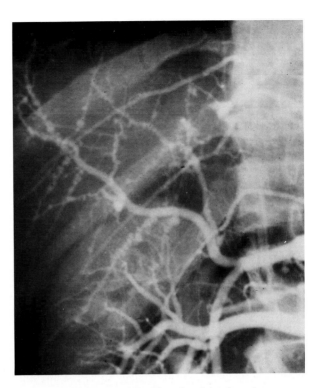

Fig. 50-22 Polyarteritis nodosa involving hepatic artery.

a recently reported syndrome of small pseudoaneurysms associated with diffuse carcinomatosis.[65] One consequence of periarteritis nodosa reported in a single case[62] was the formation of small bile duct cysts caused by small liver infarcts. This case led to experimental animal studies that confirmed the fact that small experimental liver infarcts cause changes in the bile ducts resembling Caroli's disease. In fact, these studies suggest that Caroli's disease may be the consequence of small liver infarcts, possibly occurring in utero or early in life (Fig. 50-22).

Peliosis hepatis

Peliosis hepatis is a rare lesion of the liver that has a distinctive angiographic appearance.[40,194] The disease is characterized by a myriad of small blood-filled spaces throughout the liver, which is usually enlarged. The pathogenesis is uncertain. Selective arteriography in peliosis hepatis reveals numerous small collections of contrast media throughout the liver in the late arterial phase (Fig. 50-23) and marked simultaneous opacification of hepatic veins in some cases. The abnormal vascular spaces are not visualized during the portal venous phase of the examination.

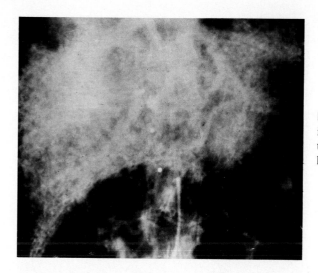

Fig. 50-23 Peliosis hepatis. In late phase of selective arterial injection there are numerous small collections of contrast media throughout enlarged liver and simultaneous opacification of hepatic veins.

INCREASED DENSITY OF THE LIVER

Deposit of sufficient concentrations of elements of high atomic number results in visualization of the liver because of its increased radiographic density. Iron, with atomic number 26, is probably the most frequent cause of this phenomenon. An excessive body burden of iron comes from three sources: (1) increased absorption in hemochromatosis,[74] (2) multiple transfusions in patients with refractory anemia, and (3) increased dietary iron.[127]

In the first form, hemochromatosis, the liver is said to be increased in density, whereas the spleen is not.[74] In transfusional hemosiderosis the density of the spleen tends to be greater,[221] but there are exceptions. Visualization of the shrunken spleen of sickle cell anemia, of course, is caused by another mechanism.[123] The third form is known as *Bantu siderosis* because it is so prevalent among the South African Bantu.[127] More than 50% of adults are affected. Excessive dietary iron stems from food preparation in iron containers, especially acid-fermented cereals and the native Kaffir beer. Greater iron losses in women because of menstruation and significantly higher beer consumption by men account for the greater incidence of siderosis in men. Increased density of both the liver and the spleen is usual in this form of hemosiderosis.[127]

Thallium intoxication has also been reported to cause increased radiographic density of the liver.[96] Most cases of thallium poisoning are caused by accidental or suicidal ingestion of rodenticides. The lethal dose is 0.2 to 1 g. Although the concentration of the element per gram of liver is relatively small, the high atomic number of 81 probably accounts for the liver opacification.

Thorium, with atomic number 90, is the other principal element causing diffuse liver opacification. Following intravascular injection of colloidal thorium dioxide (Thorotrast), about 70% is found in the liver, 30% in the spleen, and the remainder in other tissues, principally bone marrow and abdominal lymph nodes. Thorium dioxide as a reticular pattern in the liver and a stippled appearance in the spleen (Fig. 50-24). The pattern slowly changes with time. Liver density diminishes and spleen density increases, in part because of shrinkage of the spleen. Lymph nodes draining these organs become opacified. In patients given thorium dioxide to evaluate therapy for metastatic liver carcinoma, the earliest opacification of lymph nodes was noted 7 months after injection.[241] Thorium dioxide is notorious for causing liver tumors. These develop after a mean latent period of 15 years, but some take as long as 30 years.[132] About 50% of these tumors are hemangioendothelial sarcomas (Fig. 50-25), and the remainder are hepatocarcinomas and cholangiocarcinomas.[124]

LIVER CALCIFICATIONS

The reported causes of liver calcification are summarized in the box on p. 1254. Many examples given represent isolated reports of unusual cases. These conditions in which calcifications occur with any real frequency include tuberculosis, granulomatous disease of childhood, echinococcal infestation, portal venous thrombosis, metastatic adenocarcinoma, giant hemangioma, hepatoblastoma, and mixed malignant tumor. Many patterns are typical, such as the ringlike configuration of cysts and the stippled calcification of mucinous adenocarcinoma metastases. There are enough exceptions, however, that the pattern of calcification alone seldom permits a confident diagnosis.

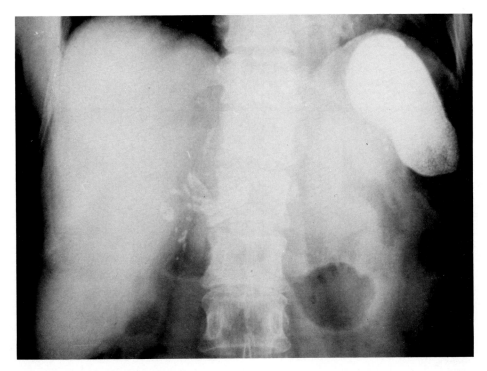

Fig. 50-24 Old thorium dioxide injection. There is reticular pattern in liver and stippled pattern in spleen and regional lymph nodes. Small dense spleen and opacified lymph nodes indicate that injection occurred several years earlier.

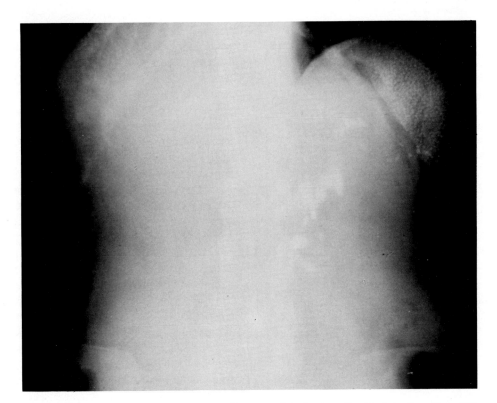

Fig. 50-25 Hemangioendothelial sarcoma 22 years after thorium dioxide injection. Very little residual thorium dioxide is present in markedly enlarged liver. Opacified lymph nodes are displaced to left by large liver tumor.

☐ **HEPATIC CALCIFICATIONS**[86,93,155,189,220] ☐

INFECTION

Tuberculosis
Histoplasmosis
Gumma
Brucellosis
Pyogenic abscess (especially in granulomatous disease
of childhood)
Amebic abscess
Echinococcus granulosus
Echinococcus multilocularis
Intrauterine infection by toxoplasmosis and herpes
simplex
Schistosomiasis japonica
Fasciola gigantica

VASCULAR

Hepatic artery aneurysm
Portal venous thrombosis

PRIMARY TUMOR

Cavernous hemangioma
Giant hemangioma
Infantile hemangioendothelioma
Hepatocellular carcinoma
Hepatoblastoma
Mixed malignant tumor
Hamartoma

METASTATIC TUMOR

Adenocarcinoma (colon, stomach, breast, ovary)
Melanoma
Mesothelioma
Osteosarcoma
Leiomyosarcoma
Carcinoid
Adrenal rest tumor
Myeloma
Hodgkin's disease
Neuroblastoma

MISCELLANEOUS

Hematoma
Intrahepatic calculi
Posteclampsia
Regenerating nodule in cirrhosis
Congenital cyst

INFLAMMATORY LESIONS
Hepatitis

In viral hepatitis radiologic findings vary with the stage and severity of the disease. In early hepatitis the liver is enlarged, and patchy uptake on liver scans is caused by scattered areas of necrosis. If the disease progresses to chronic active hepatitis or postnecrotic cirrhosis, some portions of the liver become contracted, with local arterial tortuosity reflecting this event.

Tuberculosis

The liver is regularly involved in miliary tuberculosis, but localized tuberculosis of the liver is quite rare in the western world, although sporadic cases have been reported.[77] It seems relatively frequent in the Philippines, where six to seven cases of localized hepatobiliary tuberculosis per year were encountered in a single hospital.[10] The disease was twice as frequent in males as in females, with the peak incidence being in the second decade of life. Some patients were jaundiced, but fever, weight loss, and hepatomegaly were the principal clinical findings. The liver was often hard and nodular, simulating carcinoma. Hepatic calcifications were present in 48% of these patients, and 66% had concomitant pulmonary tuberculosis.

Chronic granulomatous disease of childhood

Chronic granulomatous disease of childhood is one of the familial polymorphonuclear leukocyte dysfunction syndromes characterized by a defect in microbicidal activity, causing prolonged intracellular survival of phagocytized bacteria. Boys are affected most frequently and most severely.

The pathologic findings are those of chronic infection in which granuloma formation is common, and caseation and suppuration do occur. Pulmonary infection is almost invariable, and autopsy studies reveal a high incidence of liver involvement. An additional pathologic feature is infiltration of the reticuloendothelial system with pigmented lipid histiocytes. The infiltration is quite variable in extent and is unrelated to the site of infectious lesions.[39]

Reviews of the radiologic features of chronic granulomatous disease have stressed chronic pulmonary infections, hilar lymphadenopathy, pleural effusion, osteomyelitis, and hepatosplenomegaly as the principal findings.[237,271] Liver calcifications may be florid or rather subtle (Fig. 50-26), particularly in the early stages of this chronic disease. Sporadic case reports mention liver calcifications in chronic granulomatous disease,[145,162,186] but these have been curiously absent in the larger series.[237,271] Calcification has also been mentioned in abdominal and cervical lymph nodes, the spleen, and pul-

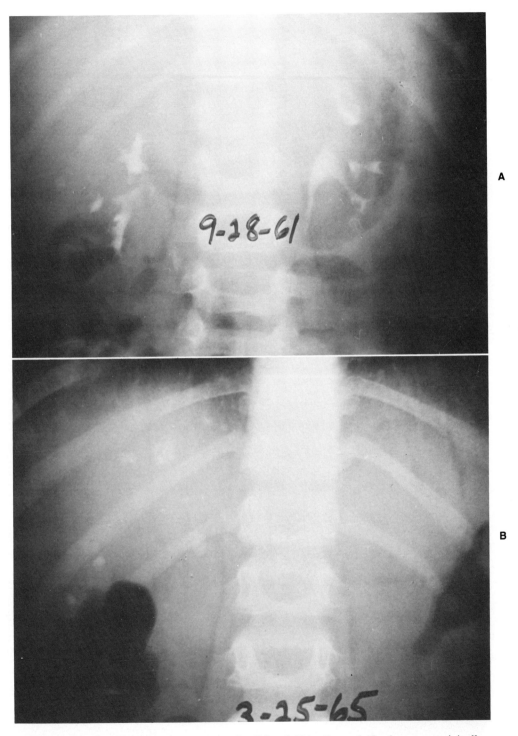

Fig. 50-26 Chronic granulomatous disease of childhood. Faint liver calcifications were originally overlooked in this little girl being evaluated for fever of unknown origin. Calcifications were clearly evident in September 1961 (**A**) and had increased in density 4 years later (**B**).

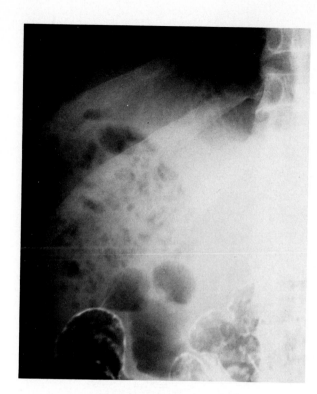

Fig. 50-27 Gas containing abscess of liver.

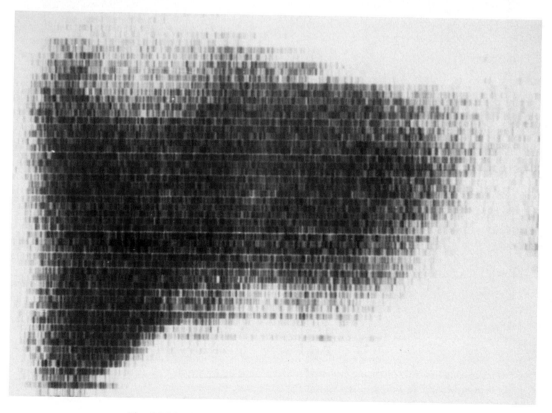

Fig. 50-28 Liver abscess. Defect high in right lobe of liver.

monary granulomas.[89] Liver scans reveal decreased uptake in regions of abscesses or granulomatous lesions,[16,186] and angiography has shown the abscesses to be avascular centrally with hypervascularity about the margins.[186]

Liver abscess: pyogenic, amebic, fungal

The mortality of unrecognized and untreated liver abscess is 100%.[8,199] In almost all cases diagnosis is possible with present radiologic techniques. An analysis of several large series reveals that abscesses are multiple in about half of the cases.[8,29,191] Most are pyogenic, about 10% are amebic, and 1% to 2% are fungal. General sepsis causes about 30% of cases, and more than 40% are caused by infection in the portal vein drainage area. About 20% are caused by bile duct disease along with some element or obstruction. Gallstones are the most common cause,[69] but some cases are caused by a tumor and a few by benign strictures. The remaining cases of liver abscess are caused by direct extension of adjacent inflammatory lesions, an infected tumor, or trauma.

Plain film findings include hepatomegaly, loss of the hepatic angle, gallbladder distention, elevation of the right diaphragm, pleural effusion, and right lower lobe atelectasis or infiltration.[213] Identification of gas in the abscess (Fig. 50-27) is a rare event usually associated with *Klebsiella* infections.[80] Abscesses cause negative defects on liver scans, and arteriography reveals displacement of arteries and avascular defects (Fig. 50-28). There may be a rim of increased vascularity about the margins of the abscess, depending on the intensity of the inflammatory reaction here. Arteriography is more sensitive than scanning in the detection of small abscesses. Amebic abscesses have the same characteristics as pyogenic lesions.[254] Most patients with amebic liver abscess do *not* have a history of intestinal amebiasis or show clinical and radiologic evidence of this.[210]

Complications of a liver abscess include septicemia, rupture into the right subphrenic space, rupture with generalized peritonitis, empyema, and common hepatic duct obstruction.[8] The less frequent lesions of the left lobe can rupture into either pleural space or the pericardium, causing acute cardiac tamponade.[38] Hemobilia caused by abscess has been recorded, and on the angiogram in one instance there was diffusion of contrast media into the abscess cavity.[252]

Sclerosing cholangitis, primary and secondary

In some cases of long-standing common bile duct stones, the intrahepatic bile ducts proximal to the lesion become narrowed, straightened, and attenuated. This is caused by a secondary sclerosing cholangitis. Primary sclerosing cholangitis is a rare lesion,[172] which, never-

theless, is an important cause of right upper quadrant pain and jaundice. Criteria for diagnosis include generalized thickening and stenosis of extrahepatic and intrahepatic ducts, absence of calculi and exclusion of previous biliary surgery, primary biliary cirrhosis, and malignancy.[53,115] It has been argued that the presence of calculi should not exclude this diagnosis when the stones are clearly a coincidental finding.[257]

Pathologically the extrahepatic ducts and to some extent the intrahepatic ducts are involved in a diffuse fibrosing process that may be patchy in some cases. The walls of extrahepatic ducts are greatly thickened by the fibrosis and nonspecific inflammatory reaction. The mucosa is usually intact. At surgery there are often adhesions about Winslow's foramen, edema of tissues in the porta hepatis, and hyperplastic lymph nodes, and the common bile duct is thickened and cordlike. Pouting of the mucosa after incision of the duct is sometimes noted.[115]

Many cases of primary sclerosing cholangitis, perhaps one half, occur in patients with chronic ulcerative colitis.[249,257] Pancreatitis has also been associated with it.[215] The cause of primary sclerosing cholangitis is unknown; speculation as to causation includes bacterial infection in the portal system and an autoimmune reaction.[53] The latter is further suggested by other associated diseases, including regional enteritis,[4,15] retroperitoneal fibrosis,[22] Riedel's struma,[22] follicular lymph node hyperplasia, and orbital pseudotumor.[260] Treatment consists of biliary decompression when feasible and corticosteroid therapy. Complete regression of the lesions may occur. The mortality, however, is significant, and some patients develop secondary biliary cirrhosis. The prognosis, though, is probably better than that of primary biliary cirrhosis.[249]

In primary sclerosing cholangitis direct cholangiography reveals either diffuse narrowing of the extrahepatic and intrahepatic ducts or multiple strictures of varying lengths, most often without much proximal dilatation.[143] Percutaneous transhepatic cholangiography usually fails when there is diffuse ductal narrowing but may succeed when the disease is patchy and focal areas of relative dilatation are present. ERCP is clearly the best procedure for making the diagnosis because of its high success rate (Fig. 50-29). When there is a single, short, segmental stricture, usually with considerable proximal dilatation, the clinical and pathologic diagnosis of primary sclerosing cholangitis is always suspect, since these cases, with very rare exceptions,[71] are eventually proved to be bile duct carcinoma.[45] Such examples are present in most series of primary sclerosing cholangitis cases.[215,249,257]

A form of biliary sclerosis quite specific in its presentation is identified in patients receiving hepatic intra-arterial floxuridine (IA-FUDR) infusions for treatment of metastatic adenocarcinoma.[223] The pathogenesis of this

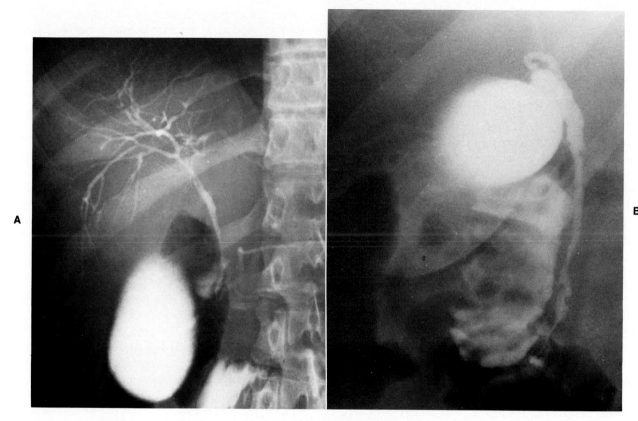

Fig. 50-29 A, Primary sclerosing cholangitis. ERCP demonstrates diffuse narrowing and irregularity of intrahepatic and extrahepatic ducts. **B,** Marginal filling defects in common duct, which are seen in some cases, are probably mucosal invaginations caused by periductal fibrosis.

process almost definitely relates to the arterial delivery of the agent. When clinical symptoms or signs of hepatic dysfunction occur in the absence of progression of metastatic disease, biliary sclerosis must be suspected.

Intrahepatic and extrahepatic bile duct changes identical to those seen in sclerosing cholangitis with strictures, focal dilatation, and thickened duct walls have also been reported in acquired immunodeficiency syndrome (AIDS).[61] There appears to be an association between cytomegalovirus and/or *Cryptosporidium* infection and acalculous inflammation of the biliary tract. Endoscopic retrograde cholangiography is the diagnostic imaging procedure of choice to demonstrate the characteristic morphologic abnormalities in the biliary tract. Endoscopic papillotomy provides variable relief of symptoms and biochemical abnormalities.

PARASITES

Other than amebic abscess, the most important parasitic diseases affecting the liver and bile ducts are schistosomiasis, echinococcal cysts, ascariasis, and infestations of liver flukes. Schistosomiasis is an important

cause of presinusoidal portal hypertension. In addition to the usual findings of portal hypertension, the hepatic fibrosis of schistosomiasis causes distortion of intrahepatic arteries and bile ducts similar to that found in cases of cirrhosis. Schistosomiasis has also been reported to cause strictures of the extrahepatic bile ducts.[135]

Echinococcal cyst

Humans are accidental intermediate hosts of the dog tapeworm, *Taenia echinococcus*. The embryos reach the body through the GI tract and are filtered through the liver and lungs, thus accounting for the more frequent involvement of these ograns. Growth of the cyst is slow, often taking years to develop. The more common *Echinococcus granulosus* tends to produce one or a few large cysts, whereas *Echinococcus multilocularis* is more invasive and produces multiple small cysts.[265] The patient's geographic and ethnic origins are important clues in the diagnosis. Eosinophilia is present in some cases. A positive result of Casoni's test usually establishes the diagnosis of echinococcal infection, although false-positive and false-negative results do occur.

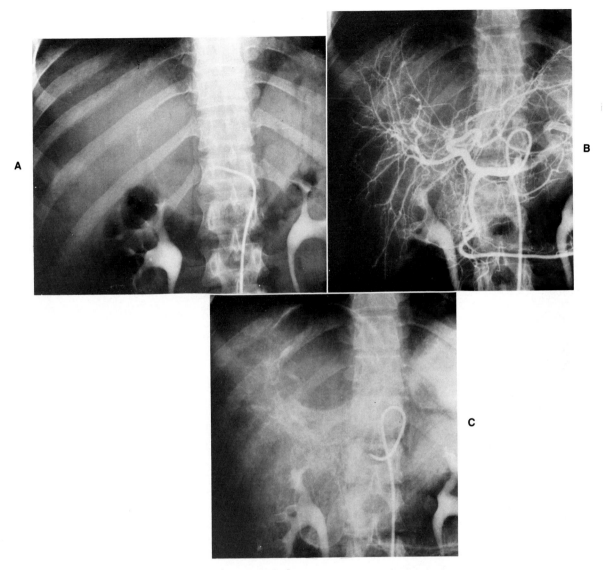

Fig. 50-30 Echinococcal cyst. **A,** There is thin arc of calcium about right side of cyst. **B** and **C,** Cyst causes negative defect on angiography with thin rim of increased vascularity about margin.

Radiologic procedures are essential for the preoperative diagnosis of echinococcal disease. The frequency of calcification of the cyst is difficult to determine but seems to be about 33%.[168,208] Very dense, irregular calcification of the entire circumference of the cyst suggests inactivity or death of the parasite. The cysts produce negative defects on liver scans. Arteriography reveals displacement of arteries and sharply circumscribed negative defects (Fig. 50-30). A well-defined rim of increased density about the margins of the cyst is a common but not invariable angiographic feature.[21,168,207] This is undoubtedly caused by the inflammatory reaction of the host, compression of liver parenchyma, or some combination of the two.

Complications of *E. granulosus* include rupture of the cyst into the lung, peritoneum, GI tract, and bile ducts. The latter is probably the most common complication. These patients have intermittent pain and jaundice because of periodic discharge of fragments of the cyst membrane or its contents.[106,158,251] When a daughter cyst can be recognized in a cavity communicating with the bile duct, the radiologic diagnosis of an echinococcal cyst is quite certain (Fig. 50-31). Passage of an intact daughter cyst may lead to total obstruction of the common duct.

Alveolar hydatid disease caused by *E. multilocularis* is quite different. The cysts are small and bud outward, causing necrosis of the adjacent liver parenchyma without the formation of a limiting capsule or pericyst. Calcifi-

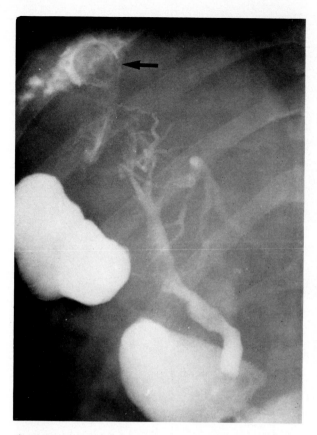

Fig. 50-31 Echinococcal cyst communicating with bile duct. Daughter cyst (*arrow*) is present in collapsed cyst cavity. Displacement of gallbladder is due to previous resection of another echinococcal cyst.
(From Berk, RN, and Clemett, AR: Radiology of the gallbladder and bile ducts, Philadelphia, 1977, WB Saunders.)

cation occurs in about two thirds of the cases[248] and is due to a combination of calcification degenerating cysts and the adjacent necrotic tissue. This results in amorphous collections of calcium that contain 2 to 4 mm radiolucencies. This pattern is quite distinctive and is believed to be diagnostic of alveolar hydatid disease.

Ascariasis

Invasion of the biliary tract by *Ascaris lumbricoides* does occur, especially with heavy infestation. Adult ascarids may be demonstrated on intravenous cholangiograms[54] and are readily recognized on direct cholangiography (Fig. 50-32). Biliary tract infestation, furthermore, is related to primary intrahepatic calculi. This disease entity is fairly prevalent in the Orient[159,261] and South America.[48] The patients tend to be younger than the usual cholelithiasis population, and many have the onset of symptoms in childhood.[48] Heavy *Ascaris* infes-

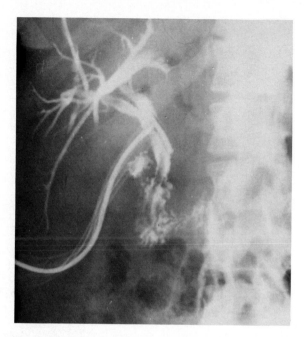

Fig. 50-32 *Ascaris lumbricoides* in common bile duct and second portion of duodenum.

tation is common, and with careful studies *Ascaris* eggs or immature worms can often be demonstrated as the nidus of the stone.[48] Such cases have been reported in the United States.[202] Investigation for parasitic infestation seems warranted in any case of primary intrahepatic calculi, particularly in youngsters.

Liver flukes

Infestation with the Chinese liver fluke *Clonorchis sinensis* is endemic in southern China and Indochina, and occasional cases are seen in Japan.[188] Most infestations are benign, since the parasites reside in small peripheral ducts, where they cause epithelial hyperplasia and periductal fibrosis. Central migration of the flukes can result in bacterial cholangitis,[83] liver abscess,[117] or choledocholithiasis.[243] The flukes themselves can cause common bile duct obstruction.[12] *Clonorchis* infestation is associated with an increased incidence of intrahepatic bile duct carcinoma.[27]

Cases seen in the United States occur in Oriental immigrants.[20] The flukes are flat, leaflike worms that have an oval or elliptic shape when viewed *en face*. They are about 10 to 15 mm long and are usually fairly uniform in size. These characteristics help distinguish them from gallstones.

Fasciola hepatica is similar in form and structure to *Clonorchis sinensis*. Its definitive host is usually a sheep or cow. It has a worldwide distribution. Accidental hu-

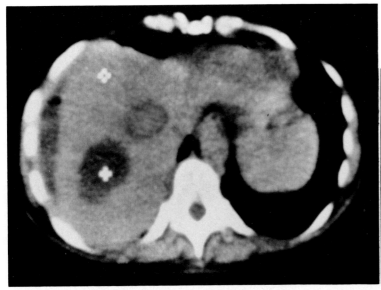
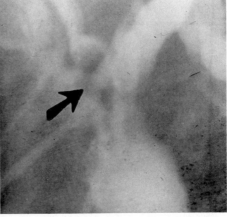

Fig. 50-33 A, CT scan of patient with long-standing peripheral eosinophilia shows focal areas of decreased attenuation caused by granulomatous hepatitis and abscess in patient with proved fasciola hepatica infestation. **B,** Cholangiogram in same patient shows another fasciola (*arrow*) at bifurcation of obstructed extrahepatic ducts.

man infestation usually is due to eating wild watercress bearing encysted metacercariae. It causes a focal granulomatous hepatitis[130] with eosinophils that appears as focal areas of decreased attenuation on CT scan (Fig. 50-33). *F. hepatica* is associated with a high incidence of choledocholithiasis.[183] The parasites themselves have been known to cause common bile duct obstruction.[26]

Clonorchis sinensis has been implicated as the cause of hepatolithiasis. In fact, only 30% to 40% of *Clonorchis sinensis* infestation is associated with ductal cholelithiasis in the Orient.[182] Also, occasional demonstration of *Ascaris* ova in intrahepatic calculi in some parts of Southeast Asia is probably incidental rather than causative.

LIVER CYSTS
Solitary liver cyst

Solitary liver cysts may be incidental findings or may be present as a right upper quadrant mass with pressure symptoms. They are said to be four times as frequent in females as in males, and the right lobe of the liver is involved twice as often as the left.[198] Most are lined by cuboidal epithelium[161]; ciliated epithelium has been noted in some[55]; and other cysts have a fibrous wall without identifiable epithelium.[198] Calcification has been noted in the wall of the cyst histologically[55] and is sometimes evident on abdominal films.[52] The diagnosis has been made by demonstration of a rounded lucent defect on

tomograms of the liver following intravenous injection of a large dose of contrast media. Angiography reveals arterial displacement about the cyst(s) and lucent defects in the sinusoidal phase. These changes, of course, are nonspecific, but CT scans demonstrating the lesions of water density are diagnostic (Fig. 50-34).

Polycystic disease of the liver

Polycystic disease of the liver is rare and generally conceded to be congenital in origin. The cysts originate from bile duct structures and contain clear fluid. The polycystic liver usually develops progressively and is rarely detected in childhood. Exceptions to this generalization are those rare cases in which the disease causes portal hypertension.[217] Polycystic liver disease usually becomes clinically evident in the fourth or fifth decade of life. This diagnosis should be suspected in the patient with hepatomegaly and multiple defects on living scanning who is clinically well and has normal liver function tests. Angiography may establish the diagnosis by demonstrating displaced arteries and sharply marginated lucent defects in the capillary phase (Fig. 50-35). CT scanning will make the definitive diagnosis.[5,232]

About half of the patients also have polycystic kidney disease,[171] and this association should help establish the diagnosis. The reverse is less frequent; only one fourth of the patients with polycystic kidney disease have polycystic liver disease.

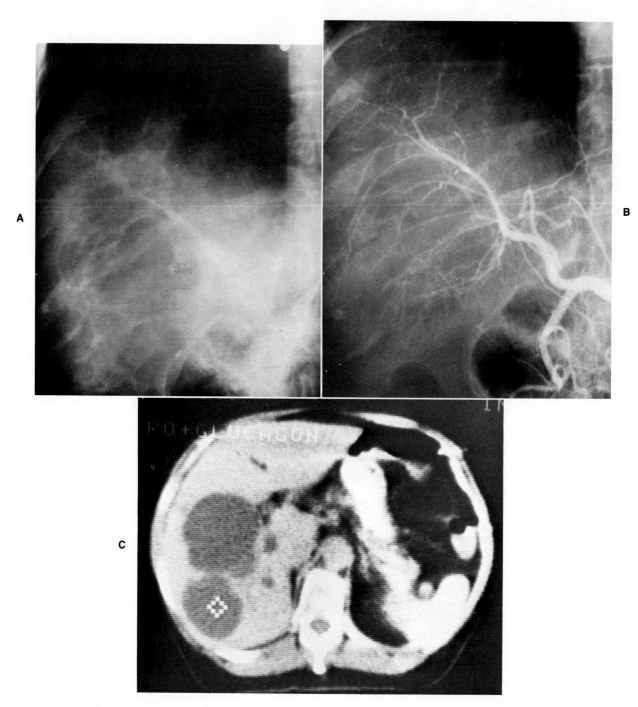

Fig. 50-34 Benign liver cysts. **A** and **B,** Angiography reveals displacement of vessels about multiple avascular defects, which could be cysts, tumors, or abscesses. **C,** Attenuation values measured by CT make specific diagnosis of cysts.

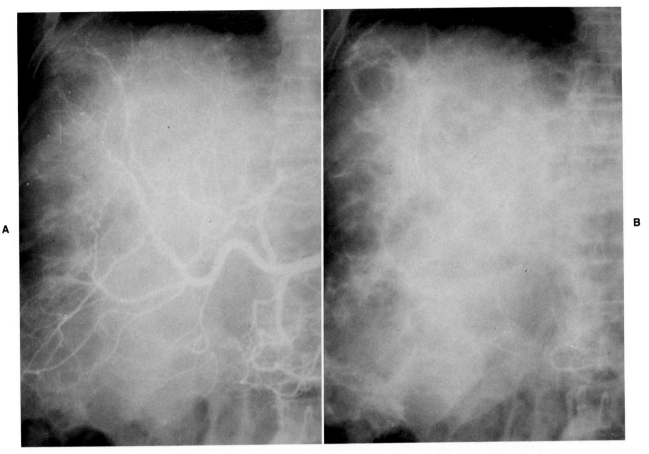

Fig. 50-35 Polycystic disease of liver. **A,** Smaller arteries are displaced by cyst. **B,** Rounded, smooth defects of varying size are present throughout liver in sinusoidal phase.

BENIGN LIVER TUMORS
Cavernous hemangioma

Cavernous hemangioma is the most common benign liver tumor.[3] Small hemangiomas are often incidental findings on angiography done for other reasons, at surgery, or at autopsy. Some are associated with the Rendu-Osler-Weber disease. They may be single or multiple. Some lesions initially appear as large hepatic masses, and calcification occurs in about 10% of these.[3] It has been stated that the calcification is characteristic in type, consisting of trabeculations or spicules of calcium radiating from a central point. This appearance (the description of which bears a striking resemblance to hemangioma of bone) is seldom found in reality. Most reproductions do not reveal any characteristic pattern to the calcifications in liver hemangiomas.[66]

Large hemangiomas produce negative defects on liver scans. Blood pool scanning has been advocated to identify hemangiomas,[81] but it is likely that this will fail in many cases because of the extensive sclerotic component of this lesion. Angiography readily demonstrates the characteristic features of cavernous hemangioma. The feeding vessels tend to be large; arteries are displaced by the tumor mass; and irregular lakes of contrast media are present and persist throughout the examination[1] (Fig. 50-36). The large number of bizarre vascular spaces at times causes confusion with hepatocarcinoma, but the displacement of arteries in hemangioma in contrast to the vessels entering the lesion in hepatoma and the persistence of contrast in the vascular lakes should readily distinguish these lesions in most instances.[167]

The dramatic complication of the lesion is spontaneous rupture with hemoperitoneum, which may be fatal.[180]

More recent reports indicate that percutaneous biopsy can be safely performed and can yield a specific histologic diagnosis in cases in which imaging data are not sufficient to determine that a liver mass is benign.[51]

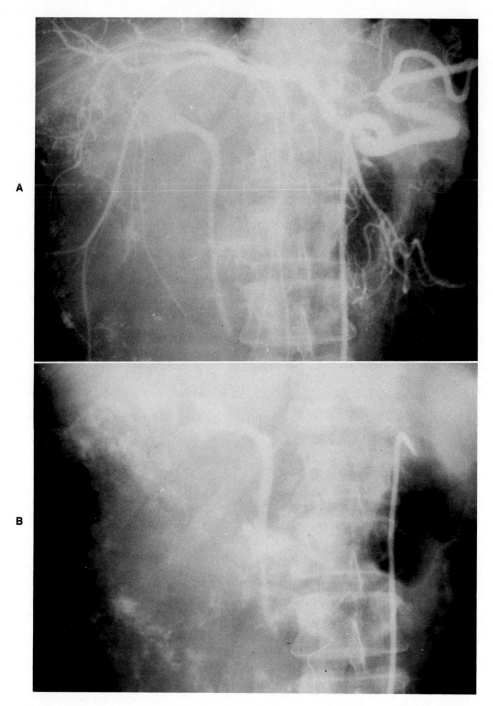

Fig. 50-36 Hemangioma of liver. **A,** Arteriogram reveals stretching of arteries about masses and filling of vascular lakes. **B,** These signs persist in late phase of examination.
(Courtesy Ray Abrams, MD)

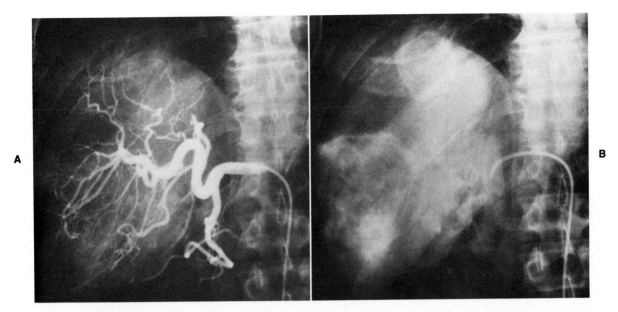

Fig. 50-37 Hamartoma of liver in 59-year-old man. **A,** Smaller hepatic arteries are displaced and distorted by tumor mass. **B,** Later film shows diffuse staining and multiple cystic lesions.

Infantile hemangioendothelioma

The cellular tumors of infantile hemangioendothelioma are also known as capillary hemangiomas of the liver.[250] They are quite rare but may cause hepatomegaly and congestive heart failure in infancy. The high output failure is caused by shunting of blood from the hepatic artery to hepatic veins. Calcification may occur in the lesion.[218] The diagnosis is established by angiography. There are large feeding vessels that are stretched and distorted and fail to taper. Fairly dense hepatic vein opacification is a characteristic diagnostic feature.[179]

If shunting is not severe or can be controlled by surgical excision or hepatic artery ligation, spontaneous involution of the tumor is the rule.[57] Some tumors have features of both the cavernous and the capillary hemangiomas.[28]

Hamartomas

Hamartomas are rather rare benign tumors that may be composed primarily of bile duct elements, liver cells, lymphatics, vascular elements, or a mixture of these.[144] Most hamartomas found in adults contain mixed elements. The patients are usually in good health and have no symptoms caused by the tumor. On arteriography these lesions may have enlarged, irregular, and tortuous feeding vessels.[5,179] A diffuse homogeneous tumor blush is usual, although irregular staining may occur because of the variable tissue components in the tumor. Cystic elements are prominent in some cases (Fig. 50-37), and a defect may be present on liver scans.

The mesenchymal cystic hamartoma of infants and children is usually present as an asymptomatic abdominal mass.[128] Most of these are avascular on angiography,[186] but some of these lesions may show areas of tumor staining reflecting their cellular and vascular components.[7]

Liver cell adenoma

Lesions in liver cell adenoma are very rare and may be encountered accidentally or cause symptoms by virtue of their size. They may be multiple. The scarce reports of liver scans indicate variable results. Uptake of ^{131}I–rose bengal and ^{99m}Tc-sulfur colloid were about the same as that in a normal liver in one case,[209] whereas a negative defect was present on an [198]Au scan in another.[193] Angiographic findings include stretching and tortuosity of small arteries, some neovascularity, and diffuse homogenous staining of the tumor (Fig. 50-38). A reticular pattern of small veins was a prominent feature in one case.[193]

Focal nodular hyperplasia

The many synonyms for focal nodular hyperplasia indicate its obscure nature. It has been called *adenoma, mixed adenoma, benign hepatoma, solitary hyperplastic nodule, focal nodular cirrhosis, solitary cirrhotic liver nodule, cholangiohepatoma, isolated nodule of regenerative hyperplasia, pseudoneoplasm,* and *focal nodular hyperplasia.*[270] This rare lesion of unknown cause occurs mostly in females. It and the liver cell adenoma have both been associated with the use of oral contraceptives.

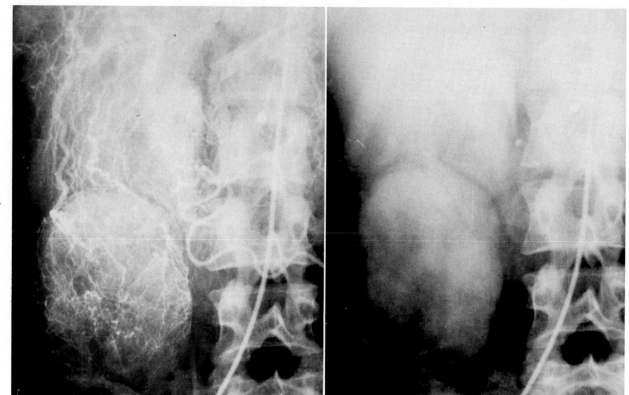

Fig. 50-38 Adenoma of liver. **A,** Feeding vessels are rather tortuous but otherwise unremarkable. **B,** Diffuse homogeneous tumor stain is present later in examination.
(Courtesy RF Colapinto, MD)

It is usually found incidentally at surgery or autopsy but occasionally may appear clinically as a relatively asymptomatic upper abdominal mass.[113,160]

Grossly the typical lesion is a circumscribed, gray-white, subcapsular nodule with many fibrous trabecular strands tending to divide the lesion into smaller nodules. At surgery it is often mistaken for a metastatic tumor. Histologically there is a pseudocapsule, and the bulk of the lesion is composed of regenerating liver nodules, with fibrosis in central and portal areas. The latter contain proliferating bile ducts and some lymphocytic infiltration. These features distinguish focal nodular hyperplasia from adenoma of the liver. The histologic features are similar to those of partial nodular transformation of the liver.[224] This entity, however, is distinctly different in that the nodules are multiple, centrally located, and encroach on major portal vein branches, causing presinusoidal portal hypertension.

The activity of the nodule on liver scans is probably rather variable. Decreased activity over the lesion has been noted with ^{131}I–rose bengal,[270] but the scan may be rather unremarkable even with a large lesion. On angi-

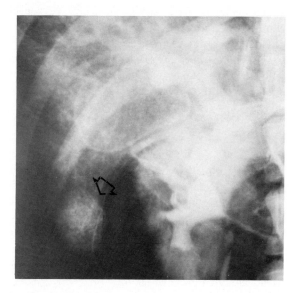

Fig. 50-39 Focal nodular hyperplasia found incidentally on arteriography done for other purposes. This late film also shows wall of gallbladder.

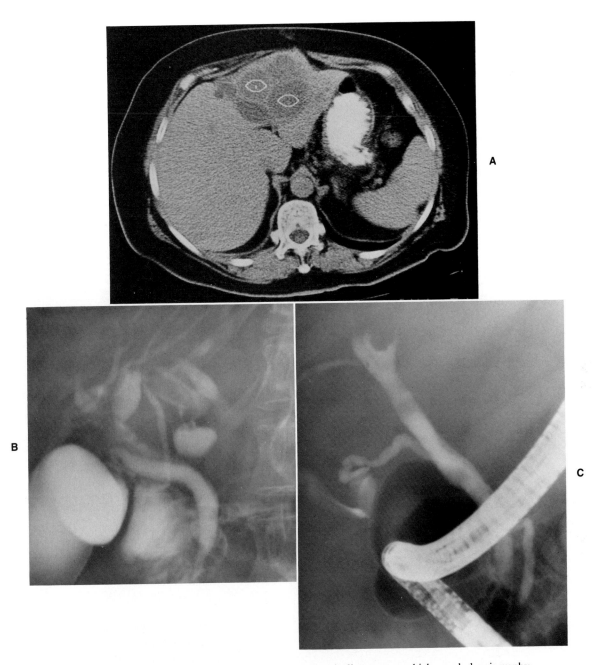

Fig. 50-40 A, CT scan demonstrates multilocular cystic liver mass, which on cholangiography exhibits communication with bile ducts (**B**) and polypoid intraluminal mass (**C**). This case of biliary cystadenoma shows histologically papillary adenoma.

ography the feeding vessels are widened and tortuous, and there is a diffuse homogeneous tumor stain (Fig. 50-39).[13] The angiographic appearance is identical to that of adenoma and of some homartomas. The absence of vascular lakes differentiates the lesion from hemangioma. Distinction from hepatocarcinoma may be difficult in some instances.

Biliary cystadenoma

Biliary cystadenoma is a relatively rare lesion of the liver or rarely the extrahepatic bile ducts. Large lesions arising in the liver are the most frequent type and are said to comprise less than 5% of nonparasitic cysts of liver origin.[79,82] There is a predilection for occurrence in middle-aged women.[82] On CT or ultrasound these tumors appear as multilocular cystic masses that may communicate with large bile ducts. Prolapse of intraluminal tumor may cause obstructive jaundice.[82] The less common type of this lesion arises in the extrahepatic bile ducts and appears initially as a polypoid intraluminal mass.[33,116] Histologically these are cystic polypoid or papillary adenomas.

A multilocular cystic liver mass that on cholangiography exhibits communication of cysts with the bile ducts plus polypoid intraluminal masses is virtually diagnostic for biliary cystadenoma (Fig. 50-40).

Biliary cystadenocarcinoma is believed to be the result of malignant transformation of a cystadenoma.[82] This is

□ **TABLE 50-1**
Classification of malignant liver tumors

Tumor	Approximate relative incidence (%)
Malignant hepatoma	
Hepatocarcinoma (cellular)	75
Hepatoblastoma	7
Cholangiocarcinoma (cellular)	6
Mixed hepatocholangiocarcinoma	12
Primary sarcomas	
Metastatic carcinoma and sarcoma	

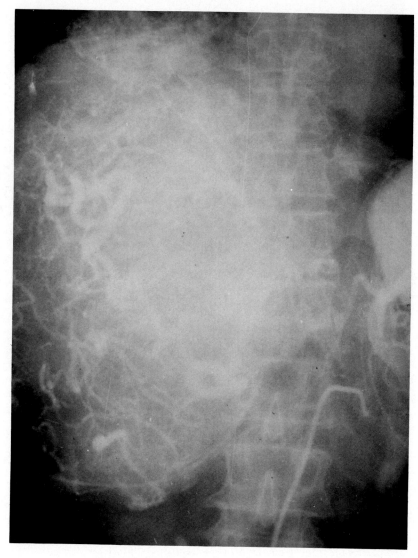

Fig. 50-41 Hepatocarcinoma, multinodular type.

a rare occurrence, and as of 1982 less than 30 cases had been reported in the English literature.[120]

MALIGNANT LIVER TUMORS

A practical classification of malignant liver tumors is given in Table 50-1.

Hepatocarcinoma

Hepatocarcinoma is much more frequent in Africa and Asia than it is in Europe and North America.[150] About 70% of cases in the United States occur in patients with cirrhosis,[126] but this association is much less frequent in Oriental countries.[150] Most patients are adults, although the tumor does occur in children, sometimes in association with biliary atresia and secondary biliary cirrhosis.[190] The major symptoms are right upper quadrant pain and weight loss, but a few patients have bone pain caused by osseous metastases,[126] shock from massive intraperitoneal hemorrhage from the tumor,[126] or obstructive jaundice caused by sloughing of necrotic tumor into the bile ducts.[87]

A large liver, sometimes with obvious irregularity, may be found on plain films. Defects caused by the tumor can be demonstrated on thorium dioxide hepatography,[30] but arteriography and scanning are the two most important diagnostic procedures.[126] On ^{99m}Tc-sulfur colloid scans the tumor causes an area of decreased or absent uptake. ^{67}Ga citrate uptake is increased in most vascular hepatomas and shows equilibrated uptake in the other hepatomas.[238] Uptake of ^{75}Se-selenomethionine is also increased in hepatocarcinoma.[68] Combinations of radioisotope scans improve diagnostic accuracy but are not specific for hepatocarcinoma, because ^{67}Ga citrate uptake and ^{75}Se-selenomethionine uptake may also be increased in some metastases, lymphosarcoma, and abscesses.[68,146,238] Exceptional hepatomas may be so well differentiated functionally that there is equilibrated uptake of ^{131}I–rose bengal.[227]

Hepatocarcinomas are very vascular tumors and with angiography show vascular proliferation, tumor staining, and arteriovenous shunting. The hypervascularity is usually massive, involving the entire tumor (Fig. 50-41), but it may be arborescent or basketlike in some cases in which there is displacement of arteries and proliferation of fine vessels at the tumor margins.[137] Angiography also differentiates the gross forms of hepatocarcinoma—uninodular or diffuse types.[85] Obstruction, deviation, or compression of the portal vein is common in hepatoma (Figs. 50-42 and 50-43) and is more likely to occur with hepatocarcinoma than with a metastatic tumor.[258] Hepatic vein invasion is also frequent, and hepatocarcinoma frequently causes the Budd-Chiari syndrome (Fig. 50-44). Some hepatomas are said to be avascular on angiography,[206] but most of these are either necrotic tumors or

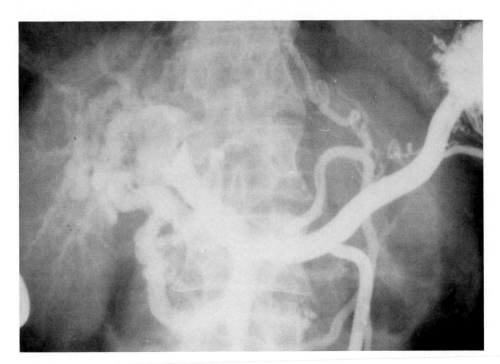

Fig. 50-42 Splenoportogram showing hepatocarcinoma invading and obstructing portal vein.

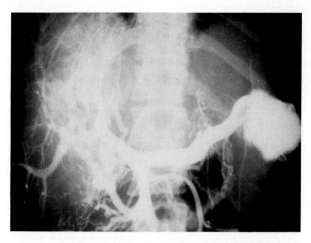

Fig. 50-43 Hepatocarcinoma. Splenoportogram shows displacement of intrahepatic portal veins and portal hypertension.

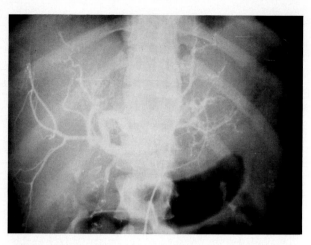

Fig. 50-44 Bulk of tumor is in left lobe with multiple nodules in right lobe of liver.

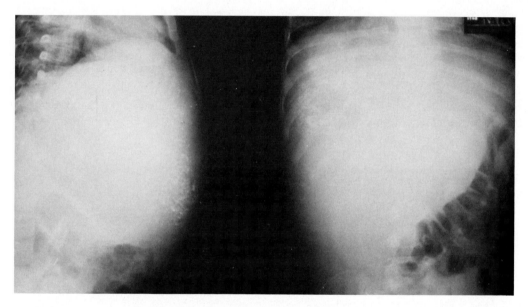

Fig. 50-45 Hepatoblastoma in 1-year-old infant.

examples of mixed hepatocellular-cholangiocellular carcinoma.

Vascular metastases can usually be distinguished from the diffuse form of hepatocarcinoma in the clinical setting. Well-differentiated hepatomas with a more normal vascularity may be difficult to distinguish from some hamartomas, adenomas, and focal nodular hyperplasia. The good health of the latter patients may aid in the distinction. The presence in serum of α-fetoglobulin aids in the diagnosis of hepatocarcinoma. This serologic test is positive in 60% to 90% of cases of hepatocarcinoma and is negative in cholangiocarcinoma.[150] It is fairly specific for hepatocarcinoma, but high titers also occur in embryonal tumors and have been noted with metastatic gastric and prostatic carcinoma,[6,141,169] as well as in Indian children with cirrhosis.[185]

Hepatoblastoma

Hepatoblastoma is an embryonal tumor that may be epithelial in type or contain mixed epithelial and meso-

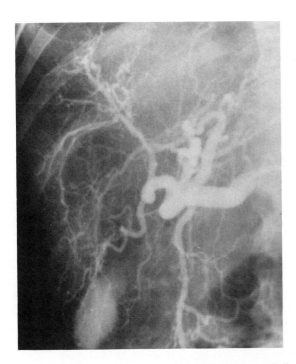

Fig. 50-46 Cholangiocellular carcinoma. Encasement and distortion of intrahepatic arteries without tumor neovascularity.

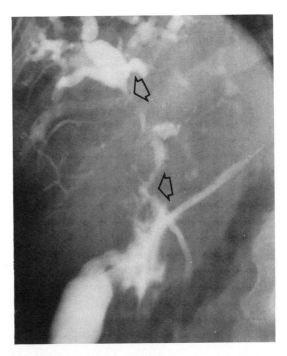

Fig. 50-47 Encasement and high-grade obstruction of intrahepatic bile ducts by large tumor between arrows.
(Courtesy Barry Held, MD)

dermal elements. It should be distinguished from hepatocarcinoma, which also occurs in children but is less frequent than hepatoblastoma in this age group.[121] Furthermore, the hepatoblastoma occurs in younger children, the usual age range being from birth to 3 years. Calcification of the tumor (Fig. 50-45) is moderately frequent (about 12%) in contrast with hepatocarcinoma, in which this does not occur. Angiography reveals tumor neovascularity and tumor staining identical to that of hepatocarcinoma.[179] The prognosis is better than with hepatocarcinoma, and about 20% of the hepatoblastomas are curable by surgical resection.[121]

Cholangiocellular carcinoma

Cholangiocellular carcinoma is the preferable term for this hepatoma of bile duct origin, since its synonyms, *cholangioma* and *cholangiocarcinoma,* have also been used to designate bile duct carcinoma, which is a quite different tumor originating from the larger bile ducts. The cholangiocellular carcinoma usually has a prominent fibrotic component and on angiography is a relatively avascular tumor showing stretched or encased arteries (Fig. 50-46). If vascular proliferation is present, it is minimal. The intrahepatic bile ducts are also encased or obstructed by the tumor (Fig. 50-47). Calcification does

occur in this tumor and may be recognized on plain films.[173]

Sarcomas

Primary sarcomas of the liver are very rare tumors arising from mesodermal elements. The hemangiosarcoma, the malignant counterpart of hemangioendothelioma, has similar angiographic features. These vascular masses have large sinusoidal pools similar to the benign tumor but differ in that encasement of arteries may also be present.[179] Primary leiomyosarcoma is a rare lesion that initially appears with hepatomegaly, shows a defect on liver scans, and rather surprisingly is a relatively avascular lesion on angiography.[269] The hemangioendotheliosarcoma, which may actually arise from Kupffer's cells, is usually associated with the administration of thorium dioxide and may be recognized as a defect in the reticular pattern of thorium dioxide in the liver.[200] Other primary sarcomas include fibrosarcoma, rhabdomyosarcoma, and malignant mesenchymoma.[200] A case of primary osteosarcoma in a patient with hemochromatosis has been reported in which tumor bone was evident histologically but not seen on radiologic examination.[164]

A few arteriograms of angiosarcomas found in vinyl

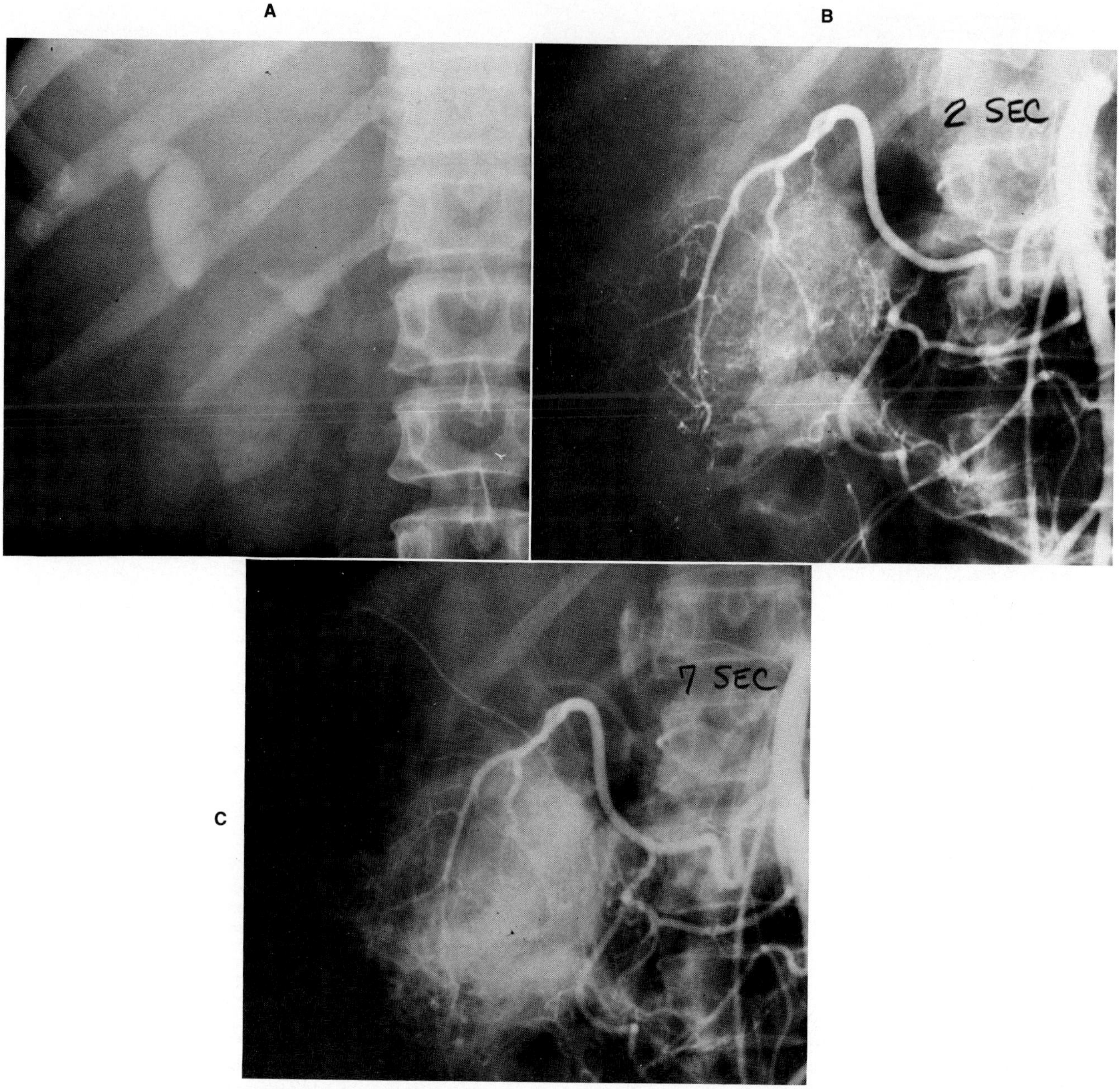

A

B

C

Fig. 50-48 Angiosarcoma of liver in vinyl chloride worker. **A,** Cholecystogram shows distortion and deformity of gallbladder by tumor in right lobe of liver. **B** and **C,** Arteriography reveals hypervascular lesion with few tumor vessels about its margin.

chloride workers have been reported.[262] These revealed a central hypovascular area with a homogeneous stain about the margins of the lesion. No tumor vessels were evident. The central avascular area was attributed to tumor necrosis. In one case typical changes of peliosis hepatis were present in the remainder of the liver. I saw one case of angiosarcoma that showed a diffuse tumor stain and a few small tumor vessels (Fig. 50-48).

Metastatic tumor

The metastatic tumor is the most common liver tumor, and metastatic disease may or may not cause hepatomegaly. Displacement and deformity of the gallbladder sometimes identifies the liver masses. Calcification, particularly in mucinous carcinoma, may aid in the specific diagnosis. The usual mucinous carcinoma calcification consists of a myriad of tiny punctate densities (Fig. 50-

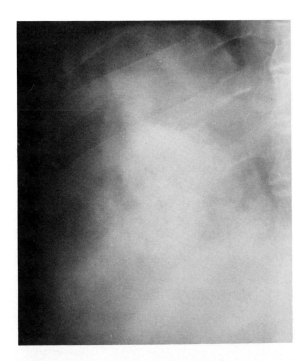

Fig. 50-49 Calcified mucinous carcinoma from colon.

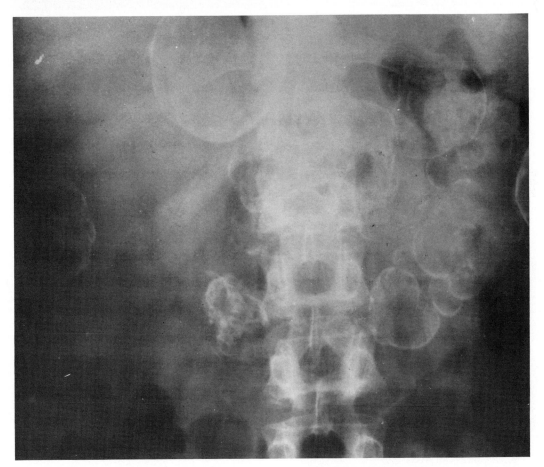

Fig. 50-50 Calcified leiomyosarcoma metastases, primarily in stomach.
(Courtesy David Inkeles, MD)

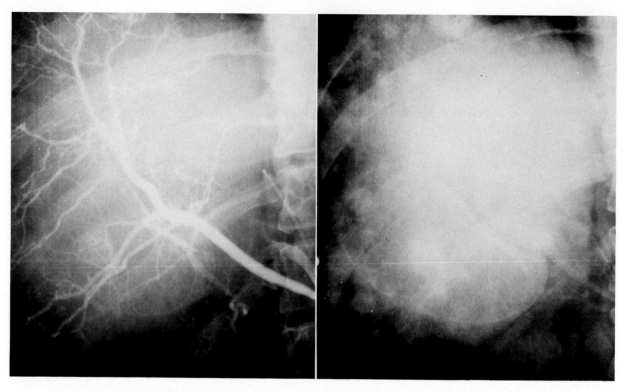

Fig. 50-51 Vascular metastases caused by metastatic carcinoid.
(Courtesy Gus Seliger, MD)

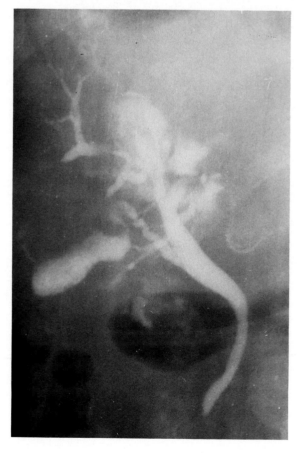

Fig. 50-52 Metastatic carcinoma shown by percutaneous chol-angiogram. Tumor is obstructing numerous intrahepatic ducts, and smaller biliary radicals failed to fill.
(Courtesy Barry Held, MD)

49) that sometimes defy certain recognition. Exceptionally, the calcification may be dense or cystic in character. Calcification also occurs in other metastatic tumors (Fig. 50-50).

If the metastases are large enough, they are readily recognized on liver scans. Angiographic findings are variable and generally reflect the arteriographic features of the primary tumor, although tumor necrosis may modify this. The usual vascular metastases are carcinoid (Fig. 50-51), islet cell carcinoma, choriocarcinoma, leiomyosarcoma, and hypernephroma,[195,206] whereas moderate vascularity may be found in seminoma, adrenal carcinoma, endometrial carcinoma, some colon and breast tumors, and rare pancreatic carcinoma.[251] Metastatic carcinoma causes displacement and distortion of bile ducts, obstruction of larger ducts, and nonfilling of smaller peripheral ducts[147] (Fig. 50-52).

BILE DUCT CARCINOMA

Bile duct carcinomas are fairly common; several cases per year may be encountered in large medical centers.[103] There are geographic variations in frequency, varying from one bile duct carcinoma for every eight pancreatic carcinomas in New Haven, Connecticut,[45] to one bile duct carcinoma for each pancreatic carcinoma in Glasgow, Scotland.[36] These tumors are most frequent in the fifth to eighth decades of life but do occur in younger individuals. There is an association with chronic ulcerative colitis. In one large series of patients with ulcerative colitis, 0.7% developed bile duct carcinoma,[203] and the youngest patients (aged 17 and 22 years) with primary bile duct carcinoma also had chronic ulcerative colitis.[103]

The tumors arise in the larger bile ducts, the site of tumor origin, determined from the combined data of two large series,[235,253] is as follows:

1. Left or right hepatic duct, 13%
2. Common hepatic duct, 37%
3. Junction of cystic and common hepatic duct, 15%
4. Cystic duct, 6%
5. Common bile duct, 33%

A few tumors are polypoid intraluminal lesions (Fig. 50-53), and some are bulky tumor masses (Fig. 50-54). When obstruction can be controlled by biliary stents, these tumors may be shown to grow along the axis of the duct system (Fig. 50-55). These types are mainly cellular adenocarcinomas. The most common lesion,

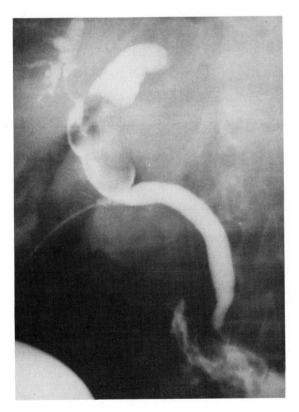

Fig. 50-53 Polypoid carcinoma of common hepatic duct.

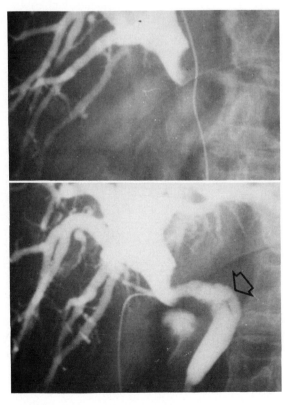

Fig. 50-54 Bulky carcinoma of common hepatic duct. Cystic duct (*arrow*) passes behind tumor.

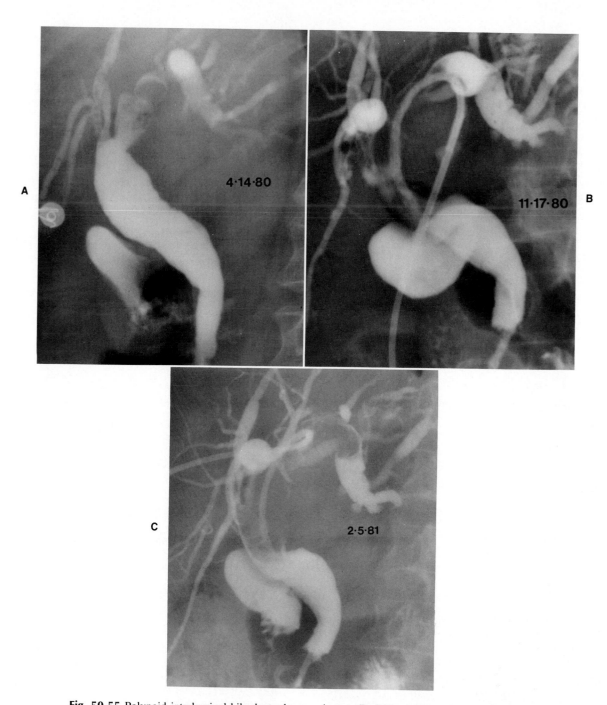

Fig. 50-55 Polypoid intraluminal bile duct adenocarcinoma. **B,** Biliary obstruction controlled by biliary stent. **C,** With intraluminal axial tumor growth as followed by cholangiography for 10 months.

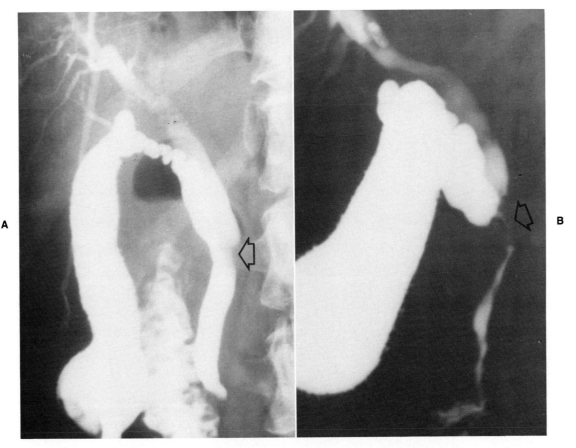

Fig. 50-56 Scirrhous carcinoma at junction of cystic and common hepatic ducts. **A,** Small defect (*arrow*) is present at junction of ducts, and there is some dilatation of common hepatic duct proximal to this. Lesion was overlooked on this injection through cholecystostomy tube. **B,** Several months later, well-defined scirrhous carcinoma with overhanging edges is present at this site (*arrows*).

however, is the small scirrhous carcinoma (Fig. 50-56).[45,263] These are often well-differentiated adenocarcinomas in which the pathologic diagnosis may be difficult because of the normal occurrence of glandular structures in the bile duct wall.

Rarely oral cholecystocholangiography may demonstrate a bile duct tumor, but oral or intravenous methods are likely to fail because of nonvisualization or poor detail when visualization does occur.[45] The diagnosis is usually easy with direct cholangiography. It is axiomatic that a short stricture of the bile ducts, in the absence of a known cause such as surgical trauma, is scirrhous carcinoma unless proved otherwise (Figs. 50-57 and 50-58). The tumor is usually slow growing and tends to extend along the axis of the ducts, resulting in some larger lesions (Fig. 50-59). Problems is differential diagnosis arise when the tumor causes total obstruction of the duct. Liver scans in cases of bile duct carcinoma may reveal patchy

or mottled uptake, which is usually caused by dilated intrahepatic bile ducts rather than by metastases.[263] Selective arteriography reveals tiny, thin tumor vessels with irregular encasement or obstruction of arteries.[136] These changes, however, can be quite subtle and may be mimicked by inflammatory lesions.

Some special features of bile duct carcinoma are of importance and deserve mention. Successful surgical resection is only rarely possible,[177] but many of these patients have long periods of good health if biliary stents or surgical measures can control biliary obstruction.[140] This is particularly true in the very slow-growing lesions, some of which have been originally and erroneously diagnosed as primary sclerosing cholangitis.[9] The other important aspect of bile duct carcinoma is the high incidence of diagnostic failure, both surgical and radiologic, in common hepatic duct tumors.[45,263] Most of these lesions high in the porta hepatis are evident only after

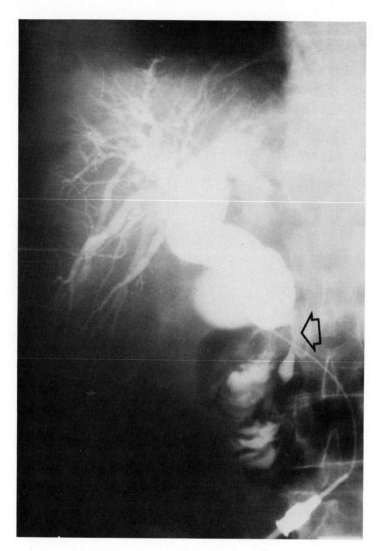

Fig. 50-57 Scirrhous carcinoma of common bile duct in head of pancreas (*arrow*).

extensive dissection (Fig. 50-58), but some of them in more accessible locations are also missed (Figs. 50-59 and 50-60). These overlooked common hepatic duct tumors present a fairly typical clinical syndrome[140] characterized by one or more unrevealing operations for obstructive jaundice, wherein the liver is found to be tense or turgid and the gallbladder and common duct are empty or collapsed. The use of preoperative percutaneous transhepatic cholangiography or ERCP prevents this error.

Differential diagnosis

Strictures or accidental surgical ligation of bile ducts can give a cholangiographic picture identical to that of the small scirrhous carcinoma (Fig. 50-61). For practical purposes, however, this is not a diagnostic problem, because the history readily reveals the nature of the lesion.

Short fibrous strictures caused by schistosomiasis have been reported from Africa, and these lesions could mimic the scirrhous tumors. Benign bile duct tumors and other primary malignant lesions such as cystoadenocarcinoma[247] and leiomyosarcoma[266] are exceedingly rare.

When there is complete obstruction of the duct, problems in differential diagnosis do arise. The configuration at the site of the obstruction seldom is specific unless there is an intraluminal mass. The location of the obstruction and the presence or absence of a mass on gastrointestinal studies usually provide a short, meaningful differential diagnosis. For instance, total obstruction of the intrapancreatic portion of the common duct some distance from Vater's papilla in the absence of a mass favors the diagnosis of primary bile duct carcinoma (Fig. 50-62). Total obstruction of the common duct at the su-

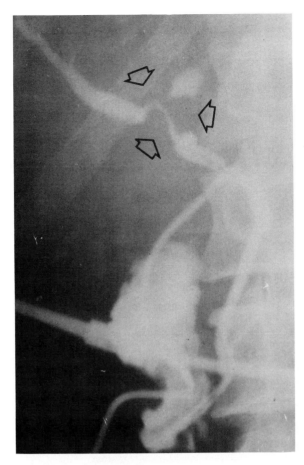

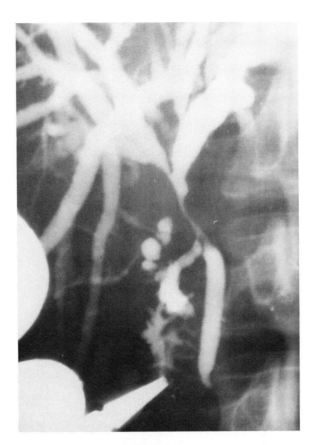

Fig. 50-59 Scirrhous carcinoma of common hepatic duct. Fistulogram demonstrates lesion involving common hepatic duct and extending to distal portions of right and left hepatic ducts. Lesion was missed at two earlier operations.

Fig. 50-58 Scirrhous carcinoma at junction of right and left hepatic ducts (*arrows*).

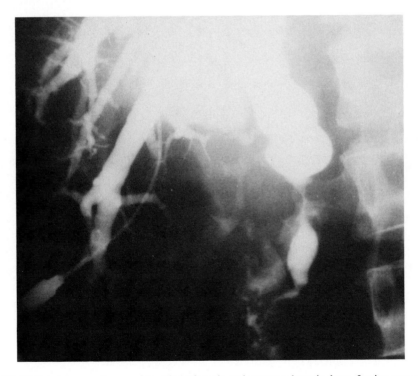

Fig. 50-60 Scirrhous carcinoma at junction of cystic and common hepatic ducts. Lesion was missed at original operation. Jaundice recurred, and percutaneous cholangiogram revealed scirrhous carcinoma.

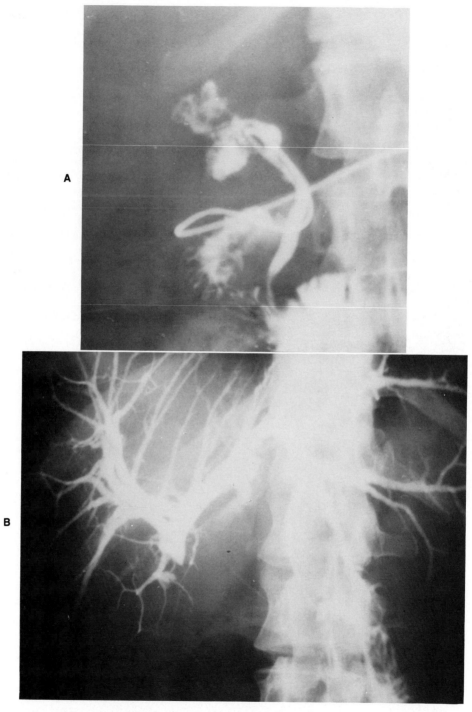

Fig. 50-61 Accidental ligation of common hepatic duct. **A,** T-tube cholangiogram. There is complete obstruction to retrograde flow in common hepatic duct with some extravasation of contrast. **B,** Following Longmire procedure, cholangiogram reveals complete obstruction of proximal hepatic duct.

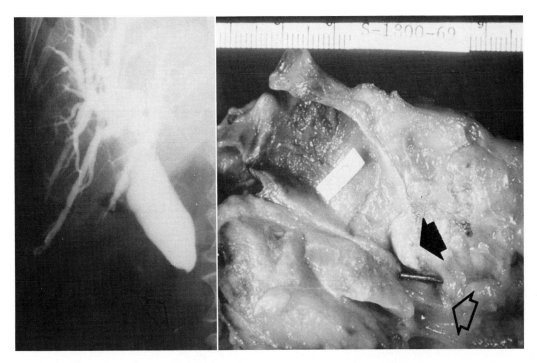

Fig. 50-62 Scirrhous carcinoma of distal common bile duct. **A,** Complete obstruction of duct about 2 cm proximal to duodenal papilla (*arrow*). There was no evidence of mass on gastrointestinal series. **B,** One-centimeter tumor (*black arrow*), 1.5 cm proximal to duodenal papilla (*open arrow*).

perior margin of the pancreas is, statistically, almost always caused by pancreatic carcinoma, even when a mass is not demonstrated on gastrointestinal examination. Total obstruction above this level results in a differential diagnostic problem between primary bile duct carcinoma, metastatic carcinoma in the porta hepatis, and gallbladder carcinoma that has extended to involve the common heaptic duct.

BENIGN BILE DUCT TUMORS

Benign tumors of the bile duct are very rare. For example, in one report of 5200 consecutive biliary operations, two adenomas of the extrahepatic bile ducts were found.[118] Adenoma is the most common benign tumor, but many other lesions have been described, including papilloma,[42] cystadenoma,[228] adenomyoma,[63] hamartoma,[63] heterotopic gastric mucosa,[268] heterotopic pancreas,[259] inflammatory gastric mucosa,[268] inflammatory pseudotumor,[81] carcinoid,[151] granular cell myoblastoma,[2,157] fibroma,[42] and neuroma.[42] Many tumors are incidental findings, but some of these lesions do cause obstructive jaundice,[101,166,259] and msssive hemobilia as the result of erosion of a benign adenoma has been reported.[244] Some cholangiograms reveal nonspecific bile duct obstruction,[101,167] whereas in others an intraluminal mass[259] or polypoid tumor[228] has been shown.

With most of these benign tumors the diagnosis depends entirely on histologic examination (Fig. 50-63). The one possible exception is granular cell myoblastoma. The several cases reported* have consistently shown that this tumor is a small subepithelial lesion that frequently causes duct obstruction. About half of the cases occur in the cystic duct and cause hydrops of the gallbladder. Tumors of the common hepatic or common bile duct cause obstructive jaundice. Radiologically this tumor causes an eccentric stricture of the duct, resulting in partial obstruction (Fig. 50-64). Although it is somewhat similar to scirrhous bile duct carcinoma, the subtle differences should suggest granular cell myoblastoma. The key to the differential diagnosis is the age, sex, and race of the patient, since most granular cell myoblastomas have occurred in black women and the average age has been 35 years.

SARCOMA BOTRYOIDES

Sarcoma botryoides is a rare bile duct tumor of late infancy or childhood.[109] The youngest patient reported was 18 months old, and the oldest was 11 years old.[109] Grossly the tumor is a bulky intraluminal mucoid-appearing mass that distends the bile ducts. Histologically

*References 41, 49, 64, 90, 139, 204, 219, 264, 267.

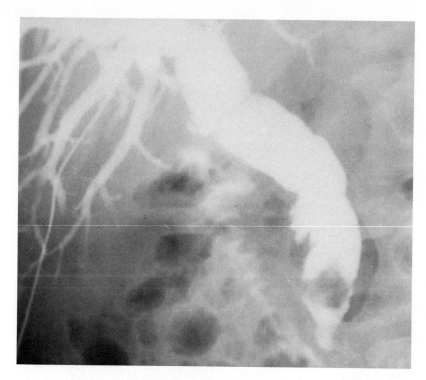

Fig. 50-63 Inflammatory polyp of distal common duct.

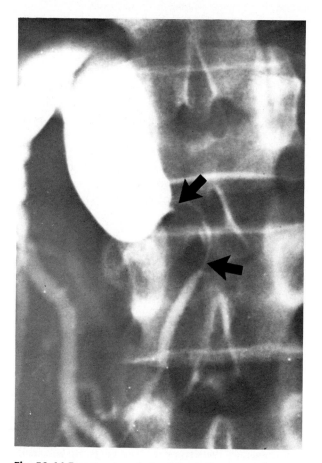

Fig. 50-64 Percutaneous cholangiogram shows smooth eccentric stenosis of common bile duct *(arrows)* caused by granular cell myoblastoma in young black woman.
(Courtesy Emil Balthazar, MD; from Berk, RN, and Clemett, AR: Radiology of the gallbladder and bile ducts, Philadelphia, 1977, WB Saunders.)

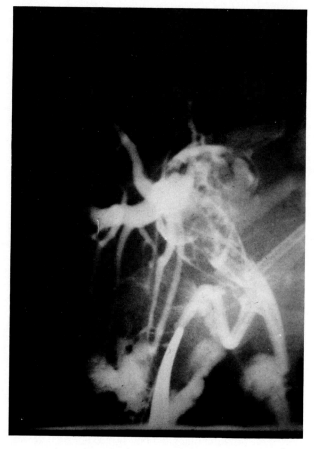

Fig. 50-65 Sarcoma botryoides.
(Courtesy Jack O'Connor, MD)

this is a subepithelial embryonal rhabdomyosarcoma.[230] The patients usually have obstructive jaundice. Extrinsic pressure defects on the second portion of the duodenum may be found on gastrointestinal series and are the same as those produced by choledochal cysts, which the lesion resembles externally. The cholangiographic findings are characteristic (Fig. 50-65) and consist of a bulky intra-luminal mass in the dilated bile ducts of a child.[56,230] This malignant tumor may decrease in size with chemotherapy or radiation, but cure by any means has not yet been reported.[56]

REFERENCES

1. Abrams, RM, et al: Angiographic features of cavernous hemangioma of liver, Radiology 92:308, 1969.
2. Abt, AB, Feinberg, E, and Kunitz, S: Granular cell myoblastoma of the extrahepatic biliary tract, Mt Sinai J Med 38:457, 1971.
3. Adam, JG, Huvos, AG, and Fortner, JG: Giant hemangiomas of the liver, Ann Surg 172:239, 1970.
4. Albo, RJ, and Obata, WG: Radiologic diagnosis of primary sclerosing cholangitis, Radiology 81:123, 1963.
5. Alfidi, RJ, et al: Hepatic arteriography, Radiology 90:1136, 1968.
6. Alpert, E, Pinn, VM, and Isselbacher, KJ: Alpha-fetoprotein in a patient with gastric carcinoma metastatic to the liver, N Engl J Med 285:1058, 1971.
7. Alpert, S, et al: Right hepatectomy for hamartoma in an eleven-month-old infant, Ann Surg 165:286, 1967.
8. Altemeier, WA, Schowengerdt, CG, and Whiteley, DH: Abscesses of the liver: surgical considerations, Arch Surg 101:258, 1970.
9. Altemeier, WA, et al: Sclerosing carcinoma of the major intrahepatic bile ducts, Arch Surg 75:450, 1957.
10. Alvarez, SZ, and Fabra, R: The clinical features of hepatobiliary tuberculosis in the Philippines. In Proceedings of the Fourth World Congress of Gastroenterology, Copenhagen, 1970.
11. Akira, T, Itai, Y, and Tasaka, A: CT of the choledochal cyst, AJR 135:729, 1980.
12. Ameres, JP, Levine, MP, and DeBlasi, HP: Acalculous clonorchiasis obstructing the common bile duct: a case report and review of the literature, Am Surg 42:170, 1976.
13. Aronsen, KF, et al: A case of operated focal nodular cirrhosis of the liver, Scand J Gastroenterol 3:58, 1968.
14. Ashby, S: Carcinoma in a choledochus cyst, Br J Surg 51:493, 1964.
15. Atkinson, AJ, and Carroll, WW: Sclerosing cholangitis, JAMA 188:183, 1964.
16. Azimi, PH, et al: Chronic granulomatous disease in three female siblings, JAMA 206:2865, 1968.
17. Babbitt, DP: Congenital choledochal cysts: new etiological concept based on anomalous relationships of the common bile duct and pancreatic duct, Ann Radiol (Paris) 12:231, 1969.
18. Babbitt, DP, Starshak, RJ, and Clemett, AR: Choledochal cyst: a concept of etiology, AJR 119:57, 1973.
19. Baker, DH, and Harris, RC: Congenital absence of the intrahepatic bile ducts, AJR 91:875, 1964.
20. Baker, MS, Baker, BH, and Woo, R: Biliary clonorchiasis, Arch Surg 114:748, 1979.
21. Baltaxe, HA, and Fleming, RJ: The angiographic appearance of hydatid disease, Radiology 97:599, 1970.
22. Bartholomew, LG, et al: Sclerosing cholangitis, N Engl J Med 269:8, 1963.
23. Bass, EM, Functon, MR, and Shaff, MI: Caroli's disease: an ultrasonic diagnosis, Br J Radiol 50:366, 1977.
24. Becker, CD, et al: Diagnosis and treatment of choledochocele complicated by choledocholithiasis (case report), Gastrointest Radiol 12:322, 1987.
25. Beker, SG, and Valencia-Parparcen, J: Portal hypertension syndrome, Am J Dig Dis 13:1047, 1968.
26. Belgrater, AH: Common bile duct obstruction due to *Fasciola hepatica*, NY State J Med 76:936, 1976.
27. Belmaric, J: Intrahepatic bile duct carcinoma and *C. sinensis* infection in Hong Kong, Cancer 31:468, 1973.
28. Berdon, WE, and Baker, DH: Giant hepatic hemangioma with cardiac failure in the newborn infant, Radiology 92:1528, 1969.
29. Block, MA, et al: Surgery of liver abscesses, Arch Surg 88:602, 1964.
30. Boijsen, E, and Abrams, HL: Roentgenologic diagnosis of primary carcinoma of the liver, Acta Radiol 3:257, 1965.
31. Boijsen, E, and Reuter, SR: Combined percutaneous transhepatic cholangiography and angiography in the evaluation of obstructive jaundice, AJR 99:153, 1967.
32. Boijsen, E, et al: Preoperative angiographic diagnosis of bleeding aneurysms of abdominal visceral arteries, Radiology 93:781, 1969.
33. Bondestam, S, et al: Sonographic diagnosis of a bile duct polyp, AJR 135:610, 1980.
34. Boyer, JL, et al: Idiopathic portal hypertension, Ann Intern Med 66:41, 1967.
35. Bron, KM, and Gajaraj, A: Demonstration of hepatic aneurysms in polyarteritis nodosa by arteriography, N Engl J Med 282:1024, 1970.
36. Brown, DB, et al: Primary carcinoma of the extrahepatic bile ducts, Br J Surg 49:22, 1961.
37. Bruwer, AJ, and Hallenbeck, GA: Aneurysm of hepatic artery: roentgenologic features in one case, AJR 78:270, 1957.
38. Burke, JF, and Scully, RE: Pulmonary disease associated with a disappearing abdominal mass, N Engl J Med 281:1004, 1969.
39. Carson, MJ, et al: Thirteen boys with progressive septic granulomatosis, Pediatrics 35:405, 1965.
40. Chopra, S, et al: Peliosis hepatis in hematologic disease, JAMA 240:1153, 1978.
41. Christensen, AH, and Isak, KG: Benign tumors and pseudotumors of the gallbladder: report of 180 cases, Arch Pathol 90:423, 1970.
42. Chu, PT: Benign neoplasms of the extrahepatic biliary ducts: review of the literature and report of a case of fibroma, Arch Pathol 50:84, 1950.
43. Clain, D, and McNulty, J: A radiological study of the lymphatics of the liver, Br J Radiol 41:662, 1968.
44. Clay, MG, and Munro, AI: Bilateral diaphragmatic hernia from blunt injury causing a Budd-Chiari syndrome, Ann Surg 173:321, 1971.
45. Clemett, AR: Carcinoma of the major bile ducts, Radiology 84:894, 1965.
46. Clemett, AR: A technique of percutaneous transhepatic cholangiography for the seventies. Paper presented at the Annual Radiologic Society of North America meeting, Chicago, December 1970.
47. Cleveland, RJ, et al: Traumatic intrahepatic hepatic artery portal vein fistula with associated hemobilia, Ann Surg 171:451, 1970.
48. Cobo, A, et al: Intrahepatic calculi, Arch Surg 89:936, 1964.
49. Coggins, RP: Granular cell myoblastoma of the common bile duct: report of a case with autopsy findings, Arch Pathol 54:398, 1952.

50. Coutinho, A: Hemodynamic studies of portal hypertension in schistosomiasis, Am J Med 44:547, 1968.

51. Cronan, JJ, et al: Cavernous hemangioma of the liver: role of percutaneous biopsy, Radiology 166:135, 1988.

52. Cummack, DH: Gastro-intestinal x-ray diagnosis: a descriptive atlas, Baltimore, 1968, Williams & Wilkins.

53. Cutler, B, and Donaldson, GA: Primary sclerosing cholangitis and obliterative cholangitis, Am J Surg 117:502, 1969.

54. Cywes, S, and Krige, H: Intravenous cholangiography and tomography in the diagnosis of biliary ascariasis, Clin Radiol 14:271, 1963.

55. Dardik, H, Gotzer, P, and Silver, C: Congenital hepatic cyst causing jaundice, Ann Surg 159:585, 1964.

56. Davis, GL, Kissane, JM, and Ishak, KG: Embryonal rhabdomyosarcoma (sarcoma botryoides) of the biliary tree, Cancer 24:333, 1969.

57. DeLorimier, AA, et al: Hepatic-artery ligation for hepatic hemangiomas, N Engl J Med 277:333, 1967.

58. Devanesan, J, et al: Congenital hepatic duct obstruction with perforate diaphragm, Arch Surg 113:1452, 1978.

59. Dodd, GD: Lymphography in diseases of the liver and pancreas, Radiol Clin North Am 8:69, 1970.

60. Doehner, GA: The hepatic venous system, Radiology 90:1119, 1968.

61. Dolmatch, BL, et al: AIDS-related cholangitis: radiographic findings in nine patients, Radiology 163:313, 1987.

62. Doppman, JL, et al: Bile duct cysts secondary to liver infarcts: report of a case and experimental production by small vessel hepatic artery occlusion, Radiology 130:1, 1979.

63. Dowdy, GS, Jr, et al: Benign tumors of the extrahepatic bile ducts: report of three cases and review of the literature, Arch Surg 85:503, 1962.

64. Duncan, JT, Jr, and Wilson, H: Benign tumor of the common bile duct, Ann Surg 145:271, 1957.

65. Easterbrook, JS: Renal and hepatic microaneurysms: report of a new entity simulating polyarteritis nodosa, Radiology 137:629, 1980.

66. Ecker, JA, and Doane, WA: Massive cavernous hemangioma of the liver, Am J Gastroenterol 52:25, 1969.

67. Ecker, JA, McKittrick, JE, and Failing, RM: Thrombosis of the hepatic veins, Am J Gastroenterol 45:429, 1966.

68. Eddleston, ALW, et al: Se-selenomethionine in the scintiscan diagnosis of primary hepatocellular carcinoma, Gut 12:245, 1971.

69. Elmslie, RG: Pyogenic liver abscess associated with common duct calculi, Med J Aust 1:800, 1965.

70. Enjoji, M, Watanabe, H, and Nakamura, Y: A case report: congenital biliotracheal fistula with trifurcation of bronchi, Ann Paediatr 200:321, 1963.

71. Evans, JA: Specialized technics in investigation of abdominal disease, Radiology 82:579, 1964.

72. Federle, MP, Filly, RA, and Moss, A: Cystic hepatic neoplasms: complementary roles of CT and sonography, AJR 136:345, 1981.

73. Feingold, ML, et al: Budd-Chiari syndrome caused by a right atrial tumor, Arch Intern Med 127:292, 1971.

74. Finch, SC, and Finch, CH: Idiopathic hemochromatosis: an iron storage disease, Medicine 34:381, 1955.

75. Fisher, MM, Chen, S, and Dekker, A: Congenital diaphragm of the common hepatic duct, Gastroenterology 54:605, 1968.

76. Flanigan, DP: Biliary cysts, Ann Surg 182:635, 1975.

77. Flemma, RJ, and Anlyan, WG: Tuberculous broncho-biliary fistula, J Thorac Cardiovasc Surg 49:198, 1965.

78. Fonkalsrud, EW, and Boles, ET, Jr: Choledochal cysts in infancy and childhood, Surg Gynecol Obstet 121:733, 1965.

79. Forrest, ME, et al: Biliary cystadenomas: sonographic-angiographic-pathologic correlations, AJR 135:723, 1980.

80. Foster, SC, Schneider, B, and Seaman, WB: Gas-containing pyogenic intrahepatic abscesses, Radiology 94:613, 1970.

81. Freeman, LM, Bernstein, RG, and Hayt, DB: Diagnosis of hepatic hemangioma with combined scanning technique, Radiology 95:127, 1970.

82. Frick, MP, and Feinberg, SB: Biliary cystadenoma, AJR 139:393, 1982.

83. Fung, J: Liver fluke infestation and cholangiohepatitis, Br J Surg 48:404, 1961.

84. Gammill, SL, et al: Filling defects on scintillation scans of the liver associated with dilatation of the bile ducts, AJR 107:37, 1969.

85. Gammill, SL, et al: Hepatic angiography in the selection of patients with hepatomas for hepatic lobectomy, Radiology 101:549, 1971.

86. Gelfand, DW: The liver: pain film diagnosis, Semin Roentgenol 10:177, 1975.

87. Gerson, CD, and Schinella, RA: Hepatoma presenting as extrahepatic biliary obstruction, Am J Dig Dis 14:42, 1969.

88. Gherardi, GJ, and MacMahon, HE: Hypoplasia of terminal bile ducts, Am J Dis Child 120:151, 1970.

89. Gold, RH, et al: Roentgenographic features of the neutrophil dysfunction syndromes, Radiology 92:1045, 1969.

90. Goldman, LI, et al: Granular cell myoblastoma of the cystic duct, JAMA 200:1185, 1967.

91. Goswitz, JT, and Kimmerling, R: Perforated choledochal cyst with bile peritonitis in an infant: case report and surgical management, Surgery 59:878, 1966.

92. Gots, RE, and Zuidema, GD: Dilatation of the intrahepatic biliary ducts in a patient with a choledochal cyst, Am J Surg 119:726, 1970.

93. Grange, D, et al: Hepatic calcification due to *Fasciola gigantica*, Arch Surg 108:113, 1974.

94. Grossman, H, Berdon, WE, and Baker, DH: Gastrointestinal findings in cystic fibrosis, AJR 97:227, 1966.

95. Grossman, H, and Seed, W: Congenital hepatic fibrosis, bile duct dilatation, and renal lesion resembling medullary sponge kidney, Radiology 87:46, 1966.

96. Grunfeld, O, and Hinostroza, G: Thallium poisoning, Arch Intern Med 114:132, 1964.

97. Gryboski, JD, and Clemett, A: Congenital hepatic artery aneurysm with superior mesenteric artery insufficiency: a steal syndrome, Pediatrics 39:344, 1967.

98. Guida, PM, and Moore, SW: Aneurysm of the hepatic artery: report of five cases with a brief review of the previously reported cases, Surgery 60:299, 1966.

99. Gundersen, AE, and Green, RM: Traumatic hemobilia: accurate preoperative diagnosis by hepatic artery angiogram, Surgery 62:862, 1967.

100. Hadad, AR, et al: Congenital dilatation of the bile ducts, Am J Surg 132:797, 1976.

101. Haith, EE, Kepes, JJ, and Holder, TM: Inflammatory pseudotumor involving the common bile duct of a six-year-old boy: successful pancreaticoduodenectomy, Surgery 56:436, 1964.

102. Halpern, M, and Citron, BP: Necrotizing angitis associated with drug abuse, AJR 111:663, 1971.

103. Ham, JM, and Mackenzie, DC: Primary carcinoma of the extrahepatic bile ducts, Surg Gynecol Obstet 118:1, 1964.

104. Han, BK, Babcock, DS, and Gelfand, MH: Choledochal cyst with bile duct dilatation: sonography and ^{99m}Tc IDA cholescintigraphy, AJR 136:1075, 1981.

105. Hanai, H, Idriss, F, and Swenson, O: Bile duct proliferation in atresia and related hepatic diseases, Arch Surg 94:14, 1967.

106. Harris, JD: Rupture of hydatid cysts of the liver into the biliary tracts, Br J Surg 52:210, 1965.

107. Hawkins, PE, Graham, FB, and Holliday, P: Gallbladder disease in children, Am J Surg 111:741, 1966.

108. Hayes, MA, Goldenberg, IS, and Bishop, CC: The developmental basis for bile duct anomalies, Surg Gynecol Obstet 107:447, 1958.

109. Hays, DM, and Snyder, WH, Jr: Botryoid sarcoma (rhabdomyosarcoma) of the bile ducts, Am J Dis Child 110:595, 1965.

110. Hays, DM, et al: Congenital cystic dilatation of the common bile duct, Arch Surg 98:457, 1969.

111. Hermann, RE, and Hawk, WA: Congenital hepatic fibrosis as a cause of portal hypertension: report of two cases, Surgery 62:1095, 1967.

112. Hermann, RE, and Shafer, WH: Aneurysm of the portal vein and portal hypertension: first reported case, Ann Surg 162:1101, 1965.

113. Hertzer, NR, Hawk, WA, and Hermann, RE: Inflammatory lesions of the liver which simulate tumor: report of two cases in children, Surgery 69:839, 1971.

114. Hirooka, M, and Kimura, C: Membranous obstruction of the hepatic portion of the inferior vena cava, Arch Surg 100:656, 1970.

115. Holubitsky, IB, and McKenzie, AD: Primary sclerosing cholangitis of the extrahepatic bile ducts, Can J Surg 7:277, 1964.

116. Hossack, KF, and Herron, JJ: Benign tumours of the common bile duct: report of a case and review of the literature, Aust NZ J Surg 42:22, 1972.

117. Hou, PC: Pathology of Clonorchis sinensis infestation of the liver, J Pathol Bacteriol 70:53, 1955.

118. Hulten, J, Johansson, H, and Olding, L: Adenomas of the gallbladder and extrahepatic bile ducts, Acta Chir Scand 136:203, 1970.

119. Hunter, FM, et al: Congenital dilation of the intrahepatic bile ducts, Am J Med 40:188, 1966.

120. Iemoto, Y, et al: Biliary cystadenocarcinoma diagnosed by liver biopsy performed under ultrasonographic guidance, Gastroenterology 84:399, 1983.

121. Ishak, KG, and Glunz, PR: Hepatoblastoma and hepatocarcinoma in infancy and childhood, Cancer 20:396, 1967.

122. Jackson, BT, and Saunders, P: Perforated choledochus cyst, Br J Surg 58:38, 1971.

123. Jacobson, G, and Zucherman, SD: Roentgenographically demonstrable splenic deposits in sickle cell anemia, AJR 76:47, 1956.

124. Janower, MJ, et al: Late clinical and laboratory manifestations of Thorotrast administration in cerebral arteriography, N Engl J Med 279:186, 1968.

125. Jarvis, L, and Hodes, PJ: Aneurysms of the hepatic artery demonstrated roentgenographically, AJR 72:1037, 1954.

126. Jewell, KL: Primary carcinoma of the liver: clinical and radiologic manifestations, AJR 113:84, 1971.

127. Joffe, N: Siderosis in the South African Bantu, Br J Radiol 37:200, 1964.

128. Johnston, PW: Congenital cysts of the liver in infancy and childhood, Am J Surg 116:184, 1968.

129. Jonasson, O, Pritchard, J, and Long, L: Intraluminal leiomyosarcoma of the inferior vena cava, Cancer 19:1311, 1966.

130. Jones, EA, et al: Massive infection with Fasciola hepatica in man, Am J Med 63:836, 1977.

131. Joseph, WL, Fonkalsrud, EW, and Longmire, WP: Cystic dilatation of common bile duct in adults, Arch Surg 91:468, 1965.

132. Kahn, D: Thorotrast-induced hemangioendothelioma of liver, Conn Med 31:557, 1967.

133. Kaiser, JA, et al: Diagnosis of Caroli disease by computed tomography: report of two cases, Radiology 132:661, 1979.

134. Kanter, DM: Hepatic infarction, Arch Intern Med 115:479, 1965.

135. Kark, AE: Bile duct strictures caused by schistosomiasis, Br J Surg 49:419, 1962.

136. Kaude, J, and Rian, R: Cholangiocarcinoma, Radiology 100:573, 1971.

137. Kido, C, Sasaki, T, and Kaneko, M: Angiography of primary liver cancer, AJR 113:70, 1971.

138. Kimura, K, et al: Choledochal cyst: etiological considerations and surgical management in 22 cases, Arch Surg 113:159, 1978.

139. Kittredge, RD, and Baer, JW: Percutaneous transhepatic cholangiography, AJR 125:35, 1975.

140. Klatskin, G: Adenocarcinoma of the hepatic duct at its bifurcation within the porta hepatis, Am J Med 38:241, 1965.

141. Kozower, M, et al: Positive alpha-fetoglobulin in a case of gastric carcinoma, N Engl M Med 285:1059, 1971.

142. Kreel, L, Freston, JW, and Clain, D: Vascular radiology in the Budd-Chiari syndrome, Br J Radiol 40:755, 1967.

143. Krieger, J, Seaman, WB, and Porter MR: The roentgenologic appearance of sclerosing cholangitis, Radiology 95:369, 1970.

144. Kwittken, J: Hamartoma of liver, NY J Med 67:3254, 1967.

145. Landing, BH, and Shirkey, HS: A syndrome of recurrent infection and infiltration of viscera by pigmented histiocytes, Pediatrics 20:431, 1957.

146. Lavender, JP, et al: Gallium 67 citrate scanning in neoplastic and inflammatory lesions, Br J Radiol 44:361, 1971.

147. Legge, DA, Carlson, HC, and Ludwig, J: Cholangiographic findings in diseases of the liver: a postmortem study, AJR 113:34, 1971.

148. Legge, DA, et al: Cholangiographic findings in cholangiolitic hepatitis, AJR 113:16, 1971.

149. Lenthall, J, Reynolds, TB, and Donovan, AJ: Excessive output of bile in chronic hepatic disease, Surg Gynecol Obstet 130:243, 1970.

150. Lin, T: Primary cancer of the liver, Scand J Gastroenterol 6:223, 1970.

151. Little, JM, Gibson, AAM, and Kay, AW: Primary common bile-duct carcinoid, Br J Surg 55:147, 1968.

152. Longmire, WP, Jr: Congenital biliary hypoplasia, Surgery 159:335, 1964.

153. Lorenzo, GA, Seed, RW, and Beal, JM: Congenital dilatation of the biliary tract, Am J Surg 121:510, 1971.

154. Ludwick, JR, Markel, SF, and Child, CG: Chiari's disease, Arch Surg 91:697, 1965.

155. Ludwig, J, et al: Calcified mixed malignant tumor of the liver, Arch Pathol 99:162, 1975.

156. MacCarty, RL, et al: Retrospective comparison of radionuclide scans and computed tomography of liver and pancreas, AJR 129:23, 1977.

157. Mackay, B, Elliott, GB, and MacDougall, JA: Granular cell myoblastoma of the cystic duct: report of a case with electron-microscope observations, Can J Surg 11:44, 1968.

158. Mackowiak, PA, et al: Pseudocholelithiasis in an elderly man with calcified hydatid cysts, Am J Med 60:707, 1976.

159. Maki, T, et al: Treatment of intrahepatic gallstones, Arch Surg 88:124, 1964.

160. Malt, RA, Hershberg, RA, and Miller, WL: Experience with benign tumors of the liver, Surg Gynecol Obstet 130:285, 1970.

161. Mandelbaum, I, and Shumacker, HB: Excision of congenital hepatic cyst of bile duct origin, Am J Surg 101:507, 1961.

162. Mandell, GL, and Hook, EW: Leukocyte function in chronic granulomatous disease of childhood, Am J Med 47:473, 1969.

163. Matsumoto, Y, et al: Congenital cystic dilatation of the common bile duct as a cause of primary bile duct stone, Am J Surg 134:346, 1977.

164. Maynard, JH, and Fone, DJ: Haemochromatosis with osteogenic sarcoma in the liver, Med J Aust 2:1260, 1969.

165. McEwan-Alvardo, G, et al: Aneurysm of the hepatic artery, Am J Dig Dis 12:509, 1967.

166. McIntyre, JA, and Cheng, P: Adenoma of the common bile duct causing obstructive jaundice, Can J Surg 11:215, 1968.

167. McLoughlin, MJ: Angiography in cavernous hemangioma of the liver, AJR 113:50, 1971.

168. McLoughlin, MJ, and Hobbs, BB: Selective angiography in the diagnosis of hydatid disease of the liver, Can Med Assoc J 103:1147, 1970.

169. Mehlman, DJ, Bulkley, BH, and Wiernik, PH: Serum alpha₁-fetoglobulins with gastric and prostatic carcinomas, N Engl J Med 285:1060, 1971.

170. Melmem, RE, and Nahra, K: Congenital diaphragm of the common hepatic duct, Br J Radiol 39:392, 1966.

171. Melnick, PJ: Polycystic liver: analysis of seventy cases, Arch Pathol 59:162, 1955.

172. Meyer, JH: Primary sclerosing cholangitis: report of a case, Ohio S Med J 58:442, 1962.

173. Meyers, MA: Calcification in cholangio-carcinoma, Br J Radiol 41:65, 1968.

174. Michels, NA: Newer anatomy of the liver and its variant blood supply and collateral circulation, Am J Surg 112:337, 1966.

175. Mikkelson, WP, et al: Extra- and intrahepatic portal hypertension without cirrhosis (hepatoportal sclerosis), Ann Surg 162:602, 1965.

176. Mistilis, SP, Green, JR, and Schiff, L: Hepatic sarcoidosis with portal hypertension, Am J Med 36:470, 1964.

177. Mistilis, S, and Schiff, L: A case of jaundice due to unilateral hepatic duct obstruction, Gut 4:13, 1963.

178. Mittelstaedt, CA, et al: Caroli's disease: sonographic findings, AJR 134:585, 1980.

179. Moss, AA, et al: Angiographic appearance of benign and malignant hepatic tumors in infants and children, AJR 113:61, 1971.

180. Muehlbauer, MA, and Farber, MG: Hemangioma of the liver: some interesting clinical and radiological observations, Am J Gastroenterol 44:355, 1966.

181. Mujahed, Z, Glenn, F, and Evans, JA: Communicating cavernous ectasia of the intrahepatic ducts (Caroli's disease), AJR 113:21, 1971.

182. Nakayama, F, et al: Hepatolithiasis in East Asia: restrospective study, Dig Dis Sci 31:21, 1986.

183. Nava, C, Metlich, A, and Marti, MM: *Fasciola hepatica*: report of a case with common duct distomiasis, Rev Invest Clin 26:181, 1974.

184. Nayak, NC, and Ramalingaswani, V: Obliterative portal venography of the liver, Arch Pathol 87:359, 1969.

185. Nayak, NC, et al: Fetoprotein in Indian childhood cirrhosis, Lancet 1:68, 1972.

186. Nebesar, RA, Tefft, M, and Colodny, AH: Angiography of liver abscess in granulomatous disease in childhood, AJR 108:628, 1970.

187. Noble, MJA: Hepatic vein thrombosis complicating polycythemia vera, Arch Intern Med 120:105, 1967.

188. Okuda, K, et al: Clonorchiasis studied by percutaneous cholangiography and a therapeutic trial of toluene-2, 4-diisothiocyanate: a case report, Gastroenterology 65:457, 1973.

189. Okuda, K, et al: Generalized calcification of the liver in advanced schistosomiasis japonica: a case report, Acta Hepatogastroenterol 22:98, 1975.

190. Okuyama, K: Primary liver cell carcinoma associated with biliary cirrhosis due to congenital bile duct atresia, J Pediatr 67:89, 1965.

191. Ostermiller, W, Jr, and Carter, R: Hepatic abscess, Arch Surg 94:353, 1967.

192. Palmer, ED: Budd-Chiari syndrome (occlusion of the hepatic veins): seven cases, Ann Intern Med 41:261, 1954.

193. Palubinskas, AJ, Baldwin, J, and McCormack, KR: Liver-cell adenoma, Radiology 89:444, 1967.

194. Pliskin, M: Peliosis hepatis, Radiology 114:29, 1975.

195. Pollard, JJ, Fleischli, DJ, and Nebesar, RA: Angiography of hepatic neoplasms, Radiol Clin North Am 8:31, 1970.

196. Porter, SD, Soper, RT, and Tidrick, RT: Biliary hypoplasia, Ann Surg 167:602, 1968.

197. Prando, A, et al: Ultrasonic pseudolesions of the liver, Radiology 130:403, 1979.

198. Prussin, G, and Schiffmann, A: Solitary nonparasitic cyst of the liver, Am J Gastroenterol 42:425, 1964.

199. Pyrtek, LJ, and Bartus, SA: Hepatic pyemia, N Engl J Med 272:551, 1965.

200. Rakov, HL, Smalldon, TR, and Derman, H: Hepatic hemangioendotheliosarcoma, Arch Intern Med 112:71, 1963.

201. Ramsay, GC, and Britton, RC: Intraparenchymal angiography in the diagnosis of hepatic veno-occlusive diseases, Radiology 90:716, 1968.

202. Raney, R, Lilly, J, and McHardy, G: Biliary calculus of roundworm origin, Ann Intern Med 72:405, 1970.

203. Rankin, JG, Skyring, AP, and Goulston, SJM: Liver in ulcerative colitis: obstructive jaundice due to bile duct carcinoma, Gut 7:433, 1966.

204. Reul, GJ, Rubio, PA, and Berkman, NL: Granular cell myoblastoma of the cystic duct: a case associated with hydrops of the gallbladder, Am J Surg 129:583, 1975.

205. Reuter, K, et al: The diagnosis of a choledochal cyst by ultrasound, Radiology 136:437, 1980.

206. Reuter, SR, Redman, HC, and Siders, DB: The spectrum of angiographic findings in hepatoma, Radiology 94:89, 1970.

207. Rizk, GK, Tayyarah, KA, and Chandur-Mnaymneh, L: The angiographic changes in hydatid cysts of the liver and spleen, Radiology 99:303, 1971.

208. Rossi, P, and Gould, HR: Angiography and scanning in liver disease, Radiology 96:553, 1970.

209. Sackett, JF, et al: Scintillation scanning of liver cell adenoma, AJR 113:56, 1971.

210. Salem, SN, and Khammash, NF: Amoebic liver abscess: a diagnostic problem in Kuwait with an obscure relationship to intestinal amoebiasis. In Proceedings of the Fourth World Congress of Gastroenterology, Copenhagen, 1970.

211. Sane, SM, Sieber, WK, and Girdany, BR: Cogenital bronchobiliary fistula, Surgery 69:599, 1971.

212. Schaffner, F, et al: Budd-Chiari syndrome caused by a web in the inferior vena cava, Am J Med 42:838, 1967.

213. Schmidt, AG: Plain film roentgen diagnosis of amebic hepatic abscess, AJR 107:47, 1969.

214. Scholz, FJ, Carrera, GF, and Larsen, CR: The choledochocele: correlation of radiological, clinical and pathological findings, Radiology 118:25, 1976.

215. Schwartz, SI, and Dale, WA: Primary sclerosing cholangitis: review and report of six cases, Arch Surg 77:439, 1958.

216. Scott, WW, Jr, Sanders, RC, and Siegelman, SS: Irregular fatty infiltration of the liver: diagnostic dilemmas, AJR 135:67, 1980.

217. Sedacca, CM, et al: Polycystic liver: an unusual cause of bleeding esophageal varices, Gastroenterology 40:128, 1961.

218. Selke, AC, and Cornell, SH: Infantile hepatic hemangioendothelioma, AJR 106:200, 1969.

219. Serpe, SJ, Todd, D, and Baruch, H: Cholecystitis due to granular cell myoblastoma of the cystic duct, Am J Dig Dis 5:824, 1960.

220. Shackelford, GD, and Kirks, DR: Neonatal hepatic calcification secondary to transplacental infection, Radiology 122:753, 1977.

221. Shanbrom, E, and Zheutlin, N: Radiologic sign in hemosiderosis, JAMA 168:33, 1958.

222. Sharp, HL, et al: Cholestyramine therapy in patients with a paucity of intrahepatic bile ducts, J Pediatr 71:723, 1967.

223. Shea, WJ, Jr, et al: Sclerosing cholangitis associated with hepatic arterial FUDR chemotherapy: radiographic-histologic correlation, AJR 146:717, 1986.

224. Sherlock, S, et al: Partial nodular transformation of the liver with portal hypertension, Am J Med 40:195, 1966.

225. Shieber, W: Lymphangiographic demonstration of thoracic duct dilatation in portal cirrhosis, Surgery 57:522, 1965.

226. Shoemaker, CP, Jr, and Baxter, JC: An extrahepatic biliary tract anomaly, Am J Surg 121:741, 1971.

227. Shoop, JD: Functional hepatoma demonstrated with rose bengal scanning, AJR 107:51, 1969.

228. Short, WF, et al: Biliary cystadenoma, Arch Surg 102:78, 1971.

229. Smith, GW, Westgaard, T, and Bjorn-Hansen, R: Hepatic venous angiography in the evaluation of cirrhosis of the liver, Ann Surg 173:469, 1971.

230. Soper, RT, and Dunphy, DL: Sarcoma botryoides of the biliary tree, Surgery 63:1005, 1968.

231. Staley, CJ, et al: Leiomyosarcoma of the inferior vena cava, Am J Surg 113:211, 1967.

232. Stephens, DH, Hattery, RR, and Sheedy, P, II: Computed tomography of the abdomen, Radiology 119:331, 1976.

233. Sterup, K, and Mosbech, J: Budd-Chiari syndrome after taking oral contraceptives, Br Med J 4:660, 1967.

234. Stigol, LC, Traversaro, J, and Trigo, ER: Carinal trifurcation with congenital tracheobiliary fistula, Pediatrics 37:89, 1966.

235. Strohl, L, et al: Carcinoma of the bile ducts, Arch Surg 87:51, 1963.

236. Sty, JR, et al: Hepatic scintigraphy in Caroli's disease, Radiology 127:732, 1978.

237. Sutcliffe, J, and Chrispin, AR: Chronic granulomatous disease, Br J Radiol 43:110, 1970.

238. Suzuki, T, et al: Positive scintiphotography of cancer of the liver with Ga^{67} citrate, AJR 113:92, 1971.

239. Tabrisky, J, and Pollack, EL: The aberrant divisional bile duct, Radiology 99:537, 1971.

240. Tadani, T, et al: Carcinoma arising in the wall of congenital bile duct cysts, Cancer 44:1134, 1979.

241. Talley, RW, et al: Laminagrams of the Thorotrast-opacified liver in evaluation of chemotherapy for metastatic cancer, Cancer 17:1214, 1964.

242. Talner, LB, Boyer, JL, and Clemett, AR: Intrahepatic portal vein occlusion, Radiology 92:1265, 1969.

243. Teoh, TB: A study of gallstones and included worms in recurrent pyogenic cholangitis, J Pathol Bacteriol 86:123, 1963.

244. Teter, LF: Massive hemorrhage from benign adenoma of biliary duct causing death, J Mich Med Sod 53:62, 1954.

245. Thistlethwaite, JR, and Horwitz, A: Choledechal cyst followed by carcinoma of the hepatic duct, South Med J 60:872, 1967.

246. Thomas, TV: Aneurysm of the portal vein: report of two cases, one resulting in thrombosis and spontaneous rupture, Surgery 61:550, 1967.

247. Thompson, JE, and Wolff, M: Intra-hepatic cystadenoma of bile duct origin, with malignant alteration: report of a case treated with total left hepatic lobectomy, Milit Med 130:218, 1965.

248. Thompson, WM, Chisholm, DP, and Tank, R: Plain film roentgenographic findings in alveolar hydatid disease: *Echinococcus multilocularis,* AJR 116:345, 1972.

249. Thorpe, MEC, Scheuer, PJ, and Sherlock, S: Primary schlerosing cholangitis, the biliary tree, and ulcerative colitis, Br Med J 8:435, 1967.

250. Touloukian, RJ: Hepatic hemangioendothelioma during infancy: pathology, diagnosis and treatment with prednisone, Pediatrics 45:71, 1970.

251. Tuttle, RJ: Cause of recurring obstructive jaundice revealed by percutaneous cholangiography: hydatid cyst, N Engl J Med 283:805, 1970.

252. Urschel, HC, Skinner, DB, and McDermott, WV, Jr: Hemobilia secondary to liver abscess, JAMA 186:797, 1963.

253. Van Heerden, JA, Judd, ES, and Dockerty, MB: Carcinoma of the extrahepatic bile ducts, Am J Surg 113:49, 1967.

254. Viana, RL: Arteriographic aspects of amoebic liver abscess and hepatosplenic schistosomiasis fibrosis. In Proceedings of the Fourth World Congress of Gastroenterology, Copenhagen, 1970.

255. Vlachos, J, Cassimos, C, and Trigonis, G: Choledochus cyst in a newborn, Arch Pathol 67:395, 1959.

256. Volpe, JA, Bergin, JJ, and Overholt, EL: Budd-Chiari syndrome caused by a web as a result of visceral thrombophlebitis migrans, Am J Dig Dis 15:469, 1970.

257. Warren, DW, Athanassiades, S, and Monge, JI: Primary sclerosing cholangitis, Am J Surg 111:23, 1966.

258. Watson, RC, and Baltaxe, HA: The angiographic appearance of primary and secondary tumors of the liver, Radiology 101:539, 1971.

259. Weber, CM, Zito, PF, and Becker, SM: Heterotopic pancreas: an unusual cause of obstruction of the common bile duct, Am J Gastroenterol 49:153, 1968.

260. Wenger, J, Gingrich, GW, and Mendeloff, J: Sclerosing cholangitis: a manifestation of systemic disease, Arch Intern Med 116:509, 1965.

261. Weyde, R, Galatius-Jensen, F, and Uhm, IK: Percutaneous transhepatic cholangiography in Korean patients, Br J Radiol 39:833, 1966.

262. Whelan, JG, Creech, JL, and Tamburro, CH: Angiographic and radionuclide characteristics of hepatic angiosarcoma found in vinyl chloride workers, Radiology 118:549, 1976.

263. Whelton, MJ, et al: Carcinoma at the junction of the main hepatic ducts, Q J Med 38:211, 1968.

264. Whisnant, JD, et al: Common bile duct obstruction by granular cell tumor (Schwannoma), Dig Dis Sci 19:471, 1974.

265. Whitcomb, FF, Jr, Parikh, NK, and Sedgwick, CE: Hydatid cyst disease, Am J Dig Dis 15:711, 1970.

266. Whitcomb, FF, et al: Leiomyosarcoma of the bile ducts, Gastroenterology 52:94, 1967.

267. Whitmore, JT: Granular cell myoblastoma of the common bile duct, Am J Dig Dis 14:516, 1969.

268. Whittaker, LD, Jr, et al: Heterotopic gastric mucosa in the wall of the cystic duct: report of a case, Surgery 62:382, 1967.

269. Wilson, SE, et al: Primary leiomyosarcoma of the liver, Ann Surg 174:232, 1971.

270. Wilson, TS, and Macgregor, JW: Focal nodular hyperplasia of the liver, Can Med Assoc J 100:567, 1969.

271. Wolfson, JJ, et al: Roentgenologic manifestations in children with a genetic defect of polymorphonuclear leukocyte function, Radiology 91:37, 1968.

272. Young, RC: The Budd-Chiari syndrome cause by *Aspergillus,* Arch Intern Med 124:754, 1969.

273. Zeegen, R, et al: Prolonged survival after portal decompression of patients with non-cirrhotic intrahepatic portal hypertension, Gut 11:610, 1970.

51 *Magnetic Resonance Imaging of the Liver*

RALPH WEISSLEDER
JACK WITTENBERG
DAVID D. STARK*

Magnetic resonance (MR) imaging (MRI) of the liver has undergone rapid technical maturation and is already acknowledged as having an important role in clinical hepatic imaging. Emerging applications include detection, characterization, and staging of a variety of tumors as well as the assessment of certain diffuse liver diseases. Major technical improvements, such as the use of motion artifact suppression techniques, fast scanning, and MR contrast agents, will undoubtedly further improve the diagnostic value of MRI. This chapter considers the current and potential role of MRI in clinical management of liver disease.

TECHNICAL CONSIDERATIONS
Tissue contrast

MR tissue contrast depends on one or more basic tissue parameters, such as relaxation times, hydrogen density, chemical shift, magnetic susceptibility, and vascular parameters (perfusion, diffusion, blood flow). In spin echo (SE) sequences, T_1 and T_2 relaxation time differences between liver and abnormal tissues are the most important parameters determining image contrast. Hydrogen density usually has the least influence, since only fat and fluids differ significantly from other tissues.[12,54] Chemical shift, magnetic susceptibility, and diffusion effects contribute little to the conventional MR image unless the pulse sequence design is altered.

Normal liver parenchyma shows rather constant relaxation times (small standard deviation); tumors display higher values and a broader range of relaxation times (large standard deviation) (Table 51-1). However, certain trends are evident and become manifest as detectable differences in MR signal intensity. Biologic variation of the same histologic tumor type can be attributed to individual variation in cellularity, necrosis, fibrosis, or fat content. As a result, MR signal intensity varies within individual lesions in a single patient and varies even more with the same tumor cell type among different patients. Note that the standard deviation for any single histologic type is greater than the difference in the means between two different histologic types (Table 51-1).

*Dr. Stark is supported by the American Cancer Society, JFRA-163 and PDT-326.

Tumor detectability improves with increasing differences in tumor-liver relaxation times. For example, tumors with long T_1 and T_2 relaxation times, such as metastases and hemangiomas, show higher tumor-liver signal intensity differences (contrast) than tumors with T_1 and T_2 relaxation times similar to liver, such as with hepatic adenoma, focal nodular hyperplasia, and hepatocellular carcinoma.

Pulse sequence performance

The selection of pulse sequence and timing parameters is a major determinant of image quality. Image quality can be defined as the product of signal-to-noise (SNR) ratio, contrast-to-noise (CNR) ratio, and spatial resolution. SNR is the mean liver signal intensity divided by the standard deviation of total background noise (SNR = S_{liver}/Noise). CNR is calculated as the difference of tumor-liver signal intensity measurements divided by the standard deviation of total background noise (CNR = $S_{tumor} - S_{liver}$/Noise).

SNR is a quantitative parameter that generally correlates with image quality or anatomic resolution. The higher the SNR, the greater is the improvement in visibility of anatomic details. Anatomic resolution can be visually assessed by inspection of the sharpness of hepatic veins in the liver (Fig. 51-1). Anatomic resolution is not to be confused with spatial resolution, which depends on voxel dimension. Inherent high SNR can be used to decrease scan time or increase spatial resolution (smaller voxel or pixel size).

CNR can be used as a quantitative parameter of tumor

☐ **TABLE 51-1**

Relaxation times (in milliseconds) of different hepatic tumors measured in vivo at 0.6 Tesla

Tissue	T_1	T_2
Primary liver tumors		
Hepatocellular carcinoma	569 ± 133	84 ± 18
Cholangio-carcinoma	654 ± 236	94 ± 37
Hemangioma	1025 ± 521	152 ± 54
Metastases (average)	876 ± 334	78 ± 32
Colon	691 ± 100	76 ± 22
Breast	723 ± 145	74 ± 12
Endocrine	921 ± 213	94 ± 21
Lymphoma	832 ± 234	84 ± 16
Liver parenchyma	460 ± 120	58 ± 11

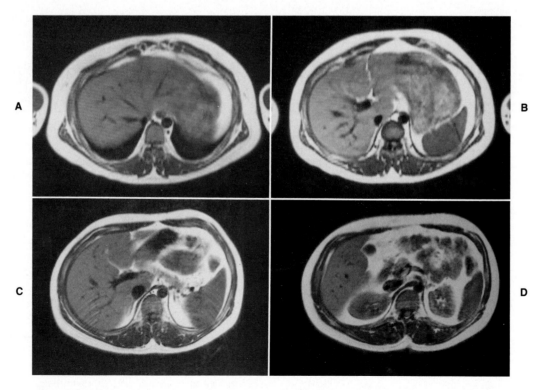

Fig. 51-1 Normal hepatic anatomy. **A** to **D,** Four contiguous 15 mm thick sections of liver. Vessels are clearly demonstrated because of signal void created by rapidly moving blood. Note absence of artifact with this T_1-weighted pulse sequence using 12 excitations (SE 275/14).

detectability. A positive CNR indicates hyperintensity and a negative CNR hypointensity of the tumor relative to liver. Deductively, therefore, detectability does not depend on whether the lesion is bright or dark relative to adjacent normal tissue, but rather on its relative numeric value. For example, a liver tumor with a CNR of -8.0 on a T_1-weighted sequence appears hypointense (dark), and a CNR of $+5.5$ on a T_2-weighted sequence appears hyperintense (bright) relative to liver. The tumor is more conspicuous on the T_1-weighted image $(8.0 > 5.5)$. Recently it has been proved that CNR correlates with increased sensitivity in lesion detection, decreased threshold for detection of small tumors, and greater accuracy in measuring tumor size.[59]

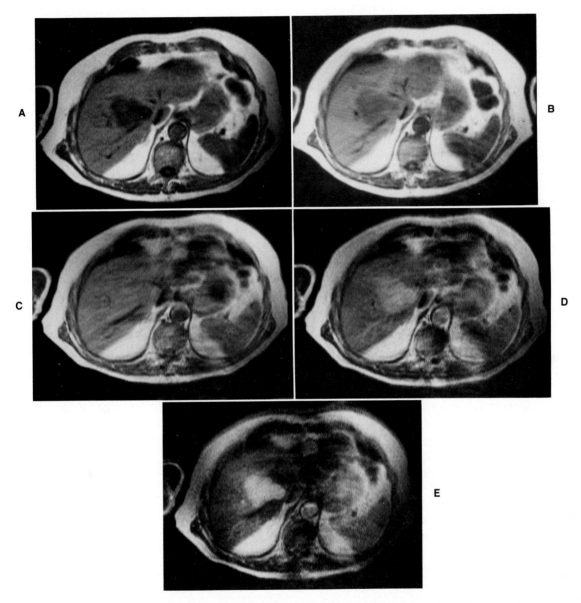

Fig. 51-2 Lesion detection. Various MR pulse sequence techniques are currently used for hepatic imaging. In this patient with colon metastasis, wide variety of pulse sequences were acquired to demonstrate dependence of tumor-liver contrast on MR pulse sequences. **A** and **B,** T_1-weighted spin echo techniques are characterized by excellent anatomic resolution, reduced motion artifacts, and excellent image contrast. Tumor is more easily detected in **A** because of high tumor-liver contrast (**A,** SE 260/14/12; **B,** SE 500/30/4). **C** to **E,** T_2-weighted spin echo techniques with TE of 30 msec do not have sufficient tumor-liver contrast to allow reliable detection of liver tumors (**C,** SE 2000/30). Increasing TE up to 90 msec increases tumor-liver contrast, but anatomic resolution is poorer and motion artifacts increase (**D,** SE 2000/60; **E,** SE 2000/90).

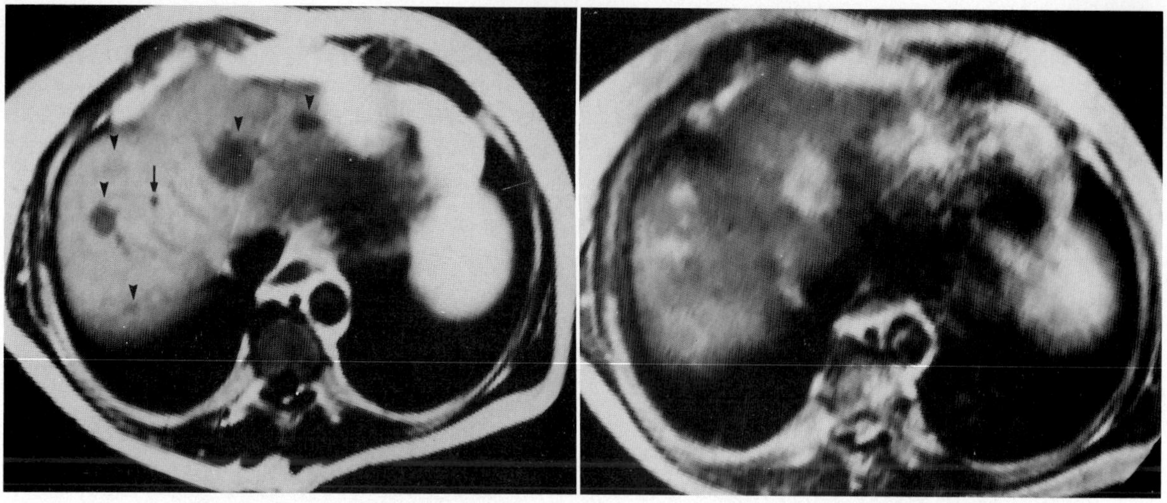

Fig. 51-3 Hepatic metastases: standard pulse sequences. For routine clinical imaging, both T_1- and T_2-weighted images are acquired for detecting hepatic metastases. Whereas T_1-weighted images show higher tumor-liver contrast, T_2-weighted images confirm presence of tumor and often contribute diagnostic information to differential diagnosis of hepatic lesions. **A,** T_1-weighted spin echo sequence (SE 275/14). Multiple masses with varying signal intensities are identified *(arrowheads)*. Structure with slightly lower signal intensity *(arrow)* is related to longitudinal course of vein, suggesting it represents a cross section of one of its branches. No distinguishing differential diagnostic signs can be seen. **B,** T_2-weighted spin echo sequence (Se 2350/120). All masses now appear with signal intensity greater than liver. Suspected venous structure is confirmed because it remains with signal intensity less than liver. Lesions have inhomogeneous appearance and irregular margins and are of intermediate signal intensity *(amorphous sign)*.

Spatial resolution is determined by the voxel size: field of view divided by the phase (*y* dimension of voxel) and frequency encoding steps (*x* dimension of voxel) and slice thickness (*z* dimension of voxel). The smaller the voxel size, the less is the SNR and therefore the poorer the anatomic resolution. The larger the voxel size, the higher is the SNR, but the lower the spatial resolution.

Spin echo pulse sequences that result in tissue T_1 difference dominating image contrast (*T_1-weighted sequences*; for example, TR < 500, TE < 30 msec) are routinely acquired in abdominal imaging because of excellent anatomic resolution (high SNR per unit time) Figs. 51-2, *A* and *B,* and 51-3, *A:* Table 51-2).[53] Many arguments can be made for imaging with as short a TR as possible. The highest contrast per unit time is achieved by shortening TR. Reductions in scan time achieved with short TR sequences can be used to average more excitations, thereby decreasing motion artifacts and further increasing SNR. T_1-weighted sequences are also characterized by excellent tumor-liver contrast (high CNR) at field strength up to 1.0 Tesla (see later discussion on field strength). Shortening of TE complements the reduction in TR by further increasing T_1-dependent image contrast (Table 51-2). Minimum TE values are set by the MR imager hardware and software.

☐ **TABLE 51-2**

Liver signal-to-noise (SNR) and tumor-liver contrast-to-noise (CNR) ratios (scan time 7 minutes, except for breath-hold gradient-recalled (GR) echo images)

Pulse sequence	SNR	CNR
SE 500/30	25.5	−6.4 ± 4.1
SE 260/30	24.8	−8.1 ± 4.6
SE 260/18	27.4	−10.3 ± 5.2
SE 1500/30	19.9	+1.9 ± 0.9
SE 1500/60	13.3	+3.5 ± 3.0
SE 1500/90	9.5	+5.5 ± 4.2
SE 2000/30	17.2	+2.4 ± 2.1
SE 2000/60	11.8	+4.7 ± 3.6
SE 2000/90	8.7	+7.5 ± 5.3
SE 2000/120	6.0	+7.7 ± 3.4
SE 2000/180	3.7	+4.2 ± 2.0
GR 100/11/10	7.1	+1.7 ± 2.4
GR 100/11/30	11.8	−0.6 ± 1.8
GR 100/11/70	12.3	−8.1 ± 4.8
GR 100/22/70	9.8	−1.4 ± 2.3

Spin echo pulse sequences with image contrast dominated by tissue T_2 differences (T_2-weighted sequences; for example, TR 2000 to 3000 msec, TE longer than 60 msec) are particularly useful for tissue characterization of liver tumors (Table 51-2). Although T_2-weighted spin echo sequences have a low anatomic resolution (low SNR), tumor-liver contrast is good (high CNR) Figs. 51-2, *C* to *E*, and 51-3, *B*). These techniques may also be used for lesion detection, particularly at field strengths higher than 1 Tesla.[16,30] However, longer TR allows fewer excitations and less averaging per unit time. Therefore T_2-weighted images are more susceptible to motion artifacts, resulting in trade-offs of SNR, as well as to decreased anatomic resolution. Metastasis-liver CNR increases with increasing TE to reach a maximum at a TE of 90 to 120 msec; further increases in TE decrease image contrast. The optimal TE depends on the difference in T_2 relaxation times between tumor, liver, and the various sources of noise affecting this type of pulse sequence. Large differences in T_2 (such as hemangioma-liver) result in higher CNR with long TE, whereas smaller differences (such as cancer-liver) result in higher CNR with shorter TE (see later discussion on differential diagnosis of tumors).

Gradient-recalled (GR) echo pulse sequence is the most widely available fast imaging technique (2 to 30 seconds/image). The major incentives for using GR techniques in abdominal MRI are to reduce respiratory artifacts by suspending respiration,[25,55] to acquire a localization scan rapidly, and to perform dynamic imaging after administration of contrast agents.[26] GR pulse sequences use gradient reversal alone to create an echo, unlike the spin echo method, which uses a 180-degree refocusing pulse coincident with gradient reversal. T_1-weighted GR sequences are obtained with a short TR (50 to 200 msec), a short TE (10 to 15 msec), and a large flip angle (40 to 90 degrees). T_2-weighted GR sequences can be acquired with a short TR, an intermediate TE, and a short flip angle (<15 degrees).[65] Although achievable T_1 contrast is similar to spin echo images, GR-generated images offer less SNR (Table 51-2). In addition, maximal T_2-dependent image contrast is lower than achievable T_1-dependent contrast.

Optimization of imaging techniques

The optimal MR pulse sequence for detecting hepatic mass lesions is the one that maximizes tumor-liver CNR, SNR, spatial resolution, and anatomic coverage per unit imaging time. Trade-offs among these parameters depend on a variety of operator-selectable and machine-limited factors.[62] A pulse sequence recommended for one imaging system may not perform as well as for another system because of varying hardware (gradient strength, field strength) and software (motion suppression techniques). Therefore pulse sequence optimization must be individually tailored for different machines.

Pulse sequence optimization can be performed theoretically and then confirmed by actual acquisition of human MR images. Mathematic calculation of signal intensity and contrast values requires that the T_1, T_2, and N(H) of the tissue pair be known. Computer-algorithms have been specifically designed to predict the optimal timing parameters for any pulse sequence (spin echo, inversion recovery, or GR echo), and three-dimensional contour plots can display theoretic SNR or CNR against TR, TE, and/or flip-angle (FA).[44a] Mathematically predicted and actually observed data can differ significantly from each other, since mathematic formulas generally do not take into account complexities such as physiologic motion and imperfections in the imaging method.

Empiric technique optimization is best accomplished in normal volunteers because long scan times are prohibitive in cancer patients.[10,65] The spleen has been noted to have proton density and relaxation times similar to adenocarcinoma and can therefore be used as an internal reference phantom to maximize cancer-liver (spleen-liver) CNR.[54] The spleen is conveniently located in the same transverse section as the liver and is large enough to allow reproducible measurements of signal intensity data. The more hypointense the spleen relative to the liver on T_1-weighted images (highest negative CNR value) and the more hyperintense on T_2-weighted images (highest positive CNR value), the better is the image contrast for detecting hepatic tumors.

Motion artifacts

Motion-related artifacts are a major determinant of image noise and significantly influence lesion detectability. Motion artifacts obscure anatomic boundaries and may even mimic the appearance of liver tumor. Artifacts are caused by physiologic motion occurring during the application of magnetic field gradients and by motion occurring between repetition of the imaging cycle.

Many techniques have been designed to reduce motion artifacts in the liver, an important testing ground for evaluation MR's adequacy for abdominal imaging. These techniques are conveniently divided into those which do or do not require respiratory monitoring (see box).[71] Techniques requiring monitoring have the disadvantage of decreased patient throughput (time required to place device), dependency on patient cooperation (continuous periodic breathing), and the necessity of additional hardware (monitor). Three techniques have emerged as being clinically superior: signal averaging, reordering of phase encoding, and rephasing.

In *signal averaging*, multiple acquisitions average random phases, a procedure that decreases artifacts.[55] Signal averaging is feasible employing short TR se-

☐ MOTION ARTIFACT SUPPRESSION TECHNIQUES ☐

NO MONITORING

    Reduction of motion
        Physical restraint
        Breath holding
    Reduction of phase-encoding errors
        Averaging
        Pseudogating
        Rephasing
    Reduction of intensity of moving structures
        STIR
        Reduction of field of view
        Spatial presaturation
        Ferrite-enhanced MR

MONITORING

    Reduction of motion
        Respiratory gating
    Reduction of phase-encoding errors
        Reordering of phase encoding

quences, but the same strategy for long TR sequences (T_2-weighted spin echo and inversion recovery techniques) is restricted by time considerations. *Reordering of phase encoding* (ROPE, respiratory-ordered phase encoding; COPE, centrally ordered phase encoding; EXORCIST) is an effective technique in reducing respiratory artifacts without significantly increasing scan time.[3] As with respiratory gating, however, effective reordered phase encoding requires monitoring of respiration. The order used for different phase-encoding steps is selected in such a way as to reduce inconsistencies in position throughout the respiratory cycle.[3,71] In rephasing techniques (MAST, motion artifact suppression technique), standard read-and-slice select gradients are modified mathematically to refocus magnetization in the imaging plane. Rephasing techniques do not increase scan time but increase the shortest TE that can be used, since the extra refocusing gradients impose additional time requirements.[42]

Field strength

T_1-weighted spin echo techniques are superior to other techniques in detecting hepatic metastases at field strength up to 1.0 Tesla.[30] Studies reporting in vivo relaxation times for metastases and surrounding liver have shown that tumor-liver T_1 differences are substantially greater than T_2 differences.[53] Although inversion recovery sequences maximize T_1 contrast, signal-averaged T_1-weighted spin echo techniques allow more time-efficient

reduction of motion artifacts in increasing SNR and anatomic resolution.

As magnetic field strength increases, T_1 differences between tumor and normal liver decrease.[16] T_2 is thought to be relatively independent of field strength.[4,36] As a result, theoretic predictions and preliminary studies have shown that T_2-weighted sequences may be superior to T_1-weighted sequences at field strength greater than 1.0 Tesla.[16,30] However, biologic variation in tumor types (and thus relaxation times) may account for larger individual differences than the issue of field strengths. In this respect certain tumors are better detected at high field strength with T_1-weighted techniques.[16]

Our own experience confirms that tumor-liver contrast is superior with motion-suppressed T_2-weighted techniques at field strengths of 1.5 Tesla (Table 51-3). Nevertheless, CNR values from optimized sequences are found to be within 20% of one another at different field strengths.[29] Therefore the major determinant of the "optimal pulse sequence" for clinical hepatic MR will be the availability of compatible, effective motion artifact suppression techniques (Table 51-3).

CLINICAL APPLICATION
Normal anatomy

Interest in segmental anatomy of the liver has increased as its relevance to hepatic tumor resection has become clearer. The liver is composed of segments that are defined by vascular cleavage planes. Arterial, portal venous, and biliary systems are located intrasegmentally, whereas the hepatic veins course intersegmentally, delineating a total of eight anatomic segments.[8] Depending on tumor localization and extension, simple segmentectomy, right or left hepatectomy, or extended hepatecomy (trisegmentectomy) can be performed.[17,38]

Hepatic vasculature is easily visualized by MR because of the flow void phenomenon. The main hepatic vein branches into the right hepatic (right intersegmental fissure), middle hepatic (interlobar fissure), and left hepatic (left intersegmental fissure) vein. The portal vein branches into the left (intersegmental fissure) and right portal vein. Other important landmarks consistently displayed by MRI include the gallbladder, interlobar fissure, and falciform ligament of the left intersegmental fissure.

Transverse MR images demonstrate hepatic and portal veins in 100% and the hepatic artery in 44% of patients.[15] Coronal images can be acquired to demonstrate the entire course of the middle hepatic or portal veins. In addition, coronal images are helpful in determining the craniocaudal extent of abdominal tumors. Sagittal sections are usually acquired to evaluate best the inferior vena cava and the aorta in their entire length. Oblique images can be acquired to display the portal triad in its anatomic course. The relationship of liver to diaphragm, lung, and

□ **TABLE 51-3**

Spleen-liver contrast-to-noise ratios in identical patients ($n = 3$) imaged at low- (0.35 Testa), middle- (0.6 Testa), and high-field (1.5 Testa) imaging systems (scan time: 8.5 minutes per scan)

Pulse sequence	0.3 Testa	0.6 Testa	1.5 Testa
T_1 weighted*	-17.8 ± 3.5	-17.4 ± 2.8	-13.4 ± 5.4
SE 500/30/8	-3.0 ± 4.2	-5.4 ± 2.3	-6.6 ± 5.5
SE 2000/30/2	$+4.6 \pm 2.7$	$+3.2 \pm 1.8$	$+3.5 \pm 3.4$
SE 2000/60/2	$+6.6 \pm 0.8$	$+8.6 \pm 2.1$	$+9.6 \pm 5.0$
SE 2000/75/2†			$+15.4 \pm 8.7$

*SE 250/15/16 at 0.3 Tesla, SE 275/14/16 at 0.6 Tesla, SE 300/20/16 at 1.5 Tesla.

†Respiratory motion suppression technique (EXORCIST).

□ **TABLE 51-4**

Sensitivity and specificity for detecting hepatic metastases

	T_1W*		T_2W†		Combined MRI	Contrast CT
	SE	IR	TE 60	TE 120		
Patients						
Sensitivity	0.86	0.89	0.82	0.77	0.82	0.80
Specificity	0.93	0.93	0.97	0.92	0.99	0.94
Individual metastases						
Sensitivity	0.60	0.64	0.43	0.43	0.64	0.51

*T_1W, T_1 weighted; SE, spin echo 260/14/12; IR, inversion recovery 1500/450/18/3.

†T_2W, T_2 weighted; TE 60, spin echo 2350/60/2; TE 120, spin echo 2350/120/2.

adjacent viscera are seen best on either sagittal or coronal sections.

Tumor detection

The excellent accuracy of computed tomography (CT) in tumor detection is well established,[1,18] and CT is the gold standard with which MRI must be compared. Despite this well-founded enthusiasm, the fallibility of CT, regardless of the technique of contrast enhancement, is well documented.* Initial studies comparing CT to MRI performed with conventional pulse sequences failed to demonstrate any superiority of MRI in lesion detection.[41] Parity of MRI with CT was found in a study of 50 patients with hepatic metastases in which inversion recovery was used for T_1 information and spin echo techniques for T_2 information.[27] In another study MRI was found to be less accurate than CT in 27 patients with hepatic metastases when T_1-weighted data were limited to SE 500/30 sequences.[22]

*References 9, 18, 19, 44, 49, and 56.

More recent experience suggests that MRI will afford superiority to enhanced CT for hepatic lesion detection when heavily T_1-weighted pulse sequences are used.[44,56] In a controlled prospective study the greater accuracy of MRI to contrast-enhanced CT for metastatic lesion detection was demonstrated in 139 patients (Table 51-4). Using MRI techniques optimized for a 0.6-Tesla imager, the sensitivity of MRI for detecting individual hepatic metastases (64%) was significantly greater ($p < 0.001$) than for CT (51%). No significant difference existed, however, in sensitivity of identifying patients with hepatic metastases (MRI 82%, CT 80%).[56] Heavily T_1-weighted sequences were more accurate than a variety of T_2-weighted sequences in lesion detection (Table 51-4). In patients without hepatic metastases the specificity of MRI was 99% versus 94% for CT ($p < 0.05$) (Table 51-4). An additional study performed on a mid-field unit (0.5 Tesla) has similarly found that heavily T_1-weighted pulse sequences are superior to both contrast-enhanced CT and T_2-weighted pulse sequences for lesion detection.[14]

☐ **TABLE 51-5**

Differential diagnosis of liver-lesion signal intensity

Criteria	Diagnosis
T_1-weighted pulse sequence	
Tumor hypointense to liver	All hepatic neoplasms
Tumor isointense to liver	Hepatocellular carcinoma
	Focal nodular hyperplasia
	Hepatocellular adenoma
	Cyst (complicated)
Tumor hyperintense to liver	Hepatocellular carcinoma
	Hemorrhagic tumors
	Melanoma
	Liver iron overload
T_2-weighted pulse sequence	
Tumor hypointense to liver	Regenerating nodules
Tumor isointense to liver	Hepatocellular carcinoma
	Hepatocellular adenoma
	Focal nodular hyperplasia
Tumor hyperintense to liver	All hepatic neoplasms
Tumor isointense to spleen	Metastases
Tumor isointense to cerebrospinal fluid	Hemangioma
	Cyst
	Cystic metastases

Data from references 6, 27, 43, 60, and 70.

Differential diagnosis of tumors

To be substantially more effective than competing techniques, MRI should allow not only improved sensitivity and specificity for lesion detection, but also offer an improved level of confidence in differential diagnosis.[14,44,56] Published reports employing numeric calculations of signal intensity data (such as T_1 and T_2 relaxation times and signal intensity ratios) for differential diagnosis have proved to be of limited use in discriminating between a variety of hepatic tumors (see Table 51-1).* These quantitative parameters are more often calculated for scientific presentations but are infrequently used to establish diagnoses in individual patients.

Tumor morphology assessed on T_2-weighted sequences provides a greater potential for tissue characterization because internal architecture is better displayed than on T_1-weighted sequences. Information obtained from multiecho T_2-weighted sequences is particularly useful to assess tumor signal intensity behavior with increasing T_2 weighting. Nevertheless, differential diagnosis of liver tumors will be most successful when diagnostic information from T_1- and T_2-weighted imaging techniques is combined (Tables 51-5 and 51-6).[69]

*References 11, 21, 45, 46, 51, and 60.

☐ **TABLE 51-6**

Differential diagnosis of hepatic tumors by morphologic criteria

Criterion	Diagnosis
Central tumor inhomogeneity	
T_1-weighted sequence	
Hypointense tumor center (doughnut sign)	Metastases (necrosis)
	Hemangioma (rapid flow)
Hyperintense tumor center	Tumor hemorrhage
Hypointense septae	Focal nodular hyperplasia (scar)
	Hepatocellular adenoma (scar)
	Hemangioma (thrombosis, scar)
T_2-weighted sequence	
Hyperintense tumor center (target sign)	Metastases (necrosis)
Hypo-/hyperintense septae	Focal nodular hyperplasia (scar)
	Hepatocellular adenoma (scar)
	Hemangioma (thrombosis, scar)
Peripheral tumor inhomogeneities	
T_1-weighted sequence	
Hypointense ring (ring sign)	Hepatocellular carcinoma (capsule)
	Hepatic adenoma (capsule)
	Displaced vasculature
Hyperintense	Peritumoral hemorrhage
T_2-weighted sequence	
Hypointense	Displaced vasculature
Hyperintense (halo sign)	Metastases (edema, congestion, hemorrhage)

Data from references 43 and 70.

Hepatic metastases

Hepatic metastases are the most common malignant liver tumor in the United States.[20,31] Correct therapy of patients with many primary tumors often depends on accurate assessment of the liver. Approximately one fourth of all patients with hepatic metastases are estimated to have potentially resectable liver disease.[17] It is critical, therefore, to detect and stage hepatic metastases and to differentiate them from common benign lesions, such as hemangiomas and cysts.

Most hepatic metastases are hypointense relative to liver on T_1-weighted images and appear hyperintense on T_2-weighted images (see Figs. 51-2 and 51-3).[69] In a retrospective review of more than 300 metastatic lesions in 98 patients, morphologic features allowed their differentiation from benign hemangiomas and cysts in 92%.[69] Morphologic criteria (descriptors) are illustrated in Fig. 51-4, and their incidence in malignant and benign hepatic mass lesions is listed in Table 51-7.

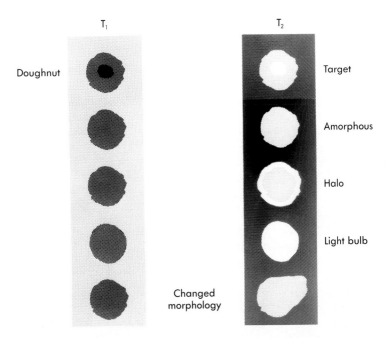

Fig. 51-4 Lesion descriptors: Morphologic and signal intensity features of characteristic lesions. Correlative T₁-weighted and T₂-weighted representations are shown. Aside from doughnut sign, remainder of lesions are indistinguishable on T₁-weighted images. On the other hand, their T₂-weighted analogs have architectural features that allow their differentiation. (From Wittenburg, J, et al: AJR, 151:79, 1988.)

□ **TABLE 51-7**

Morphologic descriptors

Sign	Metastases	Hemangiomas
Amorphous	45%	0%
Target	25%	0%
Halo	16%	0%
Changed morphology	12%	0%
Doughnut	26%	6%
Light bulb	9%	100%

Data from Reinig, JW, et al: Radiology 165 (P):202, 1987.

The *amorphous sign,* describing a featureless, in-homogeneous lesion with irregular, indistinct margins (see Figs. 51-2, *D* and *E,* and 51-3), was the most common appearance of metastases (45%) (Table 51-7). No benign lesion showed these features. The second most common morphologic descriptor for hepatic metastases was the *target sign* (25%), denoting a tumor with a hyperintense central area on T₂-weighted sequences (Fig. 51-5). The central hyperintensity is thought to result from tumor necrosis. The third most frequent specific descriptor was the *halo sign* (16%) (Fig. 51-6), characterized by a circumferential hyperintense rim on T₂-weighted

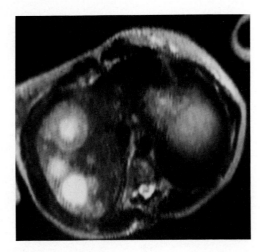

Fig. 51-5 Target sign. Three metastases have high signal intensity centrally and are surrounded by abnormal tissue whose signal intensity is somewhat less, but still greater than, normal liver (SE 2350/120).

images, possibly caused by peritumoral edema, hemorrhage, or diffuse tumor infiltration. The fourth descriptor, seen only in metastases, was the *changed morphology sign* (12%) (Fig. 51-7), an observation describing an increase in lesion size when comparing T₂- to T₁-

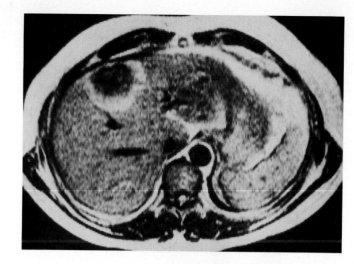

Fig. 51-6 Halo sign. Circumferential rim of tissue of high signal intensity surrounds central lesion of low signal intensity. Width of rim may vary from 3 to 15 mm (SE 2350/60).

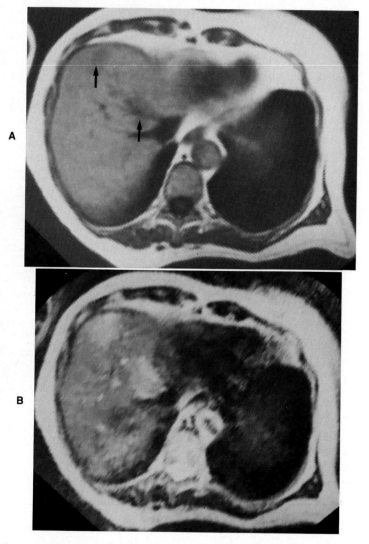

Fig. 51-7 Changed morphology sign. Size and shape of two lesions on T_1-weighted images *(arrows; A, SE 275/14)* show considerable change when imaged with T_2-weighted sequences (**B,** SE 2350/60).

weighted sequences. This "increase" is thought to be caused by an increased peritumoral water content, which is invisible on T_1-weighted sequences.

Two other morphologic features, (the doughnut and *light bulb* signs,) showed a lower specificity for hepatic metastases (Table 51-7). The *doughnut sign* (26%) (Fig. 51-8), describing a central tumor hypointensity, was the only characteristic morphologic descriptor seen on T_1-weighted pulse sequences. However, this sign was also present in 6% of hemangiomas. A mass with distinct, smooth margins and a high signal intensity (approximately that of cerebrospinal fluid or the gallbladder) was described as having a *light bulb sign* (Fig. 51-9). This sign was present in 9% of metastases but characteristic of all benign lesions.

The specificity of all these signs must be qualified by their use in patients who are suspected of having a tumor. Broadening their applications to all hepatic lesions is inappropriate, since these signs have already been seen in liver abscesses.[13]

Hepatocellular carcinoma

Hepatocellular carcinoma is the most common primary malignant liver tumor, with a worldwide incidence of more than 1 million patients per year. Pathologically there are three subtypes: solitary (50%), multifocal (25%), and diffuse hepatocellular carcinoma (25%).[24]

On T_1-weighted images hepatocellular carcinoma may appear hypointense (50%), isointense (25%), or hyperintense (25%) relative to surrounding liver (Fig. 51-10,

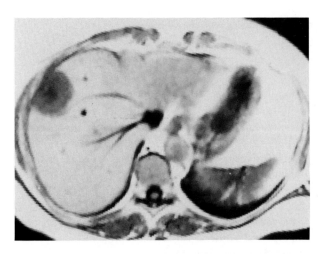

Fig. 51-8 Doughnut sign. T_1-weighted sequence demonstrates metastasis with signal intensity less than surrounding normal liver (SE 275/14). Signal intensity of metastasis is even further decreased centrally.

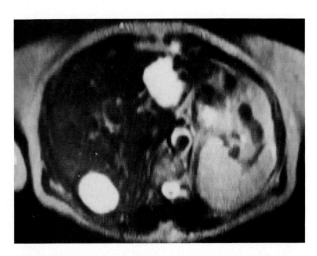

Fig. 51-9 Light bulb sign. Metastasis *(arrow)* with signal intensity similar to cerebrospinal fluid (SE 2350/180). Margin of tumor is smooth and well defined.

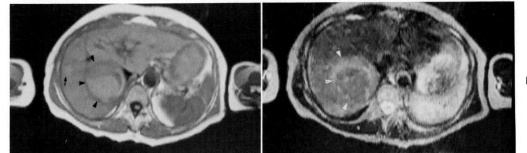

Fig. 51-10 Hepatocellular carcinoma. **A,** T_1-weighted sequence (SE 260/18) demonstrates dominant lesion primarily to have high signal intensity, which occurs infrequently in metastases. Smaller satellite mass *(arrow)* also has this high signal intensity. Narrow ring of lower signal intensity surrounds larger lesion *(arrowheads)*. **B,** T_2-weighted sequences with long TE (SE 2000/180) show larger lesion to be hyperintense with incomplete capsule *(arrowheads)*. Satellite lesion is obscured.

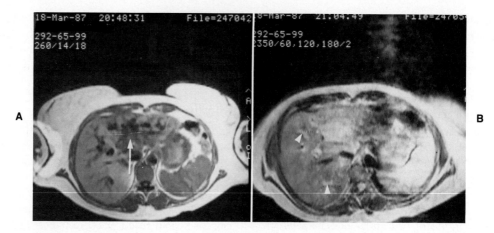

Fig. 51-11 Cholangiocarcinoma. **A,** Tubular structures are noticed to be prominent through liver, especially in periphery (SE 260/14). However, definitive differentiation of bile ducts from blood vessels is not possible. Mass with lower signal intensity is present in periportal region *(arrow).* **B,** T_2-weighted (SE 2350/60) image allows differentiation between dilated ducts *(arrowheads)* and vessels. Cholangiocarcinoma has high signal intensity, similar to that observed in metastases from other primary tumors.

*A).** The high signal intensity of some hepatocellular carcinomas on T_1-weighted images has been attributed to fatty degeneration with accumulation of triglycerides in the cytoplasm of tumor cells.[46] This appearance is sufficiently uncommon in other tumors (see Table 51-5) so that its presence warrants a serious consideration of hepatocellular carcinoma. On T_2-weighted images the tumor consistently appears hyperintense but cannot be distinguished from the common appearances of metastases (Fig. 51-10, *B*).

A tumor capsule, represented by a structure of low signal intensity circumferentially surrounding the tumor on T_1-weighted images *(ring sign)*, is another characteristic finding. Tumor capsules occur in approximately 27% of U.S. patients[46] but seem to be more common (42%) in Asia (Fig. 51-10, *A*).[44,49] On T_2-weighted images capsules can appear hypo-, iso-, or hyperintense (Fig. 51-10, *B*), depending on vascularity and the amount of T_1 (hemorrhage) or T_2 (hemosiderin) shortening substances. The ring signs can be mimicked by displaced vessels, peripheral seminecrotic tissue, and peritumoral hemosiderin deposits.

Cholangiocarcinoma

Cholangiocarcinoma is more common in Asia than in Western countries because of its association with *Clonorchis parasitosis*. Histologically, cholangiocarcinomas are either well-differentiated adenocarcinomas or infiltrating scirrhous carcinomas.[24] The most common MR

*References 11, 32, 34, 35, 46, and 61.

feature of cholangiocarcinoma is biliary dilatation (80% to 100% of cases). The tumor itself may be seen either as periductal infiltration or as a mass in the portal region in 60% of patients (Fig. 51-11). Intraductal growth is more likely visualized on T_1-weighted images because the tumor appears isointense relative to bile on T_2-weighted images.[46] Intrahepatic metastases from cholangiocarcinomas have T_1, T_2, and proton density similar to metastases from other primary tumors, and their etiology may not be suspected when the primary mass is not appreciated (see Table 51-1).

Hepatic lymphoma

Hepatic lymphoma occurs in 8% to 16% of patients with Hodgkin's disease and non-Hodgkin's lymphoma at initial presentation of the disease.[20,31] From 60% to 70% of patients with hepatic involvement show a focal pattern of disease; the remainder show diffuse or mixed patterns of hepatic infiltration. Focal patterns of hepatic lymphomas are detected with either T_1- or T_2-weighted pulse sequences and have MR features indistinguishable from other hepatic malignancies (Fig. 51-12). Mixed hepatic lymphoma, characterized by the presence of both numerous focal lymphoma deposits and diffuse panlobular infiltration, is best detected using T_2-weighted pulse sequences (Fig. 51-13).[29] Diffuse hepatic lymphoma confined microscopically to the periportal areas is not detectable by MRI.[7,29,68] Recent advances in the development of organ-specific MR contrast agents such as ferrite allow significant increases in focal lymphoma-liver CNR, allowing the detection of lymphoma deposits not visible on unenhanced MR images.[64]

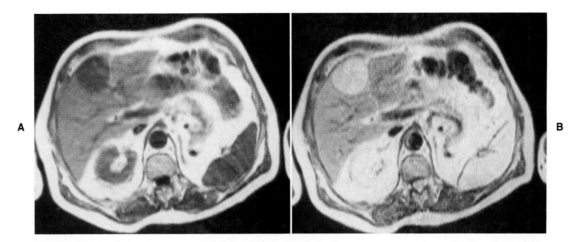

Fig. 51-12 Focal hepatic lymphoma. Signal intensity characteristics and morphologic features of focal hepatic lymphoma are indistinguishable from other hepatic malignancies. This large-cell non-Hodgkin's lymphoma is seen as a focal mass in right hepatic lobe on SE 260/14 (**A**) and SE 2350/120 (**B**) sequences.

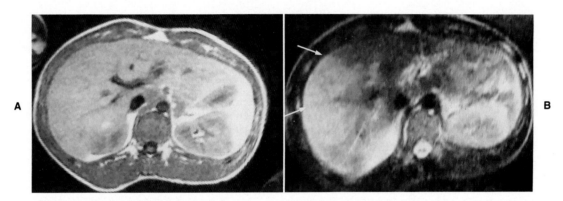

Fig. 51-13 Mixed hepatic lymphoma. **A,** T_1-weighted image (SE 260/14) demonstrates no discernible signal intensity changes. There may be slight compression of hepatic vessels in right lobe. **B,** T_2-weighted image (SE 2350/120) shows hyperintense right lobe of liver. Note geographic distribution of this Hodgkin's lymphoma *(arrows)*.

Hemangioma

Hemangioma is the most common benign liver tumor, occurring in 1% to 20% of the general population.[37,51] Although typically solitary lesions, hemangiomas are multiple in 10% to 30% of patients.[45]

Cavernous hemangiomas differ from solid liver tumors in that they have longer T_2 relaxation times (152 ± 54 msec versus 78 ± 32 msec). As a result, hemangiomas appear substantially moe hyperintense with progressive T_2 weighting (Fig. 51-14).[21,45,51] The maximal difference in signal intensities between hemangiomas and hepatic metastases has been shown to occur at a TE of 160 to 180 msec.[45] The brightness of the signal intensity of hemangiomas is comparable to the signal intensity of cerebrospinal or bile fluid. This high signal intensity on T_2-weighted pulse sequences (light bulb sign) has been found to be characteristic of hemangiomas.[45,51,69] However, 5% to 9% of metastatic tumors display this signal intensity and are otherwise indistinguishable from hemangiomas.[45,69] These mimicking tumors are more likely to originate from primary lesions of low incidence (islet cell tumors, sarcomas, vascular endocrine tumors, pseudomyxoma).

Most hemangiomas are sharply marginated and smoothly round (Fig. 51-14) or oval shaped (70%), although they may be lobulated (30%).[45] Most hemangiomas are indistinguishable from cysts on MRI. Hemangiomas more than 6 cm in diameter are more often

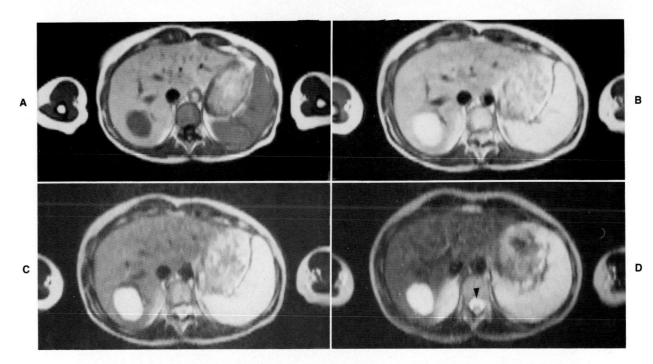

Fig. 51-14 Hemangioma. **A** to **D,** Hemangiomas demonstrating hypointensity on T_1-weighted sequence (**A,** SE 300/14) and progressive hyperintensity on T_2-weighted spin echo sequences (**B,** SE 2350/60; **C,** SE 2350/120). Further T_2 weighting decreases signal intensity of liver but not of hemangioma (light bulb effect) (**D,** SE 2350/180). Cerebrospinal or bile fluid serves as reference tissue with similar signal intensity as hemangioma *(arrowhead)*. Metastases typically show greater consistency of signal intensity with that of spleen.

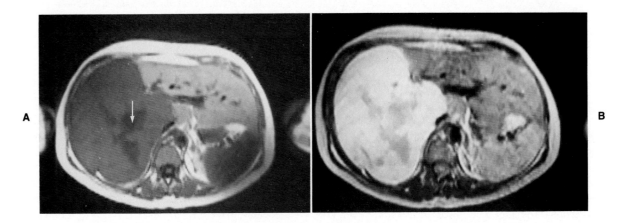

Fig. 51-15 Giant cavernous hemangioma. **A,** T_1-weighted image displays hemangioma as hypointense lesion with central area of decreased signal intensity *(arrow)* pathologically corresponding to fibrosis (SE 260/14). **B,** T_2-weighted pulse sequence demonstrates typical high signal intensity of cavernous hemangiomas to be preserved except for region of central scar (SE 2350/120). (Courtesy Dr. E. Rummeny.)

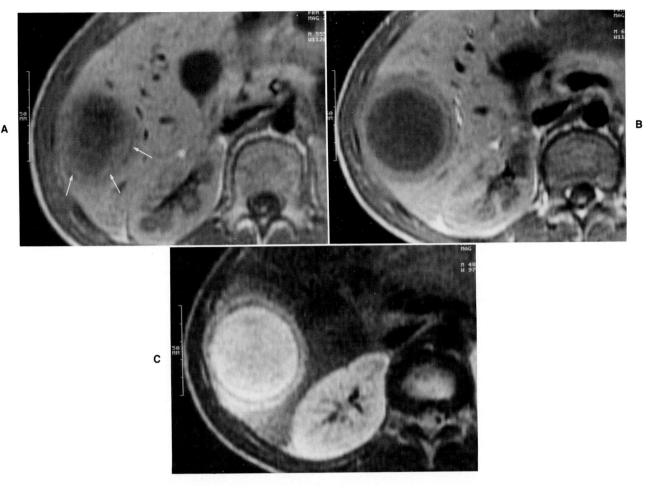

Fig. 51-16 Amebic liver abscess. **A,** Untreated amebic liver abscesses appear as heterogeneously hypointense masses on T_1-weighted image (SE 500/28). Hepatic vasculature is often deviated because of mass effect of abscesses. Incomplete rings corresponding to abscess wall can occasionally be seen *(arrows)*. **B,** After medical treatment cavity appears homogeneously hypointense relative to liver and is usually bordered by hyperintense ring surrounded by hypointense ring (SE 500/28). **C,** On T_2-weighted images (SE 2000/84) hypointense ring corresponds exactly to that seen on T_1-weighted images.

lobulated (50%) and heterogeneous (50%), with internal septations resulting from thrombosis or scar tissue (Fig. 51-15).[45]

Amebic liver abscess

Amebic liver abscesses are common in endemic areas such as Latin America and southern United States. MRI not only reliably depicts amebic abscesses, but also uniquely delineates features characteristic of the healing process. Untreated amebic liver abscesses show heterogeneous abscess cavities that appear hypointense on T_1-weighted (Fig. 51-16, *A*) and hyperintense on T_2-weighted images. Incomplete hyperintense rings can be seen at the abscess margin. With successful medical treatment hepatic edema resolves, the abscess cavity becomes homogeneous, and complete concentric rings develop (Fig. 51-16, *B* and *C*).[13] Histologic correlation has shown that these concentric rings are caused by periabscess fibrosis and hemosiderin deposits. Reparative tissue changes are seen as early as 4 days after treatment and indicate a favorable response. Abscess size, however, changes late in the healing process and seems to be a less reliable indicator of treatment response.

Pyogenic liver abscess

Pyogenic liver abscesses most often occur in older patients with cancer, biliary disease, and bacteremia. Experimentally the appearance of pyogenic liver abscesses is similar to untreated amebic abscesses, that is, hypointense on T_1-weighted images and hyperintense on T_2-

weighted images. A zone of congestion and/or edema typically surrounds the cavity and accounts for the larger lesion size depicted on T_2-weighted images. Administration of gadolinium (gd)-DTPA results in pericavitary ring enhancement comparable to the ring enhancement seen on contrast-enhanced CT.[67]

Cirrhosis

Experimental studies and clinical experience suggest that hepatic cirrhosis alone does not greatly alter T_1 and T_2 relaxation times.[50,61] Fatty liver, hepatitis, and cirrhosis frequently coexist and may either offset expected decreases in signal intensity because of T_2 shortening of collagen or actually increase hepatic signal intensity because of T_1 lengthening of water.[6,50]

Cirrhosis can be detected using conventional morphologic features applied to CT.[23] Irregular surface contour of the liver, enlargement of the caudate lobe, and distortion of intrahepatic vessels are easily identified. Secondary extrahepatic findings such as ascites, collateral veins, and splenomegaly are also readily detected by MRI. Regenerating nodules generally have the same signal intensity as normal liver on T_1- and T_2-weighted imaging techniques. However, occasionally regenerating nodules can be detected as either hyperintense (increased triglyceride content) or hypointense lesions relative to the liver.[33]

Hemochromatosis

MRI techniques have been used to detect hepatic iron overload in the range of greatest clinical significance, 1 to 10 mg iron/g liver (wet weight).[52] With deposition of hemosiderin in hepatocytes, T_2 relaxation times of hepatic parenchymal decrease. As a result, MR signal intensity decreases with increasing tissue iron concentration (Fig. 51-17). This phenomenon readily permits identification of coexisting tumor (Fig. 51-18) and forms the clinical rationale for use of ferrite as an MR contrast agent for tumor detection (see later section on hepatobiliary agents). T_2-weighted techniques are more susceptible in predicting incipient states of iron overload, whereas T_1-weighted techniques allow rough estimation of advanced states of iron overload.[52]

CONTRAST AGENTS

Intravenous contrast agents will inevitably be used to enhance the detection of hepatic tumors, improve their differential diagnosis, and assess hepatic function. Experimental liver contrast agents already available can be divided into three functional classes: perfusion, reticuloendothelial, and hepatobiliary agents.

Perfusion agents

Gadolinium-chelates (Gd-DTPA, Gd-DOTA) are paramagnetic agents, predominantly shortening T_1 relaxation times of perfused tissue, and are best imaged using T_1-sensitive pulse sequences. Gd-chelates have pharmacokinetic and biodistribution properties similar to iodinated contrast material.[70] Gd-chelates are rapidly distributed to liver tissue and are initially excluded by some (hypovascular) tumors, thereby increasing tumor-liver CNR. This biodistribution is time dependent and reverses

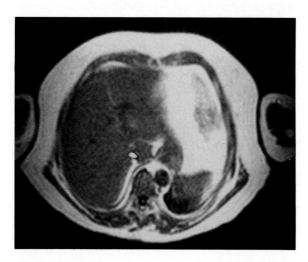

Fig. 51-17 Hemochromatosis. MR image (SE 500/28) shows decreased signal intensity of liver, spleen, and bone marrow in patient with untreated iron overload. Compare liver signal intensity to that of Fig. 51-1.

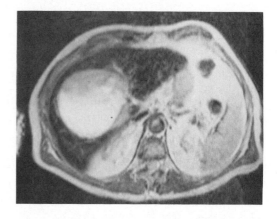

Fig. 51-18 Hemochromatosis and malignancy. Signal intensity of hepatic parenchyma is decreased because of iron overload; signal intensity of spleen is normal, however, indicating its lack of increased iron deposits (SE 1500/60). Greatly decreased signal intensity of liver provides excellent contrast to hepatocellular carcinoma, which lacks iron deposits. This principle of contrast enhancement is currently employed for ferrite-enhanced MRI.

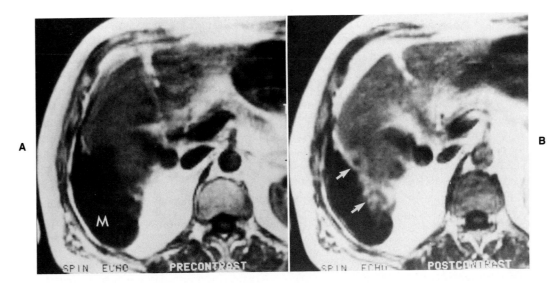

Fig. 51-19 Contrast agents: Gd-DTPA. Patient with cystic ovarian carcinoma metastatic to liver. **A,** Precontrast images show cystic metastasis in segment VI as lesion with low signal intensity, *M* (SE 400/22). **B,** Delayed imaging after administration of Gd-DTPA (0.1 mmol/kg) shows peritumoral signal intensity to be increased because of diffuse infiltration (SE 400/22; 17 minutes) *(arrows)*.
(Courtesy Dr. R. Bittner, Berlin.)

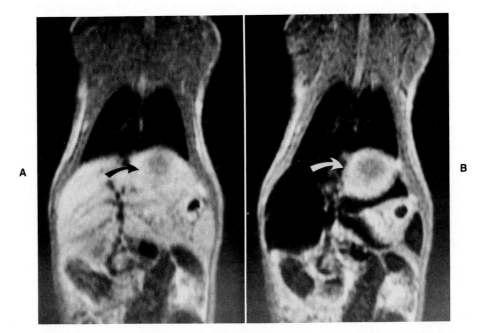

Fig. 51-20 Contrast agents: ferrite. Ferrite produces profound signal loss from hepatic tissue (**A,** before contrast; **B,** after administration of ferrite; SE 500/30). Tumor-liver contrast increases maximally, resulting in very hyperintense tumor *(arrow)* contrasted by surrounding hypointense liver.
(Courtesy Dr. G. Elizondo, Boston.)

within minutes because of washout of Gd-chelate from normal liver and retention in tumor (Fig. 51-19).[48,66] Hypervascular tumors may enhance to the same degree as normal liver and may be obscured during the initial phase.[39] Therefore perfusion MR contrast agents, as with iodinated agents used for CT, require rapid scanning for best results.

The lower SNR and CNR of rapid images, the minimal degree of enhancement at clinical doses, and the inability to perform rapid imaging on early clinical scanners have contributed to the disappointment of Gd-DTPA as a contrast agent for abdominal MRI.[5] Indeed, a decrease in tumor-liver contrast frequently was seen after intravenous bolus administration of Gd-DTPA. Rapid imaging with Gd-DTPA using fast spin echo[39] or GR echo[26] techniques have demonstrated variable degrees of enhancement.

Reticuloendothelial agents

Particulate contrast agents are selectively phagocytosed by fixed macrophages of normal spleen, lymph nodes, bone marrow, and liver tissue. Tumors, lacking reticuloendothelial cells, do not exhibit phagocytosis or specific uptake of particles. This mechanism of tissue-specific contrast enhancement has previously been exploited in sulphur colloid scintigraphy and contrast-enhanced CT using ethiodol oil emulsion (EOE-13), perfluorooctylbromide (PFOB), or radiopaque liposomes.[40,47,58]

Superparamagnetic crystalline iron oxide (ferrite) is a new reticuloendothelial-specific MR contrast agent that primarily acts to reduce T_2, decreasing hepatic signal intensity. The metabolism of intravenously administered ferrite particles and biodegradation products have recently been studied.[2,63] Within 20 minutes after intravenous administration, particles are phagocytosed by macrophages of the reticuloendothelial system (RES). The human RES consists of approximately 1800 g of reticulum cells with phagocytic ability located in liver (60%), spleen (5%), and other tissues (35%), such as lymph nodes, bone marrow, lungs, and circulatory system. Radioactively labeled ^{59}Fe-ferrite studies have shown that molecular iron of certain ferrite preparations is ultimately incorporated into hemoglobin in a time-dependent fashion. For example, using a ferrite preparation currently in clinical trials, AMI-25,* 20% of ^{59}Fe-ferrite was found in hemoglobin after 49 days.[63] No evidence of hepatic mitochondrial, microsomal, or organelle dysfunction was found. Likewise, there was no evidence of chronic hepatotoxicity.[2]

Following administration of ferrite, changes in liver SNR and tumor-liver CNR show a simple exponential

behavior (10 to 40 μmol Fe/kg). Using a SE 500/30 sequence, liver signal intensity is maximally decreased and tumor-liver contrast maximally increased 15 minutes after injection.[66] Widely available, mildly "T_1-weighted" pulse sequences such as SE 500/30 have sufficient T_2 dependence to create a T_2-weighted ferrite-enhanced image that can be signal-averaged (because of the short TR,) resulting in high contrast and low image noise. Experimental studies have shown consistent identification of hepatic lesions between 4 and 10 mm in size (Fig. 51-20).[59] This agent should also be effective with GR echo imaging techniques, which are very sensitive to magnetic susceptibility changes. Preliminary experience shows a greatly increased tumor-liver CNR using GR breath-hold imaging.[57]

Hepatobiliary agents

Hepatobiliary MR contrast agents contain a paramagnetic ion (iron, manganese, or gadolinium) bound to an organic ligand (chelate) with some degree of hepatocellular specificity. Experimental prototype hepatobiliary agents are lipophilic complexes such as iron-EHPG (ethylenebis[2-hydroxyphenyl-glycine]), iron-HBED (N,N'-bis[2-hydroxybenzyl]ethylenediamine N,N'-diacetic acid), or vitamin B_6 analogs such as manganese-DPDP (dipyridoxyl-5-diphosphate). Biliary excretion varies between 6% and 10% for iron-EHPG to 50% for iron-HBED and manganese-DPDP. The remaining fraction is distributed nonspecifically, including retention in the tumor itself. Experimentally the tumor-liver signal difference is less than optimal, although the effectiveness of these agents has not been evaluated in humans. Decreases in hepatic relaxation times as a consequence of altered excretion of Fe-HBED have been observed in experimentally induced hepatitis.

REFERENCES

1. Alpern, MB, et al: Focal hepatic masses and fatty infiltration by enhanced dynamic CT, Radiology 158:45, 1986.
2. Bacon, BR, et al: Ferrite particles: a new magnetic resonance imaging contrast agent; lack of acute or chronic hepatotoxicity after intravenous administration, J Lab Clin Med 10:164, 1987.
3. Bailes, DR, et al: Respiratory ordering of phase encoding (ROPE): a method for reducing respiratory motion artifacts in MR imaging, J Comput Assist Tomogr 9:835, 1985.
4. Bottomley, PA, et al: A review of 1H nuclear magnetic resonance relaxation in pathology: are T1 and T2 diagnostic? Med Phys 14:1, 1987.
5. Carr, DH, et al: Gadolinium-DTPA as a contrast agent in MRI: initial clinical experience in 20 patients, AJR 143:215, 1984.
6. Cherryman, GR, et al: NMR in parenchymal liver disease (abstract), Soc Magn Res Med 2:1137, 1985.
7. Cohen, MD, et al: Magnetic resonance imaging of lymphomas in children, Pediatr Radiol 15:179, 1985.
8. Couinaud, C. Le foie: etudes anatomiques et chirurgicales, Paris, 1985, Masson and Cie.

*Advanced Magnetics, Cambridge, Mass.

9. Demas, BE, et al: Magnetic resonance imaging diagnosis of hepatic metastases in the presence of negative CT studies, J Clin Gastroenterol 7:553, 1985.
10. Dousset, M, et al: Optimization of STIR imaging for abdominal MRI, Magn Reson Med, 1988. (In press.)
11. Ebara, M, et al: Diagnosis of small hepatocellular carcinoma: correlation of MR imaging and tumor histologic studies, Radiology 159:371, 1986.
12. Ehman, RL, et al: Relative intensity of abdominal organs in MR images, J Comput Assist Tomogr 9:315, 1985.
13. Elizondo, G, et al: Amebic liver abscesses: diagnosis and treatment evaluation by MRI, Radiology 165:795, 1987.
14. Ferrucci, JT: MR imaging of the liver, AJR 147:1103, 1986.
15. Fisher, MR, et al: Hepatic vascular anatomy on magnetic resonance imaging, AJR 144:739, 1985.
16. Foley, WD, et al: Contrast optimization for the detection of focal hepatic lesions by MR imaging at 1.5 T, AJR 149:1155, 1987.
17. Foster, JH, and Lundy, J: Liver metastasis, Curr Probl Surg 18:160, 1981.
18. Freeny, PC, and Marks, WM: Patterns of contrast enhancement of benign and malignant hepatic neoplasms during bolus dynamic and delayed CT, Radiology 160:613, 1986.
19. Freeny, PC, et al: Colorectal carcinoma evaluation with CT: preoperative staging and detection of postoperative occurrence, Radiology 158:347, 1986.
20. Gilbert, HA, and Kagan, AR: Metastases: incidence, detection, and evaluation without histologic confirmation. In Weiss, L, editor: Fundamental aspects of metastases, Amsterdam, 1976, North Holland Publishing.
21. Glazer, GM, et al: Hepatic cavernous hemangioma: magnetic resonance imaging, Radiology 155:417, 1985.
22. Glazer, GM, et al: Evaluation of focal hepatic masses: a comparative study of MRI and CT, Gastrointest Radiol 11:263, 1986.
23. Goldberg, HI, et al: Hepatic cirrhosis: magnetic resonance imaging, Radiology 153:737, 1984.
24. Goodman, ZD: Primary malignant neoplasms of the liver, Washington, DC, 1987, AFP course.
25. Haase, A, et al: FLASH imaging: rapid NMR imaging using low flip angles, J Magn Reson 67:217, 1986.
26. Hamm, B, Wolf, KJ, and Felix, R: Conventional and rapid MR imaging of the liver with Gd-DTPA, Radiology 164:313, 1987.
27. Heiken, JP, et al: Hepatic metastases studied with MR and CT, Radiology 156:423, 1985.
28. Hendrick, RE, Nelson, TR, and Hendee, WR: Optimizing tissue contrast in magnetic resonance imaging, Magn Reson Imaging 2:3, 1984.
29. Hendrick, RE, et al: Maximizing liver lesion detection: a comparison of pulse sequence performance at different magnetic field strengths, Radiology 165(P):182, 1987.
30. Henkelman, RM, et al: Optimal pulse sequence for imaging hepatic metastases, Radiology 161:727, 1986.
31. Horm, JW, et al: Cancer incidence and mortality in the US, 1973-1981, NIH Pub. No. 85-1837, Bethesda, MD, 1984, National Institutes of Health.
32. Itai, Y, et al: MR imaging of hepatocellular carcinoma, J Comput Assist Tomogr 10:963, 1986.
33. Itai, Y, et al: Regenerating nodules of liver cirrhosis: MR imaging, Radiology 165:419, 1987.
34. Itai, Y, et al: CT and MR imaging of fatty tumors of the liver, J Comput Assist Tomogr 11:253, 1987.
35. Itoh, K, et al: MR imaging of hepatocellular carcinoma, Radiology 164:21, 1987.
36. Johnson, GA, Herfkens, RJ, and Brown MA: Tissue relaxation time: in vivo field dependence, Radiology 156:805, 1985.
37. Karhunen, PJ: Benign hepatic tumors and tumor-like condition in men, J Clin Pathol 39:183, 1986.
38. Malt, RA: Surgery for hepatic neoplasm, N Engl J Med 313:1591, 1985.
39. Mano, I, et al: Fast spin echo imaging with suspended respiration: gadolinium enhanced MR imaging of liver tumors, J Comput Assist Tomogr 11:73, 1987.
40. Mattrey, RF, Long, DM, and Multer, F: Perfluorooctylbromide: a reticuloendothelial-specific and tumor imaging agent for computed tomography, Radiology 145:755,1982.
41. Moss, AA, et al: Hepatic tumors: magnetic resonance and CT appearance, Radiology 150:141, 1984.
42. Pattany, PM, et al: Motion artifact suppression technique (MAST) for MR imaging, J Comput Assist Tomogr 11:369, 1987.
43. Reinig, JW, et al: Comparison of liver metastasis detection at 0.5 T and 1.5 T, Radiology 165(P):202, 1987.
44. Reinig, JW, et al: Liver metastases detection: comparative sensitivities of MR imaging and CT scanning, Radiology 162:43, 1987.
44a. Ruda, H: Personal communication.
45. Rummeny, E, et al: Differential diagnosis of cavernous hemangioma and hepatic metastases, Radiology, p. 165, 1988.
46. Rummeny, E, et al: Primary malignant liver tumors, AJR 1988. (In press.)
47. Ryan, PJ, et al: Liposomes loaded with contrast material for image enhancement in computed tomography, Radiology 152:759, 1984.
48. Saini, S, et al: Dynamic spin echo MRI of liver cancer using Gd-DTPA, AJR 147:357, 1986.
49. Smith, TJ, et al: A prospective study of hepatic imaging in detection of metastatic disease, Ann Surg 195:486, 1981.
50. Stark, DD, et al: Nuclear magnetic resonance imaging of experimentally induced liver disease, Radiology 148:743, 1983.
51. Stark, DD, et al: Magnetic resonance imaging of cavernous hemangioma of the liver: tissue specific characterization, AJR 145:213, 1985.
52. Stark, DD, et al: Magnetic resonance imaging and spectroscopy of hepatic iron overload, Radiology 154:137, 1985.
53. Stark, DD, et al: Detection of liver metastasis by MR: analysis of pulse sequence performance, Radiology 159:365, 1986.
54. Stark, DD, et al: Liver metastases: detection by phase-contrast MR imaging, Radiology 158:327, 1986.
55. Stark, DD, et al: Motion artifact reduction with fast spin echo imaging, Radiology 164:183, 1987.
56. Stark, DD, et al: Hepatic metastases: Randomized, controlled comparison of detection with MR imaging and CT, Radiology 165:399, 1987.
57. Stark, DD, et al: Superparamagnetic iron oxide: clinical application as a contrast agent for magnetic resonance imaging, Radiology, 1988. (In press.)
58. Thomas, JL, et al: EOE-13 in the detection of hepatosplenic lymphoma, Radiology 145:629, 1982.
59. Tsang, YM, et al: Hepatic micrometastases in the rat: ferrite enhanced MR imaging, Radiology, 167:21, 1988.
60. Weinreb, JC, Brateman, L, and Maravilla KR: Magnetic resonance imaging of hepatic lymphoma, AJR 143:1211, 1984.
61. Weissleder, R, and Stark, DD: MRI Atlas of the abdomen, London, 1989, Dunitz Publishers.
62. Weissleder, R, and Stark, DD: MRI of the liver. In Kressel, H, editor: Magnetic resonance annual, New York, 1989, Raven Press.
63. Weissleder, R, et al: Ferrite particles: evidence for biodegradability and safety as a tissue specific contrast agent for MR imaging, Radiology 165(P):354, 1987.

64. Weissleder, R, et al: MRI of hepatic lymphoma: an experimental study in rodents using ferrite, AJR 149:1161, 1987.

65. Weissleder, R, et al: Optimization of GRASS imaging, Magn Reson Imaging, March 2, 1988, p. 56.

66. Weissleder, R, et al: Dual contrast MR Imaging: animal investigation, AJR 150:561, 1988.

67. Weissleder, R, et al: Pyogenic liver abscess: contrast enhanced MRI, AJR 150:115, 1988.

68. Weissleder, R, et al: MRI of hepatic lymphoma, Magn Reson Imaging, vol. 6, 1988.

69. Wittenberg, J, et al: Differentiation of hepatic metastases from hemangioma and cysts by MR, AJR 151:79, 1988.

70. Wolf, GL, et al: Contrast agents for magnetic resonance imaging. In Kressel, H, editor: Magnetic resonance annual, New York, 1985, Raven Press.

71. Wood, M: Overcoming motion artifacts in abdominal MR imaging, AJR 150:513, 1988.

52 *Ultrasonography*

FAYE C. LAING
ROY A. FILLY
GRETCHEN A.W. GOODING

Most would agree that the most dramatic impact of ultrasonography in abdominal imaging has been in the area of the hepatobiliary system. Dramatic strides in image improvement by manufacturers of ultrasonographic equipment now allow extrahepatic biliary structures to be displayed exquisitely.

Many disorders affecting the liver, gallbladder, and bile ducts can be imaged accurately with ultrasonography. Although information is still being gathered regarding the sensitivity and specificity for the ultrasonographic detection of various common disorders that involve this organ system, the value of ultrasonography in individual diagnostic situations cannot be denied. Its high resolution, lack of dependence on organ function, and flexibility make ultrasonography almost ideal for hepatobiliary diagnosis.

LIVER
Technical considerations

There is general agreement that the normal liver returns diffuse echo signals with an echo amplitude higher than the kidney, less than the spleen, and equivalent or less than the pancreas. The echo texture of the liver is homogeneous except for visualized vessels and ligaments (Fig. 52-1).

Technical efforts are directed at optimizing the image to display the uniform textural echogenicity of liver tissue. It is easier to detect a subtle pathologic aleration against a uniform background than against a nonhomogeneous background. Virtually all patients may be approached in the same manner. To achieve optimal homogeneity and maximal echo information, it is best to begin by balancing near- and far-field amplification employing the time-gain compensation controls. Once this is accomplished, the overall amplification or transducer power control should be progressively increased until spurious echoes begin to appear in the larger hepatic and portal veins. The overall amplification is then slightly reduced to expunge these artifacts. This method accomplishes two goals. First, it results in the maximal density of parenchymal echo dots within the hepatic tissue, which has a smoothing effect on the appearance. Second, the

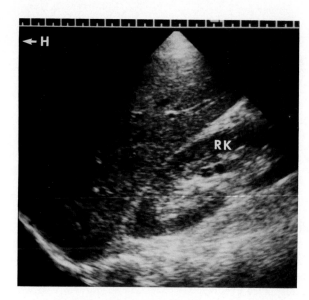

Fig. 52-1 Right parasagittal sonogram demonstrates uniform echo texture to hepatic parenchyma. Renal parenchyma is slightly less echogenic relative to hepatic parenchyma. *H,* Head; *RK,* right kidney.

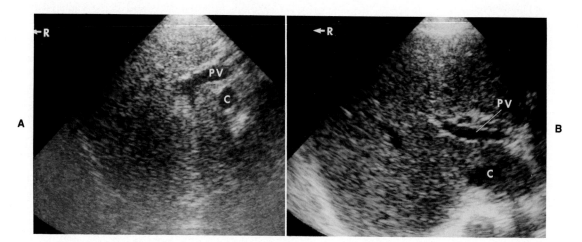

Fig. 52-2 A, Transverse scan of right lobe of liver performed with 3.5 MHz transducer. Because of fat and fibrosis within this liver, sound penetration is poor. **B,** Repeat scan using 2 MHz transducer. Note improved quality of scan, with balanced echogenicity between near, middle, and far fields. *C,* Inferior vena cava; *PV,* portal vein; *R,* right.

hepatic vessels can serve as an internal control of the signal-to-noise ratio. As long as the vessels appear echo free, one may feel confident that nondirectional echo signal noise and electronic noise have not seriously degraded the image.

Transducer selection is important. One should always select the highest frequency transducer that will allow the near- and far-field echoes to be balanced (Fig. 52-2). The two most functional transducer frequencies for this purpose are 3.5 and 5.0 MHz. One should not select a higher-frequency transducer at the expense of balanced echogenicity unless one specifically is evaluating a pos-

sible abnormality close to the transducer. The overall balance of echoes is more important.

The two most important views for visualizing hepatic tissues are the parasagittal and subcostal oblique planes. The subcostal oblique view should be considered the true transverse image of the liver, based on portal anatomy.

A more important technical aspect involves obtaining hepatic images unobstructed by bony structures or intestinal gas. Because of the overlying ribs and the rounded contour of the upper abdomen, a mechanical or electronic real-time sector transducer usually produces a more satisfactory image than does a linear array transducer. The

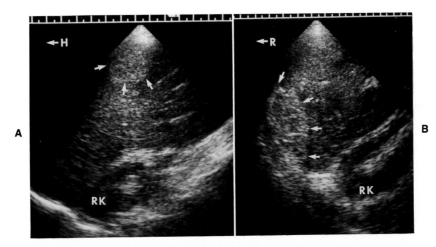

Fig. 52-3 A, Right parasagittal scan performed with the patient in left posterior oblique position and transducer placed intercostally. Subtle mass present in near field *(arrows)* could easily be missed. *H,* Head; *RK,* right kidney. **B,** Subsequent transverse scan performed with transducer positioned subcostally and pointed toward lateral aspect of right lobe of liver. Note how much easier it is to detect mass *(arrows),* which abuts lateral aspect of right lobe of liver. *R,* Right; *RK,* right kidney.

scans should be obtained with the transducer positioned inferior to the costal margin. In an effort to ensure that liver tissue descends below the costal margin, it may be useful to change the patient's position from a supine to a left decubitus or erect position. Each of these positions progressively employ gravity to assist in bringing liver tissue below the costal margin. Obviously, suspended maximal inspiration should be used regardless of the patient's position. It is unusual for satisfactory images not to be obtained with the patient in one of these positions.

In debilitated patients who may be unable to inspire deeply, suspend respiration, or assume the decubitus or erect positions, other approaches must be sought. Although every experienced ultrasonographer has individual methods, the most successful in our experience is to use a real-time sector transducer with an intercostal approach. It is important to have the patient inspire and expire as the transducer is positioned in each intercostal space in order to examine portions of liver tissue that lie behind rib shadows. This minimizes the portions of liver tissue obscured from view and maximizes the amount of hepatic parenchyma tissue that can be seen even in the worst instances.

Because the face of most real-time sector transducers is relatively small, it is easy to pivot it so that the ultrasound beam can be directed in cranial/caudal or medial/lateral directions. Using this technique, the hepatic parenchyma can be scanned rapidly and completely. Relative blind spots include the lateral aspect of the right lobe of the liver and the dome of the liver (Fig. 52-3).

The right lobe area is visualized optimally on transverse scans when the transducer is placed subcostally and pointed toward the lateral aspect of the right lobe of the liver. The dome of the liver is seen optimally on longitudinal scans with the patient erect and the transducer angled in a cranial direction.

Using these methods should result in high-quality ultrasonograms in most individuals and technically acceptable scans in the remaining patients. Fortunately, technical failures in liver imaging occur infrequently. When they do, it is usually because of a diffuse hepatic parenchymal tissue abnormality, with deposition of fibrosis or fat that results in abnormal sound attenuation.

Anatomic considerations

The normal ultrasonographic anatomy of the abdomen is covered in Chapter 11, but several points specific to the liver are important in this discussion. These involve anatomic markers that enable one to localize the lobes and segments of liver tissue.[79,83]

The liver is divided into two lobes, the right and left. Similarly, each lobe is divided into two major segments. On the right side the lobe is divided anteriorly and posteriorly, whereas on the left side the lobe is divided medially and laterally. Ultrasonography enables the visualization of several anatomic structures that serve as boundary markers for the various hepatic segments. As a general rule, *major hepatic veins course between the segments of liver tissue, whereas major portal branches enter directly into the segments.* Portal

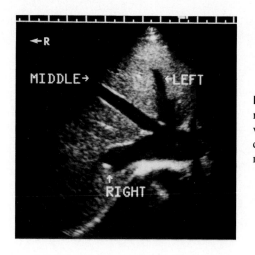

Fig. 52-4 Subcostal transverse oblique scan demonstrates normal appearance for major hepatic veins. These veins course between segments of liver, with right hepatic vein dividing anterior and posterior segments of right lobe, middle hepatic vein dividing right and left lobes, and left hepatic vein separating cephalic aspect of medial and lateral segments of left lobe. *R, Right.*

Fig. 52-5 Composite longitudinal scan contains key anatomic landmarks located in main lobar fissure. These structures include inferior vena cava *(IVC)*, gallbladder fossa *(GB)*, middle hepatic vein *(MHV)*, undivided portion of right portal vein *(PV)*, and strong linear reflection between right portal vein and gallbladder that represents visible portion of main lobar fissure *(MLF). H, Head.*

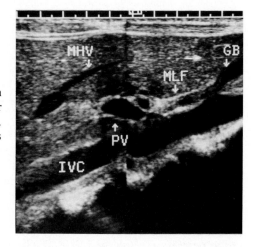

vein branches *never* violate segmental boundaries (Fig. 52-4).

Five anatomic markers can be visualized that serve to divide the right from the left hepatic lobes, or more accurately, the anterior segment of the right lobe from the medial segment of the left lobe. These markers either lie within the main lobar fissure of the liver or are visible parts of the fissure. These structures include (1) the intrahepatic inferior vena cava, (2) the gallbladder fossa, (3) the middle hepatic vein, (4) the undivided portion of the right portal vein, and (5) a strong linear reflection lying between the right portal vein and the gallbladder, representing a visible portion of the interlobar fissure (Fig. 52-5).

The caval fossa and the gallbladder fossa both are clefts in the posterior aspect of the main lobar fissure. The middle hepatic vein courses directly within the fissure. Anterior to the undivided portion of the right portal vein lies the medial segment of the left lobe, whereas

the posterior segment of the right lobe lies posterior to this vessel. The middle hepatic vein crosses anterior to the distal portion of the undivided right portal vein.

The right intersegmental fissure that divides the right lobe into anterior and posterior segments can be distinguished by identification of the longest branch of the right hepatic vein and the bifurcation point of the right portal vein. The long branch of the right hepatic vein courses within the right intersegmental fissure. From a practical point of view, this determination is relatively unimportant because surgeons do not usually attempt segmental resections of the right lobe.

The left segmental fissure that divides the left lobe into medial and lateral segments has three visible anatomic markers: one each in the cranial, middle, and caudal divisions. These markers are in order: the left hepatic vein, the ascending portion of the left portal vein, and the falciform ligament, with the teres ligament located at its free edge (Fig. 52-6)[86,110]

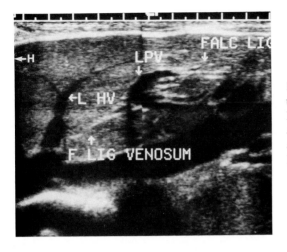

Fig. 52-6 Composite longitudinal scan contains key anatomic landmarks that denote position of left intersegmental fissure. This fissure divides left lobe into medial and lateral segments and includes left hepatic vein *(LHV)*, ascending portion of left portal vein *(LPV)*, and falciform ligament. In addition, fissure for venous ligament is seen between posterior caudate lobe and anterior left lobe of liver. *H*, Head.

The caudate lobe is often a source of confusion. Receiving its portal supply from both the left and the right portal systems, it is a portion of neither the left nor the right lobe. The fissure of the venous ligament divides the caudate lobe from the lateral segment of the left lobe. The inferior vena cava divides most of the caudate tissue from the right lobe, but the exact line of cleavage or caudate tissue from the right lobe tissue is obscure. The caudate lobe lies cephalic to the termination of the main portal vein except for the caudate process, which may insinuate posterior to this vein. The initial segment of the left portal vein as it travels to its entry position into the left intersegmental fissure (i.e., the ascending portion of the left portal vein) courses over the inferior margin of the caudate lobe.[5]

Accessory fissures of the liver, which are formed by invaginations of the diaphragm and peritoneum, are visible on computed tomography (CT) scans in approximately 25% of patients and are noted to increase with age.[4] These fissures typically occur over the superior aspect of the liver, involve the right lobe, and may exceed 2 cm in depth. When only parts of the fissures are seen on sonography, accessory fissures may be misinterpreted as echogenic liver lesions.

Understanding hepatic anatomy is becoming increasingly important as surgeons have become more aggressive in their approach to hepatic lesions.[87] The right or left lobes may be individually resected *(right* or *left lobectomy)*. The lateral segment of the left lobe may be removed *(lateral segmentectomy)*, leaving the medial segment and the right lobe intact, or conversely, the right lobe and medial segment of the left lobe may be excised *(trisegmentectomy)*, leaving only the lateral segment of the left lobe intact. It is important to recall that the lateral segment of the left lobe may be diminutive. The medial segment of the left lobe or individual segments of the right lobe are usually not surgically extirpated without removing adjoining segments. Thus the important anatomic landmarks in regard to hepatic resection are those that define the main lobar fissure and the left intersegmental fissure. Fortunately, these fissures have numerous, easily detected anatomic landmarks. This approach expands ultrasound's ability in the evaluation of hepatic malignancies and complements rather than replaces the traditional arteriographic approach.

Hepatocellular diseases

Ultrasonography has not had a great impact on the detection of diffuse hepatocellular diseases. Diffuse disease processes such as hepatitis, cirrhosis, and fatty infiltration are frequently well advanced before the liver appears unequivocally abnormal on sonograms.

In general, diffuse hepatocellular disease processes tend to increase the amplitude of reflected liver signals and sound attenuation. Unfortunately, the amplitude of returning signals from the liver varies with machine amplification settings, the type of transducer, the ultrasonic beam profile, the patient's body habitus, and acoustic coupling. For these reasons it is difficult to assess the absolute amplitude of the echo signals in individual patient diagnoses.[111] Thus it is necessary to assess the relative amplitude of echo signals by comparing liver echoes to those of adjacent organs. The usual organ for comparison is the kidney, the parenchyma of whiich is less echogenic than that of the liver in the normal adult. The detection of too great a discrepancy (i.e., the liver is significantly and therefore pathologically greater in echogenicity than the kidney) involves the experience of the examiner (Fig. 52-7). This is not a particularly easy observation to make, and thus the accuracy of the detection of diffuse disease falls. Additionally, diffuse disease processes of the kidney tend to increase the ampli-

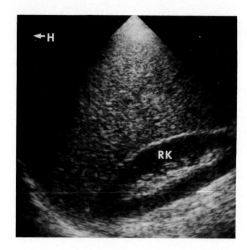

Fig. 52-7 Longitudinal scan reveals too great a discrepancy between echogenicity of liver and right kidney *(RK)*. This suggests hepatic parenchymal infiltration with either fat or fibrosis. Experience of sonographer and comparison with normal studies (see Fig. 52-1) are necessary to evaluate such disparate echogenicities. *H*, Head.

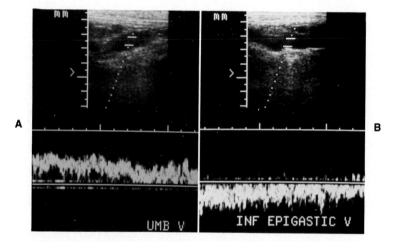

Fig. 52-8 Duplex Doppler examination of umbilical vein **(A)** and inferior epigastric vein **(B)** reveals presence of portosystemic collateral circulation. In these two veins blood is carried in opposite directions, that is, toward umbilicus.

tude of returning renal parenchymal signals. If the kidney is abnormal, therefore, the detection of increased hepatic echogenicity by comparing it to renal echogenicity becomes guesswork.

Diffuse hepatic disease also increases beam attenuation, as evidenced by difficulty in penetrating the hepatic tissue mass (see Fig. 52-2). Fibrotic processes especially tend to do this, although beam attenuation can also be observed in patients with fatty infiltration and other diffuse processes. Again, however, this is a rather subjective observation that is generally difficult to make with confidence until the disease process is relatively advanced.

Despite these difficulties, one usually can detect an altered echogenicity of the liver in patients with hepatocellular diseases.[47,88] Disease processes causing cellular infiltration, fibrosis, and fatty metamorphosis apparently

result in an increased amplitude of the echo signal. In a carefully performed although retrospective analysis, Gosink and co-workers[47] found that independent observers could correctly detect abnormal liver parenchyma in 80% of cirrhotic livers but were unable to distinguish accurately betwen cirrhosis and fatty infiltration. More recently, Needleman and associates,[88] in a comparative study of sonography and liver biopsy, were able to detect changes consistent with a fibrofatty pattern in 71 of 77 patients (92%).

In an effort to quantify liver echogenicity and attenuation, a variety of new ultrasonographic methods currently are being investigated. These include actual measurements of attenuation and backscatter amplitude, as well as modifications that correct for overlying attenuation, transducer effects, and TGC (time, gain, com-

pensation) settings.[40,117] New ways of processing the returning the ultrasound signal are also being evaluated,
such as frequency-modulated (FM) imaging and spectral
analytic techniques (microstructural sonography).[3,62]

Because ultrasound currently is not sensitive for the
detection of mild and diffuse hepatocellular disease processes, other indications have been sought. One sonographic feature that is seen often in patients with portal
hypertension is the presence of portosystemic collateral
veins, including patency of the umbilical and coronary
veins (Fig. 52-8). Some of the less frequently seen
collateral channels include the ductus venosus, splenorenal anastomoses, and splenoretroperitoneal anastomoses.[25,59,90] A second sonographic indication for portal
hypertension is abnormal dilatation of the splanchnic
(portal, splenic, superior mesenteric) veins, as well as
the diminution of the normal increase in size with respiration.[12,104,143] With the recent introduction of abdominal duplex sonography, Doppler examination may convincingly show the presence and direction of the flow in
the portal circulation as well as in collateral vasculature
(Fig. 52-8).[2,89,95]

Another approach used to detect cirrhosis was initially
suggested by Harbin and co-workers,[50] who described a
simple technique for comparing the ratio of the transverse
diameter of the caudate lobe to the right hepatic lobe.
The rationale was that in cirrhotic livers the right lobe
underwent relative shrinkage, whereas the caudate lobe
underwent relative enlargement. In the authors' experience, this technique could detect changes of cirrhosis
with the sensitivity of 84%, a specificity of 100%, and
an accuracy of 84%. A more recent investigation by
Giorgio and associates,[44] however, reported a much lower
sensitivity (43%), although their specificity and diagnostic accuracy remained high.

We disagree with those who suggest that disease processes such as acute hepatitis can result in an overall
diminution of hepatic echoes.[65] Even if this were true,
this observation would be very difficult to differentiate
from artifacts caused by many technical problems, which
can result in a spurious observation of a paucity of hepatic
echoes. In general, no specific hepatic pattern is visible
with either uncomplicated or complicated acute viral hepatitis.[43]

Probably the most important aspect of diffuse hepatocellular processes from the ultrasonographic point of
view is that they usually do not result in a disruption of
the uniformity of echogenicity. In our experience, a disruption of the architectural pattern of the liver indicates
a widespread malignant process, such as diffuse metastases or a multifocal hepatoma.[53] One notable exception
to this rule is focal fatty infiltration of the liver, which
may give the appearance of tumefactions.[61,96] In general,
focal fat deposition appears as areas of increased echo-

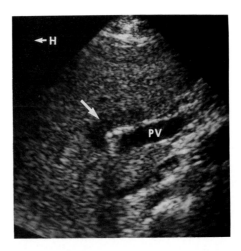

Fig. 52-9 Longitudinal scan obtained at level of portal fissure
(porta hepatis) contains hypoechoic "pseudotumor" that is
ovoid in shape *(arrow)* and caused by focal area of sparing in
patient whose liver is diffusely infiltrated with fat. *H,* Head;
PV, portal vein.

genicity. Characteristic sonographic findings that may
suggest the fatty nature of these masses include angulated, geometric margins between the normal and fatty
tissue, as well as interdigitating margins of slender fingers of normal or fatty tissue.[96] Occasionally, a hypoechoic mass may be present in patients with diffuse hepatic fatty infiltration and may be mistaken for a significant focal pathologic process. This "pseudotumor"
characteristically is located in the medial segment of the
left lobe, has an ovoid shape, and is caused by a focal
area of sparing in a patient whose liver is otherwise
generally infiltrated with fat (Fig. 52-9).[108,133] Rarely,
cirrhotic livers may contain unusual regenerating nodules
that result in architectural alterations and can be mistaken
for a focal process.[38,69,173]

Bearing in mind that these focal processes are unusual,
our opinion remains that architectural alterations should
always be considered a result of a focal disease process
and that malignancy should be first on the differential
diagnostic list until proved otherwise. This is not to say
that malignant processes may not simulate cirrhosis or
fatty infiltration, since diffuse cellular infiltration of the
liver by a lymphoma or other neoplasm can exactly mimic
their appearance.[42]

Focal hepatic lesions
General concepts

Several general features concerning the detection of
focal solid neoplasms should be considered. Although
research is ongoing regarding the development of a useful

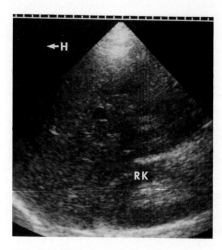

Fig. 52-10 Longitudinal scan through right lobe of liver has minimally abnormal heterogeneous echo pattern. Nonetheless, entire right lobe was infiltrated with metastatic carcinoid tumor. *RK,* Right kidney; *H,* head.

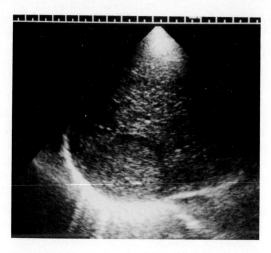

Fig. 52-11 Isoechoic metastatic deposit would be impossible to detect if it were not for hypoechoic halo that surrounds mass.

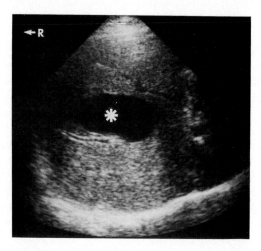

Fig. 52-12 Large simple cyst *(asterisk)* is present in right lobe of liver. Cysts are detected readily because maximal acoustic contrast exists between echogenic hepatic parenchymal tissue and anechoic cyst. *R,* Right.

sonographic parenchymal contrast agent,[80,81] at present sonographers must depend on the intrinsic contrast of a lesion for its detection. Lesions are not detected on the basis of their intrinsic echogenicity, however, but rather on the basis of their echogenicity in contrast to the background echogenicity of the liver; a lesion may be detected because it is either less or more echogenic than the surrounding hepatic tissue. The more shades of gray that distinguish the lesion from the background of liver tissue, the more conspicuous it is.[11]

The hepatic parenchyma returns relatively low-amplitude echoes. These signals are recorded in the lower gray shades of signal processing. Thus the chances of observing a highly reflective lesion are greater than the chances of observing a poorly reflective lesion because more shades of gray distinguish the dense lesion from the hepatic tissue.

In cases of masses that do not deform the contours of an organ, the contrast difference between the lesion and the liver tissue is paramount for detection. A large lesion that is isoechogenic with the liver may be quite subtle, whereas a tiny lesion that is very different in echogenicity from the liver stands out dramatically. One can never be certain that a large "quantity" of disease ensures detection (Fig. 52-10).

In an effort to increase the contrast of focal hepatic lesions relative to hepatic parenchymal tissue, the concept of contrast-enhanced ultrasound is being investigated.[80,81] Angiographically injected microbubbles containing carbon dioxide appear to be a sensitive modality for detecting small hepatic neoplasms.[80] Using this technique, Matsuda and Yabuuchi[80] were able to detect 94%

of primary hepatocellular carcinomas less than 2 cm in size. In comparison, nonenhanced ultrasound detected 75% of lesions, whereas angiography and noncontrast CT visualized 44% and 19% of lesions, respectively. Mattrey and associates[81] have used perfluorochemicals as ultrasound contrast agents to detect hepatic tumors. Fluosol allowed detection of lesions not seen before contrast medium was administered in three of seven patients.

A second consideration that contributes to the detection of focal hepatic nodules relates to the smoothness of the background against which one perceives a nodule. In general, the smoother or more homogeneous the back-

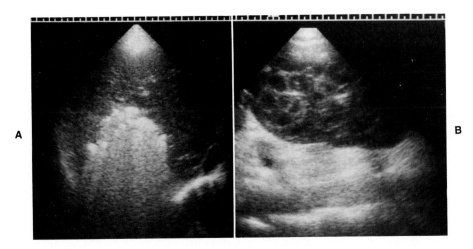

Fig. 52-13 Abscesses vary widely in their sonographic appearances. **A,** Large hepatic mass containing bright echoes that gradually fade and result in a "dirty" acoustic shadow is caused by air-containing abscess. **B,** Large multiloculated hepatic collection is caused by streptococcal abscess.

ground, the more easily a focal mass can be recognized. If the liver parenchyma were grossly nonhomogeneous in its normal state, it would be nearly impossible to detect a further pathologic nonhomogeneity against such a background (Fig. 52-11). For this reason, we have stressed the technical details for obtaining liver ultrasound images displaying a homogeneous hepatic parenchyma.

Cysts

Ultrasonography has been and continues to be one of the most sensitive diagnostic modalities for the detection and characterization of cysts. This is especially true of the liver, where the echogenicity of the hepatic parenchyma presents a good background against which one can easily recognize an anechoic cyst (Fig. 52-12).[118,126]

Cysts are characterized by two sets of criteria: (1) those related to the *physical* interaction of the sonic beam with a fluid of relatively low-protein concentration, low velocity, and low viscosity, and (2) those related to accepted *morphologic* criteria of a benign simple cyst.

Fluids tend to return no echo signals from an ultrasonic beam. Also, fluids of low viscosity and low-protein concentration tend to attenuate the beam very little, resulting in an enhanced transmission of the acoustic beam. Finally, fluids tend to be of lower velocity than the surrounding hepatic tissue, resulting in refraction at the edges of the cystic lesion. This phenomenon is noted on scans by the presence of edge shadows. The refraction phenomenon also causes the rounded cyst to act as a weakly focusing lens, thus increasing the acoustic enhancement.

In terms of the morphologic criteria, simple cysts tend

to have smooth margins and essentially imperceptible walls, and they lack septations. The presence of mural nodules, thick walls, numerous septa, or fluid levels should suggest other probably diagnoses. True cystic metastases and metastases that have undergone extensive liquefaction necrosis may be predominantly fluid filled but demonstrate wall abnormalities that suggest the correct diagnosis.[29,133] Abscesses and *Echinococcus* cysts also tend to show wall abnormalities, septations, or layering of debris that distinguish them from simple hepatic cysts.

Abscesses

The ability of ultrasonography to demonstrate hepatic abscesses has been repeatedly confirmed.[10,26,56,91,100] Ultrasound is a good modality for the detection of abdominal abscesses in general, but is is especially suited for imaging liver abscesses because bowel gas most likely will not obscure this area.

Liver abscess imaging with ultrasonography involves two important features. First, abscesses have a wide variation in appearance. Although most abscesses are sonolucent fluid collections with thick irregular walls, a relatively large percentage of abscesses deviate from this pattern (Fig. 52-13). Fluid-fluid levels, septations, a bull's-eye or target appearance, and diffuse internal echogenicity simulating a solid neoplastic mass are not unusual. In fact, abscesses have a broader spectrum of appearances on ultrasonograms than any other pathologic entity. This should not be surprising because abscesses are highly dynamic and can progress rapidly, altering their appearance as the disease progresses. The second important feature of hepatic abscesses is that they typically are multiple and occasionally exceedingly numerous. The identification of one hepatic abscess should prompt a more intensive search for others within the liver. Although microabscesses under 1 cm in diameter have been demonstrated sonographically, they are usually relatively large and do not pose a problem in detection.[16]

Amebic and echinococcal abscesses have been studied in relatively large series.[10,26,56,100] Although a spectrum of appearances is seen in both instances, ultrasound has served very well in the evaluation of these processes.

Primary hepatic neoplasms
Benign neoplasms

The most frequently encountered benign hepatic neoplasm in our experience has been the *hemangioma*.[41,84,121] Hepatic adenomas and focal nodular hyperplasia have been studied in the literatuure as well.[132] Occasionally a rarer lesion, such as a biliary cystadenoma, is detected.[39] This lesion tends to display internal septa in a manner similar to cystadenomas originating in other organs, but it is important to remember that metastases and abscesses also may demonstrate internal septations.

Hemangiomas, particularly those under 4 cm in diameter, most often generate high-amplitude reflections. However, a hemangioma may demonstrate a variety of other appearances.[84] Even small hemangiomas may appear hypoechoic. Large hemangiomas frequently display irregular internal echogenicity with patchy areas of high-, low-, and intermediate-amplitude echoes (Fig. 52-14). At times, large lesions demonstrate cystlike internal components. These may represent eithe areas of liquefaction necrosis or large, blood-filled lakes. In atypical cases, sonographically guided fine-needle biopsy can be used in an effort to obtain endothelial cells and/or agglomerates of capillaries that are thought to be diag-

nostic.[116] Follow-up examinations of adult patients with hemangiomas have shown that unlike other tumors, they do not increase in size or change in appearance over time; rarely they may decrease in size or disappear, possibly on the basis of degeneration or fibrosis.[41]

Liver cell adenomas have been demonstrated by several investigators. Our own experience tends to confirm the reported observations. Liver cell adenomas tend to be quite discrete but show a variety of echo patterns. Although the internal pattern is usually uniform, it may be either of greater or lesser echogenicity than normal hepatic tissue. The same is true of focal nodular hyperplasia, whose lesions also tend to be discrete. They also have variable echogenicity that may be greater or lesser than that of normal liver tissue.

Interestingly, well-defined lesions seen sonographically may not be perceived in nuclear or CT examinations.[132] This occurs with hemangiomas as well as focal nodular hyperplasia.

On the basis of this experience and extrapolations based on more extensive experience with hepatomas and metastases, it is unlikely that ultrasound will demonstrate specific appearances for benign neoplasms of the liver. Although variations in the echogenicity of mass lesions are obviously related to some biologically specific characteristic, the characteristic is not of a cell type.

Malignant neoplasms

More information is available regarding the ultrasonographic appearances of primary malignant hepatic neoplasms than those of their benign counterparts.[28,112,122,123] The ultrasonographic manifestations of these tumors are similar to those encountered in nuclear and CT studies. *Hepatomas* may be seen as either a large focal lesion or a diffuse disorganization of the hepatic parenchyma (multifocal lesion). As might be anticipated, some patients

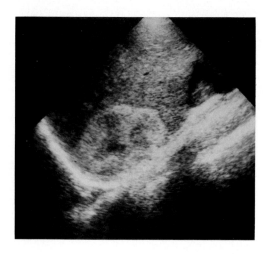

Fig. 52-14 Longitudinal scan through right lobe of liver reveals sharply marginated, primarily hyperechoic mass caused by cavernous hemangioma. As these enlarge, cavernous hemangiomas tend to become increasingly heterogeneous when compared with the well-defined, homogeneously echogenic appearance for capillary hemangiomas.

show features of both patterns. In patients with predisposing conditions such as cirrhosis, chronic hepatitis, and hemachromatosis, these patterns clearly should lead to a presumptive diagnosis of a hepatoma. However, in our and others' experience, hepatomas are relatively common even in patients without predisposing pathologic entities. Thus hepatomas should always be considered in the differential diagnosis of lesions that demonstrate the morphologic features just described.

One identifying feature that should clearly make a hepatoma a leading diagnostic consideration is tumor invasion of the portal or hepatic veins or of the inferior vena cava (Fig. 52-15).[66] Ultrasonography demonstrates these vascular structures well, and intravascular tumor thrombi can be readily detected.

Some insight into the variable sonographic appearances of hepatomas has recently been gained.[28,112,122] Sonography with histologic correlation has revealed that hypoechoic lesions correspond to solid tumors without necrosis and that complex lesions correspond to tumors with partial necrosis, whereas hyperechoic lesions correspond to either fat deposition within the lesion or pronounced sinusoidal dilatation.[122] Not surprisingly, a correlation has been shown between the size of hepatocellular carcinomas and their sonographic appearances. Small tumors (less than 3 cm) tend to be hypoechoic; as they enlarge, they progress to an isoechoic and finally a hyperechoic appearance.[28,112] Although lack of acoustic contrast theoretically would make isoechoic lesions undetectable, a peripheral halo and edge shadowing are often present and allow for their detection (Fig. 52-16).[141]

Although fine-needle aspiration biopsy generally is performed for definitive diagnosis of hepatocellular carcinoma, Taylor and co-workers[124] have recently shown that duplex Doppler ultrasound may be able to differentiate hepatocellular carcinoma from other focal liver masses. An investigation of 68 patients with focal liver lesions revealed that all 10 tumors with Doppler shifts of 5 kHz or greater proved to be primary hepatic malignancies (Fig. 52-17). In contrast, no hemangioma showed shifts greater than 7 kHz, whereas approximately

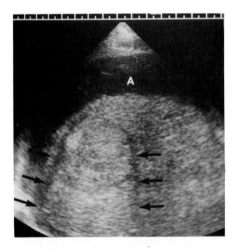

Fig. 52-16 Occasionally hepatomas can be isoechoic with surrounding hepatic parenchymal tissue. Nonetheless, peripheral halo and edge shadowing *(arrows)* are often present and allow for detection of hepatomas. *A,* Ascites.

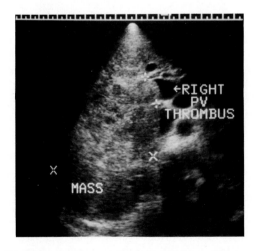

Fig. 52-15 Transverse scan through right lobe of liver reveals large mass invading right portal vein *(PV).* Venous invasion is characteristic feature for hepatoma and is readily visible by sonography.

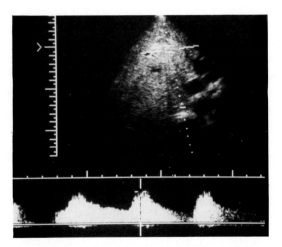

Fig. 52-17 Duplex Doppler examination over hepatoma demonstrates dramatic blood flow, which is particularly evident at periphery of lesion. Very high Doppler signals are thought to be caused by tumor vascularity with multiple arteriovenous communications.

one half of the metastatic lesions had signals up to 4 kHz (the remaining half had no Doppler signal).

The resectability of hepatomas depends on the extent of hepatic involvement as well as the presence or absence of venous invasion or metastases. In a comparative study using CT and ultrasound, LaBerge and associates[66] showed that each modality detected 29 of 30 lesions, for a sensitivity of 96%. Although CT more frequently detected extrahepatic spread of disease, ultrasound was superior for detecting venous invasion. As duplex and color Doppler systems become more available, ultrasound's ability to evaluate patients for vascular invasion should improve even further.

Metastases to the liver

Ultrasonography has been broadly employed in the detection and characterization of hepatic metastases. Individual studies have met with varying success. To our knowledge no study has yet considered ultrasound to be the procedure of choice in this pursuit. Regardless of whether one considers ultrasonography as a sensitive and specific modality for detecting focal hepatic lesions, it clearly can detect many metastases. Because ultrasound studies of the upper abdomen are performed on many patients with abdominal complaints of uncertain origin, a complete awareness of the ultrasonographic appearance of metastases is mandatory. In many of these patients ultrasound may play a pivotal role for initially detecting a neoplastic process. Hepatic metastases are common, and ultrasonographers should aways ensure that their hepatic images are of sufficient quality and sufficiently complete to detect unsuspected lesions.

Echograms display the broadest spectrum of metastatic appearances of all imaging modalities employed for this purpose. Although many terms have been used to describe the appearance of metastases on sonograms, and some authors have chosen to combine rather than split categories, the following list encompasses the variations most often encountered:

1. Echogenicity of metastases greater than that of normal liver tissue
2. Echogenicity of metastases less than that of normal liver tissue
3. Echo-dense metastases that cast an acoustic shadow
4. Metastases with areas of liquefaction (i.e., cystlike metastases)
5. Target or bull's-eye metastases
6. Diffuse disorganization of hepatic parenchyma

Subspectrums occur within these major categories. For example, lesions of greater echogenicity than surrounding hepatic tissue may vary in their relative echo intensity. The same is true of lesions less echogenic than the hepatic parenchyma. Those metastases only slightly greater or slightly less echogenic than the normal hepatic

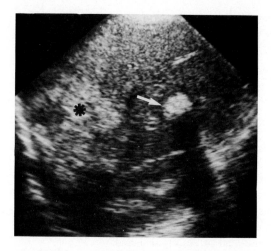

Fig. 52-18 Echogenic intrahepatic focal mass *(arrow)* that casts acoustic shadow is typical for calcium-containing metastasis. This patient also has second lesion *(asterisk)* that, although larger, does not have as pronounced an acoustic shadow.

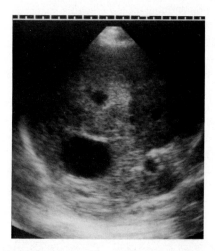

Fig. 52-19 Multiple masses with central necrosis are present in this patient's liver. Although initial perusal may interpret these masses as multiple cysts, careful inspection reveals abnormally echogenic material surrounding "cysts," suggesting that they are caused by tumor necrosis. In this case lesions resulted from metastatic carcinoid tumor.

tissue are more difficult to perceive than metastases much greater or much less echogenic. Preprocessing and postprocessing of the ultrasonic signal may enhance the contrast difference in subtle cases. Calcium-containing metastases cast an acoustic shadow, and the lesion itself is much more echogenic than the surrounding hepatic tissue (Fig. 52-18). In lesions that show an area of liquefaction, two subcategories exist: such lesions may have undergone liquefaction necrosis[137] or may represent true cystic metastases (i.e., nonnecrotic cystic metastatic deposits) (Fig. 52-19). The typical target lesion displays a dense

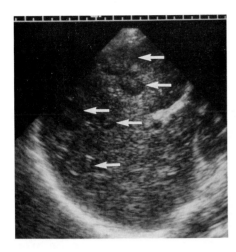

Fig. 52-20 Target lesions *(arrows)* that have dense echogenic center surrounded by rim of hypoechoic tissue frequently are caused by adenocarcinoma. In this case primary lesion was located in colon.

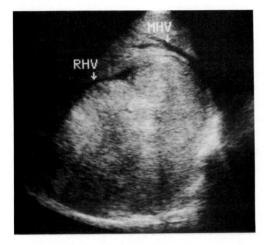

Fig. 52-21 Transverse scan obtained near dome of right lobe demonstrates fairly homogeneous mass with echo texture similar to surrounding hepatic parenchymal tissue. Nonetheless, focal displacement and indentation of right hepatic vein *(RHV)* are clearly evident and serve as clues for presence of mass. Fine-needle aspiration biopsy revealed primary hepatocellular carcinoma. *MHV,* Middle hepatic vein.

echogenic center surrounded by a rim of hypoechoic tissue (Fig. 52-20). Occasionally one encounters a lesion with a hypoechoic center and a hyperechoic rim. Additional variations of the target lesion involve differences in the depth of the surrounding rim of material, which may be thick or thin.

The most difficult hepatic sonogram to interpret is one that shows diffuse disorganization of the hepatic parenchyma. In such cases it may be difficult to pick out individual nodules within the hepatic parenchyma. Occasionally the pattern is predominantly more echogenic or less echogenic, but most often it is a mixture of the two. In evaluating these cases, one must seek ultrasonographic information confirming that the disorganization results in space-occupying nodules. This may be accomplished by carefully scanning for discrete nodules or for evidence of distortion caused by nodules. A higher frequency transducer may sometimes be successful for depicting discrete nodules, which may appear as a disorganized pattern when the lower-frequency transducer is used. Distortions may be seen on the surface of the liver or in visible fissures of the liver, such as the fissure of the venous ligament. The observation of indentations on the surface of the intrahepatic inferior vena cava, gallbladder, or intrahepatic vessels is also useful to confirm that the disorganized hepatic parenchyma is caused by multiple intrahepatic nodules (Fig. 52-21).

Originally many hoped that the numerous appearances of metastatic deposits on ultrasonograms could lead to a better prediction of the primary lesion in patients with metastases from unknown origins. Several investigations have now shown that cell type is not responsible for the acoustic appearance of metastases.[91,109] Also, however, the variety of appearances demonstrated on acoustic studies clearly is not spurious. The ultrasonogram offers some biologically specific information about hepatic lesions, but unfortunately in most instances it is still not clear what the specific information represents.

Recently Marchal and co-workers[77] have evaluated the etiology for the anechoic halo typically seen in metastatic liver lesions (see Fig. 52-20). Using microangiographic techniques and histologic correlation, they determined that in 18 of 20 lesions, the halo was extratumoral and was caused by peritumoral liver compression. In the remaining two cases the halo was caused by the tumor itself and was associated with irregular fibrosis or vascularization. In an attempt to distinguish hepatocellular carcinoma from metastatic liver disease, Yoshida and co-workers[141] have noted that a lateral shadow appears to be specific for primary hepatic malignancy and may be caused by the presence of a surrounding capsule (see Fig. 52-16).

Ultrasonography has also been useful in following the chemotherapeutic response of hepatic metastases.[9] In general, an excellent correlation has existed with ancillary imaging modalities when the ultrasonogram demonstrated no change, an improvement, or a progression. Ultrasonography is less expensive than CT, angiography, or magnetic resonance imaging (MRI) and has the advantage of being able to evaluate other complications of a malignancy that cannot be seen on nuclear scans of the liver.

Ultrasound has also been very useful as an adjunct to other imaging modalities when their results were either equivocal or indeterminate. As shown in the study of Sullivan and associates,[120] ultrasound can be used to enhance the diagnostic accuracy of liver scintigrams interpreted as equivocal for metastatic disease. In general, although nuclear scans are sensitive, ultrasound has greater specificity and diagnostic accuracy.

Ultrasound has also been shown to complement CT examinations, particularly in patients with cystic or necrotic hepatic neoplasms[29] or in those with small focal liver masses.[13] In comparison to CT, sonography is superior for determining the internal morphology of cystic hepatic lesions. Because of volume averaging, CT may also have difficulty differentiating small liver cysts (less than 2 cm) from solid hepatic lesions. In these indeterminate cases ultrasound can be used to determine the true nature of the lesions.

In our experience the perfect test for the detection of hepatic metastases clearly has yet to be devised. Ample room exists, however, for the thoughtful use of CT, ultrasonography, MRI, and nuclear scans of the liver in evaluation of a variety of patients that does not constitute a simple repetition of data gathering.

GALLBLADDER

During the past decade cholecystosonography has replaced oral cholecystography as the modality of choice for imaging the gallbladder. This is because ultrasound:

1. Lacks ionizing radiation
2. Can detect more calculi than can oral cholecystography
3. Does not require contrast material
4. Can be performed on acutely ill patients
5. Is independent of gastrointestinal, hepatic, and biliary function
6. Can image multiple other organs of the upper abdomen

Recent technologic advances, particularly in real-time imaging, allow for rapid acquisition of high-resolution images. When compared to static articulated arm equipment, real-time machines are less operator dependent and can visualize the gallbladder rapidly and in its entirety. Indications for performing an ultrasound examination of the gallbladder include signs and symptoms suggestive of acute or chronic cholecystitis, jaundice, abnormal liver functions, and pancreatitis.

Normal gallbladder

A normal gallbladder, physiologically distended following an 8- to 12-hour fast, can be visualized in virtually 100% of cases. Rarely, massive obesity or overlying distended loops of bowel may preclude visualization. In general a mechanical or electronically focused sector transducer is preferred to a linear array tranducer for examining the gallbladder, since it is easier to place the smaller face of the sector transducer subcostally or within rib interspaces. For most patients a 3.5 MHz transducer is required, but in thin patients or in those with an anteriorly positioned gallbladder, a 5.0 MHz transducer is preferable because it provides superior resolution. The gallbladder should be examined during suspended respiration, usually following a deep inspiratory effort.

The examination is usually performed with the patient lying supine or in a left posterior oblique (LPO) position.[37] Occasionally, however, an erect position or even placing the patient prone will be necessary to evaluate properly for the presence or absence of calculi.[93] Prone views may also be helpful to eliminate rib artifacts that may arise from the anterior abdominal wall or overlying bowel. A special effort should be made to examine the region of the gallbladder neck, which, because of its dependent position, is where most calculi are found. An experienced operator can complete a thorough examination of the gallbladder in 5 to 10 minutes.

Anatomic considerations

The fundus of the gallbladder has no absolute anatomic relationship with other structures in the abdomen and occasionally may be found in unusual areas. The neck of the gallbladder, however, bears a constant relationship to the undivided right portal vein or main portal

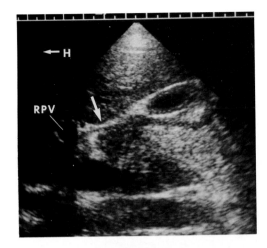

Fig. 52-22 Longitudinal scan through right hepatic lobe reveals linear echo *(arrow)* extending between right portal vein *(RPV)* and gallbladder neck. This line is caused by visible segment of interlobar hepatic fissure and serves as useful anatomic landmark for identification of gallbladder fossa region. Thickening of gallbladder wall results from physiologic contraction. *H*, Head.

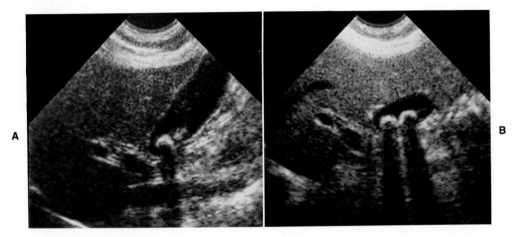

Fig. 52-23 A, Two echogenic foci are visible near gallbladder neck. Acoustic shadowing is visible behind one of these foci, consistent with calculus. Etiology for second mass is indeterminate on this scan. **B,** Repeat scan now shows acoustic shadowing behind both foci, consistent with two gallstones. It is important for gallstones to be contained within central portion of ultrasound beam in order to crease acoustic shadow.

(From Laing, FC: Ultrasonography of the biliary tree. In Sarti, DA, editor: Diagnostic ultrasound: text and cases, ed 2, Chicago, 1987, Yearbook Medical Publishers. With permission.)

vein near the origin of the left portal vein.[15,68] In approximately 70% of cases a visible segment of the interlobar hepatic fissure can be seen as an echogenic line that extends between the right portal vein and the gallbladder neck. This linear echo is a reliable indicator of the gallbladder's location (Fig. 52-22).[15] An important anatomic consideration is that the gallbladder resides in a fossa within the liver, whereas the duodenum and hepatic flexures of the colon do not. Although the normal gallbladder is easily visualized and recognized on sonograms, these anatomic features become useful when the characteristic appearance for the gallbladder is altered by various pathologic conditions.

Calculus disease

Many studies have been published that attest to ultrasound's high overall sensitivity, specificity, and accuracy and its low false-positive and false-negative rate for detecting gallstones.[20,21,24,82,119] Almost without exception, these publications report sensitivities, specificities, and accuracies greater than 95%.* Indeed, it has been shown repeatedly that ultrasound can detect gallstones not visualized with oral cholecystography despite an adequate concentration of dye.[20,21,23,64] Importantly, gastrointestinal, hepatic, and biliary function have no effect on the

---

*References 20, 21, 24, 64, 82, 119, and 136.

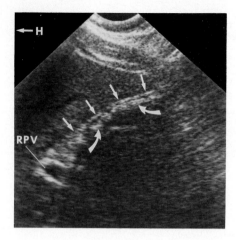

Fig. 52-24 If gallbladder is filled with multiple stones, its sonographic appearance changes such that gallbladder itself may not be visible. Instead, one may detect anterior gallbladder wall *(straight arrows)* with adjacent superficial layer of calculi *(curved arrows)*. Bile and posterior wall of gallbladder are rendered invisible because of large acoustic shadow. *RPV,* Right portal vein; *H,* head.

quality of the ultrasonic examination or its ability to detect calculi.

Intraluminal gallstones have different sonographic appearances. Some of these appearances are extremely reliable for indicating the presence of cholelithiasis, whereas others must be interpreted with caution. The most reliable features for stone detection include (1) the presence of a high-amplitude, intraluminal reflection that casts an acoustic shadow and (2) gravity-dependent movement. The second feature, which is most easily demonstrated with real-time equipment, unequivocally establishes the diagnosis. It is not mandatory, however, to demonstrate movement if a characteristic stone has been detected.

In vitro investigations have shown that all gallstones whose diameter exceeds 1 mm should cast an acoustic shadow regardless of composition, surface characteristics, and shape. Not all stones scanned in vivo, however, will have associated posterior acoustic shadowing.[32] The general rule to remember is that it is easier to detect the high-amplitude reflection caused by the stone than to demonstrate the accompanying acoustic shadow.

Nonetheless, demonstrating an acoustic shadow is more than an academic exercise. Shadowing echo densities within the gallbladder are correlated with cholelithiasis in almost 100% of cases, whereas nonshadowing echo densities are correlated with stones in one half.[21] Unfortunately, technical features can occasionally obscure visualization of an acoustic shadow (Fig. 52-23). Because posterior shadowing is best seen if the stone is situated within the central portion of a narrow beam of sound, a transducer should be used that has the highest possible frequency and is maximally focused at the depth of the stone. Aggregates of small stones acoustically behave as a larger stone in their ability to create an acoustic shadow.[17,49] In difficult cases, repositioning the patient may cause small stones to pile up on one another;

the shadow then is identified more easily. In addition, the time-gain compensation curve should be adjusted so that acoustic enhancement posterior to the gallbladder does not obliterate a faint shadow. The stone size and the velocity difference between the stone and the surrounding bile are the key factors in the ease of demonstration of an acoustic shadow. The smaller the stone and the less the velocity difference, the more difficult it is to demonstrate the acoustic shadow.

As the gallbladder progressively contracts about multiple intraluminal stones or as the lumen progressively fills with stones, the sonographic appearance of the gallbladder changes dramatically.[67] Instead of seeing a well-defined gallbladder outline, a high-amplitude echo with prominent acoustic shadowing is seen in the region of the gallbladder fossa (Fig. 52-24). The echo-shadow complex is caused by reflections and absorption of sound from the most superficial layer of stones. More deeply located stones as well as the intraluminal bile and the posterior wall of the gallbladder are rendered invisible. In most of these cases close scrutiny of the scans allows the appropriate diagnosis of cholelithiasis to be made by identifying the anterior gallbladder wall as well as the most superficial layer of calculi.[102] Other pathologic conditions that may have a similar sonographic appearance include calcification in the gallbladder wall (porcelain gallbladder)[60] or air in the gallbladder wall (emphysematous cholecystitis).[55,94] In the latter situation reverberation artifacts from the air should suggest the correct diagnosis (Fig. 52-25).

In fewer than 1% of fasting patients, one cannot identify either the gallbladder or the shadowing from its fossa. This constitutes true nonvisualization of the gallbladder by ultrasonography.[51] Even in this situation, the implication is strong that the gallbladder is abnormal. Nonetheless, nonvisualization of the gallbladder by ultrasonography should not be considered sufficiently strong

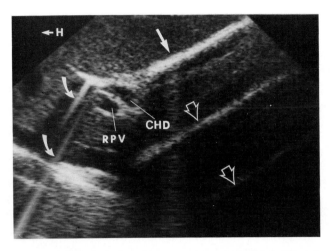

Fig. 52-25 Very bright echogenic line *(straight arrow)* present in right subhepatic space is caused by air within gallbladder. Note also presence of multiple echogenic reverberative artifacts *(open arrows)*. Comet-tail reverberations *(curved arrows)* are caused by air in common hepatic duct *(CHD)*. *RPV*, Right portal vein; *H*, head.

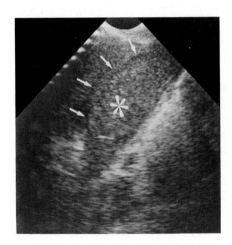

Fig. 52-26 Occasionally gallbladder may be filled with echogenic sludge *(asterisk)* such that its echo texture is similar to hepatic parenchymal tissue. Careful scanning usually can identify gallbladder wall *(arrows)*, which aids in identification of gallbladder. *H*, Head.
(From Laing, FC: Ultrasonography of the gallbladder and biliary tree. In Sarti, DA, editor: Diagnostic ultrasound: text and cases, ed 2, Chicago, 1987, Yearbook Medical Publishers. With permission.)

evidence to warrant surgical excision of the gallbladder without confirmatory studies. In patients with acute hepatitis the gallbladder occasionally may be difficult to detect because it becomes severely contracted. Presumably this results from acute hepatic dysfunction that may transiently decrease bile flow into the gallbladder.[31] After the acute phase of hepatitis the gallbladder size returns to normal.

Another unusual cause for gallbladder "nonvisualization" is when the gallbladder is filled with echogenic sludge (see later discussion) that has a similar echo amplitude to hepatic parenchymal tissue (Fig. 52-26).[105] In this situation careful real-time scanning usually can identify the gallbladder as being filled with extremely echogenic bile.

Although most gallstones behave in a characteristic fashion, atypical stones occasionally may be encountered. These include stones that are adherent or embedded within the gallbladder wall, stones that float (in the presence of either cholecystographic contrast material or in native bile) (Fig. 52-27),[140] or stones that are relatively less echogenic than usual (Fig. 52-28). Less echogenic stones have been noted primarily in patients with soft stones that have a mudlike consistency. These so-called soft stones are currently of great interest in assessing whether or not sludge may occasionally be a precursor for gallstones.[14,57]

Since real-time ultrasound has been used to detect cholelithiasis, many artifacts that were previously seen with articulated arm equipment have been eliminated. It

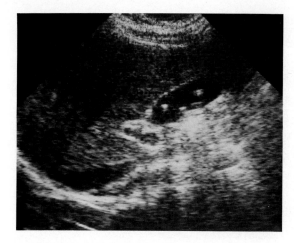

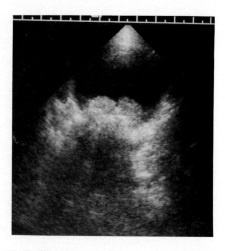

Fig. 52-27 Supine longitudinal scan reveals multiple floating gallstones in patient who has not received oral cholecystographic contrast material. Their floating appearance suggests that these stones are less dense than bile.

Fig. 52-28 Gallbladder contains two unusual gallstones that cast acoustic shadows but are less echogenic than usual. Although this appearance may be seen with soft, calcium bilirubinate pigment stones, in this patient CT suggested stones were composed primarily of cholesterol.

is important to stress the technical aspects of the examination to eliminate motion and reverberative artifacts.

One artifact that can be particularly troublesome results from shadowing that appears to arise from the neck region of the gallbladder. Because refraction can cause shadowing in this anatomic location, it is mandatory to visualize the stone and not merely an acoustic shadow before diagnosing cholelithiasis. Similarly, shadows posterior to the gallbladder that emanate from bowel should not be misconstrued as suggestive features for primary gallbladder pathology.

Acute cholecystitis

Ultrasound can be used effectively in the evaluation of patients with acute right upper quadrant pain who are suspected to have acute cholecystitis.[24,72,101,114,138] Although some tests, such as those employing ^{99m}Tc-labeled iminidiacetic acid (IDA) and IDA-like compounds, can be extremely specific for diagnosing cystic duct obstruction and acute cholecystitis,[18,106,130,131] many different pathologic entities must be considered in patients with acute right upper quadrant pain. Pathologic processes involving the liver, right kidney, bowel, pancreas, appendix, and even the ovary can cause symptoms that mimic acute cholecystitis. Only about one in three patients who have acute right upper quadrant pain are shown subsequently to have acute cholecystitis.[72] Because ultrasound can survey the entire abdomen rapidly and can diagnose acute cholecystitis as well as many other conditions that can mimic acute gallbladder disease, we believe that sonography should be the imaging modality of choice for initially evaluating these patients.

The ultrasonographic diagnosis of acute cholecystitis can be made if a patient has focal tenderness over the gallbladder fossa in association with calculi.[72,101] The presence of sludge and a thickened gallbladder wall (see following section) lend further support to this diagnosis (Fig. 52-29). Chronic cholecystitis, seen in 30% of patients clinically suspected of acute cholecystitis, can be diagnosed in patients whose gallbladders contain stones but are not focally tender. Focal pain elsewhere frequently allows ultrasound to make the appropriate diagnosis of a pathologic condition unrelated to the gallbladder in patients with incidental cholelithiasis. In the series of Laing and co-workers,[72] 35% of patients with acute right upper quadrant pain had normal gallbladders. These patients failed to exhibit pain directly over the gallbladder fossa. Not surprisingly, ultrasound was able to pinpoint the pathologic source in many of these individuals.

Gallbladder wall

Ultrasound normally perceives the gallbladder wall as a thin echogenic line whose thickness is 3 mm or less. When the gallbladder wall thickens, it usually does so in a diffuse and symmetric fashion. The wall typically becomes hypoechoic and is surrounded on either side by echogenic lines (Fig. 52-30). Although diffuse gallbladder wall thickening initially was considered to be highly specific for acute cholecystitis, it is now recognized as neither sensitive nor specific for primary gallbladder inflammation. Only 50% to 75% of patients with acute cholecystitis have thickened gallbladder walls; furthermore, fewer than 25% of patients with chronic chole-

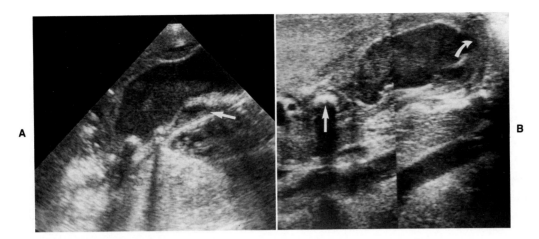

A

B

Fig. 52-29 Two longitudinal scans obtained from different patients, each of whom were proved surgically to have acute gangrenous cholecystitis. **A,** In addition to multiple gallstones, intraluminal sludge and irregular thickening *(arrow)* of the gallbladder wall are present. **B,** In addition to intraluminal stones and sludge, stone is impacted in cystic duct *(straight arrow),* and focal wall irregularity appears in fundus of gallbladder *(curved arrow)* because of impending perforation. *H,* Head.

(From Laing, FC: Ultrasonography of the gallbladder and biliary tree. In Sarti, DA, editor: Diagnostic ultrasound: text and cases, ed 2, Chicago, 1987, Yearbook Medical Publishers. With permission.)

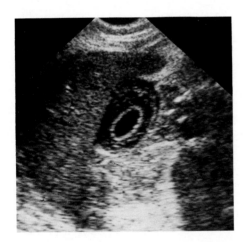

Fig. 52-30 Diffuse gallbladder wall thickening is present in this patient with severe hypoalbuminemia. No clinical evidence for acute cholecystitis was found.

(From Laing, FC: Ultrasonography of the gallbladder and biliary tree. In Sarti, DA, editor: Diagnostic ultrasound: text and cases, ed 2, Chicago, 1987, Yearbook Medical Publisher. With permission.)

cystitis display this finding.[72] Most patients with diffuse gallbladder wall thickening do not even have primary gallbladder disease. This appearance can be seen with hepatic dysfunction (associated with alcoholism, hypoalbuminemia, ascites, and hepatitis), congestive heart failure, renal disease, neoplasm, and sepsis.[36,99,113,127] Although the precise pathophysiologic mechanism that leads to diffuse gallbladder wall thickening has yet to be explained, many of these patients share decreased intravascular osmotic pressure and elevated portal venous pressure.

A more specific observation for primary gallbladder disease is focal gallbladder wall thickening. This can occur with various pathologic processes, including pri-

mary gallbladder carcinoma, polyps, cholesterolosis, papillary adenomas, metastases, adenomyomatosis, and occasionally tumefactive sludge. Primary gallbladder carcinoma has a variety of sonographic appearances (Fig. 52-31). In approximately 40% of cases carcinoma is seen either as a focal mass protruding into the gallbladder lumen or as an asymmetric thickening of the gallbladder wall.[128] Additional clues to this diagnosis include evidence for metastatic disease (liver metastases, direct hepatic invasion, adenopathy, bile duct dilatation) and cholelithiasis (80% to 90% of cases). The diagnosis of adenomyomatosis can be suggested when anechoic or echogenic foci are visible within the thickened gallbladder wall. Intraluminal diverticula (Rokitansky-Aschoff

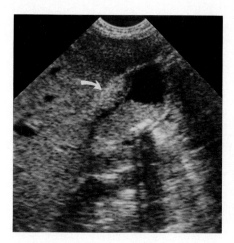

Fig. 52-31 Localized thickening is visible along anterior gall-bladder wall *(arrow)* and is caused by primary gallbladder carcinoma. In addition, sludge and multiple gallstones are present in dependent portion of gallbladder.
(From Laing, FC: Ultrasonography of the gallbladder and biliary tree. In Sarti, DA, editor: Diagnostic ultrasound: text and cases, ed 2, Chicago, 1987, Yearbook Medical Publishers. With permission.)

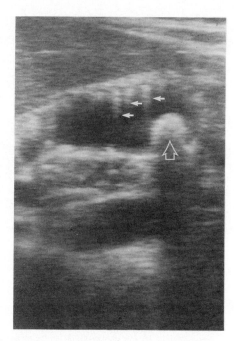

Fig. 52-32 Intramural calculi associated with adenomyomatosis are present in this patient's gallbladder. Note echogenic foci within gallbladder wall and their associated comet-tail artifacts *(closed arrows)*. Incidental gallstone *(open arrow)* is also present.

sinuses) that contain bile most likely are responsible for the anechoic areas, whereas sludge or small calculi probably are responsible for the echogenic foci (Fig. 52-32).[97]

A final cause for focal gallbladder wall changes is gangrenous cholecystitis. In approximately 50% of these patients, severe irregularity of the gallbladder wall occurs because of mucosal ulceration, hemorrhage, necrosis, or microabscess formation in the wall (see Fig. 52-29).[58]

Pericholecystic fluid

Localized pericholecystic fluid most often results from acute cholecystitis with associated gallbladder perforation and abscess formation.[76] Focal abscesses typically are located adjacent to the gallbladder fundus because of the sparse vascular supply to this region. Similar to other inflammatory fluid collections, most pericholecystic abscesses have a complex appearance and may contain linear groupings of echoes because of the high protein content within the fluid.

Another cause for a focal pericholecystic fluid collection, although rare, is pancreatitis, peptic ulcer disease, or both.[92] The etiology for this fluid is presumed to be extension of the primary inflammatory process along the hepatoduodenal ligament into the main lobar fissure, where it comes to rest adjacent to the gallbladder neck.

Sludge

Intraluminal sludge (echogenic bile) can be seen in several unrelated clinical conditions. In most cases these nonshadowing echoes are situated dependently within the

gallbladder; because echo-free bile usually layers on the sludge, a fluid-fluid level is usually visible (Fig. 52-33).[19,34] Frequently the sludge moves slowly with changes of the patient's position, indicating that it is viscous. Occasionally sludge can have an atypical appearance, since it may shift its position rapidly and mimic multiple small, nonshadowing calculi.[19] Sometimes sludge is admixed with echo-free bile, or it may settle focally within the gallbladder to simulate a mass. Occasionally sludge fills the entire lumen of the gallbladder, generating an atypical appearance of the gallbladder (see Fig. 52-26).[105] By using the specific anatomic clues previously discussed, these atypical gallbladders can usually be recognized without difficulty. In patients with gallbladder sludge one must appropriately adjust the output and time-gain compensation settings to identify small calculi that may be present within the sludge.

Artifactual echoes within the gallbladder lumen occasionally may create the false impression of sludge. Pseudosludge can occur as a result of beam thickness[35] or side-lobe artifacts.[70] A beam-thickness, also known as a slice-thickness, artifact is caused by beam averaging or a partial volume effect in the diverging portion of the ultrasound beam. This occurs when part of the ultrasound beam interacts with a fluid-filled structure while an ad-

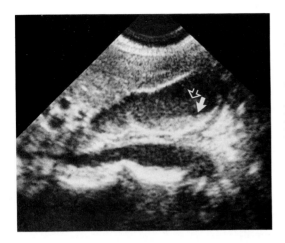

Fig. 52-33 Patient's gallbladder contains unusual appearing sludge or echogenic bile. Note two distinct fluid levels, with most dependent level composed of relatively echogenic sludge *(closed arrow)*, whereas more superficial layer is composed of slightly less echogenic sludge *(open arrow)*.
(From Laing, FC: Ultrasonography of the gallbladder and biliary tree. In Sarti, DA, editor: Diagnostic ultrasound: text and cases, ed 2, Chicago, 1987, Yearbook Medical Publishers. With permission.)

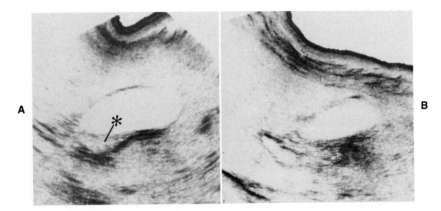

Fig. 52-34 A, Longitudinal scan through gallbladder shows what appears to be dependent sludge *(asterisk)*. In this patient, however, echoes were artifactual and caused by transducer side lobes reflecting off adjacent bowel gas. **B,** Note that artifactual echoes disappeared after decreasing transducer output and changing angulation of transducer away from adjacent gas-filled bowel loops.
(From Laing, FC, and Kurtz, AB: The importance of ultrasonic side-lobe artifacts, Radiology 145:767, 1982. With permission.)

jacent portion of the beam interacts with actual echo reflectors. Side-lobe artifacts result from the presence of transducer side lobes, which consist of multiple, lower-intensity sound beams located outside the main beam. If side-lobe echoes reflect off bowel gas located adjacent to the gallbladder, they may appear as diffuse or sludge-like echoes within the gallbladder lumen (Fig. 52-34). Both beam-thickness and side-lobe artifacts depend on transducer angulation and are independent of gravity. Changing the patient's position, changing the angulation of the transducer, or repositioning the transducer away from gas-filled structures usually eliminates these troublesome echoes.

The most frequent predisposing factor leading to true sludge is bile stasis, which can occur with an obstruction to the biliary tree at the level of the neck of the gall-

bladder, cystic duct, or common bile duct or following a prolonged fast or hyperalimentation.[19,34,47] Because sludge has been shown to be evanescent, it is thought to be a reflection of both functional and organic disease. All patients undergoing a prolonged fast do not develop sludge.

The origin of the echoes within sludge has been the subject of both speculation and more recently experimentation. Although an abnormally increased viscosity has been mentioned,[19,22] particulate matter within bile seems to be a more reasonable explanation. In vitro investigations have shown that all fluids, including those with a very high viscosity, are echo free.[33] Further in vitro work, including progressive filtration of echogenic bile, has revealed that the echoes are caused by particulate matter composed predominantly of calcium bilirubinate

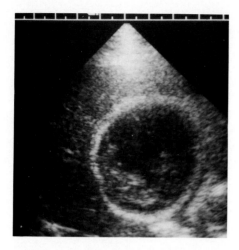

Fig. 52-35 Hemobilia secondary to complications that resulted from liver biopsy is responsible for echogenic material within this gallbladder. Note that appearance of hemorrhagic bile is almost identical to sludge.

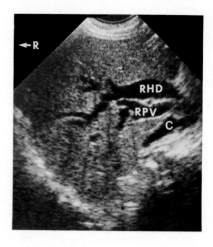

Fig. 52-36 Scan obtained parallel to long axis of right portal vein *(RPV)* demonstrates adjacent anterior tubular structure caused by dilated right hepatic duct *(RHD)*. Between these two tubular structures is a small, circular sonolucency caused by right hepatic artery. *C,* Inferior vena cava; *R,* right.
(From Laing, FC: Ultrasonography of the gallbladder and biliary tree. In Sarti, DA, editor: Diagnostic ultrasound: text and cases, ed 2, Chicago, 1987, Yearbook Medical Publishers. With permission.)

crystals and to a lesser degree of cholesterol crystals.[34,45] The particulate nature of a material and the velocity change between the crystals and the fluid that surrounds them, rather than its chemical composition, probably are responsible for echoes within the fluid. Cellular debris, pus, blood clots, and protein macroaggregates also have been associated with echogenic fluid.[1,19,125] In patients with acute cholecystitis, therefore, low-level nonshadowing echoes may result from a variety of sources, including echogenic bile, pus, and hemorrhage (Fig. 52-35).

In summary, echogenic bile usually is caused by crystalline particles that can be seen in various clinical conditions. Although bile's presence within the gallbladder suggests an underlying abnormality, this does not necessarily imply a primary gallbladder pathologic condition, since sludge frequently appears in patients with biliary stasis from different sources. The presence of sludge should not be ignored, however, because it may represent the only detectable sonographic abnormality in a patient with a primary gallbladder pathologic condition. Further investigatory work is needed to assess whether echogenic bile can be clinically harmful, that is, whether it can irritate the gallbladder mucosa or act as a precursor to stone formation.

BILE DUCTS

Ultrasonography is particularly well suited for tracking and identifying tubular, fluid-filled structures, regardless of whether these structures are blood vessels or bile ducts. Because of ultrasound's ability to detect early changes associated with intrahepatic and extrahepatic

duct dilatation, many consider this modality the procedure of choice in the initial evaluation of the jaundiced patient.

Intrahepatic bile ducts of normal caliber are below the limits of resolution of standard ultrasonographic equipment. Although they can be visualized, the normal left and right hepatic ducts do not lie within the hepatic parenchyma but are extrahepatic and course within the undivided portion of the right portal vein or initial segment of the left portal vein, respectively. Extrahepatic bile ducts of normal caliber, including the right and left hepatic ducts, common hepatic duct, and common bile duct, can be consistently visualized. For this reason methods of detection of dilatation in the intrahepatic and extrahepatic ductal systems are considered separately.

Intrahepatic bile ducts
Features of dilatation

When intrahepatic bile ducts dilate, they cross a threshold of visibility and lie parallel to the normally visible branches of the intrahepatic portal veins. Four criteria enable one to distinguish dilated intrahepatic bile ducts from portal veins.[71]

ALTERATION IN ANATOMIC PATTERN OF PORTAL VEINS

A change in the anatomy of portal veins is the most reliable feature for the identification of dilated intrahepatic ducts and can be observed in virtually all patients with generalized intrahepatic bile duct dilatation. Normally the intrahepatic segments of the portal vein are invariably seen as solitary structures because the intrahepatic components of the hepatic ducts and arteries are below the limits of resolution. When intrahepatic bile ducts dilate, two or more tubular structures can be identified in the expected location of the solitary portal veins (Fig. 52-36). This alteration of anatomy is detected most easily within the right hepatic lobe, where the dilated intrahepatic ducts accompany the divisions of the right portal vein.

IRREGULAR WALLS OF DILATED BILE DUCTS

As the intrahepatic biliary system becomes progressively more dilated, the course and caliber of the ducts become increasingly tortuous and irregular. This observation, which has long been seen with transhepatic cholangiograms, can be demonstrated sonographically as well. In contrast, the walls of the portal veins are smooth and gradually taper as the vessels proceed toward the liver periphery. Of the 50 patients reviewed by Laing and co-workers,[71] 31 showed this feature (62%).

STELLATE CONFLUENCE OF DILATED DUCTS

In patients with moderate to severe bile duct dilatation, a stellate grouping of tubular structures can be seen at points where the ducts converge (Fig. 52-37). This appearance, which has been compared to the spokes of a wheel, can be seen in approximately two thirds of patients with intrahepatic bile duct dilatation. Because portal veins at times may simulate this appearance, it should not be used as the sole diagnostic feature for distinguishing between so-called medical and surgical jaundice.

ACOUSTIC ENHANCEMENT

Enhanced transmission of sounds through dilated bile ducts is present approximately 55% to 60% of the time (Fig. 52-37)[71] and results because bile does not significantly attenuate the sound beam. Conversely, blood, because of its high protein content, has a dramatic attenuative effect on the transmission of the acoustic beam.[33] Since acoustic enhancement occasionally can be seen behind portal veins, this feature alone should not be considered as diagnostic of bile duct dilatation.

•   •   •

Of the four features just described, the anatomic alteration of the appearance of the intrahepatic portal radicles is the most reliable. The remaining three features, when present, should be considered only confirmatory findings.

Pathologic conditions

In most patients intrahepatic bile duct dilatation results from an extrahepatic obstructive lesion, usually at the level of the pancreatic head. Occasionally, however, the primary problem may be localized to the liver or may

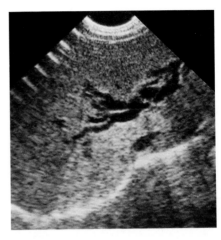

Fig. 52-37 Within substance of right lobe of liver are irregular, tortuous-appearing tubular structures that appear to converge centrally. In addition to stellate and tortuous configuration of bile ducts, enhanced sound transmission is present. These features are diagnostic for dilated intrahepatic bile ducts.
(From Laing, FC: Ultrasonography of the gallbladder and biliary tree. In Sarti, DA, editor: Diagnostic ultrasound: text and cases, ed 2, Chicago, 1987, Yearbook Medical Publishers. With permission.)

represent a combined intrahepatic and extrahepatic disease process.

Because the ultrasonographic identification of intrahepatic bile duct dilatation usually depends on the characteristic altered pattern of the portal veins in the region of the portal fissure (porta hepatis), focal and especially isolated peripheral bile duct dilatation can be easily overlooked. This pattern of dilatation can occur if a localized intrahepatic process can obstruct the bile ducts. Strategically positioned, space-occupying masses (especially primary hepatocellular carcinoma), intrahepatic calculi, and focal stricturing each can result in segmental biliary obstruction. Rarely, nonobstructive dilatation of intrahepatic bile ducts can be seen in association with Caroli's disease.[78]

Segmental biliary obstruction associated with intrahepatic calculi occurs most often in patients with recurrent pyogenic cholangiohepatitis (RPC), also known as Oriental cholangiohepatitis.[29,98] The sonograms in these patients are usually characteristic and differ in many respects from patients with typical gallstone choledocholithiasis. In these patients multiple intrahepatic stones are usually visible in both intrahepatic and extrahepatic bile ducts. Because these stones are soft and are composed primarily of bile pigment, as opposed to cholesterol, sonography may show calculi that are of only medium echo intensity and that may not be associated with acoustic shadowing. As a result these stones can form a cast of the biliary tree that can mimic sludge or even an intrahepatic bile duct neoplasm (Fig. 52-38). Occasionally, however, acoustic shadowing can predominate and

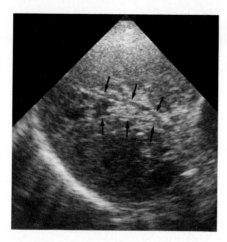

Fig. 52-38 Intrahepatic pigment stones caused by recurrent pyogenic cholangiohepatitis are creating cast within dilated right intrahepatic bile duct *(arrows)*. Note how similar echogenicity of these stones are when compared to that of sludge. (From Laing, FC: Comput Tomogr Magn Reson 8:108, 1987. With permission.)

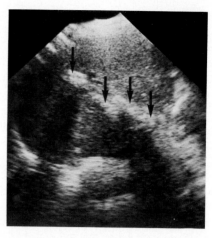

Fig. 52-39 In this patient with recurrent pyogenic cholangiohepatitis, intrahepatic calculi are much more echogenic *(arrows)* than in Fig. 52-38 and are associated with prominent acoustic shadowing. Shadowing can be so dramatic that it obliterates visualization of bile ducts in manner similar to gallbladder filled with multiple small stones.
(From Laing, FC: Comput Tomogr Magn Reson 8:107, 1987. With permission.)

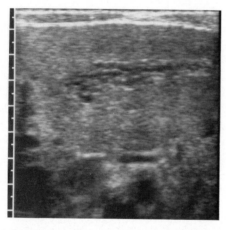

Fig. 52-40 Transverse scan over left lobe of liver obtained in patient with AIDS cholangitis. Primary finding consists of generalized periductal hypoechoic areas surrounding mildly dilated intrahepatic bile ducts.
(From Dolmatch, BL, et al: AIDS-related cholangitis: radiographic findings in nine patients, Radiology 163:314, 1987. With permission.)

in some instances can be so dramatic that it obliterates visualization of the bile ducts in a manner similar to a gallbladder that is filled with multiple small stones (Fig. 52-39).

Intrahepatic pneumobilia can also be recognized on ultrasound and should be distinguished from the appearance of intrahepatic calculi or parenchymal gas collections. The characteristic sonographic appearance of pneu-

mobilia consists of long or short echogenic foci, with associated reverberative comet-tail artifacts that are located in the distribution of the bile ducts. Because the left duct is anatomically superior and anterior to the right duct, gas tends to localize preferentially to the left duct.

Focal intrahepatic bile duct stricturing, as well as diffuse bile duct thickening can also be diagnosed by sonography. These findings may be seen with sclerosing cholangitis, primary or metastatic tumors to the biliary tract, or, as has recently been described, in patients with acquired immunodeficiency syndrome (AIDS) cholangitis.[27] AIDS cholangitis has a unique appearance in that it exhibits features common to both papillary stenosis and sclerosing cholangitis. Intrahepatic changes consist of generalized thickening of intrahepatic bile ducts as well as focally strictured areas (Fig. 52-40). The precise etiology for these findings has yet to be discovered. Nonetheless, a causal relationship appears to exist with cytomegalovirus and cryptosporidium infections and the development of cholangitis.[27]

Pitfalls in imaging

Although the appearance for dilated intrahepatic bile ducts is specific, this finding is not highly sensitive because up to 23% of patients with biliary obstruction fail to have dilated intrahepatic bile ducts.[107] This may occur in patients with early obstruction in whom only the extrahepatic bile ducts are dilated. This also may be seen in patients with intrahepatic fat or fibrosis in whom the extrinsic forces on the portal triads do not allow dilatation

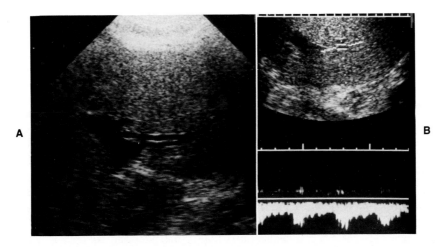

Fig. 52-41 A, Transverse scan obtained over left lobe of liver demonstrates two parallel tubular structures. Although this appearance usually denotes intrahepatic bile duct dilatation, in this patient second tubular structure resulted from abnormally large hepatic artery. **B,** Duplex Doppler examination over one of these tubular structures reveals arterial signal, which excludes diagnosis of bile duct dilatation.

to occur. Occasionally intrahepatic dilatation may be difficult to detect if the bile ducts are filled with echogenic material that is isoechoic with hepatic parenchymal tissue or if the ducts are obscured by associated shadowing (see Figs. 52-38 and 52-39). Most often recurrent pyogenic cholangiohepatitis is responsible for this appearance.

Although false-negative cases of intrahepatic bile duct dilatation are common, false-positive diagnoses are unusual. Pseudodilated intrahepatic ducts usually occur in patients with abnormally large hepatic arteries, in which case the dilated intrahepatic arteries mimic dilated intrahepatic bile ducts (Fig. 52-41).[135] This situation usually occurs in patients with cirrhosis and portal hypertension in whom increased blood flow to the liver occurs by way of the hepatic artery. Certain features distinguish pseudodilated from truly dilated bile ducts: in pseudodilated ducts the extrahepatic artery is abnormally large, the changes are primarily manifest within the left lobe of the liver, evidence of portal hypertension exists, and the extrahepatic common bile duct is of normal caliber. Duplex Doppler ultrasound can rapidly and reliably confirm that the "duct" in question is an abnormally dilated intrahepatic hepatic artery (Fig. 52-41).

Extrahepatic bile ducts
Normal anatomy

The most easily visualized portion of the extrahepatic ductal system is the common hepatic duct, which results from the union of the right and left intrahepatic bile ducts. This structure, which is visible in virtually all patients

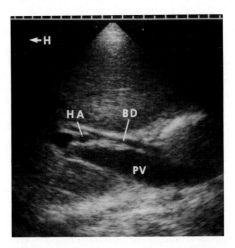

Fig. 52-42 Parasagittal oblique scan obtained over portal fissure (porta hepatis) demonstrates normal anatomic structures in this region, which consist of posterior portal vein *(PV)*, anterior bile duct *(BD)*, and interposed right hepatic artery *(HA)*. *H,* Head.

regardless of their size or body habitus, is located within the portal fissure (porta hepatis) (Fig. 52-42). The common hepatic duct's anatomic position is constant from patient to patient as it crosses anterior to the undivided right portal vein. Most often the right hepatic artery is visible in cross section as it courses between the posterior portal vein and anterior bile duct. As the common hepatic duct leaves the porta hepatis, it joins the cystic duct; the specific point of union is not usually visible by ultrasound.

As the common bile duct (CBD) descends within the hepatoduodenal ligament toward the second duodenum, it is accompanied by two other tubular structures, the main portal vein and the proper hepatic artery. Although the anatomic relationship between these three structures is somewhat confusing, they may be recognized and distinguished from one another by understanding the fixed and reproducible anatomic relationship between them. At the proximal end of the hepatoduodenal ligament, the main portal vein is posterior relative to the anterior and somewhat laterally positioned bile duct (the bile duct is positioned on the same side as the gallbladder). The proper hepatic artery is relatively anterior and medial in its relationship to the portal vein (the portal vein is on the same side as the aorta). The anatomic relationship of the CBD, portal vein, and hepatic artery changes in accordance with their sites of termination as they descend within the hepatoduodenal ligament. Because the CBD terminates in a relatively posterior position as it enters the second duodenum, it courses in a posterior direction. In contrast the portal vein descends in a relatively anterior position as it joins the superior mesenteric and splenic veins. The proper hepatic artery remains anterior as its branch, the gastroduodenal artery, enters the anterior aspect of the pancreatic head. In difficult cases Doppler ultrasound can be used to identify the vascular structures and differentiate them from the bile duct.

Scanning techniques

To evaluate the common duct optimally, it is of critical importance to use appropriate scanning techniques. Optimal transducers usually consist of mechanical or electronic sector scanners using either a 3.5 MHz (or if possible a 5 MHz) transducer focused at the level of the extrahepatic bile duct. Until recently, most ultrasound laboratories examined the CBD by performing parasagittal scans with the patient in an LPO position. This approach was first introduced in 1978 by Behan and Kazam,[7] and for years was considered the best position for examining the extrahepatic portion of the biliary tree. Although this position is acceptable for obtaining satisfactory scans of the common hepatic duct or proximal CBD, it is unacceptable for visualizing the distal CBD, the most common site for biliary obstruction. This is because in the supine or LPO position, the distal duct is frequently obscured as it passes behind the gas-filled duodenum. To obtain optimal images of both the proximal and distal portions of the CBD, each should be examined separately.

The distal duct should be examined initially by placing the patient in a semierect, right posterior oblique position, then obtaining transverse, as opposed to parasagittal, scans.[74] This position minimizes antral and duodenal bowel gas because gas tends to rise to the fundus of the stomach; in addition, retained gastric fluid will enter the antrum and duodenum. Furthermore, in the erect position the left lobe of the liver descends somewhat, allowing it to be used as an acoustic window. The transverse plane of section is superior to a parasagittal plane because it enables one to trace readily the course of the intrapancreatic distal duct. If overlying bowel gas obscures the field of view, the patient is given 6 to 12 ounces of tap water to drink, is placed in a right lateral decubitus position for 2 to 3 minutes, and then is rescanned in a semierect position. Using this technique, the distal duct can be seen in approximately 90% of cases.[74]

Although the proximal CBD also can be evaluated in this position, it is usually seen better after the patient has been repositioned into a conventional supine LPO position and parasagittal scans are obtained. In most patients a complete examination of the proximal and distal bile ducts can be complete in 5 to 10 minutes, although in difficult cases the examination may take as long as 15 to 30 minutes.

Anatomic variations

Variations in the anatomic course of the extrahepatic bile duct occur in approximately 20% of patients with common duct dilatation, in which case the duct usually courses in a primarily transverse direction. In patients with strategically located masses, that is, in the uncinate process, the distal duct may be abnormally anterior in position. Patients who have undergone biliary surgery may also have anatomic deviations in the position of their extrahepatic bile duct.

Anatomic variations in the configuration of the contiguously positioned gallbladder neck and hepatic artery occasionally can cause confusion in identifying the position of the bile duct (Fig. 52-43). In approximately 8% of patients redundancy, elongation, or folding of the gallbladder neck on itself can cause a pattern that mimics dilatation of the common hepatic duct or proximal CBD.[68] To avoid misinterpreting a redundant or elongated gallbladder neck for a dilated CBD, meticulous real-time scanning is required to define the anatomic configuration of the gallbladder neck completely. The CBD can usually be located by angling the transducer along its expected course, just medial to the gallbladder neck.

Anatomic variations in the position of the hepatic artery occur in approximately 30% of patients and also can cause diagnostic confusion. Because the diameters of both the aberrant artery and duct are usually small, it is not absolutely necessary to know which of these small

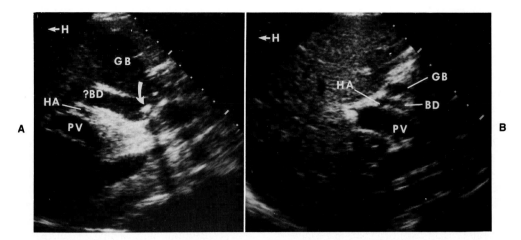

Fig. 52-43 A, Calculus with acoustic shadowing *(arrow)* is visible in what might be misconstrued for dilated bile duct *(BD)*. Gallbladder *(GB)* is situated anteriorly, whereas portal vein *(PV)* and hepatic artery *(HA)* are situated posterior to this structure. This stone actually was within redundant gallbladder neck, not in dilated bile duct. *H,* Head. **B,** Longitudinal scan obtained in slightly more medial direction reveals normal-sized bile duct *(BD)* just behind gallbladder neck *(GB)*. Also visible are more posteriorly located portal vein *(PV)* and hepatic artery *(HA)*. *H,* Head.

structures is the duct and which is the artery. Occasionally, however, the artery may dilate and be misinterpreted for a pathologically dilated bile duct. Although sonography can distinguish the bile duct from the artery in several ways, the most definitive and reliable method is to use a duplex Doppler system and note the characteristic arterial pulsations from within the hepatic artery.[8]

Size

It is generally accepted that the size of the extrahepatic bile duct is the most sensitive indicator for distinguishing obstructive from nonobstructive causes for jaundice. Normally, the diameter of the common hepatic duct or CBD is 5 mm or less, with 6 to 7 mm measurements considered equivocal, and 8 mm or greater measurements considered dilated.[107] When compared to corresponding ductal measurements made during radiographic procedures such as transhepatic cholangiography or endoscopic retrograde cholangiopancreatography, these measurements are somewhat smaller because the ultrasonograms do not include the effects of radiographic magnification or contrast agents.

The size of the common hepatic duct or CBD may be somewhat larger in patients who have previously undergone biliary surgery.[48]

Although ultrasound can distinguish medical from surgical jaundice in more than 90% of cases, atypical cases occasionally will be encountered. Infrequently, dilatation of the biliary tree can occur without jaundice.[129,142] In these patients partial or incomplete biliary obstruction

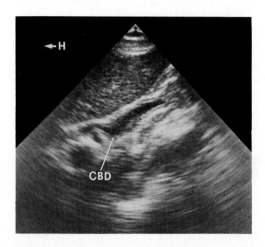

Fig. 52-44 Longitudinal scan of common bile duct *(CBD)* reveals diffuse wall thickening without dilatation. These findings resulted from AIDS cholangitis. *H,* Head.
(From Dolmatch, BL, et al: AIDS-related cholangitis: radiographic findings in nine patients Radiology 163:314, 1987. With permission.)

may be present, or only one hepatic duct may be dilated. In patients with anicteric dilatation, the ultrasound findings and the serum alkaline phosphatase level appear to be more sensitive than the serum bilirubin level for suggesting obstruction. Anicteric dilatation of the extrahepatic bile duct at times may be seen in patients following cholecystectomy or in those with prior obstruction who exhibit dilatation without obstruction.[48] Recent studies have shown that an age-dependent change occurs in the diameter of the extrahepatic duct and that the maximal duct size can be as great as 10 mm in elderly patients.[139] Finally, dilatation can also occur without obstruction in patients with conditions associated with intestinal hypomotility.[103] Recent laparotomy, parenteral hyperalimentation, and prolonged fasting have been associated with bile duct dilatation. In these situations it is postulated that extrahepatic bile duct dilatation occurs in response to factors inhibiting the relaxation or prolonging the contraction of Oddi's sphincter.

The reverse situation can also occur, in which a patient with obstructive jaundice may fail to exhibit dilatation of either the intrahepatic or extrahepatic biliary ducts.[85,107] Cholangitis (sclerosing, AIDS related) (Fig. 52-44), partial obstruction, or intermittent obstruction from choledocholithiasis are usually responsible for these cases. Rarely a patient may be encountered whose extrahepatic duct changes rapidly in size over several minutes to days.[46] These prominent fluctuations most likely relate to the elasticity and associated distensibility of the duct.

In patients with borderline or mild dilatation, biliary dynamics can be assessed by repeating the scan after administering a fatty meal.[115,134] If obstruction *is not* present, the duct should decrease in caliber following a fatty meal; if obstruction *is* present, the duct should increase in size. The literature varies regarding dilated ducts that fail to change size following a fatty meal. Willson and associates[134] consider that failure to change is not a specific indicator for obstruction, whereas Simeone and co-workers[115] believe that lack of change indicates an obstructive process.

Defining level and cause for obstruction

A wide range of accuracy has been reported with regard to ultrasound's ability to determine correctly the level and cause for biliary dilatation. Until recently many discouraging articles have been written, with the correct level of dilatation identified in only 27% to 60% of cases and the correct cause identified in only 23% to 38% of cases.[6,52,54,63] With refinements in real-time equipment and techniques of scanning, Laing and co-workers[74] more recently have been able to define the level of dilatation in 92% of cases and suggest the correct cause in 71% of cases.

The most common site for biliary obstruction is distal, at the level of the pancreatic head. In these patients the extrahepatic bile duct should be dilated throughout its course; the pancreatic duct often is dilated as well. Depending on the severity and duration of the obstruction, the intrahepatic bile ducts may or may not be dilated. Pancreatic tumors, calculi, and distal bile duct strictures most often cause distal common duct obstruction.

With optimal scanning techniques, proximal bile duct calculi can be visualized in approximately 90% of cases, whereas distal bile duct calculi can be visualized in approximately 70% of patients (Fig. 52-45).[69] Calculi most often are detected at the level of the ampulla and are seen best if the scan is performed in a transverse plane of section, with the patient in an upright right posterior oblique position. Not surprisingly, sensitivity for ultrasound diminishes dramatically if overlying bowel gas obscures the region of the pancreatic head.

Strictures, an uncommon cause for distal obstruction,

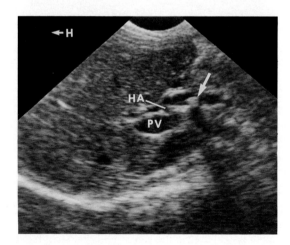

Fig. 52-45 Parasagittal scan reveals common duct stone *(arrow)* with prominent acoustic shadowing within normal-sized bile duct. *PV,* Portal vein; *HA,* hepatic artery; *H,* head.
(From Sarti, DA, editor: Ultrasonography of the gallbladder and biliary tree, Diagnostic ultrasound: text and cases, ed 2, Chicago, 1987, Yearbook Medical Publishers. With permission.)

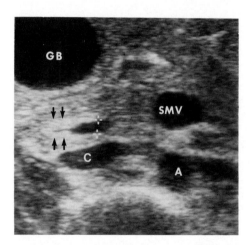

Fig. 52-46 Transverse magnified scan reveals stricture of distal common bile duct *(arrows).* In this patient AIDS cholangitis accounted for this finding. *A,* Aorta; *C,* inferior vena cava; *SMV,* superior mesenteric vein; *GB,* gallbladder.
(From Dolmatch, BL, et al: AIDS-related cholangitis: radiographic findings in nine patients, Radiology 163:314, 1987. With permission.)

are difficult to detect by sonography but occasionally can be seen in thin patients. In our laboratory a frequently observed etiology for distal common bile duct stricture is AIDS cholangitis (Fig. 52-46).[27]

Bile duct dilatation above the level of the pancreas occurs in only 10% of patients[74] and is caused by obstructive processes that are usually located either immediately above the pancreas or at the level of the porta hepatis. Malignancy, both primary and secondary, is usually responsible for these obstructions, although in unusual cases choledocholithiasis may be found.

REFERENCES

1. Alanen, A, and Kormano, M: Correlation of the echogenicity and structure of clotted blood, J Ultrasound Med 4:421, 1985.
2. Alpern, MB, et al: Porta hepatis: duplex doppler US with angiographic correlation, Radiology 162:53, 1987.
3. Aufrichtig, D, et al: Frequency-demodulated US: evaluation in the liver, Radiology 160:59, 1986.
4. Auh, YH, et al: Accessory fissures of the liver: CT and sonographic appearance, AJR 143:565, 1984.
5. Bandai, Y, et al: Sonographic differentiation between the umbilical portion of the left portal vein and intrahepatic bile ducts, J Clin Ultrasound 8:207, 1980.
6. Baron, RL, et al: A prospective comparison of the evaluation of biliary obstruction using computed tomography and ultrasonography, Radiology 145:91, 1982.
7. Behan, M, and Kazam, E: Sonography of the common bile duct: value of the right anterior oblique view, AJR 130:701, 1978.
8. Berland, LL, Lawson, TL, and Foley, WD: Porta hepatis: sonographic discrimination of bile ducts from arteries with pulsed doppler with new anatomic criteria, AJR 138:833, 1982.
9. Bernardino, ME, and Green, B: Ultrasonographic evaluation of chemotherapeutic response in hepatic metastases, Radiology 133:437, 1979.
10. Berry, M, Bazaz, R, and Bhargava, S: Amebic liver abscess: sonographic diagnosis and management, J Clin Ultrasound 14:239, 1986.
11. Black, EB, et al: Acoustic contrast enhancement: value of several system gain variations in gray scale ultrasonography, AJR 133:689, 1979.
12. Bolondi, L, et al: Ultrasonography in the diagnosis of portal hypertension: diminished response of portal vessels to respiration, Radiology 142:167, 1982.
13. Brick, SH, Hill, MC, and Lande, IM: The mistaken or indeterminate CT diagnosis of hepatic metastases: the value of sonography, AJR 148:723, 1987.
14. Britten, JS, Golding, RH, and Cooperberg, PL: Sludge balls to gallstones, J Ultrasound Med 3:81, 1984.
15. Callen, PW, and Filly, RA: Ultrasonographic localization of the gallbladder, Radiology 133:687, 1979.
16. Callen, PW, Filly, RA, and Marcus, FS: Ultrasonography and computed tomography in the evaluation of hepatic microabscesses in the immunosuppressed patient, Radiology 136:433, 1980.
17. Carroll, BA: Gallstones: in vitro comparison of physical, radiographic, and ultrasonic characteristics, AJR 131:223, 1978.
18. Cheng, TH, et al: Evaluation of hepatobiliary imaging by radionuclide scintigraphy, ultrasonography, and contrast cholangiography, Radiology 133:761, 1979.
19. Conrad, MR, Janes, JO, and Dietchy, J: Significance of low level echoes within the gallbladder, AJR 132:967, 1979.
20. Cooperberg, PL, et al: Real-time high resolution ultrasound in the detection of biliary calculi, Radiology 131:789, 1979.
21. Crade, M, et al: Surgical and pathologic correlation of cholecystosonography and cholecystography, AJR 131:227, 1978.
22. Cunningham, JJ: In vitro gray scale echography of protein-lipid fluid collections in liver tissue, J Clin Ultrasound 4:255, 1976.
23. deGraaff, CS, Dembner, AG, and Taylor, KJW: Ultrasound and false normal oral cholecystogram, Arch Surg 113:877, 1978.
24. Dempsey, PJ, et al: Cholecystosonography for the diagnosis of cholecystolithiasis, Ann Surg 187:465, 1978.
25. Di Candio, G, et al: Ultrasound detection of unusual spontaneous portosystemic shunts associated with uncomplicated portal hypertension, J Ultrasound Med 4:297, 1985.
26. Didier, D, et al: Hepatic alveolar echinococcosis: correlative US and CT study, Radiology 154:179, 1985.
27. Dolmatch, BL, et al: AIDS-related cholangitis: radiographic findings in nine patients, Radiology 163:314, 1987.
28. Ebara, M, et al: Natural history of minute hepatocellular carcinoma smaller than three centimeters complicating cirrhosis: a study in 22 patients, Gastroenterology 90:289, 1986.
29. Federle, MP, Filly, RA, and Moss, AA: Cystic hepatic neoplasms: complementary roles of CT and sonography, AJR 136:345, 1981.
30. Federle, MP, et al: Recurrent pyogenic cholangitis in Asian immigrants, Radiology 143:151, 1982.
31. Ferin, P, and Lerner, RM: Contracted gallbladder: a finding in hepatic dysfunction, Radiology 154:769, 1985.
32. Filly, RA, Moss, AA, and Way, LW: In vitro investigation of gallstone shadowing with ultrasound tomography, J Clin Ultrasound 7:255, 1979.
33. Filly, RA, Sommer, FG, and Minton, MJ: Characterization of biological fluids by ultrasound and computed tomography, Radiology 134:167, 1980.
34. Filly, RA, et al: In vitro investigation of the origin of echoes within biliary sludge, J Clin Ultrasound 8:193, 1980.
35. Fiske, E, and Filly, RA: Pseudo-sludge: a spurious ultrasound appearance within the gallbladder, Radiology 144:631, 1982.
36. Fiske, CE, Laing, FC, and Brown, TW: Ultrasonographic evidence of gallbladder wall thickening in association with hypoalbuminemia, Radiology 135:713, 1980.
37. Foster, SC, and McLaughlin, SM: Improvement in the ultrasonic evaluation of the gallbladder by using the left lateral decubitus position, J Clin Ultrasound 5:253, 1979.
38. Freeman, MP, et al: Regenerating nodules in cirrhosis: sonographic appearance with anatomic correlation, AJR 146:533, 1986.
39. Frick, MP, and Feinberg, SB: Biliary cystadenoma, AJR 139:393, 1982.
40. Garra, BS, et al: Quantitative estimation of liver attenuation and echogenicity: normal state versus diffuse liver disease, Radiology 162:61, 1987.
41. Gibney, RG, Hendin, AP, and Cooperberg, PL: Sonographically detected hepatic hemangiomas: absence of change over time, AJR 149:953, 1987.
42. Ginaldi, S, et al: Ultrasonographic patterns of hepatic lymphoma, Radiology 136:427, 1980.
43. Giorgio, A, et al: Ultrasound evaluation of uncomplicated and complicated acute viral hepatitis, J Clin Ultrasound 14:675, 1986.
44. Giorgio, A, et al: Cirrhosis: value of caudate to right lobe ratio in diagnosis with US, Radiology 161:443, 1986.

45. Glancy, JJ, Goddard, J, and Pearson, DE: In vitro demonstration of cholesterol crystals' high echogenicity relative to protein particles, J Clin Ultrasound 8:27, 1980.

46. Glazer, GM, Filly, RA, and Laing, FC: Rapid change in caliber of the nonobstructed common duct, Radiology 140:161, 1981.

47. Gosink, BB, et al: Accuracy of ultrasonography in diagnosis of hepatocellular disease, AJR 133:19, 1979.

48. Graham, MF, et al: The size of the normal common hepatic duct following cholecystectomy: an ultrasonographic study, Radiology 135:137, 1980.

49. Grossman, M: Cholelithiasis and acoustic shadowing, J Clin Ultrasound 6:182, 1978.

50. Harbin, WP, Robert, NJ, and Ferrucci, JT: Diagnosis of cirrhosis based on regional changes in hepatic morphology, Radiology 135:273, 1980.

51. Harbin, WP, et al: Nonvisualized gallbladder by cholecystosonography, AJR 132:727, 1979.

52. Haubek, A, et al: Dynamic sonography in the evaluation of jaundice, AJR 136:1071, 1981.

53. Holm, J, and Jacobsen, B: Accuracy of dynamic ultrasonography in the diagnosis of malignant liver lesions, J Ultrasound Med 5:1, 1986.

54. Honickman, SP, et al: Ultrasound in obstructive jaundice: prospective evaluation of site and cause, Radiology 147:511, 1983.

55. Hunter, ND, and Macintosh, PK: Acute emphysematous cholecystitis: an ultrasonic diagnosis, AJR 134:592, 1980.

56. Hussain, S: Diagnostic criteria of hydatid disease on hepatic sonography, J Ultrasound Med 4:603, 1985.

57. Jeanty, P, et al: Mobile intraluminal masses of the gallbladder, J Ultrasound Med 2:65, 1983.

58. Jeffrey, RB, et al: Gangrenous cholecystitis: diagnosis by ultrasound, Radiology 148:219, 1983.

59. Juttner, H-U, et al: Ultrasound demonstration of portosystemic collaterals in cirrhosis and portal hypertension, Radiology 142:459, 1982.

60. Kane, RA, et al: Porcelain gallbladder: ultrasound and CT appearance, Radiology 152:137, 1984.

61. Kawashima, A, et al: Focal fatty infiltration of the liver mimicking a tumor: sonographic and CT features, J Comput Assist Tomogr 10:329, 1986.

62. King, DL, et al: Focal and diffuse liver disease studied by quantitative microstructural sonography, Radiology 155:457, 1985.

63. Koenigsberg, M, Wiener, SN, and Walzer, A: The accuracy of sonography in the differential diagnosis of obstructive jaundice: a comparison with cholangiography, Radiology 133:157, 1979.

64. Krook, PM, et al: Comparison of real-time cholecystosonography and oral cholecystography, Radiology 135:145, 1980.

65. Kurtz, AB, et al: Ultrasound findings in hepatitis, Radiology 136:716, 1980.

66. LaBerge, JM, et al: Hepatocellular carcinoma: assessment of resectability by computed tomography and ultrasound, Radiology 152:485, 1984.

67. Laing, FC, Gooding, GAW, and Herzog, KA: Gallstones preventing ultrasonographic visualization of the gallbladder, Gastrointest Radiol 1:301, 1977.

68. Laing, FC, and Jeffrey, RB: The pseudo-dilated common bile duct: ultrasonographic appearance created by the gallbladder neck, Radiology 135:405, 1980.

69. Laing, FC, Jeffrey, RB, and Wing, VW: Improved visualization of choledocholithiasis by sonography, AJR 143:949, 1984.

70. Laing, FC, and Kurtz, AB: The importance of ultrasonic side-lobe artifacts, Radiology 145:763, 1982.

71. Laing, FC, London, LA, and Filly, RA: Ultrasonographic identification of dilated intrahepatic bile ducts and their differentiation from portal venous structures, J Clin Ultrasound 6:90, 1978.

72. Laing, FC, et al: Ultrasonic evaluation of patients with acute right upper quadrant pain, Radiology 140:449, 1981.

73. Laing, FC, et al: Noninvasive imaging of unusual regenerating nodules in the cirrhotic liver, Gastrointest Radiol 7:245, 1982.

74. Laing, FC, et al: Biliary dilatation: defining the level and cause by real-time US, Radiology 160:39, 1986.

75. Lewall, DB, and McCorkell, SJ: Hepatic echinococcal cysts: sonographic appearance and classification, Radiology 155:773, 1985.

76. Madrazo, BL, et al: Sonographic findings in perforation of the gallbladder, AJR 139:491, 1982.

77. Marchal, GJ, et al: Anechoic halo in solid liver tumors: sonographic, microangiographic, and histologic correlation, Radiology 156:479, 1985.

78. Marchal, GJ, et al: Caroli disease: high-frequency US and pathologic findings, Radiology 158:507, 1986.

79. Marks, WM, Filly, RA, and Callen, PW: Ultrasonic anatomy of the liver: a review with new applications, J Clin Ultrasound 7:137, 1979.

80. Matsuda, Y, and Yabuuchi, I: Hepatic tumors: US contrast enhancement with CO_2 microbubbles, Radiology 161:701, 1986.

81. Mattrey, RF, et al: Perfluorochemicals as US agents for tumor imaging and hepatosplenography: preliminary clinical results, Radiology 163:339, 1987.

82. McKay, AJ, et al: A prospective study of the clinical value and accuracy of gray scale ultrasound in detecting gallstones, Br J Surg 65:330, 1978.

83. Michels, NA: Newer anatomy of the liver and its variant blood supply and collateral circulation, Am J Surg 112:337, 1966.

84. Mirk, P, et al: Ultrasonographic patterns in hepatic hemangiomas, J Clin Ultrasound 10:373, 1982.

85. Muhletaler, CA, et al: Diagnosis of obstructive jaundice with nondilated bile ducts, AJR 134:1149, 1980.

86. Mukai, JK, et al: Imaging of surgically relevant hepatic vascular and segmental anatomy. Part 1. Normal anatomy, AJR 149:287, 1987.

87. Mukai, JK, et al: Imaging of surgically relevant hepatic vascular and segmental anatomy. Part 2. Extent and resectability of hepatic neoplasms, AJR 149:293, 1987.

88. Needleman, L, et al: Sonography of diffuse benign liver disease: accuracy of pattern recognition and grading, AJR 146:1011, 1986.

89. Nelson, RC, et al: Comparison of pulsed doppler sonography and angiography in patients with portal hypertension, AJR 149:77, 1987.

90. Neumaier, CE, et al: The patent ductus venosus: an additional ultrasonic finding in portal hypertension, J Clin Ultrasound 11:231, 1983.

91. Newlin, N, et al: Ultrasonic features of pyogenic liver abscesses, Radiology 139:155, 1981.

92. Nyberg, DA, and Laing, FC: Ultrasonographic findings in peptic ulcer disease and pancreatitis that simulate primary gallbladder disease, J Ultrasound Med 2:303, 1983.

93. Parulekar, SG: Sonographic findings in acute emphysematous cholecystitis, Radiology 145:117, 1982.

94. Parulekar, SG: Evaluation of the prone view for cholecystosonography, J Ultrasound Med 5:617, 1986.

95. Patriquin, H, et al: Duplex doppler examination in portal hypertension: technique and anatomy, AJR 149:71, 1987.

96. Quinn, SF, and Gosink, BB: Characteristic sonographic signs of hepatic fatty infiltration, AJR 145:753, 1985.

97. Raghavendra, BN, et al: Sonography of adenomyomatosis of the gallbladder: radiologic-pathologic correlation, Radiology 146:747, 1983.

98. Ralls, PW, et al: Sonography in recurrent oriental pyogenic chol-angitis, AJR 136:1010, 1981.

99. Ralls, PW, et al: Gallbladder wall thickening: patients without intrinsic gallbladder disease, AJR 137:65, 1981.

100. Ralls, PW, et al: Sonographic findings in hepatic amebic abscess, Radiology 145:123, 1982.

101. Ralls, PW, et al: Real-time sonography in suspected acute cho-lecystitis: prospective evaluation of primary and secondary signs, Radiology 155:767, 1985.

102. Raptopoulos, V, et al: Dynamic cholecystosonography of the contracted gallbladder: the double-arc-shadow sign, AJR 138:275, 1982.

103. Raptopoulos, V, et al: Bile-duct dilatation after laparotomy: a potential effect of intestinal hypomotility, AJR 147:729, 1986.

104. Rector, WB, Jr, et al: Utility and limitations of splanchnic venous ultrasonography in diagnosis of portal hypertension, J Clin Ul-trasound 14:689, 1986.

105. Reinig, JW, and Stanley, JH: Sonographic hepatization of the gallbladder: a cause of nonvisualization of the gallbladder by cholecystosonography, J Clin Ultrasound 12:234, 1984.

106. Rosenthan, L, et al: Diagnosis of hepatobiliary disease by ^{99m}Tc-HIDA cholescintigraphy, Radiology 126:467, 1978.

107. Sample, WF, et al: Gray-scale ultrasonography of the jaundiced patient, Radiology 128:719, 1978.

108. Sauerbrei, EE, and Lopez, M: Pseudotumor of the quadrate lobe in hepatic sonography: a sign of generalized fatty infiltration, AJR 147:923, 1986.

109. Scheible, W, Gosink, BB, and Leopold, GR: Gray scale echo-graphic patterns of hepatic metastatic disease, AJR 129:983, 1977.

110. Sexton, CC, and Zeman, RK: Correlation of computed tomog-raphy, sonography, and gross anatomy of the liver, AJR 141:711, 1983.

111. Shawker, TH, et al: B-scan echo-amplitude measurement in pa-tients with diffuse infiltrative liver disease, J Clin Ultrasound 9:293, 1981.

112. Sheu, J-C, et al: Hepatocellular carcinoma: US evolution in the early stage, Radiology 155:463, 1985.

113. Shlaer, WJ, Leopold, GR, and Scheible, FW: Sonography of the thickened gallbladder wall: a nonspecific finding, AJR 136:337, 1981.

114. Shuman, WP, et al: Evaluation of acute right upper quadrant pain: sonography and ^{99m}Tc-PIPIDA cholescintigraphy, AJR 139:61, 1982.

115. Simeone, JF, et al: The bile ducts after a fatty meal: further sonographic observations, Radiology 154:763, 1985.

116. Solbiati, L, et al: Fine-needle biopsy of hepatic hemangioma with sonographic guidance, AJR 144:471, 1985.

117. Sommer, FG, et al: Measurement of attenuation and scatterer spacing in human liver tissue: preliminary results, J Ultrasound Med 3:557, 1984.

118. Spiegel, RM, King, DL, and Green, WM: Ultrasonography of primary cysts of the liver, AJR 131:235, 1978.

119. Stoller, JL, and Cooperberg, P: Ultrasound scanning in detecting gallstones (editorial), Br J Surg 65:669, 1978.

120. Sullivan, DC, Taylor, KJW, and Gottschalk, A: The use of ul-trasound to enhance the diagnostic utility of the equivocal liver scintigraph, Radiology 128:727, 1978.

121. Taboury, J, et al: Cavernous hemangiomas of the liver studied by ultrasound, Radiology 149:781, 1983.

122. Tanaka, S, et al: Hepatocellular carcinoma: sonographic and his-tologic correlation, AJR 140:701, 1983.

123. Tanaka, S, et al: Early diagnosis of hepatocellular carcinoma: usefulness of ultrasonically guided fine-needle aspiration biopsy, J Clin Ultrasound 14:11, 1986.

124. Taylor, KJW, et al: Focal liver masses: differential diagnosis with pulsed doppler US, Radiology 164:643, 1987.

125. Thurber, LA, et al: Echogenic fluid: a pitfall in the ultrasono-graphic diagnosis of cystic lesions, J Clin Ultrasound 7:273, 1979.

126. Weaver, RM, et al: Gray scale ultrasonographic evaluation of hepatic cystic disease, AJR 130:849, 1978.

127. Wegener, M, et al: Gallbladder wall thickening: a frequent finding in various nonbiliary disorders—a prospective ultrasonographic study, J Clin Ultrasound 15:307, 1987.

128. Weiner, SN, et al: Sonography and computed tomography in the diagnosis of carcinoma of the gallbladder, AJR 142:735, 1984.

129. Weinstein, BJ, and Weinstein, DP: Biliary tract dilatation in the nonjaundiced patient, AJR 134:899, 1980.

130. Weissmann, HS, et al: Cholescintigraphy, ultrasonography and computerized tomography in the evaluation of biliary tract dis-orders, Semin Nucl Med 9:22, 1979.

131. Weissmann, HS, et al: Rapid and accurate diagnosis of acute cholecystitis with ^{99m}Tc-HIDA cholescintigraphy, AJR 132:523, 1979.

132. Welch, TJ, et al: Focal nodular hyperplasia and hepatic adenoma: comparison of angiography, CT, US, and scintigraphy, Radiology 156:593, 1985.

133. White, EM, et al: Focal periportal sparing in hepatic fatty infil-tration: a cause of hepatic pseudomass on US, Radiology 162:57, 1987.

134. Willson, SA, Gosink, BB, and vanSonnenberg, E: Unchanged size of a dilated common bile duct after a fatty meal: results and significance, Radiology 160:29, 1986.

135. Wing, VW, et al: Sonographic differentiation of enlarged hepatic arteries from dilated intrahepatic bile ducts, AJR 145:57, 1985.

136. Wolson, AH, and Goldberg, BB: Gray scale ultrasonic chole-cystography: a primary screening procedure, JAMA 240:2073, 1978.

137. Wooten, WB, Green, B, and Goldstein, HM: Ultrasonography of necrotic hepatic metastases, Radiology 128:447, 1978.

138. Worthen, NJ, Uszler, JM, and Funamura, JL: Cholecystitis: pro-spective evaluation of sonography and ^{99m}Tc-HIDA cholescintig-raphy, AJR 137:973, 1981.

139. Wu, C-C, Ho, Y-H, and Chen, C-Y: Effect of aging on common bile duct diameter: a real-time ultrasonographic study, J Clin Ultrasound 12:473, 1984.

140. Yeh, H-C, Goodman, J, and Rabinowitz, JG: Floating gallstones in bile without added contrast material, AJR 146:49, 1986.

141. Yoshida, T, et al: Ultrasonographic differentiation of hepatocel-lular carcinoma from metastatic liver cancer, J Clin Ultrasound 15:431, 1987.

142. Zeman, R, et al: Ultrasound demonstration of anicteric dilatation of the biliary tree, Radiology 134:689, 1980.

143. Zoli, M, et al: Spanchnic vein measurements in patients with liver cirrhosis: a case-control study, J Ultrasound Med 4:641, 1985.

53 *Nuclear Medicine*

LEONARD ROSENTHALL

LIVER

The liver is the largest abdominal organ, weighing approximately 1500 g in the adult. It is organized into lobules that are roughly cylindric with a central vein traveling through its long axis. Irregular interconnecting sheets of hepatic cells radiate outward from the central vein and constitute the parenchyma. Sinusoidal capillaries separate the sheets of hepatic cells and empty into the central vein. Connective tissue and components of the portal canal are seen at the periphery of the lobule. The portal canal contains the hepatic artery, portal vein, and bile-collecting ducts. Normal sinusoidal capillaries are fenestrated, and it is in these windows that the reticuloendothelial cells (Kupffer cells) are located. Kupffer cells are more plentiful in the portal than in the central vein area.[62] About 20% of the hepatic mass is formed by Kupffer cells and 80% by hepatocytes.

Radiopharmaceuticals

Radioactive tracers have been designed to exploit the properties of the Kupffer cell and the hepatocyte. Phagocytosis is a feature of the Kupffer cell, and normally 95% of colloid particles are extracted in a single pass. About 90% of the particles are trapped in the liver, and the remaining 10% are almost equally shared by the reticuloendothelial cells of the spleen and bone marrow. A variety of radiocolloids have been developed. Originally colloidal gold-198 was used, but its gamma emission of 411 KeV is not efficient for current gamma cameras. Technetium-99m (^{99m}Tc) with its 140 KeV photon is more suitable, and it has been used to label sulfur colloid, colloidal stannous phytate, tin colloid, antimony colloid, and colloidal albumin and albumin microspheres—all of which are commercially available. Other agents such as ^{99m}Tc fat emulsion,[45] ^{99m}Tc ferric hydroxide,[116] ^{113}I (OH) colloid,[39] ^{99m}TcO$_2$ colloid,[51] and others have been tried, but they are only of historical interest. The relative distribution between liver, spleen, and bone marrow may vary with the particle size. Most radiocolloids employed clinically lie within the range of 50 to 800 nm. Smaller particles have a tendency to deposit in the bone marrow, whereas larger particles tend to favor the spleen; however, the liver uptake still predominates.[9,20,56]

Iodine-131 (^{131}I) rose bengal was introduced in 1955; it was the first hepatocyte-seeking radiopharmaceutical used for studying liver kinetics.[105] Unlike the radiocolloids that are concentrated by the Kupffer cells and remain there, rose bengal is taken up by the hepatocytes and then excreted into the biliary system and gut. It is therefore used as a bile marker. Only rectilinear scanning was available in 1955, and it was not feasible to study the progress of ^{131}I rose bengal through the hepatobiliary pathways with serial images. The advent of the gamma

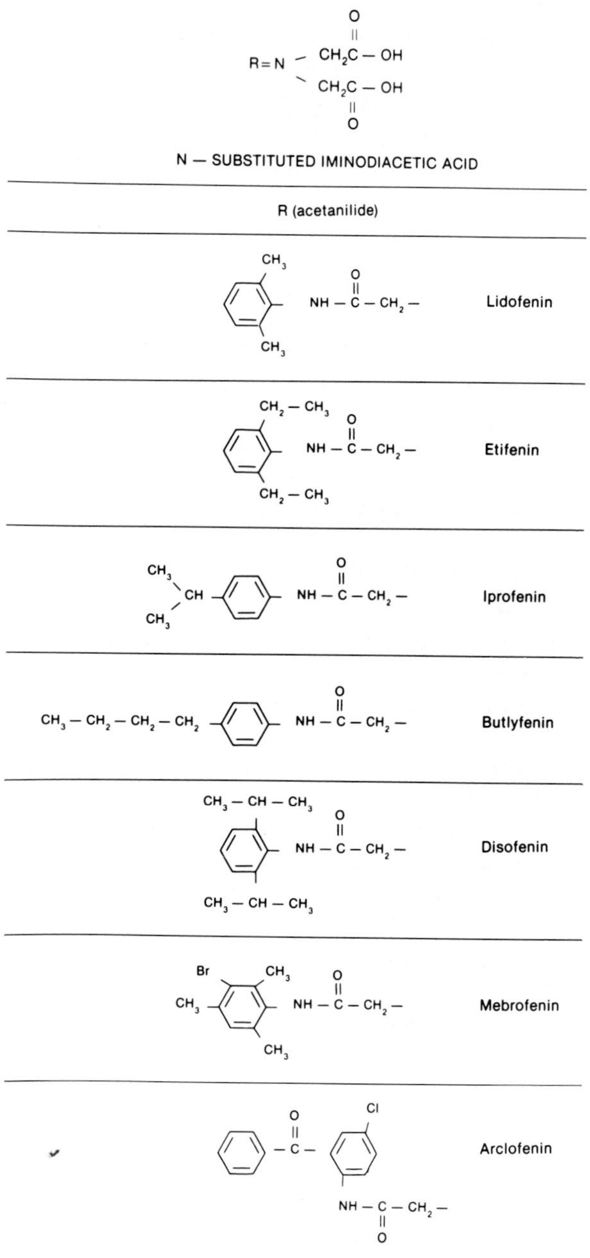

Fig. 53-1 Various analogues of acetanilide iminodiacetic acid.

camera in about 1965 made this possible. To improve image-detection efficiency ^{123}I (159 KeV) was substituted for ^{131}I (364 KeV) on the rose bengal molecule.[92] There were also some reports on the use of ^{123}I bromsulphalein and ^{123}I indocyanine green, but these received only passing interest, because cyclotron-produced ^{123}I is expensive, is not readily available, has a short physical half-life (13.2 hours), and usually requires in-house fabrication.[2,40] ^{99m}Tc, which is generator produced, is inexpensive, and has desirable physical properties for the gamma camera, went through a series of developments as ^{99m}Tc penicillamine,[106] ^{99m}Tc thiotic acid,[49] ^{99m}Tc dihydrothiotic acid,[104] ^{99m}Tc pyridoxylidene glutamate,[4] and ^{99m}Tc tetracycline[29]; it finally culminated with the introduction of the N-substituted iminodiacetic acid (IDA) derivatives[60] (Fig. 53-1). In the latter group the various agents differ in their extraction efficiency by the hepatocyte, the rate of transport from the hepatocyte to biliary tract, and the proportion of the administered dose eliminated by the kidneys. As the degree of liver damage increases, these parameters change more profoundly with some analogs than with others. The ^{99m}Tc-IDA derivatives are transported into the cell through a carrier-mediated anionic clearance mechanism.[27] Bilirubin competitively inhibits binding of the anionic radiopharmaceutical with this membrane-bound carrier, and it is for this reason that there is a continuing search for cholescintigraphic agents that will be more resistant to the competition, thereby eluding bilirubin interference.

There have also been developments in imaging hepatocytes through the mechanism of receptor binding. ^{99m}Tc-galactosyl-neoglycoalbumin binds to the hepatic protein binding receptor and is then incorporated into the hepatocyte lysosomes through endocytosis. Allegedly, the measurement of receptor concentration provides an index of functional tissue mass and improves sensitivity to liver dysfunction.[102]

Other radiopharmaceuticals that are not liver specific have been used to disclose hepatic or perihepatic disease. ^{67}Ga citrate is concentrated by hepatocytes, but also accumulates in inflammatory and tumor tissue. ^{111}In-labeled leukocytes are more specific for inflammation than tumor and are used to detect hepatic and perihepatic abscesses, and distinguish them from neoplasm. ^{99m}Tc-labeled erythrocytes are employed to assess the vascular characteristics of liver lesions.

Techniques of imaging

An adequate count rate is obtained in adults with a 5 mCi intravenous dose of radiocolloid. In children this is scaled down to 30 μCi/kg of body weight with a minimum of 300 μCi. The radiation-absorbed doses for liver and whole body in the adult are about 1.7 rads and 0.095 rad per 5 mCi, respectively. In children this will vary

applicable with normally functioning cholangiointestinal and gastroenteric anastomoses. Patients who have had a vagotomy or are on a medication that causes a transient contraction of the sphincter of Oddi (for instance, morphine) may exhibit normal liver washout and drainage into the gallbladder, but delayed gut entry: so-called preferential gallbladder filling. This should not be misconstrued as extrahepatic obstruction as long as the rate of liver washout is normal and there is no pooling of the test agent within the biliary tract.

The blood half-disappearance time of cholecystokinin (CCK) is about 2.5 minutes. It has been shown that by increasing the constant infusion rates of CCK incrementally every 15 minutes, a threshold of the normal gallbladder response was 0.010 Crick-Harper-Raper (CHR) units/kg/min.[100] Increasing the infusion rate also enhanced the rate of emptying (Fig. 53-4). There was no sex or age difference in galbladder emptying. A 15-minute infusion of 20 ng/kg sincalide produces an ejection fraction of about $75 \pm 20\%$ (mean $\pm$ SD, or standard deviation) in normal gallbladders. The lower plus-orminus standard deviation limit is therefore about 35%; a rather wide range.

LIVER IMAGING

Abnormalities of the liver may present as single or multiple focal functional defects, or as a diffuse involvement manifesting a fairly uniform or generally irregular distribution of function in a liver that may be enlarged, normal, or shrunken (Table 53-1).

Diffuse disease

Diffuse disease of the liver, whether caused by an infiltrative process or edema, is not detectable initially. It is appreciated only when the liver becomes enlarged, or when the process decreases the blood flow or interferes with Kupffer cell function to the point that radiocolloid shifts to the spleen and bone marrow. The liver may also exhibit a diffuse, heterogeneous, deposition of radiocolloid. All these signs are nonspecific and require other investigations for an etiologic diagnosis. Normally the liver and spleen show an equal concentration in the posterior view, because the number of reticuloendothelial (RE) cells per gram of tissue is approximately the same in both organs, and in this projection they are equidistant from the detector. An elevation of the spleen-to-liver ratio is not limited to liver disease alone, but can result from

☐ **TABLE 53-1**
Focal and diffuse liver diseases

Benign tumors and cysts	Malignant neoplasms	Inflammatory lesions	Trauma	Metabolic disorders	Miscellaneous
Focal liver disease					
Focal nodular hyperplasia	Metastases	Abscess	Hematoma	Amyloidosis	Postradiation therapy
Adenoma	Cholangiocarcinoma	Localized hepatitis	Laceration	Focal fatty infiltration	Cirrhosis
Regenerating nodules	Angiosarcoma	Hydatid cyst	Surgical resection		Budd-Chiari syndrome
Polycystic disease		Subphrenic abscess			Caroli's disease
Solitary cyst					Choledochal obstruction
					Infarction
					Periarteritis nodosa
Diffuse liver disease					
	Leukemia	Hepatitis	Contusion	Fatty infiltration	Cirrhosis
	Lymphoma	Mononucleosis		Amyloidosis	Drug toxicity
	Metastases	Sarcoidosis		Hemochromatosis	Subacute and chronic choledochal obstruction
		Granulomatous hepatitis		Gaucher's disease	
		Sickle cell disease		von Gierke's disease	Jejunal bypass surgery
		Schistosomiasis		Niemann-Pick disease	Alpha$_1$-antitrypsin deficiency
		Malaria		Diabetes	
		Weil's disease		Collagen vascular disease	
		Syphilis			

a grossly enlarged spleen or stimulation of RE activity in the spleen, as may occur in malignant melanoma.[55]

In cirrhosis associated with alcohol abuse there is enlargement of the liver in the early phases of the disease due to fatty infiltration. As cirrhosis advances, the liver shrinks in size, becoming less fatty and more fibrotic. This may be followed by atrophy of the right lobe with compensatory hypertrophy of the left lobe and the production of ascites. The radiocolloid depiction of the latter stages is a small liver with an irregular distribution of function and a shift of radioactivity to the spleen and bone marrow, splenomegaly and a halo caused by ascites separating the liver from the chest wall and diaphragm. In advanced stages of cirrhotic decompensation radiocolloid deposition in the lungs may also appear (Fig. 53-5). The radiocolloid end stages of other causes of cirrhosis—such as biliary cirrhosis, postnecrotic cirrhosis and hemochromatosis—may render a similar radionuclide portrayal. The hemodynamic train of events postulated for these radiocolloid patterns is that the initial fatty infiltration and subsequent scarring results in increased vascular resistence, which progresses to portal hypertension, enlargement of the spleen, and intrahepatic and extrahepatic shunting, all of which further decrease the nutritional blood flow to the liver. Superimposed on this is a decreased Kupffer cell population in regenerating nodules.[1] No satisfactory explanation has been presented for the unusual lung accretion, although migration of RE cells to lungs under the influence of estrogen, endotoxin, heparin, and other substances has been observed.[68]

Hepatitis presents a variable picture from a normal radiocolloid image to hepatomegaly with diffusely decreased concentration and a shift of radiocolloid to the spleen and bone marrow. In advanced stages it may resemble cirrhosis. ^{99m}Tc-IDA imaging is more sensitive than radiocolloid in disclosing hepatitis in the early stages, but its use is limited, since there are more specific blood tests for making this diagnosis. Fulminant hepatitis may lead to massive necrosis and shrinkage of the liver, thereby portraying a decreased or absent uptake of radiocolloid, but no increase in spleen uptake or size.[28] These necrotic lesions have been reported to concentrate the radiophosphate—the bone scanning agent.[44] Uncommonly, hepatitis may exhibit a focal defect that may be confused with a tumor.

Other causes of diffuse disease include lymphoma, leukemia, glycogen storage disease, schistosomiasis,[99] amyloidosis, chronic passive congestion by the liver in cardiac failure, alpha$_1$-antitrypsin deficiency, jejunal bypass surgery, and a variety of pharmaceuticals. All yield a nonspecific spectrum of normal to decreased, and perhaps patchy, radiocolloid deposition. A redistribution of the radiocolloid to the spleen and bone marrow may occur with chronicity. Amyloidosis in the liver, and elsewhere

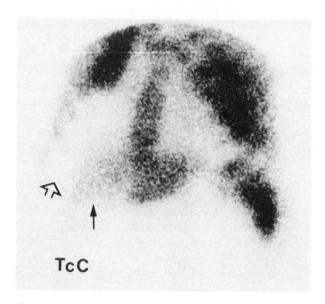

Fig. 53-5 Advanced decompensated cirrhosis. Radiocolloid scan depicts shrunken liver with atrophy of right lobe (*solid arrow*) and shift of radiocolloid (*TcC*) to the spleen, bone marrow, and lungs. Large space between liver and right lung and lateral wall (*open arrow*) is caused by massive ascites.

in the body, has been known to concentrate radiophosphate.[25] Hepatic vein thrombosis gives rise to the Budd-Chiari syndrome, and it is a posthepatic cause of portal hypertension and ascites. The characteristic radiocolloid portrayal is reduced to absent deposition in the right and left lobes, except for the caudate lobe, which has its own venous drainage and may depict a compensatory increase in size. On the other hand, this characteristic presentation is not always obtained, and the scans can be quite variable in appearance[43,77] (Fig. 53-6). Portal vein thrombosis, a prehepatic cause of portal hypertension, renders a portrayal that is similar to cirrhosis, consisting of a generalized irregular radiocolloid deposition and a shift to the spleen (Fig. 53-7).

Focal disease

The resolution of a focal lesion by the gamma camera decreases as the distance from the face of the collimator increases. Thus cold lesions 1.5 to 2 cm in diameter on the surface of the liver can be disclosed, whereas lesions of 3 cm in diameter may be missed when located in the depths of the right lobe. SPECT imaging improves the resolution and enhances the 80% to 85% sensitivity of multiprojection planar imaging to about 90%.[23] It also serves to define more clearly lesions that were equivocal under planar imaging.

Metastatic disease

In descending order of frequency, metastases to the liver emanate from primary neoplasms in the GI tract,

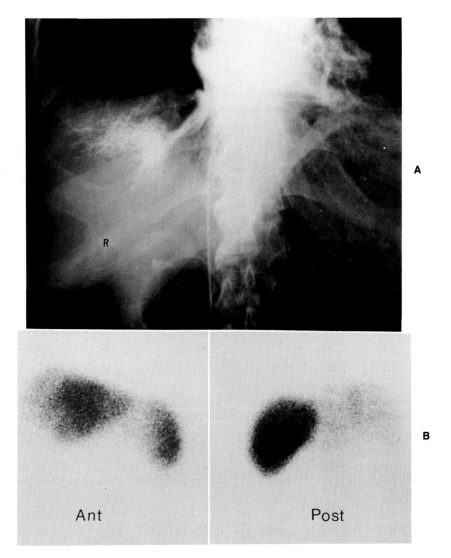

Fig. 53-6 Budd-Chiari syndrome due to thrombosis of hepatic vein. **A,** Angiogram shows typical pattern of hepatic vein thrombosis. *R,* Radiocolloid. **B,** Radiocolloid images demonstrate very little concentration in right lobe. Relatively higher concentration in medial side of liver is probably in enlarged caudate lobe, since left hepatic vein was obstructed. Note radiocolloid shift to spleen in posterior *(Post)* projection. *Ant,* Anterior.

particularly the colon, followed by the lung, the genitourinary tract, the breast, the pancreas, the cervix, and the uterus. An autopsy review indicated that 30% of patients with metastases did not have hepatomegaly, 77% had lesions in both lobes, 20% had lesions restricted to the right lobe, and 3% had lesions only in the left lobe. There were both surface and deep-seated lesions in 70% of the cases, in 19% the lesions were only on the surface, and in 2% the lesions were solitary. Approximately 30% of the lesions were less than 2 cm in diameter, but in many of these cases there were other lesions that were greater in diameter.[73]

A comparison of liver scan results and autopsy findings in 159 cases indicated a true positive rate (sensitivity) of 81% and a true negative rate (specificity) of 73%. The false negatives were caused by lesions less than 2 cm in diameter, and the false positives for tumor resulted from diffuse parenchymal disease or hilar imprints caused by dilated biliary channels.[7] Another correlation of radiocolloid liver scans and postmorten disclosure showed a sensitivity of 79% and specificity of 85%. This yielded a 93% predictive value of a positive result and a 62% predictive value of a negative result.[72]

Colon and other gastrointestinal carcinomas generally

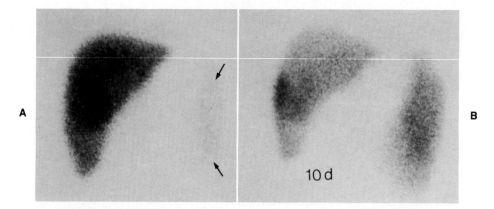

Fig. 53-7 Portal vein thrombosis; 20-year-old woman taking oral contraceptives was shown by angiography to have portal vein thrombosis. **A,** Radiocolloid scan showed enlarged liver and spleen *(arrows),* but spleen-to-liver radioactivity ratio was decreased. **B,** Repeat scan 10 days *(10d)* later, showed further enlargement of spleen, increase in spleen-to-liver ratio, and somewhat heterogeneous distribution of Kupffer cell function. If this progresses to include arteriolar thrombosis, portrayal may resemble that of focal metastatic disease.

appear as discrete focal lesions in the liver, whereas breast manifestations may be hepatomegaly, focal lesions, or a generalized patchiness, simulating cirrhosis in the extreme. One study reported a sensitivity of 67% for breast lesions if only focal lesions were considered positive, and this increased to 87% when the criteria included hepatomegaly heterogeneity or focal defects. When the latter liberal criteria were applied to colorectal cancers, there was no change in sensitivity (about 88%); however, the false positive rate increased for breast tumors from 9% to 29% and for colorectal tumors from 6% to 27%.[21] Histologically, breast lesions are known to be small, infiltrative, and associated with fibrosis, whereas colorectal lesions are discrete and large at initial presentation. Lymphomas and leukemia usually exhibit diffuse rather than focal lesions.

There is some controversy regarding liver scans for screening patients with known primary carcinomas for purposes of staging and subsequent management. In the absence of hepatomegaly and normal liver function tests, no true positive liver scans occurred in 109 bronchogenic carcinomas, whereas 23 of 154 (15%) had true positive radiocolloid liver scans when at least one clinical finding suggested liver disease.[46,80] Results of this kind prompted some investigators to conclude that it is not financially efficacious to perform preoperative liver scans routinely if there is no clinical or biochemical reason to suspect liver disease, and that high-risk patients should be screened with biochemical tests such as alkaline phosphatase, SGOT, LDH, and serum bilirubin. Others argue that baseline liver scans could disclose nonneoplastic lesions or variations in anatomic configuration, which might confuse the diagnosis when biochemical abnormalities develop later on.

Primary malignant neoplasms

Hepatomas account for 80% of primary malignancies of the liver, followed by cholangiocarcinomas and the rare Kupffer cell sarcoma. About 80% of hepatomas and 30% of cholangiocarcinomas arise in cirrhotic livers. Either one may occur as a solitary massive tumor, multiple lesions, or diffuse infiltration of the liver substance.

There are no distinguishing radiocolloid features of hepatomas or cholangiocarcinomas, and in a cirrhotic context they may resemble pseudotumors. Pseudotumors are areas of absent radiocolloid uptake caused by scarring, regenerating nodules, necrosis, and arteriovenous shunting in a cirrhotic liver. Hepatomas are often quite vascular and exhibit increased flow on first-pass perfusion studies with a ^{99m}Tc-tracer; about 90% will also concentrate ^{67}Ga, whereas pseudotumors do not express these features. However, ^{67}Ga is not specific for tumor, because avid uptakes are also obtained in liver abscess (Fig. 53-8). Hepatomas are associated with alpha$_1$ fetal protein in the serum in 50% to 70% of the patients.[61,91]

Benign tumors

Focal nodular hyperplasia and hepatic adenoma are uncommon tumors occurring in women and associated with the use of oral contraceptives or other sex steroids. Focal nodular hyperplasia features a centrally located stellate fibrous zone and hepatocytes, bile ducts, and Kupffer cells in disarray. The presence of variable numbers of Kupffer cells enables the uptake of radiocolloid, and in about 65% of the lesions the concentration is either higher or equal to that of the adjacent normal liver tissue. ^{99m}TC-IDA will be concentrated by the hepatocyte elements, but it is associated with a prolonged washout because of poorly formed biliary radicles[8,82]

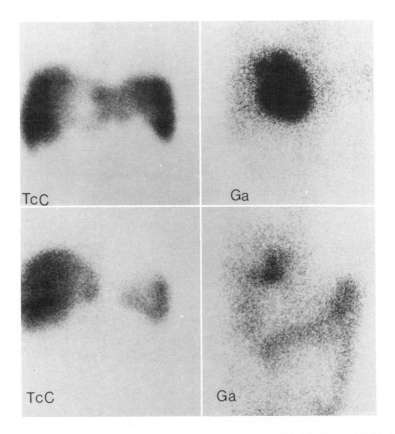

Fig. 53-8 Liver hepatoma *(upper panel)* and abscess *(lower panel)* are indistinguishable by radiocolloid *(TcC)* and ^{67}Ga imaging. Both produced photopenic lesions with radiocolloid and depicted avid uptake of [67]Ga.

(Fig. 53-9). The lesion shows normal or increased first-pass perfusion and blood pool activity with ^{99m}Tc-labeled erythrocytes.

Hepatic adenomas are characterized by a disorganized population of hepatocytes with a dense supply of small vessels around the periphery. Many lesions contain Kupffer cells, but for some unexplained reason they do not concentrate radiocolloid, and as a result the adenomas are generally photon deficient relative to normal liver tissue.[63] Hepatic adenomas are also prone to internal hemorrhage and necrosis, and this too may contribute to the photon-deficient appearance. The presence of well differentiated hepatocytes and absence of biliary structures promotes the uptake of ^{99m}Tc-IDA, but without drainage.[109]

Cavernous hemangioma is the most common benign tumor in the liver, occurring in about 3% of the population, and often found incidentally by ultrasonography. ^{99m}Tc-labeled erythrocyte imaging shows a characteristic hypoperfusion and decreased initial blood pool activity, followed by progressive accumulation of labeled erythrocytes over the next hour or two (Fig. 53-10). The rationale for these observations is that hemangiomas represent a mass of ineffectual blood spaces, and the newly injected labeled erythrocytes are slow to enter these

spaces and slow to leave. The sensitivity of detection approaches 90%.[11,24,36] Some of these lesions are too small to be seen with radiocolloid as photon-deficient zones but will be detected as hot spots with the labeled erythrocytes. SPECT imaging with ^{99m}Tc erythrocytes has been shown to detect small hemangiomas that escaped planar imaging.

Hemangiomatous lesions in the liver of infants and children, which include capillary hemangioma and infantile hemangioendothelioma, have significantly different characteristics from the adult lesion. The pediatric lesions exhibit an increase in perfusion rather than a decrease, and the immediate static blood pool images of the hemangioma show a concentration of ^{99m}Tc erythrocytes that equals the heart blood pool. These features distinguish pediatric hemangiomas from other lesions like hepatoblastoma, nodular hyperplasia, and fibromuscular hamartoma, wherein the delayed static blood pool activity is less than that of the heart.[69]

Focal fatty infiltration of the liver was virtually unknown before the advent of computed tomography (CT) and ultrasonography. The characteristics on CT scans are low density, nonspherical shape, and lack of anatomic distortion, whereas the radiocolloid image is usually normal, although low-grade inhomogeneity can occur.[3]

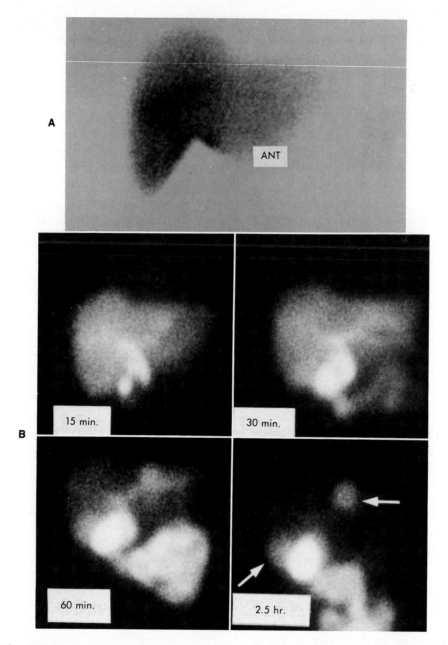

Fig. 53-9 Focal nodular hyperplasia. **A,** Anterior *(ANT)* radiocolloid image is normal except for apparent decreased uptake in upper third of right lobe caused by overlying breast attenuation in this 49-year-old woman. **B,** Serial ^{99m}Tc-IDA images showing uniform parenchymal function at 15 minutes, but with time there are two foci of prolonged parenchymal retention *(arrows)*. This is consistent with Kupffer cell and hepatocyte function within nodules.

Cysts

Solitary epithelial cysts have an occurrence of about 0.1% and are generally asymptomatic.[90] About 25% of patients with polycystic kidneys have polycystic liver disease. The radiocolloid depiction is that of hepatomegaly and multiple focal lesions, a nonspecific presentation (Fig. 53-11). The diagnosis is established by ul-trasonography, which shows well-circumscribed hypoechoic lesions.

Hydatid cysts usually occur in the right lobe of the liver, are solitary, can grow to a large size, are avascular by radionuclide perfusion, and are photon deficient by radiocolloid imaging.[50]

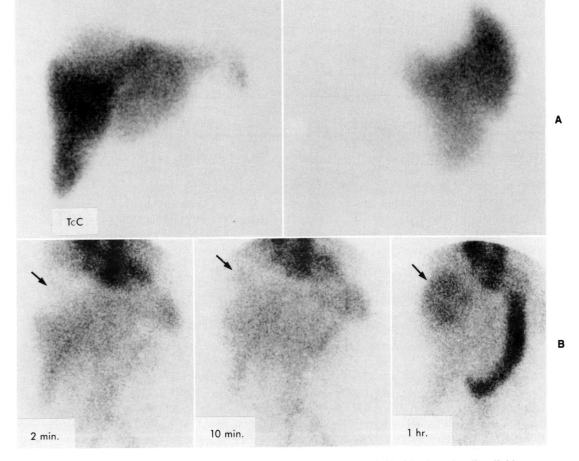

Fig. 53-10 Cavernous hemangioma in adult woman. **A,** Anterior and right lateral radiocolloid *(TcC, technetium collloid)* liver images demonstrate large solitary lesion in upper posterior part of right lobe. **B,** ^{99m}Tc-labeled red blood cell blood pool images taken at various times after administration, showing progressive accumulation within lesion. Hemangioma is not seen at 2 minutes, but early entry is observed at 10 minutes, and lesion has higher concentration than adjacent normal liver at 1 hour *(arrows)*.

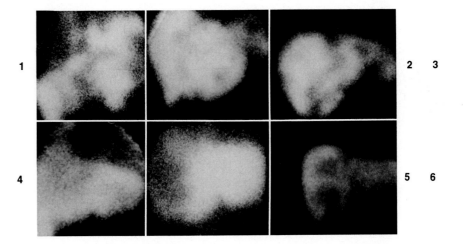

Fig. 53-11 Radiocolloid liver scans in variety of conditions, which by themselves are nonspecific in appearance. *1,* Polycystic liver; *2,* metastases from primary colonic adenocarcinoma; *3,* hemangioendothelioma in infant, which reverted to normal with steroid treatment; *4,* primary amyloidosis showing shift of colloid to lung; *5,* amebic abscess; *6,* trauma.

Abscesses

Pyogenic liver infection occurs, as a rule, after abdominal surgery. As an abscess they can be solitary or multiple, but the radiocolloid depiction is nonspecific. Within the clinical context of fever, tenderness, right upper quadrant pain, and leukocytosis, the abnormal scan will suggest sepsis. [67]Ga concentrates in abscesses, but it also has a tropism for tumors, particularly hepatoma, and therefore lacks the desired specificity (Fig. 53-8). [111]In leukocytes have greater specificity but the indium is more troublesome to prepare.

Amebic liver abscesses develop as a complication of colonic amebiasis and are solitary in 96% of the cases, with a predominantly right lobe location[17] (Fig. 53-11). This produces a photon-deficient lesion on the radiocolloid scan, but ^{67}Ga images have been reported to show a central photon deficiency surrounded by a rind of increased uptake.[37] These lesions decrease in size with successful treatment, but residual defects may remain with the patient in remission.

Perihepatic abscesses may cause a local impression on the liver due to pressure build-up, and thereby reveal its presence indirectly. Most often this is not the case, and ^{67}Ga or ^{111}In leukocytes are requested to search for a clinically suspected intraabdominal septic focus. These radiopharmaceuticals can detect the focus at the phlegmon stage, before the development of an abscess that can be aspirated. The procedure is usually combined with ultrasonography to determine the physical characteristics of the lesion.

Trauma

The liver can be affected by blunt or penetrating trauma, and the radiocolloid manifestations of decreased concentration are variable and without distinguishing features (Fig. 53-11). ^{99m}Tc-IDA images may show intrahepatic or extrahepatic bile leak as a more specific reflection of injury. An increase in intrahepatic pressure from edema and hematoma may cause a shift of radiocolloid to the spleen. A tear in the diaphragm facilitates liver herniation (Fig. 53-12). Subcapsular hematomas following needle biopsy tend to produce lentiform peripheral defects.[66] However, ultrasonography or CT is recommended for assessment of intraabdominal trauma in the initial stages of presentation, because each has a sensitivity and ability to examine other structures and search for fluid collections.

Postradiation lesions

Radiotherapy doses in the range of 3000 rad can produce a transient defect in Kupffer cell and hepatocyte function. This will be reflected in decreased uptake of radiocolloid and ^{99m}Tc-IDA within the sharp confines of the treatment portal. Higher doses may produce permanent defects as a result of vasculitis and subsequent atrophy and fibrosis.[57]

Focal hot lesions

The most common entity producing this focal increased uptake of radiocolloid above the surrounding normally functioning tissue is superior vena cava obstruc-

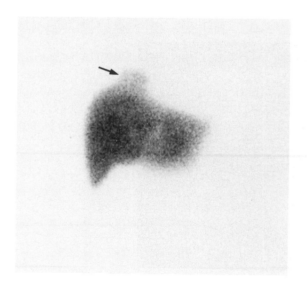

Fig. 53-12 Herniation of segment of liver through rent in right leaf of diaphragm as result of motor vehicle accident *(arrow)*.

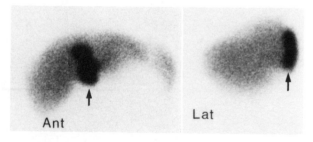

Fig. 53-13 Anterior *(Ant)* and right lateral *(Lat)* radiocolloid liver images in patient with obstruction of superior vena cava. There is increased uptake in quadrate lobe *(arrows)*.

tion. In this condition collateral channels develop between the superior vena cava and left portal vein via the umbilical vein. The branches of the left portal vein supply the quadrate lobe primarily, and this additional delivery of radiocolloid results in a focal concentration that is located anteriorly between the right and left lobes of the liver[52] (Fig. 53-13). Obstruction of the inferior vena cava has been reported to produce a similar hot spot, but it is a much rarer event.[59] Increased local vascularity has accounted for hot spots in abscesses and focal nodular hyperplasia.[13]

Hepatic artery infusion studies

Chemotherapeutic drugs and Y-90 microspheres are currently being infused through catheters placed in the hepatic artery to ablate liver metastases. It is imperative that the whole tumor is perfused and that as little as possible of the extrahepatic structures receive a direct first-pass perfusion of the cytotoxic drugs or radioactive microspheres. This requires proper placement of the catheter tip. Contrast angiography, which entails a bolus injection, does not predict the flow distribution at the slow flow rates used for treatment, nor can the amount and location of extrahepatic perfusion be determined.[54] Perfusion can be measured and located by imaging the liver after a slow infusion of ^{99m}Tc-labeled macroaggregates of albumin (MAA) through the treatment catheter. The ^{99m}Tc-MAA infusion can determine the area of the liver

receiving the treatment agent on first-pass, quantitate the amount of arteriovenous shunting by showing the lung uptake of the shunted moiety, and evaluate the presence of extrahepatic perfusion. For example, inadvertent perfusion of the gastroduodenal artery can lead to abdominal pain and gastric ulceration if it is large enough (Fig. 53-14). The amount of ^{99m}Tc-MAA deposited along this pathway can be an indicator for repositioning of the catheter tip to preclude the complications. The distribution of the catheter perfusion should be monitored periodically with ^{99m}Tc-MAA because the catheter tip can move, the tip may become clotted, or the perfused artery may thrombose—all of which may alter the territory of perfusion.[117]

BILIARY TRACT IMAGING
Cholecystitis

Obstruction of the cystic duct is the initiating cause of acute cholecystitis in about 95% of the patients. Visualization of the gallbladder with ^{99m}Tc-IDA therefore virtually excludes acute disease. Acute acalculous cholecystitis, an infrequently occurring entity, may be associated with gallbladder filling, but in that case the administration of CCK fails to induce a normal contraction. In most of these cases, however, the gallbladder is not visualized, presumably a result of cystic duct occlusion by edema.[67]

Failure to visualize the gallbladder within 4 hours or complete liver washout in the presence of normal or

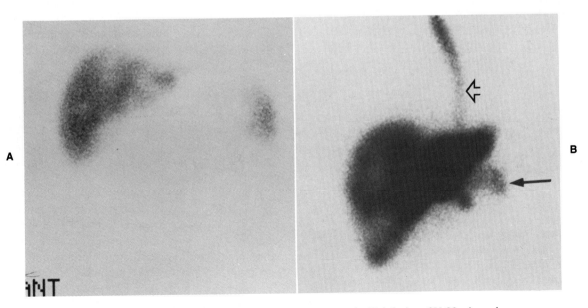

Fig. 53-14 Colorectal carcinoma with metastases to liver treated with infusion of Y-90 microspheres. Patient developed gastroduodenal ulceration as complication. **A,** Radiocolloid scan demonstrating multiple intrahepatic lesions. **B,** Overexposed ^{99m}Tc-macroaggregates of albumin scan after slow infusion into hepatic artery through treatment catheter *(open arrow)*. Solid arrow points to uptake in gastroduodenal area, site of later ulceration.

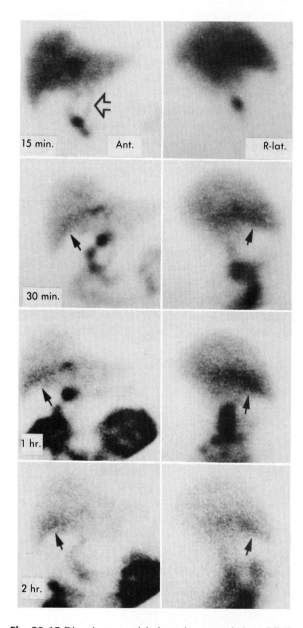

Fig. 53-15 Rim sign or pericholecystic accumulation of ⁹⁹ᵐTc-IDA in acute cholecystitis—anterior and right lateral views. At 15 minutes common duct is identified; it is deviated and bowed medially *(open arrow)*, reflecting enlarged nonvisualized gallbladder. As liver washes out, rim of relatively higher concentration develops *(solid arrows)*, but gallbladder does not visualize with time. *Ant*, Anterior; *R-Lat*, Right lateral.

mildly impaired liver function should not be considered pathognomonic of acute disease. The disease could be either acute or chronic, and the finding must be interpreted within the clinical context.[75] The frequency of nonvisualization in chronic cholecystitis varies from 0.5% to 50%.[34,81,85,113] A recent study of 101 patients who had elective cholecystectomy for chronic cholecystitis, and were documented by all clinical, surgical, and pathologic criteria to have only chronic cholecystitis, showed that 16 of 101 patients (16%) failed to have visualized gallbladders. Of the 85 gallbladders, 82 (96%) filled within 1 hour, (the same as the normal gallbladder).[81] There was no statistical difference in the duration of symptoms between those patients who had gallbladder visualization and those who did not. Whatever the incidence, it is important to recognize that abdominal distress and a nonvisualized gallbladder are not solely diagnostic of acute cholecystitis.

The rim sign, when it appears, is a diagnostic aid in the presence of nonvisualization. It consists of a faintly increased concentration of ⁹⁹ᵐTc-IDA in the liver tissue bordering the gallbladder fossa, and has been observed in acute cholecystitis, gangrenous cholecystitis, gallbladder perforation, and, rarely, in chronic cholecystitis when the gallbladder did not visualize[10,12,98] (Fig. 53-15). There is no consensus on how it is produced; delayed clearance from locally inflamed liver tissue, hepatic injury with impaired excretion into the biliary tract, and extravasation into the pericholecystic area through a gallbladder tear have all been suggested. A perfusion study with ⁹⁹ᵐTc-IDA has been advocated, because increased first-pass transit and static blood pool activity in the absence of gallbladder visualization favors acute rather than chronic cholecystitis.[16] Deviation and bowing of the common duct medially is also suggestive of an enlarged inflamed gallbladder.

The true positive frequency—that is, the sensitivity—of ⁹⁹ᵐTc-IDA nucleography for acute cholecystitis is high, varying from 95% to 100%, and with specificities ranging from 94% to 100%.[35,67,108,113] False negative results are attributed to intermittent cystic duct obstruction, partial obstruction, and acalculous cholecystitis.

It has been observed that a gallbladder that becomes visually identified after 1 hour, rather than within the first hour, is most often chronically diseased. However, in one controlled series of chronic cholecystitis this delay occurred in 3 of the 85 patients (4%), which is a rather low frequency.[81] This delayed filling is not entirely understood, but it is hypothesized that the increased diffusion gradient between the viscid gallbladder contents and the bile newly elaborated by the liver slows the usual rate of entry into the viscus. This hypothesis is supported by the observation that emptying the gallbladder with a CCK infusion may convert absent or delayed visualization beyond 1 hour to visualization in less than 1 hour.[33] It should be emphasized that gallbladder filling within 1 hour does not exclude the possibility of chronic cholecystitis, because 96% of those that fill do so within the first hour. Chronic cholecystitis is more appropriately diagnosed with ultrasonography, because the radionuclide method rarely discloses stones within the viscus because of the inherent resolution limitations of the gamma camera; nor can the method evaluate wall thickness. ^{99m}Tc-IDA imaging is essentially a dynamic appraisal of the bile flow pathways, and conclusions are drawn by inference from the observed alterations of the usual spatial and temporal relationships.

Patients on total parenteral nutrition and chronic alcoholics with liver disease are reported to have had normal gallbladders that either showed delayed visualization or no visualization at all when followed for 24 hours.[95] The gallbladder filled when oral feeding resumed. It has been suggested that the gallbladder should be emptied by an infusion of CCK before administration of ^{99m}Tc-IDA to improve chances of visualization in this group of patients. Another report implied that the false positive rate has been exaggerated in the past. It was found that 7 of 9 patients (78%) who had been on total parenteral nutrition for 5 to 27 days and 6 of 8 patients (75%) who were fasting for 5 to 11 days demonstrated gallbladder visualization.[97] The reasons for this lack of filling are not entirely clear, but it is postulated that hepatocyte damage and lack of oral intake result in a decrease in bile formation and an increase in bile viscosity. Abetted by a lack of endogenous CCK elaboration, which receives its stimulus from oral feeding, the gallbladder does not contract, its bile contents become more viscid, and the increasing intraviscus osmotic gradient deters inflow of newly formed bile. It has been suggested that patients on total parenteral nutrition who have a low serum albumin, increased alkaline phosphatase, and increased SGPT are more prone to absent gallbladder filling.[110]

It has been found that about 50% of normal gallbladders are not visualized by intravenous contrast radiography in the presence of acute pancreatitis. Only after the pancreatitis subsides can the viscus be seen.[53,111] This limitation, which could result in a fallacious presumptive diagnosis of acute cholecystitis, does not apply to ^{99m}Tc-IDA imaging. Furthermore, whereas hyperbilirubinemias of 3 mg/dl or more, seriously impair the ability of intravenous contrast radiography to visualize the gallbladder, it is not an impediment to ^{99m}Tc-IDA. In one study 13 out of 15 patients (87%) with normal and chronically diseased gallbladders coincident with acute pancreatitis were visualized, but no distinction was made between a biliary and nonbiliary origin of the pancreatitis.[31] The two patients with absent filling of the gallbladder were shown to have chronic cholecystitis by ultrasonography.

Two other reports indicated gallbladder visualization in the presence of acute pancreatitis in 16 of 21 patients (76%) and 17 of 22 patients (77%), respectively.[1,32] Failure to see the gallbladder was caused by a concommitant acute cholecystitis in both series. A large series consisting of 60 patients with acute pancreatitis, 20 of nonbiliary origin and 40 of biliary origin, showed different results in the two subgroups.[93] Of the 20 patients, 19 (95%) with nonbiliary acute pancreatitis exhibited visualization of the gallbladder and gut within 1 hour, and the remaining patient had delayed gallbladder filling; that is, all 20 patients were shown to have patent cystic ducts. In the group of 40 patients with biliary pancreatitis, only 60% of the gallbladders were seen. The failures were caused by coexisting acute or chronic cholecystitis. Normal gallbladder and gut visualization within 1 hour was achieved in only 9 of the 40 patients (23%). The other 31 patients presented with either delayed visualization or nonvisualization of the gallbladder associated with or without delayed or absent gut entry. It was concluded from these results that elevated serum amylase levels together with an abnormal ^{99m}Tc-IDA study favored biliary pancreatitis, whereas a temporally normal study implied nonbiliary pancreatitis.

Acalculous biliary pain

Biliary dyskinesia, chronic acalculous cholecystitis, and cystic duct syndrome are terms applied to abnormal gallbladder contractions associated with right upper quadrant pain in the absence of gallstone detection by radiographic cholecystography and ultrasonography.[84,107] It is alleged that these patients become symptom free following cholecystectomy.[26,58,78] Histologically the gallbladders may be normal, show evidence of cholecystitis or adenomyomatosis, or there may be fibrosis and narrowing of the lumen of the cystic duct with or without gallbladder disease. There is an ongoing debate over the criteria for selecting the patients who might benefit from cholecystectomy. It is asserted that reproduction of the pain symptoms in response to a slow infusion of CCK is sufficient indication for surgery.[58,107] A claim has been made that a CCK-induced gallbladder ejection fraction of less than 35% in the appropriate clinical setting is suggestive of chronic acalculous cholecystitis, cystic duct syndrome, or a combination of both, but there was no mention of the role of the reproduction of symptoms in this communication.[26] Some authors require both a reproduction of symptoms and an impaired ejection fraction as criteria for a positive test.[38,42] However, patients have apparently been relieved of symptoms who had normal ejection fractions, no reproduction of symptoms, or both.[78] Although CCK causes right upper quadrant pain more often in symptomatic patients than normal volunteers, the response has been too variable, and coupled with the fact that ejection fractions in chronic cholecystitis can vary from 5% to 95%,[79,81] it has been concluded by one group of investigators that the test is not predictive of clinical results and has no place in patient management.[19]

Cholestasis

Hepatobiliary scintigraphy is capable of distinguishing an extrahepatic cause of jaundice (which may be surgically remedied) from an intrahepatic or prehepatic cause (which calls for medical management). Complete extrahepatic obstruction is characterized by an absence of liver-to-bowel transit over a 24-hour-period of monitoring (Fig. 53-16). Another, secondary feature is nonvisualization of the biliary ducts and gallbladder. There is usually good hepatocyte concentration when the obstruction is of recent onset. Intrahepatic jaundice includes hepatocellular failure and intrahepatic cholestasis, which

give rise to unconjugated and conjugated hyperbilirubinemia, respectively. The ^{99m}Tc-IDA portrayal is inconstant: liver uptake is variably reduced; liver-to-bowel transit may be normal, delayed, or absent with extreme impairment; no biliary tract pooling exists to suggest dilatation, but the gallbladder may be seen sometime within the 24 hours of administration. Prehepatic jaundice (for instance, hemolytic anemia) generally shows a normal time course of liver concentration and washout. Progressive accumulation of ^{99m}Tc-IDA within the biliary tract plus gut entry beyond 1 hour is the hallmark of incomplete mechanical choledochal obstruction (Fig. 53-16). With these criteria the reported sensitivity rates for medical jaundice, complete obstruction, and incomplete obstruction are 77% to 90%, 98% to 100%, and 74% to 78%, respectively.[14,30,76]

For a given serum bilirubin level there is on average a higher initial uptake of ^{99m}Tc-IDA in mechanical ob-

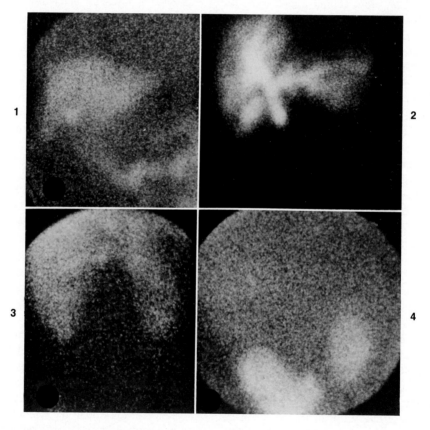

Fig. 53-16 Various causes of jaundice shown with ^{99m}Tc-IDA. *1,* Hepatitis in patient with serum bilirubin of 4.7 mg/dl. Poor liver concentration is noted, but gallbladder and duodenum are visualized. *2,* Incomplete obstruction due to carcinoma of pancreas in patient with serum bilirubin of 3.2 mg/dl. At 90 minutes there is no entry into gut, but gallbladder is visualized, and there is stasis in dilated common and intrahepatic bile ducts. *3,* Complete obstruction showing retention in liver and no bowel radioactivity at 24 hours, but kidneys are seen because they are alternate channel of excretion. *4,* End-stage liver failure in patient with serum bilirubin of 35 mg/dl. No liver uptake was seen at 8 hours, and excretion via horseshoe kidneys was demonstrated.

struction than primary hepatocellular failure. It has been reported that for bilirubin levels less than 10 mg/dl, no patient with hepatic failure had a normal uptake of the diethyl analog of ^{99m}Tc-IDA, whereas 58% of the patients with mechanical obstruction exhibited normal uptake. Normal uptake was still registered in 17% of mechanical obstructions with bilirubins between 10 mg/dl and 20 mg/dl, but within this range 42% of hepatocyte failure showed no liver uptake of diethyl-IDA compared with 8% showing mechanical obstruction. By incorporating these observations, images that do not depict the biliary tract and whose caliber cannot therefore be assessed may on occasion be correctly separated into hepatocellular failure or extrahepatic obstruction.[14,76] Certain caveats must be borne in mind. Drug-induced intrahepatic cholestasis, which is associated with obstructive biochemistries and good uptake of ^{99m}Tc-IDA, may be misconstrued as incomplete extrahepatic obstruction—a surgical disorder rather than one requiring medical management. The severity of the cholestasis may at times be so severe that there is no excretion into the gut, thereby simulating complete extrahepatic obstruction. Endotoxic shock has the potential to mimic extrahepatic obstruction by virtue of good ^{99m}Tc-IDA uptake and prolonged parenchymal transit time.[48] Massive tumor infiltration of the liver and portal vein thrombosis can also be associated with absent bile entry into the gut.

The underlying difficulty in the differential diagnosis is that the dilated biliary tract in partial common duct obstruction is not always seen as a progressive accumulation of radioactivity, a pattern that has a positive predictive value of 90% to 95%. This occurs only when the liver bile flow is adequate. The gamma-ray image of the ectatic duct is a function not only of the duct size but also of the concentration of radioactivity within it. When the bile flow is markedly reduced, as occurs in high serum bilirubin levels, the amount of radioactivity excreted into the biliary tract is low, and as a result the appearance may resemble a normal-caliber duct or it may not be seen at all. In a study consisting of 30 patients whose biliary tract was assessed by transhepatic cholangiography, ERCP, operative cholangiography, and fistulography, 10 of 13 cases (77%) of ductal dilatation secondary to incomplete obstruction were missed by ^{99m}Tc-IDA cholescintigraphy. The average serum bilirubin level in the false negative group was 7.0 mg/dl compared with 4.3 mg/dl for the true positive group, indicating a greater failure rate with more advanced liver impairment.[87] Pooling of ^{99m}Tc-IDA in the biliary tract and initial bowel entry within 1 hour does not exclude partial extrahepatic obstruction, even though it is characteristic of unobstructed dilated ducts—for instance, in Caroli's disease, choledochal cyst, oriental cholangiohepatitis,[115] congenital hepatic fibrosis,[66] and postcho-

lecystectomy with biliary tract exploration or postcholangiointestinal anastomoses (Fig. 53-17).

There is also an inherent false negative frequency common to radionuclide imaging, ultrasonography, and computed tomography: an absence of biliary tract dilatation in 5% to 10% of cases of partial mechanical obstruction.[41,89] If there is an associated delayed or absent gut entry, then the diagnosis will be suggested by cholescintigraphy. This can occur with an acute impaction of a gallstone in the common duct, because it takes about 24 hours for the intrabiliary tract pressure to build up to a level that causes detectable dilatation by ultrasonography. A group of 22 such cases has been reported.[112]

Overall, the limitations encountered with ^{99m}Tc-IDA in the differential diagnosis of jaundice weigh against its use as a primary screening procedure. Ultrasonography is preferred over CT in terms of economy, but their diagnostic efficacies are about the same. The sensitivity and specificity of ultrasound in predicting the status of the biliary tract are reported to be 85% to 100% and 75% to 100%, respectively.[65,71,89] ^{99m}Tc-IDA imaging plays an adjuvant role in patients with jaundice who have had no previous cholangioenteric reconstructive procedures, when ultrasonography is indeterminate, when the results of ultrasonography do not correspond to the clinical and biochemical parameters, or when there is a need to gain some insight into the bile flow dynamics.

Postcholecystectomy syndrome occurs in approximately 10% to 50% of patients following gallbladder resection. Causes include retained stones, biliary dyskinesia, common bile duct stricture or tumor, papillary stenosis, common bile duct obstruction secondary to pancreatitis, and cystic duct remnant. Many of these complications can be disclosed by ^{99m}Tc-IDA imaging. A cystic duct remnant occurred in 14% of one series of 125 symptomatic postcholecystectomy patients.[114] These remnants may function as small gallbladders, form stones, become inflamed, and function as a source of recurrent episodes of choledocholithiasis. On occasion the cystic duct remnant may be visualized with ^{99m}Tc-IDA.[18]

Surgically altered biliary and gastrointestinal anatomy

The technique of monitoring the bile pathway with ^{99m}Tc-IDA analogs offers an innocuous, dynamic and clinically useful procedure for clarification of postsurgical complications associated with cholecystointestinal and choledochointestinal anastomoses and gastroenteric bypasses. Normally functioning cholangiointestinal conduits exhibit bowel radioactivity within 1 hour. Extrahepatic obstruction is manifested as delayed gut entry with dilatation and stasis within the proximal biliary tract. The biliary tract is often left with residual dilatation after

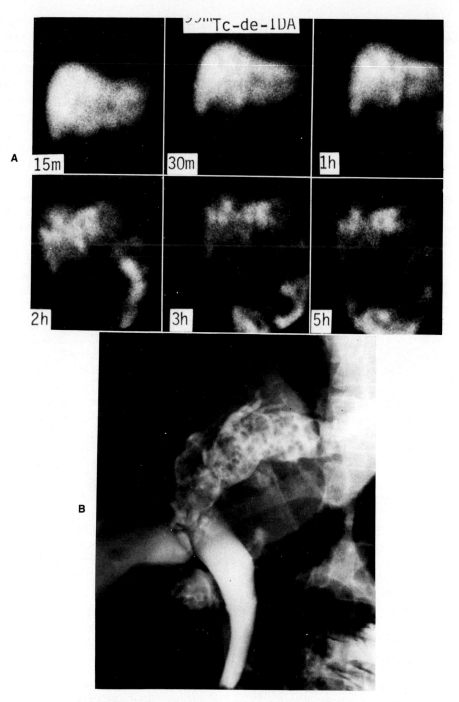

Fig. 53-17 Oriental cholangiohepatitis in Chinese male. Patient had history of repeated attacks of ascending cholangitis and jaundice. At time of examination serum bilirubin level was normal. **A,** ^{99m}Tc-diethyl-IDA (Etifenin) study exhibited good concentration in liver at 15 minutes. There was bowel entry within 1 hour, but there was also intraductal pooling within right and left lobes, persisting as long as 5 hours. **B,** ERCP portrayed innumerable stones in enlarged left biliary duct. No contrast material entered right duct.

operative intervention, but the hallmark of partial obstruction is delayed gut entry of ^{99m}Tc-IDA rather than pooling within the biliary tract per se. A patient with residual nonobstructive dilatation complicated by medical jaundice will either show a normal or a delayed intestinal entry time, and although the biliary tract will be visibly dilated, it will not show the progressive accumulation of radioactivity with time, which is characteristic of true partial obstruction. With further progressive liver impairment and decreasing bile production, gut entry will be delayed and the ductal ectasia will not be manifest because of insufficient radioactivity within it.

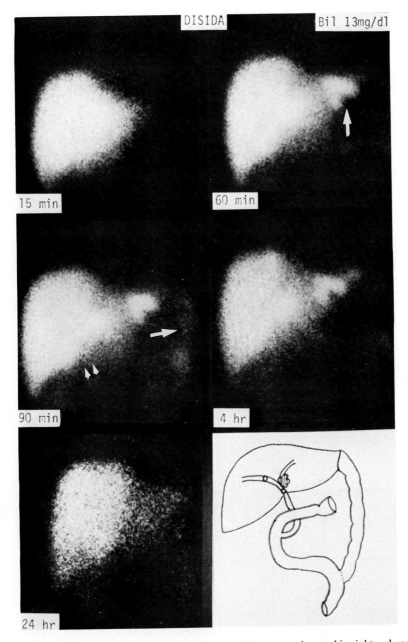

Fig. 53-18 Cholangiocarcinoma at common hepatic duct. A stent was inserted in right and common hepatic ducts to sustain biliary drainage. Additionally, partial left lobe hepatectomy and anastomosis of left hepatic duct to a Roux-en-Y segment of jejunum were effected (Longmire's procedure). The ^{99m}Tc-diisopropyl-IDA (DISIDA, Disofenin) study performed 5 days postoperatively showed drainage through this bypass *(arrow)* but no biliary flow through common duct *(twin arrows)*. Latter pathway was obstructed. Note differential drainage between right and left lobes at 24 hours as compared with 15 minutes. Serum bilirubin was 13 mg/dl at time of study.

The only conclusion that can be drawn from these conditions is that an element of patency exists. This is not as critical a limitation in the postsurgical period as it is in the unoperated patient presenting for a differential diagnosis of jaundice. The postoperative indications of cholescintigraphy are a failure of the serum bilirubin levels to normalize and clinical suspicion of bile leak. Persistent elevation of the serum bilirubin can be caused by anastomotic obstruction, anesthetic hepatotoxicity, hemolysis, or the resorption of a large volume of intraabdominal bile extravasation. In these circumstances the presence of ^{99m}Tc-IDA in the bowel indicates that the anastomosis is not completely obstructed, but it cannot distinguish partial obstruction from normal patency, because of the existing decreased bile flow (Fig. 53-18). This information is sufficient to forestall remedial surgery and keep the patient under observation. If no intestinal radioactivity is discernible over 24 hours, a potential surgical emergency exists. Bile leak is readily appreci-ated and very commonly ceases spontaneously, whether it be secondary to a tear in the biliary tract or to occlusion of the anastomosis by edema with subsequent spill through the suture sites. These patients can be monitored serially to study the changing status of the bile flow pathways (Fig. 53-19).

In patients with normally functioning gastroenteros-tomies the afferent and efferent loops are seen within 1 hour, and the afferent loop washout is usually achieved by 2 hours (Fig. 53-20). Obstruction appears as a pro-gressive accumulation of ^{99m}Tc-IDA in the segment prox-imal to the stenosis and as a delay or absence of antegrade movement (Fig. 53-21). Gastroduodenal reflux is com-monly seen with Billroth II surgery: 15 of 16 patients (94%) in one report.[88] The refluxed radioactivity nor-mally washes out of the stomach remnant in parallel with the progression from the afferent to efferent loop; failure to do so should provoke a suspicion of partial anastomotic obstruction.

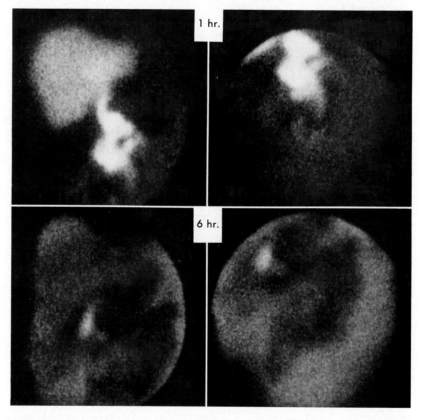

Fig. 53-19 Large-volume bile leak. This patient had cholecystectomy and common bile duct exploration with T-tube left in place. He pulled out T-tube, and assessment of bile flow pathway was requested. ^{99m}Tc-IDA images of liver and abdomen at 1 hour and 6 hours are shown. At 1 hour duodenum and adjacent amorphic collection of radioactivity were seen, with some diffusion in abdominal cavity. At 6 hours most of ^{99m}Tc-IDA had dispersed throughout abdominal cavity, and there was no entry into small intestines.

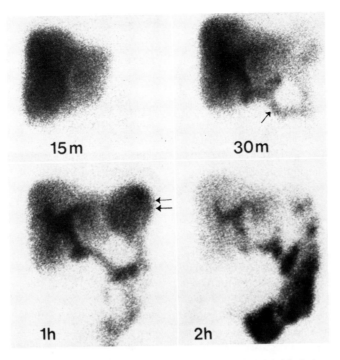

Fig. 53-20 Unobstructed dilated biliary tract and gastric reflux in patient with cholecystojejunostomy and Billroth II gastroenterostomy. Whipple's procedure for carcinoma of pancreas had been previously performed, and there was no jaundice at time of ^{99m}Tc-IDA study. Serial images demonstrate dilated hepatic and common ducts, but there was no obstruction because gut entry occurred within ½ hour of administration *(arrow)* and liver parenchyma showed normal washout. Gastric reflux is clearly seen at 1 hour *(twin arrows)*, and it progressively disappears with time. Afferent and efferent loop transit is normal, and there is no evidence of afferent loop stasis.

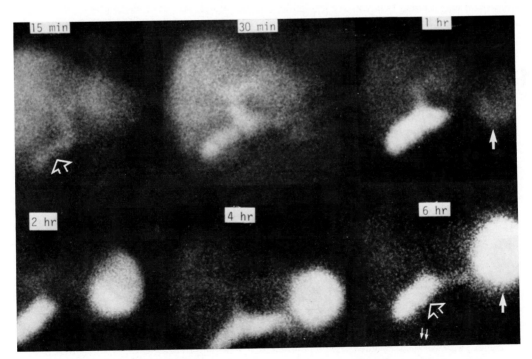

Fig. 53-21 Inlet-outlet obstruction in patient who had Whipple's procedure for papillary carcinoma of ampulla of Vater. It included partial gastrectomy, choledochojejunostomy, end-to-end pancreaticojejunostomy, and retrocolic gastrojejunostomy. Chief complaint was copious bile vomiting. ^{99m}Tc-IDA images depict efferent loop entry at 15 minutes *(open arrow)*, gastric reflux at 1 hour *(solid arrow)*, and persistent stasis in afferent loop and stomach remnant as late as 6 hours. Efferent loop entry is recorded only after 2 hours. Findings are consistent with partial inlet-outlet obstruction.

Congenital and familial defects

Biliary atresia

In neonatal jaundice that persists beyond the first month of life there exists a small group of infants who have either a conjugated or mixed conjugated-and-unconjugated bilirubinemia and inconclusive clinical and laboratory investigations. These features make the differential diagnosis of neonatal hepatitis and biliary atresia difficult at best. Some help may accrue from combined ultrasonography and hepatobiliary imaging.

The 3-day stool collection assay of parenterally administered ^{131}I–rose bengal was introduced to distinguish between neonatal jaundice and biliary atresia, but errors were introduced by the inadvertant mixing of stool and urine. It was then supplemented or replaced with serial liver and abdominal imaging. This was a qualified success, because the appearance of the test agent in the gut excluded biliary atresia, but its absence, even for as long as 96 hours, was not necessarily diagnostic of biliary atresia (Fig. 53-22). Some cases of severe intrahepatic cholestasis do not exhibit visible excretion, although the stool assay indicates that excretion has occurred.[96] Pretreating the infants with phenobarbital (5 mg/kg/day for 3 to 7 days) enhances the bile flow and increases the frequency of ^{99m}Tc-IDA visualization in the bowel of infants with neonatal hepatitis. In one small series, 4 of 5 infants demonstrated ^{99m}Tc-IDA in the bowel within 24 hours after having several days of phenobarbital pretreatment, whereas there was no visible bowel accumulation in the same group when the phenobarbital was omitted. Biliary atresia, as would be anticipated, showed no bowel

radioactivity with or without prior phenobarbital stimulation.[64]

In infants less than 3 months of age, poor liver extraction of ^{99m}Tc-IDA favors a diagnosis of neonatal hepatitis, whereas good extraction and absent bowel radioactivity support a diagnosis of biliary atresia. In biliary atresia of more than 3 months' duration the progressively developing cirrhosis tends to reduce the liver uptake of ^{99m}Tc-IDA and may resemble severe neonatal hepatitis. Ultrasonographic demonstration of a normal gallbladder is suggestive of neonatal hepatitis, whereas nonvisualization or the identification of a small gallbladder favors biliary atresia.

Gilbert's syndrome

Also known as benign unconjugated hyperbilirubinemia, it consists of diminished hepatic biliary clearance but otherwise normal liver function tests. ^{99m}Tc-IDA kinetics tend to be normal despite the hyperbilirubinemia in the few cases studied.[30]

Dubin-Johnson syndrome

It is an autosomal inherited disease of hepatic excretory function, and therefore the hyperbilirubinemia is of the conjugate type. Other compounds such as iodinated contrast material, bromsulfalein, and many metabolites are similarly affected. Intravenously administered bromsulfalein shows a characteristic initial disappearance from the blood and a later reappearance in the conjugated form. The ^{99m}Tc-IDA kinetics feature good hepatocyte uptake and prolonged parenchymal transit time, similar to drug-

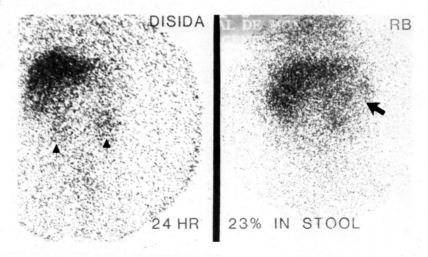

Fig. 53-22 Neonatal hepatitis. Serum bilirubin level was 6.5 mg/100 ml. At 24 hours there was no visible evidence of ^{99m}Tc-diisopropyl-IDA (DISIDA, Disofenin) in bowel; only kidneys *(arrows)* and liver were seen. With ^{131}I–rose bengal (RB), radioactivity in upper small bowel was present *(arrow)*, thereby excluding biliary artresia. Stool assay at 72 hours recovered 23% of administered dose of ^{131}I–rose bengal, which weighed against biliary atresia.

induced intrahepatic cholestasis. Four of 5 patients with this syndrome demonstrated delayed gallbladder filling, but the biliary tract was not seen, presumably a function of the slow hepatic excretion rate. Histologically the hepatocytes exhibit the presence of a brown or black pigment.[5]

Rotor syndrome

This is a rare disorder inherited as an autosomal recessive trait consisting of a defect in the transportation of organic anions from the plasma to the hepatocyte and possibly abnormalities in storage. In the few cases reported, the hyperbilirubinemia was predominantly of the conjugate type. Intravenous bromsulfalein is handled much as with Dubin-Johnson syndrome. No black pigmentation is seen in the liver. ^{99m}Tc-IDA images in this rare disorder were reported in an isolated case; it reflected the basic clearance deficiency of no visible concentration in the liver and complete elimination via the kidneys.[5]

Congenital hepatic fibrosis

Congenital hepatic fibrosis is a rare condition characterized by progressive periportal fibrosis and dilated intrahepatic biliary ducts, and is often associated with polycystic or medullary sponge kidneys. ^{99m}Tc-IDA imaging can identify these ectatic biliary radicles and preclude more invasive diagnostic techniques, which are apt to cause sepsis in these susceptible patients.[47,66,74]

REFERENCES

1. Ale, A, Turner, DA, and Fordham, EW: Tc99m-IDA cholescintigraphy in acute pancreatitis, J Nucl Med 23:867, 1982.
2. Ansari, AN, Atkins, HL, and Lambrecht, RM: I-iodocyanine green (^{123}ICG) as an agent for dynamic studies of the hepatobiliary system. In International Atomic Energy Agency: Dynamic studies with radioisotopes in Medicine (IAEA-SM-185161), vol 1, Knoxville, Tenn, 1974, IAEA.
3. Baker, MK, et al: Focal fatty infiltration of the liver: diagnostic imaging, Radiographics 5:923, 1985.
4. Baker, RJ, Bellen, JC, and Ronai, PM: Technetium-99m-pyridoxylidene glutamate: a new hepatobiliary radiopharmaceutical, J Nucl Med 16:720, 1975.
5. Bar-Meir, S, et al: Tc99m-HIDA cholescintigraphy in Dubin-Johnson and Rotor's syndromes, Radiology 142:743, 1987.
6. Beauchamp, J, Belanger, M, and Neitzschman, H: The diagnosis of subcapsular hematoma of the liver by scintigraphy, South Med J 69:1579, 1976.
7. Biersack, HJ: Accuracy of liver scintigraphy in focal liver disease: a comparison with post-mortem studies in 159 cases, Nucl Med (Stuttg) 18:177, 1979.
8. Biersack, HJ, et al: Focal nodular hyperplasia of the liver established by Tc99m sulfur colloid and HIDA scintigraphy, Radiology 137:187, 1980.
9. Boudreau, R, et al: Effect of ^{99m}Tc-Sn-colloid incubation time on in vivo distribution, Eur J Nucl Med 8:335, 1983.
10. Brachman, MB, et al: Acute gangrenous cholecystitis: radionuclide diagnosis, Radiology 151:209, 1984.
11. Bree, RL, et al: The varied appearances of hepatic cavernous hemangiomas with sonography, computed tomography, magnetic resonance imaging, and scintigraphy, Radiographics 7:1153, 1987.
12. Bushnell, DL, et al: The rim sign: association with acute cholecystitis, J Nucl Med 27:353, 1986.
13. Chayes, Z, Koenigsberg, M, and Freeman, LM: The "hot" hepatic abscess, J Nucl Med 15:305, 1974.
14. Chen, TH, et al: Evaluation of hepatobiliary imaging by radionuclide scintigraphy, Radiology 133:761, 1979.
15. Chervu, LR, Nunn, AD, and Loberg, MD: Radiopharmaceuticals for hepatobiliary imaging, Semin Nucl Med 12:5, 1982.
16. Colletti, PM, et al: Acute cholecystitis: diagnosis with radionuclide angiography, Radiology 163:615, 1987.
17. Cuaron, A, and Gordon, F: Liver scanning: analysis of 2500 cases of amebic hepatic abscesses, J Nucl Med 11:435, 1970.
18. D'Alonzo, W, and Velchik, MG: Postcholecystectomy syndrome due to a cystic duct remnant diagnosed by hepatobiliary scintigraphy, Clin Nucl Med 9:719, 1984.
19. Davis, GB, et al: Cholecystokinin, cholecystography, sonography and scintigraphy: detection of chronic acalculous cholecystitis, AJR 139:1117, 1982.
20. Dobson, EL, and Jones, HB: The behaviour of intravenously injected particulate material: its rate of disappearance from the blood stream as a measure of blood flow, Acta Med Scand (Suppl 144) 273:1, 1952.
21. Drum, DE, and Beard, JM: Scintigraphic criteria for hepatic metastases from cancer of the colon and breast, J Nucl Med 17:677, 1976.
22. Eikman, EA: Computer-assisted liver mass estimation from gamma-camera images, J Nucl Med 20:144, 1979.
23. Ell, PJ, and Kahn, O: Emission computerized tomography: clinical applications, Semin Nucl Med 11:50, 1981.
24. Engel, MA, et al: Differentiation of focal intrahepatic lesions with Tc99m red blood cell imaging, Radiology 146:777, 1983.
25. Ferraro, EM, et al: Hepatic amyloidosis in an intravenous drug abuser detected by bone scintigraphy, Clin Nucl Med 12:274, 1987.
26. Fink-Bennett, D, et al: Cholecystokinin cholescintigraphic findings in the cystic duct syndrome, J Nucl Med 26:1123, 1985.
27. Fitzberg, AR, Whitney, WP, and Klingensmith, WC: Hepatobiliary transport mechanism of Tc-99m-N2-(2,6 diethyl-acetanilide)–iminodiacarboxylic acid (diethyl-IDA). J Nucl Med 20:642, 1979.
28. Fleicher, MR, Sharpstone, P, and Osborne, SB: Liver scintiscanning in acute hepatic necrosis, Br J Radiol 44:401, 1971.
29. Fliegel, CP, Dewanjee, MK, and Holman, BL: Tc-99m tetracycline as a kidney and gallbladder imaging agent, Radiology 110:407, 1974.
30. Fonseca, C, et al: Differential diagnosis of jaundice by Tc99m-IDA hepatobiliary imaging, Clin Nucl Med 4:135, 1979.
31. Fonseca, C, et al: 99mTc-IDA in the differential diagnosis of acute cholecystitis and acute pancreatitis, Radiology 130:525, 1979.
32. Frank, MS, et al: Visualization of the biliary tract with Tc99m-HIDA in acute pancreatitis [abstract], Gastroenterology 78:1167, 1980.
33. Freeman, LM, Sugarman, LA, and Weismann, HS: Role of cholecystokinetic agents in Tc99m-IDA cholescintigraphy, Semin Nucl Med 11:186, 1981.
34. Freitas, JE, and Fink-Bennett, DM: Asymptomatic cystic duct obstruction in chronic cholecystitis (abstract), J Nucl Med 21:17, 1980.
35. Frietas, JE, et al: Suspected acute cholecystitis: comparison of hepatobiliary imaging versus ultrasonography, Clin Nucl Med 7:364, 1982.
36. Front, D, et al: Scintigraphy of hepatic hemangiomas: the value of Tc99m-labeled red blood cells, J Nucl Med 22:687, 1981.

37. Geslien, GE, Thrall, JH, and Johnson, MC: Gallium scanning in acute hepatic amebic abscess, J Nucl Med 15:561, 1974.

38. Goldberg, HI: Cholecystokinin cholecystography, Semin Roentgenol 11:175, 1976.

39. Goodwin, DA, Stern, HS, and Kramer, HH: A new radiopharmaceutical for liver scanning, Nucleonics 24:65, 1966.

40. Goris, ML: ^{123}I-iodo-bromsulfthalein as a liver and biliary scanning agent, J Nucl Med 14:820, 1973.

41. Greenwald, RA, Periras, R, and Morris, SJ: Jaundice, choledocholithiasis and non-dilated common duct, JAMA 240:1983, 1978.

42. Griffin, WO, et al: Cholecystokinin cholecystography in the diagnosis of gallbladder disease, Am Surg 191:636, 1980.

43. Gupta, S, et al: Comparison of ultrasonography, computed tomography and 99mTc-colloid liver scan in the diagnosis of Budd-Chiari syndrome, Gut 28:242, 1987.

44. Hakim, S, Joo, KG, and Baeumler, GR: Visualization of acute hepatic necrosis with a bone imaging agent, Clin Nucl Med 10:697, 1985.

45. Harper, PV: Improved liver scanning with 6-hour 99mTc in fat emulsion, J Nucl Med 16:56, 1969.

46. Hooper, RG, Beechler, CR, and Johnson, MC: Radioisotope scanning in the initial staging of bronchogenic carcinoma, Am Rev Resp Dis 118:272, 1978.

47. Howlett, SA, et al: Cholangitis complicating congenital hepatic fibrosis, Dig Dis 20:790, 1975.

48. Hughes, KS, et al: Endotoxic shock and its effect on hepatobiliary scanning in dogs, Radiology 148:823, 1983.

49. Jackson, RA, Bolles, TF, and Kubiatowicz, DO: Technetium-mercaptide complexes and their potential application as a liver specific agent, J Nucl Med 14:411, 1973.

50. Jain, AN, Ramanathan, P, and Ganatra, RD: Scan appearance in hydatid cysts of the liver: analysis of 55 cases, Clin Nucl Med 5:25, 1980.

51. Johnson, AE, and Gollan, F: 99mTc-technetium dioxide for liver scanning, J Nucl Med 11:564, 1970.

52. Joyner, JT: Abnormal liver scan (radiocolloid "hot spot") associated with superior vena cava obstruction, J Nucl Med 13:849, 1972.

53. Kaden, VG, Howard, JM, and Doubleday, JC: Cholecystographic studies during and immediately following acute pancreatitis. Surgery 38:1082, 1955.

54. Kaplan, WD, Ensminger, WD, Come SE, et al: Radionuclide angiography to predict patient response to hepatic artery chemotherapy, Cancer Treat Rep 64:1217, 1980.

55. Klingensmith, WC: Resolution of increased splenic size and uptake of 99mTc-sulfur colloid following removal of a malignant melanoma, J Nucl Med 15:1203, 1974.

56. Kloiber, R, Damtew, B, and Rosenthall, L: A crossover study comparing the effect of particle size on the distribution of radiocolloid in patients, Clin Nucl Med 6:204, 1981.

57. Kurohara, SS, et al: Response and recovery of liver to radiation as demonstrated by photoscans, Radiology 89:129, 1967.

58. Lennard, TWJ, Farndon, JR, and Taylor, RMR: Acalculous biliary pain: diagnosis and selection for cholecystectomy using the cholecystokinin test for pain reproduction, Br J Surg 71:368, 1984.

59. Lin, MS, Fletcher, JW, and Donati, RM: Local colloid trapping in the liver in the inferior vena cava syndrome, J Nucl Med 22:344, 1981.

60. Loberg, MD, et al: Development of new radiopharmaceuticals based on N-substitute iminodiacetic acid, J Nucl Med 17:633, 1976.

61. Lomas, F, Dibos, PE, and Wagner, HN: Increased specificity of liver scanning with the use of gallium-67 citrate, N Engl J Med 286:1323, 1972.

62. Lough, J, et al: Kupffer cell depletion associated with capillarization of liver sinusoids in carbon tetrachloride—induced rat liver cirrhosis, J Hepatology 5:190, 1987.

63. Lubbers, PR, et al: Accumulation of technetium 99m colloid by hepatocellular adenoma AJR 148:1156, 1987.

64. Majd, M, Reba, RC, and Altman, RP: Hepatobiliary scintigraphy with Tc99m-PIPIDA in the evaluation of neonatal jaundice, Pediatrics 67:140, 1981.

65. Malini, S, and Sabel, J: Ultrasonography in obstructive jaundice, Radiology 123:429, 1977.

66. Masuda, Y, Sawa, H, and Kim, OH: A case of congenital hepatic fibrosis: usefulness of hepatic biliary scintigraphy, Clin Nucl Med 5:339, 1980.

67. Mauro, MA, McCartney, WH, and Melmed, R: Hepatobiliary scanning with 99mTc-PIPIDA in acute cholecystitis, Radiology 142:193, 1982.

68. Mikhael, MA, and Evans, RG: Migration and embolization of macrophages to the lung: a possible mechanism for colloid uptake in the lung during liver scanning, J Nucl Med 16:22, 1975.

69. Miller, JH: Technetium 99m-labeled red blood cells in the evaluation of hemangiomas of the liver in infants and children, J Nucl Med 28:1412, 1987.

70. Mould, RF: An investigation of variations in normal liver shape, Br J Radiol 45:586, 1972.

71. Neiman, HL, and Mintzer, RA: Accuracy of biliary duct ultrasound: comparison with cholangiography, AJR 129:979, 1977.

72. Ostfeld, DA, and Meyer, JE: Liver scanning in cancer patients with short-interval autopsy correlation, Radiology 138:671, 1981.

73. Ozarda, A, and Pickren, J: The topographic distribution of liver metastases: its relation to surgical and isotope diagnosis, J Nucl Med 3:149, 1962.

74. Padhy, AK, et al: Hepatobiliary scintigraphy in congenital cystic dilatation of biliary tract, Clin Nucl 10:703, 1985.

75. Pare, P, Shaffer, EA, and Rosenthall, L: Nonvisualization of the gallbladder by 99mTc-HIDA cholescintigraphy as evidence of cholecystitis, Can Med Assoc J 118:384, 1978.

76. Pauwels, S, et al: Tc99m-diethyl imaging: clinical evaluation in jaundiced patients, J Nucl Med 21:1022, 1980.

77. Picard, M, et al: Budd-Chiari syndrome: typical and atypical scintigraphic aspects, J Nucl Med 28:803, 1987.

78. Pickleman, J, et al: The role of sincalide cholescintigraphy in the evaluation of patients with acalculous gallbladder disease, Arch Surg 120:693, 1985.

79. Pomerantz, IS, and Shaffer, EA: Abnormal gallbladder emptying in a subgroup of patients with gallstones, Gastroenterol 88:787, 1985.

80. Ransdell, JW, et al: Multiorgan scans of staging lung cancer, J Thorac Cardiovasc Surg 73:653, 1977.

81. Raymond, F, Lepanto, L, and Rosenthall, L: Tc99m-IDA gallbladder kinetics and response to CCK in chronic cholecystitis, Eur J Nucl Med (In press).

82. Rogers, JV, et al: Hepatic focal nodular hyperplasia angiography, CT, sonography and scintigraphy, AJR 137:983, 1981.

83. Rollo, FD, and Deland, FH: The determination of liver mass from radionuclide images, Radiology 91:1191, 1968.

84. Rose, JD: Serial cholecystography: a means of preoperative diagnosis of biliary dyskinesia, Arch Surg 78:56, 1959.

85. Rosen, PR, et al: 99mTc-PIPIDA cholescintigraphy in the diagnosis of gallbladder disease, Am J Med Sci 284:23, 1982.

86. Rosenfield, AT, and Schneider, PB: Rapid evaluation of hepatic size on radioisotope scan, J Nucl Med 15:237, 1974.

87. Rosenthall, L: Cholescintigraphy in the presence of jaundice utilizing Tc-IDA, Semin Nucl Med 12:53, 1982.

88. Rosenthall, L, et al: Tc99m-IDA hepatobiliary imaging following upper abdominal surgery, Radiology 130:735, 1979.

89. Sample, WF, Sasti, DA, and Goldstein, LI: Gray-scale ultrasonography and the jaundiced patient, Radiology 128:719, 1978.

90. Sanfelippo, R, Beahrs, O, and Weiland, L: Cystic disease of the liver, Ann Surg 179:933, 1974.

91. Sazuki, T, et al: Serum alphafetoprotein and gallium-67 citrate uptake in hematoma. AJR 120:627, 1974.

92. Serafini, AN, Smoak, WM, and Hupf, HB: Iodine-123 rose bengal: an improved hepatobiliary imaging agent, J Nucl Med 16:629, 1975.

93. Serafini, A, et al: Biliary scintigraphy in acute pancreatitis, Radiology 144:591, 1982.

94. Seymour, E, Puchette, S, and Edwards, J: Pseudoabnormal liver scans secondary to residual barium in the bowel, AJR 107:54, 1969.

95. Shuman, WP, et al: PIPIDA scintigraphy for cholecystitis: false positives in alcoholism and total parenteral nutrition, AJR 138:5, 1982.

96. Silverberg, M, Rosenthall, L, and Freeman, LM: Rose bengal excretion studies as an aid in the differential diagnosis of neonatal jaundice, Semin Nucl 3:69, 1973.

97. Sippo, WC, et al: The effect of prolonged fasting and total parenteral nutrition on hepatobiliary imaging with Tc99m-DISIDA, Clin Nucl Med 12:169, 1987.

98. Smith, R, et al: Pericholic hepatic activity in cholescintigraphy, Radiology 156:797, 1985.

99. Sostre, S, Silva, F, and Zaidi, M: Liver scintigraphy in chronic hepatosplenic schistosomasis: a predictor of disease severity, Clin Nucl Med 12:277, 1987.

100. Spellman, SJ, Shaffer, EA, and Rosenthall, L: Gallbladder emptying in response to cholecystokinin, Gastroenterology 77:115, 1979.

101. Spencer, RP, and Antar, MA: Radionuclides in the investigation of liver disease. In Poppen, H, and Schaffner, F, editors: progress in liver disease, vol 4, New York, 1972, Grune & Stratton.

102. Stadalnik, RC, et al: Technetium-99m NGA functional hepatic imaging: preliminary clinical experience, J Nucl Med 26:1233, 1985.

103. Strauss, LG, et al: Single photon emission computerized tomography (SPECT) for estimates of liver and spleen volume, J Nucl Med 25:81, 1984.

104. Tonkin, AK, and Deland, FH: Dihydrothioctic acid: a new polygonal cell imaging agent, J Nucl Med 17:362, 1976.

105. Toplin, GY, Meredith, OM, and Kade, H: The radioactive (^{131}I-tagged) rose bengal uptake: excretion test for liver function using external gamma-ray scintillation counting technique, J Lab Clin Med 45:665, 1955.

106. Tubis, M, Krishnamurthy, GT, and Endow, JS: ^{99m}Tc-penicillamine, a new cholescintigraphic agent, J Nucl Med 13:652, 1972.

107. Valberg, LS, et al: Biliary pain in young women in the absence of gallstones, Gastroenterol 60:1020, 1971.

108. Velasco, J, et al: Hepatobiliary scanning in cholecystitis, Eur J Nucl Med 7:11, 1982.

109. Vincent, LM, et al: Hepatic adenoma: demonstration of discordant uptake with Tc99m sulfur colloid and Tc99m-DISIDA, Clin Nucl Med 9:415, 1984.

110. Warner, BW, et al. The value of hepatobiliary scans in fasted patients receiving total parenteral nutrition. Paper presented at the Central Surgical Association meeting, Louisville, March 1987.

111. Weens, HS, and Walker, LA: The radiologic diagnosis of acute cholecystitis and pancreatitis, Radiol Clin North Am 2:89, 1964.

112. Weismann, HS, et al: The role of nuclear medicine in evaluating cholestasis, Ultrasound 1:131, 1980.

113. Weismann, HS, et al: Spectrum of 99mTc-IDA cholescintigraphic patterns in acute cholecystitis, Radiology 138:167, 1981.

114. Weismann, HS, et al: Evaluation of the postoperative patient with Tc99m-IDA cholescintigraphy, Semin Nucl Med 12:27, 1982.

115. Yeh, SH, Lui, OK, and Huang, MJ: Sequential scintiphotography with technetium 99m pyridoxylidene glutamate in the detection of intrahepatic lithiasis, J Nucl Med 21:17, 1980.

116. Yeh, SH, Ohlsen, J, and Kountz, SL: Distribution and scintiphotography studies of ^{99m}Tc-iron colloid in the rabbit, J Nucl Med 10:56, 1969.

117. Ziessman, HA, et al: Atlas of hepatic arterial perfusion scintigraphy, Clin Nucl Med 10:675, 1985.

54 *Endoscopy*

PREMYSL SLEZAK

GENERAL CONSIDERATIONS

Endoscopic cannulation of Vater's papilla was first described by McCune and co-workers[64a] in 1968 in the United States, but it was developed as a clinical tool in Japan and Europe. In spite of enormous advances in noninvasive imaging of the biliary tree and the development of the "skinny" Chiba needle, endoscopic retrograde cholangiopancreatography (ERCP) remains an important technique for evaluation of patients with pancreatic or biliary diseases. It is usually necessary to perform a direct cholangiography to define the site and cause of obstruction in the biliary tree or to exclude biliary disease with confidence. Unnecessary surgery may be spared in 10% to 15% of jaundiced patients by preoperative cholangiography.[108]

ERCP in expert hands is a relatively safe method with high success and accuracy rates. The diagnostic and therapeutic potential of ERCP is much broader than that of percutaneous transhepatic cholangiography (PTC). It includes the esophagus, stomach, duodenum, and pancreas. ERCP is either a cooperative venture between the radiologist and skilled endoscopist or a one-man job for a radiologist who is also a skilled endoscopist and performed in a sophisticated radiology unit. ERCP is a difficult technique to master, and proficiency can be achieved only by personal experience. ERCP is impossible in patients with obstruction in the gastrointestinal (GI) tract above the papilla, is difficult in patients with Billroth II partial gastrectomy, and may be impossible when the duct is blocked at the papilla. The most important indications for ERCP are obstructive jaundice, postcholecystectomy syndrome (a particularly important indication for ERCP as the primary method of examination), to elucidate the cause of pancreatitis and cholangitis (even in acute cases),* and suspected iatrogenic biliary damage from surgery. ERCP has no absolute contraindications. However, in my experience patients with α_1-antitrypsin deficiency should be selected for ERCP with caution.[119]

---

*References 77, 78, 79, 99, 101, 134.

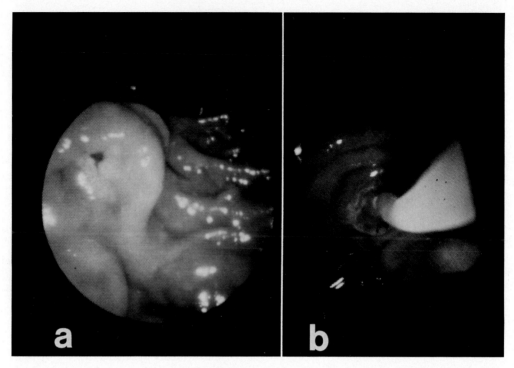

Fig. 54-1 Duodenoscopy. **A,** Vater's papilla and its punctiform orifice. **B,** Cannula entering orifice angled slightly upward for cannulation of biliary duct.

ENDOSCOPIC RETROGRADE CHOLANGIOPANCREATOGRAPHY
Technique and anatomy

ERCP is performed with the patient under sedation and preferably in the left lateral decubitus position. A side-viewing duodenoscope is passed to the papilla for cannulation under direct vision. Induced hypotonia of the duodenum is helpful with intermittent intravenous injection of hyoscine-N-butylbromide (Buscopan) 20 to 40 mg, or glucagon, 0.2 to 0.5 mg. Cannulation should not be attempted until the operator is fully familiar with the lateral-viewing endoscope. For cannulation experts favor a straight endoscope, achieved by hooking the tip of the instrument in the second part of the duodenum and bringing the lens up the medial wall of the duodenum to the longitudinal fold and papilla. Often the longitudinal fold is first seen and not the papilla per se. The papilla can be found at the lower end of the longitudinal fold and is generally situated in the middle third of the second part of the duodenum (in 54% of cases).[60] The papilla minor (orifice of Santorini's duct) is classically 2 to 3 cm above Vater's papilla and has no longitudinal fold. The papillary orifice is generally punctiform but can be linear or polygonal. The color of the orifice in the close-up view differs slightly from the surroundings. In exceptional cases there may be two separated orifices (seen in 2% of cases).[60] In general, the pancreatogram is more likely to be successful if the papilla is entered *en face* and the cholangiogram by angling the cannula upward (Fig. 54-1). In 55% of cases the main pancreatic duct (PD) and the common biliary duct (CBD) form a common duct a few millimeters long.[2] The CBD and the PD open separately into the papillary orifice in 42% of patients,[2] which demands a separate cannulation of each of the ducts. Lower concentrations of contrast media (25% to 30%) should be used. The volume of injected contrast agent depends on the duct size. When Oddi's sphincter is intact, the contrast medium remains long enough in the biliary tree for the instrument and the cannula to be completely removed and the most suitable patient posture to be arranged for radiography. The interpretation of the intramural part of the CBD on radiographs may be difficult. The appearance of the lower 2 cm of the CBD varies from patient to patient, and the diagnosis of abnormality in this area should be made with great caution. The appearance of the intramural portion is influenced by Oddi's sphincter, which consists of the choledochus sphincter, pancreatic sphincter, and sphincter ampullas.[93] Another difficulty in interpretation of the cholangiogram is the normal variation in size of the CBD. The size depends on the method of cholangiography (for example, the normal maximal diameter of the CBD in intravenous cholangiography (IVC) is reported to be 7 to 8 mm and for ERCP and PTC, 10 to 11 mm),[81] taking into account the magnification factor. Recording the size of CBD without stating the technique and magnification factor is of limited value.[80] Knowledge of biliary tree anatomy is of practical importance for the surgeon both before and after hepatobiliary surgery in case iatrogenic damage in the biliary tree occurs. Descriptions of ductal radiologic anatomy of the biliary tree have been published elsewhere.[42,44,82]

Diagnostic accuracy and success rate

ERCP has the very high diagnostic accuracy, sensitivity, and specificity of direct cholangiography and in experienced hands a very high success rate of cannulation. The diagnostic accuracy stated in the literature varies from 67%[129] to 100%.[86] The overall accuracy rate has been reported to be 90%,[127] 80% to 95%,[31,72,86] and more than 95%[31,86,127] (see Table 54-1). The range of success rates is reported from 50%[110] to 98%.[113] The 50% success rate is not representative, as it includes Billroth II–operated cases. For an experienced endoscopist the success rate is higher than 90% (my cannulation success rate is 95%).

Complications

ERCP is currently the least invasive technique for obtaining detailed images of the pancreatic and biliary ductal system. ERCP performed by an expert is now an acceptably safe procedure. However, it may be followed by serious complications and even death. The most common and important of these complications are acute pancreatitis (injection pancreatitis), cholangitis, cholangitic sepsis, and pancreatic sepsis. Complications from instrumentation or medication are very rare. Of all the complications following ERCP, the most common and most important is acute pancreatitis, which is the killer.

Injection pancreatitis varies in severity from slight hyperamylasemia, appearing in as many as 75% of patients undergoing ERCP,[33,55,108] to a fatal necrotizing pancreatitis. In most patients serum and urine amylase levels return to normal in 1 to 4 days. However, 1% to 5% of injection pancreatitis cases are resistant to therapy and fatal.[45] No correlation exists between the incidence of acute pancreatitis and underlying abnormality of pancreas. Pathologic conditions of the pancreas before ERCP have been found in only 25% of those who developed injection pancreatitis.[51] The incidence of fatal necrotizing pancreatitis after ERCP has been reported in 0.1% of patients subjected to ERCP.[28] My two patients who developed lethal necrotizing pancreatitis following ERCP had normal pancreatograms and cholangiograms. Acinar contrast filling is observed in 45% of patients with injection pancreatitis.[10] On the other hand, injection pancreatitis is reported even without injection of contrast media into the papillary orifice in 5.9% of patients.[51,130]

The cause of injection pancreatitis is poorly understood. Factors generally assumed to play a role include *speed* and *pressure* of injection and *volume* of contrast media. An important pathogenic factor could be the rise of intraductal pressure. On the other hand, experimental contrast infusion of diatrizoate meglumine and diatrizoate sodium (Renografin) into the PD did not generate an increase of intraductal pressure.[75] Kasugai[49a] believes that acute pancreatitis can be almost abolished by monitored control of pressure, volume, and speed of pancreatic injection. Fluoroscopic control during PD injection is recommended to prevent overfilling. The contrast injection should be stopped as soon as a large branch filling is recognized on the fluoroscopic screen. Despite careful fluoroscopic monitoring of the PD injection, acute pancreatitis still occurs. Some authors[38] suggest that repeated injections into the PD during the attempts to cannulate the CBD is of major importance in the development of pancreatitis. This is reasonable, and it can be easily avoided by using a cannula with a metallic tip seen on the fluoroscopy without contrast injection. Pain during contrast filling of the PD or during manipulations with the cannula in the PD is in my experience an important sign, warning of a high risk for the development of acute pancreatitis. The *chemical properties* of the contrast media may be important in the development of hyperamylasemia.[23,116] Other authors have not been able to verify this hypothesis nor to find any advantage in the use of nonionic, low-osmolar contrast media.[40,96] Pancreatitis develops more often after the selective contrast filling of the PD than the CBD.[51,55] The level of *experience of the endoscopist* is also an important factor. The inexperienced examiner has four times the failure rate in cannulation and twice the rate of complications compared with an expert.[10] However, acute pancreatitis occurs even in expert hands. *Deficiency of α_1-antitrypsin* may play a role. One of my patients who developed necrotizing pancreatitis following ERCP suffered this defect. ERCP should be avoided in patients with this deficiency, or one should be more restrictive before accepting these patients for ERCP.[119]

One cannot totally avoid cases of acute pancreatitis after ERCP, but some mechanical and pharmacologic measures can be taken, albeit with doubtful preventive effects. Mechanical measures include prevention of overpressurizing or overfilling of the PD by using a simple injection pistol* for volume control[142] and metal-tipped cannulas.[1] Pharmacologic measures include the use of substances inhibiting pancreatic secretion and pancreolytic enzymes. (The use of inhibitors is based on the hypothesis that the pathogenesis of injection pancreatitis involves the activation of trypsinogen to trypsin, which in turn activates prophospholipase A_2 to phospholipase A_2, which turns lecithin into lysolecithin—an extremely tissue-toxic substance).[35] Trasylol and glucagon have no preventive effect. Synthetic protease inhibitor FOY-gabexat-mesilate, with membrane-stabilizing and trypsin-inhibiting effects, decreases hyperamylasemia after ERCP according to some researchers.[90,133] Somatostatin, among others, has a pancreas-inhibiting effect; some authors have reported a favorable effect,[16,121,125] and others have reported no effect at all.[12,132]

Cholangitis, cholangitic sepsis, and pancreatic sepsis, although less frequent, are not entirely uncommon after ERCP and can be very serious. The pathogenesis is bacterial and occurs most commonly in obstruction of the CBD. Lately, *Pseudomonas aeruginosa* sepsis has been reported after ERCP, even without known underlying abnormality.[24,43,61] The incidence of transient bacteremia after ERCP is estimated to be as high as 14%.[33] The cause is instrument contamination. Mortality from cholangitis and cholangitic sepsis is reported to be 10% and 20%, respectively.[33] Pseudocysts of the pancreas are no longer a contraindication for ERCP, previously feared because of sepsis. Ninety-one percent of patients with pseudocysts were free of complications after ERCP.[10]

ERCP is a safe technique even in patients with a previous history of allergic reactions to iodized contrast media,[54] despite the fact that the contrast media is absorbed primarily from the PD,[54] as seen by the pyelography in ERCP, in as many as 35% of cases.[100] Allergic reactions

are very rare (0.03%),[100] probably because of the slow rate of absorption.

Rare complications in ERCP include impaired oral glucose tolerance after ERCP[131]; emphysematous cholecystitis[5]; intramural duodenal hematoma[88]; and pancreatic duct disruption.[115]

Incidence of the more important complications

The overall rate of complications after ERCP ranges from 0.38%[73] to 12%[13] (see Table 54-1). Incidences reported have been less than 1%,[73,87,95] between 1% and 3%,* and more than 3%.[33,87,108,117] The overall incidence may be considered to be 3% to 5%. Acute injection pancreatitis has been reported in 0.1%[84] to 17%[96] of patients. Incidences of less than 1%,[33,73,84,87,108] between 1% and 3%,† and more than 3%‡ have been reported. The overall incidence may be regarded as 2% to 5%. Overall mortality ranges from 0%[87] to 2.9%.[104] Incidences of less than 0.1%,[33,73,87,95,108] between 0.1% and 0.2%,§ and more than 0.2%[51,84,117,120] have been reported. Cholangitis has been reported in 0.06%[33] to 20% of cases.[19] Incidences in this range have been reported by several authors.[19,33,73,114] The mortality from cholangitis is considered to be 10%.[33] The incidence of cholangitic sepsis ranges from 0.65%[108] to 1%.[33] Incidences in this range have been reported.[33,87,108] The mortality from cholangitic sepsis is 20%.[33] Pancreatic sepsis occurs in 0.3%[87,108]—a rare but serious complication.

Cost-benefit analysis

A comparison of the costs and benefits of ERCP and other diagnostic modalities is shown in Table 54-1. Two

---

*References 10, 33, 45, 84, 87, 108, 114, 120.
†References 10, 19, 33, 51, 87, 96, 108, 114, 117.
‡References 33, 50, 51, 55, 96, 108.
§References 10, 50, 51, 87, 108, 117, 120.

---

*Wilson-Cook Medical, Inc., Winston-Salem, N.C.

☐ **TABLE 54-1**

Risk-benefit analysis: comparison of ERCP with other diagnostic modalities

Modality	Diagnostic accuracy (%)	Success rate of cannulation (%)	Overall complication rate (%)	Mortality (%)
ERCP	67-100	50-98	0.38-12	0-2.9
PTC	69-99.7[53]	84-100[46](D)* 33-95[46](ND)	1.8-29[9]	0.25-6.9[9,143]
Ultrasonography	13-45[83,110]	—	—	—
CT	43-90[47,86]	—	—	—

*D, Dilated ducts; *ND*, nondilated ducts.

questions must be asked in a cost-benefit analysis. First, is one diagnostic procedure more beneficial than another—that is, more precise and/or less risky? Second, to what extent will a more precise diagnosis benefit the patient?

The following conclusions could be drawn:

1. Diagnostic accuracy is comparable in ERCP and PTC and is significantly higher than in ultrasonography or computed tomography (CT).
2. Success rate is also comparable in ERCP and PTC. PTC has a slightly lower success rate in nondilated biliary ducts and ERCP in Billroth II–operated cases.
3. The complication rate is slightly more than twice as high in PTC as in ERCP.
4. The mortality is slightly more than twice as high in PTC as in ERCP.

Thus direct cholangiography (ERCP and PTC) allows a more certain diagnosis than noninvasive diagnostic modalities. It also has a therapeutic potential. ERCP has half the morbidity and mortality of PTC (as well as the advantages of simultaneous endoscopy of the esophagus, stomach, and duodenum; biopsy; and pancreatography).

RADIOLOGIC DIAGNOSIS AND DIFFERENTIAL DIAGNOSIS

This section focuses on the radiologic interpretation of the contrast-filled biliary ducts from a radiologist's point of view, not from a clinician's or pathologist's. The most important radiologic findings are stenosis, dilatation, contrast defects in the biliary duct and leakage of contrast medium outside the biliary duct, and functional signs. These findings are rarely isolated; they most often occur in combination (for example, stenosis with dilatation). It is often not particularly difficult to find a primary cause that is the basis for classification. The value of ERCP in the diagnosis of these abnormalities is summarized in Table 54-2.

Stenosis
Intrahepatic and combined intrahepatic, and extrahepatic stenosis

Although stenoses are easily visualized on ERCP, its sensitivity—its ability to reveal an intrahepatic lesion that can cause a stenosis—is low, with a high incidence of false-negative diagnoses. On the contrary, the specificity of ERCP is high, with a low incidence for false-positive diagnoses. The differential diagnosis is very difficult and often impossible.

Cirrhosis involves generalized crowding of the intrahepatic ducts and zigzagging and corkscrewing of the fine radicles (because of the collapse of the hepatic parenchyma).[30,97,109] *Infiltrative parenchymatous process* (fatty liver, myeloproliferative disorders, hepatitis, and so on) shows straightening and elongation of intrahepatic ducts that are spread apart (because of enlargement of the liver).[30,97] *Hepatic tumors* involve mass lesions causing displacement of the intrahepatic ducts but even signs of invasion, such as enveloping, compressing (Fig. 54-2), and stenosing to complete block of intrahepatic ducts.[30,97] The radiographic signs in these diseases are generally similar, but they are present in only a minority of cases,[39,109] demonstrating the low sensitivity of cholangiography in the diagnosis of these diseases. *Iatrogenic lesions* following biliary surgery are more common in the extrahepatic part of biliary tract, but they occur even in the intrahepatic system (Fig. 54-3). *Recurrent pyogenetic cholangitis and hepatolithiasis* involve strictures and stones in both the intrahepatic and extrahepatic bile ducts.[15,74] *Primary sclerosing cholangitis (PSC)* is an uncommon disease of unknown cause characterized by inflammation and fibrosis of the biliary tree with diffuse stricture formation. It is usually associated with ulcerative colitis (in 1% to 4% of patients with ulcerative colitis).[70] Conversely, ulcerative colitis is present in 50% to 70% of patients with PSC,[70,111] and rarely in those with Crohn's disease, vasculitis, retroperitoneal fibrosis,

□ **TABLE 54-2**
Diagnostic value of ERCP

Abnormality	Sensitivity	Specificity	Differential diagnosis
Intrahepatic and combined intrahepatic and extrahepatic stenosis	Low	High	Very difficult
Extrahepatic stenosis	High	High	Neither particularly difficult nor easy
Dilatation	High	High	Easy
Contrast medium defects	High	High	Very difficult to impossible
Leakage of contrast medium outside biliary tract	High	High	Easy

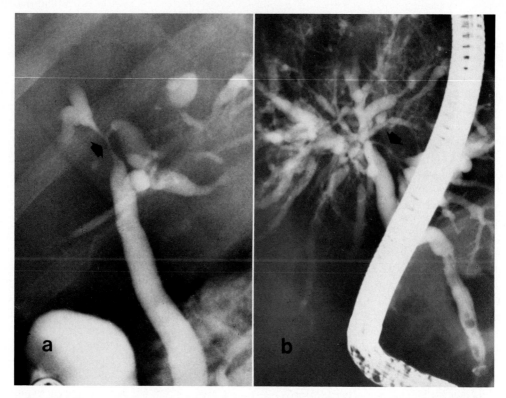

Fig. 54-2 Two cases of metastatic liver tumor (primary pancreatic carcinoma). **A,** Tumor causes severe stenosis in bifurcation of common hepatic duct at hilum of liver *(arrow)*. **B,** Periductal spreading of tumor around left hepatic duct *(arrow)*.

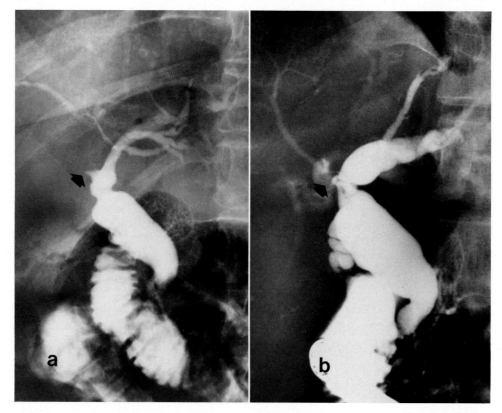

Fig. 54-3 Two cases of iatrogenic stricture of intrahepatic biliary tree. **A** and **B,** Total occlusion of right hepatic duct close to hilum of liver *(arrow)*. Almost identical finding in both patients on ERCP performed 2 and 4 years, respectively, after cholecystectomy.

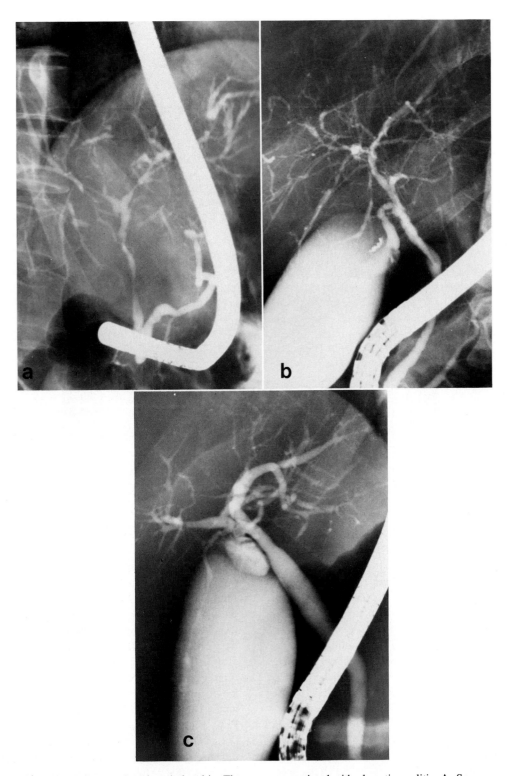

Fig. 54-4 Primary sclerosing cholangitis. Three cases associated with ulcerative colitis. **A,** Severe changes in intrahepatic bile ducts (pruning and beading), as well as in extrahepatic bile duct. **B,** Severe changes in intrahepatic and extrahepatic biliary ducts. **C,** Moderate changes mainly in intrahepatic biliary tree. Only slight narrowing of common hepatic duct close to hilum of liver can be seen.

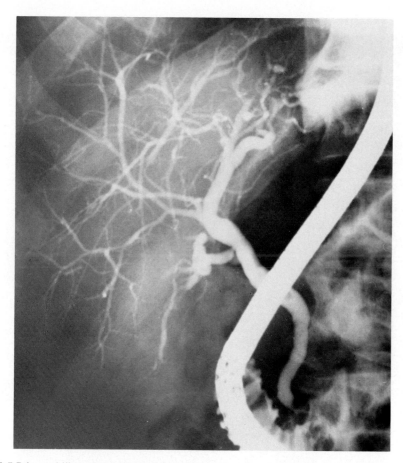

Fig. 54-5 Primary biliary cirrhosis. Moderate changes—corkscrewing and zigzagging of radicles—in left liver lobe and very discrete diffuse changes in ducts of right liver lobe. Extrahepatic biliary ducts are normal in PBC, unlike in most cases of PSC.

mediastinal and orbital fibrosis, Riedel's thyroiditis,[63] reticulum cell lymphoma,[122] and familial immunodeficiency syndrome.[122] Cellular immune response to biliary antigens have been found in 80% of patients with PSC.[139] PSC is a progressive obliterative process involving the intrahepatic and extrahepatic biliary tree. The *cholangiographic appearance* (Fig. 54-4) is characterized by pruning (decreased arborization) and beading (short circular stenosis with intervening slight dilatations) of the intrahepatic and extrahepatic bile ducts. Isolated involvement of intrahepatic ducts does occur in 20% of patients.[62] Isolated extrahepatic duct involvement can also occur.[111] The extrahepatic bile ducts may show shaggy margins. When there is only intrahepatic involvement, the most prominent findings are stenoses of the bile ducts without intervening dilatation.[52]

In isolated intrahepatic involvement it is difficult to distinguish PSC from *primary biliary cirrhosis (PBC)*. However, the negative mitochondrial antibody test can distinguish PSC from PBC.[66,111] The major extrahepatic ducts are normal in PBC (Fig. 54-5). *Cholangiocarcinoma* (diffuse sclerosing carcinoma) of the bile ducts may mimic PSC, and the differential diagnosis between PSC and carcinoma is extremely difficult, sometimes impossible. The combination of PSC and cholangiocarcinoma is not unusual (Fig. 54-6).[111] The distinction may, in spite of biopsy, remain obscure.[57,139] The tumor kills by its site rather than by its malignancy,[111] and about 20% are resectable.[111] Since decompression plus drainage seem to be the proper treatment for both PSC and cholangiocarcinoma,[139] the demand for exact differential diagnosis is not absolute. *Histiocytosis* may simulate PSC.[111] *Hepatocellular carcinoma* may cause bile duct obstruction. In the Klatskin type of tumor there is a dilatation of one half of the biliary tree, while the other half is normal.[41] In *cholangitis associated with acquired immunodeficiency syndrome* (AIDS) ERCP often reveals all classic signs of PSC in the intrahepatic and extrahepatic bile ducts. The cause is biliary infection by cytomegalovirus, cryptosporidia, or *Campylobacter* spe-

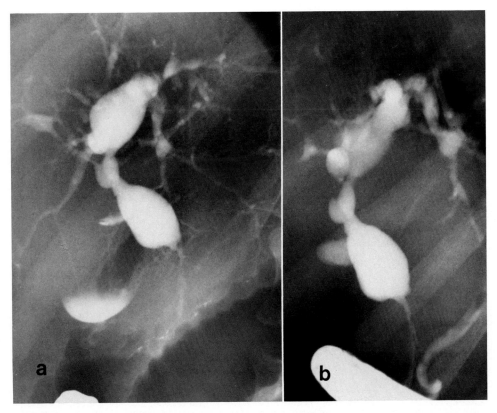

Fig. 54-6 A and **B,** Patient with PSC associated with ulcerative colitis combined with cholangio-carcinoma. Intrahepatic biliary tree reveals changes of PSC. Long stenosis of lower CBD with prestenotic dilatation is not usual finding in PSC and is highly suggestive of malignancy.

cies.* *Lymphoma* (Hodgkin and non-Hodgkin) may cause encasement of the intrahepatic and extrahepatic bile ducts.[107] In *iatrogenic cholangitis* following hepatic artery cytostatic infusion therapy, direct chemotoxic effect on the biliary ductal mucosa or a toxic effect on the vascular system with secondary ischemia of the biliary ducts leads to fibrosis. Cholangiography reveals smooth tapering of the proximal common hepatic duct and changes characteristic of PSC.[3] Rare causes of bile duct obstruction include hepatobiliary tuberculosis,[118] Watson-Alagille syndrome (in which ERCP reveals no evidence of intrahepatic bile ducts),[6,111] eosinophilic cholangitis,[14] and rupture of hydatid cyst.[20]

Extrahepatic stenosis

Many differential diagnostic possibilities must be considered in a case of stenosis of the extrahepatic bile duct. *Cholangiocarcinoma* may arise at any point, but the anatomic sites of preference are common hepatic duct (CHD) and CBD.[89] More than half of the lesions appear

*References 1, 18, 26, 32, 91, 106, 123.

in the upper third of the CBD, classically at the hepatic hilum. It may be associated with ulcerative colitis with or without PSC. Colitis-associated tumors of CBD represent only 1.6% of all cholangiocarcinomas.[136] All members of the congenital fibropolycystic family, including congenital hepatic fibrosis, Caroli's disease, choledochal cysts, polycystic liver, and von Meyenberg complexes such as microhamartoma, as well as liver fluke infestations may be complicated by cholangiocarcinoma.[111] Most of the tumors are annular scirrhous infiltrating lesions[89] with a great tendency to infiltrate extensively in the submucosal plane.[122] They may be classified into three groups[58]: type I (70%)—obstructive (with smooth or irregular contours); type II (24%)–short or long stenoses, most frequently in the hilum; and type III (6%)–filling defect. Type III is very often a curable lesion. *Strictures in the mid duct must be presumed to be malignant if there has been no prior biliary surgery or trauma* (Fig. 54-7). Those caused by cholangiocarcinoma generally have an abrupt cutoff or rat-tailed appearance.[109] Distinguishing between benign and malignant stenoses radiographically is difficult or impossible

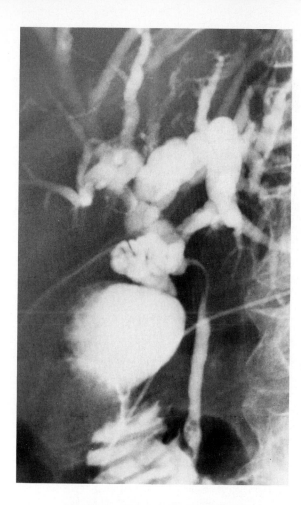

Fig. 54-7 Cholangiocarcinoma causing severe circular stenosis of mid duct—usual localization of CBD tumors.

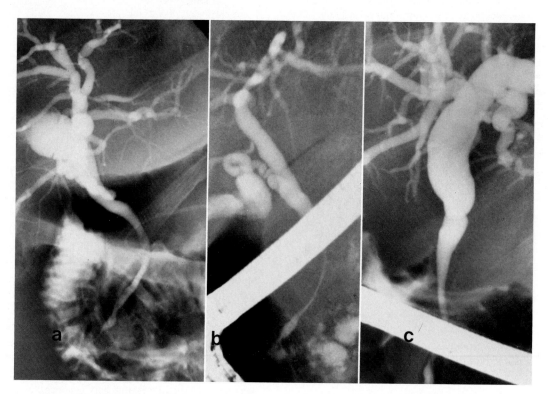

Fig. 54-8 Three cases of severe stenosis of lower part of CBD. **A,** Cholangiocarcinoma. **B,** Pancreatitis (calcifications in head of pancreas). **C,** Pancreatic cyst. Radiologic distinction between benign and malignant stenosis is often impossible.

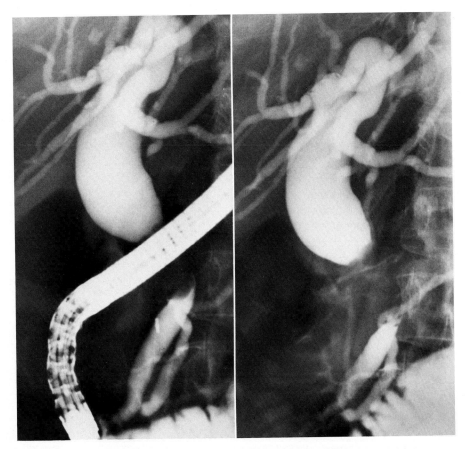

Fig. 54-9 Case of malignant stenosis in middle part of CBD caused by carcinoma of head of pancreas. Pancreatogram was normal.

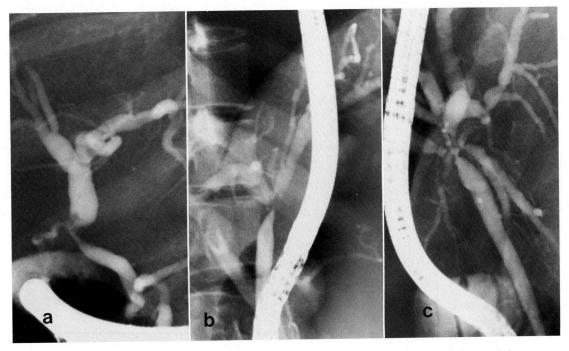

Fig. 54-10 Three cases of biliary duct stenoses. **A,** Classic localization of postsurgical stenosis in CBD at level of cystic duct. **B,** Severe iatrogenic stenosis of common hepatic duct at hilum. ERCP was performed 6 months after cholecystectomy. **C,** Severe stricture of common hepatic duct at hilum without previous history of biliary surgery. This stenosis was due to cholangiocarcinoma. Differential diagnosis between benign and malignant stenosis may be very difficult.

(Fig. 54-8). A normal pancreatogram does not exclude a pancreatic malignancy as a cause of CBD involvement (Fig. 54-9).[58] *Pancreatic carcinoma* classically involves the lower part of the CBD and generally leaves no or extremely little of the lumen of the CBD patent at the time of ERCP. Complete obstruction of CBD in the pancreatic head area is pathognomonic of pancreas cancer. In *pancreatitis* some patency of the CBD in the stenosis generally is left, but differential diagnosis from pancreatic malignancy based on cholangiography is impossible (see Fig. 54-8). These stenoses have a reported incidence of 22% of all CBD stenoses.[58] *Postsurgical stenosis* is usually localized in the common hepatic duct (74%) (Fig. 54-10) and at the junction of the CBD and cystic duct, sometimes in the common hepatic duct just below the bifurcation.[140] Long-standing strictures may result in cholangitis, calculus formation, and biliary cirrhosis (Fig. 54-11). Although histologically benign, the clinical course may be pernicious. Ninety percent of benign strictures result from surgery.[122] One in 400 to 500 cholecystectomies result in bile duct injury.[122] Only 15% of major bile duct injuries are recognized at the time of operation.[122] A major injury to the bile duct is usually suggested by the onset of jaundice, cholangitis, and biliary fistula formation. ERCP can delineate the extent of injury. Another kind of iatrogenic stenosis of the CBD is stenosis of the supraduodenal part, which may be ischemic and follow hepatic transplantation or pancreatic resection.[111] *Stenosis in the papillary region* is generally characterized by dilatation of the CBD and delayed emptying of the contrast media (more than 45 minutes).[17] *Primary papillary stenosis* has no causative or concomitant disease in the neighboring organs. *Secondary papillary stenosis* (PS) with underlying pathologic changes in the biliary tract is most common, choledocholithiasis or cholelithiasis being present in 90%.[17] Other causes are tumors and previous surgical manipulations of the papilla. A combination of papillary stenosis and intrahepatic ductal strictures appears unique to AIDS-related cholangitis.[26]

The differential diagnosis of benign and malignant stenosis of Vater's papilla may be difficult. Sphincterotomy can be performed to obtain biopsies, but the histologic diagnosis is reported to be possible in only 60% of cases.[17] Tumors of the papillary region[11,94,111] are almost all carcinomas. Their frequency is estimated to be 9% of all bile duct cancers, and they comprise 2% of all digestive tract cancers.[64] Carcinoma of the ampulla is about one tenth as common as a tumor of the pancreas.[94] It has the highest rates of resectability (60% to 96%) and a 5-year survival rate of 34%, with a 10-year incidence of surgical cure rate of 20% of all cancers encountered at upper gastrointestinal endoscopy.[11]

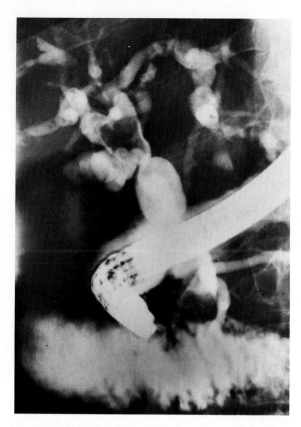

Fig. 54-11 ERCP 10 years after cholecystectomy. Appearance of long-standing iatrogenic stricture of common hepatic duct resulting in calculus formation.

The *intraduodenal form* of tumor in the papillary region (75%) are endoscopically easily identifiable. The polypoid form seems to be the most frequent and can have a central ulceration. The *intraampullary form* (25%) (Fig. 54-12) is difficult to discover endoscopically, as they do not deform the duodenal outline. The papilla may sometimes be enlarged, with an appearance of a cylindrically shaped mass. It is usually difficult to find the site of origin (it may arise from the papilla, duodenum, bile duct, or pancreas and constitutes a *periampullary carcinoma*). A cholangiogram often reveals a filling defect (Fig. 54-13). The CBD and/or PD are usually dilated. Drainage of contrast media from the ducts may be delayed. Radiographs are seldom diagnostic for malignant tumor. The sensitivity of histologic study is only 60%.[135] Despite the difficulty of finding the exact origin of the tumor when the tumor is resectable, the outcome is the same, regardless of origin.[11]

In *dysfunction of Oddi's sphincter* it is always possible to see the contraction of the sphincter on fluoroscopy and the relaxation of the narrow sphincter zone as opposed to an organic stenosis. *Nonvisualized gallbladder during*

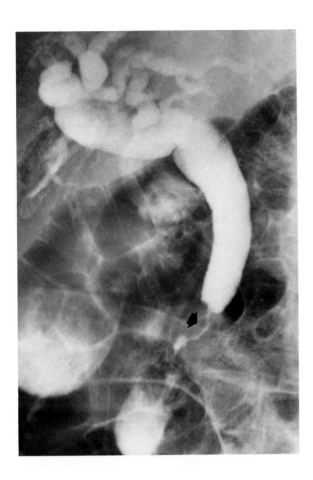

Fig. 54-12 Intraampullary carcinoma. Duodenoscopy did not reveal any abnormality of Vater's papilla. Intraampullary carcinoma causes severe stricture of intramural part of CBD *(arrow)*. Narrowing of such long segment of CBD, as well as irregular outline of stenotic segment, is abnormal finding. Prestenotic dilatation of CBD.

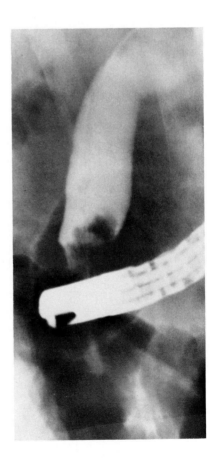

Fig. 54-13 Filling defect in lower part of dilated CBD above Vater's papilla caused by periampullary carcinoma. Radiologic differential diagnosis between calculus and tumor may be quite difficult.

ERCP[85,98] has been called a sign of undetermined meaning.[98] If the extrahepatic system is of normal caliber without evidence of obstruction, nonfilling of the gallbladder is highly predictive of abnormality.

Dilatation

The most common dilatations of the bile ducts are *prestenotic,* or secondary, and will therefore not need any further analysis. Of the remaining dilatations, most are represented by congenital malformations. According to Sherlock,[111] the various dilatations belong to the same family of *fibropolycystic diseases.* They do not exist as single entities but are found in various combinations. Fibropolycystic diseases consist of polycystic liver disease, microhamartoma, congenital hepatic fibrosis, congenital intrahepatic biliary dilatations (Caroli's disease), and choledochal cysts. There are three clinical manifestations present in varying proportions: (1) space-occupying lesions, (2) portal hypertension, and (3) cholangitis. For the purpose of cholangiography the heterogeneous group of choledochal cysts is the most important. Other entities of the fibropolycystic disease lie outside the diagnostic potential of cholangiography and will be disregarded here. Todani's classification of choledochal cysts[21,128] is most used. It divides the cysts into five types. Type I, the most common (80% to 90%), is subdivided into (a) choledochal cyst, (b) segmental choledochus dilatation, and (c) diffuse cylindrical dilatation. Type II, which is rare (2%), is a diverticulum anywhere in the extrahepatic ducts. Type III, also rare (1% to 5%), is a choledochocele. Type IV is not common (19%) and is subdivided into (a) multiple cysts of the intrahepatic and extrahepatic ducts and (b) multiple cysts in the extrahepatic ducts only. Type V is intrahepatic bile duct cyst (single or multiple), also known as Caroli's disease.

The choledochal cyst is a dilatation of the CBD. The gallbladder, cystic duct, and hepatic ducts above the cyst are normal. It may obstruct the portal vein, leading to portal hypertension.[111] There is an increased incidence of carcinoma associated with choledochal cyst, estimated at 2% to 5%[112,126] (in a normal population, 0.012% to 0.4%).[126] Clinically there is an intermittent jaundice, pain, and palpable abdominal tumor. Complications are biliary obstructions, sludge and stone formation, infection, perforation, bleeding, biliary cirrhosis, and malignancy. Most patients are girls under 10 years of age, and there is a preponderance among Oriental people (Fig. 54-14).

Choledochocele is defined as a prolapse of the intramural segment of the CBD into the duodenum. Major endoscopic differential diagnoses include papillary (ampullary) tumor and papillitis from an impacted stone. Radiographic features are characteristic—the terminal end of the CBD is clubbed and appears as a round cystic contrast-filled structure adjacent to the termination of the CBD, often protruding as a smooth round defect in the duodenum (see Fig. 54-14). There may be delayed drainage of contrast media from the CBD, which must not be

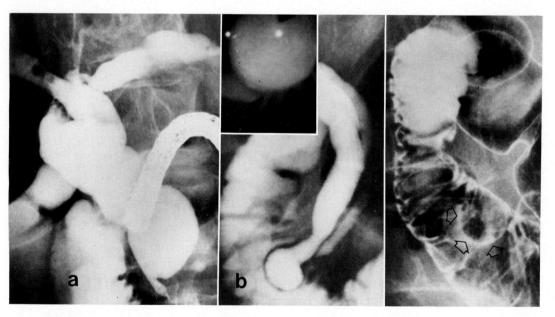

Fig. 54-14 A, Case of choledochal cyst classified as either type Ia or IVa according to Todani.
B, Case of choledochocele. Duodenoscopy revealed enlarged papilla covered by normal mucosa.
(insert). Radiograph is characteristic, showing clubbing of terminal end of CBD, producing contrast
defect in descending part of duodenum *(open arrows).*

dilated. Choledochoceles are classified into five variants on the basis of ERCP findings, depending on the anatomic relationship between the CBD, pancreatic duct, and choledochocele.[49] Clinically it exists in association with recurrent obstructive jaundice, cholangitis, and even pancreatitis.

Caroli's disease is a hereditary autosomal recessive disease often associated with nephrospongiosis.[68] The intrahepatic bile ducts are ectatic and form rounded or oval dilatations 2 to 10 cm in size. The surrounding parenchyma is normal. There is no portal hypertension (unless it is associated with other entities of fibropolycystic disease). Caroli's disease leads to intrahepatic biliary lithiasis and infection. Hepatolithiasis is invariably present.[68] The normal course of the disease consists of suppurative cholangitis, septicemia, and intrahepatic or subphrenic abscess formation. Its onset is most common between the fourth and sixth decades of life. The prognosis depends on the extent of the lesion. Caroli's disease is possibly a precancerous condition. The incidence of a biliary carcinoma in Caroli's disease is 20 times that in the normal population.[25]

Contrast medium defects

Sensitivity of ERCP is very high but depends on the size of the defect and density of contrast media used;

false-negative diagnoses are uncommon. Specificity of ERCP is very high. Few false-positive diagnoses are made (and of these, most are due to air bubbles). Differential diagnosis is often very difficult or impossible, especially when the defect occludes the biliary duct. Only a few defects have a typical diagnostic appearance (see Fig. 54-18).

Stones are in general the most common cause of filling defects in the biliary ducts. The radiologic appearance of the stone is a clue to its chemical composition, which may be important to medical treatment, since only cholesterol stones can be dissolved by chenodeoxycholic acid. Pure cholesterol stones are large and usually solitary. Mixed cholesterol stones (70% to 90%)[124] are usually smooth and faceted; pigment stones are usually small and multiple. Bile duct stones are found in 2% to 10% of the patients after cholecystectomy. In differentiating stone from air bubble in the CBD, apart from change in size, number, and shape of air bubbles during the examination, the traditional remedy is the upright position of the patient when stones move down and air up in the biliary duct. This maneuver is, however, not reliable, as stones may sometimes move in the opposite direction (Fig. 54-15). It is good to be aware of the possibility of spontaneous stone passage through Vater's papilla: stones of less than 7 mm in size are able to pass without causing

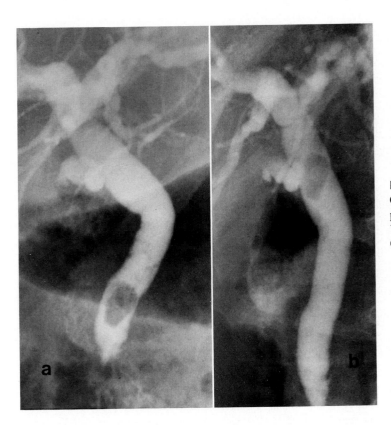

Fig. 54-15 Paradoxical movement of biliary stone in CBD. **A,** Cholangiogram with patient in horizontal position. Calculus is seen in lower part of CBD above Vater's papilla. **B,** Same patient in upright position. Calculus has moved cranially.

any significant symptoms.[120] In differential diagnosis two functional phenomena may simulate a concrement in the lowest part of the CBD—an inconstant clawlike concavity from a juxtapapillary diverticulum[59] and contractions of Oddi's sphincter, which is sometimes referred to as a pseudocalculus sign. The differential diagnosis is easy, however; fluoroscopic control will detect the real cause of these defects.

Hepatolithiasis is a quite specific group of biliary lithiasis. This disease is very rare in Western countries (with an incidence of 0.6%),[74] but East Asia has been reported to have an incidence of 51%.[74] Soft brown calcium-bicarbonate stones are present in the dilated intrahepatic ducts proximal to a stricture. Stricture of the left hepatic duct at the hilum is common. The left liver lobe is more often involved. Affected bile ducts are dilated and form cystic structures filled with brown stones and sludge. The liver parenchyma becomes fibrous. Bile stasis and infection are the main factors responsible for the clinical signs, which are often pain in the right upper quadrant (RUQ), fever, and jaundice. Cholangiography is the diagnostic method of choice. If left alone, this disease leads ultimately to cholangiohepatitis and death, usually from multiple liver abscesses and hepatic failure. The treatment is surgical. The disease is complicated further by concomitant intrahepatic cholangiocarcinoma (inci-

dence, 3.3% to 5.7%),[141] which may be difficult to detect by ERCP simply because of the presence of stones in the ducts. *Large stones* may appear in an unusual manner. Stones with a size of 3 cm and more are not an unusual finding, especially in elderly persons. Stones of this size that are located in the cystic duct or neck of the gallbladder may lead to *Mirizzi syndrome or Bouveret's syndrome*.[22,108,137] Mirizzi syndrome is characterized by large stone impaction in the gallbladder neck, erosion into and obstruction of the common hepatic duct, and proximal biliary tree dilatation. It leaves the CBD undilated. In Bouveret's syndrome there is a gastric outlet obstruction, another uncommon manifestation of large gallstones. The stone penetrates into the pyloric part of the stomach or duodenal cap and can be seen at endoscopy. Before endoscopy was introduced, the preoperative diagnosis was made in only 37% of patients, and the operative mortality was 33%.[92] Most patients with correct preoperative diagnosis recover after operation. ERCP of Mirizzi syndrome reveals a dilated common hepatic duct and smooth large well-demarcated filling defect in the cystic duct and/or gallbladder with narrowing of common hepatic duct at the same level. The radiographic differential diagnosis includes acute cholecystitis, gallbladder carcinoma, pancreatic tumor, pancreatic pseudocyst, primary hepatic tumor, and porta hepatis lymphadenopathy.[137]

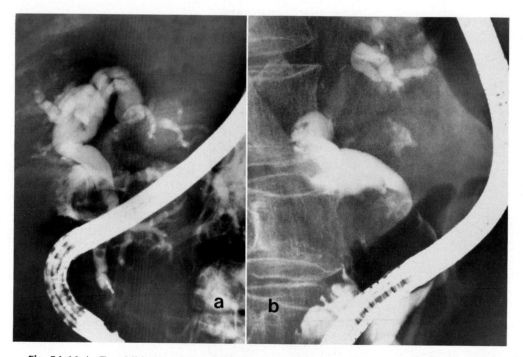

Fig. 54-16 A, True Mirizzi syndrome. Calculus in neck of gallbladder causing stricture of CBD. Dilatation of biliary tree above gallbladder as opposed to normal size of lower CBD. **B,** False Mirizzi syndrome caused by carcinoma of gallbladder—almost same radiologic appearance as in **A.** Radiologic differential diagnosis between true and false Mirizzi syndrome may be very difficult.

The true Mirizzi syndrome is due to gallstones, but similar features may be seen in cystic duct or gallbladder carcinoma (Fig. 54-16).[92]

The most frequent manifestation of cholangiocarcinoma is stenosis. Only the rare exophytic bile duct carcinomas (type III)[58] may cause a filling defect in the biliary duct (Fig. 54-17). A less common type of biliary carcinoma—the papillary adenocarcinoma—causes multiple defects in the biliary ducts. *Intrahepatic biliary papillomatosis*, which is both uncommon and histologically benign, produces multiple filling defects in the biliary tree. This tumor discharges large quantities of mucus.[69] *Hepatocellular carcinomas* may sometimes produce lobulated irregular filling defects in the major

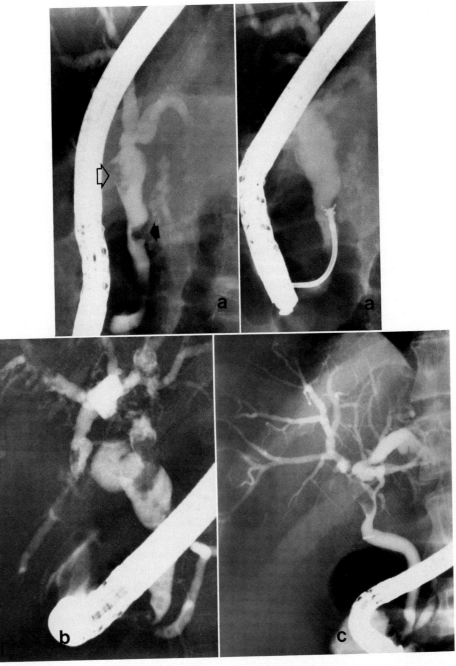

Fig. 54-17 Defects in contrast-filled CBD caused by several kinds of tumor. **A,** Protuberant type of cholangiocarcinoma (type III according to Liguory and Canard). Tumor is visualized in upper portion of CBD *(open arrow)* as well as in mid portion *(arrow),* from where biopsies are taken during ERCP. **B,** Highly differentiated papillomatous adenocarcinoma of CBD and CHD. **C,** Hepatocellular tumor invading CHD and producing contrast defect in duct.

bile ducts (see Fig. 54-17).[15] *Intrabiliary tumor embolus* is demonstrated by ERCP as a free-floating filling defect in the biliary duct.[4] This is a rare cause of defects.

Hemobilia is hemorrhage arising from pathologic changes in the intrahepatic biliary tract. Its main causes include iatrogenic and noniatrogenic trauma, cholangitis, tumors, and coagulopathies.[102] It occurs in 2% of hepatic injuries. After diagnostic and therapeutic interventions, such as PTC, percutaneous transhepatic biliary drainage, and endoscopic papillotomy, hemobilia occurs in 4% to 13%.[36] It usually appears as a clinical triad of colicky RUQ pain, jaundice with fluctuating intensity, and acute upper gastrointestinal hemorrhage. ERCP reveals longitudinal defects in the biliary ducts. The defects have a quite typical appearance, as they are often casts of the lumen (Fig. 54-18), and in contrast to other filling defects, the diagnosis is not particularly difficult.

Parasites in the biliary tract may cause defects of various shapes and sizes, some of them with quite diagnostic appearance. Infestation of the biliary tract by adult helminths or their ova may produce recurrent pyogenic cholangitis, hepatic abscess, stones, and biliary obstruction. There is a preponderance in Southeast Asia.[65] Organisms most commonly involved are trematodes or flukes, including *Clonorchis sinensis, Opisthorchis* species, and *Fasciola hepatica,* as well as duct migration of *Ascaris* species or a rupture of the hydatid cyst produced by *Echinococcus* species. Cholangiography may reveal defects as well as stenoses and dilatations in the biliary ducts. *Ascaris* species may produce a typical longitudinal strip sign or spaghetti sign[67] or round bull's eye defects.[67] Ruptured hydatid cysts produce round defects representing daughter cysts.[27] Chinese liver fluke appears as small elliptic or filamentous defects.[15] *Ascaris* worms are large and can produce bile duct obstruction.[111]

Rare causes of defects include posttraumatic obstructive jaundice from foreign body.[29] *Cirrhosis* may cause a tumor simulating filling defect in the biliary duct, most probably because of focal hypertrophy compressing the CBD (in my experience) (Fig. 54-19). In *cystic fibrosis* multiple defects throughout the biliary tree represent thickened bile and mucus or stones.[8]

Leakage of contrast medium outside the biliary tract

Leakage is most often the result of injury to the biliary tree during surgery. Noniatrogenic injury as a cause of contrast medium leakage is rare. Clinically postoperative jaundice, fever, and/or biliary fistula formation is highly suggestive of iatrogenic biliary damage. An early and accurate location of the damage is important. Recognition of bile leaks is facilitated by the detection of fluid with ultrasonography or CT, but the exact anatomy of the

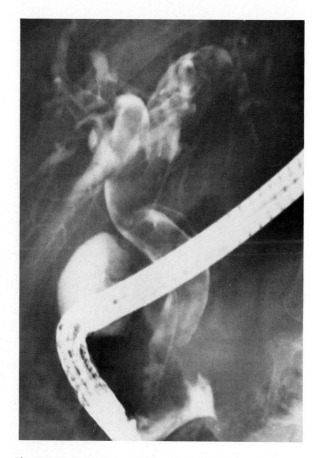

Fig. 54-18 Case of hemobilia after endoscopic papillotomy. ERCP performed 5 days later shows large contrast defects with typical appearance of casts in lumen of intrahepatic and extrahepatic biliary tree.

damage will be revealed by cholangiography, allowing for endoscopic decompression, which achieves an immediate relief of symptoms and rapid healing of the fistulas. A common cholangiographic finding is leakage from the cystic duct (Fig. 54-20). Injury to extrahepatic bile ducts from blunt abdominal trauma is uncommon.[48] Partial or complete tears may appear at any location. ERCP reveals extravasation of contrast media from bile duct, which is not visualized higher than to the point of extravasation, indicating a complete transsection. The most frequent site of bile duct injury from blunt trauma is the pancreaticoduodenal junction. The next most frequent sites are the bifurcation of the common hepatic duct and origin of the left hepatic duct.[48]

There are two main types of biliary fistulas[76]: the more common fistulas developing on the basis of calculous disease and the rare traumatic fistulas (0.4% to 2.6% of liver trauma cases). There are several reports on the visualization of *hepatic abscesses*.[37,103,105,124,138] The ERCP appearance is of an irregular extravasation of contrast

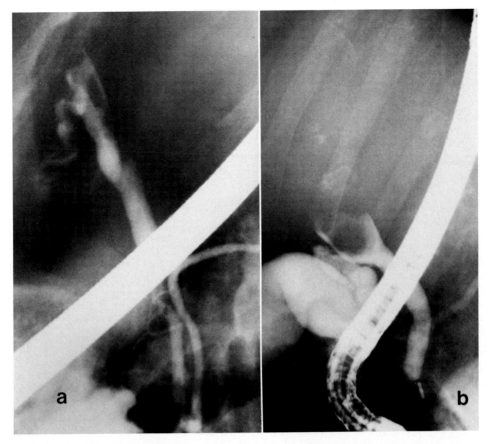

Fig. 54-19 Rare cause of filling defect in biliary tree. **A,** Cirrhosis causing defect in CHD from focal hypertrophy compressing biliary duct. **B,** Radiographically similar to **A** but caused by cholangiocarcinoma. Both cases illustrate enormous radiologic differential diagnostic difficulty when defect totally occludes lumen.

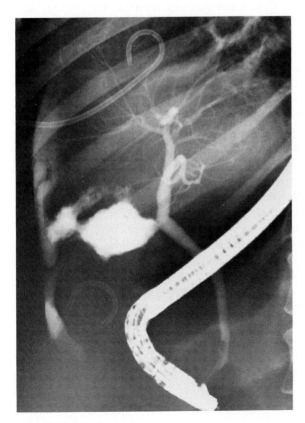

Fig. 54-20 Contrast leakage from CBD at level of cystic duct. ERCP performed 5 days after cholecystectomy. Contrast media has spread around right liver lobe and in subhepatic space.

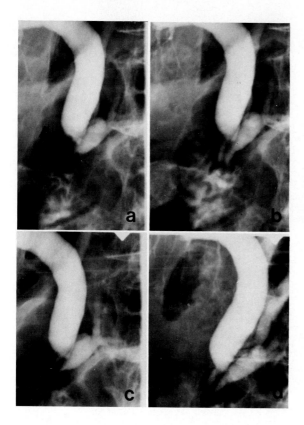

Fig. 54-21 A, Pseudocalculus sign caused by deep contraction of Oddi's sphincter *(arrow).* **B, C,** and **D,** Serial films in same case showing change of shape and relaxation of intramural part of CBD, making differential diagnosis of stone easy.

media into the liver parenchyma. In patients with subphrenic and subhepatic abscess ERCP can reveal a communication between the biliary tree and the abscess cavities.[103,124] In *hepatic hydatid disease*[27] rupture of the cyst into the biliary tree produces the cholangiographic appearance of filling defects in the bile ducts as well as direct cystobiliary communication. In patients with *rupture of the gallbladder* complicating acute cholecystitis has been diagnosed with ERCP.[71]

Functional signs

Functional signs on ERCP can only be observed in the sphincter zone—that is, in the intramural portion of the CBD. Even manometry will not detect abnormal changes in the CBD above the sphincter zone, which therefore appears to be a passive conduit for bile. Functional signs can mimic organic changes, such as defects in the CBD, and give an indication of the drainage capacity of the biliary tree to the duodenum. The latter is a very controversial subject. For a more accurate interpretation of the functional factors, ERCP is performed in combination with manometry of Oddi's sphincter.

Several functional signs can be observed. *The pseudocalculus sign* is very often seen as a deep and vigorous contraction of Oddi's sphincter, which may mimic a stone

in the intramural portion of the CBD. Serial films, however, show a change in the shape of the sphincter zone with relaxation and subsequent filling of the duodenum (Fig. 54-21). Occasionally, antispasmodics are necessary to achieve relaxation. In *dysfunction of Oddi's sphincter and papillary stenosis,*[135] at the most distal end of the CBD, a high-pressure zone of 4 to 6 mm length is noted—a so-called SO zone. Its basal pressure lies around 5 mm Hg above the CBD pressure. CCK-octapeptide and glucagon decrease sphincter pressure. A basal pressure of 15 ± 3 mm Hg has been measured in control subjects.[34] Sphincter dysfunction results in a hindrance of biliary and pancreatic flow at the level of the sphincter.[135] Two types of Oddi's sphincter dysfunction are found[135]: (1) *papillary stenosis* from structural abnormality of the sphincter, which may be caused by chronic inflammation, fibrosis following migration of gallstones through the papilla, trauma, or adenomyosis, and (2) *biliary dyskinesia,* which is a functional blockage at the sphincter zone because of spasm, hypertrophy, or denervation of the sphincter. ERCP with manometry is the most valuable investigative modality for the diagnosis of Oddi's sphincter dysfunction. Radiographic abnormalities include dilatation of the CBD above an apparently normal sphincter segment, delayed contrast me-

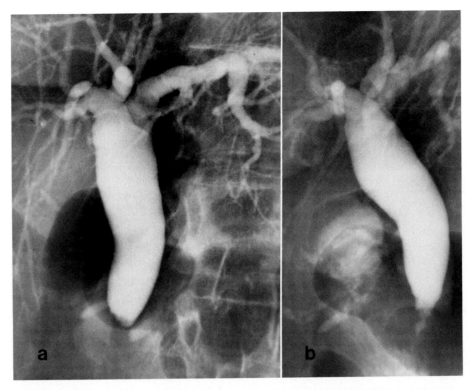

Fig. 54-22 Papillary stenosis—biliary dyskinesia. **A,** Cholangiogram immediately after withdrawal of cannula. **B,** Cholangiogram of same patient 45 minutes later. Dilatation of CBD, delayed contrast emptying, and absence of other causes of bile duct obstruction.

dium emptying to the duodenum (more than 45 minutes), and absence of other causes of bile duct obstruction (Fig. 54-22). Manometric measurements appear to be helpful in determining which patient will benefit from sphincterotomy.[7,34] A value of 44 ± 8 mm Hg is highly suggestive of dysfunction of Oddi's sphincter, whereas the value of 61 ± 11 mm Hg is equivalent to a definite dysfunction.[34] The study of functional disturbances using an invasive technique can be associated with certain errors of interpretation, and one may argue that the emptying capacity can be better studied using a noninvasive method. Some positive reports have been published on the use of hepatobiliary imaging,[56] which can be used both for the diagnosis of stenosis-dysfunction and the evaluation of the effect of sphincterotomy.

REFERENCES

1. Agha, FP, et al: Cytomegalovirus cholangitis in a homosexual man with acquired immune deficiency syndrome, Am J Gastroenterol 81:1068, 1986.
2. Anacker, H, Weiss, HD, and Kramann, B: Endoscopic retrograde pancreatico-cholangiography (ERCP), New York, 1977, Springer-Verlag.
3. Anderson, SD, et al: Causes of jaundice during hepatic artery infusion chemotherapy, Radiology 161:439, 1986.
4. Auld, RM, and Weiss, JB: Intrabiliary tumor embolus: demonstration by ERCP, Gastrointest Endosc 33:130, 1987.
5. Baker, JP, et al: Emphysematous cholecystitis complicating endoscopic retrograde cholangiography, Gastrointest Endosc 28:184, 1982.
6. Balli, F, et al: Endoscopic retrograde cholangiopancreatography in the diagnosis of Alagille's syndrome, Pediatr Med Chir (Med Surg Pediatr) 6:831, 1984.
7. Bar-Meir, S, et al: Manometric study during endoscopic retrograde cholangiopancreatography: a new technique for the evaluation of pathology in the pancreatic and biliary systems, Isr J Med Sci 18:769, 1982.
8. Bass, S, Connon, JJ, and Ho, CS: Biliary tree in cystic fibrosis: biliary tract abnormalities in cystic fibrosis demonstrated by endoscopic retrograde cholangiography, Gastroenterology 84:1592, 1983.
9. Baumgartner, F, Williams, RA, and Wilson, SE: Patient selection and complications of transhepatic cholangiography, Surg Gynecol Obstet 165:199, 1987.
10. Bilbao, MK, et al: Complications of endoscopic retrograde cholangiopancreatography (ERCP), Gastroenterology 70:314, 1976.
11. Blackstone, MO: Endoscopic interpretation: normal and pathologic appearances of the gastrointestinal tract, New York, 1984, Raven Press.
12. Börsch, G, et al: Der Einfluss von Somatostatin auf die Amylasespiegel und Pankreatitisrate nach ERCP, Medwelt 35:109, 1984.
13. Brandes, J-W, et al: ERCP: Komplikationen und Prophylaxe—eine kontrollierte Studie, Z Gastroenterol 19:242, 1981.

14. Butler, T, Feintuch, TA, and Caine, WP, Jr: Eosinophilic chol-angitis, lymphadenopathy, and peripheral eosinophilia: a case report, Am J Gastroenterol 80:572, 1985.

15. Choi, TK, and Wong, J: Endoscopic retrograde cholangiopan-creatography and endoscopic papillotomy in recurrent pyogenic cholangitis, Clin Gastroenterol 15:393, 1986.

16. Cicero, GF, et al: Effects of somatostatin on clinical, biochemical and morphological changes following ERCP, Ital J Gastroenterol 17:265, 1985.

17. Classen, M, Leuschner, U, and Schreiber, HW: Stenosis of the papilla Vateri and common duct calculi, Clin Gastroenterol 12:203, 1983.

18. Costel, EE, Wheeler, AP, and Gregg, CR: *Campylobacter fetus* ssp fetus cholecystitis and relapsing bacteremia in a patient with acquired immunodeficiency syndrome, South Med J 77:927, 1984.

19. Cotton, P, and Salmon, PR: Potential complications of ERCP. In Schiller, KFR, and Salmon, PR, editors: Modern topics in gastrointestinal endoscopy, London, 1976, Heinemann.

20. Cottone, M, Amuso, M, and Cotton, PB: Endoscopic retrograde cholangiography in hepatic hydatid disease, Br J Surg 65:107, 1978.

21. Crittenden, SL, and McKinley, MJ: Choledochal cyst: clinical features and classification, Am J Gastroenterol 80:643, 1985.

22. Cruz, FO, et al: Radiology of the Mirizzi syndrome: diagnostic importance of the transhepatic cholangiogram, Gastrointest Radiol 8:249, 1983.

23. Cunliffe, WJ, et al: A randomised, prospective study comparing two contrast media in ERCP, Endoscopy 19:201, 1987.

24. Davion, T, et al: *Pseudomonas aeruginosa* liver abscesses fol-lowing endoscopic retrograde cholangiography: report of a case without biliary tract disease, Dig Dis Sci 32:1044, 1987.

25. Dayton, MT, Longmire, WP, and Tompkins, RK: Caroli's dis-ease: a premalignant condition? Am J Surg 145:41, 1983.

26. Dolmatch, RL, et al: AIDS-related cholangitis: radiographic find-ings in nine patients, Radiology 163:313, 1987.

27. Dyrszka, H, Sanghavi, B, and Peddamatham, K: Hepatic hydatid disease: findings on endoscopic retrograde cholangiography, Gas-trointest Endosc 29:248, 1983.

28. Ebner, F, et al: Pankreasnekrose nach endoskopisch retrograder Pankreatikographie, Dtsch Med Wschr 107:453, 1982.

29. Edwards, FH, and Davies, RS: Late post-traumatic obstructive jaundice secondary to a biliary tract foreign body, J Trauma 22:336, 1982.

30. Falkenstein, DB, et al: The endoscopic intrahepatic cholangio-gram, Invest Radiol 10:358, 1975.

31. Frederic, N, et al: Comparative study of ultrasound and ERCP in the diagnosis of hepatic, biliary and pancreatic diseases: a prospective study based on a continuous series of 424 patients, Eur J Radiol 3:208, 1983.

32. Galloway, PG: Widespread cytomegalovirus infection involving the gastrointestinal tract, biliary tree, and gallbladder in an im-munocompromised patient, Gastroenterology 87:1407, 1984.

33. Geenen, JE: ERCP and the problem of sepsis, Gastrointest Endosc 28:197, 1982.

34. Geenen, JE: New diagnostic and treatment modalities involving endoscopic retrograde cholangiopancreatography and esophago-gastroduodenoscopy, Scand J Gastroenterol 17 (Suppl 77):93, 1982.

35. Goebell, H: Trends in der modernen Behandlung der akuten Pan-kreatitis. In Grözinger, K-H, Schrey, A, and Wabnitz, RW, ed-itors: Foy Workshop: proteinasen-inhibition, Munich, 1982, Ver-lag Dr C Wolf & Sohn.

36. Goldberg, ME, and Waye, JD: Traumatic hemobilia, Am J Gas-troenterol 71:605, 1977.

37. Hall, RI, Venables, CW, and Lendrum, R: ERCP diagnosis of multiple hepatic abscesses due to portal pylephlebitis, Br J Surg 72:439, 1985.

38. Hamilton, I, et al: Acute pancreatitis following endoscopic ret-rograde cholangiopancreatography, Clin Radiol 34:543, 1983.

39. Hamilton, I, et al: The endoscopic retrograde cholangiogram and pancreatogram in chronic liver disease, Clin Radiol 34:417, 1983.

40. Hannigan, BF, et al: Hyperamylasemia after ERCP with ionic and non-ionic contrast media, Gastrointest Endosc 31:109, 1985.

41. Harary, AM, et al: Hepatocellular carcinoma presenting as biliary colic and unilateral bile duct obstruction: demonstration by ERC, Gastrointest Endosc 30:350, 1984.

42. Healey, JE, Jr, and Schroy, PC: Anatomy of the biliary ducts within the human liver, Arch Surg 66:599, 1953.

43. Helm, EB, et al: Pseudomonas-Septikämie nach endoskopischen Eingriffen am Gallengangsystem, Dtsch Med Wschr 109:697, 1984.

44. Hjortsjö, C-H: The topography of the intrahepatic duct systems, Acta Anat 11:599, 1951.

45. Ihre, T, and Hellers, G: Complications and endoscopic retrograde cholangio-pancreatography, Acta Chir Scand 143:167, 1977.

46. Irish, CR, and Meaney, TF: Percutaneous transhepatic cholan-giography: comparison of success and risk using 19- versus 22-gauge needles, AJR 134:137, 1980.

47. Jeffrey, RB, et al: Computed tomography of choledocholithiasis, AJR 140:1179, 1983.

48. Jones, KB, and Thomas, E: Traumatic rupture of the hepatic duct demonstrated by endoscopic retrograde cholangiography, J Trauma 25:448, 1985.

49. Kagiyama, S, et al: Anatomic variants of choledochocele and manometric measurements of pressure in the cele and the orifice zone, Am J Gastroenterol 82:641, 1987.

49a. Kasugai, T, Kuno, N, and Kizu, M: Manometric endoscopic retrograde pancreatocholangiography: technique, significance, and evaluation, Am J Dig Dis 19:485, 1974.

50. Kessler, RE, et al: Indications, clinical value and complications of endoscopic retrograde cholangiopancreatography, Surg Gy-naecol Obstet 142:865, 1976.

51. Koch, H, Schneider, A, and Demling, L: Pankreatitis nach en-doskopisch-retrograder Cholangio-Pankreatikographie (ERCP) und endoskopischer Papillotomie (EPT). In Lindner, H, editor: Fortschr der Gastroenterol Endoskopie, Gräselsing, 1977, De-meter-Verlag.

52. Kolmansskog, F, et al: Cholangiographic findings in ulcerative colitis, Acta Radiol Diagn 22:151, 1981.

53. Kreek, MJ, and Balint, JA: "Skinny needle" cholangiography: results of a pilot study of a voluntary prospective method for gathering risk data on new procedures, Gastroenterology 78:598, 1980.

54. Ladas, SD, et al: Absorption of iodized contrast media during ERCP, Gastrointest Endosc 32:376, 1986.

55. LaFerla, G, et al: Hyperamylasaemia and acute pancreatitis fol-lowing endoscopic retrograde cholangiopancreatography, Pan-creas 1:160, 1986.

56. Lee, RG, et al: Sphincter of Oddi stenosis: diagnosis using he-patobiliary scintigraphy and endoscopic manometry, Radiology 156:793, 1985.

57. Lefton, HB, and Winkelman, EI: Endoscopic retrograde cholan-giographic evaluation of sclerosing cholangitis, Cleve Clin Q 41:143, 1974.

58. Liguory, C, and Canard, JM: Tumours of the biliary system, Clin Gastroenterol 12:269, 1983.

59. Lintott, DJ, Ruddell, WSJ, and Axon, ATR: Pseudostone at ERCP due to juxtapapillary diverticulum, Clin Radiol 32:173, 1981.

60. Ljunggren, B, et al: Contribution of endoscopic retrograde cholangiopancreatography to the study of endoscopic and radiological anatomy of Oddi's sphincter. In Delmont, JS, editor: The sphincter of Oddi: Third Gastroenterology Symposium, Nice, 1976, Basel, 1976, Karger.

61. Low, DE, et al: Infectious complications of endoscopic retrograde cholangiopancreatography: a prospective assessment, Arch Intern Med 140:1076, 1980.

62. MacCarty, RL, et al: Primary sclerosing cholangitis: findings on cholangiography and pancreatography, Radiology 149:39, 1983.

63. Mairose, UB, Wurbs, D, and Classen, M: Das Krankheitsbild der primär sklerosierenden Cholangitis, Med Klin 74:453, 1979.

64. Martin, ED: Tumors of the Oddian region: pathological aspects. In Delmont, JS, editor: The sphincter of Oddi: Third Gastroenterology Symposium, Nice, 1976, Basel, 1976, Karger.

64a. McCune, WS, Shorb, PE, and Moscovitz, H: Endoscopic cannulation of the ampulla of Vater: a preliminary report, Am Surg 167:752, 1968.

65. McPhee, MS, and Greenberger, NJ: Diseases of the gallbladder and bile ducts. In Braunwald, E, et al, editors: Harrison's principles of internal medicine, vol 2, New York, 1987, McGraw-Hill.

66. Mendel, R, et al: Zwei Fälle einer primär sklerosierenden Cholangitis: ERCP-Dokumentation eines 3-jährigen Verlaufs unter immunsuppressiver Therapie, Radiologe 25:83, 1985.

67. Mensing, M, et al: Biliary ascariasis, Röntgenblätter 39:151, 1986.

68. Mercadier, M, et al: Caroli's disease, World J Surg 8:22, 1984.

69. Mercadier, M, et al: Papillomatosis of the intrahepatic bile ducts, World J Surg 8:30, 1984.

70. Mir-Madjlessi, SH, Farmer, RG, and Sivak, MV, Jr: Bile duct carcinoma in patients with ulcerative colitis, Dig Dis Sci 32:145, 1987.

71. Morgan, TR, et al: Demonstration of free rupture of the gallbladder by endoscopic retrograde cholangiography, Arch Surg 121:1213, 1986.

72. Myllylä, V, et al: Sensitivity of ultrasonography in the demonstration of common bile duct stones and its ranking in comparison with intravenous cholangiography and endoscopic retrograde cholangiopancreatography, Fortschr Roentgenstr 141:192, 1984.

73. Myren, J: Risk of cannulation of the papilla of Vater, Scand J Gastroenterol 12(suppl 47):22, 1977.

74. Nakayama, F, and Koga, A: Hepatolithiasis: present status, World J Surg 8:9, 1984.

75. Nebel, OT, et al: Complications associated with endoscopic retrograde cholangiopancreatography, Gastrointest Endosc 22:34, 1975.

76. Nelson, AM: Demonstration of a traumatic biliary fistula by ERCP, Gastrointest Endosc 30:315, 1984.

77. Neoptolemos, JP, et al: A prospective study of ERCP and endoscopic sphincterotomy in the diagnosis and treatment of gallstone acute pancreatitis: a rational and safe approach to management, Arch Surg 121:697, 1986.

78. Neoptolemos, JP, et al: The role of clinical and biochemical criteria and endoscopic retrograde cholangiopancreatography in the urgent diagnosis of common bile duct stones in acute pancreatitis, Surgery 100:732, 1986.

79. Neoptolemos, JP, et al: Acute cholangitis in association with acute pancreatitis: incidence, clinical features and outcome in relation to ERCP and endoscopic sphincterotomy, Br J Surg 74:1103, 1987.

80. Nichols, DM, and Burhenne, HJ: Magnification in cholangiography, AJR 142:947, 1984.

81. Niederau, C, Sonnenberg, A, and Mueller, J: Comparison of the extrahepatic bile duct size measured by ultrasound and by different radiographic methods, Gastroenterology 87:615, 1984.

82. Norman, O: Studies on the hepatic ducts in cholangiography, Acta Radiol (Suppl) 84, 1951.

83. O'Connor, HJ, et al: Ultrasound detection of choledocholithiasis: prospective comparison with ERCP in the postcholecystectomy patient, Gastrointest Radiol 11:161, 1986.

84. Oi, I: Complications. In Takemoto, T, and Kasugai, T, editors: Endoscopic retrograde cholangiopancreatography, Tokyo, 1979, Igaku-Shoin.

85. Okada, K, et al: Study on cases of nonvisualized cholecystogram by the use of ERCP, Jap J Surg 10:115, 1980.

86. Okada, K, et al: Diagnostic evaluation of CT and ERCP based on a retrospective analysis of hepato-biliary and pancreatic diseases, Jap J Surg 11:277, 1981.

87. Ott, DJ, and Gelfand, DW: Complications of gastrointestinal radiologic procedures. II. Complications related to biliary tract studies, Gastrointest Radiol 6:47, 1981.

88. Patel, R, and Shaps, J: Intramural duodenal hematoma: a complication of ERCP, Gastrointest Endosc 28:218, 1982.

89. Pereiras, R: Special radiologic procedures in liver diseases. In Schiff, L, and Schiff, ER, editors: Diseases of the liver, ed 5, Philadelphia, 1982, JB Lippincott.

90. Phillip, J, et al: Einfluss des synthetischen Proteasen-Inhibitors FOY auf die Trypsinkonzentrationen nach ERCP. In Grözinger, K-H, Schrey, A, and Wabnitz, RW, editors: Foy Workshop: proteinasen-inhibition, Munich, 1982, Verlag Dr C Wolf & Sohn.

91. Radin, DR, Cohen, H, and Halls, JM: Acalculous inflammatory disease of the biliary tree in acquired immunodeficiency syndrome: CT demonstration, J Comput Assist Tomogr 11:775, 1987.

92. Rajender Reddy, K, et al: The unusual presentation of "large" gallstones, J Clin Gastroenterol 8:171, 1986.

93. Rappaport, AM: Physioanatomic considerations. In Schiff, L, and Schiff, ER, editors: Diseases of the liver, ed 5, Philadelphia, 1982, JB Lippincott.

94. Read, AE: Periampullary cancer: clinical introduction. In Delmont, JS, editor: The sphincter of Oddi: Third Gastroenterology Symposium, Nice, 1976, Basel, 1976, Karger.

95. Reiertsen, O, et al: Complications of fiberoptic gastrointestinal endoscopy: five years' experience in a central hospital, Endoscopy 19:1, 1987.

96. Reimer Jensen, A, et al: A randomized trial of iohexol versus amidotrizoate in endoscopic retrograde pancreatography, Scand J Gastroenterol 20:83, 1985.

97. Rohrmann, CA, Jr, et al: Endoscopic retrograde intrahepatic cholangiogram: radiological findings in intrahepatic disease, AJR 128:45, 1977.

98. Rohrmann, CA, Jr, et al: Significance of the nonopacified gallbladder in endoscopic retrograde cholangiography, AJR 132:191, 1979.

99. Rosseland, AR, and Solhaug, JH: Early or delayed endoscopic papillotomy (EPT) in gallstone pancreatitis, Ann Surg 199:165, 1984.

100. Sable, RA, et al: Absorption of contrast medium during ERCP, Dig Dis Sci 28:801, 1983.

101. Safrany, L, et al: Endoskopische Papillotomie bei akuter, biliär bedingter Pancreatitis, Dtsch Med Wschr 105:115, 1980.

102. Sandblom, P, Saegesser, F, and Mirkovitch, V: Hepatic hemobilia: hemorrhage from the intrahepatic biliary tract—a review, World J Surg 8:41, 1984.

103. Sassaris, M, et al: ERCP demonstration of biliary fistula and subphrenic abscess, Endoscopy 14:151, 1982.

104. Satake, K, et al: Evaluation of cholangiographic procedures in diagnosis of obstructive jaundice, Am Surg 47:387, 1981.

105. Sauerbruch, T: Endoskopische retrograde Cholangiographie (ERC) zur Abklärung von Lebererkrankungen, Z Gastroenterologie 22:21, 1984.

106. Schneiderman, DJ, Cello, JP, and Laing, FC: Papillary stenosis and sclerosing cholangitis in the acquired immunodeficiency syndrome, Ann Intern Med 106:546, 1987.

107. Severini, A, et al: Lymphomatous involvement of intrahepatic and extrahepatic biliary ducts, Acta Radiol Diagn 22:159, 1981.

108. Shamir, M, and Schuman, BM: Complications of fiberoptic endoscopy, Gastrointest Endosc 26:86, 1980.

109. Shapiro, HA: Endoscopic diagnosis and treatment of biliary tract disease, Surg Clin North Am 61:843, 1981.

110. Shea, JA: Preoperative evaluation of the biliary tract, Surg Clin North Am 65:47, 1985.

111. Sherlock, S: Diseases of the liver and biliary system, ed 7, Oxford, 1985, Blackwell.

112. Siedek, M, et al: Kongenitale intrahepatische Gallengangszysten (M Caroli), Leber Magen Darm 4:242, 1974.

113. Siegel, JH: Endoscopy and papillotomy in diseases of the biliary tract and pancreas, J Clin Gastroenterol 2:337, 1980.

114. Silvis, SE, et al: Endoscopic complications, JAMA 235:928, 1976.

115. Sisley, JF, Bowden, TA, and Mansberger, AR, Jr: Pancreatic duct disruption and duodenal hematoma associated with endoscopic retrograde cholangiopancreatography, South Med J 80:1441, 1987.

116. Skude, G, et al: Hyperamylasaemia after duodenoscopy and retrograde cholangiopancreatography, Gut 17:127, 1976.

117. Standerskjöld-Nordenstam, CG, and Fräki, OI: Endoscopic retrograde cholangiopancreatography in a surgical unit, Ann Clin Res 10:30, 1978.

118. Stanley, JH, Yantis, PL, and Marsh, WH: Periportal tuberculous adenitis: a rare cause of obstructive jaundice, Gastrointest Radiol 9:227, 1984.

119. Svenberg, T, et al: Haemorrhagic pancreatitis after ERCP in patients with alpha₁-antitrypsin deficiency, Lancet, 1988. (Submitted for publication.)

120. Takemoto, T, and Kasugai, T: Endoscopic retrograde cholangiopancreatography, Tokyo, 1979, Igaku-Shoin.

121. Tamás, G, Jr, et al: Effect of somatostatin on the pancreatitis-like biochemical changes due to endoscopic pancreatography: preliminary report, Metabolism 27:1333, 1978.

122. Tan, EC, and Warren, KW: Diseases of the gallbladder and bile ducts. In Schiff, L, and Schiff, ER, editors: Diseases of the liver, ed 5, Philadelphia, 1982, JB Lippincott.

123. Teixidor, HS, et al: Cytomegalovirus infection of the alimentary canal: radiologic findings with pathologic correlation, Radiology 163:317, 1987.

124. Teplick, SK: Biliary tract investigations by imaging modalities. In Teplick, JG, and Haskin, ME, editors: Surgical radiology, vol 1, Philadelphia, 1981, WB Saunders.

125. Testoni, PA, Masci, E, and Tittobello, A: Somatostatin in prevention of pancreatic reaction following endoscopic papillosphincterotomy, Ital J Gastroenterol 18:169, 1986.

126. Thatcher, BS, et al: ERCP in evaluation and diagnosis of choledochal cyst: report of five cases, Gastrointest Endosc 32:27, 1986.

127. Tobin, RS, et al: A comparative study of computed tomography and ERCP in pancreaticobiliary disease, J Comput Assist Tomogr 11:261, 1987.

128. Todani, T, et al: Congenital bile duct cysts, Am surg 134:263, 1977.

129. Triller, J, et al: CT and ERCP als Kombinationsuntersuchung bei Erkrankungen der Gallenwege, ROFO 142:138, 1985.

130. Tulassay, Z, and Papp, J: Akute Pankreatitis nach endoskopischer retrograder cholangiographie, Dtsch Z Verdau Stoffwechselkr 40:133, 1980.

131. Tulassay, Z, et al: Changes in glucose tolerance after endoscopic retrograde cholangiopancreatography, Gut 22:575, 1981.

132. Tydén, G, et al: Effect of somatostatin on hyperamylasemia following endoscopic pancreatography, Acta Chir Scand Suppl 530:43, 1986.

133. Tympner, F: Einfluss von FOY (Gabexat mesilat) auf die Serumamylasespiegel nach endoskopisch retrograder Pankreatikographia. In Grözinger, K-H, Schrey, A, and Wabnitz, RW, editors: Foy Workshop: proteinasen-inhibition. Munich, 1986, Verlag Dr C Wolf & Sohn.

134. Van Husen, N: Endoskopische Sphinkterotomie der Vaterschen Papille bei akuter biliärer Pankreatitis, Schweiz Rundschau Med (PRAXIS) 75:249, 1986.

135. Venu, RP, and Geenen, JE: Diagnosis and treatment of diseases of the papilla, Clin Gastroenterol 15:439, 1986.

136. Warren, GH, and Kern, F, Jr: The biliary tract in inflammatory bowel disease, Clin Gastroenterol 12:255, 1983.

137. Weiss, SL, et al: Mirizzi syndrome simulating a tumor by ERC, Dig Dis Sci 31:100, 1986.

138. Weizel, A, and Czygan, P: Demonstration of a liver abscess by ERC, Endoscopy 8:110, 1977.

139. Williams, LF, Jr, and Schoetz, DJ, Jr: Primary sclerosing cholangitis, Surg Clin North Am 61:951, 1981.

140. Wurbs, D: Operationsfolgen an der Gallenwegen: analyse mit der ERCP, Internist 26:9, 1985.

141. Yoshimoti, H, et al: Intrahepatic cholangiocarcinoma associated with hepatolithiasis, Gastrointest Endosc 31:260, 1985.

142. Zimmon, DS: Injection pistol for volume control of contrast injection during endoscopic retrograde cholangiopancreatography, Gastrointest Endosc 33;238, 1987.

143. Zimmon, DS, and Clemett, AR: Visualization of the bile ducts. In Popper, H, and Schaffner, F, editors: Progress in liver diseases, vol 6, New York, 1979, Grune & Stratton.

55 *Magnetic Resonance Spectroscopy*

DIETER J. MEYERHOFF
MICHAEL W. WEINER

GENERAL CONSIDERATIONS

METABOLIC PATHWAYS DETECTED BY MAGNETIC
RESONANCE SPECTROSCOPY

PRINCIPLES OF MAGNETIC RESONANCE
SPECTROSCOPY

ANIMAL STUDIES

HUMAN STUDIES
Localization
^{31}P-NMR studies
Clinical studies
Other nuclei

GENERAL CONSIDERATIONS

A major function of the liver is regulation of carbohydrate, lipid, and nitrogen metabolism. Food is absorbed by the intestines and transported to the liver by the portal circulation. Substrates are metabolized and stored in the liver to maintain optimal blood concentrations of glucose and lipids. Ammonia generated in the gastrointestinal tract is converted to urea in the liver by the urea cycle.

Various forms of liver disease are associated with disorders of carbohydrate, fat, and nitrogen metabolism. Therefore the ability to characterize liver metabolism noninvasively is of potential diagnostic value. Magnetic resonance spectroscopy (MRS) provides information about tissue metabolism by measuring concentrations of metabolites. However, to determine the anatomic location from which spectroscopic signals are derived, MRS could be performed in conjunction with MRI. This chapter summarizes the current experience with spectroscopy in animal models of human disease and reviews the clinical experience with hepatic MRS to date.

METABOLIC PATHWAYS DETECTED BY MAGNETIC RESONANCE SPECTROSCOPY

Fig. 55-1 depicts metabolic pathways that can be detected by MRS. Cellular energy in the form of ATP derives from two pathways—glycolysis converts glucose to lactate, generating small amounts of adenosine triphosphate (ATP); aerobically pyruvate and fatty acids are metabolized by the citric acid cycle within mitochondria, producing CO_2. ATP, derived from mitochondrial oxidative phosphorylation, is transported to the cytoplasm where it can be used for cellular work. In the liver, most ATP is used for sodium transport by the enzyme sodium potassium ATPase. In addition, ATP is used in the urea cycle, for biosynthetic reactions including gluconeogenesis, for lipogenesis, and in the synthesis of protein and nucleic acids. In most cases, hydrolysis of ATP produces adenosine 5^l-diphosphate (ADP) and inorganic phosphate (Pi). However, in some synthetic reactions, ATP is hydrolyzed to adenosine monophosphate (AMP) and pyrophosphate. ADP and Pi reenter the mitochondria and are resynthesized to ATP. Alternatively, ATP may be

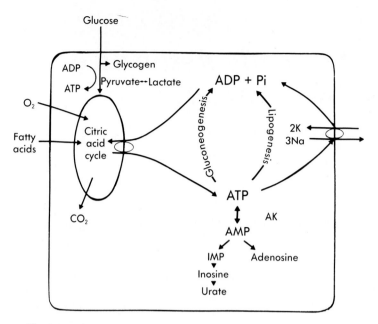

Fig. 55-1 Metabolic pathways in hepatocytes as observed by MRS.

converted to AMP, adenosine, inosine, and ultimately to uric acid. The liver lacks the enzyme creatine kinase, which in muscle and brain generates the storage form of high-energy phosphates, phosphocreatine. Thus no phosphocreatine is present within the liver.

PRINCIPLES OF MAGNETIC RESONANCE SPECTROSCOPY

Nuclear magnetic resonance (NMR) is the property whereby certain nuclei absorb and emit radio frequency (rf) radiation when placed in a magnetic field.[57] To perform MRS, the sample is placed within a magnetic field and pulsed with FM radio waves using a wire rf coil. The wide-frequency band rf pulse excites the nuclei, which subsequently emit a characteristic rf signal that is detected by the coil (antenna). The resonance frequency of a given nucleus is affected by the molecular environment of the nucleus, especially its electrons and those of adjacent atoms. The change, or shift, of the resonance frequency as a consequence of the chemical environment of the nucleus is called the chemical shift. Because every chemically distinct nucleus of a given species is in a different chemical environment, it resonates at a slightly different frequency, resulting in distinct NMR peaks. This property allows the spectroscopist to detect a wide variety of individual chemicals.

MRS may be performed on many nuclei. ^{1}H, ^{31}P and ^{13}C are most frequently used for in vivo MRS. ^{31}P MRS (or ^{31}P NMR) detects various phosphates including ATP and Pi. Inorganic phosphate is a buffer at physiologic pH, and the resonance frequency of Pi can be used to measure pH.[27,28] ^{31}P MRS also detects phospholipid metabolites. The precursors of phospholipid synthesis, such as phosphorylcholine and phosphorylethanolamine, are present in the phosphomonoester (PME) peak. Phosphodiesters, such as phosphatidylcholine and phosphoenolpyruvate are present in the phosphodiester (PDE) peak.

The most abundant carbon nucleus in the body is ^{12}C, but only the ^{13}C nucleus is detectable by MRS, though its natural abundance is only 1.1%. Therefore ^{13}C signals can only be detected from abundant glycogen and fat. However, when ^{13}C-labeled substrates are introduced in the body, their metabolism can be monitored as a function of time.

^{1}H MRS detects water, lipids, and a variety of metabolites with nonexchangeable protons. Under most circumstances, the very large signal from water (concentration about 100 M) obscures signals from protons in other molecules present in smaller concentrations. If lipid signals, for example, originate from lipid in concentrations greater than approximately 20 mM, they can be detected without the use of "water suppression" techniques. However, to detect protons of metabolites (for example, lactate) water suppression techniques must be used to eliminate or markedly reduce the signal from protons in water. These techniques allow observations of lactate and a variety of amino acids.

Fig. 55-2 shows a typical ^{31}P MR spectrum from rat liver as obtained with a surface coil. Each peak represents signals from individual metabolites resonating at different frequencies or "chemical shifts" around the basic spectrometer frequency (in this case 81 MHz for ^{31}P).

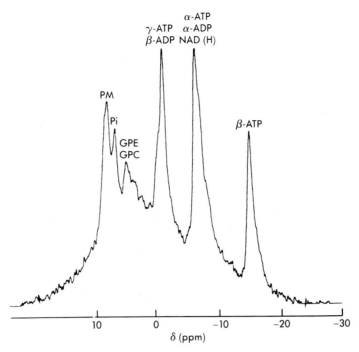

Fig. 55-2 Spectrum recorded at 81 MHz is sum of 1000 data accumulations over 34 minutes. *PM*, phosphomonoesters (mainly phosphocholine with small amounts of phosphorylated monosaccharides, e.g., glycerol-1-phosphate): *GPE*, glycerophosphoethanolamine; *GPC*, glycerophosphocholine.

(Reprinted by permission from Biochemical Journal, 229:141, copyright © 1985, The Biochemical Society, London.)

The chemical shift is given in parts per million (ppm) and is derived from the difference in hertz between the observed signal and a reference signal divided by the absolute resonance frequency of the reference signal in MHz. The area of each peak is roughly proportional to the number of nuclei detected. However, peak intensities are affected by spin-lattice (T_1) and spin-spin (T_2) relaxation of the individual nuclei. Relaxation is a characteristic property of nuclei placed in a magnetic field and irradiated with rf energy. Relaxation effects have to be taken into account if absolute concentrations are derived from MRS spectra.

ANIMAL STUDIES

Animal experiments illustrate the type of diagnostic information that will ultimately be obtained clinically. Cohen[13] reviewed ^{13}C and ^{31}P MRS of liver metabolism in animals.

^{31}P MRS has been used to measure phosphate metabolites in isolated rat liver cells,[21] perfused livers,[14,36,45,59,63] and livers of intact animals.* Several investigators have used the sugar fructose to investigate factors that regulate hepatic metabolism. Fig. 55-3 depicts schematically the effects of fructose on liver me-

tabolism. Fructose is rapidly phosphorylated to fructose-1-phosphate (F-1-P) by the enzyme fructokinase. F-1-P is slowly converted to triosephosphate by aldolase B; thus F-1-P accumulates in liver cells. Because Pi is trapped as F-1-P, cytosolic liver phosphate is depleted and may become rate limiting in respiration. Low intracellular concentration of Pi activates the enzyme AMP deaminase, which depletes ATP and leads to increased levels of inosine and uric acid. These effects have been studied in isolated perfused livers[36] and intact animals,[40] as well as in humans (discussed later). The metabolic consequences of fructose loading suggest that it may be used as a "metabolic stress test" to perturb liver metabolism and monitor metabolic reserve.

^{13}C MRS has been used to study the regulation of metabolic pathways in isolated liver cells[19,22] and perfused rate livers.[14-18,20,22,61] Natural abundance ^{13}C can be used to monitor hepatic glycogen,[3,12] and glycogen depletion induced by glucagon can be rapidly detected.[55a,60b] Glycogen synthesis can be monitored following incorporation of ^{13}C label into glycogen.[2,55a,60a,60b] Stimulation of the fed rat liver by physiologic glucagon levels led to rapid glycogenolysis, which could be detected spectroscopically. The time course of glycogenolysis in perfused rat liver as measured by natural abundance ^{13}C MRS is shown in Fig. 55-4. It clearly demonstrates the possibility

---

*References 23, 30, 31, 34, 37, 39-41, 54, 60.

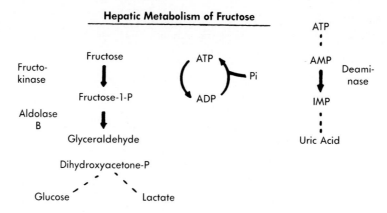

Fig. 55-3 Effects of fructose on liver metabolism. See text for details. P_i, inorganic phosphate; *ATP*, adenosine triphosphate; *IMP*, inosine monophosphate; *AMP*, adenosine monophosphate. (From Oberhaensli, RD, et al: Br J Radiol 59:695, 1986.)

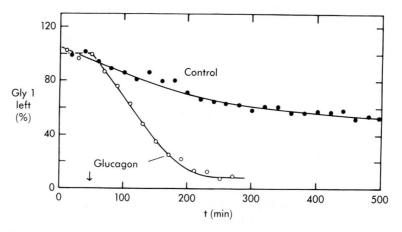

Fig. 55-4 Time course of glycogenolysis in situ from livers of ad lib fed rats perfused in spectrometer. Data are plotted as percent change in area of glycogen C_1 signal. Filled circles are control data taken without addition of 20 nM glucagon to perfusate, and open circles are with addition. (Reprinted with permission from Sillerud, LO, and Shulman, RG: Biochemistry 22:1087. Copyright 1983 American Chemical Society.)

of ^{13}C MRS to monitor glycogen content of the liver in real time. ^{13}C MRS is currently being used for biochemical studies in animal livers but may be ultimately applied to investigation in humans of diabetes and other disorders of carbohydrate metabolism and the effects of various nutritional perturbations.

HUMAN STUDIES
Localization

Clinical MRS of the liver became possible when large-aperture magnets with a field strength of at least 1.5 T became available. To obtain meaningful metabolic information from the liver by MRS, it is important to ensure that NMR signals arise solely from the liver. If the rf detector is simply placed on the body wall over the liver, signals will also be detected from the fat and muscle surrounding the liver. To avoid this "contamination," a

localization technique that acquires signal from a defined volume of interest (VOI) must be used. (For a review of localization techniques see Reference 65.) The first approach to localization used in human liver studies was topical magnetic resonance (TMR)[29] by Radda and co-workers.[48] They used a "field profiling" technique, allowing signal only to be acquired from a homogeneous static magnetic field region, focused on the liver. Fig. 55-5 demonstrates the effect of magnetic field profiling. The upper spectrum was obtained without any localization profile; the lower spectrum was obtained with the TMR technique. This approach provides only signals from the liver (ATP, phosphodiesters, inorganic phosphate, phosphomonoesters) without significant phosphocreatine contamination from surrounding muscle.

Blackledge and co-workers[6] also used the rotating-frame depth selection approach[9] to obtain localized spec-

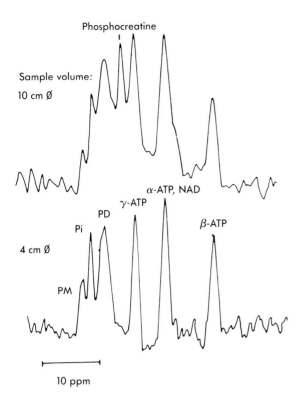

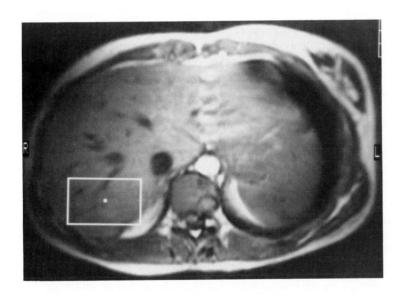

Fig. 55-5 Effect of magnetic field profiling. Radiofrequency coil was positioned on thoracic wall in region of liver. Top panel shows ^{31}P spectrum before magnetic field profiling. Spectrum contains signals from intercostal muscle and liver. Pulse repetition rate 2s^{-1} and 64 scans. Bottom panel shows normal P-31 spectrum of liver after magnetic field profiling. Pulse repetition rate 2s^{-1} and 1024 scans. *PM*, phosphomonoesters (e.g., sugar phosphates); *Pi*, inorganic phosphate; *PD*, phosphodiesters; *ATP*, adenosine triphosphate.
(Reprinted with permission from Oberhaensli, RD, Magn Reson Imaging. 4:413, copyright 1986, Pergamon Press, Inc.)

Fig. 55-6 Proton image (1.5 T) of normal human liver showing typical position of volume of interest used to obtain ^{31}P magnetic resonance spectra.
(From Meyerhoff, DJ, et al: Non-invasive quantitation of human liver metabolites using image-guided ^{31}P magnetic resonance spectroscopy. Submitted for publication.)

tra from human liver. This technique takes advantage of the nonhomogeneous magnetic field produced by a surface coil for spatial localization. However, neither of these techniques used the three-dimensional information provided by MRI for localization. Bottomley[10] introduced the DRESS technique which selectively excites a slice defined from a MRI image and then further defines the VOI by using a surface coil for acquisition. MRI-guided three-dimensional ^{31}P MRS (ISIS)[53] was used by

Meyerhoff and co-workers[46] to obtain localized NMR spectra from human liver. The spatial definition of this method allows the derivation of absolute molar concentrations of hepatic phosphates, assuming uniform distribution of each metabolite throughout the VOI.

^{31}P-NMR Studies

A ^{1}H MRI scan of the liver of a normal subject is shown in Fig. 55-6. The white rectangle indicates the

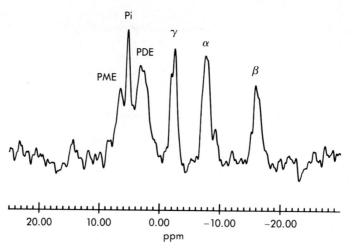

Fig. 55-7 ^{31}P ISIS spectrum (25.89 MHz) of normal human liver. VOI of 150 ml was used. Pulse repetition rate 2s and 256 scans. Processing was convolution difference with line broadening factor of 300 Hz and convolution scaling factor of 0.8; exponential multiplication with line broadening factor was 10 Hz. Peak assignments were *PME*, phosphomonoesters; *Pi*, inorganic phosphate; *PDE*, phosphodiesters; *ATP*, α, β, and δ-phosphate of adenosinetriphosphate.
(From Meyerhoff, DJ, et al: Non-invasive quantitation of human liver metabolites using image-guided ^{31}P magnetic resonance spectroscopy. Submitted for publication.)

position of the VOI in the posterior segment of the right lobe of the liver from which ^{31}P MRS ISIS spectra were typically acquired.[46]

Fig. 55-7 shows a localized liver ^{31}P NMR spectrum obtained using the ISIS technique with a surface coil placed under the normal subject over the right lobe of the liver. The spectrum is a result of data acquisition from a volume of 100 ml of liver tissue in 15 minutes. The Pi signal probably originates from intracellular[21,52] and extracellular Pi.[36] In the human liver, nicotinamide adenine dinucleotide (NAD) resonates at almost the same frequency as α-ATP. Therefore the peak labeled α-ATP has contribution of about 20% NAD.[47] The phosphomonoester (PME) peak is composed of sugar phosphates such as F-1-P and glucose-6-phosphate, as suggested by human biopsy results.[7,8] Phosphorylcholine, AMP, and 3-phosphorylglycerate also contribute to the PME resonance of isolated perfused rat liver.[14] Whether these compounds also contribute to PME resonance in human liver is not known. It is also uncertain whether the same compounds as in rat liver (glycerophosphorylethanolamine, glycerophosphorylcholine and phosphoenolpyruvate[14,21,52]) contribute to the PDE region in human liver spectra. Resonances from ADP are not visible in the spectra, because ADP is present only at low concentrations. In addition, its resonance signal may be extremely broadened[1,26,34,35,37] because of compartmentation in the mitochondria,[52] binding to proteins or both.[13]

Meyerhoff and co-workers[46] measured T_1 relaxation times for phosphorus-containing metabolites in human liver. ^{31}P T_1 relaxation times in rat liver were shown to be independent of static magnetic field strength and most likely obscured by signals from paramagnetic cations that accumulate in the liver (manganese, nickel, cobalt, iron).[25,62] T_1 relaxations obtained for human liver are shorter than those for the corresponding metabolites in human muscle and brain as obtained by Hubesch and co-workers[32] and Roth and co-workers[58] in the same laboratory. This may reflect the great affect of hepatic paramagnetic material on T_1 relaxation. Surprisingly, ATP and PME line widths, which are mainly determined by T_2 relaxation, do not significantly differ from corresponding line widths in muscle and brain.[58] This suggests that the paramagnetic compounds in the liver do not contribute to broadening of ^{31}P MR signals by affecting ^{31}P T_2 relaxation. The broader line widths and irregular shapes observed for the PDE and Pi resonances in spectra of liver compared with those of muscle and brain are probably[46] caused by the contribution of multiple unresolved components such as intracellular and extracellular Pi[6,36] and the various diesters mentioned previously.

Ratios of hepatic ^{31}P metabolite concentrations corrected for T_1 saturation are depicted in Table 55-1. In addition, ratios obtained with a repetition time of 1 second are compared with ratios obtained with the same T_1 saturation by Oberhaensli and co-workers.[48] Both studies showed a PDE/ATP ratio of about 2.5 and a PME/ATP ratio of 0.6 under saturating conditions. The Pi/ATP ratio

☐ **TABLE 55-1**

Ratios of ^{31}P metabolite concentrations in normal human liver (mean ± standard deviation)

| | T₁-corrected* (Meyerhoff and co-workers) | Repetition time = 1 s† | |
		(Meyerhoff and co-workers)	(Oberhaensli and co-workers)
PME/ATP	0.51 ± 0.17	0.62 ± 0.22	0.62 ± 0.27
PDE/ATP	3.13 ± 0.67	2.58 ± 0.58	2.30 ± 0.30
Pi/ATP	1.10 ± 0.45	1.28 ± 0.44	0.92 ± 0.21
PME/PDE	0.16 ± 0.10	0.24 ± 0.18	0.27 ± 0.17

Data from Meyerhoff, DJ: Non-invasive quantitation of human liver metabolites using image-guided ^{31}P magnetic resonance spectroscopy. Submitted for publication; and Oberhaensli, RD: Magn Reson Imaging 4:413, 1986.
*n = 8.
†n = 4.

☐ **TABLE 55-2**

Absolute ^{31}P metabolite concentrations in normal liver in mmol/kg wet weight (mean ± standard deviation)

| | Human liver | | Rat liver* | |
	In vivo†	Freeze-clamping	In vivo	Freeze-clamping
PME	1.05 ± 0.38	<0.3‡	—	—
Pi	2.31 ± 0.60	5.13 ± 1.33§	1.25	5.14 ± 0.29
PDE	6.51 ± 1.41	—	—	—
γ-ATP	2.61 ± 0.59			
α-ATP	2.05 ± 0.30	2.50 ± 0.60‡	3.50 ± 0.19‖	3.50 ± 0.19
β-ATP	1.21 ± 0.13¶			

*Data from Iles, RA, et al: Biochem J 229:141, 1985; values recalculated for 80% tissue water content.
†Data from Meyerhoff, DJ, et al: Non-invasive quantitation of human liver metabolites using image-guided ^{31}P magnetic resonance spectroscopy. Submitted for publication; n = 3; assuming uniform distribution of metabolites over VOI.
‡Data from Hultman, E, Nilsson, LH, and Sahlin, K: Scan J Clin Lab Invest 35:245, 1975; n = 9.
§Data from Bode, JC, et al: Eur J Clin Invest 3:436, 1973.
‖Assumed to be the same as freeze-clamping value.[37]
¶Reduced by chemical-shift-effect.[46]

of 1.1 obtained by Meyerhoff and co-workers using the ISIS localization technique[46] was about 30% higher than reported by Oberhaensli and co-workers.[48]

Almost all human liver ATP in mitochondria and cytosol appears to be visible by MRS,[46] assuming that the freeze-clamping studies of biopsied human liver[37] yielded valid hepatic ATP concentrations without losses caused by hydrolysis. This is in contrast to ATP in rat liver[16] and isolated rat liver mitochondria that produces broad signals because of its compartmentation. In contrast to ATP, the Pi concentration obtained with the ISIS experiment (2.3 mmol/kg wet weight) was less than half the concentration obtained from freeze-clamp studies of human and rat liver. According to Meyerhoff and co-workers[46] and others[37] this is probably because MRS detects free Pi, whereas freeze-clamping extraction tech-

niques yield total Pi, free and bound. (In rat liver, for example, only 25% of Pi is free[37] and detectable by MRS.)

Measurement errors that affect absolute quantitation[46] mainly result from inaccurate integration of overlapping peaks, low signal-to-noise ratio of analyzed spectra, and inaccurate measurements of T₁ relaxation times. Therefore, there is a 25% uncertainty of PME, Pi and PDE concentrations given in Table 55-2. The uncertainty of ATP concentration is about 9%.

Spectroscopic imaging (SI) techniques,[64] using phase encoding pioneered by Maudsley and co-workers[44] and Brown and co-workers,[11] have recently been shown by Young and colleagues[4,24,56,66] to provide spectra from multiple volumes of human liver. Fig. 55-8 shows SI spectra taken from the liver regions marked.

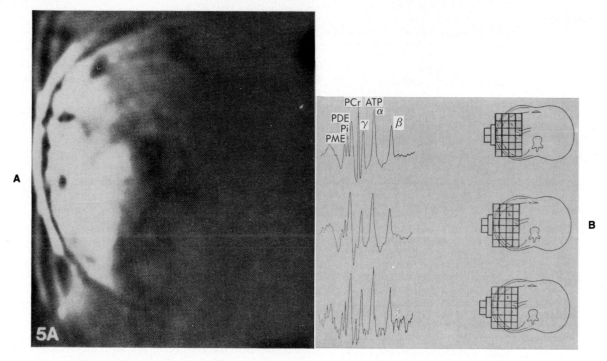

Fig. 55-8 A, Low-resolution (64 × 64 matrix) image of abdomen taken at 68 MHz as one of pair used in producing phase map to help shim and correct three-dimensionally encoded set of spectra. Note substantial motion artifact in image, which is likely also to affect spectra. **B,** Spectra (31 P MRS of normal human liver) taken from regions marked show improvement in resolution as localization is increasingly tightened.
(From Young, IR: Diagn Imag 9:119-131, 1987.)

Clinical Studies

The first investigators to use ^{31}P MRS for clinical studies were Maris and co-workers.[42,43] They placed a surface coil over the liver of a three-month-old infant and obtained ^{31}P NMR spectra in a 26 cm bore magnet. Fig. 55-9 shows six such spectra obtained from an infant with neuroblastoma demonstrating alterations in metabolic content as a function of therapy. Note the presence of phosphocreatine in these spectra. This is a property of the neuroblastoma itself, since cell culture of this tumor shows a similar PCr/ATP value. Because of the large tumor mass, no localization method was used. The time course of the metabolic changes are illustrated in Fig. 55-10 (case 2). Changes in the spectra, especially in the fall of PME/ATP ratio, appeared to be correlated with successful therapeutic intervention. With other cases of infant neuroblastoma[12a] Chance and Northrop showed that ^{31}P MRS was able to predict response to chemotherapy (as expressed in PME/β-ATP ratios) within 24 hours.

The greatest experience using ^{31}P MRS to study the human liver has been reported by Radda and co-workers[55]

and by Oberhaensli and co-workers.[47-51] The spectrum of one patient with longstanding hemochromatosis showed marked decrease of ATP and Pi resonance intensity attributed to T_2 shortening, which results in broadening of peaks.[48] Another patient with glucose-6-phosphatase deficiency was studied after overnight fasting showing an increased PME/β-ATP and PME/PDE ratio. The ratios of Pi/β-ATP, Pi/PDE and β-ATP/PDE were decreased.[55] The authors attributed the increase in sugar phosphates to the accumulation of gluconeogenic intermediates, the result of the block in glucose release.

Intravenous fructose was administered to stress hepatic adenine nucleotide metabolism by Oberhaensli and co-workers.[47] Five minutes following intravenous injection of 250 mg fructose/kg, sugar phosphates increased sevenfold, while Pi and ATP decreased by three or four times. The time course of these metabolic changes followed by ^{31}P MRS is given in Fig. 55-11, together with the results of enzymatic analysis of Pi and fructose levels in blood plasma. Metabolism of sugar phosphates could be followed with a temporal resolution of 5 minutes.

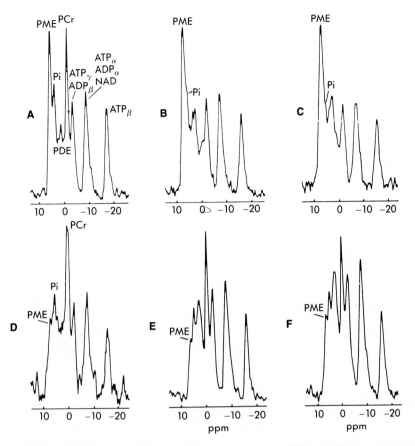

Fig. 55-9 ^{31}P NMR spectra of infant neuroblastoma as function of time. **A** Shows spectrum in first study, **B** and **C** 4 and 8 weeks later, **D** 16 weeks after the initial response to treatment, and **E** and **F** 24 weeks after initial response to treatment at edge of liver *(E)* and anterolateral to edge *(F)*. *PME*, phosphomonoesters; *Pi*, inorganic phosphate: *PDE*, phosphodiesters; *PCr*, phosphocreatine; *ATP*, adenosine triphosphate; *ADP*, adenosine diphosphate, *NAD*, nicotinamide adenine dinucleotide, and *ppm*, parts per million.

(Reprinted, by permission of The New England Journal of Medicine, from Maris, JM, et al: ^{31}P nuclear magnetic resonance spectroscopic investigation of human neuroblastoma in situ, N Engl J Med 312:1500, 1985.)

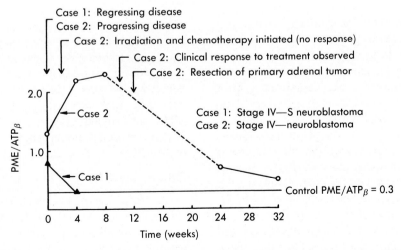

Fig. 55-10 Phosphomonoester/ATP$_\beta$ as function of time. Time course of changes in PME:ATP ratio in cases 1 and 2. Note increase in ratio during tumor progression and decrease during tumor regression. Abbreviations are explained in Fig. 55-9.

(Reprinted, by permission of The New England Journal of Medicine, from Maris, JM, et al: ^{31}P nuclear magnetic resonance spectroscopic investigation of human neuroblastoma in situ, N Engl J Med 312:1500, 1985.)

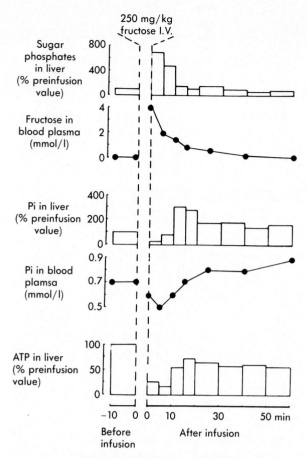

Fig. 55-11 Time course of effects of intravenous fructose load on liver metabolism of healthy subject. Changes in hepatic content of sugar phosphates, inorganic phosphate (Pi) and ATP were followed by ^{31}P MRS. Parallel blood samples were taken for determination of Pi and fructose.
(From Oberhaensli, RD, et al: Br J Radiol 59:695, 1986.)

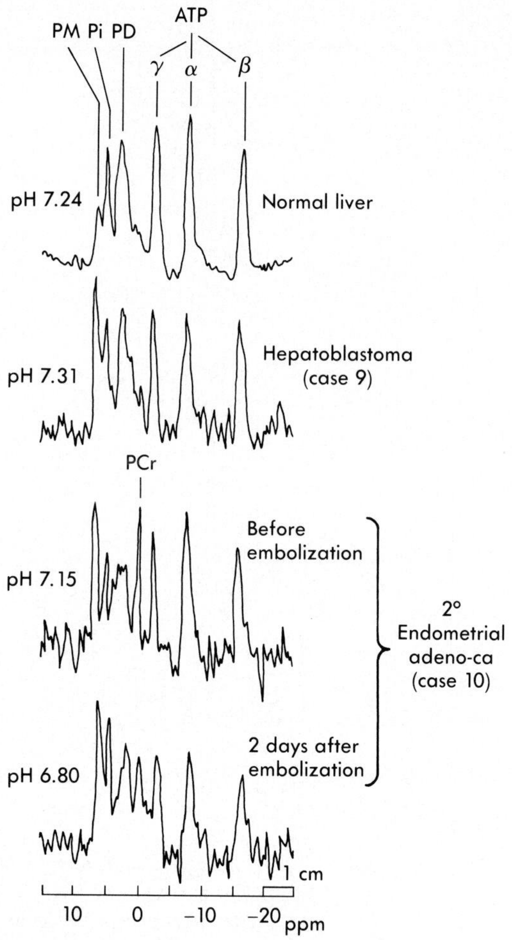

Fig. 55-12 ^{31}P spectra of normal liver and liver tumors.
(From Oberhaensli, RD, et al: Lancet 5:8, 1986.)

Oberhaensli and co-workers[50] have recently reported that individuals who are heterozygous for fructose intolerance also show reversible changes of hepatic phosphates as a result of the fructose ingestion.

The ability to characterize liver lesions using MRS was investigated by Oberhaensli and co-workers[49] who reported spectra from hepatoblastoma and endometrial adenocarcinoma (Fig. 55-12). The pH of these tumors was 7.31 and 7.15, respectively. The adenocarcinoma contained increased phosphocreatine and PME compared to normal controls but relatively little phosphodiester. After embolization this tumor had an increase in the Pi/ATP ratio and a fall of pH from 7.15 to 6.8.

The liver of a patient with Caroli syndrome examined by Ross[56] showed higher amounts of PME throughout the liver but especially around the porta hepatis corresponding to the region of thickened bile ducts. The ap-

plication of spectroscopic imaging as a "multiple-volume" technique facilitated the construction of a phosphorous metabolite map of this patient's entire liver.

Hepatic cirrhosis was recently studied by ^{31}P MRS by Ban and co-workers.[5] They were not able to detect definite differences between spectral patterns in normal adults and cirrhotic patients.

A review of the current state of clinical MRS is given by Ross.[56]

Other Nuclei

Studies of human liver metabolism using ^{13}C MRS have not been undertaken so far, probably because the isotope is not abundant. However, Jue and co-workers[38] recently observed the natural-abundance ^{13}C signal from C-1 glycogen, making possible noninvasive study of glycogen metabolism in humans.

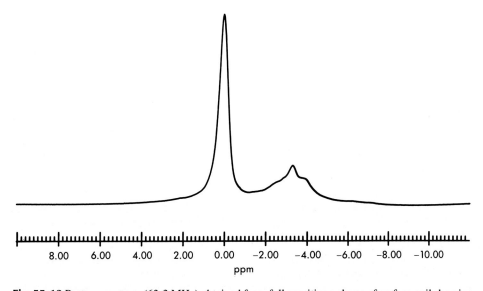

Fig. 55-13 Proton spectrum (63.3 MHz) obtained from full sensitive volume of surface coil showing resonances from water set at 0 ppm and lipids. Lipid peaks are due to $-OCH_{2-}$, $-CH_{2-}$, and $-CH_3$ functions at -2.5, -3.3 and -3.9 ppm, respectively.
(From Meyerhoff, DJ, et al: Non-invasive quantitation of human liver metabolites using image-guided ^{31}P magnetic resonance spectroscopy. Submitted for publication.)

To date, ^{1}H MRS studies on humans are also limited because of the difficulties mentioned previously. Fig. 55-13 shows a typical nonlocalized ^{1}H spectrum with a 9 cm surface coil placed over the liver.[46] Major resonances were from adipose tissue composed of water and three lipid components. The major lipid resonance at -3.3 ppm is that of methylene ($-CH_2-$) groups. Intensity and line shape of the lipid resonances usually vary with the sensitive volume of the surface coil, magnet shimming, and the individual. Localization techniques also have to be employed in the future to get metabolic information from the liver only.

Clinical use of MRS for assessment of liver disease is at a very early stage. However, studies of animal models show that alterations of hepatic metabolism can readily be detected by MRS. Now that MRI and MRS are available for clinical use, it can be expected that MRS will have an increasing role in medical investigation and clinical diagnosis.

REFERENCES

1. Ackerman, JJH, et al: Mapping of metabolites in whole animals by ^{31}P NMR using surface coils, Nature 283:167, 1980.
2. Alger, JR, et al: In vivo carbon-13 nuclear magnetic resonance studies of mammals, Science 214:660, 1981.
3. Alger, JR, et al: Natural-abundance carbon-13 NMR measurement of hepatic glycogen in the living rabbit, J Magn Reson 56:334, 1984.
4. Bailes, DR, et al: Localized phosphorus-31 NMR spectroscopy of normal and pathological human organs in vivo using phase-encoding techniques, J Magn Reson 74:158, 1987.
5. Ban, N, et al: In vivo P-31 MR spectroscopic studies of liver in cirrhotic patients. Presented at the annual meeting of the Society of Magnetic Resonance in Medicine, New York, August 1987.
6. Blackledge, MJ, et al: Measurement of in vivo ^{31}P relaxation rates and spectral editing in human organs using rotating-frame depth selection, J Magn Reson 71:331, 1987.
7. Bode, JC, et al: Depletion of liver adenosine phosphates and metabolic effects of intravenous infusion of fructose or sorbitol in man and in the rat, Eur J Clin Invest 3:436, 1973.
8. Bode, JC, et al: Loss of hepatic adenosine phosphates and metabolic consequences following fructose or sorbitol administration in man and in the rat. In Lundquist, F, and Tygstrup, N, editors: Regulation of hepatic metabolism. Copenhagen, 1974, Munksgaard.
9. Boehmer, JP, Metz, KR, and Briggs, RW: One-dimensional spatial localization of spin-lattice relaxation times using rotating frame imaging, J Magn Reson 62:322-327, 1985.
10. Bottomley, PA: Noninvasive study of high-energy metabolism in human heart by depth-resolved ^{31}P NMR spectroscopy, Science 229:769, 1985.
11. Brown, TR, Kincaid, BM, and Ugurbil, K: NMR chemical shift imaging in three dimensions, Proc Natl Acad Sci USA 79:3252, 1982.
12. Canioni, P, Alger, JR, and Shulman, RG: Natural-abundance carbon-13 nuclear magnetic resonance of liver and adipose tissue of the living rat, Biochemistry 22:4974, 1983.
12a. Chance, B, and Northrup, J: How MR spectroscopy is deployed depends upon intended goal, Diagn Imaging 11:311, 1986.
13. Cohen, SM: Application of nuclear magnetic resonance to the study of liver physiology and disease, Hepatology 3:738, 1983.
14. Cohen, SM: Simultaneous ^{13}C and ^{31}P NMR studies of perfused rat liver: effects of insulin and glucagon and a ^{13}C NMR assay of free Mg^{++}, J Biol Chem 258:14294, 1983.
15. Cohen, SM: Effects of insulin on perfused liver from streptozotocin-diabetic and untreated rats: ^{13}C NMR assay of pyruvate kinase flux, Biochemistry 26:573, 1987.

16. Cohen, SM: ^{13}C and ^{31}P NMR study of gluconeogenesis: ultilization of ^{13}C-labeled substrates by perfused liver from streptozotocin-diabetic and untreated rats, Biochemistry 26:563, 1987.

17. Cohen, SM: ^{13}C and ^{31}P NMR studies of hepatic metabolism in two experimental models of diabetes, Ann NY Acad Sci 508:109, 1987.

18. Cohen, SM, Glynn, P, and Shulman, RG: ^{13}C NMR study of gluconeogenesis from labeled alanine in hepatocytes from euthyroid and hyperthyroid rats, Proc Natl Acad Sci USA 7:60, 1981.

19. Cohen, SM, Ogawa, S, and Shulman, RG: ^{13}C NMR studies of gluconeogenesis in rat liver cells: utilization of labeled glycerol by cells from euthyroid and hyperthyroid rats, Proc Natl Acad Sci USA 76:1603-07.

20. Cohen, SM, Shulman, RG, and McLaughlin, AC: Effects of ethanol on alanine metabolism in perfused mouse liver studied by ^{13}C NMR, Proc Natl Acad Sci USA 76:4808, 1979.

21. Cohen, SM, et al: ^{31}P nuclear magnetic resonance studies of isolated rat liver cells, Nature 273:554, 1978.

22. Cohen, SM, et al: A comparison of ^{13}C nuclear magnetic resonance and ^{14}C tracer studies of hepatic metabolism, J Biol Chem 256:3428, 1981.

23. Cosby, RL, Shapiro, JI, and Chan, L: Phosphorus NMR study of acute biliary obstruction in the rat, Hepatology. Submitted for publication.

24. Cox, IJ, et al: Imaging of phosphorus metabolites of the human liver using phosphorus-31 magnetic resonance spectroscopy. Presented at Conference of the Society of Magnetic Resonance in Medicine, New York, August 1987.

25. Evelhoch, JL, et al: ^{31}P spin-lattice relaxation times and resonance linewidths of rat tissue in vivo: dependence upon the static magnetic field strength, Magn Reson Med 2:410, 1985.

26. Freeman, DS, et al: Energetics of sodium transport in the kidney: saturation transfer ^{31}P-NMR, Biochem Biophys Acta 762:325, 1983.

27. Gadian, DG, et al: pH measurements of cardiac and skeletal muscle using ^{31}P-NMR. In Liss, AR, editor: Intracellular pH: its measurement, regulation, and utilization in cellular functions, New York, 1982, Academic Press.

28. Gillies, RJ, et al: Intracellular pH measured by NMR: methods and results. In Liss, AR, editor: Intracellular pH: its measurement, regulation, and utilization in cellular functions, New York, 1982, Academic Press.

29. Gordon, RE, Hanley, PE, and Shaw, D: Topical magnetic resonance, Prog NMR Spec 15:1, 1982.

30. Gordon, RE, et al: Localization of metabolites in animals using P-31 topical magnetic resonance. Nature 287:736, 1980.

31. Helzberg, JH, et al: Metabolic state of the rat liver with ethanol: comparison of in vivo ^{31}Phosphorus nuclear magnetic resonance spectroscopy with freeze clamp assessment, Hepatology 7:83, 1987.

32. Hubesch, B, et al: Quantitation of metabolites in human organs from ^{31}P NMR spectra obtained with surface coils. Presented at conference of the Society of Magnetic Resonance in Medicine, New York, 1987.

33. Hultman, E, Nilsson, LH, and Sahlin, K: Adenine nucleotide content of human liver: normal values and fructose-induced depletion, Scand J Clin Lab Invest 35:245, 1975.

34. Iles, RA, and Griffiths, JR: Hepatic metabolism by ^{31}P NMR, Biosci Rep 2:735, 1982.

35. Iles, RA, Stevens, AN, and Griffiths, JR: NMR studies of metabolites in living tissue, Prog NMR Spectrosc 15:49, 1982.

36. Iles, RA, et al: Effects of fructose on the energy metabolism and acid-base status of the perfused starved-rat liver, Biochem J 192:191, 1980.

37. Iles, RA, et al: Phosphorylation status of liver by ^{31}P-NMR spectroscopy, and its implications for metabolic control, Biochem J 229:141, 1985.

38. Jue, T, et al: Natural abundance ^{13}C NMR spectrum of glycogen in humans, Magn Reson Med 5:377, 1987.

39. Karczmar, GS, and Weiner, MW: ^{31}P NMR saturation transfer in vivo. Submitted for publication.

40. Karczmar, GS, et al: Hepatic fructose metabolism studied in vivo using ^{31}P NMR, in preparation.

41. Koretsky, AP, et al: ^{31}P NMR spectroscopy of rat organs, in situ, using chronically implanted radiofrequency coils, Proc Natl Acad Sci USA 80:7491, 1983.

42. Maris, JM, et al: Analysis of the metabolism of lipid precursors in human neuroblastome by ^{31}P NMR spectroscopy. In Allen, PS, Boisvert, DPJ, Lentle, BC: Magnetic Resonance in Cancer: proceedings of the International Conference on Magnetic Resonance in Cancer, Banff, Canada, Elmsford, NY, 1985, Pergamon Press.

43. Maris, JM, et al: ^{31}P nuclear magnetic resonance spectroscopic investigation of human neuroblastoma in situ, N Engl J Med 312:1500, 1985.

44. Maudsley, AA, et al: Spatially resolved high resolution spectroscopy by "four-dimensional" NMR, J Magn Reson 51:147, 1983.

45. McLaughlin, AC, Takeda, H, and Chance, B: Rapid ATP assays in perfused mouse liver by 31P NMR, Proc Natl Acad Sci USA 76:5445, 1979.

46. Meyerhoff, DJ, et al: Non-invasive quantitation of human liver metabolites using image-guided ^{31}P magnetic resonance spectroscopy. Submitted for publication.

47. Oberhaensli, RD, et al: Assessment of human liver metabolism by phosphorus-31 magnetic resonance spectroscopy, Br J Radiol 59(703):695, 1986.

48. Oberhaensli, RD, et al: First year of experience with P-31 magnetic resonance studies of human liver, Magn Reson Imaging 4:413, 1986.

49. Oberhaensli, RD, et al: Biochemical investigation of human tumours in vivo with phosphorus-31 magnetic resonance spectroscopy, Lancet 5:8, 1986.

50. Oberhaensli, RD, et al: Study of hereditary fructose intolerance by use of ^{31}P magnetic resonance spectroscopy, Lancet 24:931, 1987.

51. Oberhaensli, RD, et al: The study of human organs by phosphorus-31 topical magnetic resonance spectroscopy, Br J Radiol 60:367, 1987.

52. Ogawa, S, et al: High-resolution ^{31}P nuclear magnetic resonance study of rat liver mitochondria, Proc Natl Acad Sci USA 75:1796, 1978.

53. Ordidge, RJ, Connelly, A, Lohman, JAB: Image-selected in vivo spectroscopy (ISIS): a new technique for spatially selective NMR spectroscopy, J Magn Reson 66:283, 1986.

54. Quistorff, B, Engkagul, A, and Chance, B: 31P-NMR in the study of liver metabolism in vivo, Pharmacol Biochem Behav 18:241, 1983.

55. Radda, G, Oberhaensli, RD, and Taylor, DJ: The biochemistry of human diseases as studied by ^{31}P NMR in man and animal models, Ann NY Acad Sci. (Submitted for publication.)

55a. Reo, NV, Siegfried, BA, and Ackerman, JJH: Direct observation of glycogenesis and glucagon-stimulated glycogenolysis in the rat liver in vivo by high-field carbon-13 surface coil NMR, J Biol Chem 259:13664, 1984.

56. Ross, BD: The current state of clinical magnetic resonance spectroscopy with phosphorus-31: a view from Hammersmith, Magn Reson Med Biol 1:81, 1988.

57. Roth, K: NMR-tomography and -spectroscopy in medicine: an introduction, Berlin, 1984, Springer-Verlag.

58. Roth, K, et al: Non-invasive quantitation of phosphorous metabolites in human tissue by NMR spectroscopy, J Magn Reson. In press.

59. Salhany, JM, et al: ^{31}P-nuclear magnetic resonance of metabolic changes associated with cyanide intoxication in the perfused rat liver, Biochem Biophys Res Commun 86:1077, 1979.

60. Schmidt, HC, et al: Comparison of in vivo ^{31}P-NMR spectra of the brain, liver, and kidney of adult and infant animals, Pediat Radiol 16:144, 1986.

60a. Shalwitz, RA, et al: Visibility of mammalian hepatic glycogen to the NMR experiment, in vivo, Magn Reson Med 5:462, 1987.

60b. Siegfried, BA, et al: Effects of hormone and glucose administration on hepatic glucose and glycogen metabolism in vivo: a ^{13}C NMR study, J Biol Chem 260:16137, 1985.

61. Sillerud, LO, and Shulman, RG: Structure and metabolism of mammalian liver glycogen monitored by carbon-13 nuclear magnetic resonance, Biochemistry 22:1087, 1983.

62. Thiers, RE, and Vallee, BT: Distribution of metals in subcellular fractions of rat liver, J Biol Chem 226:911, 1957.

63. Thoma, WJ, and Ugurbil, K: Saturation-transfer studies of ATP-P_i exchange in isolated perfused rat liver, Biochim Biophys Acta 893:225, 1987.

64. Twieg, D, et al: ^{31}P Spectroscopic imaging of human organs. Manuscript in preparation.

65. Weiner, MW: The promise of magnetic resonance spectroscopy for medical diagnosis, Invest Radiol 23:253, 1988.

66. Young, IR: Phase-dependent techniques offer new direction in MRI, Diagn Imag 9:119, 1987.

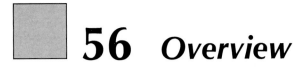

56 *Overview*

H. JOACHIM BURHENNE

GENERAL CONSIDERATIONS

Radiology of the liver and biliary tract has made further strides in the past decade. No other anatomic region has benefited more from technical and imaging innovations. The addition of ultrasound and computed tomography (CT) has changed the diagnostic approach to almost all pathologic conditions in the liver and biliary tract. These new biliary imaging modalities have resulted in a decrease in more conventional radiographic techniques such as oral cholecystography and have almost completely eliminated intravenous cholangiography.

Radiologists have taken great care to sort out the advantages and shortfalls of different imaging techniques, reassessing indications for transhepatic and endoscopic retrograde cholangiography (ERC) and comparing interventional radiologic therapy to surgical therapy. In designing algorithmic flow charts, radiologists have considered the sensitivity and specificity of various diagnostic techniques, identified their place in the diagnosis of biliary tract disease, and taken into account the availability and difficulty of these imaging procedures, including the cost of health care.[73] Studies of the cost efficiency of the ever-increasing armamentarium of biliary imaging procedures have been accepted as the radiologist's responsibility. This cost factor undoubtedly will become more important in future investigations, particularly now that magnetic resonance imaging (MRI) has become more widely available.

In the discussion of effective algorithms for various biliary abnormalities, many presume that all new techniques are available in the institution. Often this may not be the case, and available equipment then alone determines what pathways to follow to determine the diagnosis. Experience and expertise in nuclear medicine, endoscopic retrograde cholangiopancreatography (ERCP), and CT and ultrasound are usually not at the same levels in the institution. In the definitive diagnosis of jaundice, for instance, the least expensive and most widely available technique is percutaneous cholangiography. This procedure certainly requires the least amount of additional equipment for small institutions, and the associated risk is low.

In the detection and differentiation of focal hepatic masses, the choice of the initial imaging procedure and the advantages of different modalities to identify different disease entities in the liver is ongoing between ultrasound, CT, and MRI. Scanning with multiple techniques has significant cost implications, and it is hoped that future randomized studies will bring new answers and clarity.

CHOLELITHIASIS

The Graham-Cole test has been the time-honored radiologic approach for the diagnosis of gallstones for more than 50 years. This test demonstrates the number, size, and position of stones in the gallbladder. Additional radiographs can determine if gallstones are floating within contrast and if the gallbladder is able to contract. For the diagnosis of cholecystolithiasis, however, all that is required is to identify the presence or absence of stones in the gallbladder. This answer can be obtained just as accurately and with far greater ease through the use of ultrasonography, particularly high-resolution, real-time ultrasonography. Using this technique, the radiologist can examine the gallbladder and related anatomy thoroughly in less than 5 minutes. Real-time is easier to learn and perform than gray scale ultrasonography.

We believe that real-time ultrasonography is the diagnostic technique of choice for calculous gallbladder disease.[14] Compared to oral cholecystography in terms of technicians' time, room use, and use of film and contrast material, real-time ultrasonography is considerably less expensive.

With the developing techniques of cholelitholysis and cholelithotripsy, information about the size and number of stones is required to determine if patients are eligible for nonsurgical therapy. Real-time ultrasonography is

most accurate for identification of stone size but is less helpful in identifying the number of stones, particularly if multiple stones are present. Oral cholecystography is therefore required at present for patient selection if chemical stone dissolution or lithotripsy is contemplated.

If ultrasonography has negative results in patients suspected clinically of cholecystolithiasis, oral cholecystography may be used as a second approach. Previously reported low figures for gallbladder visualization with this technique and second-dose cholecystography can be avoided in both outpatients[8] and inpatients[9] with the technique of single-visit oral cholecystography. Preliminary plain film radiography routinely performed with oral cholecystography carries an unacceptably low diagnostic yield.[2]

In expert hands and with state-of-the-art ultrasound equipment, even gallbladder pathologic conditions such as tumor or adenomyomatosis can be detected (Fig. 56-1).

CHOLECYSTITIS

Sonography has also an important role in the evaluation of patients suspected of having acute cholecystitis.[4,45,66] The demonstration of gallstones supports this diagnosis, but patients carrying silent gallstones may have clinical signs and symptoms caused by another pathologic condition in the right upper quadrant. The same is true of other indirect sonographic signs of cholecystitis, such as thickening of the gallbladder wall and the sonographic Murphy's sign. Tenderness in the region of the gallbladder fossa may be caused by hepatitis, pyelonephritis, pancreatitis, or other abnormalities.[59]

The presence of sonographically detected gallbladder

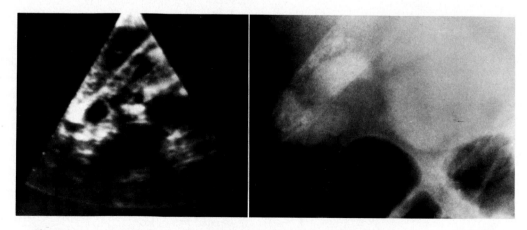

Fig. 56-1 Adenomyomatosis of gallbladder as seen on ultrasonography and subsequent oral cholecystography. Contracted area of gallbladder body with thickening of wall and with presence of Rokitansky-Aschoff sinuses are demonstrated with both imaging techniques.

wall thickening is suggestive of but not pathognomonic for acute cholecystitis. One investigator found that 87% of normal patients had a wall thickness of 5 mm or less, whereas only 45% of patients with acute cholecystitis had gallbladder walls thicker than 5 mm.[58] The gallbladder wall may be thicker than 5 mm in patients with chronic cholecystitis or a history of ascites or alcoholism. Caution is urged in making the diagnosis of cholecystitis on the basis of wall thickening alone.[60] Hypoalbuminemic patients also show a significantly thickened gallbladder wall in comparison with volunteers.[52] Wall thickening is also a major sonographic finding in patients affected with acquired immunodeficiency syndrome (AIDS) of the gallbladder.[54] Ultrasonic evaluation typically is used as the initial modality to evaluate patients with suspected acute cholecystitis, even though other causes are more common in patients with acute right upper quadrant pain.[37]

Persistent dense visualization 36 hours after oral cholecystography in an otherwise normal-appearing gallbladder is not diagnostic of acute cholecystitis.[3]

A specific radiologic diagnosis of acute cholecystitis is obtained by the demonstration of cystic duct obstruction. Nuclear medicine studies are the method of choice today for this diagnosis (Fig. 56-2). If the extrahepatic ducts are visualized but not the gallbladder, acute cholecystitis is the diagnosis of choice. Cholescintigraphy with ^{99m}Tc-labeled iminidiacetic acid (IDA) derivatives has proved to be extremely reliable in the evaluation of suspected acute cholecystitis.[72] The length of the examination can be shortened by the use of radionuclide angiography.[13] Frequent false-positive studies with the use of hepatobiliary scintigraphy[45] can be decreased with the intravenous injection of morphine if the gallbladder is not demonstrated within 40 minutes.[12] A rim of increased activity adjacent to the gallbladder fossa suggests the presence of acute gangrenous cholecystitis.[6]

If nuclear medicine cholecystoscintigraphy is not available in the medical setting, intravenous cholangiography remains the conventional method of choice for identifying cystic duct obstruction in cases of cholecystitis. Intravenous cholangiography, however, has never been a designated method for the diagnosis of gallbladder stones.[30]

Total body opacification has been considered a diagnostic sign of obstructive cholecystography. The opacification of the gallbladder wall depends on inflammatory hypervascularity, and thus the diagnosis of acute cholecystitis cannot be rendered if the gallbladder wall is gangrenous. The diagnosis of emphysematous cholecystitis can readily be made with plain film radiography and has also been described with CT.[51] An 11% concomitant common duct calculi rate in cases of cholecystitis has been demonstrated,[50] indicating clearly that routine operative cholangiography is recommended in all patients undergoing surgery for acute cholecystitis.[35]

The diagnostic accuracy of cholecystokinin cholecystography has not been confirmed in patients with acalculous biliary tract disease. Patients with abnormal test results undergoing surgery usually show histologic evi-

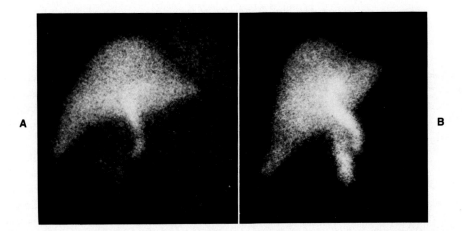

Fig. 56-2 Transient common bile duct obstruction demonstrated. **A,** by hepatobiliary imaging 30 minutes after ^{99m}Tc–diethyl-IDA. Stasis in hepatic and upper common duct and no progression into duodenum. Nonvisualization of gallbladder indicates cystic duct obstruction. Total serum bilirubin level was 5.1. One week later, following relief of right upper quadrant pain and return of serum bilirubin to normal, comparable 30-minute image, **B,** shows normal progression of bile activity from common duct into duodenum, but again there is no visualization of gallbladder.
(Courtesy Dr. J.G. McAfee.)

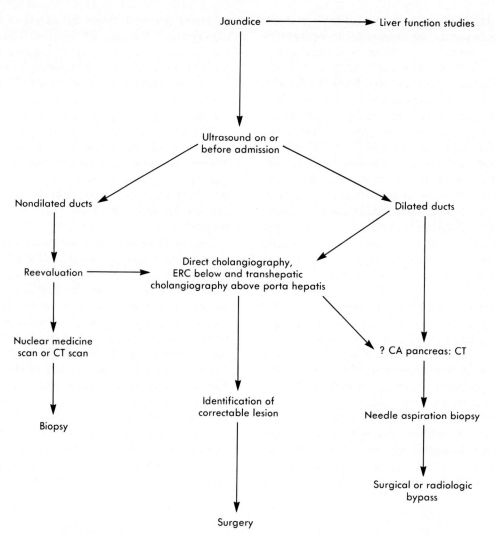

Fig. 56-3 Algorithm for jaundice.

dence of chronic cholecystitis.[32] This finding carried little significance, however, because gallbladder walls with a chronic infiltrate are typically present in older patients.

The role of MRI in the diagnosis of cholecystitis is as yet undetermined, and more experience is required.[43]

JAUNDICE

Extrahepatic ductal dilatation is the earliest change occurring with biliary obstruction. Dilatation precedes elevation of the serum bilirubin level.[79] The radiologic diagnosis of extrahepatic bile duct distention therefore can be obtained before the clinical onset of jaundice. The early diagnosis of jaundice is clearly in the domain of the radiologist (Fig. 56-3).

Ultrasonography is the accepted first imaging modality in cases of biliary obstruction and jaundice.[29] Its sensi-

tivity for detecting distention of the common hepatic duct is as high as any other test, and the technique is noninvasive and widely available. An ultrasonic measurement of 4 mm is considered normal for the common hepatic duct.[15]

The accuracy of ultrasound in the detection of distended intrahepatic ducts is equal to that of CT, but this technique is not as sensitive for detecting common hepatic duct distention. One must remember that jaundice can be present in the absence of distended intrahepatic biliary ducts. When gas within the biliary tree prevents evaluation by ultrasound, biliary IDA scans are useful in a patient following biliary-enteric anastomosis.

Although the sensitivity of ultrasonography for detecting hepatic bile duct distention is high, visualization of the distal common duct may be more difficult to

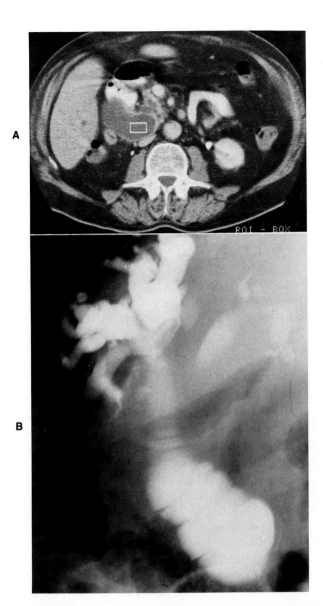

Fig. 56-4 A, Very large distal common duct is demonstrated in region of head of pancreas *(marker)* with carcinoma of pancreas. **B,** Subsequent transhepatic cholangiography demonstrates extensive dilatation of biliary tract with "rat tail" at distal end, consistent with carcinoma of pancreas.

achieve because of overlying gas in the duodenum. Whereas ultrasound is not very sensitive for the detection of common duct stones, it is of great diagnostic help if a pancreatic mass is demonstrated. With improvement in ultrasound equipment and technique, the detection rate of choledocholithiasis by ultrasonography is now 45% to 55%.[16,47] Direct cholangiography must follow ultrasonography for the definitive diagnosis of choledocholithiasis.

An early differentiation between hepatocellular and obstructive jaundice greatly influences good patient care. The prompt surgical relief of a bile duct obstruction prevents further hepatocellular damage and lowers the operative risk of complications such as superimposed cholangitis. Thus ultrasonographic evaluation is best performed in jaundiced patients on or before admission.

CT is the initial imaging procedure for identifying distended intrahepatic bile ducts if state-of-the-art ultrasound equipment is not available. CT is most specific in determining the cause of obstruction in suprapancreatic neoplasm.[53] Distention of intrahepatic bile ducts can also be evaluated with MRI.[20]

The next diagnostic procedure in the evaluation of the jaundiced patient after ultrasonography should be direct cholangiography. This technical sequence is indicated even if the initial imaging procedure shows no distended bile ducts in patients suspected of having a biliary duct obstruction and even if the level of the obstruction has been identified by ultrasound.[38] The choice between transhepatic cholangiography and ERC depends on the expertise available. Most institutions use transhepatic cholangiography for intrahepatic lesions and lesions at the portal fissure (porta hepatis). Transhepatic cholangiography is also added if ERC is inconclusive or demonstrates only the distal extent of the lesion. A 76% diagnostic accuracy rate with percutaneous cholangiography was reported already in 1965 before the more widespread use of a finer and more flexible needle.[21] Recent reports indicate that successful examinations can be obtained in 99% of cases with dilated intrahepatic ducts and in 85% if the bile ducts are normal (Fig. 56-4). This high rate of success in nondilated systems can be attributed to the number of passes; it is not unusual to make as many as 15 passes to opacify a nondilated biliary system.[11]

There is no significant change in the internal diameter of the common hepatic duct in normal subjects in response to an intravenous dose of a cholecystogogue.[22] An increase in caliber of a normal or slightly dilated common duct after a fatty meal, however, is a strong indicator of biliary obstruction, whereas a decrease in caliber virtually excludes obstruction.[76]

Cholescintigraphy is useful in the evaluation of postoperative patients.[71] The common bile duct in postcholecystectomy patients may remain dilated, which may be misleading with other imaging modalities. Cholescintigraphy, however, presents functional evaluation to demonstrate the patency of the duct. The patency of a biliary-enteric bypass can be demonstrated with the same nuclear medicine approach.

Intravenous cholangiography is of no diagnostic help if jaundice is present. Although this technique is only

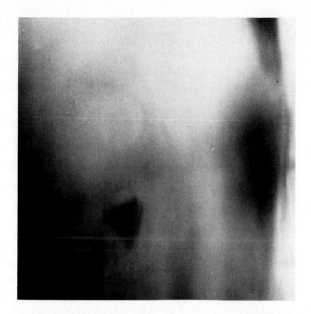

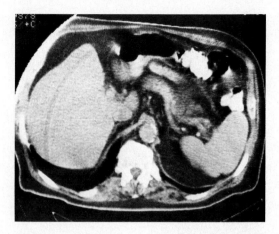

Fig. 56-6 Congenital absence of lateral segment of left lobe of liver is well demonstrated with CT. This was called a mass lesion on nuclear medicine scan.

Fig. 56-5 Large gallstone impacted in neck of gallbladder deviating common hepatic duct in patient with intermittent jaundice. Only tomographic studies of intravenous cholangiograms demonstrated surgically confirmed abnormality, the so-called Mirizzi syndrome.

rarely performed in North America today, intravenous cholangiography is reported to give excellent results in several European centers where it still is in common use (Fig. 56-5).[1,31,40]

TRAUMA

Liver injury is less common than splenic laceration, but it carries a higher mortality. Plain film radiography should not be neglected because about one half of these patients have associated rib fractures.[28] CT and arteriography are the methods of choice for detecting subcapsular hematomas. Serial abdominal CT studies have become an integral part of conservative treatment of blunt hepatic injuries and are useful in monitoring resorption of hemoperitoneum and the pattern of healing of intrahepatic hematomas, lacerations, and fractures.[23]

Hepatobiliary scintigraphy imaging has been successful in detecting gallbladder perforation, fractured liver, and fluid leakage following blunt abdominal trauma.[44] In comparison to other imaging techniques, nuclear medicine studies are able to detect liver injury if the collection represents an active bile leak. Radiation injuries to the liver are detectable with CT.[36] Arteriography can demonstrate arteriovenous fistulas or active bleeding. Even injuries deep within the hepatic parenchyma are demonstrated with this technique.

LOCALIZED IMAGING DEFECTS

New and improved imaging modalities are changing the approach to screening for focal hepatic lesions. Radionuclide scans are no longer considered as the initial approach because of rapid further development of new and improved CT techniques (Fig. 56-6). These involve the incremental bolus dynamic scan,[27] CT arteriography,[25,42] and delayed iodine scanning.[5] An even more recent report on hepatic metastasis detection by MRI, on the other hand, suggests increased overall accuracy in detection of focal hepatic lesions by MRI when compared to contrast-enhanced CT.[63] Plain films are still indicated for the differentiation of liver abscess (Fig. 56-7).

The most common benign liver tumors represent hemangiomas, and the most common malignant focal lesions are metastases. Differentiation of these lesions therefore serves as a good example of our present approach to the radiologic detection of focal lesions in the liver.

Benign lesions

Hemangiomas are the most common benign hepatic tumor and have been found at autopsy at a rate of 4% to 6%,[26] although other studies suggest a worldwide incidence as high as 15%.[62] Most lesions are silent and are discovered incidentally on abdominal sonography, CT scanning, or nuclear scintigraphy. Technetium-99m red blood cell (RBC) scanning, angiography, CT, or MRI may then be required. The diagnosis of hemangioma, however, can be only confirmed in approximately 55% of patients with dynamic bolus CT.[26] MRI has been described as quite accurate for the diagnosis of hepatic hemangioma,[62] but RBC scintigraphy is probably as ac-

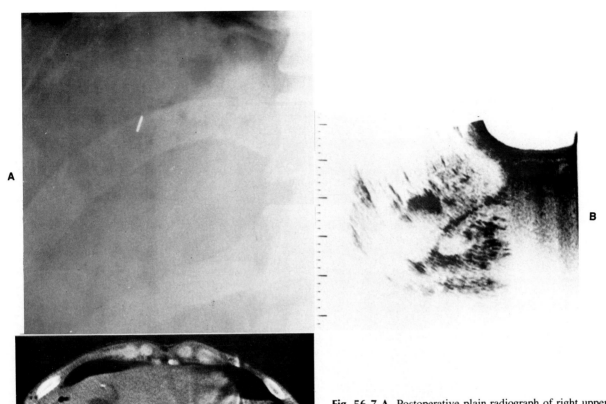

Fig. 56-7 A, Postoperative plain radiograph of right upper quadrant after surgery shows presence of air in liver. **B,** Ultrasonography demonstrates fluid collection with air-filled level. **C,** CT again shows air and also pyogenic postoperative liver abscess.

curate and certainly more cost effective. If inconclusive, hepatic angiography remains the best technique,[24] and fine-needle aspiration may provide cytologic diagnosis.[61]

This multimodality imaging approach to the diagnosis of hemangiomas exemplifies our predicament for cost containment, particularly since hemangiomas may overlap in their imaging appearance with hepatic neoplasms. We limit ourselves to ultrasonography followed by scintigraphy and interval follow-up in most cases. The search for a specific imaging technique continues.

Malignant lesions

Liver metastases are present in 41% of all malignancies, and the frequency of spread to the liver is superseded only by that to lymph nodes. Patients suspected of primary or metastatic hepatic neoplasms must be imaged

preoperatively. Again, patients often undergo a sequence of imaging procedures with ultrasonography, nuclear medicine studies, CT, angiography, and MRI.[41] A more cost-effective approach appears in a recent report of randomized control comparison for the detection of hepatic metastases with CT versus MRI.[63] The report claims a higher sensitivity for the detection of metastases and a slightly higher overall accuracy with MRI. The ongoing debate, however, is demonstrated by a 1988 publication concluding that CT results in a higher detection rate for focal hepatic lesions than MRI.[46] Further studies with comparable state-of-the-art technology are needed to compare ultrasound, CT, and MRI.[17] It is hoped that a single imaging technique can be suggested in the future for a more economic diagnostic approach. At present, most institutions such as ours use ultrasonography fol-

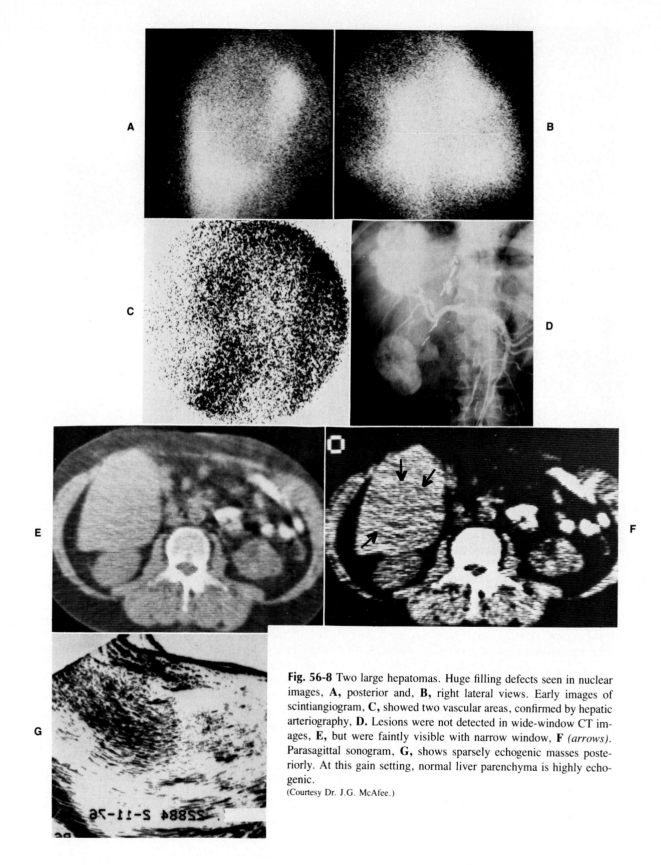

Fig. 56-8 Two large hepatomas. Huge filling defects seen in nuclear images, **A,** posterior and, **B,** right lateral views. Early images of scintiangiogram, **C,** showed two vascular areas, confirmed by hepatic arteriography, **D.** Lesions were not detected in wide-window CT images, **E,** but were faintly visible with narrow window, **F** *(arrows).* Parasagittal sonogram, **G,** shows sparsely echogenic masses posteriorly. At this gain setting, normal liver parenchyma is highly echogenic.
(Courtesy Dr. J.G. McAfee.)

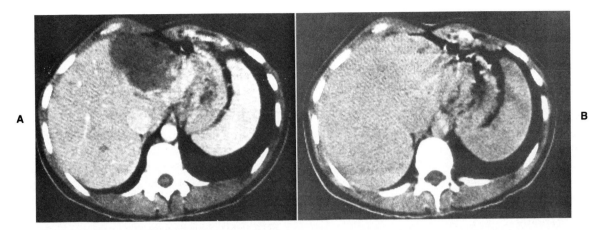

Fig. 56-9 Large focal mass in left lobe of liver shown on CT, **A,** before disappearing after contrast injection, **B.** Specific diagnosis by CT avoids risk of liver biopsy with possible complication of hemorrhage.

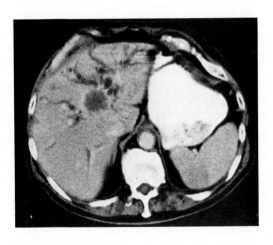

Fig. 56-10 Obstructing cholangiocellular carcinoma with dilatation of bile ducts in liver but not of extrahepatic ducts, as shown on CT after contrast injection.

lowed by dynamic contrast CT scanning for the evaluation of focal liver lesions (Figs. 56-8, 56-9, and 56-10).

Another significant advance has been fine-needle aspiration biopsy, which is now well established as a method for diagnosing malignant disease. The sensitivity of the technique has been given as 77.5% for pancreatic tumors and 60% for biliary malignancy.[33]

NEWLY DEVELOPING FIELDS

Radiologists must familiarize themselves not only with new technical developments affecting imaging of the liver and biliary tree, but also with new areas of therapy for lesions in the liver and biliary tract requiring radiologic support.

Liver transplants

Rejection is the leading cause of liver allograft dysfunction. Rejection is usually detected by liver biopsy,

but good correlation between angiographic findings and histologic evidence of rejection has been demonstrated. Angiography, however, is not advocated at this time as a test for transplant rejection.[68,74] The periportal collar sign on CT of the allograft is helpful in the early diagnosis and confirmation of rejection.[69] CT also provides data on the hepatic parenchyma, vasculature, and biliary system and identifies the presence of intraabdominal fluid.[39]

Starzl performed the first human liver transplant in 1963. His group has demonstrated that radiographic assessment of the biliary tract is often essential in patients who have undergone liver transplantation. Complications diagnosed by cholangiography include obstruction, bile leaks, and problems with tube drainage that sometimes require transhepatic biliary drainage or balloon catheter dilatation of strictures to restore drainage tube patency.[77] Bile sludge formation may also be a problem. Familiarity with the postoperative appearance of the common bile duct anastomosis and its complications is necessary for proper assessment of transplant patients.[48] Preoperative information on anatomic variants of the hepatic arteries and detailed analysis of the sectional anatomy of the porta hepatis and the hepatoduodenal ligament are readily obtained by radiographic techniques in the preoperative patient.[56,70] Because the hepatic artery provides the only blood supply to the biliary tree of the liver allograft, posttransplantation arterial occlusion will result in a complication. Liver transplant recipients who exhibit nonanastomotic contrast leakage or nonanastomotic strictures on cholangiography should be evaluated for occlusion of the hepatic artery as the probable cause.[78]

Duplex scanning

Duplex Doppler techniques have been used for the qualitative assessment of splanchnic venous hemodynamics in patients with portal hypertension. The direction of blood flow in splenic, superior mesenteric, portal and intrahepatic portal, and portasystemic collaterals can be assessed.[49] MRI cannot be used to grade the blood flow in the portal vein but accurately detects portable vein thrombosis and the patency of surgical shunts.[65] Duplex sonography is also a valuable portable technique for evaluating patients before and after liver transplants and can be used with patients requiring angiography.[64] In one study MRI of portal venous thrombosis demonstrated a slight increase in sensitivity when compared to CT and sonography.[80]

Biliary lithotripsy

Extracorporeal shock wave lithotripsy shows promise for the treatment of cholelithiasis in selected cases as an alternative to surgery, endoscopic or radiologic intervention, and chemolitholysis.[7,67] Stone fragmentation with cholelithotripsy is only the first step of therapy, whereas fragment passage into the intestinal tract is the realistic endpoint of successful gallstone treatment. Fragment passage requires more time than after lithotripsy with renal stones. Ninety percent of fragments are shown to clear from the biliary tract after gallbladder stone fragmentation within 12 to 18 months for a 90% success rate.[57]

The experience with choledocholithotripsy is more encouraging. Interventional access to the biliary tract is available either transhepatically, endoscopically, by way of a T-tube tract or cholecystostomy. As opposed to fragment passage after cholecystolithotripsy, stone fragments will readily pass through a sphincterotomy or may be amenable for fragment clearing by basket extraction.[10]

The patient selection for shock wave therapy of gallbladder stones is therefore different than for common duct stones. Adjuvant chemolitholysis is probably required for cholecystolithotripsy. Efficient lithotripsy equipment should have both ultrasonography and fluo-

roscopy for stone targeting. The imaging aspects of extracorporeal shock wave lithotripsy are the difficult part of the procedure and are best accomplished under the radiologist's direction.

Magnetic resonance imaging

Although MRI of the liver and biliary tract is in its beginnings, this new modality already shows great promise for the detection of hepatic metastases and other focal lesions.[17,63] More randomized studies with comparable equipment are required to evaluate whether contrast-enhanced CT or MRI is the imaging procedure of choice for these lesions.

MRI is also being compared to other radiologic modalities in the investigation of gallbladder carcinoma,[55,75] cholangiocarcinoma,[19] and gallbladder physiology.[18,34]

REFERENCES

1. Alinder, G, et al: Pre-operative infusion cholangiography compared to routine operative cholangiography at elective cholecystectomy, Br J Surg 73:383, 1986.
2. Anderson, JF, and Rorbaek, PER: The value of plain radiographs prior to oral cholecystography, Radiology 133:309, 1979.
3. Banner, MP, Bleshman, MH, and Speckman, JM: Persistent gallbladder opacification after iopanoic acid cholecystography: diagnostic implications for acalculous cholecystitis, Am J Roentgenol 132:51, 1979.
4. Becker, CD, Burckhardt, B, and Terrier, F: Ultrasound in postoperative acalculous cholecystitis, Gastrointest Radiol 11:47, 1986.
5. Bernardino, ME, et al: Delayed hepatic CT scanning: increased confidence and improved detection of hepatic metastases, Radiology 159:71, 1986.
6. Brachman, MB, et al: Acute gangrenous cholecystitis: radionuclide diagnosis, Radiology 151:209, 1984.
7. Burhenne, HJ: Perspective: the promise of extracorporeal shockwave lithotripsy for the treatment of gallstones, Am J Roentgenol 149:233, 1987.
8. Burhenne, HJ, and Obata, WG: Single-visit oral cholecystography, N Engl J Med 292:627, 1975.
9. Burhenne, HJ, Morris, DC, and Graeb, DA: Single-visit oral cholecystography for inpatients, Radiology 140:505, 1981.
10. Burhenne, HJ, et al: Biliary lithotripsy by extracorporeal shockwaves: an integral part of nonoperative intervention, Am J Roentgenol 150:1279, 1988.
11. Butch, RJ, and Mueller, PR: Fine-needle transhepatic cholangiography: state of the art, Semin Intervent Radiol 2:1, 1985.
12. Choy, N, et al: Cholescintigraphy in acute cholecystitis: use of intravenous morphine, Radiology 151:203, 1984.
13. Colletti, PM, et al: Acute cholecystitis: diagnosis with radionuclide angiography, Radiology 163:615, 1987.
14. Cooperberg, PL, and Burhenne, HJ: Real-time ultrasound: diagnostic technique of choice in calculous gallbladder disease, N Engl J Med 302:1277, 1980.
15. Cooperberg, PL, et al: Accuracy of common hepatic duct size in the evaluation of extrahepatic biliary obstruction, Radiology 135:141, 1980.
16. Cronan, JJ: US diagnosis of choledocholithiasis: a reappraisal, Radiology 161:133, 1986.

17. Curati, WL, et al: Ultrasound, CT and MRI comparison in primary and secondary tumors of the liver, Gastrointest Radiol 13:123, 1988.

18. Demas, BE, et al: Gallbladder bile: an experimental study in dog using MR imaging and proton MR spectroscopy, Radiology 157:453, 1985.

19. Dooms, GC, et al: Cholangiocarcinoma: imaging by MR, Radiology 159:89, 1986.

20. Dooms, GC, et al: MR imaging of the dilated biliary tract, Radiology 158:337, 1986.

21. Drake, CT, and Beal, JM: Percutaneous cholangiography, Arch Surg 91:558, 1965.

22. Fein, AB, et al: Intravenous cholecystokinin octapeptide: its effect on the sonographic appearance of the bile ducts in normal subjects, Radiology 153:499, 1984.

23. Foley, WD, et al: Treatment of blunt hepatic injuries: role of CT, Radiology 164:635, 1987.

24. Freeny, PC: Angiography of hepatic neoplasms, Semin Roentgenol 18:114, 1983.

25. Freeny, PC, and Marks, WM: Computed tomographic arteriography of the liver, Radiology 148:193, 1983.

26. Freeny, PC, and Marks, WM: Hepatic hemangioma: dynamic bolus CT, Am J Roentgenol 147:711, 1986.

27. Freeny, PC, et al: Colorectal carcinoma evaluation with CT: preoperative staging and detection of postoperative recurrence, Radiology 158:347, 1986.

28. Gelfand, DW: The liver: plain film diagnosis, Semin Roentgenol 10:177, 1975.

29. Gibson, RN, et al: Bile duct obstruction: radiologic evaluation of level, cause, and tumor resectability, Radiology 160:43, 1986.

30. Goodman, MW, et al: Is intravenous cholangiography still useful? Gastroenterology 79:642, 1980.

31. Göransson, A-M: Cholegraphy, its applicability and reliability in connection with gallstone operations: a follow-up study of 534 patients operated on because of cholelithiasis, Acta Chir Scand Suppl 496:1, 1980.

32. Griffen, WO, Jr, et al: Cholecystokinin cholecystography in the diagnosis of gallbladder disease, Ann Surg 191:636, 1980.

33. Hall-Craggs, MA, and Lees, WR: Fine-needle aspiration biopsy: pancreatic and biliary tumors, Am J Roentgenol 147:399, 1986.

34. Hricak, H, et al: Work in progress: nuclear magnetic resonance imaging of the gallbladder, Radiology 147:481, 1983.

35. Jacobs, JK, Cebul, RD, and Adamson, TE: Acute cholecystitis: evaluation of factors influencing common duct exploration, Am Surg 52:177, 1986.

36. Jeffrey, RB, Jr, et al: CT of radiation-induced hepatic injury, Am J Roentgenol 135:445, 1980.

37. Laing, FC, et al: Ultrasonic evaluation of patients with acute right upper quadrant pain, Radiology 140:449, 1981.

38. Laing, FC, et al: Biliary dilatation: defining the level and cause of real-time US, Radiology 160:39, 1986.

39. Letourneau, JG, et al: Liver allograft transplantation: postoperative CT findings, Am J Roentgenol 148:1099, 1987.

40. Marions, O, Pyk, E, and Wiechel, K-L: Iotroxamide, iodipamide and ioglycamide-image quality and side-effects, Läkartidningen 77:1948, 1980.

41. Marks, WM, and Freeny, PC: Hepatic masses. In Eisenberg, RL, editor: Diagnostic imaging, an algorithmic approach, Philadelphia, 1988, JB Lippincott.

42. Matsui, O, et al: Dynamic sequential computed tomography during arterial portography in the detection of hepatic neoplasms, Radiology 146:721, 1983.

43. McCarthy, S, et al: Cholecystitis: detection with MR imaging, Radiology 158:333, 1986.

44. Mettler, FA, Jr, Wicks, JD, and Christie, JH: Biliary imaging: a new look, Curr Probl Diagn Radiol 9:1, 1980.

45. Mirvis, SE, et al: The diagnosis of acute acalculous cholecystitis: a comparison of sonography, scintigraphy, and CT, Am J Roentgenol 147:1171, 1986.

46. Nelson, RC, et al: Focal hepatic lesions: detection by dynamic and delayed computed tomography versus short TE/TR spin echo and fast field echo magnetic resonance imaging, Gastrointest Radiol 13:115, 1988.

47. O'Connor, HJ, et al: Ultrasound detection of choledocholithiasis: prospective comparison with ERCP in the postcholecystectomy patient, Gastrointest Radiol 11:161, 1986.

48. Olutola, PS, Hutton, L, and Wall, WJ: Radiologic assessment of bile duct complications in liver transplantation: initial experience, J Can Assoc Radiol 37:276, 1986.

49. Patriquin, H, et al: Duplex Doppler examination in portal hypertension: technique and anatomy, Am J Roentgenol 149:71, 1987.

50. Pitluk, HC, and Beal, JM: Choledocholithiasis associated with acute cholecystitis, Arch Surg 114:887, 1979.

51. Poleynard, GD, and Harris, RD: Diagnosis of emphysematous cholecystitis by computerized tomography, Gastrointest Radiol 4:153, 1979.

52. Ralls, PW, et al: Gallbladder wall thickening: patients without intrinsic gallbladder disease, Am J Roentgenol 137:65, 1981.

53. Reiman, TH, Balfe, DM, and Weyman, PJ: Suprapancreatic biliary obstruction: CT evaluation, Radiology 163:49, 1987.

54. Romano, AJ, et al: Gallbladder and bile duct abnormalities in AIDS: sonographic findings in eight patients, Am J Roentgenol 150:123, 1988.

55. Rossmann, MD, et al: MR imaging of gallbladder carcinoma, Am J Roentgenol 148:143, 1987.

56. Rygaard, H, et al: Anatomic variants of the hepatic arteries, Acta Radiol Diagn 27:425, 1986.

57. Sackmann, M, Delius, M, and Sauerbruch, T: Shockwave lithotripsy of gallbladder stones: the first 175 patients, N Engl J Med 318:393, 1988.

58. Sanders, RC: The significance of sonographic gallbladder wall thickening, J Clin Ultrasound 8:143, 1980.

59. Sherman, M, et al: Intravenous cholangiography and sonography in acute cholecystitis: prospective evaluation, Am J Roentgenol 135:311, 1980.

60. Shlaer, WJ, Leopold, GR, and Scheible, FW: Sonography of the thickened gallbladder wall: a nonspecific finding, Am J Roentgenol 136:337, 1981.

61. Solbiati, L, et al: Fine-needle biopsy of hepatic hemangioma with sonographic guidance, Am J Roentgenol 144:471, 1985.

62. Stark, DD, et al: Magnetic resonance imaging of cavernous hemangioma of the liver: tissue-specific characterization, Radiology 145:213, 1985.

63. Stark, DD, et al: Hepatic metastases: randomized, controlled comparison of detection with MR imaging and CT, Radiology 165:399, 1987.

64. Taylor, KJW, et al: Liver transplant recipients: portal duplex US with correlative angiography, Radiology 159:357, 1986.

65. Torres, WE, et al: The correlation between MR and angiography in portal hypertension, Am J Roentgenol 148:1109, 1987.

66. Ulreich, S, et al: Acute cholecystitis: comparison of ultrasound and intravenous cholangiography, Arch Surg 115:158, 1980.

67. vanSonnenberg, E, and Hofmann, AF: Perspective: horizons in gallstone therapy—1988, Am J Roentgenol 150:43, 1988.

68. Viamonte, M, Jr: Emerging technologies for the diagnosis of portal hypertension, Am J Roentgenol 148:1113, 1987.

69. Wechsler, RJ, et al: The periportal collar: a CT sign of liver transplant rejection, Radiology 165:57, 1987.

70. Weinstein, JB, et al: High resolution CT of the porta hepatis and hepatoduodenal ligament, RadioGraphics 6:55, 1986.

71. Weissmann, HS, et al: Role of ^{99m}Tc-IDA cholescintigraphy in evaluating biliary tract disorders, Gastrointest Radiol 2:215, 1980.

72. Weissmann, HS, et al: Spectrum of 99m-Tc-IDA cholescintigraphic patterns in acute cholecystitis, Radiology 138:167, 1981.

73. Whalen, JP: Radiology of the abdomen: impact of new imaging methods, Am J Roentgenol 133:585, 1979.

74. White, RM, et al: Liver transplant rejection: angiographic findings in 35 patients, Am J Roentgenol 148:1095, 1987.

75. Wilbur, AC, Gyi, B, and Renigers, SA: High-field MRI of primary gallbladder carcinoma, Gastrointest Radiol 13:142, 1988.

76. Wilson, SA, Gosink, BB, and vanSonnenberg, E: Unchanged size of a dilated common bile duct after a fatty meal: results and significance, Radiology 160:29, 1986.

77. Zajko, AB, et al: Cholangiography and interventional biliary radiology in adult liver transplantation, Am J Roentgenol 144:127, 1985.

78. Zajko, AB, et al: Cholangiographic findings in hepatic artery occlusion after liver transplantation, Am J Roentgenol 149:485, 1987.

79. Zeman, RK, et al: Acute experimental biliary obstruction in the dog: sonographic findings and clinical implications, Am J Roentgenol 136:965, 1981.

80. Zirinsky, K, et al: MR imaging of portal venous thrombosis: correlation with CT and sonography, Am J Roentgenol 150:283, 1988.

PART XI

SPLEEN

57 *Pathology*

EDWARD A. SMUCKLER
HARLAN J. SPJUT

The spleen is one of the largest units of the reticuloendothelial system in the human body. As such, it serves as a major filtration site for blood, removing erythrocyte inclusions and culling dammed and effete erythrocytes.[5,6] The spleen is also an immunologically competent organ, with both T and B cells present in the white pulp. Many systemic human diseases are associated with splenic enlargement, for example, systemic inflammatory diseases, generalized hematopoietic disorders, and a variety of metabolic disturbances (some genetic in origin).

EMBRYOLOGY AND HISTOLOGY

The spleen is derived from a mass of mesenchymal cells within the dorsal mesogastrium, which forms the capsule, the connective tissue framework, and the splenic pulp. The splenic artery arises from the celiac axis and penetrates into the mesenchyme, and this penetration carries with it fibrous tissue investments forming the trabeculae. The finer divisions of the vessel constitute the central artery in the white pulp. When the arteriolar branches of the splenic artery leave the connective tissue core, a sheath of lymphocytes surrounds the vessel. The lymphatic structures with the enclosed artery can be seen on the cut surface of the spleen as malpighian bodies, or lymphatic follicles, and vary from 0.1 to 1 mm in diameter. The arterioles empty into the splenic sinusoid. There are spaces between the cells of the sinusoids that permit permeation of the blood plasma between these reticuloendothelial elements. The spleen has two major cell populations, lymphoid and reticuloendothelial.[2,9] Splenic functions include phagocytosis, hematopoiesis, erythrocyte and platelet storage, and immunologic reactions.

Phagocytosis

The cells of the reticuloendothelial system lining the sinusoids of the spleen constitute one of the largest collections of phagocytic cells of the human body. They function to remove effete red blood cells, damaged red blood cells, and aggregated particulate matter including bacteria, cell debris, and abnormal macroglobulins. Specific examples of inborn errors of metabolism in which these phagocytic cells may collect abnormal cell products include Gaucher's disease and Niemann-Pick disease.

Hematopoiesis

In the human fetus from the fourth month onward the spleen is a major site of hematopoiesis, a function that continues into the immediate postpartum period. In the child and the adult the white pulp contains immunologically competent lymphocytes and is also believed to participate in the formation of mononuclear cell population for blood and other connective tissues, macrophages, and lymphocytes.

Cell storage

The spleen is capable of storing erythrocytes and platelets. It has been suggested that it contains 30% to 40% of the total platelet mass of the body.

Immunologic responsiveness

Under conditions of antigenic stimulation, proliferation of splenic macrophages and increased lymphopoiesis take place.

CONGENITAL ANOMALIES

Accessory spleens (spleneculi) are particularly common, occurring in 30% of some autopsy populations. They occur most frequently along the route of the vascular supply and within the derivatives of the primitive mesogastrium (the lienorenal ligament and the greater omentum). These frequently can be identified by computed tomography, radionuclide injection, and angiography. Therapeutic intervention involving splenic removal without the identifying and removal of accessory spleens is not effective.

HYPERSPLENISM

The most common presenting symptom of splenic disease is splenic enlargement, often accompanied by upper abdominal pain or discomfort. From the standpoint of pathologic processes, the increase in organ size can represent reactive alterations to systemic diseases, hemopoietic diseases, hemodynamic changes, and the many lesions described in this section.

Neoplastic involvement, either primary or secondary, can produce splenic enlargement, the former as total gland enlargement and the latter as discrete masses[11] (Figs. 57-1 and 57-2). Malignant neoplasms of the reticuloendothelial and/or lymphoproliferative systems are the most common primary splenic cancers,[15] though primary lymphomas of the spleen are rare.[1] Other malignant neoplasms primary in the spleen are most uncommon.

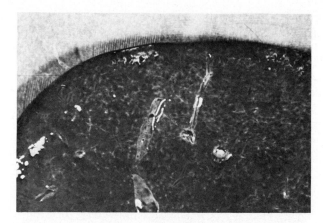

Fig. 57-1 Cut surface of enlarged spleen (1200 g) diffusely infiltrated with Hodgkin's disease. Note bulging surface and discernible gray infiltrates.

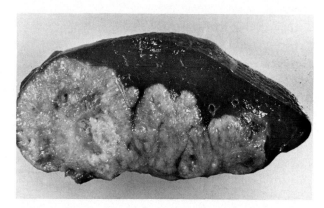

Fig. 57-2 Massive involvement of spleen by metastatic squamous cell carcinoma arising in vocal cord.

Angiosarcomas, fibrosarcomas, and malignant fibrous histiocytomas have been described.[14] These tumors often result in enlargement of the spleen to over 1000 g. The few angiosarcomas seen have been particularly aggressive. Benign tumors that arise include fibromas, lymphangiomas, hamartomas, and hemangiomas. The spleen rarely is involved in lymphangiomatosis, that is, splenic enlargement concomitant with lymphangiomas elsewhere in the body.[10]

Hodgkin's disease commonly arises in the spleen or lymph nodes. This malignant neoplasm may be present either as a single mass in the spleen or diffuse lymph node disease with splenic enlargement. Secondary involvement of the spleen by other cancers whose primary site is elsewhere in the body produce single or multiple discrete metastatic nodules. As they grow, these nodules may coalesce to form large areas of replacement (Fig. 57-2). A critical survey of patients with diffuse carcinomatosis reveals that 50% show splenic metastases. The malignant neoplasms with most common secondary splenic seeding are melanomas, bronchogenic carcinomas, and carcinomas of the pancreas and the breast. These metastatic lesions may be single large masses or they may be minute small lesions peppering the splenic substance.

Splenic enlargement may also result from infection, vascular congestion (as in portal hypertension), lympho-proliferative benign disorders, immunologic inflammatory states (autoimmune states), storage disease, and inflammatory pseudotumors.[4]

Calcification in the spleen may result from a number of conditions such as tuberculosis, histoplasmosis, cysts, and vascular aneurysms. Splenic cysts are usually lined by stratified squamous epithelium. Pseudocysts may result from trauma or inflammation and do not have an epithelial lining.[3]

Splenic abscesses are diagnosable with modern imaging techniques, yet a small number still rupture spontaneously. Often bacterial endocarditis or an immunosuppressed disease underlies the abscess. These may be multilocular.[13]

INFECTIOUS OR REACTIVE SPLENITIS

Enlargement of the spleen as a result of inflammatory or immunologic inflammatory disease can be up to twice its normal size (200 to 300 g). The pulp is softened, and reticuloendothelial hyperplasia and numerous macrophages are commonly found. Lymphoid follicles are also readily apparent and enlarged. The spleen is uniformly enlarged. Histologic verification of specific infections is performed by microbiologic rather than histologic techniques in most instances. Immunologic diseases can be recognized by their clinical pattern and often by histologic patterns such as the onion skin alteration of blood vessels as in cases of lupus erythematosus.

Even greater splenic enlargement, up to 10 times the normal size (1000 to 2000 g), is commonly seen in immunologic inflammatory conditions such as rheumatoid arthritis, lupus erythematosus, and infectious mononucleosis.[7] Here too there is a hyperplastic change in splenic follicles as well as in the reticuloendothelial cells. This type of splenic enlargement is often associated with splenic rupture.

Vascular congestion, specifically associated with increased portal venous pressure (portal hypertension), is associated with massive splenic enlargement, the weight reaching as high as 5000 g. In these instances there is a particular prominence to the vascular channels, which are readily recognized by microscopy. The sinusoidal blood spaces are widened and distinct, outlining the follicular structure.

These different diseases appear similar in computed tomography images, but the difference in the vascularity between nonspecific splenitis and passive congestion permits differential diagnosis.

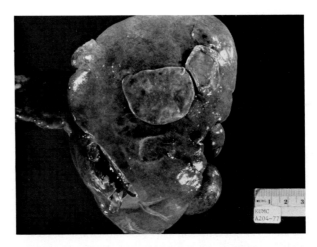

Fig. 57-3 Several areas of infarction manifested on surface by gray patches in black male with sickle cell disease.

Systemic lymphoproliferative disease, including Hodgkin's disease, involves a diffuse infiltration of the spleen by neoplastic cells. In large part this is a uniform process, commonly leading to massively enlarged splenic structures. There is a diffuse enlargement, often accompanied by an encroachment of vascular channels. The histologic pattern of the cells and the presence or absence of Reed-Sternberg cells permit the histologic confirmation of specific neoplasms.

SPLENIC INFARCTS

Enlargement of the spleen, particularly with a compromise of the vascular structure, may lead to localized splenic infarcts. These areas fail to perfuse via the normal vascular channels, resulting in localized tissue necrosis. The infarcts stand out against the darker red background of the spleen as lighter pale areas (Fig. 57-3). With resolution the tissue is replaced by nonvascular collagenous connective tissue, becomes smaller and fibrotic, and forms contracted scars.

In cases of sickle cell disease, "log jamming" by deformed red blood cells produces focal infarcts. This process, however, is recurrent, and coalescense of the infarcts often leads to obliteration of the spleen—an autosplenectomy.

MYELOID METAPLASIA

The most striking change in the spleen in cases of myeloid metaplasia is massive extramedullary hematopoiesis. A spleen thus affected may enlarge to as much as 4000 g, a diffusely enlarged structure in which there is remarkable addition of hematopoietic cells. This increase represents an increase in the overall density of the spleen with a relative reduction in vascular components.[8]

REFERENCES

1. Burke, JS: Surgical pathology of the spleen: an approach to the differential diagnosis of splenic lymphomas and leukemias, Am J Surg Pathol 5:551, 1981.
2. Burke, JS, and Simon, GT: Electron microscopy of the spleen, Anat Microcirculation 58:127, 1970.
3. Carpenter, G, Cotter, PW, and Davidson, JRM: Epidermoid cyst of the spleen, Aust NZ J Surg 56:365, 1986.
4. Cotelingam, JD, and Jaffe, ES: Inflammatory pseudotumor of the spleen, Am J Surg Pathol 8:375, 1984.
5. Crosby, W: Hyposplenism: an inquiry into normal functions of the spleen, Ann Rev Med 14:349, 1963.
6. Crosby, WH: Splenic remodelling of red cell surfaces, Blood 50:643, 1977.
7. Epstein, MA, and Achong, BG: Pathogenesis of infectious mononucleosis, Lancet 2(8051):1270, 1977.
8. Lazlo, J: Myeloproliferative disorders: myelofibrosis, myelosclerosis, extramedullary hematopoiesis and hemorrhagic thrombocythemia. Semin Hematol 12:409, 1975.
9. Li, CY, Yam, LT, and Crosby, WH: Histochemical characterization of the cellular and structural elements of the human spleen. J Histochem Cytochem 20:1049, 1972.
10. Marymont, JV, and Knight, PJ: Splenic lymphangiomatosis: a rare cause of splenomegaly, J Pediat Surg 22:461, 1987.
11. Marymount, JH, and Gross, S: Patterns of metastatic carcinoma in the spleen, Am J Clin Pathol 40:58, 1963.
12. Morgenstern, L, et al: Hamartomas of the spleen, Arch Surg 119:1291, 1984.
13. Nelken, N, et al: Changing clinical spectrum of splenic abscess, Am J Surg 154:27, 1987.
14. Wick, MR, et al: Primary nonlymphoreticular malignant neoplasms of the spleen, Am J Surg Pathol 6:229, 1982.
15. Wolf, DJ, Silver, RT, and Coleman, M: Splenectomy in chronic myeloid leukemia, Ann Intern Med 89:684, 1978.

General reference

Kissane, JM, and Anderson, WAD, editors: Pathology, ed. 8, St. Louis, 1985, The C.V. Mosby Co.

58 *Ultrasonography*

FAYE C. LAING
ROY A. FILLY
GRETCHEN A. W. GOODING

METHOD OF EXAMINATION

SIZE

CONTOUR

CONSISTENCY

PITFALLS

Although ultrasonography has not been in the forefront of diagnostic modalities insofar as the spleen is concerned, it can offer useful information, particularly in patients with splenic pathologic conditions. Although exact volume measurements may be difficult to obtain, ultrasound permits ready visualization of splenomegaly and can easily be used to determine changes in the spleen's size with serial examinations.

The normal spleen is difficult to examine with either palpation or ultrasonography because of its posterior and superior location in the left upper quadrant and because of the interposition of the ribs. Although the spleen's size may vary somewhat depending on the amount of blood it contains, the average adult spleen measures approximately 12.5 cm in length, 7.5 cm in transverse diameter, and 3.5 cm in thickness. Its normal weight is about 150 g, with a range of about 50 to 250 g.[24]

When the spleen becomes involved in any of a number of pathologic processes, it enlarges. Under these circumstances it is more easily examined with either palpation or ultrasonography. Often the sonographic appearance of splenomegaly is nonspecific. However, ultrasound is usually able to determine whether a mass in the left upper quadrant represents an enlarged spleen as opposed to a mass arising from a neighboring organ. Occasionally, focal pathologic processes affect the spleen, in which case ultrasound can be extremely useful in assessing the consistency of the lesion and suggesting the cause.

METHOD OF EXAMINATION

The ultrasonographic examination of the spleen varies depending on its size and to some degree on the body habitus of the patient. In individuals who have normally sized spleens the easiest way to visualize the spleen is to place the patient in a right lateral decubitus position and to scan obliquely along the axis of the spleen—that is, between the tenth and eleventh ribs. Occasionally the examination must be performed one interspace higher or lower to obtain a satisfactory image. In all cases the sonograms should be obtained with suspended, deep inspiration.

A 3.5 MHz high-resolution real-time mechanical or electronic sector transducer usually produces the most satisfactory image. When sonograms are obtained over the upper portions of the spleen, a slight cranial angulation of the transducer is normally required for best results; conversely, sonograms that image the more caudal portions of the spleen may require that the transducer be angled slightly toward the patient's feet (Fig. 58-1). The anteroinferior portion of the spleen is usually best seen by obtaining the sonogram from an anterior subcostal position.

Longitudinal scans of the spleen are usually coronal and are obtained with the patient lying in a right lateral decubitus position. The transducer is usually placed either intercostally or subcostally (Fig. 58-2). Occasionally, satisfactory images of the spleen may result from placing the patient in an erect or sitting position and obtaining longitudinal sonograms from posterior and posterolateral approaches. When studies are performed in

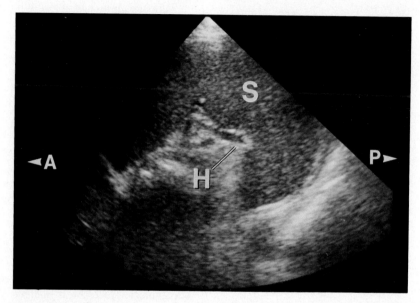

Fig. 58-1 Normal transverse scan over spleen shows homogeneous low-level echoes throughout splenic parenchyma *(S)*. Hilus of spleen *(H)* normally contains stronger echoes than remainder of spleen because of entry of vascular pedicle into this region. Patient is lying in right lateral decubitus position. *A*, Anterior; *P*, posterior.

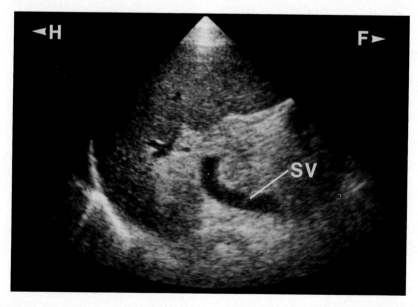

Fig. 58-2 Longitudinal subcostal sonogram shows normal contour of spleen with entry of splenic vein *(SV)* at splenic hilus. *H*, Head; *F*, feet.

this manner, the patient is instructed to lean forward. This change of position elevates the rib cage while gravity causes both kidney and spleen to descend away from the ribs. This method of scanning has proved to be extremely useful in examining patients with pleural effusions.[13] Frequently, however, normal aerated lung in the posterior costophrenic sulcus prevents the ultrasound beam from reaching the most superior portion of the spleen, which is situated immediately beneath the diaphragm.

The shielded position of the spleen often makes it difficult to obtain successful sonograms of normally sized spleens. As one author has declared, "If you have trouble seeing it, it is unlikely to be abnormal."[3] It is fortunate for the sonographer that most abnormal spleens are enlarged. As splenomegaly becomes increasingly pronounced, the spleen becomes progressively easier to visualize ultrasonographically. The enlarged spleen descends beneath the left costal margin and displaces the gas-filled stomach medially. When this occurs, the spleen may be satisfactorily visualized sonographically even with the patient in a supine position. Longitudinal and transverse scans are performed through the spleen in a manner identical to that used in hepatic ultrasonographic examinations.

SIZE

A variety of diagnostic methods are available for determining a spleen's size. Radiographic examination can usually visualize the splenic shadow, primarily because of its juxtaposition to gas in the stomach and splenic flexure of the colon. In patients with abnormal left upper quadrant masses, however, radiographs are usually not helpful in discerning whether the mass arises from the

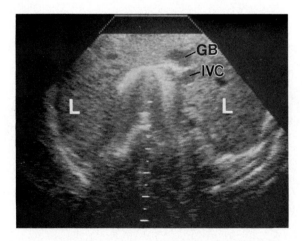

Fig. 58-3 Transverse sector scan over upper abdomen of neonate with congenital heart disease. Midline position of liver *(L)* suggested appropriate diagnosis of asplenia. *IVC,* Inferior vena cava; *GB,* gallbladder.

spleen or an adjacent organ. Radionuclide imaging is another useful procedure for estimating the spleen's size. The accuracy of this method depends, however, on the vascular integrity and function of the spleen. Angiographic methods, although very accurate, subject the patient to radiation and the risks inherent in any invasive procedure. Computed axial tomography and magnetic resonance imaging are not limited by the overlying ribs or aerated lung and thus do not suffer several of the technical difficulties encountered by ultrasound when imaging small spleens.

Ultrasound has been of value in assessing the spleen's size, particularly in patients with splenomegaly. Occasionally asplenia may be suggested, especially in neonates with congenital heart disease and a liver situated in the midline (Fig. 58-3). The normally sized spleen may sometimes be seen on transverse sonograms of the abdomen (with the patient erect or lying supine). If the spleen is not visualized from this position, it is not enlarged. When seen, the normally sized spleen does not usually extend more than 2 cm anterior to an imaginary line drawn tangentially to the anterior border of the aorta and parallel to the back. Leopold and Asher[14] and Asher et al.[2] evaluated over 3000 patients and found this to be a generally reliable index for determining whether splenomegaly existed. Occasionally body habitus affects the shape of the spleen, or masses adjacent to the spleen may displace it and give the false impression of splenomegaly. Several authors have employed more sophisticated methods for determining the spleen's volume, using serial transverse sections and computed analysis for determining the area of individual spleen slices.[11,22] In general, these ultrasonic volume measurements have tended to overestimate the size of the spleen (as determined following splenectomy) by about 12%.[10,11] This inaccuracy may arise because of blood flow and other physiologic factors that differ between in situ and excised states.

Because of its noninvasive nature, ultrasound can be used sequentially in the evaluation of patients with primary or secondary diseases involving the spleen. In a study of Koga and Morikawa[12] serial changes in the spleen's size in patients with various types of liver disease were reported. They found that useful information regarding the prognosis of liver pathologic processes could be obtained by observing serial changes in the sectional area of the spleen. Ultrasound can also be useful in assessing the response of the spleen to radiotherapy and chemotherapeutic regimens in patients with a variety of lymphatic and hematologic disorders.

When the spleen enlarges, it frequently causes displacement of adjacent organs, particularly the left kidney. Anterior or posterior displacement of the kidney may occur (Fig. 58-4). Ultrasound can easily assess whether

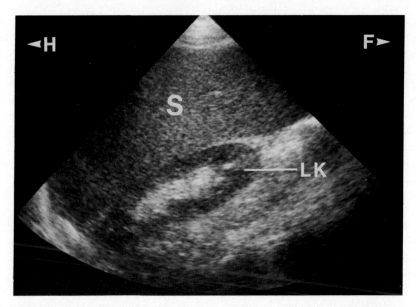

Fig. 58-4 Longitudinal sonogram in patient with moderate splenomegaly *(S)*, showing some compression of left kidney *(LK)*. Normally spleen does not extend over considerable portion of left kidney, as in this case. *H,* Head; *F,* feet.

the renal displacement is secondary to an enlarged spleen, an intrinsic renal pathologic process, or a mass arising in another contiguous organ.

CONTOUR

The spleen is normally well defined and smooth along its superior and lateral borders, both of which have a convex margin. The undersurface and medial aspect of the spleen are more lobulated because of focal impressions made on its surface by surrounding viscera. Occasionally a medial lobulation arising from the spleen can be observed projecting between the tail of the pancreas and the left kidney. This variant is seen in approximately 10% of patients with splenomegaly and should not be confused with lesions arising in the tail of the pancreas or adrenal gland.[8]

The hilar region is normally umbilicated or lobulated because of the entry of the vascular pedicle at this point. A highly reflective group of echoes is frequently seen within the spleen in this region, in part secondary to acoustic reflections from the wall of the splenic vasculature as well as surrounding fibrous and fatty tissue. Splenic echoes in this area of the spleen may be particularly prominent in patients with splenomegaly and should not be misinterpreted as an abnormal focus or a pathologic condition (see the section on pitfalls).

The medial surface of the spleen is normally well defined and has an overall concave configuration. In the evaluation of patients with left upper quadrant masses it is important to note whether the mass in question is concave medially. In the great majority of patients with splenomegaly the shape and contour of the spleen remain normal despite its large size. This is particularly true if there is a hematologic disorder or passive congestion of the spleen. The enlarged spleen may lose its normal contour, however, if there is a space-occupying lesion within it, such as a hematoma or cyst (Fig. 58-5).

In approximately 10% of individuals a single accessory spleen is present. Ultrasonographic identification is based on (1) its appearance, which is usually round or

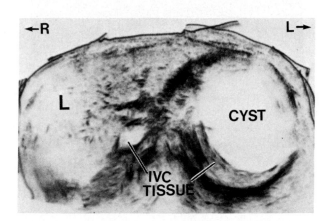

Fig. 58-5 When space-occupying lesion is present, spleen may lose its normal contour. In this patient with splenic cyst, normal splenic tissue can be identified posteriorly. *IVC,* Inferior vena cava; *R,* right; *L,* liver.

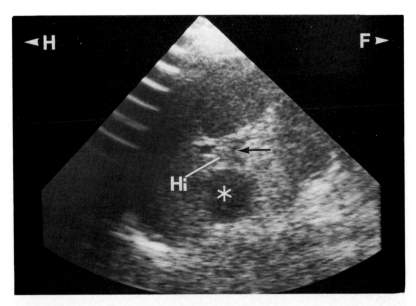

Fig. 58-6 Longitudinal scan showing accessory spleen (*) near splenic hilus *(Hi)*. Branch of splenic artery *(arrow)* is seen entering accessory spleen. *H,* Head; *F,* feet.

oval with an echo texture identical to that of the main spleen; (2) its location at or near the splenic hilum, or in relation to the gastrosplenic and splenocolic ligaments; and (3) demonstration of its vascular supply from the splenic atery or vein[28] (Fig. 58-6).

CONSISTENCY

The internal consistency of the spleen normally causes a very homogeneous echo pattern to be displayed. Although several investigators have suggested that echoes from the normal splenic parenchyma are of lower intensity than those from normal hepatic parenchyma[6,9,25] recent evidence suggests that normal splenic tissue is of greater echo texture than hepatic tissue.[1,15]

Attempts to classify splenic pathologic conditions according to echo texture have led to considerable confusion in the ultrasound literature. Lymphomatous nodules within the spleen are usually hypoechoic[5,6,9,19,29] (Fig. 58-7). Several authors state that diffuse involvement may be associated with hypoechogenicity, whereas others state that it may be associated with normal or increased echogenicity.[23,25] In general, splenic congestion and enlargement in cases of hepatocellular disease most often cause a hyperechoic pattern within the splenic parenchyma.[6,18,29] Recent work by Sommer and co-workers suggests that measuring ultrasonic waveforms that are back scattered from splenic parenchymal tissue is a more sensitive method for detecting diffuse splenic involvement with Hodgkin's lymphoma than is visual assessment of altered echogenicity.[27] In their preliminary report, a

significantly increased numerical value was obtained from spleens involved with a variety of infiltrative processes, including lymphoma, leukemia, infection, and congestion.

Normal splenic parenchyma displays a remarkably uniform pattern. Unlike that of the liver, its internal vasculature cannot ordinarily be identified. In patients with splenomegaly, however, enlarged splenic vessels can frequently be clearly identified, particularly in the region of the splenic hilus (Fig. 58-8).

With continued improvement in transducers, scanning techniques, and equipment, small areas of intrasplenic focal pathology have become increasingly visible to the sonographer. Multiple low- or high-density echoes can be observed in patients with a variety of pathologic processes, both benign and malignant[5,6,18,19] (Fig. 58-9).

Although ultrasound is sensitive for detecting focal splenic lesions, similar to other noninvasive imaging modalities, it often lacks information enabling one to make a specific diagnosis. Inflammatory, neoplastic, and even posttraumatic processes can appear remarkably similar.[26] Furthermore, the ultrasonographic appearances for a particular pathologic process can vary greatly. Even lymphamatous nodules, which are characteristically sonolucent, may contain large focal echogenic deposits.[26] Splenic metastases, which are most often caused by melanoma, are also typically hypoechoic (but of higher echo amplitude than lymphoma); occasionally, these lesions are also predominantly echogenic.[19] Other, less common tumors that metastasize to the spleen include carcinoma

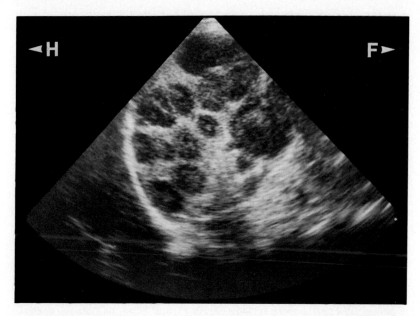

Fig. 58-7 Longitudinal sonogram reveals multiple hypoechoic splenic masses in patient with lymphoma. *H*, Head; *F*, feet.

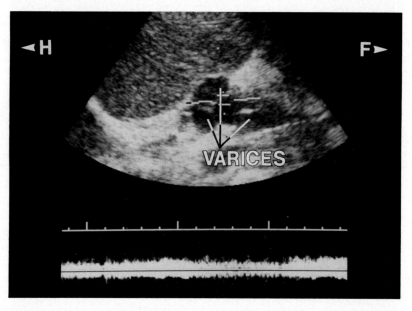

Fig. 58-8 Splenic varices are evident in region of splenic hilus in this patient with portal hypertension. Doppler signal confirms patency of vessels and displays typical venous flow pattern. *H*, Head; *F*, feet.

of the lung, breast, stomach, ovary, and choriocarcinoma. To obtain a precise tissue diagnosis, ultrasound can be used as a guide for fine-needle aspiration biopsy[26] (Fig. 58-10).

Predominantly fluid-filled splenic masses are usually caused by splenic cysts (Fig. 58-5). These lesions are classified as true cysts when they are lined by a specific secreting membrane, or as false cysts when they contain serous, hemorrhagic, or inflammatory fluid or are caused by a degenerating infarct.[26]

The contents of splenic cysts sometimes contain considerable particulate material because of either cholesterol crystals[7] or blood products.[20] These impart low-level echoes to the fluid and can cause confusion in that the

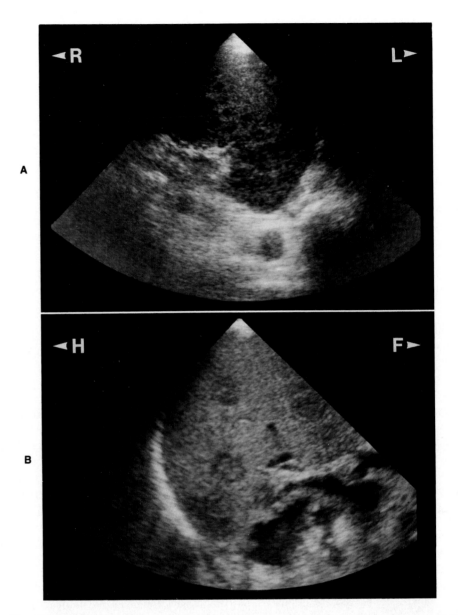

Fig. 58-9 Spleens of these two patients each contain multiple focal hypoechoic lesions. **A,** Patient had metastatic adenocarcinoma (primary unknown). *R,* Right; *L,* left. **B,** Patient had multiple tuberculous abscesses. Correct diagnosis was made in each case following percutaneous fine-needle aspiration. *H,* Head; *F,* feet.

lesion may be misinterpreted as solid.[7] Septations and fluid levels are also occasionally seen in patients with atypical cystic masses.

Other focal nonmalignant splenic lesions may be caused by granulomas, infarcts, abscesses, and hematomas. Granulomas, when calcified, are easily recognized because they appear as small collections of high-amplitude echoes with prominent posterior acoustic shadowing.

Acute splenic infarction typically appears as a well-demarcated wedge-shaped hypoechoic area with its apex directed toward the splenic hilus and its base directed toward the periphery of the spleen.[30] Not infrequently, splenic infarcts are atypical in appearance: they may be rounded, multiple, or echogenic. Most likely these variations can be accounted for by the age of the lesion the pathophysiologic changes that occur with time.[17] During acute splenic infarction, when edema, inflammation, and necrosis predominate, the ultrasonographic appearance is primarily hypoechoic. As the infarct becomes more chronic and is associated with fibrosis and shrinkage, the ultrasonographic pattern gradually changes toward in-

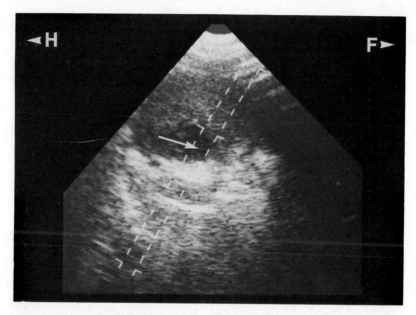

Fig. 58-10 Using ultrasound guidance it is possible to pass needle between parallel lines to obtain tissue or fluid for diagnostic purposes. In this patient sonolucent mass *(arrow)* was proven to be splenic abscess. *H,* Head; *F,* feet.

creased echogenicity and reduction in the size of the lesion. An old healed infarct is characteristically seen as a dense, hyperechoic focus.

Although splenic abscesses are uncommon, they are associated with a very high mortality if the diagnosis is delayed or missed. Predisposing conditions include endocarditis, trauma, sickle cell disease, and infection in a contiguous organ.[21] Similar to abscesses elsewhere in the body, the ultrasonographic appearance for a splenic abscess varies greatly with respect to number, size, echo texture, wall definition, and sound penetration (Figs. 58-9 and 58-10). The most expeditious way to diagnose a splenic abscess is to direct a needle into the suspicious lesion (Fig. 58-10).

Traumatic splenic injuries are a leading cause of morbidity in patients who have sustained splenic trauma. Although computed tomography is the modality of choice for detecting and diagnosing intrasplenic and perisplenic traumatic processes, occasionally a history of trauma may be withheld or remote, in which case ultrasound may be performed because of vague left upper quadrant symptoms. The ultrasound findings are based on the age of the hematoma, its size, and its location (intrasplenic, perisplenic, or both) (Figs. 58-11 and 58-12). The ultrasonographic appearances for clotted blood have been shown to vary greatly and depend primarily on the age of the hematoma.[4] An acute hematoma is a highly echogenic lesion that may be well or poorly defined, depending on its location (Figs. 58-11 and 58-12, *A*). Evolution of the hematoma is associated with clot lysis. On

ultrasonography this may be reflected initially as enlargement of the hematoma with the development of a progressively sonolucent pattern (Figs. 58-12, *B*, and 58-13). Intrasplenic hematomas most often appear as focal masses, whereas perisplenic collections are caused by subcapsular hematomas. In our experience, precise identification of a site of splenic laceration is the exception and not the rule.

Because it is becoming increasingly common to adopt a nonsurgical approach to patients with injured spleens, ultrasound has gained acceptance as an ideal modality for monitoring these individuals and observing the natural progression of splenic morphology as the hematoma evolves.[16]

PITFALLS

Many other masses can occur in the left upper quadrant that unwary ultrasonographers and even those with experience may mistake for the spleen. It is a good rule of thumb to try to distinguish the spleen from the mass in question. This may present quite a challenge to the ultrasonographer, who frequently is required to scan the patient from unusual angles and in unconventional positions. Radionuclide scans, computed tomography, or both may be of immeasurable assistance in defining the position of the spleen and in determining whether the mass seen ultrasonographically represents the spleen.

Occasionally it is difficult to discern whether or not a cystic mass in the left upper quadrant is splenic in origin. For example, fluid in the stomach may sometimes

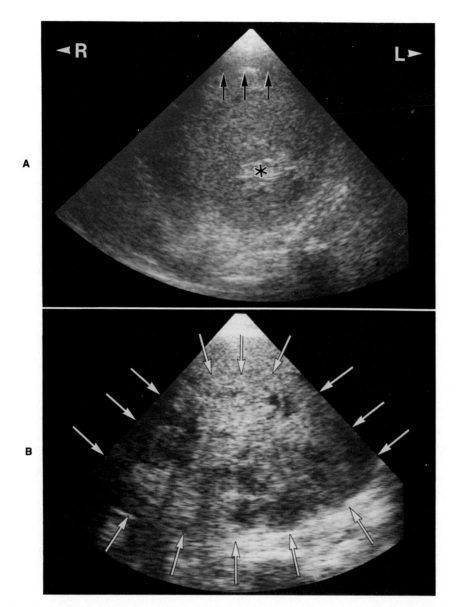

Fig. 58-11 Each of these patients had sustained remote splenic trauma that was not clinically evident at their presentation. **A,** Small echogenic intrasplenic focus (*) is caused by small parenchymal hematoma. Note also presence of subtle sonolucent area superficial to spleen that was caused by small subcapsular hematoma *(arrows). R,* Right; *L,* left. **B,** Much larger hematoma *(arrows)* with varying echogenicity occupying large portion of spleen *(arrows).*

be mistaken for a splenic lesion. This dilemma can be readily resolved in several ways. First, the anatomic position of the stomach relative to the spleen is more medial and anterior to the left kidney. Second, the ingestion of a small amount of tap water by the patient causes echoes to appear within the stomach because of the presence of microbubbles.[31] Third, scans obtained with an erect posterior longitudinal approach are usually able to separate the sonolucent spleen from the fluid-filled stomach. Pathologic fluid collections in the left upper quadrant may

also challenge the ultrasonographer. Pseudocysts in the tail of the pancreas and left subphrenic fluid collections are two situations that may be difficult to sort out and separate from splenic fluid collections. Repeat scans performed after repositioning the patient and the identification of a displaced spleen frequently aid the ultrasonographer in correctly evaluating these conditions.

Solid left upper quadrant masses of nonsplenic origin may also be confused with the spleen. As previously mentioned, in the majority of patients with splenomegaly,

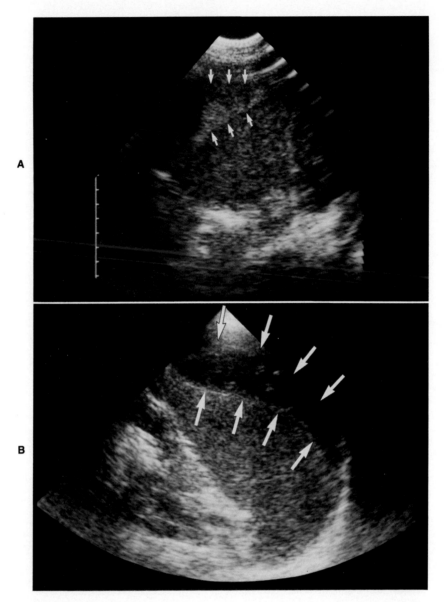

Fig. 58-12 These two patients demonstrate subcapsular hematomas that have markedly different sonographic appearances. **A,** Hematoma *(arrows)* is echogenic, suggesting that it is acute. **B,** Hematoma *(arrows)* is largely sonolucent, consistent with hematoma that has undergone clot lysis.

the spleen maintains its normal contour and shape. Occasionally, however, masses resulting from other causes mimic the shape of the spleen. Actively searching for another structure that may represent a normal but displaced spleen and obtaining a radionuclide scan may prevent the occurrence of an embarrassing error.

Because primary and metastatic neoplasms of the spleen are rare, it is unlikely that a rounded left upper quadrant solid mass represents an abnormal spleen. In most of these patients an extrinsic abnormality is present. As shown in Fig. 58-5, however, splenic cysts frequently cause the spleen to assume a round shape.

It is also worth mentioning that two other normal anatomic structures can occasionally be confused for splenic or perisplenic pathologic conditions. The first problem area involves the splenic hilus being confused for an echogenic intrasplenic abnormality. This occurs in patients with marked splenomegaly in whom normal hilar echoes become unusually pronounced. Because of the lobulation and concavity of the hilar area, these echoes may be confused on longitudinal sonograms with an intrasplenic focal abnormality (Fig. 58-14). In addition, a prominent splenic hilus, because of highly reflective fibrofatty tissue, can occasionally cause a pseudomass in

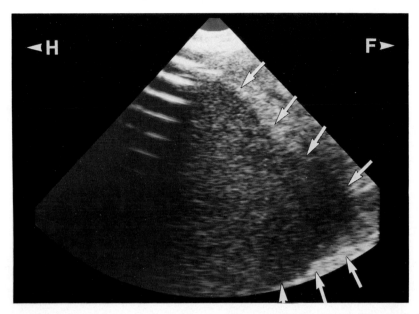

Fig. 58-13 This large sonolucent intrasplenic mass *(arrows)* was caused by evolving intrasplenic hematoma. *H,* Head; *F,* feet.

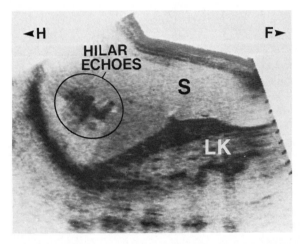

Fig. 58-14 This longitudinal ultrasonogram demonstrates markedly echogenic focus with focal acoustic shadowing that appears to be intrasplenic in location. Scans performed in other positions (right lateral decubitus and supine transverse), however, proved that echoes were caused by prominent splenic hilus. *S,* Spleen; *LK,* left kidney; *H,* head; *F,* feet.

the posterior aspect of the spleen (Fig. 58-15). Careful scanning and the use of longitudinal, transverse, and right lateral decubitus positions with appropriate acoustic windows should enable one to avoid these pitfalls.

The second normal anatomic structure that can cause confusion is the left lobe of the liver, which in some individuals extends between the spleen and left hemidiaphragm and can resemble a perisplenic (subcapsular) fluid collection[1,15] (Fig. 58-16). This pitfall can be avoided if one carefully observes during the real-time examination that the "perisplenic abnormality" appears

to move independently of the spleen during shallow respiration. In addition, it is frequently possible to identify small blood vessels within the pseudolesion that are caused by tributaries of the left portal venous system (their identification will undoubtedly become easier as deep and colored Doppler scans become increasingly available). Finally, a subcapsular pseudohematoma can be distinguished from a true hematoma by the fact that the pseudolesion is predominantly situated superior to the spleen, whereas a true subcapsular hematoma is localized primarily lateral to the spleen.

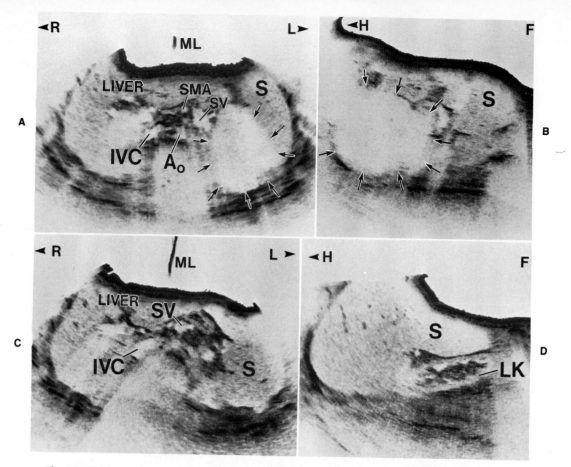

Fig. 58-15 Transverse, **A,** and longitudinal, **B,** scans in patient with splenomegaly *(S)* suggest presence of large sonolucent mass within spleen *(arrows)*. Repeat scans, **C** and **D,** performed with different angulation of transducer avoided scanning over fibrofatty tissues within hilar region of spleen. Pseudomass is no longer evident. *R,* Right; *L,* left; *ML,* midline; *LK,* left kidney; *IVC,* inferior vena cava; *Ao,* aorta; *SV,* splenic vein; *SMA,* superior mesenteric artery.

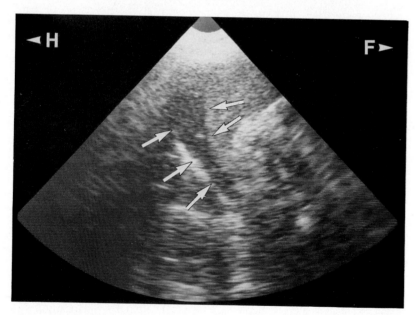

Fig. 58-16 This longitudinal sonogram demonstrates relatively sonolucent crescentic region *(arrows)* superior to spleen. Although this appearance can mimic subcapsular hematoma, it was subsequently shown to be left lobe of liver that extended superior to spleen. *H,* Head; *F,* feet.

REFERENCES

1. Arenson, AM, and McKee, JD: Left upper quadrant pseudolesion secondary to normal variants in liver and spleen, J Clin Ultrasound 14:558, 1986.
2. Asher, WM, et al: Echographic evaluation of splenic injury after blunt trauma, Radiology 118:411, 1976.
3. Bartrum, RJ, and Crow, HC: Gray scale ultrasound: a manual for physicians and technical personnel, Philadelphia, 1977, WB Saunders.
4. Coelho, JCU, et al: B-mode sonography of blood clots, J Clin Ultrasound 10:323, 1982.
5. Cunningham, JJ: Ultrasonic findings in isolated lymphoma of the spleen simulating splenic abscess, J Clin Ultrasound 6:412, 1978.
6. De Graaff, CS, Taylor, KJW, and Jacobson, P: Gray scale echography of the spleen, Ultrasound Med Biol 5:13, 1979.
7. Glancy, JJ: Fluid-filled echogenic epidermoid cyst of the spleen. J Clin Ultrasound 7:301, 1979.
8. Gooding, GAW: The ultrasonic and computed tomographic appearance of splenic lobulations: a consideration in the ultrasonic differential of masses adjacent to the left kidney, Radiology 126:719, 1978.
9. Hunter, TB, and Haber, K: Unusual sonographic appearance of the spleen in a case of myelofibrosis, AJR 128:138, 1977.
10. Kardel, T, et al: Ultrasonic determination of liver and spleen volumes, Scand J Clin Lab Invest 27:123, 1971.
11. Koga, T: Correlation between sectional area of the spleen by ultrasonic tomography and actual volume of the removed spleen, J Clin Ultrasound 7:119, 1979.
12. Koga, T, and Morikawa, Y: Ultrasonographic determination of the splenic size and its clinical usefulness in various liver diseases, Radiology 115:157, 1975.
13. Laing, FC, and Filly, RA: Problems in the application of ultrasonography for the evaluation of pleural opacities, Radiology 126:211, 1978.
14. Leopold, GR, and Asher, WM: Fundamentals of abdominal and pelvic ultrasonography, Philadelphia, 1975, WB Saunders.
15. Li, DKB, et al: Pseudo perisplenic "fluid collections": a clue to normal liver and spleen echogenic texture, J Ultrasound Med 5:397, 1986.
16. Lupien, C, and Sauerbrei, EE: Healing in the traumatized spleen: sonographic investigation, Radiology 151:181, 1984.
17. Maresca, G, et al: Sonographic patterns in splenic infarct, J Clin Ultrasound 14:23, 1986.
18. Mittelstaedt, CA, and Partain, CL: Ultrasonic-pathologic classification of splenic abnormalities: gray-scale patterns, Radiology 134:697, 1980.
19. Murphy, JF, and Bernardino, ME: The sonographic findings of splenic metastases, J Clin Ultrasound 7:195, 1979.
20. Propper, RA, et al: Ultrasonography of hemorrhagic splenic cysts, J Clin Ultrasound 7:18, 1979.
21. Ralls, PW, et al: Sonography of pyogenic splenic abscess, AJR 138:523, 1982.
22. Rasmussen, SN, et al: Spleen volume determination by ultrasonic scanning, Scand J Haematol 10:298, 1973.
23. Rochester, D, et al: Ultrasound in the staging of lymphoma, Radiology 124:483, 1977.
24. Romanes, CJ: Cunningham's textbook of anatomy, ed 10, London, 1964, Oxford University Press.
25. Siler, J, et al: Increased echogenicity of the spleen in benign and malignant disease, AJR 134:1011, 1980.
26. Solbiati, L, et al: Focal lesions in the spleen: sonographic patterns and guided biopsy, AJR 140:59, 1983.
27. Sommer, FG, et al: Spleen structure in Hodgkin disease: ultrasonic characterization, Radiology 153:219, 1984.
28. Subramanyam, BR, Balthazar, EJ, and Horii, SC: Sonography of the accessory spleen, AJR 143:47, 1984.
29. Taylor, KJW, and Milan, J: Differential diagnosis of chronic splenomegaly by grey-scale ultrasonography: clinical observations and digital A-scan analysis, Br J Radiol 49:519, 1976.
30. Weingarten, MJ, et al: Sonography after splenic embolization: the wedge-shaped acute infarct, AJR 142:957, 1984.
31. Yeh, HC, and Wolf, BS: Ultrasonic contrast study to identify stomach tap water microbubbles, J Clin Ultrasound 5:170, 1977.

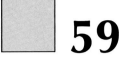

59 *Magnetic Resonance Imaging*

RALPH WEISSLEDER
PETER F. HAHN
DAVID D. STARK

MR1 TECHNIQUES
Pulse sequences
Imaging plane

BENIGN DISEASE
Hemorrhage
Iron overload
Infarction
Benign splenomegaly

TUMOR
Detection
Lymphoma
Leukemia
Metastases
Benign tumors

FUTURE DEVELOPMENT
Contrast agents

□ **TABLE 59-1**
Tissue composition and relaxation times

Parameter	Spleen		Liver	
Water (%)	77%	(72%-79%)	71%	(64%-74%)
Lipid (%)	1.6%	(1%-3%)	7.9%	(1%-11%)
Protein (%)	19%	(18%-20%)	18%	(16%-22%)
Blood content (ml)	60-120		250	
Iron (mg/g wet tissue)	0.049	(0.02-0.12)	0.32	(0.13-0.58)
T_1 (msec, 20 MHz)	805 ± 263		499 ± 140	
T_2 (msec, 20 MHz)	70 ± 20		48 ± 11	
N(H)	481 ± 143		583 ± 151	

Magnetic resonance imaging of the spleen has been difficult for many reasons. Most important, motion artifacts can severely decrease image quality in the abdomen and commonly result in nondiagnostic MRI. New techniques to suppress motion artifacts are currently in clinical investigation and have been shown to improve image quality. Second, splenic neoplasms have been difficult to detect because of the small difference in tumor-spleen relaxation times and proton densities. Administration of particulate MRI contrast agents, such as ferrite, has proved to increase tumor-spleen contrast greatly and thus increase tumor detectability. Although the spleen has not been studied as extensively as other abdominal organs, these recent advances are expected to increase the utility of MRI for detecting splenic disease.

MRI TECHNIQUES
Pulse sequences

A routine technique of MRI of the spleen includes acquisition of images with different contrast dependencies. Spin echo (SE) pulse sequences with T_1-dependent contrast ("T_1-weighted sequences": TR < 500, TE < 30 msec) are routinely acquired in abdominal imaging because of excellent anatomic resolution (high SNR). Reduction of TR to less than the tissue T_1 (Table 59-1) increases SNR per unit time and allows extensive signal averaging to reduce motion artifacts. Shortening of TE complements reductions in TR by increasing SNR and T_1-dependent image contrast and by further suppressing ghost artifacts.[22]

Spin echo pulse sequences with T_2-dependent image contrast ("T_2-weighted sequences": TR = 2000 to 3000 msec, TE > 60 msec) techniques are usually acquired to detect splenic lesions with a long T_2 (necrosis) and to characterize lesions with different T_2 (cysts versus solid tumors). Although increasing TR and TE increases T_2-weighted contrast, images are more susceptible to motion artifacts, resulting in trade-off in anatomic resolution. The optimum TE depends mostly on the difference in T_2 relaxation times of tumor and spleen. Large differences

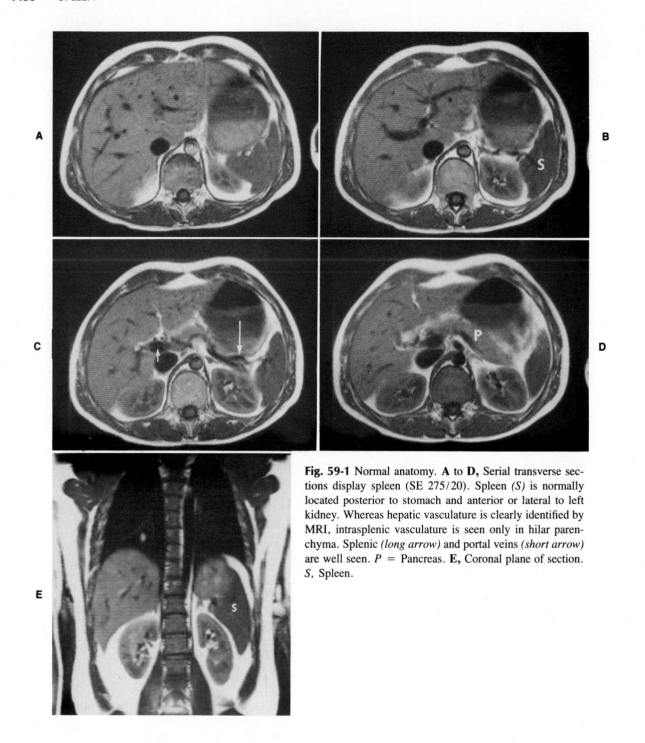

Fig. 59-1 Normal anatomy. **A** to **D,** Serial transverse sections display spleen (SE 275/20). Spleen *(S)* is normally located posterior to stomach and anterior or lateral to left kidney. Whereas hepatic vasculature is clearly identified by MRI, intrasplenic vasculature is seen only in hilar parenchyma. Splenic *(long arrow)* and portal veins *(short arrow)* are well seen. *P* = Pancreas. **E,** Coronal plane of section. *S,* Spleen.

in T$_2$ (such as cyst-spleen) result in higher CNR with long TE, whereas smaller differences (such as metastasis-spleen) result in lower CNR.

The spleen is readily displayed with routine abdominal MRI techniques. Transverse planes of section demonstrate the upper third of spleen posterior to the stomach, the middle third posterior to small bowel loops, and the inferior third lateral to the left kidney (Fig. 59-1). Splenic

contour is well delineated by intraperitoneal fat of a high signal intensity on motion artifact–resistant T$_1$-weighted pulse sequences. On T$_2$-weighted pulse sequences splenic parenchyma and perisplenic fat may have similar signal intensities. Despite having well-defined histologic architecture, this intrasplenic anatomy is not visible by MRI. The splenic vein is seen on transverse images in 90% to 100% of patients. However, intrasplenic vasculature is

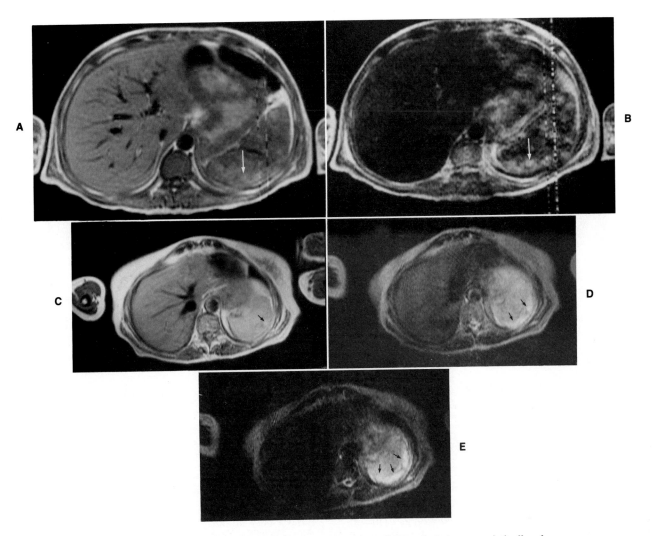

Fig. 59-2 Hemorrhage. Intrasplenic hemorrhage occurs most frequently in hematopoietic disorders (increased clotting times) or after trauma. **A** and **B,** Patient with lymphoma, multiple blood transfusions, and increased clotting time (**A** = SE 500/28, **B** = SE 2000/84/2). Multiple blood transfusions have led to iron overload with decrease in hepatic and splenic MRI signal intensity. Multiple intrasplenic areas of hyperintensity are seen on both T_1 and T_2 weighted images. **C** to **E,** T_1-weighted images (**C** = SE 300/20) show small zone of splenic hyperrintensity. T_2-weighted images (**D** = SE 2000/120; **E** = SE 2000/180) display subcapsular hematoma *(arrows)* as linear region of hyperintensity. Electronic image windowing is optimized to differentiate spleen and hematoma.

visible by MRI only in the central (hilar) third of splenic parenchyma.

Imaging plane

Abdominal organs are best imaged either in or perpendicular to their anatomic axis. Transverse planes of section routinely demonstrate the spleen and splenic vasculature and seem to be sufficient for diagnostic purposes in most cases. However, images in coronal planes of section may be acquired to evaluate the diaphragmatic portion of the spleen. Changing the plane of section can also prove advantageous in displacing motion artifacts.

BENIGN DISEASE
Hemorrhage

Splenic hemorrhage occurs most frequently after trauma and in patients with coagulopathy. Trauma commonly leads to subcapsular bleeding, and if the splenic capsule remains intact, blood accumulates under pressure, changing the normally convex splenic contour (Fig. 59-2). Coagulopathy-induced splenic hemorrhages most commonly cause intraparenchymal bleeding (Fig. 59-2).

Hemorrhage can be distinguished from normal splenic parenchyma because of its prolonged T_2. Furthermore, blood undergoes a complex transformation into para-

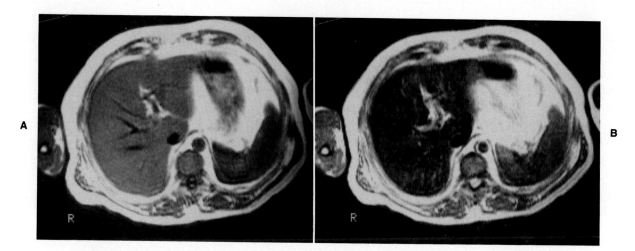

Fig. 59-3 Hemochromatosis. Iron overload reduces splenic and hepatic tissue relaxation times and thus MRI signal intensity. Although liver shows slight reduction in signal intensity on SE 260/18 images **(A)**, spleen still appears hypointense relative to liver. With T_2-weighted SE 2000/120 sequence **(B)** normal spleen would appear hyperintense relative to liver. In this case both spleen and liver signal intensities are decreased because of iron overload.

magnetic degradation products after extravasation. Acute hematomas (<24 hours) consist predominantly of oxyhemoglobin and deoxyhemoglobin and are still isointense, with splenic parenchyma on T_1 and T_2-weighted images. Subacute (>3 days) and chronic hematomas (>14 days) contain predominantly methemoglobin (T_1 shortening) and hemosiderin (T_2 shortening). Chronic hematomas become markedly hyperintense on T_1- and T_2-weighted pulse sequences (T_1 shortening of methemoglobin) and show a peripheral hypointense ring (T_2 shortening of hemosiderin).

Iron overload

Unlike hereditary hemochromatosis, which preferentially causes hepatocellular iron deposition, hemolysis initially causes greater concentration of excess iron in the spleen. However, chronic iron overload leads to massive iron deposition (hemosiderin, ferritin) in both liver and spleen. Regardless of the underlying pathologic process, iron overload shortens T_2 and reduces image signal intensity (Fig. 59-3).

Patients with sickle cell anemia (hemolysis of rigid and deformed erythrocytes) show an abnormally low spleen signal intensity on T_1- and T_2-weighted pulse sequences.[1] Masses of relatively hyperintense splenic tissue may represent infarcts.[1]

Infarction

Splenic infarcts most commonly occur in hemoglobinopathies (sickle cell disease, myeloproliferative disease) or in systemic embolism (endocarditis, septum de-

fects). Other causes of splenic infarcts (splenic artery aneurysm, local atherosclerosis) are rare. Infarcts vary in size but rarely involve the entire organ. Infarcts are peripherally located and have a wedge-shaped appearance in 33% of cases. In the remainder of cases infarcts appear as multiple heterogeneous (42%) or massive (25%) lesions replacing normal splenic tissue.[3]

The MRI appearance of splenic infarcts has been described only in sickle cell disease[1] and lymphoma.[13] In all cases iron overload was present and probably facilitated detection by MRI. Infarcts appeared on both T_1 and T_2 images as structures of high signal intensity against the abnormally reduced signal from the iron-overloaded splenic parenchyma. In non–iron overloaded spleens the infarct-spleen contrast is probably lower, and small infarcts may not be detectable by MRI. In analogy to CT[3] the signal intensity of splenic infarcts is expected to vary in histologic stages of congestion, hemorrhage, inflammation, organization, and fibrosis.

Benign splenomegaly

Congestion is the most common cause of benign splenomegaly. Whether vascular obstruction arises in the portal vein, in the venous channels within the liver, or in the hepatic veins, the effect on the spleen is the same. MRI signal intensity of congested spleens is similar to that of normal spleens (Fig. 59-4). Portosystemic collaterals are demonstrated by MRI as structures of low signal intensity on SE images (Fig. 59-4) and of high signal intensity on gradient-echo images.

Inflammatory and hyperplastic benign splenomegaly

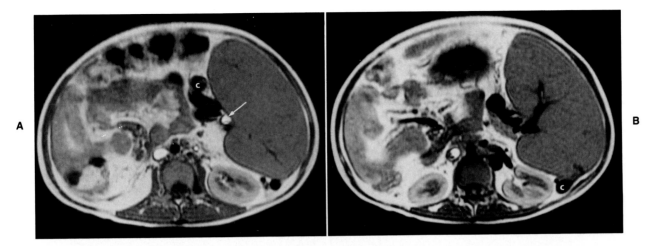

Fig. 59-4 Portal hypertension. **A** and **B,** Patient with hepatic cirrhosis and portal hypertension (SE 500/28/6). There are prominent venous collaterals in splenic hilum *(C)* and posterior pole of spleen. High signal intensity in one collateral *(arrow)* is due to entry slice phenomenon. Spleen appears homogeneous. Intrasplenic vasculature is well seen because of venous dilatation.

☐ **TABLE 59-2**

Relaxation times and tumor-spleen and tumor-liver contrast

	Spleen	Tumor	Liver
T_1 (msec)	805 ± 263	876 ± 334	499 ± 140
T_2 (msec)	70 ± 20	78 ± 32	48 ± 11
N(H)	481 ± 143	519 ± 239	583 ± 151
T_1 contrast	0.042	—	0.274
T_2 contrast	0.054	—	0.238
N(H) contrast	0.038	—	0.058

T_1 contrast: $|T_1$ tissue $- T_1$ tumor$|/T_1$ tissue $+ T_1$ tumor. T_2 contrast: $|T_2$ tissue $- T_2$ tumor$|/T_2$ tissue $+ T_2$ tumor. N(H) contrast: $|$N(H)tissue $-$ N(H) tumor$|/$N(H) tissue $+$ N(H) tumor.

has been studied experimentally by MRI.[27] These experimental results[27] and clinical observation[25] indicate that MRI does not allow differentiation of various forms of benign splenomegaly or even differentiation from malignant splenomegaly.

TUMOR
Detection

Detection of focal splenic tumors by MRI has been disappointing for many reasons. Normal splenic parenchyma and tumor tissue have similar relaxation times and similar proton densities, resulting in low tumor-spleen contrast (Table 59-2).[9] Second, motion from stomach, bowel, or heart frequently blurs anatomic boundaries of the spleen and casts ghost artifacts onto the spleen (Fig. 59-5). Third, splenic anatomy varies considerably among individuals and even in the same individual. Splenic lobulations may thus be mistaken for tumor, and tumor may be misdiagnosed as a normal variant. Fourth, inability to observe intrasplenic anatomy on MRI has added to the insensitivity of MRI in detecting focal splenic tumors. Deviation of hepatic vasculature is a useful sign of mass lesions that is not applicable to the spleen. Fifth, the most common splenic tumors (lymphoma) often show a diffuse or miliary pattern of spread, with tumor nodules measuring less than 1 cm.

Despite the insensitivity of MRI in diagnosing splenic tumors, detection is possible under certain circumstances. Necrotic tumors show T_1 and T_2 relaxation times longer than those for spleen and are best detected on either heavily T_1- or heavily T_2-weighted pulse sequences (Fig. 59-6). Unfortunately tumor necrosis is a late event of tumor outgrowing its vascular supply. Distortion of splenic anatomy has occasionally been found useful in diagnosing spenic tumors (Fig. 59-7).[9] Hemochromatosis decreases the relaxation times of normal spenic tissue, and in vivo signal intensity is reduced. Since a tumor does not take up T_2-shortening hemoglobin degradation products, its signal intensity remains unchanged, tumor-spleen contrast is increased, and lesions become more conspicuous (Fig. 59-8). Tumor-induced hemorrhage (see the section on hemorrhage and Fig. 59-2) can be detected by MRI as lesions of high signal intensity on both T_1- and T_2-weighted pulse sequences.

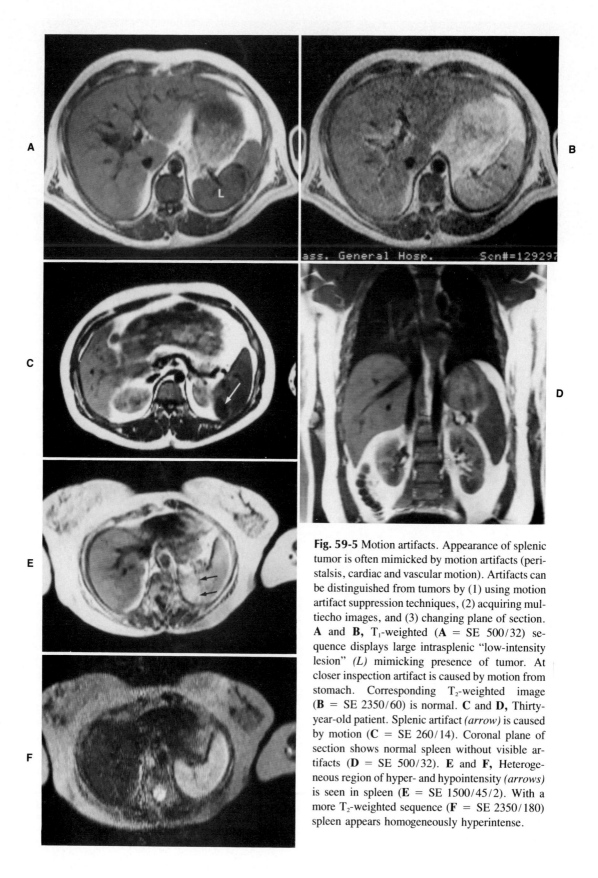

Fig. 59-5 Motion artifacts. Appearance of splenic tumor is often mimicked by motion artifacts (peristalsis, cardiac and vascular motion). Artifacts can be distinguished from tumors by (1) using motion artifact suppression techniques, (2) acquiring multiecho images, and (3) changing plane of section. **A** and **B,** T_1-weighted (**A** = SE 500/32) sequence displays large intrasplenic "low-intensity lesion" *(L)* mimicking presence of tumor. At closer inspection artifact is caused by motion from stomach. Corresponding T_2-weighted image (**B** = SE 2350/60) is normal. **C** and **D,** Thirty-year-old patient. Splenic artifact *(arrow)* is caused by motion (**C** = SE 260/14). Coronal plane of section shows normal spleen without visible artifacts (**D** = SE 500/32). **E** and **F,** Heterogeneous region of hyper- and hypointensity *(arrows)* is seen in spleen (**E** = SE 1500/45/2). With a more T_2-weighted sequence (**F** = SE 2350/180) spleen appears homogeneously hyperintense.

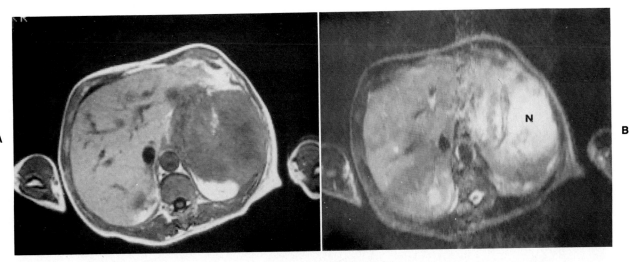

Fig. 59-6 Tumor necrosis. Tumor hemorrhage and necrosis are readily detectable by MRI. Central foci of hemorrhage or necrosis are often only clue to presence of splenic neoplasm. **A,** Gastric adenocarcinoma with hepatosplenic metastases. Entire spleen is replaced by inhomogeneous low-intensity tumor. Hilar vessels are displaced (SE 300/14). **B,** Corresponding SE 2350/180 image. Splenic tumor necrosis *(N)* is now identified as irregular zone of hyperintensity. Intrahepatic infiltration is appreciated. Note multiple hepatic metastases.

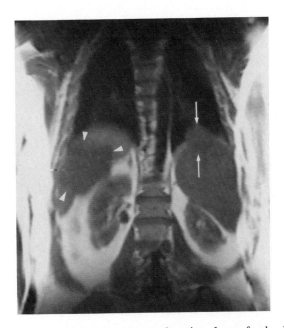

Fig. 59-7 Splenic morphologic features and tumor detection. Large focal splenic tumors cause contour changes of spleen that can be detected by MRI. T_1-weighted coronal image shows that focal lymphoma arises from dome of spleen *(arrows)*. Tumor is isointense with adjacent spleen and invisible on transverse T_1-weighted and T_2-weighted images. Because lymphoma has lower signal intensity than has liver, concurrent liver lesions are more easily detected *(arrowheads)*.

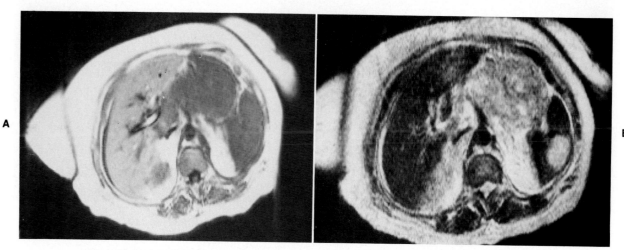

Fig. 59-8 Hemochromatosis and splenic tumor. **A,** Heavily T_1-weighted magnetic resonance images (SE 260/14/12) are insensitive in demonstrating incipient changes of hepatosplenic iron overload. Signal intensities of spleen and liver appear normal. Splenic tumor is not detected. **B,** T_2-weighted images are more sensitive in detecting incipient hemochromatosis (predominant T_2 shortening of liver and spleen) (SE 2350/60). Splenic tumor is clearly seen because of decreased signal intensity of iron-overloaded spleen.

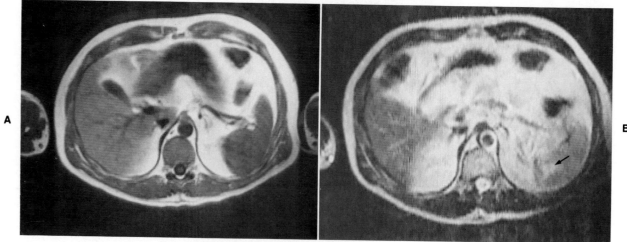

Fig. 59-9 Focal splenic lymphoma. **A,** Non-Hodgkin's lymphoma (SE 300/14). No abnormality is seen. **B,** Corresponding SE 2350/180 image. Small region of high signal intensity *(arrow)* is due to tumor necrosis. True size of lymphoma is underestimated.

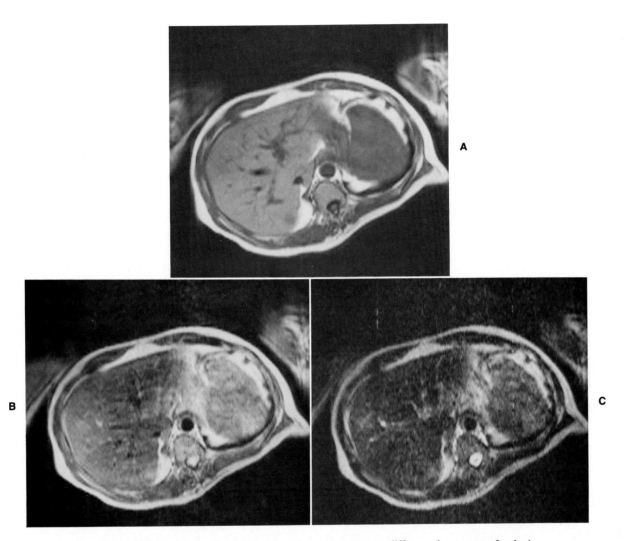

Fig. 59-10 Diffuse splenic lymphoma. Lymphoma presents as diffuse enlargement of splenic parenchyma in approximately half of all cases. Since many patients with splenic lymphoma have spleens of normal size and many patients without splenic lymphoma have splenomegaly, sensitivity of splenomegaly as diagnostic criterion of lymphoma is only 35%. **A,** SE 275/14 of diffusely enlarged spleen in patients with stage IV lymphoma. No focal abnormality is seen. Signal intensity of spleen appears normal. **B** and **C,** Corresponding SE 2350/60 (**B**) and SE 2350/180 (**C**).

Lymphoma

The cut sectional surface of lymphomatous spleens reveals three patterns of tumor distribution: (1) diffuse homogeneous spread, not visible macroscopically (Fig. 59-9); (2) multinodular ("miliary") form with nodules less than 1 cm in diameter; and (3) nodular pattern with masses often several centimeters in diameter (Fig. 59-10 and Table 59-3).* Histiocytic, large cell non-Hodgkin's lymphoma often produces large focal splenic masses several centimeters in diameter, whereas 30% to 65% of patients with Hodgkin's disease show tumor nodules approximately 1 cm in diameter. Lymphocytic non-Hodgkin's lymphoma most commonly shows a "miliary" pattern of distribution, with tumor deposits of less than 1 cm in diameter.

Splenic lymphoma has been studied by MRI only in small series of patients, by means of different imaging techniques.* Prospective clinical trials using pathologic

---

*References 2, 6, 7, 10, 14, 17, 20, 28.

*References 5, 9, 11, 13, 15, 18, 26.

☐ **TABLE 59-3**

Pattern of spread of splenic lymphoma[2,4,7,10,14,17,20]

Lymphoma	Size	Frequency
Hodgkin's disease		
Diffuse	Not visible*	14% (0%-33%)
Multinodular	<1 cm	29% (23%-38%)
Focal	>1 cm	55% (33%-64%)
Non-Hodgkin's lymphoma		
Diffuse	Not visible*	30% (0%-36%)
Multinodular	<1 cm	40% (30%-55%)
Unifocal	>1 cm	30% (9%-70%)
Leukemia, histiocytosis		
Diffuse	Not visible*	100%

*Not visible macroscopically; splenomegaly may be present (60% to 80%) or absent (20% to 40%).

correlation as the "gold standard" have not been reported. As a result, reported sensitivity for detecting splenic lymphoma varies from 10% to 87% (Table 59-4). Splenic size as a diagnostic criterion of splenic lymphoma has a poor correlation unless the spleen is greatly enlarged. Focal splenic lesions are seen more commonly in Hodgkin's disease than in non-Hodgkin's lymphoma (Tables 59-3 and 59-4). Focal splenic lymphoma can appear as lesions of low or high signal intensity on T_1- or T_2-weighted pulse sequences.[13,18] The varying signal intensity is most likely attributable to concomitant presence of iron overload, hemorrhage, and fibrous lymphoma components.

Leukemia

The MRI appearance of leukemic spleens has been reported only in case presentations.[25] Our initial experience suggest that only massively infiltrated leukemic spleens have a higher in vivo MRI signal intensity than have normal spleens (Fig. 59-11). With a SE technique SNR of grades III and IV leukemic spleens was 43.3 ± 4.3 (normal 25.8 ± 7.1) for an SE of 500/28 and 29.1 ± 7.1 (normal 24.5 ± 9.4) for an SE 1500/84. Grades I and II leukemic spleens showed characteristics of MRI signal intensity identical to those of normal spleens. Indications for performing MRI on leukemic patients are the same as for CT and ultrasonography; evaluation of pain in the left upper quadrant and exclusion of focal spenic lesions (infarct, abscess).

Metastases

The most common primary sources of splenic metastases are melanoma and breast and lung cancer. Despite the insensitivity of MRI, four distinct patterns of metastases have can be detected by MRI: necrotic tumors (long T_2), hemorrhagic tumors (short T_1), tumors that cause gross splenic deformity, and focal splenic tumors in the presence of transfusional iron overload.[9]

Benign tumors

Benign splenic tumors are most commonly incidental findings detected on routine MRI. Cysts are the most common benign tumors, with a predominance in the young age group (younger than 30 years). True cysts (primary cysts, 20%) have a cellular lining and are congenital in origin, whereas false cysts (secondary cysts, 80%) do not have a cellular lining and are traumatic in origin. The average cyst size is 10 cm, ranging from 2 to 27 cm.[8] Hemangiomas are the second and lymphangiomas the third most common benign tumors of the spleen.

The T_1 and T_2 relaxation times of benign cysts are longer (increased water content) than those of solid splenic tumors. As a result cysts are well visualized on both T_1-weighted (hypointense relative to spleen) and T_2-weighted pulse sequences (hyperintense relative of spleen) (Fig. 59-12). However, with T_2-weighted short TE (<60 msec) sequences, cyst content and splenic parenchyma may appear isointense and the lesions are not detectable. It is unlikely that MRI will aid in the differential diagnosis of true and false splenic cysts, since they exhibit similar relaxation times. One fourth of cysts have calcified walls that appear as hypointense rings on T_1- and T_2-weighted images (Fig. 59-13).

Splenic hemangiomas have the same features on MRI as hemangiomas in other parts of the body.[8,16,19,21,25] On T_1-weighted SE sequences hemangiomas appear hypointense, and on T_2-weighted sequences they are markedly hyperintense relative to spleen. Small hemangiomas are homogeneous and have a smooth, well-defined contour. Giant hemangiomas may exhibit some heterogeneity caused by hemorrhage, thrombosis, fibrosis, and hemosiderin deposition.

FUTURE DEVELOPMENT

The most important clinical applications of splenic imaging are detection of splenic involvement in patients with lymphoma, differential diagnosis of splenomegaly, and staging of metastatic cancer. Routine MRI techniques used for splenic imaging have shown considerable motion artifact degradation and low lesion-spleen contrast, resulting in no or only marginal diagnostic benefit of splenic MRI. Preliminary clinical and experimental experience suggests that two major advances, the implementation of motion artifact suppression techniques and the use of tissue-specific contrast agents, will greatly modify the role of MRI for diagnosing splenic disease.

☐ **TABLE 59-4**

MRI of splenic lymphoma

Type	Reference	MRI technique	Sensitivity (%)	Specificity (%)
Hodgkin's lymphoma	31	T_1-weighted, T_2-weighted SE	71	
	30	T_1-weighted, T_2-weighted SE	67	100
Non-Hodgkin's lymphoma	31	T_1-weighted, T_2-weighted SE	10	
Combined	31	T_1-weighted, T_2-weighted SE	35	
	32	T_1-weighted, T_2-weighted SE	38	
	10	T_1-weighted, T_2-weighted GR	87	50
	29	T_1-weighted, T_2-weighted SE	81	50

MRI techniques: 52:SE 500/30, SE 900/30, SE 1500/30, 60, 90, SE 2000/120; 53:SE 275/14, SE 2350/60, 120, 180; 39: SE 800/30, 60, 90, 120; 5*: flash 80/16/ 60°, flash 80/16/30°; 40: SE 300/20, SE 800/25, SE 2000/40, 80.

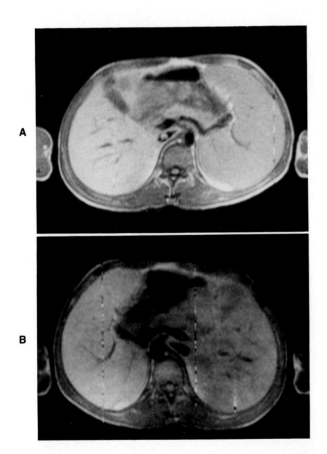

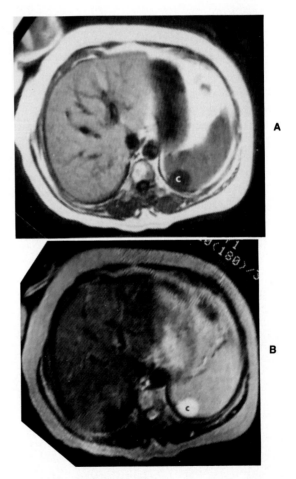

Fig. 59-11 Splenic leukemia. Leukemia often causes diffuse massive splenomegaly. In patients with left flank pain, MRI can be indicated to rule out splenic infarcts or necrosis and measure extent of splenic enlargement. **A,** Acute lymphocytic leukemia (SE 500/28). Massive splenomegaly is typical finding of acute lymphocytic leukemia. Spleen usually appears homogeneous, and few hilar vessels are seen. **B,** Corresponding SE 1500/42.

Fig. 59-12 Cyst *(C)*. Splenic cysts show signal intensity similar to that of liver cysts; that is, they are as hyperintense as bile and cerebrospinal fluid on T_2-weighted images. **A,** Note that cyst has signal intensity lower than that of splenic and hepatic parenchyma on T_1-weighted images (SE 260/14). **B,** Corresponding T_2-weighted SE 3000/120 sequence. Signal intensity of cyst behaves in manner similar to that of other fluid-filled structures with long T_2 relaxation times (cerebrospinal fluid).

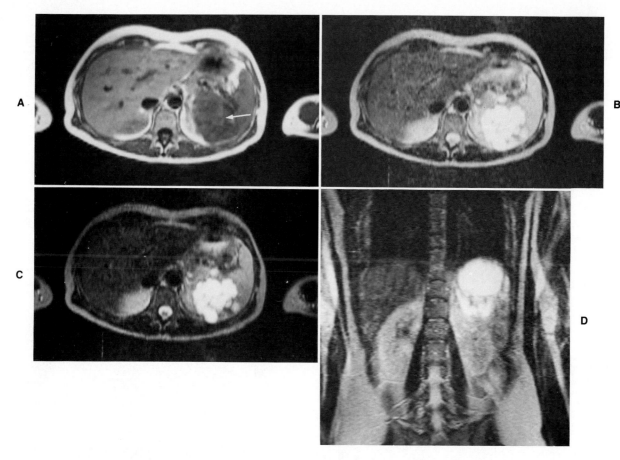

Fig. 59-13 Multiple calcified cysts. **A,** Mass lesions of low signal intensity are seen in posterior part of spleen *(arrow)*, distorting normal anatomy (SE 320/20). T₁-weighted images do not allow differential diagnosis of splenic mass lesions. **B** and **C,** T₂-weighted images (**B** = SE 2350/120, **C** = SE 2350/180) show multiple lesions of high signal intensity. With heavily T₂-weighted sequences cysts have signal intensity similar to that of cerebrospinal fluid. **D,** SE 2350/120 coronal image.

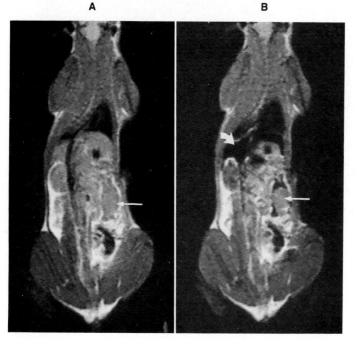

Fig. 59-14 Ferrite-enhanced tumor detection. Routine MRI techniques are not sufficiently sensitive to be useful in detection of splenic tumors. Ferrite has been shown to increase tumor-spleen contrast significantly in animal models. Clinical studies to assess efficacy of ferrite-enhanced MRI are currently underway. **A,** Coronal image (SE 500/32) of tumor-bearing animal before administration of ferrite. Note poor tumor-spleen contrast *(solid arrow)*, which does not allow detection of intrasplenic mass. **B,** Coronal image (SE 500/32) after administration of ferrite. Administration of ferrite increases tumor-spleen contrast 43-fold; normal splenic tissue is seen as dark rim surrounding tumor. *Curved arrow,* Liver.

☐ **TABLE 59-5**

Splenectomy performed for splenomegaly of unknown cause[12]

Disease	Frequency (%)	
Lymphoma	31	
Lymphocytic lymphoma		69
Other malignant lymphoma		19
Hodgkin's disease		6
Leukemia		6
	25	
Congestive		
Inflammatory	19	
Infiltrative		15
Histiocytosis		50
Lipogranulomatosis		25
Plasmacytoma		12.5
Myeloid metaplasia		12.5
Cysts	6	
Other	4	

Contrast agents

Magnetic resonance imaging enhanced by crystalline iron oxide (ferrite) shows the greatest promise in MRI of the spleen. As a particulate contrast agent, ferrite exploits the RE function of the spleen and therefore acts as a tissue–specific rather than a nonspecific contrast agent. Ferrite particles are phagocytosed by macrophages located in the red pulp but not splenic tumor. As a result, relaxation times and MRI signal intensity of spleen decrease profoundly, whereas tumor remains unaffected. Initial experience shows at least three different clinical advantages of ferrite-enhanced MRI of the spleen: (1) increased tumor detection, (2) improved differential diagnosis of splenomegaly, and (3) reduction of motion artifacts as a result of reduced signal intensity.

Detectability of focal intrasplenic lesions increases after administration of ferrite (35-fold increase in CNR; Fig. 59-14),[23] and splenic tumors as small as 2×3 mm can be detected in humans by means of widely available imaging techniques.[24] Use of high-resolution techniques (increase in phase encoding steps, surface coils) is expected to improve splenic tumor detectability further.

Differential diagnosis of splenomegaly is of considerable clinical importance. Approximately one third of enlarged spleens of unknown origin are caused by lymphoma. Conversely, one third of enlarged spleens in patients with lymphoma are of benign origin (Table 59-5). Investigation in animals has shown that ferrite-enhanced MRI can significantly improve the differential diagnosis of malignant and benign splenomegaly.[27] In malignant splenomegaly (for example, diffuse splenic lymphoma) macrophages located in the red pulp are displaced by lymphoma cells. After administration of ferrite, fewer particles are taken up per unit weight of tissue, resulting in little or no change in spleen relaxation times and in vivo MRI signal intensity. In benign splenomegaly (reactive hyperplasia, congestion) the red pulp/white pulp ratio remains the same, phagocytosis is not impaired, and spleen signal intensity decreases in a fashion similar to that in normal spleens. Clinical trials of ferrite-enhanced MRI for the detection of diffuse splenic lymphoma and differential diagnosis of splenomegaly are in progress.

References

1. Adler, DD, Glazer, GM, and Aisen, AM: MRI of the spleen: normal appearance and findings in sickle cell anemia, AJR 147:843, 1986.
2. Ahmann, DL, Kiely, JM, Harrison, EG, et al: Malignant lymphoma of the spleen: a review of 49 cases in which the diagnosis was made at splenectomy, Cancer 19:461, 1966.
3. Balcar, I, et al: CT patterns of splenic infarction: a clinical and experimental study, Radiology 151:723, 1984.
4. Burke, JS: Surgical pathology of the spleen: an approach to the differential diagnosis of splenic lymphomas and leukemias. Part II. Diseases of the red pulp, Am J Surg Path 5:681, 1981.
5. Cohen, MD, et al: Magentic resonance imaging of lymphomas in children, Pediatr Radiol 15:179, 1985.
6. Davey, FR, Skarin, AT, and Moloney, WC: Pathology of splenic lymphoma, Am J Clin Pathol 59:95, 1973.
7. Farrer-Brown, G, et al: The diagnosis of Hodgkin's disease in surgically excised spleens, J Clin Pathol 25:294, 1972.
8. Garvin, DF, and Kling, FM: Cysts and non-lymphomatous tumors of the spleen, Pathol Annu 16:61, 1981.
9. Hahn, PF, et al: MRI of splenic tumors, AJR, 150:823, 1988.
10. Harris, NL, et al: Diffuse large cell (histiocytic) lymphoma of the spleen, Cancer 54:2460, 1984.
11. Heelan, RT, et al: Magnetic resonance imaging of the spleen in Hodgkin's disease, New York, Society of Magnetic Resonance Imaging Annual Meeting, 1987, p. 85.
12. Herman, RE, DeHaven, KE, and Hawk, WA: Splenectomy for the diagnosis of splenomegaly, Ann Surg 168:896, 1968.
13. Hess, CF, et al: Splenic involvement by malignant lymphoma: improved detection by MR imaging compared with US and dynamic CT scanning, Radiology 161(P):207, 1986.
14. Kim, H, and Dorfman, RF: Morphological studies of 84 untreated patients subjected to laparatomy for the staging of non-Hodgkin's lymphoma, Cancer 33:657, 1974.
15. Kurdziel, JC, et al: MR imaging of the spleen and bone marrow in hemopathies, Radiology 165(P):201, 1987.
16. Levine, E, Wetzel, LH, and Neff, JR: MR imaging and CT of extrahepatic cavernous hemangiomas, AJR 147:1299, 1986.
17. Lowenbraun, S, et al: Diagnostic laparatomy and splenectomy for staging Hodgkin's disease, Ann Intern Med 72:655, 1970.
18. Nyman, R, et al: Magnetic resonance imaging, chest radiography, computed tomography and ultrasonography in malignant lymphoma, Acta Radiol 28:253, 1987.
19. Ross, PR, et al: Hemangioma of the spleen: radiologic-pathologic correlation in 10 cases, Radiology 162:74, 1987.
20. Skarin, AT, Davey, FR, and Moloney, WC: Lymphosarcoma of the spleen, Arch Intern Med 127:259, 1971.

21. Stark, DD, et al: Magnetic resonance imaging of cavernous hemangioma of the liver: tissue specific characterization, AJR 145:213, 1985.

22. Stark, DD, et al: Motion artifact reduction with fast spin echo imaging, Radiology 164:183, 1987.

23. Weissleder, R, et al: MR imaging of splenic metastases: ferrite-enhanced detection in rats, AJR 149:723, 1987.

24. Weissleder, R, Hahn, PF, Stark, DD, et al: Ferrite enhanced MRI of focal splenic tumors, Radiology. (Submitted for publication.)

25. Weissleder, R, and Stark, DD: MR atlas of the abdomen, London, 1989, Martin Dunitz Publisher. (In press.)

26. Weissleder, R, et al: MRI of hepatic lymphoma, Magn Reson Imaging 6(S):77, 1987.

27. Weissleder, R, et al: Splenic lymphoma: ferrite-enhanced MRI in rodents, Radiology 166:423, 1988.

28. Wick, MR, et al: Primary nonlymphoreticular malignant neoplasms of the spleen, Am J Surg Pathol 6:229, 1982.

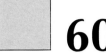

60 *Nuclear Medicine*

DAVID C. PRICE

ANATOMY AND PHYSIOLOGY

The spleen is a sinusoidal vascular filter that is an integral part of the reticuloendothelial system and is the largest single lymphoid organ in the body. Thus it has important scavenging and immunologic functions in humans. It is also a site for normal hematopoiesis in humans during the third to sixth months of gestation. Splenic hematopoiesis does occur normally in adult animals of other species (for instance, mouse, rat, rabbit), but it is seen postnatally in humans only when they have certain hematologic disorders such as myelofibrosis with myeloid metaplasia and severe hemolytic anemias.

Other normal functions of the spleen include its role as a reservoir for blood and for platelets and granulocytes, and the active process of cleaning up or removing from circulation any cells that are immature, damaged or senescent, particularly erythrocytes.[52] The spleen is a part of the portal circulation, receiving approximately 2% of the cardiac output through the celiac and splenic arteries and draining through the splenic vein into the portal circulation. Thus splenomegaly is frequently associated with diseases affecting portal venous drainage.

The spleen normally increases in size through childhood to a maximum in the early teens or early twenties,[6] then diminishes somewhat in size thereafter. In one adult series the average spleen's weight ranged from 146 g at age 20 to 78 g at age 79, with a distinct sexual differential.[9] Ordinarily the spleen must be enlarged two to three times before it can be palpated clinically below the left anterior costal margin. As a result, noninvasive methods for quantitating spleen size can be useful in the evaluation of certain diseases, such as in confirming the diagnosis of polycythemia vera.[57]

In its role as a reticuloendothelial organ the adult human spleen serves as a vascular scavenger. Arterial blood filters through a network of arterioles, cords, and sinuses in a closed system that requires the blood cells to be pliable and brings them into intimate contact with macrophages suspended on the reticulin stroma of the cords.[56] Erythrocyte culling and pitting functions as described by Crosby[7] result in a transient retention of immature circulating erythroid cells until residual intracellular nuclear fragments have been extruded. The increased risk for overwhelming infection in children and adults whose spleen has been removed for reasons other than acute trauma would appear to be caused by the loss of both its phagocytic and its immunologic (antibody-producing) contributions to the monitoring of the circulating blood.[4]

The ability of the spleen to phagocytose intravascular foreign particles and to recognize and destroy damaged erythrocytes is the basis for the current use of radiopharmaceuticals in spleen scintigraphy.

RADIOPHARMACEUTICALS
Radiolabeled damaged erythrocytes

Following the initial description of erythrocyte labeling with chromium-51 by Gray and Sterling[17] in 1950, Johnson et al.[23] first established the ability to image the spleen using chromium-51-labeled erythrocytes "damaged" with incomplete anti-D antibodies. Winkelman et al.[59] then extended this principle to the now-traditional method of damaging erythrocyte membranes by heating them. The quality of chromium-51 scintigraphic images is considerably compromised by its 320-keV gamma emission and 9% gamma abundance. More recently, therefore, technetium-99m(^{99m}Tc) has been used to label autologous erythrocytes[11] with cell membranes damaged either by heat or by an excess of tin.[12] The recommended degree of heat damage to labeled erythrocytes for effective splenic scintigraphy is 49° to 50° C for 15 to 45 minutes.[2,10] Such procedures are still complex in that one must label, sensitize, and wash autologous erythrocytes in vitro before reinfusion and imaging. The use of mercury-203– or mercury-197–labeled MHP (1-mercury-2-hydroxypropane) has waned because of the considerable radiation dose to the spleen, even though with this method the necessity for in vitro labeling and damaging of erythrocytes is eliminated.

Radiocolloids

Since the original description of its production by Harper et al.[20] in 1965, ^{99m}Tc–sulfur colloid has been the most widely used radiopharmaceutical for spleen scintigraphy. In fact, the routine use of this radiopharmaceutical for hepatic scintigraphy has led to the incidental scintigraphic evaluation of thousands of spleens, with relatively few splenic pathologic conditions other than mild splenomegaly being uncovered in the process. This rare occurrence of incidental splenic pathologic conditions is reflected also in the relative rarity with which a nuclear medicine laboratory is asked to image the spleen as a routine clinical procedure.

Commercial kits are available for the production of ^{99m}Tc–sulfur colloid, using the principle of the release of free sulfur from sodium thiosulfate by heating. Free sulfur in a hot acid solution aggregates into colloidal particles that trap ^{99m}Tc (as pertechnetate) quantitatively. These particles are approximately 200 μm in average diameter. Bubbling hydrogen sulfide through a hot acid

solution creates sulfur colloid particles that are considerably smaller in diameter and free of charge and that therefore can pass through a Millipore filter. Because the spleen tends to phagocytize large particles, the latter radiopharmaceutical results in a lower intensity of spleen labeling compared to liver labeling.

^{99m}Tc–sulfur colloid leaves the circulation with a rapid disappearance half-time of 1.5 to 4.2 minutes.[31] In normal humans approximately 80% to 90% of the radiopharmaceutical goes to the liver, 5% to 10% to the spleen, and 3% to 5% to the bone marrow. Imaging can begin 10 to 15 minutes after the injection of 2 to 5 mCi of the radiocolloid. Routine spleen views consist of an anterior and posterior view of the left upper quadrant and a lateral view of the spleen and left lobe of the liver. When the liver is enlarged, a left anterior oblique view is often important to separate the spleen from the left lobe of the liver for proper evaluation. The left posterior oblique view of the spleen can also be extremely useful in the characterization of size, configuration, and focal pathology.

Numerous other radiocolloids have been used in splenic scintigraphy, such as ^{99m}Tc–microaggregated albumin and ^{113}In–ferric hydroxide colloid.[10] Gold-198 colloid has disappeared from routine use because of the high patient radiation exposure. In addition, because of its small particle size and reduced spleen uptake, spleen images with gold-198 were often inadequate for good clinical evaluation.

Because of the cellular reservoir function of the spleen, excellent scintigraphic images are generally seen in studies performed with radiolabeled erythrocytes, granulocytes, or platelets. In current practice this particularly occurs with ^{99m}Tc RBCs used for cardiac wall motion and gastrointestinal bleeding, ^{111}In WBCs for abscess detection, and ^{111}In platelets for platelet kinetics or thromboscintigraphy. In each case, unexpected information regarding the spleen may be of considerable clinical importance; for example, accessory spleens can be seen on ^{111}In platelet scans.[8]

CLINICAL INDICATIONS FOR SPLEEN SCINTIGRAPHY
Spleen size

Several authors have described external measurement techniques for estimating spleen weight in vivo.[25,40,44] These appear to be quite accurate except in the extremes of spleen size. However, there are very few clinical situations in which the accurate determination of spleen size influences the diagnosis or management of a given patient.

The simplest single measurement correlated with spleen weight is the posterior spleen length, normally 10.7 ± 1.7 cm with a maximum normal length of 14

☐ **TABLE 60-1**

Causes of splenomegaly

Massive splenomegaly (over 1000 g)	Moderate splenomegaly (500-1000 g)	Mild splenomegaly (150-500 g)
Malaria	Early stages of those at left	Acute febrile disorders (infection, toxemia)
Chronic myelogenous leukemia	Portal vein thrombosis	Malignancy (involving or not involving spleen)
Myelofibrosis with myeloid metaplasia	Chronic liver disease, portal hypertension	Collagen-vascular disorders
Kala-azar, schistosomiasis	Infectious mononucleosis	Chronic infections
Gaucher's and Niemann-Pick diseases	Polycythemia vera	Idiopathic thrombocytopenic purpura
Thalassemia major	Malignant lymphomas	
Some spleen cysts	Chronic hemolytic anemias	
	Acute leukemias	
	Early sickle cell anemia (childhood)	
	Tuberculosis, sarcoid	

cm.[44] Spleen weight can be approximated by the following formula[25]:

$$W = 71L - 537$$

in which W is the spleen weight in grams and L is the posterior length in centimeters. More complex formulas exist for multiple views and measurements.[25,40] Image dimensions must be determined with each study utilizing some form of precalibrated source phantom or distance markers. Highly accurate estimates of spleen (and liver) volume may also be obtained by single photon–emission computerized tomography (SPECT).[51]

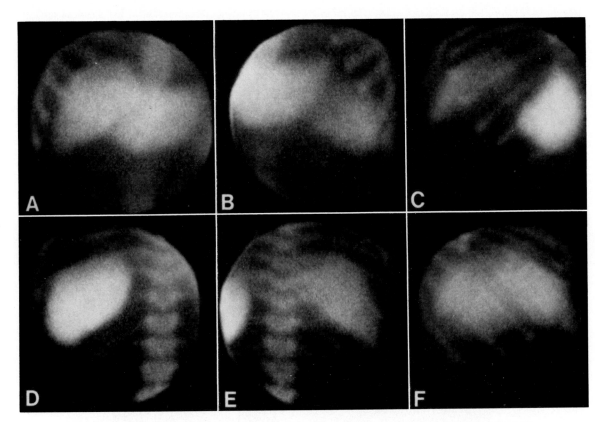

Fig. 60-1 Severe cirrhosis (⁹⁹ᵐTc–sulfur colloid). Note small, irregular liver with its negative halo caused by ascites. Spleen is mildly enlarged and bright, and bone marrow in ribs and vertebrae is unusually prominent as result of reduced hepatic radiocolloid uptake. **A,** Right anterior; **B,** left anterior; **C,** left lateral; **D,** left posterior; **E,** right posterior; **F,** right lateral.

Splenomegaly

Table 60-1 lists the common causes of splenomegaly according to degree: mild (150 to 500 g), moderate (500 to 1000 g), or massive (over 1000 g). Mild splenomegaly is a common finding in patients with a wide variety of disorders, possibly representing an attempt at immunologic response by that organ to such foreign systemic processes as infection and malignancy. The mild splenomegaly frequently seen in patients with malignant melanoma is a particularly good example of this phenomenon. Hepatocellular disease is another common mechanism for mild to moderate splenomegaly (Fig. 60-1). As previously mentioned, mild to moderate splenomegaly occurs in patients with polycythemia vera[57] and is considered by some hematologists to be an absolute requirement for the diagnosis. In many diseases with moderate to massive splenomegaly, recurrent episodes of splenic infarction may occur, with the result that spleen labeling may be considerably reduced in intensity and irregular in distribution (Fig. 60-2). As catalogued by Groshar et al.,[18] the causes of splenomegaly can also be considered in terms of their frequency of occurrence rather than the degree of splenic enlargement.

Small or absent spleen

Asplenia may be congenital, in which case it is commonly associated with situs inversus or other midline developmental abnormalities (Fig. 60-3). More commonly asplenia is iatrogenic, the result of splenectomy during some form of upper abdominal surgery, or splenectomy specifically treating idiopathic thrombocytopenic purpura, autoimmune hemolytic anemia, hereditary spherocytosis, Hodgkin's disease, and so on. Radiocolloid or heat-damaged Tc-RBC scintigraphy is the most effective means for documenting the presence of accessory spleens (Fig. 60-4). The small autoinfarcted spleen occurring in cases of adult sickle cell disease does not label with radiocolloids, although if calcified it may sometimes be seen in the routine bone scan[14] (Fig. 60-5).

If the spleen is not visualized in its normal location, the possibility of a "wandering" or displaced spleen should be considered, and searched for with scintiphotographs over the entire torso.[19]

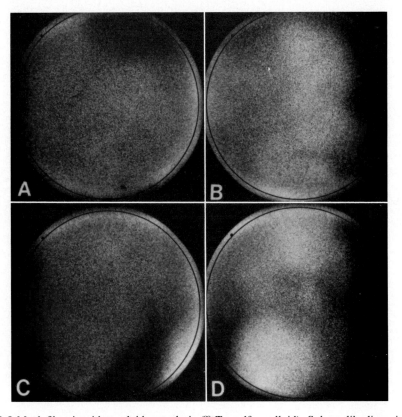

Fig. 60-2 Myelofibrosis with myeloid metaplasia (^{99m}Tc–sulfur colloid). Spleen, like liver, is massively enlarged, because of its hematopoietic function. Marked irregularity of spleen labeling results at least in part from repeated episodes of infarction with fibrous scarring. **A,** Right upper anterior; **B,** left upper anterior; **C,** right lower anterior; **D,** left lower anterior.

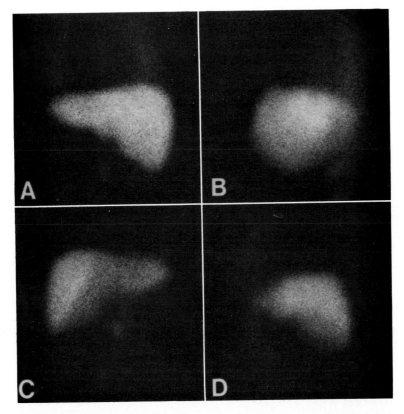

Fig. 60-3 Situs inversus with asplenia (^{99m}Tc–sulfur colloid). **A,** Anterior; **B,** left lateral; **C,** posterior; **D,** right lateral.

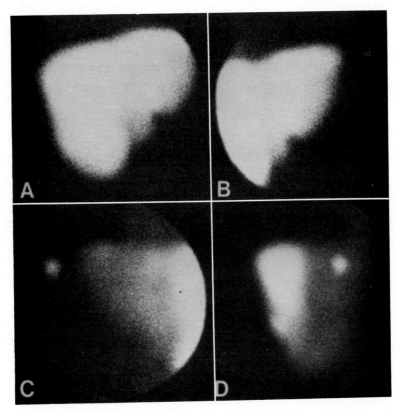

Fig. 60-4 Accessory spleen (^{99m}Tc–sulfur colloid) found incidentally after splenectomy. Intensities are increased to demonstrate finding. **A,** Right anterior; **B,** left anterior; **C,** left posterior; **D,** left lateral.

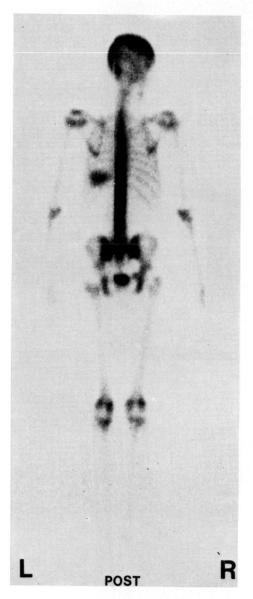

L   **POST**   R

Fig. 60-5 Positive sickle cell spleen labeling in bone scan (^{99m}Tc–methylene diphosphonate) in young adult with sickle cell disease and autoinfarcted spleen that does not label with ^{99m}Tc–sulfur colloid.

Left upper quadrant mass

Evaluation of patients with a left upper quadrant mass should include spleen scintigraphy to differentiate an enlarged spleen (with or without focal pathologic condition) from an extrasplenic mass (gastric or colonic carcinoma, renal or adrenal neoplasm, or so on). For example, in cases of myelofibrosis with myeloid metaplasia the spleen may be so firm and scarred from repeated infarctions that it feels like a hard, irregular tumor mass. Left upper quadrant masses may be well characterized by combining the spleen scan with renal scintigraphy, an intravenous pyelogram, or abdominal CT scanning or ultrasound. The combination of a spleen scan, gallium scan, and abdominal CT scan has proved to be very effective in characterizing subphrenic abscesses.[43]

BENIGN LESIONS
Cysts

Splenic cysts may be parasitic or nonparasitic in origin and are relatively rare.[21,52] They are seen as clearly defined focal defects in the spleen on scintigraphy associated with an absence of perfusion when a flow study is performed. They are sometimes discovered incidentally during liver scintigraphy. Fig. 60-6 demonstrates a large intrasplenic "chocolate" cyst in a 20-year-old woman with an asymptomatic enlarging left upper quadrant mass. Parasitic cysts may occur in patients with an echinococcal infection (hydatid disease), again being seen as a left upper quadrant mass that may be asymptomatic.

Abscesses

Splenic abscesses may occur in patients with a bloodstream infection, especially subacute or acute bacterial endocarditis. If sufficiently large, they appear as focal defects in the spleen, although multiple small abscesses may be below the resolution limits of the scintillation camera (2 to 2.5 cm in vivo). With small splenic abscesses, a ^{67}Ga scan will probably be more useful.[54] Dual radionuclide subtraction imaging of ^{99m}Tc–sulfur colloid with ^{111}In-WBC or ^{67}Ga may be essential for proper identification of intrasplenic or subphrenic abscesses.[41] Fig. 60-7 illustrates a patient with acute bacterial endocarditis leading to a septic infarct and subsequently a mycotic aneurysm of the spleen.

Infarcts

Splenic infarcts occur occasionally in patients with bacterial endocarditis and are generally seen as peripheral defects in the spleen image. They frequently also occur concomitantly with massive splenomegaly such as occurs in patients with myelofibrosis with myeloid metaplasia (Fig. 60-2). Fig. 60-8 illustrates the spleen scan in a black patient with sickle cell trait who had no relevant symptomatology throughout his life until vacationing for 3 weeks in the mountains of California at at altitude of 6000 feet. Multiple splenic infarcts are evident in the study. Splenic infarcts occur occasionally but rarely in patients with other hemoglobinopathies such as hemoglobin SC disease[42] or hemoglobin S-thalassemia.

Hematomas

Subcapsular splenic hematomas generally occur as a result of blunt abdominal trauma, which may or may not be spontaneously recalled by the patient at the time of medical presentation with left upper quadrant pain. An

Static views

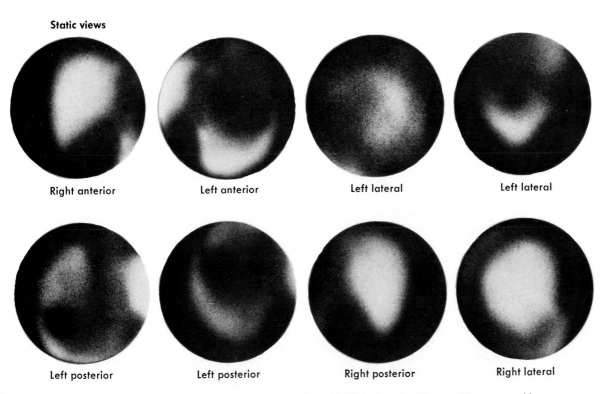

Right anterior	Left anterior	Left lateral	Left lateral
Left posterior	Left posterior	Right posterior	Right lateral

Fig. 60-6 Huge benign splenic cyst (^{99m}Tc–sulfur colloid) in healthy 20-year-old woman with progressive painless upper abdominal enlargement. This was "chocolate" cyst, presumably caused by ectopic endometrial cyst.

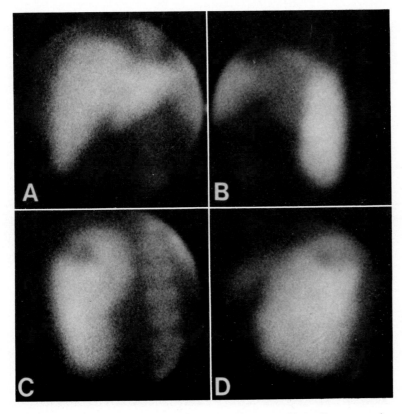

Fig. 60-7 Splenic abscess (septic infarct) in acute bacterial endocarditis leading to mycotic aneurysm (^{99m}Tc–sulfur colloid). Patient was young heroin addict with recurrent history of fever and left upper quadrant pain. **A,** Right anterior; **B,** left anterior; **C,** left posterior; **D,** left lateral.

Continued.

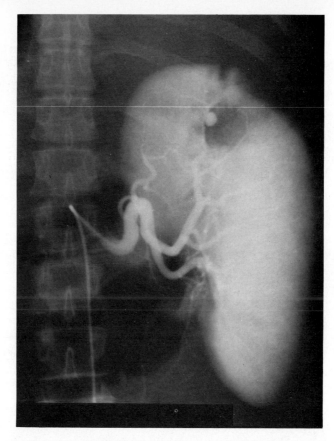

Fig. 60-7, cont'd. E, Celiac angiogram on same patient, demonstrating mycotic aneurysm and peripheral perfusion defect.

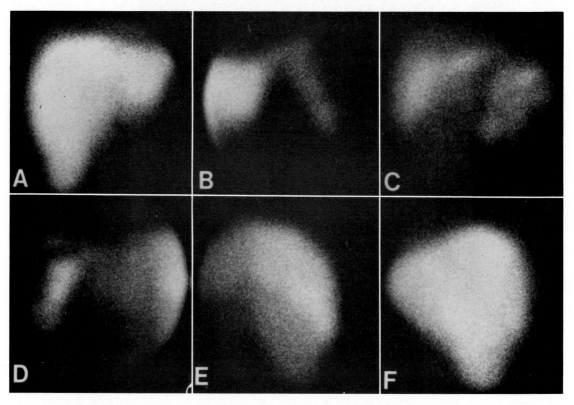

Fig. 60-8 Splenic infarcts (^{99m}Tc–sulfur colloid). Patient was 45 years of age with sickle cell trait and 3 weeks of recurrent left upper quadrant pain while vacationing in mountains. **A,** Right anterior; **B,** left anterior; **C,** left lateral; **D,** left posterior; **E,** right posterior; **F,** right lateral.

acute traumatic rupture of the spleen is a surgical emergency that rarely comes to scintigraphy. A spontaneous rupture may occur during the acute splenic enlargement in cases of infectious mononucleosis or acute leukemia. Left upper quadrant pain and tenderness are usually the presenting features.

Scintigraphic spleen visualization is a sensitive technique for the diagnosis of subcapsular and intrasplenic hematomas.[27,48] Gilday and Alderson,[16] reviewing several publications, indicated no false-negative results and five (7%) false-positive results in 69 cases. The accurate diagnosis of splenic hematomas is essential because of the substantial risk of a delayed rupture (20%)[58] and the increased risk of mortality with a delayed rupture.[47] Generally a focal lesion is seen within or adjacent to the spleen image, at times even transecting the spleen. The greatest difficulty occurs with subcapsular hematomas that may have little effect on the overall spleen image but may displace the entire spleen medially or anteriorly. Fig. 60-9 shows a spleen that has only slight irregularity at the lower pole in the left anterior oblique projection.

This patient had just been in an automobile accident and at surgery was found to have an acute splenic rupture with 500 ml of blood in the abdomen and only a small subcapsular hematoma.

A combination of the radiocolloid spleen study with either lung scintigraphy or a flow study may convincingly demonstrate a negative space between the spleen and left lateral body wall (Fig. 60-10). In clinical situations of significant uncertainty, abdominal CT scanning can provide definite information as well. Early splenic hematomas have the same CT number as normal spleen tissue but do not enhance with contrast, whereas later hematomas have progressively lower CT numbers, again without enhancement.[30] In a prospective comparison of scintigraphy with ultrasound in 32 patients, Froelich et al.[15] found the two modalities to be essentially identical in sensitivity and specificity for subcapsular hematoma after trauma, although a substantial proportion of the patients could not be properly studied by ultrasound because of injuries or pain. For this reason they recommend scintigraphy as the primary screening procedure.

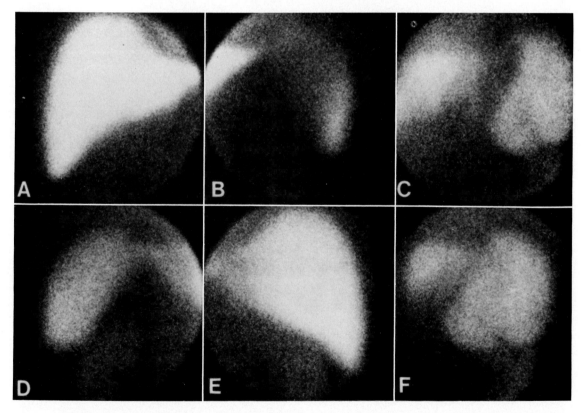

Fig. 60-9 Splenic hematoma (^{99m}Tc–sulfur colloid). This patient had just been in motor vehicle accident and was seen with left upper quadrant pain and 8-point drop in hematocrit. Note that only slight distortion of spleen image is noted at its anterior tip. At surgery anterior tip of spleen was found to be ruptured, with small subcapsular hematoma present as well as 500 ml of blood in peritoneal space. **A,** Right anterior; **B,** left anterior; **C,** left anterior oblique; **D,** left posterior; **E,** right posterior; **F,** left lateral.

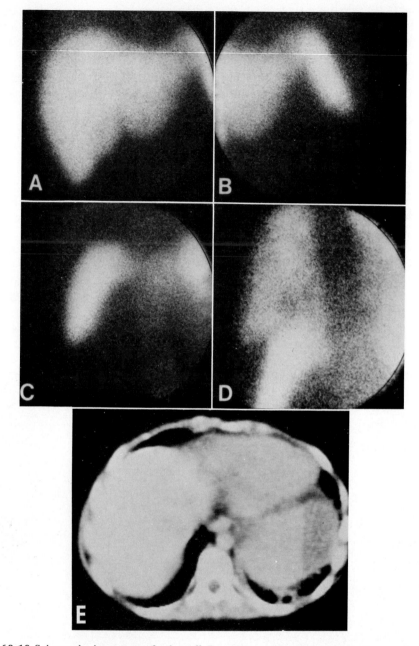

Fig. 60-10 Subcapsular hematoma of spleen (^{99m}Tc–sulfur colloid) in child with history of recent abdominal trauma. Note medial displacement of spleen, best evaluated with combined lung image— **D,** in this case. Lateral aspect of spleen is unusually flattened. **A,** Right anterior; **B,** left anterior; **C,** left posterior; **D,** left posterior, after labeling lungs with ^{99m}Tc-MAA. **E,** Body CT scan in same patient, demonstrating lower CT number hematoma accounting for lateral one third of spleen volume.

Benign tumors

Benign tumors of the spleen are extremely rare. They include hemangiomas, fibromas, myomas, and hamartomas. If sufficiently large, benign tumors are seen as discrete focal defects involving the spleen.

MALIGNANT LESIONS
Primary tumors

Primary tumors of the spleen are rare, with the exception of splenic involvement by lymphoreticular malignancies. Scintigraphic abnormalities include splenic

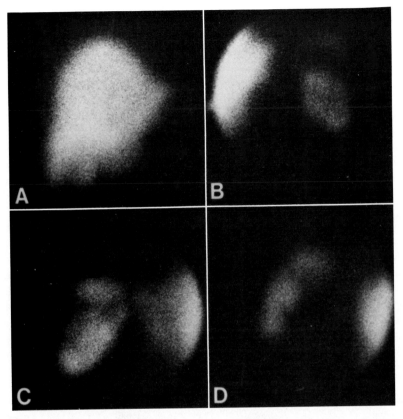

Fig. 60-11 Focal lesions of spleen caused by Hodgkin's disease (^{99m}Tc–sulfur colloid). **A,** Right anterior; **B,** left anterior; **C,** left posterior; **D,** right posterior oblique.

enlargement without direct spleen involvement by the tumor, splenic enlargement with cellular infiltration that does not appear as a focal abnormality on scans, and focal lesions caused by large tumor deposits[26,45] (Fig. 60-11). Hodgkin's disease is the most common type of lymphoma, although lymphosarcomas and reticulum cell sarcomas also may produce a focal pathologic condition in the spleen. Chronic lymphocytic leukemia causes splenic enlargement with diffuse cellular infiltration and sometimes a diffuse decrease in radiocolloid labeling but no focal defects. Sarcomas and fibrosarcomas may also occur in the spleen.

Secondary tumors

Solid tumor metastases to the spleen are rare but may occasionally be found with widely disseminated metastatic neoplasms such as malignant melanoma or breast carcinoma. Occasionally local primary tumors such as a gastric carcinoma or colonic carcinoma extend directly to involve the spleen.

Several authors[1,24] have described the findings of increased spleen labeling (or a "hot spleen") in patients with malignant melanoma—a shift in radiocolloid to the spleen, which at least in Stage 1 and 2 patients appears to correlate with a poor prognosis.

ACCESSORY SPLEENS

Accessory spleens are stated to occur in approximately 10% of the normal population[5], although two studies of nontraumatic postsplenectomy patients have demonstrated the incidence of accessory spleens in this setting to be as high as 43%.[1,32] Accessory spleens are commonly associated with other congenital abnormalities (53% of cases). They usually are located in the splenic hilus or along the associated ligaments and vessels. Ordinarily accessory spleens remain small, do not present clinical problems, and are rarely seen on routine spleen scintigraphy. Their presence may be of great importance in patients with autoimmune hemolytic anemias, idiopathic thrombocytopenic purpura, or hereditary spherocytosis who initially responded well to splenectomy but then relapsed. The presence and growth of accessory spleens must be ruled out in such patients. The simplest scintigraphic technique is that utilizing ^{99m}Tc–sulfur colloid, including views of the entire abdomen and pelvis. If clinical suspicion is high and this study is negative, it should be repeated using autologous tin- or heat-damaged red blood cells labeled with [99mTc], which has been demonstrated to be more sensitive for the identification of small accessory spleens.[13]

SPLEEN RESPONSE TO THERAPY

It is possible to follow the response of an enlarged spleen (or a spleen containing a tumor, cysts, or abscesses) to specific therapy such as radiation or chemotherapy.[28] Spleen sizing should be carried out as detailed in the earlier section. Such information is of value only in occasional clinical situations.

FUNCTIONAL ASPLENIA

In 1969 Pearson et al.[33] first described functional asplenia as the presence of palpable splenomegaly associated with absence of radiocolloid spleen labeling in young patients with sickle cell disease. The peripheral blood smear in these patients showed the red cell changes characteristic of absence of the spleen including pleomorphism, normoblasts, Howell-Jolly bodies, and pitted erythrocytes. In adult life the spleens of these patients

autoinfarct to a small fibrous remnant, and the term "functional asplenia" is no longer applicable. Characteristically, the failure of labeling with radiocolloids is reversible by transfusion with normal (hemoglobin A) blood, possibly because normal cells interpose between sickling cells in the relatively hypoxic spleen and permit a better sinusoidal flow of blood. Although the entity is seen predominantly in young sickle cell patients, it has been described in patients with other disease states such as those who have received chronic Thorotrast irradiation to the spleen, some cases of celiac disease, hemoglobin SC disease and S-thalassemia syndromes, splenic artery or vein occlusion, and so on.[2,35,49]

Fig. 60-12 illustrates the spleen studies in a 12-year-old girl with sickle cell disease and functional asplenia. The reduced spleen blood flow in comparison to that of the kidneys and the failure of the spleen to label with radiocolloid are noted. We have also noted the failure of such a spleen to label with heat-damaged chromium-51–labeled autologous red cells.

Spencer et al[50] have recently described a syndrome called "splenic overload syndrome," in which the pe-

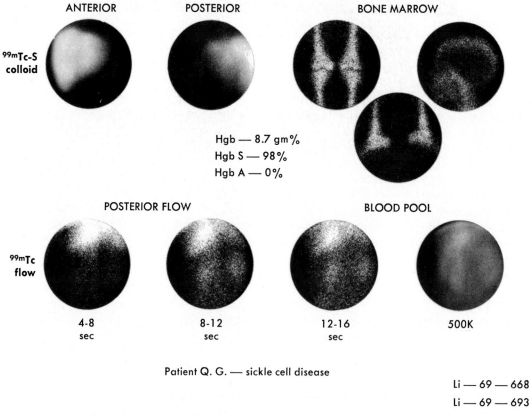

Patient Q. G. — sickle cell disease

Li — 69 — 668
Li — 69 — 693

Fig. 60-12 Functional asplenia in 12-year-old girl with sickle cell disease ([99mTc]–sulfur colloid). Note failure of spleen labeling in spite of palpably enlarged spleen. Also of interest is reduced spleen perfusion (compared to kidneys) in posterior flow study and marked peripheral extension of bone marrow into feet caused by chronic anemia.

ripheral blood morphology is typical of the postsplenectomy pattern, but spleen scintigraphy demonstrates good labeling of a distinctly small spleen. In this instance it appears that the spleen is not of sufficient size to handle the peripheral blood needs for splenic RES function, resulting in a relative shortfall in spleen function, or splenic overload.

BORN-AGAIN SPLEEN

It has been known for many years that children who have undergone splenectomy for traumatic rupture of the spleen do not have the same high risk of infections as children whose spleen had been removed for other reasons.[3,46] Pearson et al.[34] evaluated this phenomenon in 22 such patients and observed markedly reduced evidence of splenic hypofunction in the form of red cell "pitting." The liver-spleen scan performed in several patients demonstrated splenosis, a condition of multiple small loci of splenic tissue scattered throughout the abdominal and pelvic cavities, which apparently originate from seeding throughout these spaces by scattered spleen cells released at the time of splenic rupture. They termed this regrowth of scattered spleen cells into functionally effective splenic nodules the "born-again spleen." Spleen scanning in such patients can be an effective way of estimating the risk of infection following posttraumatic splenectomy.

Jacobson and DeNardo[22] first described the effective use of spleen scintigraphy in the evaluation of splenosis. It may occur in as many as 65% of patients undergoing splenectomy for trauma.[60] Fig. 60-13 illustrates the typical findings on ^{99m}Tc–sulfur colloid imaging.[37] As one might expect, spleen scintigraphy can be equally useful

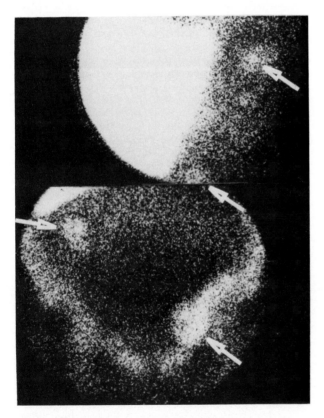

Fig. 60-13 Multiple splenic foci, the "born-again spleen," in 29-year-old man following posttraumatic splenic rupture and splenectomy 7 years previously. Splenic tissue released at time of rupture has settled throughout abdominal and pelvic cavities *(arrows)* and then grown into discrete nodules.
(From Price, DC: The hematopoietic system. In Harbert, J, and DaRocha, AFG, editors: Textbook of nuclear medicine, ed 2, vol 2 (Clinical applications), Philadelphia, 1984, Lea & Febiger.)

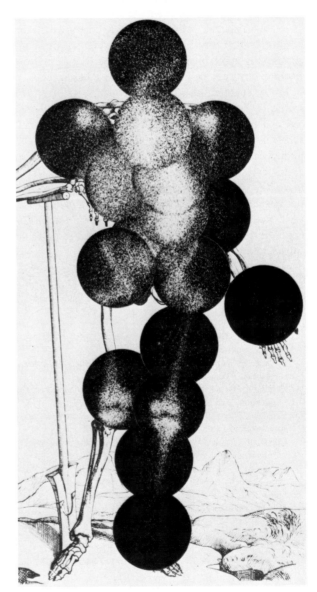

Fig. 60-14 ^{52}Fe positron camera study in patient with myelofibrosis and active hematopoiesis in markedly enlarged spleen. Study performed at Donner Laboratory, University of California at Berkeley.

in evaluating patients who have undergone splenic autotransplantation to minimize long-term risk of overwhelming postsplenectomy infection.[53]

NONIMAGING RADIONUCLIDE STUDIES

Several probe-counting techniques exist for the evaluation of the spleen's role in the production and destruction of circulating blood elements. A ferrokinetics study performed with iron-59 involves probe determinations of the radioiron kinetic patterns seen over the spleen, liver, bone marrow, and precordium to evaluate sites of hematopoiesis. This can be very important in evaluating the splenic contribution to extramedullary hematopoiesis (myeloid metaplasia) and to a lesser extent the destruction of in vivo–labeled erythrocytes.[36] In centers where the positron emitter iron-52 and a positron camera are availabe, scintigraphic imaging of splenic as well as marrow erythropoiesis can be effectively achieved (Fig. 60-14).

Probe counting of chromium-51 kinetics over the spleen is a routine procedure in the evaluation of red cell and platelet survival. In the evaluation of red cell survival, a progressive rise in the spleen-liver ratio through one blood disappearance half-life of labeled erythrocytes indicates a probable benefit from splenectomy.[29] In our own experience, however, a progressive rise in spleen chromium-51 activity during a platelet survival study for idiopathic thrombocytopenic purpura is not correlated with a significantly improved response to splenectomy.[38,39]

REFERENCES

1. Ambriz, P, et al: Accessory spleen compromising response to splenectomy for idiopathic thrombocytopenic purpura, Radiology 155:793, 1985.
2. Armas, RR: Clinical studies with spleen-specific radiolabeled agents, Semin Nucl Med 15:260, 1985.
3. Balfanz, JR, et al: Overwhelming sepsis following splenectomy for trauma, J Pediatr 88:458, 1976.
4. Bohnsack, JF, and Brown, EJ: The role of the spleen in resistance to infection, Ann Rev Med 37:49, 1986.
5. Cahalane, SF, and Kiesselbach, N: The significance of the accessory spleen, J Pathol 100:139, 1970.
6. Coppoletta, JM, and Wolbach, SB: Body length and organ weights of infants and children, Am J Pathol 9:55, 1933.
7. Crosby, WH: Normal functions of the spleen relative to red blood cells: a review, Blood 14:399, 1959.
8. Davis, HH, et al: Detection of accessory spleens with indium-111–labeled autologous platelets, Am J Hematol 8:81, 1980.
9. DeLand, FH: Normal spleen size, Radiology 97:589, 1970.
10. Desai, AG, and Thakur, ML: Radiopharmaceuticals for spleen and bone marrow studies, Semin Nucl Med 15:229, 1985.
11. Eckelman, W, et al: Technetium-labeled red blood cells, J Nucl Med 12:22, 1971.
12. Eckelman, W, et al: Visualization of the human spleen with 99mTc-labeled red blood cells, J Nucl Med 12:310, 1971.
13. Ehrlich, CP, et al: Splenic scintigraphy using Tc-99m–labeled heat-denatured red blood cells in pediatric patients: concise communication, J Nucl Med 23:209, 1982.
14. Fischer, KC, Shapiro, S, and Treves, S: Visualization of the spleen with a bone-seeking radionuclide in a child with sickle-cell anemia, Radiology 122:398, 1977.
15. Froelich, JW, et al: Radionuclide imaging and ultrasound in liver spleen trauma: a prospective comparison, Radiology 145:457, 1982.
16. Gilday, DL, and Alderson, PO: Scintigraphic evaluation of liver and spleen injury, Semin Nucl Med 4:357, 1974.
17. Gray, SJ, and Sterling, K: The tagging of red blood cells and plasma proteins with radioactive chromium, J Clin Invest 29:818, 1950.
18. Groshar, D, Israel, O, and Front, D: Spleen imaging: enlargement of the spleen, Semin Nucl Med 13:295, 1983.
19. Groshar, D, et al: The value of scintigraphy in the evaluation of a wandering spleen, Clin Nucl Med 11:42, 1986.
20. Harper, PV, et al: Technetium-99m as a scanning agent, Radiology 85:101, 1965.
21. Hartshorne, MF, et al: The place of liver-spleen scanning in the workup of giant secondary cysts of the spleen, Clin Nucl Med 11:4, 1986.
22. Jacobson, SJ, and DeNardo, GL: Splenosis demonstrated by splenic scan, J Nucl Med 12:470, 1971.
23. Jonson, PM, and Herior, JC, and Morring, SL: Scintillation scanning of the normal spleen utilizing sensitized radioactive erythrocytes, Radiology 74:99, 1960.
24. Koh, HK, et al: Prognosis in stage 1 malignant melanoma: seven-year follow-up study of splenic radiocolloid uptake as predictor of death, J Nucl Med 25:1183, 1984.
25. Larson, SM, et al: Dimensions of the normal adult spleen scan and prediction of spleen weight, J Nucl Med 12:123, 1971.
26. Lindfors, KK, et al: Scintigraphic findings in large-cell lymphoma of the spleen: concise communication, J Nucl Med 25:969, 1984.
27. Lutzker, LG: Radionuclide imaging of the injured spleen and liver, Semin Nucl Med 13:184, 1983.
28. Mathews, J, et al: Rapid response of intrasplenic lesions to steroids in non-Hodgkin's lymphoma, Int J Nucl Med Biol 12:155, 1985.
29. McCurdy, PR, and Roth, GE: Splenectomy in hemolytic anemia: results predicted by body scanning after injection of 51Cr-tagged red cells, N Engl J Med 259:459, 1958.
30. Moss, AA, et al: Computed tomography of splenic subcapsular hematomas: an experimental study in dogs, Invest Radiol 14:60, 1979.
31. Mundschenk, H, Hromec, A, and Fischer, J: Phagocytic activity of the liver as a measure of hepatic circulation: comparative study using 198Au and 99mTc–sulfur colloid, J Nucl Med 12:711, 1971.
32. Orda, R, et al: Developmental pattern of splenic dysfunction in sickle cell disorders, Pediatrics 76:392, 1985.
33. Pearson, HA, Spencer, RP, and Cornelius, EA: Functional asplenia in sickle-cell anemia, N Engl J Med 281:923, 1969.
34. Pearson, HA, et al: The born-again spleen: return of splenic function after splenectomy for trauma, N Engl J Med 298:1389, 1978.
35. Pearson, HA, et al: Developmental pattern of splenic dysfunction in sickle cell disorders, Pediatrics 76:392, 1985.
36. Pollycove, M: Iron metabolism and kinetics, Semin Hematol 3:235, 1966.
37. Price, DC, and McIntyre, PA: The hematopoietic system. In Harbert, J, and DaRocha, AFG, editors: Textbook of nuclear medicine, ed 2, vol 2, (Clinical applications), Philadelphia, 1984, Lea and Febiger.
38. Ries, CA: Platelet kinetics in autoimmune thrombocytopenia: relation between splenic platelet sequestration and response to splenectomy [editorial], Ann Intern Med 86:194, 1977.
39. Ries, CA, and Price, DC: (51Cr) Platelet kinetics in thrombocytopenia, Ann Intern Med 80:703, 1974.
40. Rollo, FD, and DeLand, FH: The determination of spleen mass from radionuclide images, Radiology 97:583, 1970.

41. Rosenberg, RJ, Sziklas, JJ, and Rich, DA: Dual radionuclide subtraction imaging of the spleen, Semin Nucl Med 15:299, 1985.

42. Sears, DA, and Udden, MM: Splenic infarction, splenic sequestration, and functional hyposplenism in hemoglobin S-C disease, Am J Hematol 18:261, 1985.

43. Shimshak, RR, et al: The complementary role of gallium citrate imaging and computed tomography in the evaluation of suspected abdominal infection, J Nucl Med 19:262, 1978.

44. Sigel, RM, Becker, DV, and Hurley, JR: Evaluation of spleen size during routine liver imaging with ^{99m}Tc and the scintillation camera, J Nucl Med 11:689, 1970.

45. Silverman, S, et al: Evaluation of the liver and spleen in Hodgkin's disease. II. The value of splenic scintigraphy, Am J Med 52:362, 1972.

46. Singer, DB: Postsplenectomy sepsis, Perspect Pediatr Pathol 1:285, 1973.

47. Sizer, JS, Wayne, ER, and Frederick, PL: Delayed rupture of the spleen, Arch Surg 92:362, 1966.

48. Spencer, RP, and Gupta, SM: Radionuclide studies of the spleen in trauma and iatrogenic disorders, Semin Nucl Med 15:305, 1985.

49. Spencer, RP, Pearson, HA, and Binder, HA: Identification of cases of "acquired" functional asplenia, J Nucl Med 11:763, 1970.

50. Spencer, RP, et al: Splenic overload syndrome: possible relationship to a small spleen, Int J Nucl Med Biol 11:291, 1984.

51. Strauss, LG, et al: Single photon emission computerized tomography (SPECT) for estimates of liver and spleen volume, J Nucl Med 25:81, 1984.

52. Sty, JR, and Conway, JJ: The spleen: development and functional evaluation, Semin Nucl Med 15:276, 1985.

53. Szasz, IJ, and Nagy, A: Scintigraphic demonstration of viable splenic autotransplant, Clin Nucl Med 11:209, 1986.

54. Vasquez, TE, et al: Fungal splenic abscesses in the immunosuppressed patient. correlation of imaging modalities, Clin Nucl Med 12:36, 1987.

55. Wagstaff, J, et al: The "hot spleen" phenomenon in metastatic malignant melanoma: its incidence and relationship with the immune system, Cancer 49:439, 1982.

56. Weiss, L: A scanning electron microscopic study of the spleen, Blood 43:665, 1974.

57. Westin, J, et al: Spleen size in polycythemia, Acta Med Scand 191:263, 1972.

58. Willox, GI: Nonpenetrating injuries of the abdomen causing rupture of the spleen, Arch Surg 90:498, 1965.

59. Winkelman, JW, et al: Visualization of the spleen in man by radioisotope scanning, Radiology 75:465, 1960.

60. Zwas, ST, et al: Scintigraphic assessment of ectopic splenic tissue localization and function following splenectomy for trauma, Eur J Nucl Med 12:125, 1986.

61 *Overview*

WERNER WENZ

GENERAL CONSIDERATIONS

The spleen is a lymphoid organ located in the left side of the abdominal cavity under the diaphragm. In human beings the spleen is about the size of a fist and has an abundant blood supply. It serves as a temporary storage site for blood and removes from the circulation degenerated blood cells. The splenic parenchyma or pulp is largely composed of vascular sinuses, which are large channels of lymphatic tissue carrying venous blood. The organ is enclosed in a thin membranous capsule of elastic tissue. Fibrous cords called trabeculae run from the capsule to the depth of the pulp to give the organ a firm structural framework.

Infections from other parts of the body spread readily to the spleen, but splenic abscesses are infrequent infections. Splenic tumors are very rare and usually cause splenic enlargement. Splenomegaly may appear in several diseases, including systemic syndromes, hematologic diseases, inherited splenic disorders, sequelae of trauma, or impaired flow through the splenic vein.

Only the enlarged spleen can be palpated below the left rib cage. The methods of choice for examining the normal and diseased spleen are ultrasound and computed tomography (CT). Earlier roentgenographic techniques, such as plain film radiography, visualization of the adjacent organs by barium meal, barium enema, or selective or superselective angiography, have lost relevance. Ultrasonography, CT, magnetic resonance imaging (MRI), and in some cases radionuclear scintigraphy give optimal information about the spleen and surrounding organs.

ALGORITHMIC PATHWAYS OF MODERN IMAGING

At present, abdominal ultrasonographic screening is the method of choice to investigate upper abdominal disorders. Therefore many splenic lesions are readily detected by ultrasound in clinically asymptomatic patients (Fig. 61-1). Kremer and co-workers[17] reported 5720 patients in whom they routinely performed ultrasound of the upper abdomen. Pathologic ultrasonic findings were reported in 47.1%, but most were not clinically relevant. Splenomegaly appeared in 147 patients (2.5%). The enlargement of the spleen was either caused by viral infections or existing liver disease. In no instance could hematologic or lymphatic systemic disease be proved.

Ultrasonographic screening is often followed by other

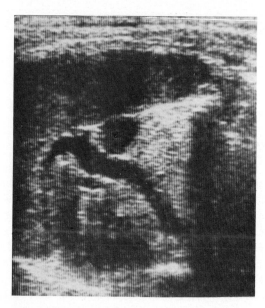

Fig. 61-1 Abdominal ultrasound image of accessory spleen close to hilum.

imaging modalities. In suspected splenic disturbances, sonography gives information about the organ size, shape, location, and the presence or absence of focal lesions within the parenchyma. Plain film radiography is primarily helpful in the detection of splenic calcifications, which are listed in the following outline.[7]

A. Solitary calcifications
  1. Common
    a. Splenic artery aneurysm
    b. Splenic artery atherosclerosis
  2. Uncommon
    a. Abscess
    b. Ascites
    c. Cysts
    d. Granuloma
    e. Hematoma
    f. Hemangioma (phleboliths)
    g. Previous infarction
B. Multiple calcifications
  1. Common
    a. Hemangiomatosis
    b. Histoplasmosis (healed)
    c. Tuberculosis
  2. Uncommon
    a. Brucellosis
    b. Hamartoma
    c. Hemosiderosis
    d. Infarction
    e. Parasites
    f. Sickle cell anemia

Thorotrast, which is no longer used because it is an α-particle emitter, is picked up by the reticuloendothelial cells and opacifies the spleen (Fig. 61-2).

As with ultrasound, CT examination also allows visualization of focal and diffuse splenic lesions with simultaneous demonstration of pathologic changes in nearby areas. CT scans can demonstrate splenic lesions with great detail and are particularly useful when compared to previous examinations (Fig. 61-3). CT dynamic studies are essential to study the arterial perfusion and easily evaluate portal blood flow in liver disease.

MRI has indications similar to those of CT. MRI can

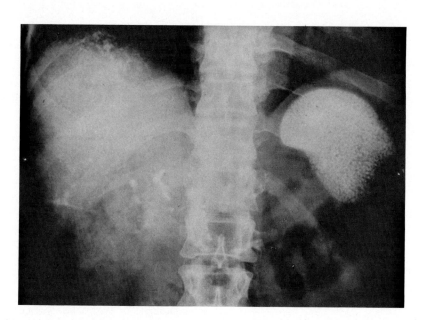

Fig. 61-2 Abdominal plain film shows thorotrastosis of spleen, liver, and periportal lymph nodes.

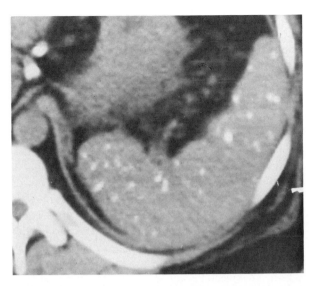

Fig. 61-3 Computed tomogram of splenic calcifications in tuberculosis.

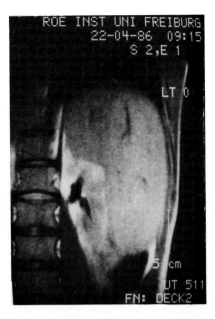

Fig. 61-4 Magnetic resonance tomogram of enlarged spleen in acute lymphatic leukemia. Histologically proved infiltrates could not be visualized.

demonstrate arteries and veins in the various planes without the need for injection of contrast media. The fatty tissue of the adjacent organs allows recognition of pathologic changes in surrounding areas. Anomalies of shape and location of the organ are relatively easy to identify with MRI (Fig. 61-4).[31]

Angiography by way of the splenic artery had been the diagnostic method of choice for many years. Vascular mapping by contrast injections into the celiac trunk or the splenic artery is still indicated in primary vascular lesions such as aneurysm, arterioportal fistula, hemangioma, and splenic vein thrombosis and in preoperative demonstration of the vascular system after trauma. Splenic arteriography is also a prerequisite for interventional procedures such as those involving visceral transcatheter embolization.

Isotope studies are indicated for detecting ectopic spleens and accessory organs or for the verification of the asplenia syndrome. Barium-air double contrast studies of the stomach and the small bowel are rarely needed for the delineation of splenic lesions.

In summary, the following algorithmic pathway is suggested for the examination of the human spleen:

1. Ultrasonography
2. Abdominal plain film
3. Computed tomography
4. Magnetic resonance imaging
5. Nuclear scintigraphy
6. Arteriography, portography

THE NORMAL SPLEEN

Ultrasonography can rapidly and reliably help to determine the size of the spleen. In 95% of patients the length of the spleen is less than 11 cm, the width less than 7 cm, and the depth less than 5 cm. The weight, as determined by the rotation ellipsoid formula, is less than 190 g in 95% of patients.[22] Sonographic biometry in children reveals an almost linear increase of these parameters during development and a good correlation with the body height.[6,19] In 1987 Markisz[19] and co-workers also performed scintigraphic tomography evaluation of the spleen of normal children. Plain film radiographs of the normal-size spleen are of no value.

Dimensions of the normal spleen[8]

Clinical	7 cm (by percussion)
Anatomic	12 × 8 × 3 cm
Scintigraphic	8 × 12 cm
Sonographic	10 × 6 × 14 cm

The splenic size diminishes with age and is slightly smaller in women compared to men. The organ moves 2 to 3 cm with normal breathing and as much as 7 cm with deep inspiration.

SPLENIC ABNORMALITIES

In 1927 Lubarsch idenitified anatomic abnormalities of the spleen as follows[36]:

1. Lien accessorius, or ectopic spleen: no contact with the main organ.

2. Lien succenturiatus: accentuation of the splenic fissures.

3. Lien lobatus: multiple lobes with absence of main or central spleen.

Absence of the spleen (asplenia syndrome, Ivemark's syndrome)

Splenic agenesis is often associated with cardiac anomalies, disturbances of the pulmonary circulation, trilobed left lung (dextroisomerism) with horseshoe kidney, malrotation of the gastrointestinal tract, and liver anomalies. In addition to the juxtaposition of the abdominal aorta and inferior vena cava, two additional abnormalities can be demonstrated sonographically: absent splenic vein and midline portal vein.[14] However, the method of choice for outlining the features of Ivemark's syndrome is isotopic scan.

Polysplenia

Polysplenia is a syndrome characterized by multiple individual splenules, cardiac anomalies, atypical confluence of the pulmonary veins, and the presence of biliary, urogenital, and bronchial disorders. Chest radiogaphs and abdominal CT[32] demonstrate multiple masses consistent with splenules in association with partial visceral heterotaxia and concomitant levoisomerism (bilateral left-sidedness).

Autotransplantation of splenic tissue following trauma is called *splenosis* and can be detected by ^{99m}Tc-labeled, heat-damaged autologous erythrocytes.[5] Moncada and co-workers[21] reported nine cases of left-sided thoracic splenosis appearing as single or multiple pleural-based soft tissue masses. Failure to include splenosis in the differential diagnosis of thoracic masses has unfortunately resulted in unnecessary surgery. Although the localization of heterotopic splenic tissue has been made by CT, radioisotopic uptake similar to that of the normal spleen provides definitive proof of the problem. Accessory spleens can also be identified by isotopic scan in the workup of abdominal masses. Nishitani and associates[23] were able to detect accessory spleens as small as 10 mm in diameter in the left upper quadrant.

Ectopic spleen

The diagnosis of ectopic spleen can be subject to severe errors. Pedicle torsion of a "wandering" spleen is a rare phenomenon that can cause lower abdominal symptoms such as those of twisted hemorrhagic ovarian cyst.[24] Chronic splenic pedicle torsion may result in subcapsular hematoma[12] or ileus of unknown origin.[29] Wandering spleen should always be suspected when examination of the left upper quadrant indicates absence of the spleen. Definitive diagnosis of ectopic spleen can be made by radioisotope examination or angiography. Vascular studies also have been done in cases of splenogonal fusion.[15]

Upside-down spleen

Upside-down spleen is a rare positional anomaly unrelated to wandering spleen.[35]

Splenomegaly

Measurements of spleen size based on abdominal palpation and percussion are inaccurate because a palpable spleen can be normal. Niederau and co-workers[22] established normal, average spleen dimensions and found good correlation between splenic size and sex, age, weight, height, and body surface area. Correct delineation of "borderline" splenomegaly is very difficult. Often only serial studies showing progressive enlargement of the organ establish a definitive diagnosis. In case of overlying ribs, hyperaerated lung, or excessive stomach and colonic air precluding ultrasound, CT allows precise sizing of the spleen.

The following outline lists a complete differential diagnosis of splenomegaly, as provided by Felson and Reeder.[7]

A. *Blood dyscrasia*
   1. Anemia
   2. Dysgammaglobulinemia
   3. Extramedullary hematopoiesis
   4. Hemochromatosis
   5. Myelofibrosis (hypersplenism)
   6. Osteoporosis
   7. Polycytopenic purpura
B. *Infection*
   1. Bacterial
   2. Fungal
   3. Parasitic disease
   4. Viral
C. *Neoplasm*
   1. Cyst
   2. Hemangioma, lymphangioma
   3. Lymphoma
   4. Metastases
   5. Neoplasm (benign)
   6. Sarcoma (especially angiosarcoma)
D. *Portal hypertension*
   1. Congestive splenomegaly
   2. Nutritional or alcoholic cirrhosis
   3. Schistosomiasis
   4. Splenic or portal vein obstruction
E. *Storage diseases*
   1. Gaucher's disease
   2. Glycogen storage disease
   3. Histiocystosis X
   4. Mucopolysaccharidosis
   5. Niemann-Pick disease
   6. Wilson's disease
F. *Trauma*
   1. Hematoma
   2. Hemorrhagic pseudocyst
G. *Other*
   1. Antitrypsinase deficiency

2. Amyloidosis
3. Collagen disease
4. Congenital syndrome
5. Congestive heart failure
6. Infarction
7. Juvenile rheumatoid arthritis (Still's disease)
8. Sarcoidosis

Other forms of splenomegaly are part of congenital syndromes, including the rare Aase-Smith syndrome, Felty's syndrome, and many others.

In trying to establish an approximate diagnosis by considering only the size of the spleen, a good rule of thumb is:

1. Slight splenomegaly suggests infection.
2. Moderate splenomegaly may be related to portal hypertension.
3. Marked splenomegaly suggests hematologic disease (leukemia?).

Ultrasound is the predominant imaging method for the determination of splenic morphometry and recently has also been used to assess splenic size in fetuses. Normal ultrasound values for longitudinal, coronal, and transverse dimensions; perimeter; and calculated volume have been established.[27] Since sonographic examination can be regarded as reliable, nomograms can be used to detect growth disorders of the fetal spleen, thus providing a method to identify genetic disorders involving splenomegaly in utero.

Inflammatory disorders

The spleen is a very sensitive indicator for inflammatory processes. A palpable spleen, for example, is typical of subacute endocarditis. Other disorders with variable degrees of splenomegaly include histoplasmosis, infectious mononucleosis, malaria, kala azar, and tuberculosis. Fungal infections of the spleen are seen with increasing frequency among patients with hematopoietic malignancies.[16]

Candidiasis in some cases causes focal lesions of the spleen, as detected by CT and ultrasound. Occasionally, spontaneous subcapsular hematoma may be detected in infectious mononucleosis,[28] thus providing an important diagnostic clue.

Abscesses

Splenic abscess occurs infrequently. When it does, the abscess causes symptoms and signs that often do not suggest the diagnosis because of the nonspecific nature of the patient's complaints. Abdominal ultrasound allows precise diagnosis by showing sonolucent areas within an enlarged spleen. On CT, low-density areas with air bubbles and absent contrast enhancement are typical findings. In immunosuppressed patients, CT and ultrasound examinations suggestive of splenic cyst or hematoma must be followed by needle aspiration to rule out abscess.

Bacterial and chemical analyses of the needle aspirate give definitive information.

^{111}In-labeled leukocytes and ^{67}Ga scintigraphy can be used to differentiate splenic abscess from infarction.[2] Ultrasound and CT are the imaging methods of choice in the workup of drug addicts with fever and abdominal pain caused by splenic abscesses.

Cysts

Primary splenic cysts are rare. Almost all are the result of previous splenic trauma and evolve from a subcapsular hematoma that has not ruptured. Parasitic and nonparasitic cysts can be easily identified as sonolucent images with echo enhancement behind them. They are seen as focal defects in radionuclide scintigraphy, but the scan does not help in differentiating a cystic from a solid lesion.

In some cases plain film studies reveal calcification of the cystic wall. CT and MRI are more precise by clearly outlining the fluid collection. The angiographic appearance of a cyst is a rounded, avascular area surrounded by normal splenic parenchyma. The artery branches are stretched around the cyst, but no abnormal vessels are present.

Ultrasound- or CT-guided puncture offers the possibility of cytologic and chemical examination of the aspirate. In rare cases a suspected splenic mass, as seen in ultrasound or CT studies, is actually of pancreatic origin. In addition to detection of amylase in the aspirate, needle aspiration is helpful in the recognition of a primary pancreatic pseudocyst mimicking an intrasplenic cyst.[9] A rare cause of multiple splenic cysts is cystic lymphangioma.

Tumors

Primary neoplasms of the spleen are rare; exceptions are malignant lymphoma and plasmacytoma. Other tumors, listed here in decreasing order of frequency, have been observed[20]:

Hemangioma
Lymphangioma
Hamartoma
Fibroma
Myxoma
Chondroma
Osteoma
Hemangiosarcoma
Fibrosarcoma

Metastases to the spleen are only seen in terminal stages. Tumors that often metastasize to the spleen are those of the lung, breast, ovary, colon, prostate, and skin (melanoma).

Splenic tumors do not necessarily cause splenomegaly and will easily be shown on sulfur colloid scintigraphy. Ultrasound, however, is the best screening method for

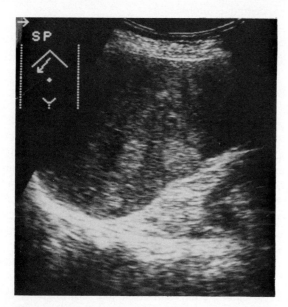

Fig. 61-5 Abdominal ultrasound image of non-Hodgkin's lymphoma of spleen. Splenomegaly is present with hypoechogenic areas bulging the contours.

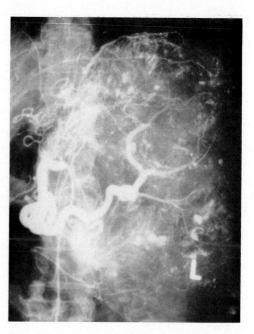

Fig. 61-6 Selective splenic arteriography shows hemangiomatosis of spleen with multiple contrast pools and massive splenic enlargement.

this purpose and demonstrates whether the lesion is cystic or solid (Fig. 61-5).

Despite the numerous publications about the CT appearances of lymphatic disorders of the spleen, especially in Hodgkin's disease and non-Hodgkin's lymphoma, no specific imaging criteria exist besides the presence of low-attenuation areas, circumscript or generalized enlargement of the organ, and possible infiltration into adjacent organs.[10] Even in a case of primary angiosarcoma, CT showed no contrast enhancement.[33]

Angiography reveals a characteristic hypervascular network in hemangioma and hamartoma. Vascular lakes and malignant tumor vessels can be seen in hemangiosarcomas. In the rare hemangiomatosis of liver and spleen, selective arteriography of the celiac trunk gives excellent information (Fig. 61-6).

Almost all modern imaging techniques provide accurate localization of benign or malignant splenic tumors but indicate little information about their nature. Ultrasound- or CT-guided needle biopsies are indispensable for definitive diagnosis in most cases.

More recently, efforts have been made to correlate the splenic volumes, based on CT measurements, with histologic findings in Hodgkin's disease. The "splenic index" presented by Strijk and co-workers[30] in 1985 was controversial. Magnetic resonance spectroscopy may provide more information about neoplastic changes in the future.

Perisplenic masses

The distance from the spleen to the diaphragm is normally variable. This should not be considered in the diagnosis of space-occupying masses whenever ultrasound and CT do not reveal subdiaphragmatic fluid collections or masses in the adjacent organs. Occasionally, omentum extending to the left upper quadrant may mimic tumors in the splenic hilum. Tumors of the left upper renal pole, the left adrenal gland, or in some cases the pancreatic tail are difficult to differentiate from primary splenic neoplasms. In vascular tumors angiography may demonstrate the vascular supply to the tumor, thereby establishing the origin of the lesion. Since lymphomas are usually hypovascular, attempts to image left upper quadrant vessels are ineffective. Needle biopsy or even exploratory laparotomy, in cases of very extended malignancies, are sometimes unable to indicate the origin of the tumor.

Pseudocysts of the pancreatic tail penetrating the spleen occasionally mimic splenic cysts. Likewise, a large gastric ulcer penetrating into the spleen can be best seen during a barium meal as a filling defect surrounded by splenic tissue.[3] When the left liver lobe is seen draped around the spleen, CT or ultrasound differentiation of the two organs may be impossible[4]; angiography may be indicated in such cases (traumatized spleen, splenic tumor and so on).

The development of left suprarenal masses following

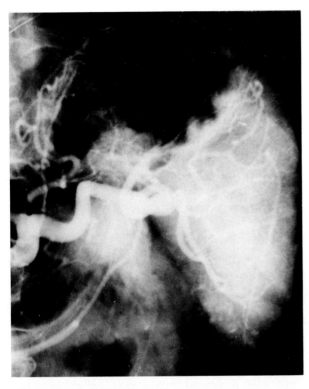

Fig. 61-7 Selective splenic arteriography shows missing parenchymal staining caused by separate vascularization of upper pole by aberrant aortic branch.

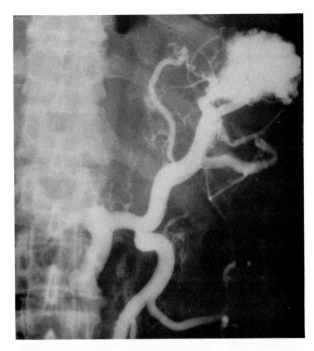

Fig. 61-8 Splenoportography demonstrates occlusion of splenic vein close to hilum, with multiple collaterals present.

splenectomy has been related to splenosis or accessory spleens. [99m]Tc sulfur colloid imaging shows uptake in such masses, confirming the splenic origin.[25]

Vascular diseases

Atherosclerotic changes of the splenic artery can be detected frequently in older patients on plain film studies of the abdomen. The tortuous, calcified vessel sometimes even shows aneurysmal dilatation. Celiac or superselective splenic angiography are indicated when occlusive disease is suspected. Stenosis of the splenic artery causes collaterals to develop through the tail of the pancreas, through the gastroepiploic arteries, and over the left and short gastric arteries.[34]

Occlusion of one of the segmental arterial branches leads to infarction. The diagnosis is easily made by demonstration of occluded branches and a wedge-shaped parenchymal defect. One should be careful to avoid mistaking absence of opacification caused by an aberrant vessel for an infarct (Fig. 61-7). The diagnosis can be made noninvasively by isotope studies or dynamic CT.

Chronic pancreatitis causing repeated exposure of the splenic artery to pancreatic enzymes during acute attacks may cause aneurysm formation.[26] Noncalcified aneu-

rysms may rupture spontaneously, especially in pregnant women.

Arterioportal shunts, causing portal hypertension, can be congenital in origin or may be acquired traumatically.[34]

Arteriography demonstrates rapid contrast filling of the splenic vein and poor parenchymal opacification.

Splenic vein occlusion by thrombosis or compression leads to marked splenomegaly. The diagnosis can be made by ultrasound, angiography and CT, or arteriography. Larger than usual amounts of contrast material are necessary for the visualization of the patent portions of the splenic vein. The contrast material bypasses the obstruction through the left and right gastroepiploic, the short gastric, and left gastric veins.

Direct measurement of the portal pressure is possible after splenic puncture for splenoportography. Only in very rare cases is the examination justified in order to clarify preoperatively the venous anatomy (Fig. 61-8).

Trauma

The spleen is the most frequently injured organ in blunt abdominal trauma. Clinical examination and plain film findings of lower rib fractures, elevation of the left

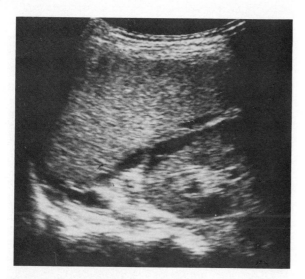

Fig. 61-9 Abdominal ultrasound image of small subcapsular and pericapsular fluid accumulation. Bleeding from capsular injury caused by blunt abdominal trauma.

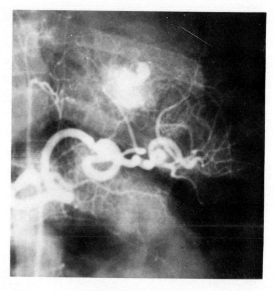

Fig. 61-10 Selective splenic arteriography demonstrates intrasplenic hematoma after traffic accident.

hemidiaphragm, and splenic enlargement are insufficient criteria to indicate surgical exploration. Currently, splenic trauma is not always followed by liberal surgical removal, and a more conservative trend exists in the surgical management.[36]

Ultrasound is the basic imaging method in blunt abdominal trauma, since it may demonstrate free intraperitoneal fluid as well as a splenic lesion. As little as 50 to 100 ml of free blood could be recognized in our own studies.[13] Paracentesis has not been necessary in any of our cases to rule out bloody peritoneal fluid. Ultrasound examinations give information about the size of the organ, subcapsular or pericapsular hematoma, parenchymal contusion, or rupture with concomitant bleeding (Fig. 61-9).

Resolution of lesions within the traumatized spleen can be confirmed by sonographic investigation. In children, evidence of splenic laceration and intrasplenic, perisplenic, and intraperitoneal fluid collections may disappear within 2 to 4 weeks, as demonstrated by serial ultrasound examinations. Intrasplenic hematomas and contusions are usually resorbed over a few months to a year.[11]

Not limited by bowel gas or ribs, CT gives better information about details of splenic injury. Angiography and CT can also recognize vascular damage with ensuing infarction.

Radionuclide studies are not useful in acute phases of splenic trauma. Conversely, angiography is valuable for the detailed visualization of acute traumatic changes, ranging from a small, focal hematoma to total organ avulsion (Fig. 61-10). In addition, angiographic tech-

niques may be lifesaving by using transcatheter embolization when massive bleeding is evident and emergency surgery is contraindicated.

The algorithmic pathway for rapid evaluation of splenic trauma is as follows:
1. Thoracic and abdominal plain films
2. Ultrasound and/or CT
3. Angiography

INTERVENTIONAL RADIOLOGY

As already mentioned, transcatheter embolization of splenic artery branches or the main splenic artery can be lifesaving. Using Gianturco coils, detachable balloons, Gelfoam, or other occlusive agents, acute posttraumatic bleeding can be stopped.

The intrasplenic branches are end arteries and do not anastomose with each other. Therefore complete embolization obviously leaves no opportunity for development of an anastomotic blood supply. Splenic infarction or abscess formation may develop after complete or partial therapeutic embolization.[1] Embolization of the spleen should only be undertaken in extreme cases and should be used judiciously.

A rare indication for splenic artery embolization is a bleeding splenic artery aneurysm in high-risk patients so as to avoid emergency surgery. In some hematologic disorders with clinical evidence of hypersplenism, partial embolization of the spleen may result in an increase in the platelet count.[1] We have seen five patients in our experience who had these symptoms.

Abscess formation within the spleen or under the diaphragm can be treated by percutaneous ultrasound- or CT-guided needle puncture and drainage. Needle biopsy of the spleen may be followed by peritoneal bleeding. A special instrument that consists of a spring-loaded system has been recommended to avert this complication.[18]

REFERENCES

1. Allison DJ: Interventional radiology. In Grainger, GR, and Allison, DJ: Diagnostic radiology, vol 3, New York, 1986, Churchill Livingstone.
2. Bihl, H, Breivogel, B, and Hofmann, W: Zur Wertigkeit von Leukozyten- und Galliumszintigraphie bei der Differentialdiagnose Milzabszess/infarkt, Digitale Bilddiagnostik 7(1):47, 1987.
3. Chńg, JLC, Owen, MC, and Heller, CA: Radiological gastric filling defect due to penetration into the spleen by a large gastric ulcer, Br J Radiol 56:488, 1983.
4. Cholankeril, JY, Zamora, BO, and Ketyer, S: Left lobe of the liver draping around the spleen: a pitfall in computed tomography diagnosis of perisplenic hematoma, J Comput Tomogr 8(3):261, 1984.
5. Denin, H, et al: Detection of splenosis of radionuclide scanning, Br J Radiol 60:873, 1987.
6. Dittrich, M, et al: Sonographic biometry of liver and spleen size in childhood, Pediatr Radiol 13:206, 1983.
7. Felson, B, and Reeder, M: Gamuts in radiology, Cincinnati, 1987, Audivisual Radiology.
8. Frank, K, et al: Sonographische Milzgrößenbestimmung: Normalmaße beim Milzgesunden Erwachsenen, Ultraschall Medizin 7:134, 1986.
9. Garnic, JD, et al: Pancreatic masses that angiographically simulate intrasplenic lesions, Cardiovasc Intervent Radiol 8(3):146, 1985.
10. Gilbert, T, and Castellino, RA: Critical review—the spleen in hodgkin disease: diagnostic value of CT, Invest Radiol 21(5):437, 1986.
11. Greenbaum, EI: Radiology of the emergency patient, New York, 1982, John Wiley & Sons.
12. Grenier, N, et al: Volvolus chronique d'une rate ectopique avec hêmatome souscapsulaire, Radiologie 68:615, 1987.
13. Hauenstein, KH, et al: Die Rolle der Sonographie beim stumpfen Bauchtrauma, Radiologe 22(2):106, 1982.
14. Hausdorf, G: Das sonographische Bild des Asplenie-Syndroms, Fortschritte Röntgenstrahlen 138(5):553, 1983.
15. Heloury, Y, et al: Spleno-gonadal fusion: anatomic and angiographic study of a case, Surg Radiol Anat 8(2):147, 1986.
16. Helton, WS, et al: Diagnosis and treatment of splenic fungal abscesses in the immune-suppressed patient, Arch Surg 121(5):580, 1986.
17. Kremer, H, et al: Abdominal ultrasonic screening, Ultraschall Medizin, 5:272, 1984.
18. Lindgren, PG, et al: Excision biopsy of the spleen by ultrasonic guidance, Br J Radiol 58:853, 1985.
19. Markisz, JA, Treves, ST, and Davis, RT: Normal hepatic and splenic size in children, Pediatr Radiol 17:273, 1987.
20. Meyer, JE, et al: Large-cell lymphoma of the spleen: CT appearance, Radiology 148(1):199, 1983.
21. Moncada, R, et al: thoracic splenosis, Am J Roentgenol 144(4):705, 1985.
22. Niederau, C, et al: Sonographic measurements of the normal liver, spleen, pancreas, and portal vein, Radiology 149(2):537, 1983.
23. Nishitani, H, et al: Computed tomography of accessory spleens, Radiat Med 2(4):222, 1984.
24. Pundaleeka, SK, Zimmers, TE, and Nassos, TP: Splenic torsion presenting as a twisted hemorrhagic ovarian cyst, Ann Emerg Med 14(1):64, 1985.
25. Rao, KG, and Fitzer, PM: Left suprarenal mass following splenectomy: case reports, J Urol 132(2):323, 1984.
26. Reuter, SR, and Redman, HC: Gastrointestinal angiography, Philadelphia, 1977, WB Saunders.
27. Schmidt, W, et al: Sonographic measurements of the fetal spleen: clinical implications, J Ultrasound Med 4(12):667, 1985.
28. Shirkhoda, A: CT findings in hepatosplenic and renal candidiasis, J Comput Assist Tomogr 11(5):795, 1987.
29. Smevik, B, and Monclair, T: Torsion of a wandering spleen in an infant, Acta Radiol (Diagn) (Stockh) 27(6):715, 1986.
30. Strijk, SP, et al: Critical review—the spleen in Hodgkin's disease: diagnostic value of CT, Radiology 154(2):753, 1985.
31. Turnheer, S, et al: MR Bildgebung der Milz, Freiburg, 1988, Dt Röntgenkongress.
32. Vossen, PG, et al: Computed tomography of the polysplenia syndrome in the adult, Gastrointest Radiol 12(3):209, 1987.
33. Wafula, JMC: Ultrasound and CT demonstration of primary angiosarcoma of the spleen, Br J Radiol 58:903, 1985.
34. Wenz, W: Abdominal angiography, New York, 1974, Springer Publishing.
35. Wenz, W, and Mathias, K: Die "Upside-Down" Milz, Deutsche Medizinische Wochenschrift 102:20, 1977.
36. Wenz, W, and Bodendörfer, G: Modern imaging procedures of splenic diseases, Radiologe 27:11, 1987.

PART XII

INFECTIOUS DISEASES

62 *Infections and Infestations*

MAURICE M. REEDER
PHILIP E.S. PALMER

GASTROINTESTINAL TUBERCULOSIS[1-29]

Tuberculosis of the alimentary tract is now a rare disease. It is clear from the radiologic, surgical, and pathologic literature before 1950 that tuberculosis of the alimentary tract used to be much more common. Although the general decrease in tuberculosis since adequate chemotherapy became available must account in part for this decline, other factors are probably involved. Tuberculosis of the lungs and skeleton is still extremely common in many parts of the world, and yet, with few exceptions, tuberculosis of the alimentary tract has become very uncommon. Only from India have significant series been reported in the last 20 years (one hospital reported 400 cases in 5 years, which amounted to 15% of all gastrointestinal studies). In North America and Europe it is a very rare disease. Wherever it occurs, it most commonly affects the lower small bowel, cecum, and ascending colon. It is much less frequent in the esophagus, stomach, and upper small bowel. In this respect there has been little change over the years; the ileocecal region has always been the most common site of occurrence of tuberculosis. However, both previously and currently, peritonitis is a common manifestation of tuberculosis within the abdomen.

As elsewhere in the body, tuberculosis in the alimentary tract forms granulomas. These may present clinically and radiologically as an ulcer, a mass, or a hypertrophic tumor (tuberculoma). If the infection is chronic or the patient's immunity is sufficient, there will be fibrosis, leading to a stricture or malfunction of the normal alimentary peristalsis. When the peritoneum is involved, the eventual result may be adhesions.

Apart from symptoms and signs similar to those of tuberculosis anywhere, that is, loss of weight, general malaise, "feeling unwell," there is no specific findings that may lead to the clinical diagnosis of alimentary tract tuberculosis. Nausea, vomiting, diarrhea, or, in some cases, constipation can occur.[1] Distention due to intestinal obstruction, when there is a stricture or adhesions, may be the presenting symptom. Clinical examination of the patient with peritonitis may be helpful, but this is the only aspect of alimentary tract tuberculosis in which the clinical diagnosis is likely to be correct. In fact, depending on the site of the lesion, the initial clinical impression will nearly always suggest malignant disease. In the esophagus or stomach benign peptic ulceration may occasionally be suspected. In the small bowel the clinical findings may suggest acute or chronic low-grade gastroenteritis. In the large bowel any pattern of colitis may be suggested. The whole clinical picture is essentially vague and ill defined. Wherever the lesion and whatever the findings, the determining factor will be histologic.

There are no specific laboratory tests. It is difficult to recover the mycobacteria from gastric washings when there is tuberculous esophageal or gastric ulceration. It is equally difficult to recover them from the feces when the colon or rectum is involved, but should *Mycobacterium tuberculosis* be found in the stool, it is of considerable significance. Most patients will be anemic, and some will have blood in the stool. Many will be underweight. The vast majority of patients will have a positive tuberculin skin reaction (Mantoux or purified protein derivative [PPD]), but the laboratory findings will be of little guidance to the correct diagnosis.

Much has been written about the incidence of pulmonary tuberculosis in patients with alimentary tract infection, and vice versa. The reports are conflicting. Although it is not unusual to find a pulmonary tuberculous lesion associated with alimentary tract tuberculosis (in one series 20% of such patients had active pulmonary tuberculosis), it is by no means consistent.[1,15,24] Many patients who have tuberculosis of the alimentary tract will have normal findings on a chest radiograph, and the absence of pulmonary infection should not in any way negate the diagnosis.[19] On the other hand, many thousands of patients have active pulmonary tuberculosis and swallow sputum containing active mycobacteria but do not develop a clinical alimentary tract infection. It has proved impossible to reproduce alimentary tract tuberculosis in animals even when they are fed large quantities of tuberculous bacilli. Nevertheless, the finding of pulmonary tuberculosis may influence the diagnosis. For example, an unusual ulcer in the rectum seen at proctoscopy in a patient who has pulmonary tuberculosis must raise a high index of suspicion that the rectal ulceration is tuberculous also. Yet, if the findings on the chest radiograph are normal, tuberculosis cannot be excluded, and suspicion of a tuberculous ulcer must remain. Perhaps the presence of a known pulmonary tuberculous infection may be an added reason for including tuberculosis in the differential diagnosis of an alimentary tract lesion, but in practice it will seldom make the diagnosis more accurate.

It is not difficult to demonstrate most alimentary tract tuberculous lesions radiologically, but it is much more difficult, if not impossible, to recognize their cause. The histologic findings will almost always be a surprise and will often provide a relief that the lesion is not malignant.

Tuberculosis of the esophagus

Tuberculosis of the esophagus initiates an inflammatory reaction that results in ulceration, thickening of the esophageal wall, or, least commonly, a tumor. Direct spread from caseating tuberculous lymph nodes in the mediastinum may involve the esophagus. All these varieties may cause fistulas between the esophagus and the mediastinum or occasionally into the trachea or a bronchus. Almost all heal by fibrosis so that a stricture is the most common presentation (Fig. 62-1).

The upper half of the esophagus is most frequently affected, and no age is exempt. Patients complain of difficulty in swallowing, which may be of slow onset or relatively acute. When there is an obvious stricture or ulcer, the clinical history and appearance strongly resemble those associated with malignancy. Tuberculous ulcers are usually flat and partially surround the esophagus. When there is intramural thickening, there will be disruption of normal peristalsis.

Although the upper part of the esophagus is most frequently affected, tuberculous ulceration and strictures also occur in the lower third of the esophagus, with the same differential diagnosis between benign or malignant stricture or ulceration. In some cases the narrowing in the region of the cardia may result in a dilated esophagus, resembling achalasia or the stricture of peptic esophagitis;

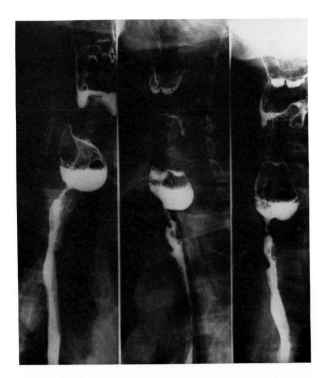

Fig. 62-1 Tuberculous stricture in upper third of esophagus with marked proximal dilatation above narrow, elongate, irregular stricture. Histologic confirmation would be necessary to distinguish this from other inflammatory strictures or from carcinoma.
(From Reeder, MM, and Palmer, PES: The radiology of tropical diseases, Baltimore, 1981, Williams & Wilkins).

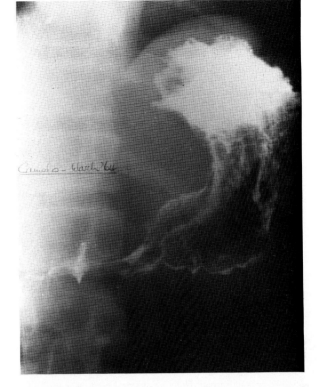

Fig. 62-2 Tuberculous gastritis causes thickening of wall of stomach and narrowing of pyloric antrum in African patient. Duodenal bulb and C loop are also distorted and narrowed.
(From Reeder, MM, and Palmer, PES: The radiology of tropical diseases, Baltimore, 1981, Williams & Wilkins.)

it may also be mistaken for a neoplasm in the region of the cardia.

The radiologic differential diagnosis between a tuberculous lesion and malignancy is impossible. Because dilatation of the esophagus occurs above the stricture, there will often be a "rat-tail" appearance on the barium study that is indistinguishable from carcinoma. Tuberculous ulcers have no distinguishing features radiologically. If there is an active pulmonary tuberculous lesion, the possibility of tuberculosis should be considered, but even this is not easy. In more than one patient the spread of miliary tuberculosis throughout the lungs has been confused with multiple small metastatic lesions, and the associated stricture of the esophagus was accordingly labeled malignant rather than tuberculous. Biopsy is essential.

Tuberculosis of the stomach

Tuberculosis may cause the stomach to ulcerate or become fibrotic and resemble malignant infiltration (as in linitis plastica), or, less commonly, tuberculosis may occur as a hypertrophic "mass" (Fig. 62-2). The radiologic and pathologic variations are considerable. Even an erosive tuberculous gastritis has been reported, with numerous small mucosal defects, almost a type of miliary disease.

The clinical symptoms are those of peptic ulceration or neoplasm and cannot be distinguished. If there is active pulmonary tuberculosis, this as a cause may at least be suggested. The most common site for a tuberculous ulcer is close to the pylorus. Some tuberculous ulcers are very shallow but can be quite extensive.[13,26] They are unlikely to be mistaken for malignancy. Others have induration around the ulcer, the edge of which is undermined; this will not be mistaken for benign peptic ulceration. A not infrequent presentation is pyloric obstruction, which may be due to tuberculous ulceration, fibrosis subsequent to appearance of such an ulcer, severe submucosal thickening, or in some cases extrinsic pressure from tuberculous lymphadenopathy. If these lymph nodes caseate,

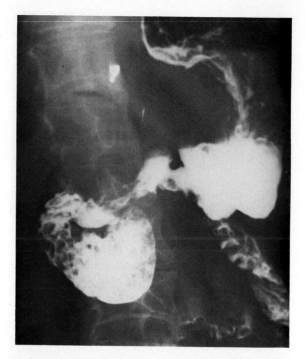

Fig. 62-3 Tuberculosis involving stomach and duodenum. Infiltration along lesser curvature has narrowed stomach. Duodenal bulb is deformed. Nodular mucosal contour is evident in duodenum. Partial obstruction of third portion of duodenum is caused by tuberculous celiac lymph nodes.

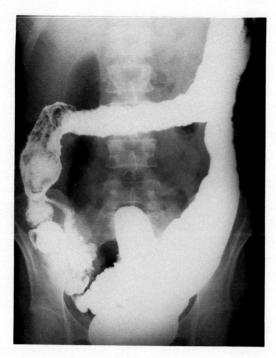

Fig. 62-4 Tuberculous ileocolitis manifested by narrowed ileum and cecum, narrowing of right and transverse portions of colon with loss of haustra, and extensive ulceration. Left portion of colon is normal. Crohn's disease and occasionally amebiasis may produce this radiographic pattern.

the pylorus or greater curvature of the stomach may become directly involved. However, as with most cases of marked pyloric obstruction, the true cause cannot be diagnosed radiologically.

Tuberculosis of the duodenum and small bowel

Tuberculosis affects all parts of the small bowel, the jejunum very infrequently, the duodenum occasionally, and the lower part of the ileum more commonly. There may be ulceration, granulomatous thickening, or, occasionally, hyperplastic nodules or tuberculoma. Any part of the small bowel, but particularly the duodenum, can be distorted by tuberculous lymphadenopathy (Fig. 62-3). It is unlikely that the correct diagnosis will be made either clinically or radiologically.

The common clinical presentation for tuberculosis of the duodenum and small bowel is obstruction, either high in the duodenum or jejunum or, most commonly, in the lower part of the ileum. Supine and erect films of the abdomen may show dilated loops of small bowel with fluid levels, depending on the position of the obstruction.

Tuberculosis of the duodenum most commonly occurs either as ulceration or as strictures, both most frequently in the third part of the duodenal loop. Thick, hypertrophic mucosa, almost resembling polyps, has been reported; granulomatous infiltration along short lengths of the duodenum may cause loss of peristalsis or even narrowing of the lumen. Isolated tuberculous involvement of the duodenum is uncommon; it will be associated either with lesions elsewhere in the small bowel or, quite frequently, with gastric tuberculosis. One series reports that 11% of patients with gastric tuberculosis also have duodenal infection.[11] Where there is ulceration, the ulcers are frequently multiple and associated with considerable thickening of the duodenal wall. Perforation with fistula formation can occur. As healing takes place, the result is almost always contraction and stenosis leading to duodenal obstruction.

In the ileum tuberculosis causes transverse ulcers in the Peyer's patches, with typically undermined edges. This is usually a chronic condition, and there may be considerable dilatation of the small bowel above the narrow areas. Accurate demonstration of lower small bowel tuberculosis is enhanced by use of a small bowel enema, which will show the exact site and the characteristics of the stricture or strictures. However, even with this technique, differentiation from Crohn's disease is very difficult radiologically (Fig. 62-4). Tuberculosis may form fistulas similar to those of regional ileitis. They may occur at multiple levels and can be insidious in onset and chronic in duration. It is helpful to remember that Crohn's disease is rare in many parts of the world, for instance, India, and a knowledge of geography may provide more help than will radiology in the differential diagnosis.

A small bowel obstruction due to tuberculous peritonitis is not uncommon. Adhesions may also result from tuberculous enteritis.[8,19]

Pressure on the duodenal loop from tuberculous lymphadenopathy may cause extrinsic distortion and even obstruction. This may be in the acute stage or, as the lymphadenopathy heals, may result from fibrosis. It will be impossible to differentiate the distortion from malignant lymphadenopathy or in some cases from enlargement of the pancreas. The clinical and the radiologic diagnosis is likely to be lymphoma or malignancy, tuberculous lymphadenopathy in the abdomen being uncommon and unrecognizable unless there is generalized tuberculous peritonitis.

Ileocecal tuberculosis

The ileum-cecum is and always has been the most common site for tuberculosis of the alimentary tract and because of the marked local reaction has been called "hyperplastic" tuberculosis of the gastrointestinal tract[10,11] (Fig. 62-5). In some series it is said to account for 80% to 90% of all patients with gastrointestinal tuberculosis. This figure is probably too high as an overall average. Similarly, it is claimed that correlation with an autopsy series will show that about 80% of gastrointestinal tuberculous infection are not shown by radiologic investigation. Although this figure may be true, it is unlikely that many of the "missed" infections would have caused significant clinical findings. Certainly the radiologic accuracy of diagnosis of pathologic conditions in the ileocecal region is high, although the accuracy of recognition that the disease is tuberculosis may well be very much less. The clinical symptoms are ill defined and include diarrhea or constipation, vague cramping pain, and often a palpable mass. Histologically there will be granulomatous proliferation followed by fibrosis until the size and lumen of the cecum shrink, distorted by the inflammatory mass and the resulting fibrosis.

The classic radiographic appearance of ileocecal tuberculosis has been described on barium enema examination as a conical, shrunken, retracted cecum associated with a narrow ulcerated terminal ileum[2] (Fig. 62-5). The cecal deformity is the result of spasm early in the disease and transmural infiltrate with fibrosis in more advanced

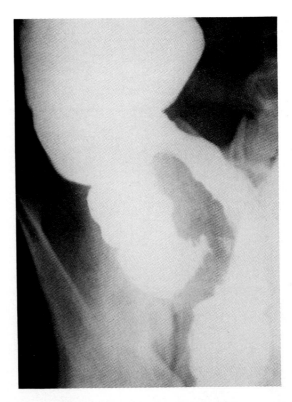

Fig. 62-5 Typical, narrowed, shrunken, conical cecum and narrowed ulcerated terminal ileum of ileocecal tuberculosis. Note gaping ileocecal valve.

phases. Narrowing of the terminal ileum may be caused by persistent irritability with rapid emptying of the narrowed segment when filling retrograde or antegrade (Stierlin's sign) from a barium enema. This narrowing corresponds to the acute inflammatory phase of the disease. It may be the result of stricture with thickening and ulceration of the bowel wall in advanced ileocecal tuberculosis. The ileocecal valve has been described as "gaping,"[14] similar to that in chronic ulcerative colitis (Fig. 62-5). In the more advanced ileal lesions, deep fissures and ulcers develop, as well as enterocutaneous fistulas.[16] Circumferential deep ileal ulcers may progress to perforation at those times when clinical and pulmonary response to antitubercular drugs is seen. Most perforations, however, are of the walled-off type rather than of the free intraperitoneal type.

Because the mesocolon contracts, the cecum may be pulled out of the iliac fossa, while at the same time it is reduced in size by fibrosis. Similarly, the hepatic flexure may be pulled downward. There may be a partial stricture of the ileocecal junction, also resulting from fibrosis. The terminal ileum therefore dilates and, as viewed by barium enema, may seem to be suspended and hanging

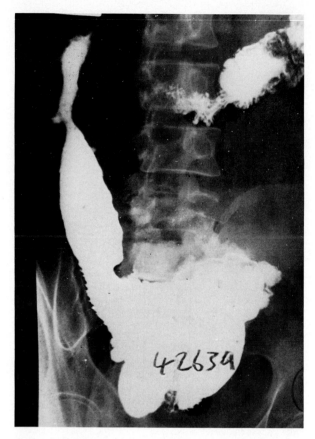

Fig. 62-6 Contracted cecum of tuberculosis. There is ulceration of terminal ileum and minimal obstruction. Ileum is dilated and seems to hang from small contracted cecum.
(From Reeder, MM, and Palmer, PES: The radiology of tropical diseases, Baltimore, 1981, Williams & Wilkins.)

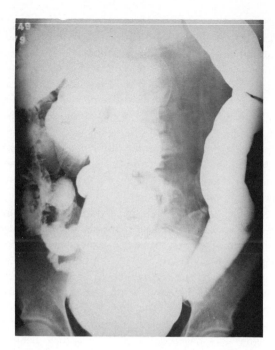

Fig. 62-7 Deep penetrating ulcers and fissures of cecum and ascending colon cause extensive narrowing and deformity of right portion of colon in patient with ileocecal tuberculosis.

from the cecum (Fig. 62-6). Movement of the cecum, both clinically and radiologically, is restricted in every direction. Spontaneous sinus formation is not common, but fistulas between various loops of bowel may result, particularly after surgical interference, if the correct diagnosis has not been realized at the time of surgery. Pericecal abscesses are not common but may occur and resemble an appendiceal or an amebic abscess.

Although it is essential to use a barium enema for examination of the large bowel in tuberculosis, a follow-through upper gastrointestinal study should be part of the investigation. The lower part of the cecum may appear to be obliterated, and reflux of an enema into the ileum may not be obtained or may be incomplete. The follow-through study helps exclude other sites of small bowel infection and delineate the exact involvement of the terminal ileum and the ileocecal junction. In about 20% of cases of ileocecal tuberculosis there are other small bowel strictures, particularly in the distal ileum. In other patients the granulomatous infiltration of the bowel wall

may produce an appearance similar to the rigid "tube" of Crohn's disease. When these findings are added to those of the granulomatous cecal mass and the overall fibrosis, the distortion at the ileocecal region may be considerable.

In the hypertrophic variety (or perhaps "stage" is a better term, because most hypertrophic tuberculous infections will eventually fibrose) the hypertrophic masses may be shown on barium study projecting into the lumen of the cecum and ascending colon. Because there is almost always some associated contraction, it may be possible to suggest the correct (tuberculous) cause when this combination is seen. As the hypertrophic granulomas progress, the cecum radiologically becomes conical, and stenosis occurs, both at the ileocecal junction and in the ascending colon.[2] Eventually only a strip of barium may be left to outline the affected area, particularly at the junction of the cecum and ascending colon (Fig. 62-7).

The differential diagnosis of such distortion radiologically will include an appendix abscess and an amebic abscess (Fig. 62-8). Other cases will resemble Crohn's disease. In many reports reflux from the cecum into the ileum is uncommon in tuberculosis when compared with amebiasis or a malignant tumor. However, at some stages a patulous ileocecal valve is seen,[14] particularly in series reported from India. This may perhaps be a reflection of the slower development of fibrosis when the infection is more of the acute, overwhelming pattern. To make the

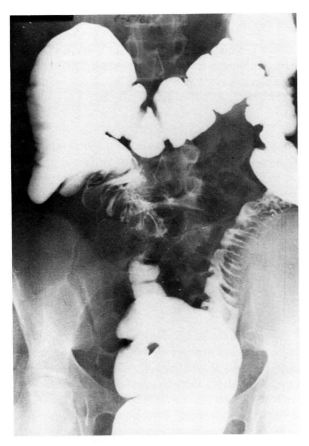

Fig. 62-8 Tuberculosis of cecum and colon. Cecum is displaced upward by lymphadenopathy; mucosa is edematous and swollen. Mass was palpable and clinically suggested malignancy. Marked mucosal changes in sigmoid colon led to alternative diagnosis of amebiasis or lymphoma. Tuberculosis was not considered. Combination of matting and adhesions of small bowel, fixation of ileocecal junction, and contracted cecum suggests correct diagnosis of tuberculosis. Massive lymphadenopathy seen here is unusual in tuberculosis alone.
(From Reeder, MM, and Palmer, PES: The radiology of tropical diseases, Baltimore, 1981, Williams & Wilkins.)

differential diagnosis more difficult, amebiasis can also occasionally be a fibrosing condition. However, amebiasis seldom affects the small bowel above the terminal ileum. Finding amebas in the stool may solve the radiologic dilemma.

Bone infection in the ilium has resulted from a tuberculous abscess in the region of the cecum. As with other tuberculous infections, it tends to be chronic and may even be mistaken for actinomycosis.

Tuberculosis of the colon

Below the cecum, tuberculous granulomas occur in the colon either as colitis or strictures; either may be multifocal.[6,16] Ulceration also occurs, usually in the early

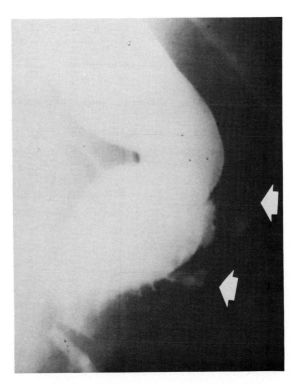

Fig. 62-9 Deep penetrating rectal ulcers and fissures with production of perirectal *(arrows)*—result of tuberculosis. This patient also had pulmonary tuberculosis.

stages, but is seldom seen radiologically. Tuberculous infection usually spreads over short distances, 5 to 7 cm, and tuberculosis seldom involves extensive areas of the colon.

The clinical presentation of these strictures is usually that of incomplete obstruction without severe pain. The most likely clinical diagnosis will be malignant disease or, in appropriate areas, an ameboma. Making the differential diagnosis radiologically can be extremely difficult. Similarly, tuberculous colitis may resemble amebiasis, affecting short lengths of bowel and occasionally occurring at several sites. Perforation and fistulas are not often seen in tuberculosis, but both may occur, and a pericolic abscess may be formed.

A barium enema will show the constricted and often edematous area of bowel and only occasionally will show that other lengths of bowel are involved. The stricture is seldom as marked as the "apple-core" narrowing of malignancy and seldom as extensive as an ameboma. However, tuberculosis of the colon is not a diagnosis that will be made radiologically with great accuracy.

Tuberculosis of the rectum

Tuberculous infection seldom involves the rectum, although it may rarely present as an ulcerating proctitis (Fig. 62-9). Fistulas may result, and rectal strictures have been reported. Chronic sciatic-rectal abscesses may be tuberculous in origin. There are no distinguishing radiologic characteristics.

Enteroliths

Intestinal calculi are not common but may occur above any bowel stricture. When the stricture is high within the small bowel, the enteroliths are usually nonopaque. They are then composed of choleic acid. In the lower bowel, with a more alkaline medium and a higher concentration of calcium salts, enteroliths often become radiologically opaque. Some are completely opacified, whereas others have translucent centers with a ring of calcification. Such calcified enteroliths may be found in the lower ileum or colon in 3% to 4% of cases of intestinal tuberculosis. They vary from multiple small stones to single large lamellated calculi. They must be differentiated from renal stones or gallstones and, less commonly, from vesical stones. It is seldom difficult to differentiate them radiologically from calcified granulomas within the lymph nodes. Although tuberculosis is not unique in occurring with enterolithiasis, this possibility should be raised whenever such calculi are seen.

Peritoneal tuberculosis

Peritonitis is the most common presentation of tuberculosis within the abdomen. In some countries the peritoneum may be the most common single nonpulmonary site of infection. In every case there is associated abdominal lymphadenopathy, and in the majority there will be ascites. It is seldom possible, even histologically, to locate the primary tuberculous focus.

The patient usually complains of abdominal distention and pain, but many of the findings are nonspecific: weight loss, tiredness, and ill health. About one third of the patients are afebrile. The tuberculous skin reaction (either Mantoux or PPD) is usually positive but can be negative. The result on the chest radiograph is usually normal. Thorough clinical examination may reveal lymphadenopathy outside the abdomen, most commonly in the neck. Within the abdomen the liver and spleen may be enlarged but difficult to palpate. The abdomen is doughy to palpation and is often tender. Abdominal distention may be due to ascites or in some cases to subacute obstruction. In some patients it is possible to palpate a mass of enlarged lymph nodes, particularly in the right iliac fossa.

Routine supine and erect radiographs of the abdomen confirm the clinical suggestion of ascites and often show distended loops of small bowel, with thickened intestinal walls. The dilated loops suggest ileus rather than mechanical obstruction. As healing progresses, adhesions form and may later cause subacute obstruction at various levels. There is no indication for barium studies during

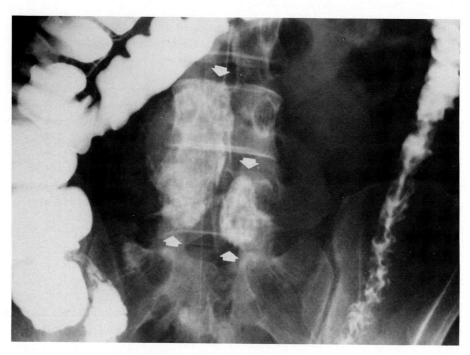

Fig. 62-10 Irregular patchy calcifications distributed throughout large tuberculous mesenteric lymph nodes (arrows). This patient had inactive pulmonary tuberculosis.

the acute stage, but later they can be used to determine whether the bowel has become fixed or remains mobile. There is seldom any intrinsic abnormality in the small bowel in cases of tuberculous peritonitis, but the lymphadenopathy may cause distortion.

The typical calcified tuberculous lymph nodes tend to cluster, with lobulated contours and spotty calcification throughout (Fig. 62-10). These nodes vary in size from 0.5 to 10 cm. Calcification of mesenteric lymph nodes 1 to 2 years after the onset of intestinal infection has been reported.[22]

DIFFERENTIAL DIAGNOSIS

Gastric tuberculosis must be differentiated radiographically from gastric carcinoma, lymphoma, and syphilis.

Intestinal tuberculosis is a granulomatous disease that involves all layers of the bowel wall. As in other granulomatous processes, it produces deep ulcers and may progress to formation of fistulas and strictures. Crohn's disease must be the first entity considered in the differential diagnosis, particularly when the ileocecal region is involved. These two processes may be indistinguishable radiographically. Definite apical pulmonary infiltrates seen on the chest radiograph in cases of typical ileocecal deformity suggest a tuberculous granulomatous process rather than Crohn's disease. Periappendiceal abscess may also produce the cecal deformities and narrowing of the terminal ileum that are suggestive of tuberculosis. Cecal diverticulitis has produced similar cecal and ileal narrowing. Although amebiasis may produce the typical shrunken cecum seen in tuberculosis, associated small bowel involvement with this infestation is rare. Lymphoma and carcinoma of the cecum may produce a short truncated cecal tip. Cecal carcinoma that crosses the ileocecal valve and involves the ileum is rare, however. Also, the margins of a carcinoma do not ordinarily taper but tend to be sharply demarcated.

More extensive tuberculosis that involves the colon must be differentiated from ulcerative colitis, Crohn's disease, the colitis of bacillary dysentery, amebic colitis, ischemic colitis, and pseudomembranous colitis. Idiopathic ulcerative colitis does not produce deep ulcerations and fistulas as does tuberculous colitis. However, the other forms of ulcerating colitis may be radiographically indistinguishable from tuberculous colitis.

SALMONELLA INFECTIONS[30-44]

Many species of Salmonella organisms may be responsible for food poisoning that originates from the ingestion of contaminated foods.[36,38,44] This infectious type of food poisoning, in which the salmonellae produce a thermostabile endotoxin that irritates the mucosa of the stomach and small and large bowels, must be differentiated from the toxin type of food poisoning caused by enterotoxin-producing organisms such as staphylococci.[39]

Infected carrier animals or their by-products, such as eggs, meat, and milk, are principal sources of Salmonella infections in humans. Chronic or temporary human carriers, especially those engaged in food handling, can play a significant role in the transmission of the disease, as can flies, cockroaches, and other insects.[39,41]

Once ingested, Salmonella organisms incubate for 7 to 30 hours before causing gastroenteritis. Infected persons may have headache, pyrexia, nausea, vomiting, and diarrhea with fluid stools that contain mucus and occasionally a small amount of blood. Patients with Salmonella food poisoning usually recover in about 5 days, although occasionally they may become extremely toxic and advance into a typhoid state. Mortality from this fulminant form of the disease is about 1%.[39]

Necropsy on the rare individuals who die of Salmonella food poisoning shows the mucosa of the stomach and small and large bowels to be inflamed and hyperemic and covered with a slimy exudate, small hemorrhages, and superficial ulcers, especially in the colon.[36,39] Peyer's patches are usually swollen, and the spleen may be enlarged and soft in patients with septicemia. In infants complications such as osteomyelitis, purulent arthritis, intraperitoneal abscess, subacute bacterial endocarditis, and meningitis may result from septicemia.

Reports of radiologic evaluation of patients with Salmonella gastroenterocolitis are virtually nonexistent. Golden[36] observed rapid transit of barium through the intestine with hypertonicity in one patient with probable food poisoning. The case illustrated here with diffuse ulcerations of the colon may be unique in the radiologic literature (Fig. 62-11).[41]

TYPHOID FEVER[30-44]

Typhoid fever, caused by Salmonella typhi, and the paratyphoid fevers, caused by the paratyphi A, B, and C bacilli of the Salmonella group, are specifically human diseases. They are transmitted by the excreta of one infected person to another, usually through polluted drinking water. Occasionally organisms are transmitted through dairy products or other food items that are contaminated by chronic carriers of the organism. Although flies and contaminated shellfish may also act as intermediaries, the enteric fevers are primarily water-borne diseases. This fact explains the explosive onset of epidemics in military or civilian populations.[39] After the bacilli enter the gastrointestinal tract, they invade the intestinal lymphatics and multiply, eventually entering the bloodstream. In the bloodstream they are phagocytized by reticuloendothelial cells, liver, and spleen. A

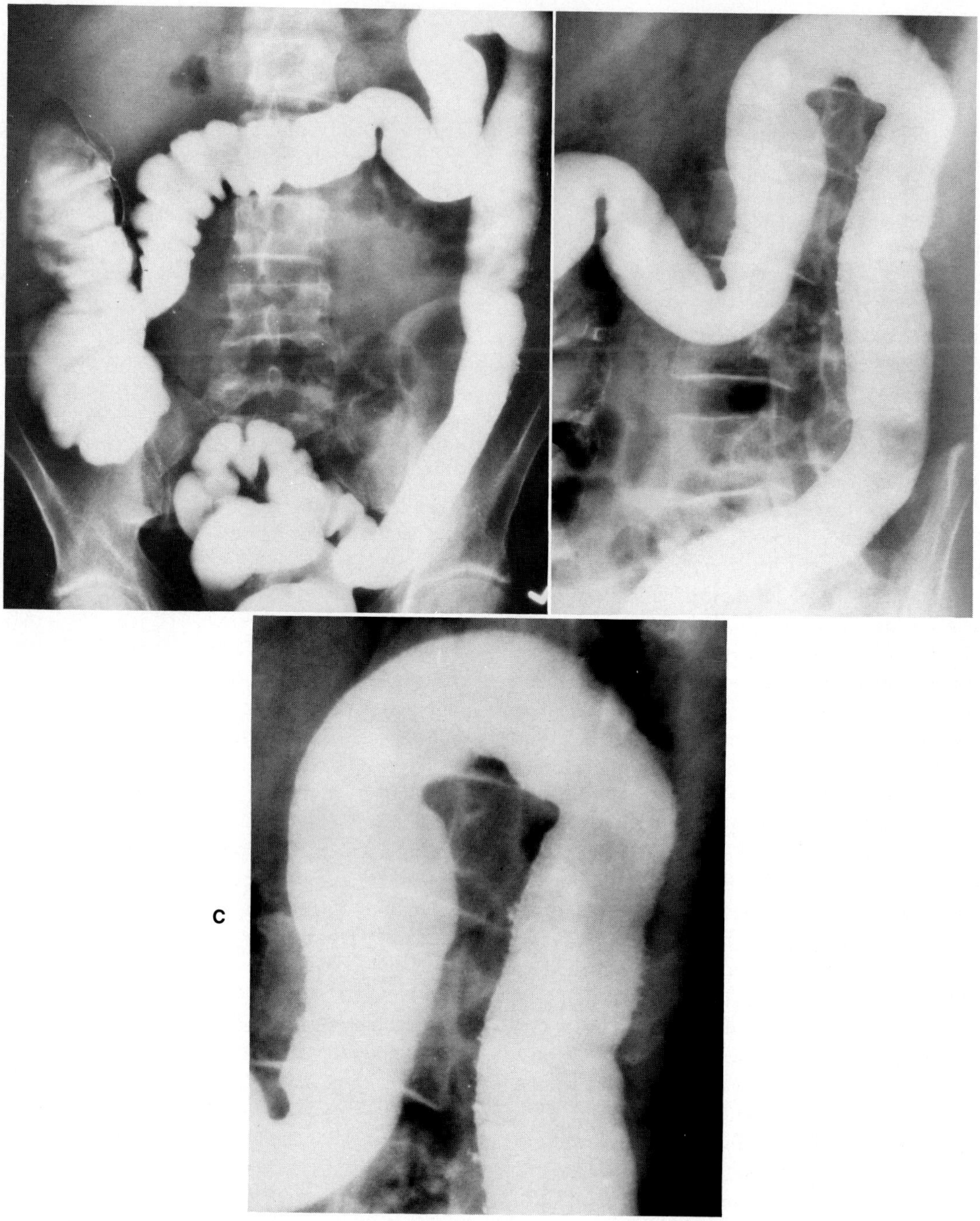

Fig. 62-11 *Salmonella* colitis. Numerous collar-button ulcerations are seen along both borders of sigmoid. **A,** and along descending and transverse colon, with diffuse loss of haustrations, **B** and **C.** Rectal valves and sigmoid haustra are enlarged and edematous, **A.** Sigmoidoscopy revealed friable, ulcerated mucosa. *Salmonella* organisms were cultured from feces and from scraping of rectal mucosa. Radiographic findings of this type of colitis are indistinguishable from those of idiopathic ulcerative colitis.
(Courtesy Dr. Proper.)

secondary bacteremia develops when the bacilli are re-leased from the liver and spleen. This release coincides with the beginning clinical manifestations of the dis-ease.[39]

The incubation period for typhoid fever is usually 10 to 15 days. Characteristic lesions develop in the intestinal lymphatic tissues, especially in the terminal ileum. The colon is involved in only one third of patients, although not extensively.[39] The involvement includes hyperplasia of Peyer's patches, hyperemia and edema of the follicles, and mucosal inflammation. The inflammatory changes are maximal about the tenth day, after which they may resolve or, more commonly, progress to necrosis of the hyperplastic lymphoid tissue. This necrosis results in sloughing of overlying mucosa, leaving ulcers of various extent and depth.[30,39] The oval-shaped ulcers situated on the long axis of the intestinal lumen on the antimesenteric margin of the distal ileum coincide with the distribution of Peyer's patches.[30,41] The ulcers are deepest near the ileocecal valve, where perforation is most frequent. To-ward the end of the second week or during the third week of illness, further sloughing of necrotic ulcerating tissue may lead to intestinal perforation and hemorrhage.[30]

Radiographic findings

Because the pathologic anatomy and clinical course of typhoid and paratyphoid fevers are well known, ra-diographic examination is rarely indicated except when perforation of a typhoid ulcer is suspected. Such perfo-ration in the distal ileum is a complication in 2% to 4% of all such ulcers and is the cause of 25% to 40% of deaths from typhoid fever.[30] Most investigators agree that perforation occurs between the end of the second week and the fourth week of clinical illness.[37,44] Others have noted perforation earlier, sometimes after only 3 to 7 days of clinical symptoms.[30,37] The clinical severity of the typhoid illness is apparently not related to the oc-currence of perforation.[30]

The main radiographic finding in patients with typhoid fever but *without intestinal perforation* is accumulation of gas produced by a paralytic ileus in distended loops of bowel, especially in the small bowel.[30,35,37] Fluid levels are uncommon. By contrast, peritonitis resulting from other diseases typically produces a generalized paralytic ileus with gaseous distention of the entire intestine, with the colon more distended than the small bowel. In typhoid fever, distention of the small bowel primarily may be explained by paresis and functional obstruction before perforation. Mechanical obstruction from kinking, edema, and adhesions may further distend the small bowel after perforation.[30,37]

The presence of free intraperitoneal gas in typhoid patients *with perforation* is believed uncommon by some investigators,[52] whereas others have reported that up to 65% of patients with free perforation have evidence of free gas.[30] In Bohrer's study[30] of 12 Nigerian patients with perforation resulting from typhoid ulcers, six showed free gas, and in five of these the accumulation was marked, producing a double contour sign of the bowel wall on supine films. In virtually all patients with perforation and clinical evidence of peritonitis, there are also radiographic findings of peritonitis, consisting of loss of the properitoneal fat lines, free abdominal fluid, and elevation of the diaphragm. Distention of the gas-filled bowel, especially the small intestine, is commonly seen, as is the presence of either resting or hoop-shaped fluid levels within the small bowel. Segments of the distal small bowel may be irregularly narrowed and fixed, as outlined by intraluminal gas[30] (Fig. 62-12). When com-bined with paralytic ileus from generalized peritonitis, inflammatory hyperplasia of the ileocecal valve may add to the radiographic appearance of a mixed paralytic and obstructive ileus.[30]

Large amounts of free intraperitoneal gas after per-foration in some patients may be explained by excessive gas that distends the small bowel before perforation. The absence of free intraperitoneal gas in other instances may be the result of insidious perforations walled off by adhe-sions before radiographic examination.[30]

Reports of barium studies of the small intestine and colon in patients with typhoid fever are rare. Chérigié and associates[31] reported the results of examinations of the small bowel in 32 patients studied during a typhoid epidemic in France in 1950. They found the caliber of the jejunum to be dilated to two or three times its normal size, with enlargement and edema of the valves of Kerckring, suggesting a "stacked-plate" appearance. The barium in the ileum appeared segmented as a result of multiple areas of spasm. Small pea-sized mucosal nod-ules were found in the distal ileum, which represented hypertrophy of the Peyer's patches. Small ulcerations of the distal ileum were seen in only three of their patients. The ileum, however, was the least well-opacified portion of the small bowel. Transit of barium through the small intestine required about 5 hours, with delay noted in the dilated areas.

Schinz and co-workers[52] noted that, as in tuberculosis, typhoid bacilli tend to invade the lower ileum because of the greater abundance of lymphatic tissue in that lo-cation. In the initial stages the dominant pathologic and radiographic appearances are those of mucosal edema with thickening of the folds, narrowing of the lumen, and mural rigidity. During the advanced stage of typhoid fever, the extensively ulcerated intestinal surface appears as a ragged ill-defined contour on radiographs[41] (Fig. 62-13). Because of the disturbed motility of the small bowel,

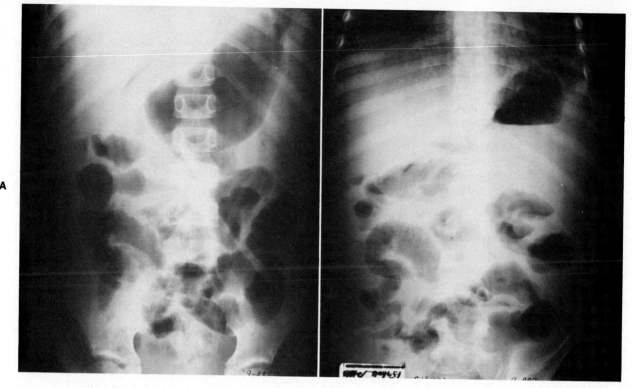

Fig. 62-12 Typhoid fever with perforation. **A,** Note multiple loops of distended, gas-filled small bowel on supine view. **B,** In upright projection, multiple resting fluid levels are seen. Properitoneal fat lines are lost, and several of the small bowel loops, especially those in right lower quadrant, appear fixed on two projections. Free gas can be seen below liver margin on both views. Radiograph of chest in erect position showed free air beneath right hemidiaphragm.
(Courtesy Dr. Stanley Bohrer.)

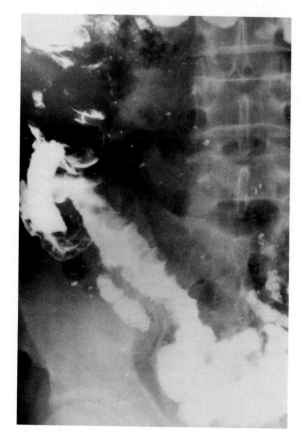

Fig. 62-13 Straightening and rigidity of terminal ileum with pronounced edema and irregularity of lumen—result of typhoid fever. Numerous ulcers that project from both sides of ileum produce spiked, ragged bowel contour. There are several lucent areas near ileocecal area that represent hypertrophied Peyer's patches. Cecum and ascending colon are incompletely filled.

aperistalsis may alternate with hyperperistalsis. In a still later stage, if perforation has not occurred, the ulcerations may disappear, indicating healing of the diseased area. Healing of ulcers by granulation tissue may begin about the fourth week of the disease. When healing is complete, a slightly depressed, smooth scar remains, which does not cause stricture or intestinal obstruction.[39]

A chronic typhoid infection of the intestinal tract of 4 years' duration has been described.[40] Serial radiographs of the small bowel revealed extensive segmentation and puddling of barium throughout the ileum, with loss of normal mucosal folds and dilatation of loops of bowel. Hypermotility of the intestine was observed with barium reaching the cecum in 1 hour. Similar findings have been reported as the result of paratyphoid fever caused by *Salmonella schottmülleri* (paratyphi B).[42] Paratyphoid fevers usually do not produce extensive lymphatic invasion and ulceration, as does typhoid fever. More often, on postmortem studies of intestinal specimens in paratyphoid fever, little or no change is noted, although the entire intestine may be acutely inflamed.[44] In the paratyphoid fevers and some other forms of salmonellosis, ulceration of the large intestine is more frequent than in typhoid fever.

The differential diagnosis of terminal ileal spasticity and ulceration, and later luminal rigidity, includes regional enteritis, tuberculous ileitis, histoplasmosis, lymphosarcoma, radiation vasculitis, ischemia, and periarteritis nodosa. Regional enteritis and tuberculosis in particular may resemble the radiographic findings of typhoid fever.

BACILLARY DYSENTERY[45-53]

Bacillary dysentery, or shigellosis, is an acute or chronic inflammatory disease involving the colon and occasionally the distal ileum. Epidemics of dysentery have occurred throughout all recorded history whenever large groups living in close contact in crowded communities, armies, prisons, or mental institutions have neglected the cardinal rules of sanitation. Whether in early or modern civilizations, failure to prevent the spread of the bacilli by the sanitary disposal of feces, control of flies, and strict personal hygiene has resulted in epidemics of dysentery. Great wars have been won or lost as a result of outbreaks of dysentery among the opposing armies. The disease is worldwide in distribution but is most frequent and severe in those developing countries of the wet, humid tropics where poor sanitation and primitive conditions still exist.

The disease is named for members of the genus *Shigella*, the dysentery bacilli, which vary markedly as to their antigenicity and pathogenicity. *Shigella dysenteriae*, the Shiga bacillus, produces a potent endotoxin that

accounts for epidemics of severe diarrhea in the tropics and subtropics. *Shigella* of the Flexner, Sonne, and Boyd subgroups are not endotoxin producers and are generally less pathogenic, causing less serious disease and a lower incidence of chronic dysentery. The Flexner and Sonne subgroups are the most common causes of bacillary dysentery in the United States, England, Europe, Egypt, and the Orient. The Boyd subgroup is found in India and Egypt. However, strains of any of the four *Shigella* subgroups may be found in North America, where bacillary dysentery is primarily an institutional disease seen in nursery schools, mental institutions, prisons, and military compounds. Sonne dysentery has been prevalent in America, England, and Europe in recent winters, occurring especially in children.[51]

Bacillary dysentery occurs almost exclusively in humans. Human carriers are common where the disease is prevalent and are the only important reservoir of shigellosis. Pollution of water supply by feces, contamination of food by infected food handlers, or transfer of the bacilli by flies are the principal modes of transmission.[46,50] Epidemics commonly occur after mild cases are overlooked. In epidemics positive cultures may be obtained from up to 25% of apparently healthy contacts. About 3% of those who recover from an attack of shigellosis become asymptomatic carriers for variable periods.[50]

Clinically the incubation period may vary from 24 hours to a week. The disease may begin suddenly or insidiously; it commonly occurs as a simple diarrhea but may be quite varied in its severity, leading to classification of cases into the following clinical types: mild (catarrhal), acute, fulminating, relapsing, and chronic dysentery.

Shiga dysentery may be acute and fulminating. The chief clinical symptoms are manifestations of the colitis and include gripping abdominal pain, tenesmus, and frequently passage of loose stools that may vary greatly in number and character. The abdomen is often rigid early in the disease. High fever to 104° F and vomiting may be present with leukocytosis. In severe cases of shigellosis the stools eventually may consist only of frequently evacuated blood-stained mucus containing a characteristic purulent, cellular exudate and great numbers of dysentery bacilli. There may be 20 to 40 involuntary evacuations per day accompanied by intense tenesmus and abdominal pain, resulting in the patient remaining literally "glued" to the toilet.

A swollen, diffusely inflamed rectal mucosa, often covered with mucus and pus, may be seen through the proctoscope. Underlying this exudate is a granular mucous membrane that oozes blood freely. Shallow ulcerations, irregular in size and shape and covered with pus, may be present.

Pathologically shigellosis is characterized by acute, diffuse inflammation of the colon with initial hyperemia of the mucosa, followed by edema, hemorrhage, and leukocytic infiltration. This process often extends into the submucosa and causes marked thickening of the intestinal wall. Epithelial necrosis and desquamation with formation of a diphtheritic membrane is followed by ulceration that may extend deep into the submucosa and occasionally into the muscularis[45,50]; perforation is rare. Inflammation is usually not distributed uniformly throughout the colon but is most severe in the rectosigmoid and descending colon. The terminal ileum is occasionally involved. Secondary bacterial infection occurs once ulcerative lesions have developed and may be important in the development of the chronic stage of the disease in which adjacent lesions may be joined by ulcerating channels beneath bridges of hyperplastic mucosa. Mucosal retention cysts may harbor *Shigella* bacilli, which are intermittently discharged in the chronic carrier state.[45,50]

In chronic bacillary dysentery there is characteristically extensive scarring and fibrosis of the colon, indolent ulceration, and a continued subacute or chronic inflammation that periodically becomes acute. The disease resembles chronic idiopathic ulcerative colitis, both clinically and pathologically, including a tendency to undergo exacerbation and remission. During periods of active disease, the patient may have fever and diarrhea with varying amounts of blood, mucus, and cellular exudate in the stools.[50]

Radiographic findings

The radiographic findings are influenced by the severity and stage of the disease. Many radiographic features of bacillary dysentery are similar to those seen in other inflammatory diseases of the small and large bowel. On plain film examination of the abdomen a considerable amount of gas may be seen in the small intestine and colon. Barium examination of the small intestine may show mucosal edema, segmentation, loss of normal fold pattern, hypersecretion, and especially hypermotility with rapid transit time.[48,52]

Many patients with bacillary dysentery show no radiologic changes in the colon on barium enema examination. However, in active, moderately advanced disease, edema of the mucosa with spasm and irregularity of outline of the bowel wall may be present.[53] Complete filling of the colon and distal ileum is difficult because of spasmodic contractions and tenesmus. Postevacuation films usually show complete elimination of the barium.[48]

In more severe cases of *Shigella* dysentery, focal ulcerations may be present, which usually are not deep and rarely extend into the muscularis. These superficial ulcers are most prevalent in the rectosigmoid colon but may be found throughout the colon in advanced cases[51] (Figs. 62-14 and 62-15). At this stage the ulcerated appearance of the colon radiologically may resemble acute ulcerative colitis with irregular bowel contour, marked spasm, and eventual partial cicatricial stenoses.[52,53]

In chronic cases transient spasmodic emptyings and reflux fillings may take place, and the colon may be rigid and tubelike in some segments with loss of haustrations. Postevacuation films show segmental puddling of barium with lack of haustral markings.[48]

The radiographic differential diagnosis of bacillary dysentery includes acute and chronic idiopathic ulcerative colitis, *Salmonella* enterocolitis, pseudomembranous enterocolitis, and amebiasis. All are inflammatory diseases that produce edema, spasm, and ulceration of the small bowel or colon. Crohn's disease and tuberculosis may produce similar radiologic findings, although these inflammatory diseases tend to be more segmental and eccentric in distribution, and show deeper ulcerations and, at times, fistula formation and stenoses.

PSEUDOMEMBRANOUS ENTEROCOLITIS[54-65]

Necrotizing enterocolitis of the newborn and in Hirschsprung's disease are discussed in Chapter 69. Pseudomembranous enterocolitis is a disease that involves both the small and large bowel. It derives its name from the fact that a pseudomembrane composed of necrotic debris adherent to ulcerated mucosa follows necrosis of the intestinal mucosa. Of the many causes, the one most frequently associated with the name pseudomembranous enterocolitis is antibiotic-induced change in intestinal flora.[59] Penicillin,[61] lincomycin,[54] streptomycin,[57] chlortetracycline, and chloramphenicol[64] have been known to alter the normal *Escherichia coli* and *Bacteroides* flora of the intestine. The result may be an overgrowth of pathogenic organisms, the most common being *Staphylococcus aureus*.[57,61,65] Mixed gram-positive and gram-negative rods have been reported, as well as *Proteus* infections.[54,57] Enterocolitis after antibiotics, however, has been associated with no definable bacterial overgrowth.[61] Intestinal vascular insufficiency,[55] sometimes associated with intestinal surgery, is thought to initiate acute pseudomembranous enterocolitis, either from hypoperfusion, arteriosclerotic disease, or bleeding disorders. Many cases of pseudomembranous enterocolitis have been reported in patients with debilitating diseases, such as lymphosarcoma and leukemia, or after irradiation for malignant disease.[55,59] Long-term steroid therapy has also been implicated.[56,60] A similar form of colitis has been noted in patients with intestinal obstruction proximal to the site of obstruction.[60,63]

The onset of pseudomembranous enterocolitis is usu-

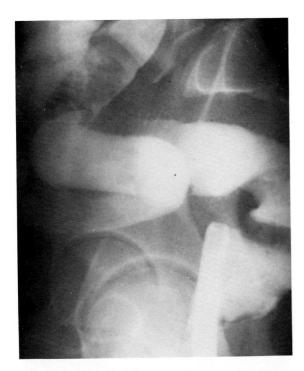

Fig. 62-14 Multiple, shallow, collar-button ulcerations are present in sigmoid colon of this patient with bacillary dysentery *(shigellosis)*. Presacral space is widened and rectal valves thickened because of inflammatory process in rectosigmoid colon.

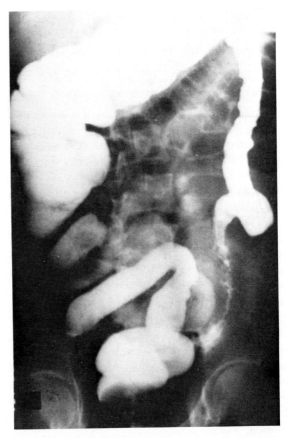

Fig. 62-15 Bacillary dysentery. There is tubular narrowing of descending and proximal sigmoid colon, with multiple small ulcerations and irregularity of the mucosal pattern. Rectum and distal sigmoid colon appear normal on this study.
(From Reeder, MM, and Palmer, PES: The radiology of tropical diseases, Baltimore, 1981, Williams & Wilkins.)

ally heralded by severe diarrhea with or without blood.[57,61] In drug-induced *S. aureus* infections the organism is capable of producing an enterotoxin that is itself diarrheagenic.[57,65] Abdominal cramps and abdominal tenderness, and sometimes signs of peritonitis,[57,61,63] are associated with the diarrhea. Hypoproteinemia with peripheral edema and ascites has also been reported.[61]

Proctoscopic examination demonstrates a friable and erythematous mucosa with yellowish green exudate or patchy, adherent, elevated yellow mucosal plaques, which may progress to become a confluent purulent pseudomembrane.[54,57,61,63]

In the gross specimen of bowel involved with pseudomembranous colitis, the bowel wall is markedly thickened, a yellow-green patchy or confluent pseudomembrane is present, and the mucosa is ulcerated.[61,63] Histologically the pseudomembrane is composed of mucus, fibrin, leukocytes, occasional gram-positive or gram-negative rods, and frequently identifiable *S. aureus*.[57,65] Shallow mucosal ulcerations are present, although occasionally ulceration may extend into the submucosa. Goblet cell hypertrophy of the mucosa may be seen. The lamina propria and submucosal area are edematous and filled with cellular infiltrate. These histologic changes are

nonspecific, however, and may be seen with many other forms of enteritis, such as typhoid fever, bacillary dysentery, septicemia, and uremia.[62]

Radiographic findings

Plain radiographs of the abdomen are usually the first obtained in patients with the sudden onset of severe diarrhea. An adynamic ileus pattern with distention of the small and large bowel may be seen.[57] The ileus may be caused by associated peritonitis, by electrolyte disturbances because of severe diarrhea, or possibly by release of enterotoxin by offending bacteria. Frequently, the colon is greatly distended, and its contour is irregular. Thumbprintlike indentations in the gas-filled transverse colon may simulate the appearance of toxic megacolon of chronic ulcerative colitis[56,57] or ischemic colitis. In severe advanced colitis air in the bowel wall may be seen.[57]

Because of these colonic findings extreme caution should be exercised before a barium enema is performed. A markedly dilated colon with an irregular contour in a febrile patient with bloody diarrhea contraindicates a barium enema examination. The high pressure from the barium enema examination is conducive to perforation of the necrotic megacolon. With some resolution of the acute colonic dilatation, however, and a change in symptoms, barium enema examination may be performed with caution under low pressure. Thumbprintlike indentations in the contour of the colon may be seen; there are most prominent in the transverse colon. These indentations are believed to be the result of hematoma formation in the bowel wall from mesenteric and submucosal bleeding.[57] Extensive vascular involvement with occlusion of small vessels and lymphatics has been reported in pseudomembranous colitis and may be reversible.[57] An irregular, ragged, polypoid contour to the colon wall is seen on barium enema examination.[54,58] An alteration of the mucosa-barium interface is the cause of this irregularity. The pseudomembrane itself ordinarily covers a vast area of the mucosa and accounts for the irregular appearance on barium enema examination[54] (Fig. 62-16). Ulcerations, although present, are usually shallow and often are covered by pseudomembrane. These findings are similar, both histologically and radiographically, to those of ischemic colitis.

The small bowel may also be involved.[60,61] Its involvement is indicated by edema of the valvulae conniventes and of the bowel wall, with thickening and separation of loops. Ulceration and complete loss of the fold pattern may be seen in more severely involved areas.

Treatment by supportive measures, discontinuation of the offending antibiotic, and addition of *E. coli* to re-establish the bacterial flora may result in healing to such an extent that follow-up radiographs may have a normal appearance. Pseudomembranous enterocolitis may resolve so that a smooth atrophic-appearing colon without haustra remains, which simulates inactive chronic ulcerative colitis.[56] Stenosis and strictures of both the large and small bowel may also take place.

Differential diagnosis

Many other diseases may produce radiographic similarities. Ulcerative colitis, both in the active and healed phases, may resemble pseudomembranous enterocolitis on plain radiographs (toxic megacolon) and on barium enema examination.[60] The distribution of pseudomembranous enterocolitis may be more patchy than that of ulcerative colitis. Identifiable pseudopolyps, as seen in some instances of ulcerative colitis, are rarely produced by pseudomembranous enterocolitis. However, any form of ulcerating colitis may produce radiographic findings

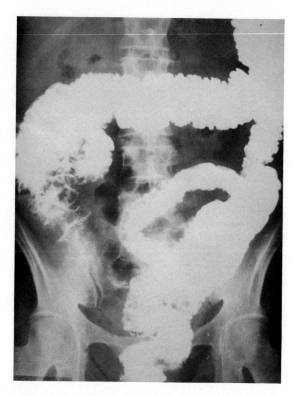

Fig. 62-16 Irregular, ragged contour of entire colon with loss of haustra, and thumbprintlike indentations in cecum—result of extensive pseudomembranous colitis in patient receiving antibiotics for suppurative otitis. *Staphylococcus aureus* organisms were cultured from stools.

similar to those of pseudomembranous enterocolitis. These findings include Crohn's disease, amebiasis, *Salmonella-Shigella* colitis, and particularly ischemic colitis. When the small bowel is involved, ischemia, radiation enteritis, regional enteritis, periarteritis nodosa, and lymphoma should be considered in the differential diagnoses.

ACUTE GASTROENTERITIS[66,67]

Acute nonspecific gastroenteritis is the most frequent gastrointestinal disease and yet one in which a cause has rarely, if ever, been proved. So-called traveler's diarrhea, acute epidemic gastroenteritis, or "mal de turista" may be caused by enteropathic *E. coli* (EEC),[67] by intestinal viruses, such as enteric cytopathogenic human orphan (ECHO) and coxsackie A and B, or by mixed flora.[66] The disease is a self-limiting pathophysiologic process of altered water and electrolyte absorption, increased intestinal motility, or in some instances ileus of small and large bowel.

Radiographic findings in acute gastroenteritis are nearly always confined to the plain radiographs of the

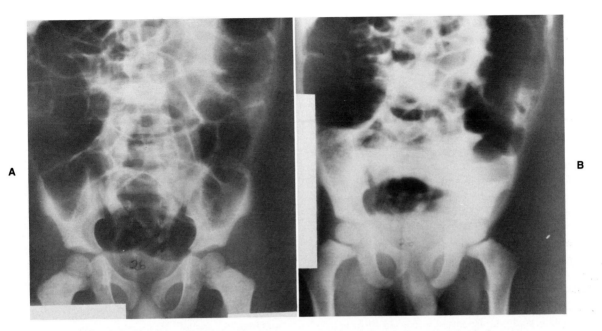

Fig. 62-17 Acute gastroenteritis in child who had sudden onset of diarrhea and abdominal cramps with one episode of vomiting. Although acute gastroenteritis was epidemic in community, no specific etiologic agent was found in this child. Note dilatation, **A,** and air-filled levels, **B,** in small and large bowel.

abdomen. Air-fluid levels may be seen in dilated loops of small and large bowel (Fig. 62-17). Dilatation and fluid may become so prominent as to simulate mechanical obstruction of the large bowel. Outpouring of large amounts of water and electrolytes into the small bowel results in dilatation, air-fluid levels, and increased but often incoordinate motor activity. Electrolyte loss may also produce adynamic ileus pattern. Some experimental evidence exists that in EEC diarrhea a toxin may be produced, further potentiating the ileus.[66] Air-fluid levels in distended large and small bowel, coupled with the history of diarrhea of acute onset, permit differentiation from mechanical obstruction.

On those rare occasions when barium meals are administered or barium enema examination is performed on patients with acute diarrhea, no specific radiographic findings are noted. The small bowel is dilated, but the mucosal pattern is normal. Motility may be increased during fluoroscopic examination, producing rapid changes in the location and extent of air-fluid levels. When ileus is pronounced, little activity is noted. On barium enema examination mucosal edema is best demonstrated on the postevacuation radiograph (Fig. 62-18). The mucosal pattern remains coarse in the partially collapsed colon and haustra, and septa are often not present. These changes may be seen in any cause of acute diar-

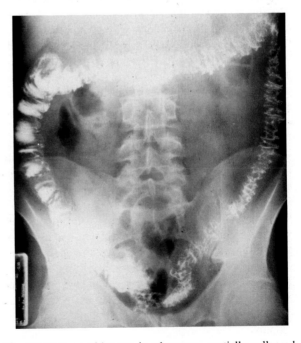

Fig. 62-18 Loss of haustra in edematous, partially collapsed colon of man with acute gastroenteritis, which resolved without treatment after 4 days.

rhea, for example, food poisoning, bacillary dysentery, cholera, and ulcerative and amebic colitis.

LYMPHOGRANULOMA VENEREUM[68-79]

Lymphogranuloma venereum (LGV), also known as lymphopathia venereum, is a venereal disease especially common in the tropics among black women of the lower socioeconomic group with poor sexual hygiene.[68-70] The disease has been reported in all races and in most countries and is especially common in prostitutes, sodomists, and other sexually promiscuous individuals. It is most common in seaports of Africa, South India, Indonesia, the southern United States (for example, New Orleans), Latin America, Jamaica, and other Caribbean islands. In some areas it assumes epidemic proportions and constitutes an important public health problem. The disease must be considered in the differential diagnosis of any inflammatory process or stricture involving the rectosigmoid colon.

Lymphogranuloma venereum is caused by a species of the genus *Chlamydia*, long considered to be viruses and previously designated *Bedsonia*. These obligate intracellular organisms measure 300 μ in their infectious stage and are now morphologically classified as bacteria occupying a position between the rickettsiae and viruses. LGV is acquired almost exclusively by sexual contact. The organisms can be recovered from the primary genital lesions, involved lymph nodes, and the inflammatory lesions of the rectosigmoid colon and pelvic soft tissues. The initial herpetiform lesion develops about 2 weeks after infection and is usually a tiny, painless papule, vesicle, or ulcer located on the penis in men and on the vulva, posterior vaginal wall, or cervix in women, where it usually escapes detection. Since *Chlamydia trachomatis* is markedly lymphotrophic, the regional lymph nodes are rapidly invaded, producing an acute purulent lymphadenitis (bubo formation) 4 to 8 weeks after coitus.

In men the secondary stage of the disease develops insidiously and pursues a chronic indolent course with the inguinal lymph nodes becoming enlarged, matted together, and fluctuant, with draining sinuses. In women there are usually no localizing symptoms until the pelvic lymph nodes (especially the anorectal group) are invaded, with subsequent involvement of the rectum and discharge of blood and pus in the stools.[68,74] The different lymphatic drainage in the two sexes is responsible for the much greater involvement of the rectosigmoid colon in women and its relative rarity among men, except when the organism has been directly implanted into the rectum by sodomy.

The pathologic changes in the rectum are the result of invasion and blockage of the rectal lymphatics by *Chlamydia*. There is subsequent lymphangitis, lymphatic stasis, rectal edema, cellular infiltration in the submucosa and muscularis, endarteritis and phlebitis, and eventually mucosal destruction.[72,74] The sequence of pelvic lymphadenitis, lymphatic stasis, and secondary infection leads to ulcerative proctocolitis, elephantiasis of the genitalia, and perirectal fistulas and abscesses. Rectal biopsy may show granulomas in the rectal wall. Later in the disease fibrosis leads to the development of rectal or rectosigmoid strictures. In women involvement of the rectovaginal septum often results in a large rectovaginal fistula in the center of the posterior vaginal wall above the anorectal ring and distal to the stricture.[68-70]

Clinically the initial genital lesion often goes undetected, especially in women. In the secondary stage of the disease there is often a seropurulent discharge from the inguinal buboes in men. The onset of proctocolitis in women, and occasionally in men, is accompanied by diarrhea, constipation, rectal bleeding, and discharge of pus and blood in the stools. The mucosa feels coarse and granular on rectal examination, and sigmoidoscopy shows an acute proctitis with intense inflammation and a pseudomembrane covering a bleeding friable mucosa.

The third stage of LGV is most striking in women and is characterized by chronic proctitis and extensive fibrosis with development of a rectosigmoid stricture. Rectal pain, tenesmus, constipation, and narrow stools are now the dominant clinical features. Rectovaginal fistula with passage of feces through the vagina frequently develops, as may perianal abscess and vulvar elephantiasis. In this stenotic phase the rectal ampulla is severely narrowed by scarring, and proctoscopy often shows a friable, bleeding, ulcerated mucosa overlying the stricture. The perianal skin is thickened and edematous, and there may be a characteristic lymphorrhoid present. The lower edge of the stricture can usually be palpated 1 to 2 inches from the anal orifice; it is never further than 5 inches from the anus. The stricture varies in diameter from slight narrowing to almost complete stenosis of the rectal lumen.

The diagnosis of LGV may be confirmed by the complement fixation test, by the Frei intradermal test, or by recovery of *Chlamydia* organisms from the blood, feces, or buboes.

Radiographic findings

The radiographic features of lymphogranuloma venereum have been well documented by several investigators,[68-73,75-79] especially Annamunthodo and Marryatt[68,69] in their review of 144 black patients from Jamaica, 90% of whom were female. Two distinct stages of the disease were recognized by those authors: 34 cases with generalized proctocolitis and 113 chronic cases with anorectal stricture. Thus the findings on barium enema

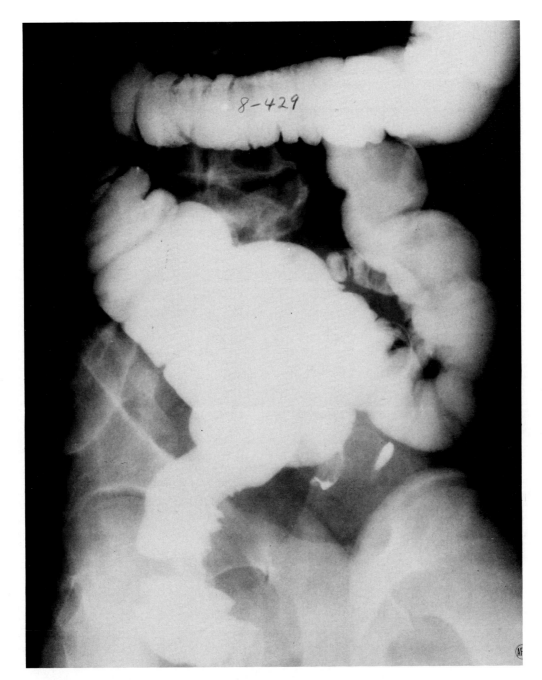

Fig. 62-19 Ulcerative proctitis, with localized rectal narrowing, deep ulcerations, and thickened rectal valves caused by lymphogranuloma venereum.

examination depend largely on the phase and activity of the disease.

In the prestenotic phase the rectal ampulla is narrowed and spasm is present with loss of the normal haustral and mucosal pattern in the rectum and occasionally in the sigmoid colon.[68,71,72] The contour of the narrowed rectum is irregular and ulcerated (Fig. 62-19). Fistulous tracts

and perirectal abscesses may be present, as well as widening of the presacral space with anterior displacement of the rectosigmoid colon[72,77] (Fig. 62-20). The fistulas may extend to the buttocks and occasionally upward to involve the parametrium, peritoneum, sigmoid colon, and rarely the small bowel.[76]

As the disease progresses to fibrosis, strictures of var-

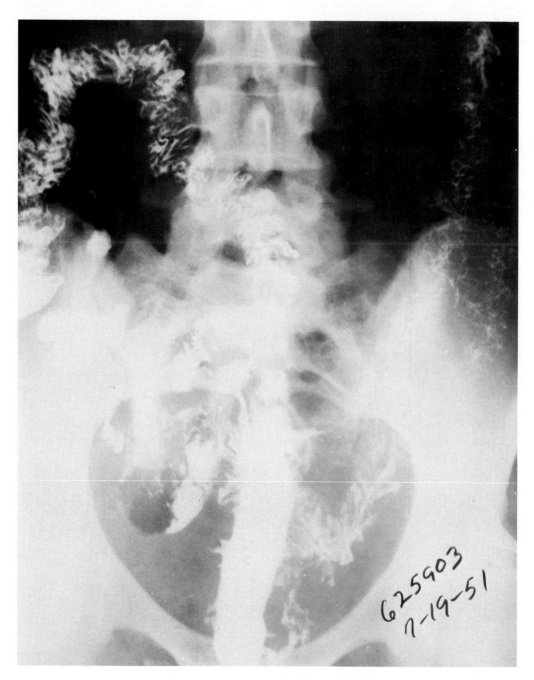

Fig. 62-20 Narrowed, rigid rectosigmoid colon resulting from lymphogranuloma venereum. Rectosigmoid junction is straightened because of large perirectal abscess. Multiple deep and shallow perirectal sinuses extend laterally and downward to perineum.

ied lengths may develop.[68] LGV strictures are usually long and tubular with a tapering proximal (and sometimes distal) edge (Fig. 62-21). They may involve the anorectal area, the entire rectum and sigmoid colon, or occasionally areas higher in the colon. Strictures as long as 25 cm have been noted.[72] Many are palpable within 3 to 5 cm of the anus and are readily identified on barium enema examination. Distal rectal strictures arising just above the anorectal junction may extend to narrow the entire rectal ampulla[74] (Fig. 62-22).

The strictures of the rectum and colon are usually in continuity, but occasionally there are separate skip areas

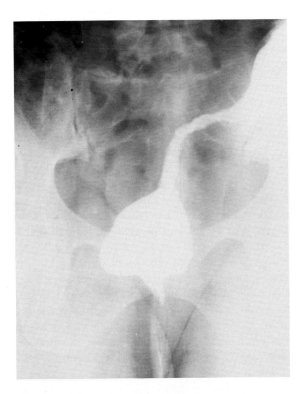

Fig. 62-21 Woman with rectosigmoid stricture caused by lymphogranuloma venereum. Note sparing of distal rectum and ulcerated appearance of stricture lumen. Both proximal and distal margins taper smoothly. Dilatation and loss of haustration above stricture impart conical appearance to cecum.

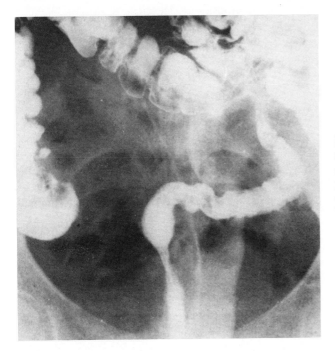

Fig. 62-22 LGV in black man from South Africa. There is marked narrowing of entire rectum and irregular ulcerated contour of moderately narrowed and shortened sigmoid colon. Rectal wall is considerably thickened, rigid, and fibrotic.
(From Reeder, MM, and Palmer PES: The radiology of tropical diseases, Baltimore, 1981, Williams & Wilkins.)

with apparently normal intervening colon, similar to those seen in Crohn's disease and tuberculous colitis.[68] The rectal lumen may be severely narrowed with a string-like or filiform appearance, resulting in obstruction. Dilatation and loss of haustration of the bowel proximal to a stricture often give a conical appearance to the recto-sigmoid colon.

The contour of the narrowed rectosigmoid colon may be smooth, but frequently it is irregular as a result of mucosal ulceration and occasional fistulous tracts.[72] In Annamunthodo and Marryatt's series,[68.69] the major complications were rectovaginal fistula (34 patients), perianal sinuses, fistulas and abscesses (26 patients), and elephantiasis of the vulva (9 patients). Short or long perirectal sinuses may extend outward at right angles or downward from the rectum to the perineum, always at or below the site of the stricture. These fistulous tracts may extend into large perirectal abscesses, reenter the bowel, or connect with the vagina, perineum, or anterior surface of the abdomen. Lateral and oblique radiographs of the rectum are necessary to best demonstrate recto-vaginal fistulas and retrorectal sinuses when present.[75] Because an extensive retrorectal inflammatory reaction or abscess is invariably present, causing an increased thickness of the presacral soft tissue space, the rectosigmoid colon frequently is straightened on the frontal projection and is displaced forward and upward on the lateral view.

Differential diagnosis

With the radiographic finding of rectal stricture, many inflammatory diseases of the colon such as idiopathic chronic ulcerative colitis and, especially, granulomatous diseases such as Crohn's disease, tuberculosis, schistosomiasis, amebiasis, and actinomycosis must be considered, since they may produce radiographic findings similar to those of LGV.[75] In many of these diseases rectal biopsies may show granulomas similar to those seen in LGV.

Amebiasis and tuberculosis can cause proctocolitis, rectal narrowing, and perianal fistulas. Actinomycosis, although a rare disease, can produce fistulous tracts. All can occasionally simulate LGV. Schistosomiasis may cause diffuse irregular narrowing and ulceration of the rectosigmoid colon, often with a large pelvic abscess. However, fistulous tracts, which are so common in LGV, do not occur in schistosomiasis. Conversely, colonic granulomatous polyps may be seen in schistosomiasis, especially in Africa and the Orient, but they do not occur in LGV.

Posttraumatic strictures caused by foreign bodies or by sclerosing agents used in hemorrhoid treatment may cause smooth rectal strictures that radiographically may

appear similar to those of LGV; however, they seldom cause fistulas or ulceration. Colitis cystica profunda may cause nodular rectal lesions, but the rectal narrowing does not extend into the sigmoid colon; sigmoidoscopy and rectal biopsy easily differentiate the two diseases. Perirectal abscess or tumor may cause rectal narrowing, but usually in these instances the mucosa overlying the narrow rectal wall is not ulcerated.

A scirrhous infiltrating type of carcinoma can also produce a lengthy rectal stricture, but the mucosa is usually not ulcerated as it so often is in LGV, and sinus tracts and fistulas do not often develop in cancer.

TROPICAL SPRUE[80-90]

Depending largely on the geographic area in which the patient is encountered, there are two varieties of sprue. There is little to differentiate the nontropical from the tropical variety, and it is possible for the radiologist to differentiate the various causes that may produce the spruelike syndrome. Both varieties of sprue are usually classified under "idiopathic steatorrhea." However, abnormalities of the pancreas or of biliary flow, or changes in the bowel wall or mesentery due to amyloidosis, scleroderma, mesenteric thrombosis, and various poisons such as arsenic and some antibiotics can all produce the radiologic appearance of sprue. Many intestinal parasites, particularly *Giardia, Ancylostoma, Capillaria,* and *Strongyloides,* produce similar appearances, and there has been much debate whether the parasites are the cause or the result of the intestinal disturbance.

Malabsorption through the small bowel can therefore occur in many different diseases. The clinical symptoms are similar and the radiologic findings almost identical. The main difference between nontropical and tropical sprue is that the latter is almost always negaloblastic and will respond to antibiotic and vitamin therapy; nontropical sprue is difficult to treat and seldom shows a megaloblastic bone marrow. Most authorities believe that tropical sprue is at least in large part infectious in etiology, although the organism has not yet been found. Both varieties of sprue result in malabsorption, alteration of the bacterial flora of the gut, and dysfunction of normal bowel movement. However, pathologic correlation with the radiologic findings in sprue is not consistent. In some patients there are remarkably few histologic abnormalities, whereas in others there is edema of the bowel wall, atrophy of the villi or other layers of the mucosa, and degeneration of the intramural plexus. In tropical sprue there is almost always a chronic inflammatory reaction in the lamina propria with a varying degree of edema; this may be followed by atrophy. Eventually all layers of the small bowel may become atrophic and thin, and the full length of the gastrointestinal tract, including the

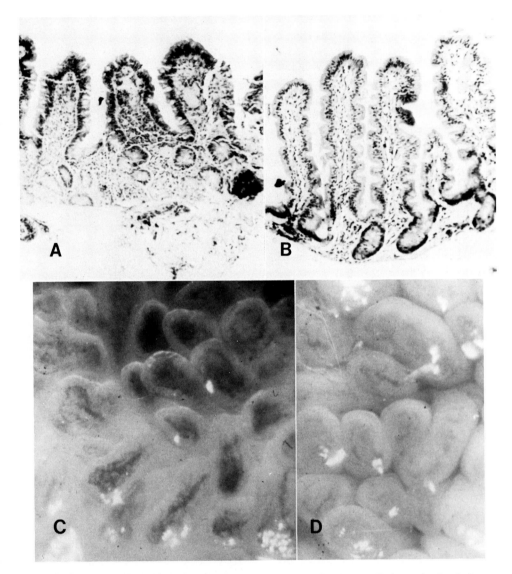

Fig. 62-23 Tropical sprue. Jejunal biopsy before, **A,** and after, **B,** therapy. Endoscopic view before, **C,** and after, **D,** therapy.
(From Reeder, MM, and Palmer, PES: The radiology of tropical diseases, Baltimore, 1981, Williams & Wilkins.)

tongue (filiform papillae), may be affected. It is debatable whether the loss of the surface epithelium is the result of the vascular and neurologic damage that is found or whether it is the cause of these changes. In both varieties of sprue there may be some regeneration, but it is most marked in tropical sprue, where there is often a dramatic response to antibiotic therapy with folate and vitamin B_{12} replacement (Fig. 62-23).

Many biochemical tests may help to differentiate the various types of malabsorption, including the fecal fat content, the serum carotene level, the ^{131}I-labeled olein absorption test, and various carbohydrate absorption tests. The excretion of D-xylose, the vitamin A absorption test, and the 24-hour fecal fat estimation are perhaps the

most reliable, but much will depend on the skill and experience of the individual laboratories. The oral glucose tolerance test is nonspecific. There is usually a macrocytic anemia in patients with tropical sprue, but this is a much less consistent finding in other varieties.

Clinically, the disease may be very mild and almost asymptomatic, or it may become severe, with all the complications of malabsorption. Estimation of the severity of the disease must be based on the combination of the clinical picture, biochemical tests, jejunal biopsy, radiologic examination of the small bowel, and eventually the response or otherwise to appropriate therapy.

Diarrhea is almost always present, accompanied by fatigue and lassitude. Remissions and exacerbations are frequent, with progressive ill health, steatorrhea, and eventually abdominal pain with explosive defecation of bulky, foul-smelling stools. Bleeding may occur, and evidence of vitamin deficiency, particularly the vitamin B complex, becomes evident in the skin, tongue, mouth, and eyes. There may be peripheral neuropathy. The severity of the illness and the enteric disturbance may lead to loss of appetite with dehydration, which can progress to cardiac and adrenal failure.

Radiographic findings

The radiologic evidence of sprue depends largely on the duration of the disease. In mild or moderate cases plain films of the abdomen are normal. As the disease progresses and becomes more severe, there may be evidence of mild ileus with air-fluid levels scattered throughout the abdomen on the erect film.

Barium studies must be carried out with micropulverized, nonflocculating barium. The diagnosis of a "sprue" pattern is invalid unless this type of barium is used. Abnormalities have been reported in the esophagus, stomach, and occasionally the large bowel, but these findings are minimal and play no part in the diagnosis.

In the early stages of sprue there is a significant difference between various small bowel segments because of a difference in tone. Because there is also some inflammatory reaction, there is edema and therefore thickening of the mucosal folds. This, too, alters the segmental appearance of the bowel. None of these early changes will be appreciated accurately unless there is sequential fluoroscopy with manual palpation to separate the various loops of the small bowel and to record the changes in appearance. In sprue there is an increase in the poorly saturated fatty acids in the lumen of the gut, with increased secretion of mucin. This is one of the main causes of the irritation and diarrhea seen in sprue and also of the flocculation that occurs during barium studies. As the edema progresses and the mucosa becomes more swollen, there is also dilatation of the small bowel. Attempts have been made to differentiate the cause of this pattern by describing the variation in the degree of mucosal swelling, but this is probably erroneous. There is so much individual variation between patients and considerable variation in the same patient between different examinations that it is better for the radiologist to offer the diagnosis of a "malabsorption pattern" rather than try to indicate its cause.

Although there will be marked variation in each group of findings within individual patients, the radiologic findings in the established case can be divided into (1) changes in tone, caliber and peristalsis, (2) changes in the amount of secretion, and (3) changes in the mucosa, both in the surface and in the mucosal folds.

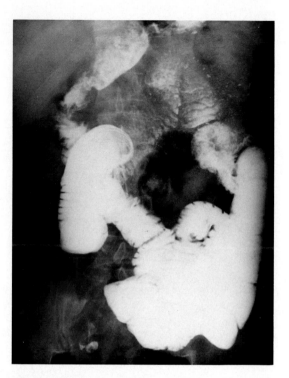

Fig. 62-24 Tropical sprue shows generalized dilatation of proximal small bowel loops as well as smudging and dilution of barium in left upper quadrant caused by excess fluid in several loops of proximal jejunum. Moulage sign is produced by barium reaching such dilated, fluid-filled, hypotonic segments. Note normal-sized, but widely spaced and therefore sparser, folds in jejunum.
(From Reeder, MM, and Palmer, PES: The radiology of tropical diseases, Baltimore, 1981, Williams & Wilkins.)

Segmentation is one of the hallmarks of the sprue syndrome. This may be seen as bowel segments in which there is diminished peristalsis, to the extent that it is almost absent, or as segments in which there is rapid passage of the contents. The rapid movements are nearly always followed immediately by slowed movements. At the same time, there is usually considerable loss of bowel tone, with dilatation and stagnation of the contrast material (Fig. 62-24). This does not in any way respond to the injection of carbachol. The variation in the emptying time of the small bowel may be considerable, increasing to as much as 12 hours or more. It is probable that the changes are more marked in the midportion of the small bowel than elsewhere, and the distal ileal loops are frequently relatively normal.

Because of the disordered motility, intussusception may occur in sprue, which may be transient as the part of the bowel that is moving actively proceeds into an inactive segment. The degree of dilatation is nonspecific, although it is a definite indication of abnormality. It prob-

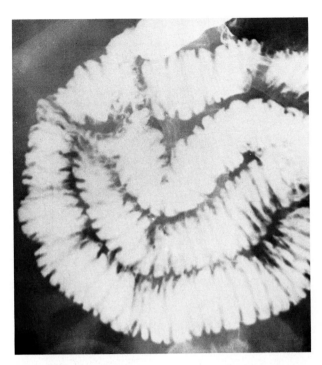

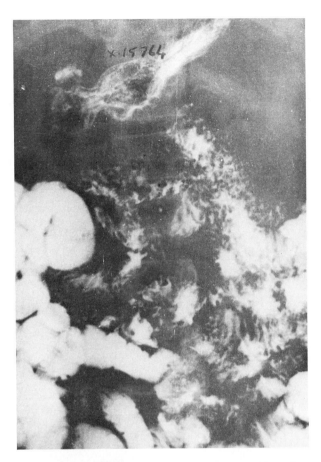

Fig. 62-25 Tropical sprue. Thickening of valvulae conniventes (primary and secondary mucosal folds, valves of Kerckring) produces cogwheel mucosal appearance of proximal small bowel. There is also increase in caliber of these loops due to loss of tone and slowing of peristalsis.
(From Reeder, MM, and Palmer, PES: The radiology of tropical diseases, Baltimore, 1981, Williams & Wilkins.)

Fig. 62-26 Segmentation of barium column is noted in patient from India with tropical sprue. Scattered boli of barium remain in same loops for significant time. There is also coarse clumping and fragmentation of barium within affected loops.
(From Reeder, MM, and Palmer, PES: The radiology of tropical diseases, Baltimore, 1981, Williams & Wilkins.)

ably occurs in as many as 80% of patients who have sprue symptoms. It is usually persistent, or at least recurrent, and involves a lengthy segment of bowel—often multiple, involved, dilated loops. Because there is such variation in the normal pattern, it is essential to restrict the diagnosis of dilatation to those patients in whom the changes are persistent and involve more than one localized segment.

The changes in the mucosa are of different varieties. The general pattern of the mucosa shows less flexibility and less mobility. There is thickening of the transverse mucosal folds presenting the rigid "cogwheel" appearance instead of the normal feathery pattern (Fig. 62-25). These folds may measure 4 or 5 mm thick. Later, atrophy may occur and the mucosal folds may disappear altogether. These changes are, like the other changes of sprue, extremely variable.

Excess secretion is shown by the presence of flocculation, particularly if standard barium sulfate is used. In the lower small bowel there is often coarse clumping of the barium column, which fragments into various sections. This segmentation may be quite marked, partic-

ularly in tropical sprue, and some of the segments show considerable stasis (Fig. 62-26). Because of the mucosal changes, the normally clear outline of the mucosal pattern may be smudged and may be made worse if excess bowel secretions cause dilution of the barium mixture. In extreme cases this leads to the "moulage sign," resulting in a faint outline to that specific segment. This finding is as changing and variable as the others in sprue, which is part of the diagnostic evidence.

Late in the disease the bowel wall becomes considerably thinned, as can be identified by the lessened interval between two adjacent loops of bowel. When this is seen radiologically, it is unwise to perform per oral biopsy, since there is considerable risk of perforation.

It is impossible to determine the specific cause of the malabsorption pattern radiographically. The diagnosis of tropical sprue may be suggested by the combination of

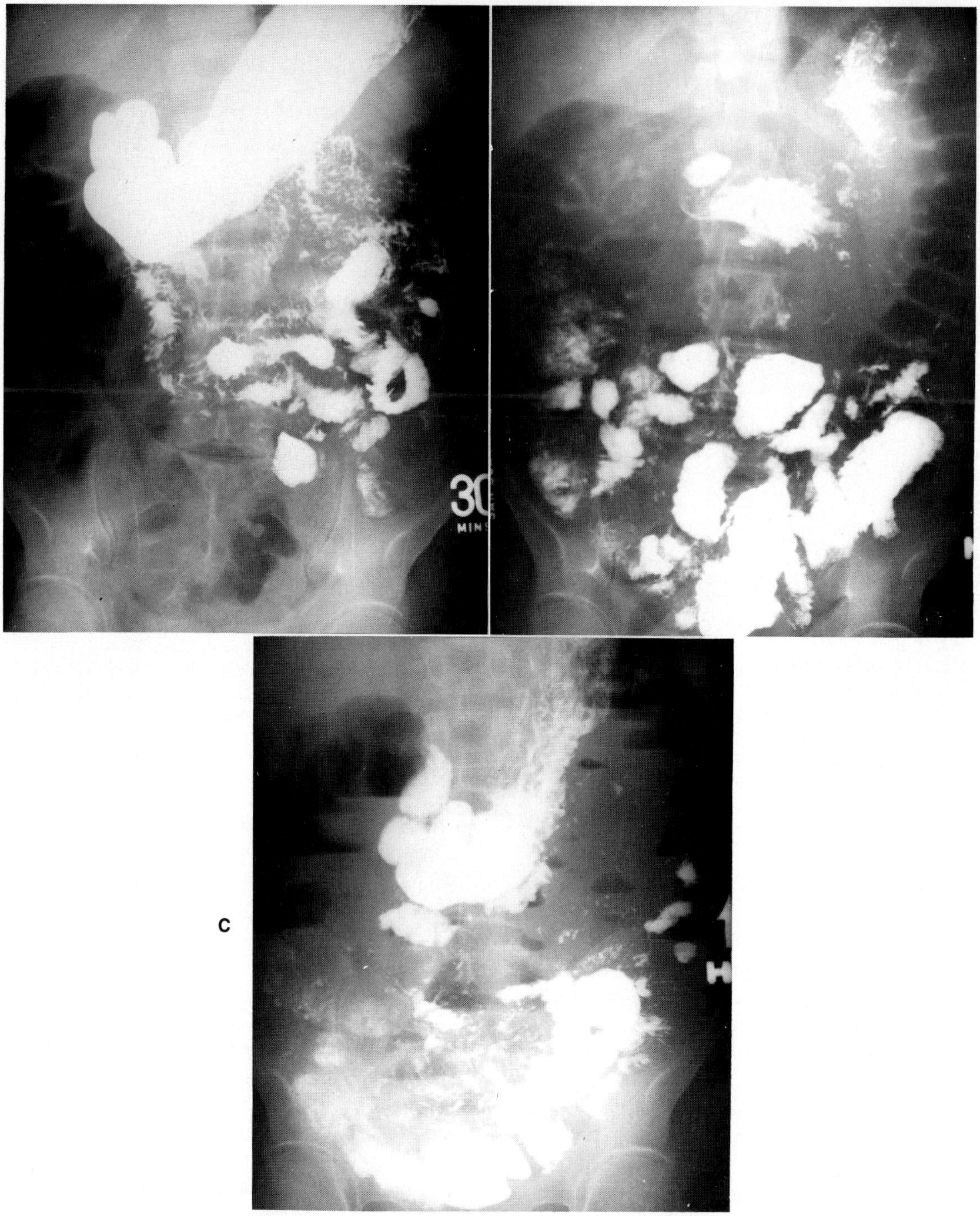

Fig. 62-27 Tropical sprue. Multiple films at varying time intervals during small bowel series on patient with tropical sprue, illustrating changing patterns during single examination. **A,** At 30 minutes there is no dilatation of proximal small bowel loops, but normal feathery mucosal pattern in duodenum and proximal jejunum is lost, whereas many of midjejunal loops show sparse or absent valvulae conniventes. There is also some flocculation and segmentation of barium column. **B,** At 1 hour there is marked degree of segmentation, with barium stagnant in multiple hypotonic and dilated loops of distal jejunum and ileum. Some coarse clumping of barium is also noted, and no normal mucosal folds are seen. **C,** At 1 hour erect film of abdomen shows multiple air-fluid levels in small bowel and colon. Rather marked early flocculation and segmentation of the barium column are undoubtedly related to presence of excessive fluid within bowel, as well as disordered motility. Involvement of colon with slightly dilated hypotonic loops of large bowel containing air-fluid levels is well demonstrated in this patient.

(From Reeder, MM, and Palmer, PES: The radiology of tropical diseases, Baltimore, 1981, Williams & Wilkins.)

the findings as described, along with their very inconstancy (Fig. 62-27). The length of the bowel involved, the restriction to the small bowel in the vast majority of patients, and, of course, the clinical condition of the individual and pertinent laboratory tests confirm the diagnosis. Barium can be used as a method of serial evaluation of the success or otherwise of treatment, although improvement will lag behind the endoscopic biopsy findings. It may be some time after histologic healing that there is complete restoration of the bowel to its normal peristalsis, tone, and function.

GASTROINTESTINAL CANDIDIASIS[91-99]

Gastrointestinal candidiasis or moniliasis is caused by the fungus *Candida albicans*. This commensal organism is found in the mouth and upper respiratory and gastrointestinal tracts of many normal persons. It nearly always becomes pathogenic as a result of an underlying debilitating state, such as may be caused by prolonged antibiotic therapy[98,99] that alters the gastrointestinal flora, malignancy, and chemotherapy for neoplastic disease (immunosuppressive agents, steroids, and antimetabolites). Blood dyscrasias, such as sickle cell disease[97] and especially leukemia,[92] advanced tuberculosis or diabetes, drug addiction, and malnutrition (either dietary or resulting from abnormal intestinal absorption) are other underlying causes. Candidal infections of the gastrointestinal tract are frequently accompanied by oral thrush or ulcerations of the buccal mucosa, but this relationship is not absolute.[96] Although all sites in the gastrointestinal tract may be invaded by *C. albicans,* the oral cavity, pharynx, and esophagus are most commonly involved. Dysphagia is therefore the most common presenting symptom.

In children vomiting and dehydration from esophagitis is common and may lead to aspiration and pulmonary infection.[99] Plaquelike white patches on the gums and pharyngeal mucosa indicate oral involvement.

In the esophagus the lesions are ulcerative or membranous and can extend deep into the muscular coat. Both yeast and pseudohyphal fungal colonies occur. The yeast form produces surface granulomas and membranes, whereas the hyphal form penetrates into the esophageal coats and causes deep microabscesses and ulcers. Similar changes are seen in other affected mucosal surfaces. Esophagoscopy may reveal erythematous and ulcerated esophageal mucosa, sometimes with a visible pseudomembrane. When these plaques or membranes are removed, they leave a raw, granulating base.

The diagnosis of candidal gastrointestinal lesions is more difficult. Identification of mycelia in the feces is important for diagnosis. Mycelia are thought to be evidence of invasion of mucosa rather than of simple saprophytic activity, as may be the case when only yeast cells are found in the feces.[99] The ultimate diagnosis is established by demonstration of mycelia in material from the gastrointestinal ulcerations or on histologic section. Gram's stains and periodic acid–Schiff stain are necessary to show the fungi in caseating foci or abscesses. Invasion of the gastrointestinal tract by *Candida* organisms may be followed by septicemia.[98,99] The ulcerating gastrointestinal lesions provide a portal of entry for *Candida* organisms into the intestinal venules and thus into the circulation. Specific antibody titers have been found in the blood and are of diagnostic value.[98]

Radiographic findings

Radiographic abnormalities resulting from *C. albicans* are most frequently seen in the esophagus. A long segment, particularly the lower half of the esophagus, is involved, although short plaquelike lesions have been seen. The esophageal lumen may be wide and remain distended because of involvement of the deeper layers. The tone is partially lost, and both primary and secondary peristalsis are sluggish because of the muscular involvement. On the other hand, esophageal spasm as well as atony, have been noted in candidal esophagitis.[95,97]

Because of the granulomas and ulceration, the mucous membrane seen on barium studies is irregular, ragged, and shaggy, like a carpet (Fig. 62-28). This appearance is produced by mucosal ulceration and by a pseudomembrane covering areas of ulceration.[93-95] The pseudohyphae trap the barium and retain it for a long period, whereas normally the mucosal coating is lost soon after the bolus travels down the esophagus. Multiple small smooth nodules caused by edema and infiltrate accompanied by granuloma formation, but without ulceration of the esophagus, may produce a cobblestone pattern[93] (Fig. 62-29). The radiographic findings reverse rapidly when antibiotics and steroids are stopped and antifungal drugs are administered.

C. albicans esophagitis must be differentiated from esophagitis that results from other causes, such as caustic agents and reflux esophagitis. A history of ingestion of caustics or long-standing heartburn is helpful in the differentiation. Reflux esophagitis is usually not as extensive, and the ulcerations are not as prominent as in candidal esophagitis. At times esophageal varices may be confused with candidal esophagitis, but the contour irregularity is smooth and not ragged, and varices will be most prominent in the lower third of the esophagus.

Upper gastrointestinal candidal infection occurs most frequently in very ill infants or in the aged.[95,99] Both present technical difficulties radiologically, and it may be impossible to obtain the mucosal studies that are required. Candidiasis in the stomach and small bowel is thus usually revealed only at autopsy without signs having been demonstrated radiographically. In one large series[91] no specific gastrointestinal radiograph abnormality below the esophagus was reported.

When seen, changes in the stomach and small bowel result from extensive ulceration and invasion by the fungus. Peristalsis is sluggish. The main mucosal folds are partly preserved, but there is effacement of the minor folds, with prolonged retention of barium in a shaggy, carpetlike pseudomembrane over the mucosal lining. This secondary pseudomembranous formation may result in a ragged, irregular-appearing ulcer with associated edema. The pseudomembrane may be proliferative and contain many mycelia that produce irregular intraluminal filling defects (Fig. 62-30). A repeat gastrointestinal study after treatment shows return of peristalsis and mucosa to normal and lack of retention of contrast on the mucosa, a process that takes several weeks.

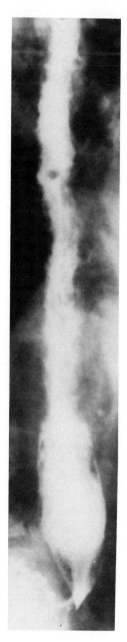

Fig. 62-28 Irregular, shaggy, esophageal contour—result of ulcerating candidal esophagitis.

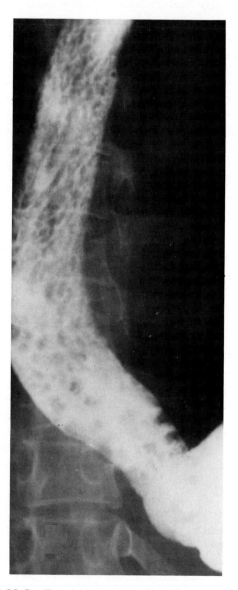

Fig. 62-29 Small nodular contour defects from candidal invasion without ulceration (cobblestone esophagus).
(From Goldberg, HI, and Dodds, WJ: Am J Roentgenol 104:608, 1968.)

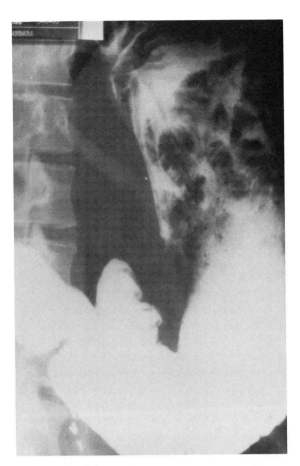

Fig. 62-30 Amorphous, irregular, filling defects in body that persisted in location and appearance—result of massive candidal invasion with ulceration and pseudomembranous formation.
(Courtesy Dr. Harold Jacobson.)

There are no specific changes of candidiasis in the small intestine. An irritable colon pattern may be seen in the large bowel.[95]

GASTROINTESTINAL HISTOPLASMOSIS[100-107]

Gastrointestinal involvement by the fungus *Histoplasma capsulatum* produces clinical and radiographic findings similar to those of tuberculosis. As in tuberculosis, the lung is the main portal of entry and the site of primary infection.[105] Occasionally primary intestinal infection has been reported.[100] More often, however, radiographic evidence of pulmonary histoplasmosis is present in patients with gastrointestinal involvement.[105,107]

The swallowing of organism-laden sputum results in mucosal involvement, whereas hematogenous spread involves the submucosa of bowel.[107] Dissemination to the gastrointestinal tract is accompanied with symptoms in only 20% of patients. These symptoms consist of weight loss, anorexia, abdominal pain, and watery diarrhea with involvement of colon. Gastrointestinal hemorrhage with perforation, peritonitis, and intestinal obstruction have also been initial manifestations.[105]

Histoplasmosis has been reported in nearly all areas of the gastrointestinal tract. Ulcerating granulomatous lesions of the pharynx[107] and anus have been noted, as have lesions of more common areas of disease, such as the ileum, cecum, jejunum, and colon.[101-105] The esophagus may be involved after spread from involved mediastinal lymph nodes.

Radiographic findings

Plain radiographs of the abdomen in patients with gastrointestinal histoplasmosis may frequently show

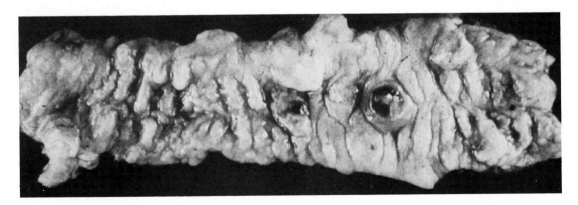

Fig. 62-31 Section of colon from child with disseminated histoplasmosis, showing thickened indurated mucosal folds. Nodular lesions resulted from microabscesses in colon wall, which were filled with fungi that had become necrotic and ulcerated.
(From Silverman, FN, et al: Am J Med 19:410, 1955.)

small, round, calcified granulomas in the spleen. Hepatosplenomegaly caused by frequent involvement of the reticuloendothelial system by histoplasmosis may also be present.[107]

Gastrointestinal histoplasmosis involves lymphoid aggregates in the submucosa and causes a granulomatous infiltrate with transmural involvement. A radiographic pattern is produced, similar to that of tuberculosis. Three types of radiographic findings are seen:

1. The mucosal pattern may be distorted by either small nodules or ulcerations from underlying granulomatous reaction[101,104-106] (Fig. 62-31). The ulcers are generally shallow and difficult to see radiographically.
2. A mass in the area of the terminal ileum and cecum, the result of involvement of Peyer's patches and regional nodes, may indent the cecal tip.[101] In a later phase of the disease scarring and fibrosis may cause stricture and deformity.[101,105]
3. Generalized widening of mucosal folds of small bowel by edema of protein-losing enteropathy, with underlying intestinal histoplasmosis, has been reported.[100]

The differential diagnoses are identical to those of tuberculosis: Crohn's disease, tuberculosis, periappendiceal abscess, carcinoma, and lymphoma.

HELMINTHOMA[108-113]

A helminthoma is an inflammatory tumor of the bowel wall caused by penetration of the wall of the cecum or colon by an intestinal worm. In theory this can occur with many of the intestinal parasites and in any part of the world, but although penetration of the gut occurs occasionally, particularly in heavy *Ascaris* infections, the usual result is peritonitis rather than the marked inflammatory reaction known as helminthoma. Such "tumors" have been reported most commonly from West ad East Africa but have occurred in South America, and one case has been reported from Indonesia.

The parasites most commonly responsible are *Strongyli: Oesophagostomum apiostomum, Oesophagostomum stephanostomum,* and rarely, the hookworm *Ancylostoma duodenale* and *Oesophagostomum brumpti.* Although it is difficult to assess the frequency of *Oesophagostoma* in humans, they are common parasites in the colon of many animals, particularly sheep, goats, pigs, cattle, apes, and monkeys, in whom they cause serious illness with dysentery, peritonitis, and malnutrition. The worms are found not only throughout Africa but in Brazil, Indonesia, the Philippines, and parts of China. The ova resemble those of the hookworm. In many patients the worms cause relatively little general reaction until the bowel wall is entered. Then there is abdominal pain, usually localized to the affected bowel segment, most commonly in the right lower quadrant. Seldom is there nausea, dysentery, or vomiting. There may be a low-grade fever, but this is not constant. The history is usually vague, nonspecific, and brief, often of only 2 to 5 days' duration. Children may have a somewhat longer attack, lasting 2 or 3 weeks and simulating intussusception. Clinical examination usually shows an easily palpable tender mass, often smooth and well localized but sometimes more diffuse. The white blood cell count is elevated, and there may be some eosinophilia. The usual clinical diagnosis is an appendiceal or pericecal abscess or amebiasis. In children perforation of the cecal wall can occur anteriorly, and an abdominal wall abscess may be the presenting finding.

What happens next depends on the sequence of events. After the acute phase, the mass may subside, with resolution and absorption of the inflammatory reaction and calcification of the worm. This may become visible on plain film of the abdomen and may be an incidental finding at some later date. Alternatively, the abscess may perforate into the bowel lumen or into the peritoneal cavity to cause peritonitis, or the abscess may become adherent to the abdominal wall. In many cases the whole process is more chronic, resulting in a large granulomatous mass in which specific identification of the worm has become impossible, extensive adhesions to neighboring structures have occurred, and central caseous necrosis or calcified fibrotic nodules may be found. Both clinical and histological differentiation from amebiasis, tuberculosis, and schistosomiasis must be made. Surgical resection is usually required, and it is probable that the actual cause of many of these cases has been missed once they have entered the chronic stage. (There are only some 50 cases in the literature.)

Radiologic investigation of such cases seldom occurs, because the patients usually have an obvious indication for surgery. The essential finding on barium enema is a mass within the wall of the bowel. The helminthoma seldom encircles the bowel lumen but narrows it eccentrically, since the mass is partially intramural and largely extramural. Distortion is caused by extrinsic pressure and by the mass within the bowel wall (Fig. 62-32). The most common localization is in the region of the cecum or ascending colon, but helminthomas have also been demonstrated in the transverse and descending colon. Air contrast studies will show that the mucosa is intact but stretched over the underlying intramural tumor, the edge of which is usually reasonably well defined. There is usually too much edema to allow demonstration of the tiny perforation that follows the route of the worm. As the tumor enlarges and nearby tissue becomes involved, the bowel wall becomes thick. Contraction, so

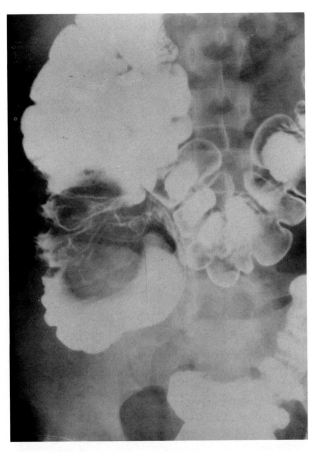

Fig. 62-32 Helminthoma of cecum. This large granulomatous tumor caused by worm burrowing into wall of cecum must be distinguished from ameboma, tuberculosis, and carcinoma in patients from the tropics.
(From Reeder, MM, and Palmer, PES: The radiology of tropical diseases, Baltimore, 1981, Williams & Wilkins.)

common in amebiasis and tuberculosis, is unlikely to occur.

The tumor is most likely to be mistaken for a colon carcinoma, partially encircling the bowel wall. The helminthoma differs in that it seldom produces mucosal ulceration or destruction (and there is seldom melena clinically), and the outline of the mass is often well defined. In the more acute case the most likely diagnosis will be an appendiceal abscess or even an amebic abscess of the ileocecal region. A high index of suspicion is *most important* in making the diagnosis preoperatively.

Localized bowel granulomas have been caused by other parasites. *Anisakiasis* may occasionally cause ileal or cecal nodules. Similarly, *Angiostrongyles costaricensis* has been known to deposit eggs in the cecal and ileal wall, causing nodular granulomas. Such masses may cause subacute intestinal obstruction or infarction of the bowel after death of the parent intravascular parasite. As the name would suggest, this organism is most frequently seen in Costa Rica and Honduras and is most common in children. Parasitic embolism has also been reported from Australia as a result of *Spriurida physalopteridae,* causing eosinophilic granulomas in the distal small bowel. None of these appears to have been demonstrated radiologically, and, if they were seen, it would be impossible to make a differential diagnosis.

CHAGAS' DISEASE[114-125]

Although Chagas' disease (American trypanosomiasis) occurs only in the central and southern half of the American continent from Texas to Argentina, the World Health Organization estimated in 1960 that there were at least 7 million infected individuals and another 35 million exposed to infection.[125] It is thus an important public health problem in many South American nations, especially in rural eastern Brazil where more than 30% of all adults with clinical evidence of chronic Chagas' disease die as a result of their infection.[115,117,119]

Despite research since 1909, when it was first described by Carlos Chagas, the disease remains a baffling one with many unresolved problems and many different manifestations in both its acute and chronic stages. In the acute phase it may lead to extensive myocarditis and encephalitis; in its chronic form, in addition to severe myocardiopathy, there is a decrease in the number of ganglion cells in the central and peripheral autonomic nervous system, which may lead to marked enlargement of the heart, esophagus, colon, and hollow viscera. The heart is the organ most commonly involved, and in both the acute and chronic phases myocarditis accounts for greater morbidity and mortality than does involvement of all other organs. Chronic Chagas' disease accounts for tens of thousands of cases of cardiomyopathy in hyperendemic areas such as Argentina, Uruguay, Chile, and Venezuela and is a special problem in eastern Brazil where megaesophagus and megacolon are commonly seen in addition to the cardiac involvement.

Chagas' disease is primarily an infection of children and young adults living in mud huts in rural areas. The causative organism, *Trypanosoma cruzi,* is a tiny pleomorphic protozoon that inhabits the blood and tissues of humans and animals. It is transmitted by several species of reduviid or triatome bugs, which become infected after feeding on humans and on armadillos, or other animal hosts. These bloodsucking bugs have a predilection for biting sleeping children on the face at night. Infection results from contamination of the punctured skin by the insect's feces, which are loaded with trypanosomes. Once introduced into the body, the protozoa travel within the bloodstream as flagellated trypanosomal C- or U-shaped forms. Once they invade tissue cells, especially reticuloendothelial cells, muscle, and glia, they undergo transformation to leishmanial forms. These divide by binary fission to form intracellular colonies that fill and rupture the invaded cells. The fact that *T. cruzi* multiplies within the host cell's cytoplasm and not in the blood makes Chagas' disease especially difficult to treat.

Once the cell has ruptured, liberated organisms either invade adjacent cells or are destroyed by macrophages releasing a neurotoxin that attacks and over a period destroys the ganglion cells in the myenteric plexi of the affected organ.[117,119] The heart, brain, esophagus, and colon are the principal sites of involvement, although the spleen, liver, lymph nodes, bronchi, ureters, and salivary glands may also be affected.

In the acute phase of the infection, which is most commonly seen in children, there may be fever, edema, anemia, lymphadenitis, meningoencephalitis, and especially myocarditis.[123] The mortality rate from acute myocarditis or meningoencephalitis varies from 2% to 10%.

The pathogenesis of Chagas' disease involves at least three distinct phases, each with its own pathologic processes. Once defense mechanisms have developed during the acute phase, the disease passes into a latent phase of many years' duration, during which time the parasites are difficult to demonstrate either in the blood or in body tissues.

The third, or chronic (late), stage of the disease gives rise to the Chagas' syndromes that are the end result of the destruction of ganglion cells in the central or peripheral nervous system that occurred during the acute phase. The lesions may be widespread but are most severe in the heart, muscles, nervous system, and gastrointestinal tract, particularly the esophagus and colon.

The three stages of the disease, although of one cause, are clinically and radiologically distinct. The middle or latent period is clinically silent, whereas the acute and late stages can be severe and dramatic in their clinical and radiologic manifestations.

Thus, after a period of as many as 10 to 20 years and probably after repeated infections with the trypanosome, the systemic changes of the chronic stage may develop, especially involving the heart, esophagus, and rectosigmoid colon. Several Brazilian investigators[116-120] have clearly established that aperistalsis and dilatation of the esophagus and colon are common late sequels to infection with *T. cruzi*, in addition to the more common chronic chagasic cardiomyopathy. In Ferreira-Santos' large series[117] the complement fixation text for trypanosomiasis was positive in 95% of a large group of autopsied or surgically treated patients with esophageal and colonic aperistalsis. The age range in this series was 2 to 75 years, with an average of 33 years. Brasil[116] suggested

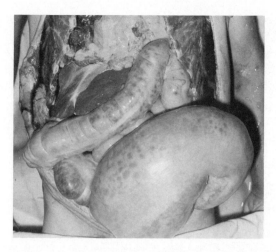

Fig. 62-33 Chronic Chagas' megacolon at necropsy. Note massive distention and elongation of rectosigmoid colon, with less marked dilatation of more proximal portion of colon. (Courtesy Dr. Clovis Simão.)

that the name "aperistalsis" be applied to chronic Chagas' disease to denote the pathophysiologic disturbances of motor incoordination, defective esophageal and colonic motility, and disturbed or absent peristalsis without propulsive efficiency, which characterize advanced cases. Köberle[119,120] demonstrated that the quantitative and qualitative reduction in the number of ganglia throughout the entire gastrointestinal tract, especially in the colon and esophagus, is responsible for the production of the aperistalsis and atony, which in turn results in dilatation of these hollow viscera. Although ganglia deficiency may be seen throughout the entire gastrointestinal tract, clinically and radiographically the esophagus and the rectosigmoid colon show the greatest distention, probably because they are subjected to greater mechanical pressure and stasis (Fig. 62-33).

Radiographic findings

The earliest radiographic manifestations of Chagas' disease in the esophagus relate only to motor dysfunction. Tone is maintained in the early stages, and there may be little or no dilatation. Gradually increasing disturbances in tone, rhythm, and motility over several years give the appearance of bizarre, dysrhythmic contractions on barium swallow. Hypercontractility, increased tone, and hypertrophy of circular muscle layers are manifestations of motor dysfunction often resulting in dysphagia. Later, as denervation progresses, hypotonia, aperistalsis, stasis, and dilatation occur. The transverse diameter of the flaccid esophagus may reach 7 cm or more, and contractions may be weak and uncoordinated or absent[117] (Fig. 62-34).

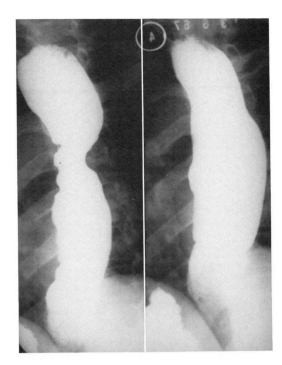

Fig. 62-34 Megaesophagus in Brazilian patient with chronic Chagas' disease. Considerable esophageal dilatation and altered peristalsis denote advanced disease. Local, incoordinate, nonpropulsive contractions are present.
(From Reeder, MM, and Hamilton, LC: Semin Roentgenol 3:62, 1968.)

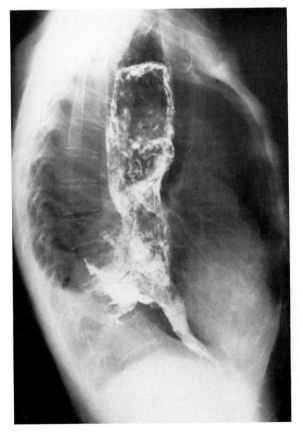

Fig. 62-35 Chagas' megaesophagus in adult Brazilian man with development of carcinoma in distal third of esophagus with perforation to form large abscess extending into right lower lobe and pleural space.
(From Reeder, MM, and Palmer, PES: The radiology of tropical diseases, Baltimore, 1981, Williams & Wilkins.)

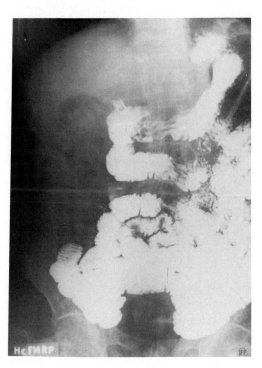

Fig. 62-36 Chagas' megaduodenum and megajejunum in 57-year-old Brazilian man. At surgery duodenum was dilated throughout its length. Neither ulcers nor obstruction by aortic mesenteric vessels was present.
(Courtesy Dr. Clovis Simão.)

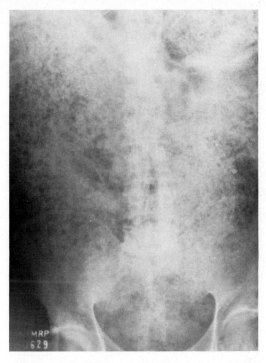

Fig. 62-37 Chronic Chagas' megacolon with massive amount of retained feces throughout grossly dilated colon, opacifying virtually the entire abdomen. This 51-year-old Brazilian man had progressive intestinal constipation for more than 14 years, despite two previous partial resections of colon. Following this examination, entire colon was removed after it was emptied of fecalomas. Colon measured 10 cm in diameter and contained numerous small mucosal ulcers and secondary inflammation. Wall was not thickened uniformly; it was thin in some places and thick in others.
(Courtesy Dr. Clovis Simão.)

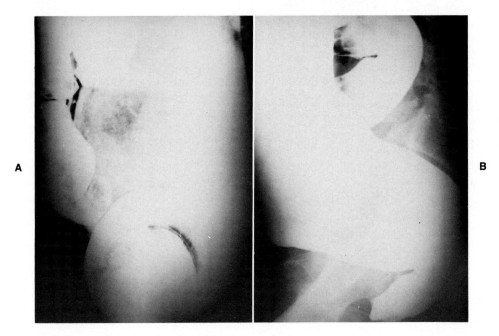

Fig. 62-38 Chagas' disease of colon in 56-year-old Brazilian woman with chronic trypanosomiasis. Anteroposterior, **A,** and lateral, **B,** views show massive dilatation of entire left colon. Note large fecaliths within colon. Rectum is not dilated to same degree as sigmoid and descending colon because of action of pelvic musculature. Follow-up radiograph 47 days later showed marked retention of barium from this examination.
(From Reeder, MM, and Hamilton, LC: Semin Roentgenol 3:62, 1968.)

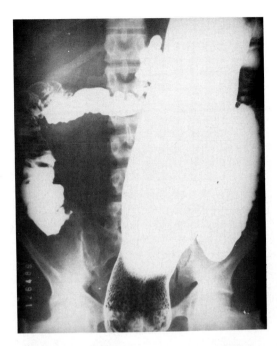

Fig. 62-39 Chagas' disease of colon. Severe distention and elongation of the rectum, sigmoid, and descending colon with normal caliber of proximal portion of colon in Brazilian man. Cobblestone mucosal pattern is seen in rectum similar to pattern seen with mucosal hives from hypersensitivity phenomenon. (From Reeder, MM, and Hamilton, LC: Semin Roentgenol 3:62, 1968.)

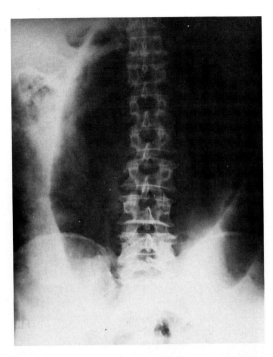

Fig. 62-40 Volvulus of sigmoid colon in 59-year-old Brazilian man with Chagas' disease who had abdominal colic, distention, and obstipation for 15 days. A 180-degree torsion of mesosigmoid was discovered at surgery. (From Reeder, MM, and Hamilton, LC: Semin Roentgenol 3:62, 1968.)

The appearance of advanced megaesophagus on plain film radiographs of the chest and on barium swallow is remarkably similar to that of achalasia. In both entities the dilated esophagus will appear on frontal films as a vertical density along the entire right paramediastinal border, usually distended with air and sometimes showing an air-fluid level if the patient has recently ingested liquids. There often is tapering of the distal esophageal segment down to the cardiac sphincter, and the radiologic picture may be indistinguishable from achalasia, although of quite different cause. There may be a delay in passage of food or barium through this area because of failure of relaxation and motor incoordination at the level of the sphincter, as well as lack of propulsive peristalsis throughout the esophagus. Food may become lodged in the esophagus and cause local irritation leading to inflammation, ulceration, bleeding, perforation, and fistulas. Carcinoma develops in 7% of patients with megaesophagus, sometimes with rupture into the mediastinum and abscess formation[117,123] (Fig. 62-35).

There are usually no radiographic changes in the stomach or small bowel other than occasional cases of megastomach, megaduodenum, or megajejunum (Fig. 62-36).

In patients with megacolon the predominant symptom is chronic obstipation, with bowel movements occurring at intervals from 8 days to several months. Large boluses of desiccated feces may become impacted in the dilated, atonic rectosigmoid colon, leading to inflammation and stasis ulceration. Sigmoid volvulus, which occurs in 10% of patients, is often the presenting manifestation that causes the patient to finally seek medical attention.[118]

On plain radiographs of the abdomen, multiple large coproliths may be seen within a dilated, often redundant colon[121-123] (Fig. 62-37). A dilated splenic flexure or elongated sigmoid colon may sometimes be seen beneath an elevated left hemidiaphragm, simulating the splenic flexure syndrome.[123] The striking elongation and dilatation of the rectosigmoid and descending colon are best illustrated by barium enema (Fig. 62-38). The haustral markings of the colon are diminished or absent, and colonic contractility and evacuation are poor, with most of the barium and retained feces still present on postevacuation films.[118] A cobblestone mucosal pattern is occasionally seen within a portion of the dilated distal colon or rectum; the pattern is similar to that seen with mucosal hives caused by hypersensitivity phenomenon[123] (Fig. 62-39). Rarely a diffusely ulcerated distal colon may be seen.[123]

Occasionally the dilatation of the colon is not uniform

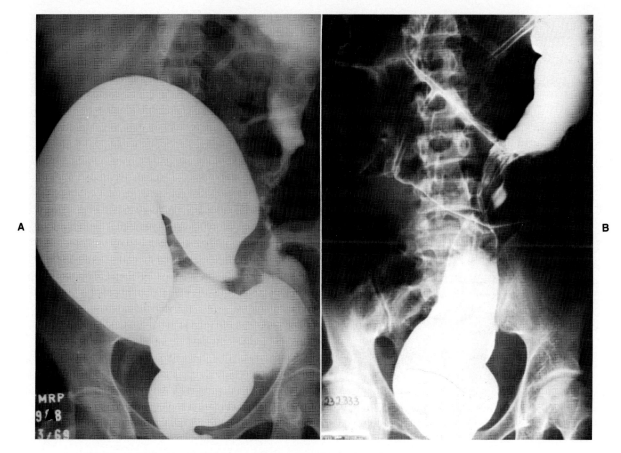

Fig. 62-41 Sigmoid volvulus in two different Brazilian patients with Chagas' megacolon. **A,** There is typical beaklike appearance of barium column as it reaches point of volvulus in proximal sigmoid colon. **B,** Classical twisted appearance of sigmoid is well seen with slight amount of barium passing beyond area of volvulus in midsigmoid colon. Note considerable distention of entire large bowel caused by underlying chagasic aganglionosis.

(From Reeder, MM, and Palmer, PES: The radiology of tropical diseases, Baltimore, 1981, Williams & Wilkins.)

throughout. A less distended, short segment of the colon, where loss of ganglia and subsequent dilatation are less pronounced when compared with the dilated adjacent bowel, may predispose to sigmoid volvulus. A massively dilated loop of sigmoid colon is seen, often with a prominent air-fluid level on erect view (Fig. 62-40). Barium enema may show the typical beaklike or twisted appearance of the colon at the site of the volvulus (Fig. 62-41).

In most cases of advanced chronic Chagas' disease, a generalized enlargement of the heart is present with weak pulsations resulting from chronic myocardiopathy[114,120,123,124] (Fig. 62-42). The lungs are clear, and no pleural fluid is present until the end stages of cardiac failure. In rare cases the bronchi, ureters, and gallbladder may be dilated.[123]

TRICHURIASIS[126-134]

Trichuriasis is an infection of the human cecum and colon and rarely the distal ileum that is caused by the whipworm *Trichuris trichiura*. This nematode is cosmopolitan in distribution but thrives chiefly in the warm, moist tropics, where several hundred worms may be present in a severely infected patient. In 1947 more than 350 million persons were estimated to be infested with whipworms, and in some hyperendemic areas 90% of the population is infected.[134] In the United States trichuriasis is found chiefly in the southern Appalachian Mountains and rural Louisiana, where fecal pollution, dense shade near the houses, and heavy rainfall favor growth of the parasite. In Brazil it is the most common parasite in large cities, with an incidence of up to 40%, and in Costa Rica it is found in almost 100% of patients with chronic diarrhea.[132-134]

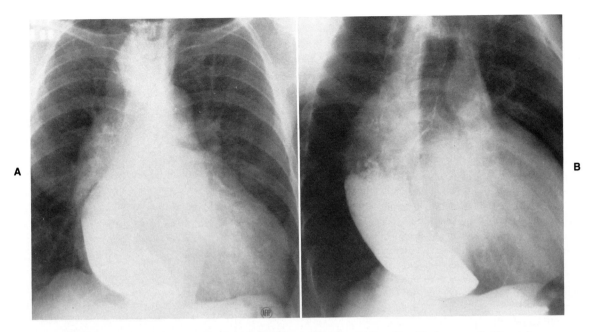

Fig. 62-42 Megaesophagus and myocardiopathy in 58-year-old Brazilian black man with Chagas' disease. **A,** Posteroanterior view shows prominent soft tissue density along entire right mediastinal border caused by greatly dilated esophagus partially filled with barium. Convexities of right and left sides of heart are prominent because of enlargement of both sides of heart. Left atrial enlargement produces bulge along left upper cardiac border and upward displacement of left main bronchus. No pulmonary vascular congestion is noted. **B,** Right oblique view shows posterior displacement of megaesophagus by grossly dilated left atrium.
(From Reeder, MM, and Simão, C: Semin Roentgenol 4:374, 1969.)

Humans become infected by ingesting contaminated vegetables, soil, or water that contain infective *T. trichiura* eggs previously passed in feces. Small children are more likely to develop heavy worm burdens, since they often play with contaminated soil. After ingestion, the eggs hatch into larvae, which attach briefly to the villi of the proximal small bowel for about a week before they pass on into the cecum (the usual habitat of *trichuris* organisms) or elsewhere in the large bowel to develop over a 2- to 3-month period into adult worms attached to the mucosa. In severe infestations *T. trichiura* may be found throughout the entire colon, including the rectum and appendix, and rarely in the terminal ileum.

The adult *T. trichiura* has a characteristic whiplike shape, the anterior three fifths of the worm being long and threadlike and containing the mouth and esophagus. The broader posterior position or "handle" of the whip contains the reproductive organs and is spirally coiled in the male parasite but describes a semilunar arc in the female worm. The parasites are attached to the cecum and colon by means of their slender anterior ends, which transfix superficial folds of mucosa. They lie embedded beneath the surface epithelium between intestinal villi amid considerable mucus; their blunt posterior portions are either coiled or project freely into the bowel lumen as semilunar arcs (Fig. 62-43). There is usually no inflammatory reaction at the site of attachment, although liquefaction necrosis of adjacent cells, ulcerations, and some bleeding may occur in severe infections.

Diagnosis depends on identification of adult worms, usually by sigmoidoscopy, or finding *T. trichiura* eggs on stool concentration tests. Eosinophilia is common in patients with heavy worm burdens. An iron-deficiency anemia is often present as a result of chronic blood loss. Mild infections are usually asymptomatic and are often discovered incidentally during evaluation of a patient concomitantly infected with *Ascaris*, hookworms, or *Entamoeba histolytica*, since they have a similar geographic distribution.

A heavy infestation with *T. trichiura*, however, especially in poorly nourished children, can cause severe chronic diarrhea or dysentery lasting from 6 months to 3 years, with blood and excess mucus in the stools, tenesmus, abdominal pain, rectal prolapse, weakness,

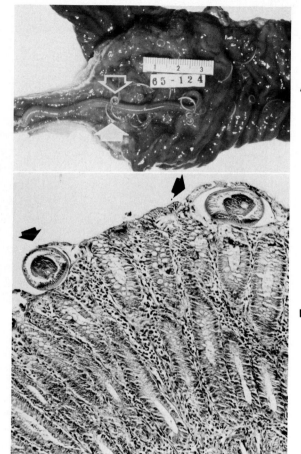

Fig. 62-43 A, Photograph of gross specimen of cecum and appendix of patient from San Salvador shows coexistent whipworm and *Ascaris* infection, a frequent combination. Glistening mucosal surface is not inflamed or ulcerated. It is coated with thick mucus secreted in vicinity of numerous whipworms, especially near appendix. Note typical coiled appearance of male parasites *(open arrow)* and curved semilunar configuration of female worms *(solid arrow),* as their posterior portions protrude into lumen of bowel. **B,** Anterior portions of two whipworms are seen in cross section as they lie embedded in their typical location beneath surface epithelium of colonic mucosa *(arrows).* Note lack of any significant inflammatory reaction in vicinity of worms. (Hematoxylin and eosin; ×40.)
(From Reeder, MM, Astacio, JE, and Theros, EG: Radiology 90:382, 1968.)

pallor, anorexia, irritability, dehydration, and weight loss.[129] Occasional deaths from profuse hemorrhage or intussusception have been reported.[128,132] *T. trichiura* has also been associated with appendicitis in the tropics; in one series from Colombia and parasite was found in 16 of 20 patients with appendicitis.[123] Allergic manifestations such as urticaria, rhinitis, and eosinophilia are frequently seen. Radiology rarely plays a significant role in the diagnosis of trichuriasis, and case reports in the literature are rare.[127,132] However, the worms may be found during barium enema examination as part of an investigation for rectal bleeding or other colon disease. The radiographic appearance of the colon in trichuriasis was described in 1968 by Reeder and associates,[132] who based their findings on barium enema examination of a 7-year-old San Salvador boy (Fig. 62-44). A routine barium enema may be unremarkable or may show a granular mucosal pattern throughout the colon. The excess mucus surrounding hundreds of small whipworms may occasionally cause flocculation of the barium (most modern barium preparations will not flocculate). An air contrast

barium enema is definitive and will demonstrate clearly the wavy radiolucent outlines of numerous small trichurids against the air-barium background of the colon and rectum.[127,132-134] The characteristic uncurled, crescentic, or whiplike pattern of the female parasite and the tightly coiled "pinwheel" or "target" pattern of the male worm can be recognized (Fig. 62-45). Subsequently patients from South Africa,[27] Brazil, and elsewhere have shown identical findings on air contrast examinations. These pathognomonic radiographic features should be kept in mind when patients from areas of high prevalence and poor socioeconomic background are examined.

GIARDIASIS[135-153]

Giardia lamblia is one of the most common intestinal parasites of humans and is worldwide in distribution. It is found in 4% to 16% of inhabitants of tropical countries and in 3% to 20% of children in parts of the southern United States.[149] The organisms is found most often in children, especially those in large families and in institutions such as shcools and orphanages. The reported

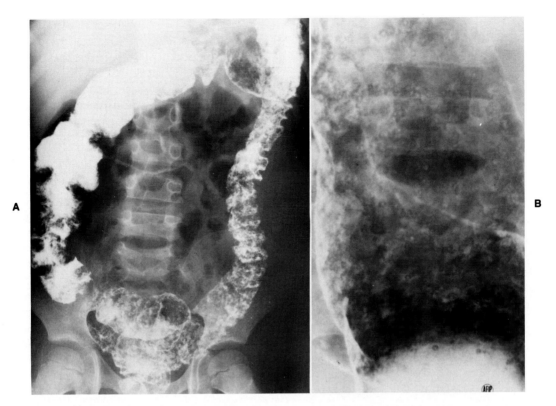

Fig. 62-44 A, Trichuriasis in 7-year-old boy with profuse rectal bleeding. Innumerable whipworms were seen to be attached to rectal mucosa at proctoscopy. Granular mucosal pattern was noted on barium enema examination, similar in appearance to cystic fibrosis. Flocculation of barium and poor mucosal coating are produced by excessive mucous secretions surrounding numerous whipworms. **B,** Magnified view of rectosigmoid colon on air contrast barium enema examination shows outlines of many tiny whipworms attached to mucosa, with their posterior portions either tightly coiled or unfurled in whiplike configuration.
(From Reeder, MM, Astacio, JE, and Theros, EG: Radiology 90:382, 1968.)

incidence of infestation in institutionalized people ranges from 2% to 50%. Occasional epidemics have occurred in cities such as Aspen, Colorado, where leakage of sewage into part of the town's water supply was responsible for the outbreak. Until two decades ago it was thought that this ubiquitous organisms did not invade the mucosa of the duodenum and jejunum (its usual habitat) and that there were no specific radiologic manifestations of giardiasis.[142] Recent studies have shown that neither of these prior assumptions is true, and giardiasis is now recognized as a significant cause of diarrhea, malabsorption, and inflammatory changes in the proximal small bowel in many patients throughout the world, especially in children or those with immunoglobulin deficiencies.[139,151] It must be remembered, however, that the vast majority of people infected with *G. lamblia* have no clinical or radiographic manifestations of their infestations.

The organisms are usually harmless protozoa attached to the mucosal surface of the duodenum and jejunum by their sucking disks. There are two stages in the life cycle of *G. lamblia*: the trophozoite (an actively moving flagellated form) and the cyst, which may be passed in the stool. Humans acquire giardiasis by ingesting contaminated food or water containing viable cysts, which pass unharmed through the gastric juices and undergo excystation in the duodenum, with each cyst giving rise to two trophozoites. These flagellates are usually found in the mucus between intestinal villi and rarely in intestinal crypts. They may attach to the mucosal epithelium of the duodenum and jejunum and rarely the ileum by their sucking disks and may actually invade the mucosa and occasionally produce a mild, inflammatory reaction in the lamina propria of the crypts.

In a number of patients with symptomatic giardiasis, electron microscopy study of small bowel biopsies has

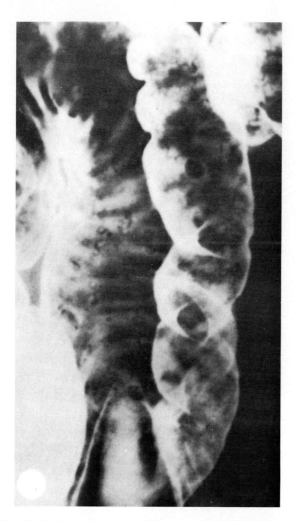

Fig. 62-45 Massive *Trichuris* infestation in Brazilian child. Air contrast examination of colon identifies typical wavy outlines of innumerable trichurids in rectosigmoid colon; some are tightly coiled in "target" pattern typical of male parasites, whereas others are unfurled in whiplike configuration of female parasites.

(From Reeder, MM, and Palmer, PES: The radiology of tropical diseases, Baltimore, 1981, Williams & Wilkins.)

shown acute and chronic inflammatory changes, abnormal villi, and damage to the epithelial cells with increased mitoses.[144,153] The villi are short and thickened, with increased cellular infiltrate in the lamina propria.

Malabsorption is often associated with giardiasis and is thought to result from irritation, inflammatory reaction, and altered epithelial function caused by cellular damage and distrubed epithelial cell maturation. Other theories suggest there may be a mechanical barrier to the absorption of nutrients caused by massive numbers of parasites attached to the mucosal surface or that overwhelming number of *Giardia* organisms compete with the host

for nutrients.[150] However, the exact mechanism of malabsorption in giardiasis remains unproved, since there appears to be no direct correlation between malabsorption and the severity of underlying mucosal changes in many patients.[145] The diagnosis of giardiasis may be established by discovery of cysts or trophozoites in stool specimens or in duodenal aspirates. In some cases examinations of serial sections and impression smears from intestinal biopsies may be necessary.

The vast majority of people infected with *G. lamblia* have no symptoms. In a minority of individuals with giardiasis, usually children or persons with suppressed immunologic systems, there may be a variety of symptoms ranging from mild abdominal discomfort to nausea, anorexia, fever, weight loss, flatulence, recurrent diarrhea, malabsorption, and steatorrhea.[136,140] The stools and clinical manifestations in children may resemble those of sprue or celiac disease.[140] The individual response of a patient to infection with *G. lamblia* varies, depending on the number of organisms present, age, nutrition, associated bacterial infection, and immunoglobulin deficiency.[145,153]

Radiographic findings

Until the mid-1960s reports of radiographic changes in giardiasis were rare. In 1944 Welch[152] described irritability of the duodenal cap with coarsening of the mucosal pattern in 22 of 29 patients with giardiasis. Later Peterson[147] described a deficiency pattern in patients with *G. lamblia* infestation that consisted of pronounced segmentation, a moderate degree of dilatation of small bowel loops, coarsening of the mucosal folds in the midportion of the small bowel, and prolonged transit time. Since those early reports, Marshak et al.,[145] Reeder and Palmer[148,150] and Basu[137] have described radiographic changes of an inflammatory nature, usually localized to the duodenum and jejunum in patients with giardiasis. The proximal ileum is rarely involved; the lower ileum and the colon appear normal.

The changes in the mucosa may be quite marked, with thickening, blunting, distortion, and spiking of the folds (Fig. 62-46). There is marked spasm and irritability of the bowel, resulting in rapid change in configuration of the valvulae conniventes[146,150] (Fig. 62-47). Rapid transit of barium is noted through the affected area, with narrowing of the bowel lumen because of the spasm. Because of the resultant poor filling of the duodenum and jejunum with barium, fluoroscopic spot filming is difficult unless the patient is given large amounts of barium. Secretions are often increased, causing blurring of the mucosal folds that is sometimes associated with fragmentation and segmentation. Cure or clinical improvement of the patient is associated with return to a normal

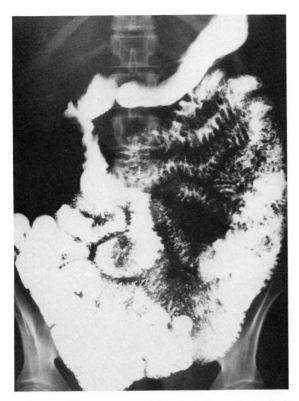

Fig. 62-46 Giardiasis. Second portion of duodenum is markedly irregular, and considerable spasm is noted within duodenal sweep and proximal jejunum. These loops are poorly filled because of irritability and are separated from each other. Mucosal folds are thickened, and secretions are increased. Lumen of bowel is slightly rigid and narrowed. Changes suggest actual inflammatory reaction rather than malabsorption pattern. They disappeared after quinacrine hydrochloride therapy for giardiasis.
(Courtesy Dr. Richard H. Marshak.)

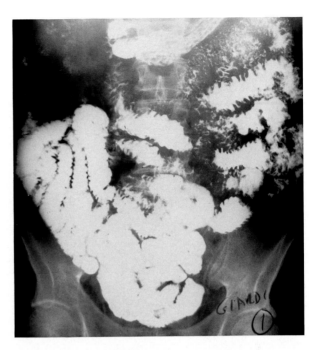

Fig. 62-47 Giardiasis. There are spasm and irritability of proximal small bowel and normal-appearing ileum. Mucosal folds in duodenum and jejunum are thickened and spiked, and there is segmentation and fragmentation of barium column resulting from combination of irritability, mucosal edema, and increased secretions.
(Courtesy Dr. Richard H. Marshak.)

intestinal pattern after the organisms are eradicated by quinacrine hydrochloride (Atabrine), usually within a month.[145]

In addition to the above inflammatory changes, there may also be a small bowel malabsorption or deficiency pattern, especially in children as part of a spruelike syndrome.[140] Although malabsorption may be present clinically and to some extend radiographically, the radiographic appearance in giardiasis (as well as in some patients with strongyloidiasis and hookworm disease) is chiefly the result of inflammation, at least in the proximal small bowel[146,150]; a spruelike pattern may also be present in the distal jejunum and ileum of some of these patients.[150]

There is an unusually high incidence of giardiasis in patients with the syndrome of dysgammaglobulinemia, nodular lymphoid hyperplasia, recurrent respiratory and urinary tract infections, chronic spruelike diarrhea, and other clinical and radiographic evidence of malabsorption[142,143,148] (Fig. 62-48). The generally lowered resistance of these patients permits the usually innocuous *Giardia* organisms to flourish in the small bowel. The innumerable, tiny, uniform 2 to 3 mm nodular lesions found throughout the small intestine are not related to giardiasis but represent hypertrophy of the lymphoid follicles in an effort to produce as much gamma globulin as possible (Fig. 62-49).

Localization of the pathologic and radiologic changes in giardiasis to the duodenum and jejunum is of great importance in differential diagnosis, since many other gastrointestinal diseases are thereby excluded. The principal differential considerations include other parasitic diseases, such as strongyloidiasis and hookworm disease, as well as other inflammatory diseases of the proximal small bowel, such as Whipple's disease and eosinophilic enteritis.[150] Intestinal lymphagiectasia, lymphoma, amyloidosis, vascular diseases, and pancreatitis are unlikely to be confused with giardiasis, since they show more pronounced changes in the mucosal fold pattern but less

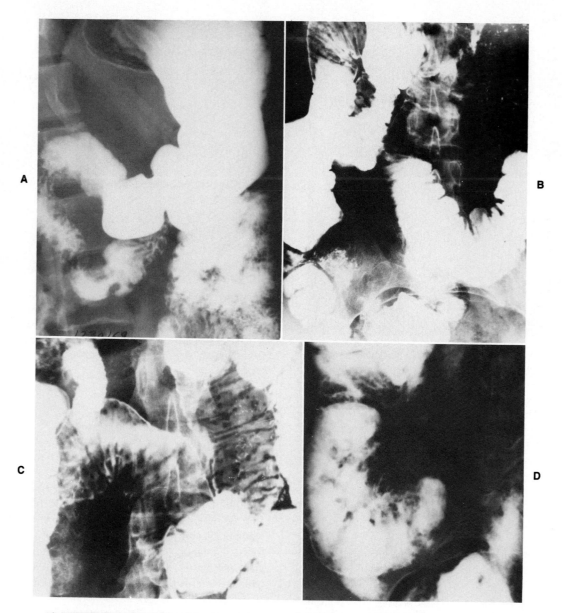

Fig. 62-48 Giardiasis and nodular lymphoid hyperplasia of small intestine in 24-year-old woman with dysgammaglobulinemia, recurrent respiratory infections, and constant spruelike diarrhea. **A,** Mucosal pattern within duodenal bulb and C loop is coarse, with some edema of folds. Duodenal sweep failed to fill out normally as seen on multiple spot films, indicating slight spasm. **B,** Abnormal motor activity with dilatation of multiple loops of jejunum and ileum, together with segmentation of barium column and coarsening of the mucosal folds, is seen in some areas. **B** and **C,** Mucosa of entire jejunum and ileum is uniformly studded with numerous, tiny, round polypoid lesions, 1 to 3 mm in diameter. These nodules are especially well outlined in areas of air-barium contrast. **D,** Nodules are also present in terminal ileum and right portion of colon.
(From Reeder, MM: Radiology 93:427, 1969.)

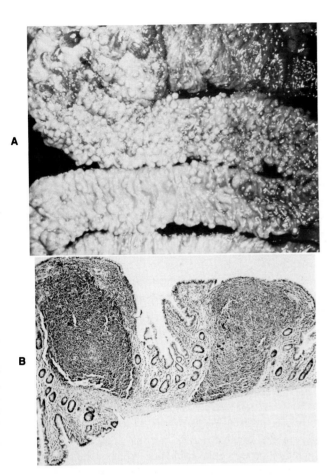

Fig. 62-49 A, Gross specimen of small intestine from patient with nodular lymphoid hyperplasia, in which innumerable small, uniform polypoid lesions studded mucosal surface. These tiny nodules account for multiple round filling defects noted on radiographs of small bowel. **B,** Photomicrograph from jejunal biopsy of patient with dysgammaglobulinemia and nodular lymphoid hyperplasia. Lymphoid follicles within lamina propria are greatly enlarged, elevating mucosal surface to produce polypoid appearance. Overlying villi appear flattened. (Hematoxylin and eosin; ×50.)

extensive spasm, fragmentation, and secretions than are seen in giardiasis. In cases of giardiasis where the "deficiency pattern" is prominent, the differential diagnosis will include other causes of malabsorption, but these only rarely simulate the overall radiographic pattern seen in giardiasis, especially when the prominent inflammatory changes and spasm in the duodenum and jejunum are recognized.

PARASITIC INFECTIONS[154-189]

Parasites vary as widely as the human primates and the other animals in which they live. They are not a new problem. Alimentary worms were recognized in ancient Egypt (in the Ebers Papyrus about BC 1500), and it is probable that the biblical description of the plague of fiery serpents (in the book of *Numbers*) refers to guinea worms, and we have not bettered the method of extraction recommended then, winding the worm around a piece of stick. The best of the early descriptions of worms was by Avicenna (980-1037 AD), who described the symptoms produced by tapeworms, roundworms, and threadworms and knew the different ways of treating patients who had them. References to roundworms have been found in Greek texts and in the writings of Mesopotamia, Rome, and China. Yet in spite of their ancient lineage their life cycle was not unraveled until 1916.

The history of parasitic infections is as diverse as are the life cycle and pathologic characteristics of the parasites: whereas echinococcosis (hydatid disease) was well known to Hippocrates and Galen, intestinal capillariasis was recognized only in 1963. It is not only their histories that vary, but their sizes: tapeworms may be 30 feet long, but even more harmful parasites can be seen only with a high-power microscope.

War has always stimulated medical research. Strongyloidiasis was first recognized in 1876 in French soldiers who had been in Cochin-China (now Vietnam). New knowledge about filariasis, malaria, paragonimiasis, amebiasis, and other parasitic diseases was gained as recently as World War II and the Korean and Vietnam conflicts. In war or peace, parasites continue to plague mankind and are an enormous source of morbidity, mortality, and economic distress.

Parasites are found worldwide—they are not confined to the tropics or to the poor. They flourish where sanitation and hygiene are inadequate and may easily be acquired even by fastidious travelers. Although geography, social status, cultural practices, and education play a large part in parasitic epidemiology, outbreaks of giardiasis have occurred in sophisticated ski resorts, and gourmet diners in Japan have been infected with anisakiasis from the slices of raw fish that they favor.

The number of people infected with parasites throughout the world is almost unimaginable, but a few examples will suffice. Perhaps 25% of the world's population harbor roundworms, and in many parts of the tropics the incidence may be well over 90%.[186] In 1968 it was estimated that 10% of the world's population harbored the ameba. In 1978 the estimate was increased to 20%, although perhaps only 5% or 6% developed invasive and therefore clinical amebiasis.[189] The number of patients with schistosomiasis is difficult to assess, but in 1981 it was thought that 600 million were infected.[173] This represents approximately 90% of the population of the less developed countries, and yet it is probably an underestimate. Figures for ancylostomiasis (hookworm) suggest that 900 million people, almost one quarter of the world's population, are infected.[186] There is wide variation in its prevalence among countries, particularly in the tropics. Because parasites can be found in the most unlikely patients, whose clinical states may vary from normal health to severe illness, the recognition of the presence of the parasite in the alimentary tract is essential, even when least expected. Knowledge of where the patient lived or traveled is as important in diagnosis as laboratory tests and images. The reaction of those with chronic infection may differ considerably from the often acute reaction of a first infection. Parasites and the diseases they cause tend to be unpredictable.

Pathophysiology

Parasitism has been defined as "a physiologic association between two organisms belonging to different species, one of which (the parasite) is smaller and weaker and lives within or on the surface of the body of the larger and stronger one (the host) from which it obtains its food and on which it generally inflicts some degree of injury."[177a] Parasites often live in symbiosis for many years until some change occurs, and the host starts to suffer. Parasites are not confined to humans, and many wild animals die of their parasitic infections. The king of beasts, the lion, who survives the territorial imperative and lives to fight another day, will often die ignominiously of worms. Many animals are an essential part of the life cycle of the parasites so that eating infected animals, walking on contaminated ground, and swimming in contaminated water are the most common of the many ways in which parasites enter their hosts. The cost to the world's economy is beyond estimation. It involves not only human illness or inability to perform daily tasks satisfactorily but the loss of food when animals die of parasitic infection.

There is such variation in the pathophysiology that the only logical way to review those parasites that inhabit the alimentary tract is to describe each separately.

Nevertheless it must be remembered that in many parts of the world and in many immigrants who come to the United States or Europe, multiple parasitism will be the rule rather than the exception. Three or four different infections may lie hidden, either unnoticed or even accepted as normal by the patient. In many cases the parasite will not be the reason the patient comes to the doctor, and finding a parasite does not always mean that the cause of the patient's ill health has been discovered. There may well be another problem. The opposite is also true, particularly in the immigrant and those from poorly developed rural areas. Finding a positive cause for ill health, such as tuberculosis, should not end the search for concomitant parasites in the alimentary tract or elsewhere.[163]

Helminthic Infections—Roundworms (Nematodes)
Ascariasis (roundworms)

Ascaris lumbricoides is the most common roundworm, particularly in children; infections by *Toxocara canis* and *T. cati* and by *Ascaris suum* are rare. In 1979 it was estimated that between 800 million and 1 billion persons were infected with *Ascaris,* making it third among the 10 most common human infections.[189] Whereas infection is commonest where temperatures are warm and there is high humidity, any area with overpopulation and poor sanitation is at risk, and there are probably several million hosts to this parasite in North America. *Ascaris* infection is acquired by ingesting food, water, or soil that has been contaminated with embryonated eggs. Self-contamination, particularly by children, is common. Uncooked vegetables (particularly where night soil is used for a fertilizer) and polluted drinking water are other important sources of infection.

The *Ascaris* eggs become infective in about 3 weeks in shady, moist soil. A minimum temperature exceeding 70° F is necessary. When swallowed, the outer shell of the ova is digested by the gastric juices, and the ova hatch in the small bowel to become free tiny larvae, which then penetrate the epithelium of the intestinal mucosa. They then pass either through the portal system into the liver or via the intestinal lymphatics to the thoracic duct. By either route they can reach the lungs via the right heart, and a few days later they perforate the alveoli. After molting twice and growing in size in the lungs, they travel up the bronchi and trachea and are swallowed. They then mature as worms within the lumen of the small intestine, reaching 35 cm in about 2 months. Copulation occurs in the small intestine, and in 6 months a single female may produce millions of eggs. A new generation of ova appears in the feces at the end of the 2- to 3-month cycle.

The clinical symptoms are first seen as the larvae lodge in the lungs, and they include those of bronchitis or pneumonia, particularly in children. Pyrexia of 99° to 105° F with chills and vomiting, coughing, and even hemoptysis can occur. There is usually a high blood eosinophilia during this state (50% or more for a short period). Asthma may result, particularly in Asian Indians. In the next stage, as the worms mature in the intestinal tract, there may be few or even no symptoms. Sometimes there is nausea, vomiting or abdominal discomfort, or perhaps colicky pain. Distention and tenderness and, surprisingly, constipation may result. Some patients become hypersensitive and present with men-

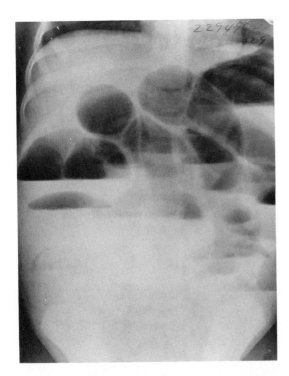

Fig. 62-50 Ascariasis can cause mechanical small bowel obstruction because of large number of worms, usually forming bolus in ileum. Sometimes worm can be recognized, but this is common cause of obstruction in childhood and should be remembered even if worms cannot be seen.
(From Reeder, MM, and Palmer, PES: The radiology of tropical diseases, Baltimore, 1981, Williams & Wilkins. Armed Forces Institute of Pathology, photographic negative No. 67-10130-1.)

ingism, idiopathic epilepsy, or febrile convulsions. Then, as the worm population grows, there may be partial or complete intestinal obstruction. Children may harbor more than 2000 worms, which can be entwined and form a large bolus; this is not an uncommon complication.[179] The most common site of obstruction is the ileocecal region, but blockage can occur anywhere in the small or large bowel; gastric outlet obstruction is also reported (Fig. 62-50). Intussusception and volvulus occur but much less commonly. In one series 13% of all acute abdominal emergencies in children were caused by ascariasis.[190]

The worms may find their way into the biliary tract, one of the commonest causes of jaundice in children, particularly in China, South Africa, and South America. When the infection is chronic, cholecystitis, cholangitis, pancreatitis, and even liver abscess may occur. Biliary ascariasis has been found in persons of all ages and most of these patients respond to conservative treatment. Reports from China, Japan, and Colombia suggest an eti-

ologic relationship in the development of gallstones.[165]

The laboratory diagnosis depends on the identification of adult worms or eggs in the stool, vomit, sputum, or small bowel aspirates, aided by very characteristic radiologic or ultrasound findings. Blood eosinophilia fluctuates and is especially high in the pulmonary phase. When the worms are in the intestine, it usually ranges from 5% to 12%. Immunodiagnostic tests are unreliable, since there is a cross-reaction with antigens from other helminths. Immunoglobulin E may be found in fecal extracts.

RADIOLOGIC DIAGNOSIS

Large collections of worms are often identifiable on a plain film of the abdomen, contrasted against the gas in the bowel and resembling a tangled group of thick cords. They can be seen on ultrasonograms. There also may be evidence of partial or complete mechanical intestinal obstruction. After the patient swallows barium, the outline of the individual worm is shown as an elongated radiolucent filling defect that is most common in the jejunum and ileum but may be anywhere in the alimentary tract from the esophagus to the rectum (Figs. 62-51 and 62-52). If the patient has not eaten for about 12 hours, the worms ingest the barium. In this case a thin white thread will be seen running the length of the worm's body, which is itself outlined by the surrounding barium in the bowel. The position and shape of the worm may indicate which way it is moving or if it is reacting favorably to an anthelmintic agent. There may be an associated disordered pattern of the small bowel mucosa, with thickening of the mucosal folds. The mass of worms can be well demonstrated by ultrasonography and, if in sufficient numbers, by computed tomography (it is hoped, as a chance finding).

Ultrasonography is the easiest way to demonstrate the worm in the biliary tract, where it may be seen either in cross section or lengthwise.[165] If ultrasound is not available, the worm can be seen on intravenous cholangiograms and can also be demonstrated by T tube or transhepatic cholangiograms. In the pancreatic duct the worm can be seen by ultrasonography or on endoscopy, which will also allow removal if anthelmintics are unsuccessful.

Rarely the worm will escape from the bowel and form a "tumor." This may lie free in the peritoneal cavity, and the differential diagnosis, even at operation, can be very difficult (see the section on helminthoma).

In the larval stage, particularly in children, the chest radiograph may show soft, patchy, ill-defined asymmetric densities that are often transient (Löffler's pneumonia). These are due to localized pulmonary reaction or even necrosis and hemorrhage and may progress to bronchopneumonia. If the adult worm is aspirated into

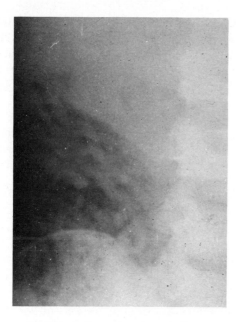

Fig. 62-51 Soft tissue film of abdomen of child shows multiple ascarides in loop of bowel.

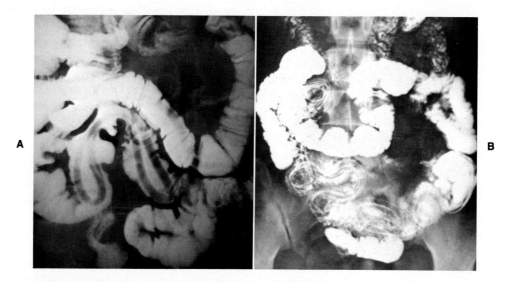

Fig. 62-52 A, *Ascaris* in mid small bowel outlined with barium. **B,** *Ascaris* in small bowel with alimentary tract of *Ascaris* demonstrated.
(Courtesy Dr. JP Balikian.)

the lung, there can be collapse of the lobe or entire lung. Eventually, where the larvae die, pulmonary granulomas and fibrosis may form and even appear as a solitary pulmonary nodule.

DIFFERENTIAL DIAGNOSIS

The appearances in the gastrointestinal and biliary tracts are so characteristic either on barium examination or by ultrasonography that they are not likely to be mis-interpreted. On the chest radiograph, the most important factor in diagnosis is to remember the possibility. The transient nature of the lung densities is very helpful, because very seldom does an ordinary bacterial infection change so rapidly in size, position, and shape. However, the pulmonary changes are very nonspecific. When the patient has a high possibility of *Ascaris* infection and eosinophilia is demonstrated, examination of the stools and treatment for worms may produce a remarkable cure in the patient with suspected bronchopneumonia or pulmonary tuberculosis.

Ancylostomiasis (hookworm disease)

Ancylostomiasis is infection with one or more species of the ancylostomidae. Most common are *Ancylostoma duodenale* and *Necator americanus,* which may occur together. Geographically *Ancylostoma* extends through the Mediterranean, the Middle East, Eastern Europe, Pakistan, and North India. *Necator* extends through Central and South America, the West Indies, sub-Saharan Africa, India, and Sri Lanka. Mixed infections are found in Asia, particularly in Burma, Malaysia, Vietnam, Laos, Cambodia, Taiwan, China, and Japan. In the United States *Necator* occurs in the south and in Puerto Rico. Thus *N. americanus* is predominant in the tropics and *A. duodenale* in the temperate climates. Intensive efforts have reduced the incidence during the last 50 years, particularly in North America, but infection is still extremely common in the tropics, exceeding 90% in some parts of Latin America, Asia, and Africa.[186,189] Agriculture is important in the spread of hookworm, particularly in areas such as coffee and cocoa plantations where there is high humidity in the shade and a very fertile soil. The use of human night soil for fertilization maintains the disease in many parts of the Orient; indeed man may be the primary factor in the epidemiology. It is common in workers in mines and tunnels and wherever people walk unshod. Hookworms are also found in other primates and animals varying from the rhinoceros to rodents. Those ancylostomes *(A. braziliense, A. caninum,* and *A. malayanum)* that occur in animals only occasionally invade man, in whom they seldom undergo full development but can cause a localized skin eruption.

The small hookworms, measured in millimeters, firmly attach themselves to the intestinal mucosa in man, sucking blood, tissue, and intestinal juices to obtain nourishment; within the intestine they may live for 6 or more years and produce 50 million eggs per female during that time. The eggs develop as they travel in the intestine, and if deposited in warm, moist soil, the embryos become visible within 24 hours, double their size within the next 48 hours, and become infective within another week. They are active and can swim, wriggle, or climb a moist surface, being capable of going through as much as 1 m (3 feet) of light soil. They remain viable for up to 6 weeks.

The larvae usually enter man through the skin of the foot or ankle and occasionally through the mouth. The normal site of penetration is through a hair follicle. They then move into the lymphatic or blood circulation. From the lung capillaries and alveoli they migrate up the bronchi and are swallowed, to mature again in the small intestine, usually the jejunum. Other more complex methods of infection are uncommon but can occur.

Whereas there may be intraalveolar and interstitial hemorrhage in the lungs, most of the pathologic changes occur in the second and third portions of the jejunum, where there are minor mucosal changes that can disappear with therapy. On intestinal biopsy there is a marked eosinophilia with other findings resembling sprue. Laboratory diagnosis is made by recognizing the eggs in a fresh sample of feces, but at least 20 eggs are needed to suggest a clinical rather than a subclinical infection, and differentiation from *Strongyloides* may be difficult. A skin test antigen is available for screening populations. Anemia can result, because there may be a loss of 100 ml of blood per day if there is a heavy infestation. The anemia is usually hypochromic and microcytic, but there may be a hypoplastic bone marrow. Peripheral eosinophilia is often found.

Clinically it is important to differentiate between hookworm carriers and hookworm disease; in the former there are no symptoms, whereas hookworm disease is recognized by anemia and symptoms that result from malnutrition and concomitant illness. There are two clinical phases. In the first, during migration and development of the larvae, there can be pruritus and vesiculation where the larvae have penetrated the skin. These sites may become infected. Pulmonary symptoms develop within 2 weeks, and are often mild and transient. The chest x-ray results will be normal. At this stage there will be a marked peripheral eosinophilia. When *A. duodenale* reaches the small bowel, there can be severe diarrhea with foul stools. Thereafter the patient often has no symptoms for prolonged periods, although dyspepsia, nausea, and pain may occur. As the anemia worsens, the general symptoms of tiredness, weakness, and palpitations develop. Hemoglobin levels of 1 gm/100 ml have been reported and eosinophilia has been 90% to 100%. Concomitant cardiac disease and nephritis can occur.

On a chest radiograph the most common finding is mild cardiac enlargement because of the anemia and hypoproteinemia. In most patients the results of barium examinations are normal. In others there may be some abnormality of the small intestine pattern, resembling a deficiency pattern with coarsening and irregularity of the mucosa. The changes are usually proportional to the severity of the infection, and the ileum is usually normal unless infection is severe. Radiologically attention should be focused on the jejunum, where there is likely to be thickening of the mucosal folds and distortion of the loops, with either dilatation or contraction. The differential diagnosis includes other parasitic infections, particularly giardiasis and strongyloidiasis, and any other cause of the malabsorption pattern. The differentiation between hookworm disease and steatorrhea of another cause may be very difficult. There seems to be some geographic variation in the incidence of steatorrhea-like findings.

Hookworms have rarely been found in bone and soft tissues, especially in fibrosarcomas.[182]

Strongyloidiasis

Immunosuppression is of particular importance when considering *Strongyloides* parasites. Although some patients may have no symptoms, the immunosuppressed patient may develop very severe disease. Until recently strongyloidiasis was considered to be a disease of the small bowel, but in severe cases very acute ulcerating colitis can occur.[166]

Strongyloides stercoralis occurs worldwide, but it is most common in the tropics. No age-group is exempt, although it is more common in adults. Man is the major host, but dogs and chimpanzees have been infected. The female parasite, usually residing in the duodenum or upper jejunum, can reproduce without a male parasite and may deposit 30 to 50 eggs per day for several months. When discharged in the feces, the larvae feed on the soil and require 4 months to develop. In tropical countries multiplication can occur on the ground, which becomes heavily contaminated. Where conditions are unfavorable, filariform larvae develop, and these remain mobile and can infect man, penetrating the skin on contact. However, in this form larvae die within a few days unless in contact with a host. Penetration in man is usually through the sole of the foot or hands and causes mild local reaction. The larvae travel through blood vessels and lymphatics to the heart, then into the lungs, entering the alveolar sacs, where they molt and become worms. There may at this stage be a bleeding, inflammatory response in the lungs and some eosinophilia. If there is a very heavy infestation, pulmonary hemorrhage, eosinophilic nodules, and bronchopneumonia with damage to the pulmonary tissue can result.

Further migration through the bronchial tree and down the esophagus allows the worms to reach the duodenum and jejunum, where they burrow into the mucosa to establish themselves. Invasion can occur in any other part of the gastrointestinal tract, from the stomach to the anus, but usually the female parasites mature in the crypts of the small intestine and invade only the superficial layers of the mucosa without penetrating the muscularis. Some filariform larvae penetrate the mesenteric venules and start the cycle again by endoautoinfection. Autoinfection can also occur through the anal and perianal skin so that the cycle of infection can persist for 10 years or more, even when there is a change of environment and no external reinfection.

In the bowel there may be only a catarrhal enteritis,

with increased mucosal congestion and mucous secretion, but this may progress to an edematous phase, with thickening of the intestinal wall, swelling of the folds, and then flattening and atrophy of the mucosa. At this stage the appearance may resemble sprue, and by then parasites will be in all layers of the intestinal wall. The most severe stage is that of ulcerative enteritis, with thickening of the intestinal wall by edema and fibrosis, producing a rigid tubelike intestine. The mucosa will then be atrophied and ulcerated, with granulomas in the mucosa and submucosa and marked eosinophilic infiltration. Ulcers of up to 7 mm in diameter may be seen in the large bowel, and when the patient is immunosuppressed, clinically there may be severe paralytic ileus.

These three varieties of pathologic response cause a wide variation in gastrointestinal symptoms and radiologic findings. In the first two phases reversal can be complete, but in the ulcerative stage there will be residual fibrosis. The hyperinfective stage, with involvement of the colon, occurs almost always in patients who are immunosuppressed for natural or therapeutic reasons.[166] Histologically it can be difficult to identify the *Strongyloides* or ova in the mucosa of the colon, but larvae may be seen throughout the intestinal wall and lymphatics and in mesenteric lymph nodes in severe cases. Jaundice has resulted when the biliary tract has been invaded but is more commonly due to obstruction resulting from edema and spasm of the ampulla of Vater. The damage to the gut can be so severe that septicemia from *E. coli* or other organisms occurs, with metastatic abscesses in almost any part of the body.

Laboratory diagnosis is by identification of the larvae or the adult worm in fresh stools or sometimes by stool culture. Multiple stool specimens may have to be examined, and it is not usual to find ova. The larvae can also be found by duodenal aspiration, probably a more accurate method than stool examination; duodenal or jejunal biopsy will often confirm the diagnosis. There is a complement fixation test that is nonspecific and of little help in diagnosis. There is usually a significant eosinophilia, but if this starts to fall during an infection, it may indicate a suppressed immune reaction and a poor prognosis.

Clinically patients may complain of irritation at the site of penetration or around the anus during autoinfection, and if the larvae move under the skin, there can be a severe pruritus. Pulmonary symptoms vary from an innocuous cough and mild hemoptysis to frank pneumonia and asthma; bronchopneumonia can be present, as in other parasitic infections. However, the changes in the chest are usually less than might be expected. Abdominal symptoms depend on the intensity of the infection; some patients may have no complaints, and others may have gastritis or mild crampy abdominal pain. Food

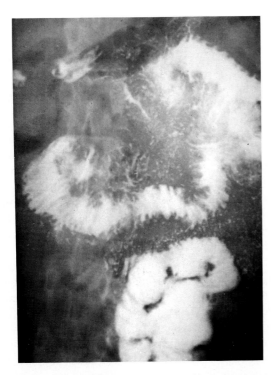

Fig. 62-53 Malabsorption pattern in upper jejunum in strongyloidiasis.
(Courtesy Prof. P. Cockshott.)

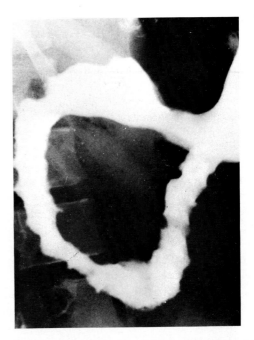

Fig. 62-54 Duodenal loop in gross case of strongyloidiasis shows pipe-stem rigidity.
(Courtesy Dr. J. Barton.)

tends to exacerbate the problem. Later the pain becomes more diffuse and the abdomen more distended. Diarrhea, often watery and with mucus, can develop. As the infection becomes more chronic, there are weight loss, anorexia, and a clinical presentation that may resemble peptic ulceration, other parasitic infections, or sprue. When the host is immunosuppressed, overwhelming rapid malnutrition and death, with gross abdominal distention, may occur.

The correct diagnosis may be suspected radiologically in patients who are referred with a clinical diagnosis of peptic ulceration or other gastrointestinal disease, because barium studies show prominent mucosal folds with an irritable, tender duodenum. There may be excess mucous secretion, with rapid peristalsis and irritability, and such rapid transit that the proximal small intestine may be difficult to evaluate. The ileum may be widened and show a coarse mucosal pattern. At this stage the findings are reversible and will return to normal. In the more severe cases the inflammatory process is much more widely spread in the duodenum and jejunum, with a malabsorption (Fig. 62-53) or spruelike pattern, delayed gastric emptying, hypomotility with slow transit times, and an increase in the diameter of the small intestine. Return to normal is still possible at this stage. However, in the third and most severe stage of infection, plain films

of the abdomen will show multiple dilated small bowel loops, suggesting paralytic ileus or even partial obstruction. If this mistake is made, a laparotomy may have an unfortunate result, since surgery should be avoided. There will be marked hypotonia and rigidity of multiple segments of the small bowel as a result of the severe inflammatory and fibrotic response to the larvae. The stomach may be small, with mucosal atrophy. Peristalsis in the duodenum and proximal jejunum may be absent; appearance lower in the bowel may suggest regional ileitis, with alternating segments of constriction and dilatation. There is complete loss of the mucosa, where a narrow pipe-stem segment will eventually develop (Fig. 62-54), with thickening of the bowel wall and mesenteric lymphadenopathy. Where there is immunosuppression, severe *Strongyloides* colitis has developed and resulted in hemorrhage, sepsis, and death. Barium examination in these cases shows an extensive ulcerating colitis, with both small and large ulcers and sinus formation, especially in the left colon. From the cecum to the rectum the bowel may be nodular, with almost complete loss of haustration. This is a very severe state, irreversible and often fatal.[166]

The differential diagnosis includes other parasitic infections, especially giardiasis, but as the disease progresses, malabsorption and regional ileitis will have to be considered. In the severe cases ulcerative colitis (from any cause) may be suspected. In most cases the difficulty is to exclude small bowel obstruction and to avoid surgery during the course of the severe infection. In the chest the pattern may be indistinguishable from Löffler's syndrome, presenting with patchy areas of pneumonia as is the case in other parasitic diseases. When the patient is immunosuppressed, there will be pulmonary edema, hemorrhage, and generalized infection.

Oesophagostomum (helminthoma)

There are three strongyli in this group of nematode worms: *O. apiostomum*, *O. stephanostomum*, and the rare *O. brumpti*. All are parasitic in many different primates, including man, throughout Africa, India, the Philippines, and China. *O. apiostomum* affects man most frequently (Fig. 62-55). These nematodes can be about 2 cm long, and one report stated that they were found in 4% of prisoners in the jails of northern Nigeria some years ago.[177] However, primates are not the only animals infected, since these parasites are common in sheep, goats, pigs, and cattle and cause severe illness in all of them. The ova are very difficult to distinguish from those of the hookworm.

Eggs are passed in feces, and the larvae hatch in the soil until ingested by new hosts feeding on grass. Man becomes accidentally infected. When the larvae reach the lower small bowel, they penetrate the wall and molt. In 5 days they return to the lumen and move down into the cecum and colon, molt again, and become adults. They penetrate the intestinal mucosa once more and provoke an extensive inflammatory reaction that causes a sterile abscess, which contains the live worm. This is called a helminthoma. Although in theory a helminthoma could be caused by any type of worm that penetrates the bowel, such granulomatous tumors are uncommon in hookworm infections and rare in ascariasis, since these worms do not provoke the same marked granulomatous reaction.

These inflammatory granulomas and sterile abscesses enlarge and extend into the mesocolon but usually do not obstruct the bowel. The worm may calcify within the mass and occasionally be visible on the plain film. Because there are adhesions of the small bowel and omentum, there can be a large palpable tender mass that may later resolve and be almost completely absorbed. Alternatively the abscess may perforate into the bowel or into the peritoneal cavity. Adhesions to the abdominal wall may occur, and the whole process may become chronic.

At any stage, helminthoma is a major diagnostic problem, most likely to be mistaken, even at surgery, for an amebic or appendiceal abscess. The nodular tumors can occur anywhere in the bowel, particularly in the large bowel where they may resemble a carcinoma or a perforated diverticulum. The exact diagnosis may be missed at surgery, because the worm may not be recognized in the midst of the severe and sometimes large inflammatory reaction.[154] Histologically there is nearly always a zone of eosinophilic necrosis and, around the track of the worm, a zone of lymphocytes, plasma cells, and fibroblasts with collagen.

It is not surprising that the clinical history is vague, very nonspecific, and often of only a few days' duration. In children intussusception may be suspected. Only in

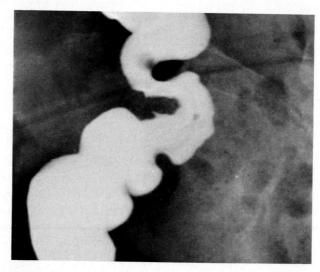

Fig. 62-55 Crypt in narrow segment of colon in patient infected with *Oesophagostomum apiostomum*.
(Courtesy Dr. M. Welchman.)

countries where there is a high incidence of infection is the true nature likely to be suspected clinically.

The essential radiologic finding is a mass of variable size in the wall of the bowel. It seldom encircles the bowel completely but may cause eccentric narrowing, which is often mistaken for extrinsic pressure. It is most common in the cecum and ascending colon but can be found elsewhere in the colon or occasionally in the small bowel. There may very rarely be multiple helminthomas. Usually a contrast enema will show intact mucosa stretched over the underlying intramural mass. Sometimes a small perforation may be demonstrated, but usually there is too much edema. The picture is that of distortion, without true invasion of the bowel. As the mass increases in size, that part of the bowel will become fixed.[188]

It is helpful to remember when considereing the differential diagnosis of helminthoma that malignant disease of the bowel is very rare in many parts of the world, as is diverticulitis. Amebiasis, which is common in such countries, will present the principal problem in differential diagnosis. A high index of suspicion is the examiner's most important single asset.

Anisakiasis

The full name of this parasite, *Anisakis marina*, indicates its habitat. The adult stage is found in whales and dolphins, whereas the larvae are found in many species of fish, including herring, mackerel, cod, salmon, and squid. Man becomes infected by eating raw fish, because the larvae, which are normally in the peritoneum of the fish, may migrate into the muscles.[176]

In man the larvae burrow into the gastric mucosa and cause ulceration, but they have also been found in the small bowel, colon, and rectum. Perforation into the human peritoneum is possible, with resulting irritation, fluid, and associated lymphadenopathy. Histologically there is a marked eosinophilic reaction in the tissue around the site of perforation, suggesting that the ulcer is a local, presensitized reaction to the parasite. The reaction is far more than would be expected if it were due merely to the burrowing of the parasite. There is some geographic variation in the site of the lesion. Patients from Holland who had eaten lightly salted herring had ulcers mainly in the ileum. In 92 Japanese patients the stomach was mainly involved, and the ileum was involved in only 30%. Another Japanese series reported 12 small bowel infections.[191]

A history of eating raw fish is very significant, and symptoms may occur in 24 hours. These usually resemble subacute peptic ulceration, but when the small bowel is infected, the complaints suggest gastroenteritis or even appendicitis. In some patients there may be severe pain and evidence of ileus. Laboratory examinations are dif-

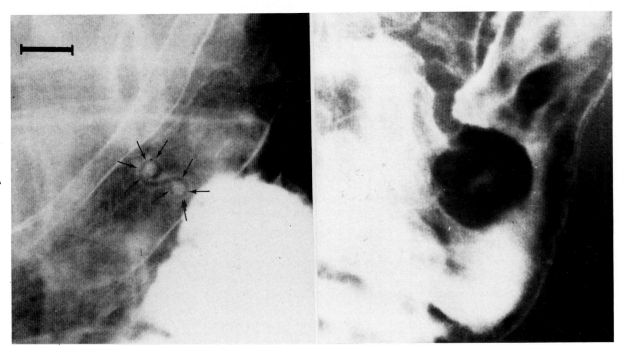

A

B

Fig. 62-56 A, *Anisakis* worm outlined in double contrast barium meal in stomach of adult patient. **B,** Well-defined antral phlegmon causes intramural inflammatory mass.
(Courtesy Dr. Masayoshi Namiki.)

ficult; stool examination usually produces negative results. Specific antibodies for the larvae can be detected within 1 to 60 days after they are ingested. Radiologically a careful double contrast barium study of the stomach may show a submucosal mass, and the worm may be seen (Fig. 62-56). It can also be seen on endoscopy and can be removed in some cases. In the small bowel the appearance simulates Crohn's disease.[183] There is irregular thickening of the jejunum, ileum, or colon, with mucosal edema, luminal narrowing, and dilatation of the proximal intestine. In some cases threadlike filling defects suggesting tiny worms can be seen on the barium study. The plain radiographs may show evidence of ileus. Surgery is seldom indicated.

Trichuriasis (whipworm infection)

Millions of people in the tropics, in endemic areas up to 90% of the population, are affected with *Trichuris trichiura*, often in association with *Ascaris*. Yet radiologic demonstration is extremely rare. One female organism may produce up to 10,000 ova daily; these can develop in warm soil in 2 to 4 weeks or remain latent for 5 or more years. Man is infected by ingesting contaminated soil, food, or water. Small children are infected more often than adults. Within the bowel the ovum is softened by intestinal juices, and the larva escapes and gains nourishment from the small bowel. It migrates to the cecum, or sometimes lower in the large bowel, and takes 2 or 3 months to develop to full adult form. In severe *Trichuris* infections the entire colon, including the rectum and appendix, may be infected, but the organism is uncommon in the ileum and may be totally unsuspected clinically. If there is no reinfection, the cycle will be complete within 3 years.

The worms attach themselves to the bowel with very little inflammatory reaction, but sometimes cause excessive mucous secretion. Only in severe infections will there be bleeding, ulceration, and inflammatory reaction, which seldom extend beyond the muscularis mucosa. The laboratory diagnosis depends on the identification of the worms during sigmoidoscopy or on stool concentration studies. An eosinophilia is common, with a heavy whipworm infection, and there may be an iron-deficiency anemia. Heavily infected children may have severe chronic diarrhea lasting for years, with resulting ill health; however, even in patients with diarrhea, trichuriasis may be a coincidental finding.

Radiologic examination is not necessary to make the diagnosis but may provide a chance finding with barium enema when, particularly in double contrast studies, the wavy outlines of the numerous small "whips" may be seen, often amid considerable mucus (Fig. 62-57). A tightly coiled target pattern identifies the male *Trichuris*, whereas the uncurled whip indicates the female worm.[169]

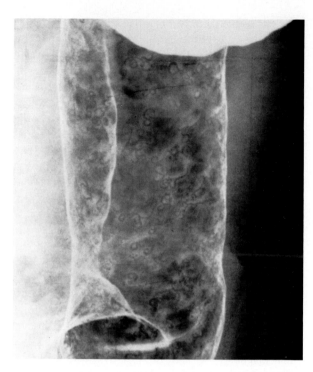

Fig. 62-57 Double contrast enema shows *Trichuris trichiura* worms outlined in descending colon.
(Courtesy Prof. BJ Cremin.)

Dracunculus Medinensis (guinea worm infestation)

This deserves only brief mention, since it is not an alimentary tract disease even though infection occurs through oral ingestion of the larvae. The adult dead worm frequently calcifies with a typical long linear serpiginous or whirl appearance that may be found anywhere in the soft tissues and thus be seen superimposed on films of the abdomen or the pelvis. Such calcified worms are much more common in the limbs (Fig. 62-58).[182]

Cestodes
Tapeworms

Tapeworms are among man's oldest companions and may grow to 30 feet in length. Their existence has been known for millennia. The two commonest are *Taenia saginata* and *T. solium*. Although many other tapeworms infect man, most do not have any radiologic significance; among these, heavy infestation of the fish tapeworm, *Diphyllobothrium latum* (found in freshwater fish and crustaceans), may cause mechanical intestinal obstruction and a background eosinophilia and anemia. None of the others has gastrointestinal significance.

The beef tapeworm, *T. saginata* (Figs. 62-59 and 62-60) occurs throughout the world, sometimes in a high proportion of the population (as in Ethiopia). The pork

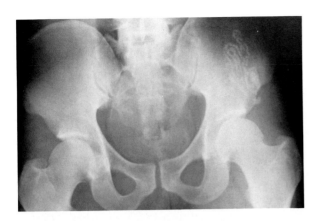

Fig. 62-58 Calcified (dead) adult female *Dracunculus* in soft tissues overlying left ileum—chance finding in patient being examined for injury. Faint calcification, caused by schistosomiasis, can be seen in bladder, another unexpected finding.
(From Reeder, MM, and Palmer, PES: The radiology of tropical diseases, Baltimore, 1981, Williams & Wilkins.)

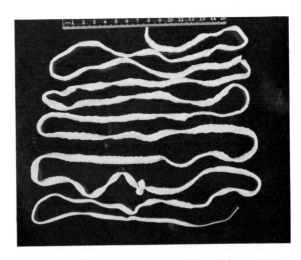

Fig. 62-60 Adult *Taenia saginata*. Head is at bottom of picture, and worm gradually widens into hundreds of individual proglottid segments. Worms 20 to 30 feet in length have been recorded.
(From Reeder, MM, and Palmer, PES: The radiology of tropical diseases, Baltimore, 1981, Williams & Wilkins.)

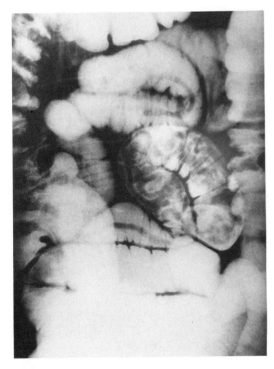

Fig. 62-59 Negative shadow of adult *Taenia saginata* in ileum of 25-year-old Lebanese complaining of acute abdominal pain. When worm was passed after treatment, it was 210 cm in length.
(Courtesy Dr. Lawrence E. Fetterman.) (From Reeder, MM, and Palmer, PES: The radiology of tropical diseases, Baltimore, 1981, Williams & Wilkins.)

tapeworm, *T. solium*, although widespread, is much less common. Mixed infections may occur. The life cycles of the worms are similar, but the intermediate host of *T. saginata* is cattle and of *T. solium* is pigs. The adult worm lives in the alimentary tract of humans, attached by its scolex to the mucosa, usually in the mid small bowel. The worms have no alimentary tract, and they absorb nutrition from the content of the intestine through their surfaces. The eggs pass in the feces and are ingested by grazing cattle or pigs, where they hatch in the intestine of the intermediate host. Burrowing through the intestinal wall to reach a blood vessel or lymph channel, they enter striated muscles. There the larva develops into *Cysticercus bovis* in cattle and *C. cellulosae* in the pig. If the meat is eaten insufficiently cooked or raw, the life cycle in man starts again. Cysticerci can also be found in cats, rats, monkeys, dogs, giraffes, buffaloes, llamas, and some antelope.

The laboratory diagnosis depends on the recognition of the ova or proglottids in the stools. Eosinophilia is common. Clinically many patients show no significant illness. Others may complain of abdominal discomfort, loss of weight and appetite, indigestion, or diarrhea. Multiple worms may occasionally cause obstruction, and pruritus ani is not uncommon.

The adult *T. saginata* is very seldom demonstrated radiologically, because it does not ingest contrast material. When seen, there is a long and gradually widening radiolucent line within the barium pattern, usually in the jejunum or ileum. At its neck it may be 1 to 2 mm wide, but distally it may be 12 mm or more.[171] It is often folded and reduplicated but is always continuous and may reach 20 or more feet in length.

The eggs of *T. solium,* the pork tapeworm, may accidentally be ingested by humans, who when unwittingly become the intermediate host for the disease cysticercosis. The *C. cellulosae* cyst is an irritant to the host; it becomes encapsulated and surrounded by fibrous tissue and may eventually calcify, a process that can take 5 years. Whether it affects the host depends on the number and the location of the cysts. They are very common in muscle and usually produce no symptoms, but cysts in the brain may cause epilepsy, and those in the spinal canal may cause obstruction to the flow of cerebrospinal fluid. There are no gastrointestinal symptoms, but the typical calcified linear or oval cyst, 4 to 10 mm in length, may be found superimposed on the abdomen, particularly when there is heavy infestation of the muscles of the back, flanks, or abdominal wall.[182]

Armillifer *(tongue worm)* infestation—Pentastomides

Two tongue worms infect man, gaining entry through the alimentary tract but causing no gastrointestinal symptoms. When dead, they often become calcified within the peritoneum, liver, or spleen and should be easily recognized and differentiated from calculi or calcified lymph nodes.

Armillifer armillatus and *A. moniliformis* cause porocephaliasis or pentastomiasis in man. These parasites live in the trachea and bronchi of snakes, particularly pythons, adders, and cobras. *A. armillatus* is most common in West Africa and much less common elsewhere on that continent. *A. moniliformis* occurs in the python and other snakes of India, Malaysia and Southeast Asia, China, Indonesia, and the Philippines. The eggs may be ingested with contaminated water or by eating snakes. The larvae are freed in the intestine and lie under the peritoneum, molting to become nymphs. They may migrate across the diaphragm to the pleural cavity. They can be found within the liver or spleen, but their route is not understood.

The presence of *Armillifer* may have some diagnostic significance if there is a heavy infestation, because the larvae may cause such acute peritoneal irritation that an abdominal emergency such as appendicitis or perforated viscus may be suspected. These organisms have been seen at laparotomy moving beneath the peritoneum. The radiologic findings of curved calcified nymphs scattered throughout the peritoneum, pleura, liver, and spleen are characteristic (Fig. 62-61).[155,161] They are not found in muscle and should be easily distinguished from cysticercosis (which is predominantly in peripheral muscles).

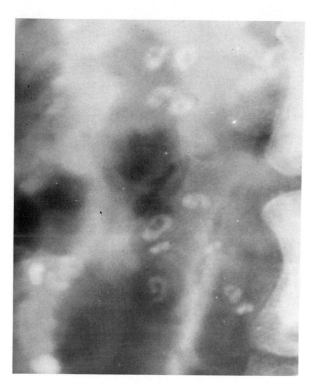

Fig. 62-61 Calcified *Armillifer armillatus* in peritoneum.

Liver flukes (trematodes)—Clonorchiasis, fascioliasis, and opisthorchiasis

Of the flukes that infect the biliary tract, three are most important. The Oriental liver fluke, *Clonorchis sinensis,* occurs throughout East Asia, Japan, Korea, coastal China, Taiwan, and Southeast Asia. The liver fluke *Fasciola hepatica* is found in Europe, the U.S.S.R., the Middle East, Asia, Africa, Australia, and Central and South America. *Opisthorchis felineus* occurs in man in central, eastern, and southern Europe, with isolated cases in India, Vietnam, North Korea, Japan, and the Philippines. *O. viverrini* is important in northeast Thailand and in Laos, where it is surprisingly common.

Clonorchis

This parasite inhabits the bile ducts of man, mammals, and birds. It is about 10 to 20 mm long, flat, and somewhat pointed. Eggs are laid in the small biliary ducts and pass through the common bile duct into the duodenum and then the colon. Excreted in the feces, hatching occurs when the eggs are ingested by a snail of the family Bulimidae. Further development of the miracidia within the snail takes 4 or 5 weeks. The resulting freeswimming cercariae penetrate the muscles of freshwater fish, particularly carp, and after several weeks of further development are once again infective when the fish is eaten raw or poorly cooked. The larvae move up to the biliary tree using their suckers and mature into adult flukes. Secondary bacterial infection is common, but the clinical significance of clonorchiasis depends entirely on the extent of the infection. The flukes can persist for up to 20 years, and more than 21,000 have been found in some patients. It is not surprising that the pancreatic duct also becomes infected and that the flukes may be found in the stomach and duodenum or gallbladder.

So much irritation within the biliary tract leads to the development of calculi, acute suppurative cholangitis, recurrent pyogenic cholangitis, and acute pancreatitis and is probably significant in the causation of carcinoma of the liver. Biliary stasis and incomplete obstruction occur, and infection iwth *E. coli* or salmonellae is not uncommon. Multiple abscesses that start in the biliary system may progress and cause a severe febrile illness with jaundice. Secondary infection with *Ascaris* is not uncommon.

Clonorchiasis should be considered in any patient with liver disease, particularly from the endemic areas of the Far East. The laboratory diagnosis is by detection of the eggs in feces or in bile or fluid after incubation. There is often an associated leukocytosis (over 30,000) and up to 40% eosinophilia. Surprisingly the majority of infections are at first asymptomatic. Patients may then develop fever, indigestion, and pain in the right upper quadrant. This may progress to diarrhea, anorexia, and liver tenderness and enlargement. In the more advanced cases the liver becomes cirrhotic, and there may be ascites and marked jaundice. The cause of death is usually severe repeated infection or cholangiocarcinoma.

The flukes can be demonstrated by operative or transhepatic cholangiography and occasionally by intravenous cholangiography, showing as 1 to 2 cm curved or crescentic filling defects within dilated bile ducts.[182] Far more easily recognized are the characteristics of severe cholangitis with biliary stasis, sludge, and stones accompanied by dilatation and constriction of the bile ducts. Hepatic abscesses may be demonstrated by ultrasonography, computed tomography, and magnetic resonance imaging.[162] There are no characteristic findings for the abscess except the associated cholangitis. In the chest nonspecific pulmonary alveolar densities have been described but have no diagnostic characteristics.

Another liver fluke, *Fasciola*, although it is common and causes clinical symptoms, has not been recognized reliably on radiologic examination. However, the changes in the liver imaged with computed tomography have been described as characteristic. There are nodular intrahepatic lesions of diminished attenuation, ranging in size from 4 to 10 mm but sometimes as large as 2 cm. In addition, branching lesions have been seen. Contrast CT examination provides better definition of the nodules. After treatment there can be partial disappearance of the lesions, or in some cases they disappear completely; however, spontaneous decrease in the size of one low-density area on a scan has also been reported as occurring before treatment, in spite of the patient's continuing symptoms. CT scanning is therefore useful not only for diagnosis but for follow-up of patients with fascioliasis. There is no proven relationship between fascioliasis and carcinoma of the liver.

Opisthorchiasis

These liver flukes are usually found in cats or fish-eating animals. *O. felineus* is the most common, but infection with *O. viverrini* is more readily recognized radiologically—especially in Southeast Asia, where it is so prevalent. Similar infections have been recorded in New Guinea and Ecuador. Man is the accidental host, probably by way of eating infected pigs or fish. The life cycle is the same as that of *C. sinensis* and lasts about 4 months. The irritation in the biliary tract is more severe, with hypertrophy and thickening of the mucosa and duct walls and marked dilatation of the bile ducts up to 5 to 6 mm. There may be numerous parasites (8000 flukes), and these can cause mechanical obstruction and biliary stasis. Large cysts may develop, up to 7 cm or more in diameter, depending very much on the severity of the infection. Ascending cholangitis may often develop, spreading to cause hepatitis or multiple abscesses. Rupture of such an abscess has been described. There is little doubt that opisthorchiasis predisposes to the development of cholangiocarcinoma, but somewhat surprisingly there is no further evidence that there is an increased incidence of cirrhosis of the liver. Chronic cholecystitis has occurred, but opisthorchiasis does not predispose to biliary calculi. Jaundice is common and is especially likely where there is hepatic malignancy.

Cholangiography and ultrasonography, or CT scanning may show multiple small dilatations of the intrahepatic bile ducts, with diffuse saccular changes as the condition progresses. Eventually there will be marked cystic dilatation, and this combination of large areas of cystic dilatation with multiple small cysts is pathognomonic.[168] Where there is cholangiocarcinoma there is likely to be massive hepatomegaly, and such tumors are frequently multiple. Although cholangiography can sometimes demonstrate long slender filling defects in the bile ducts, the differential diagnosis of the actual parasite can be made only when the flukes have been recovered and examined.

Vascular flukes—Schistosomiasis

Four species of *Schistosoma* cause significant infection in man: *S. haematobium, S. mansoni,* and *S. japonicum* are the most common; *S. intercalatum* is less frequently found. Other schistosomes are parasitic for cattle or birds and occasionally have been found in man, but they seldom cause significant symptoms and have not been described radiologically.

Bilharziasis, one of the synonyms for schistosomiasis, has been known for 5000 years and infects about 200 million persons worldwide. Strict hygiene would eliminate the infection within a generation. *S. haematobium* is common throughout Africa, the Mediterranean, and Southwest Asia. *S. mansoni* (Fig. 62-62) is found more commonly in North Africa, Arabia, the West Indies, and the northern parts of South America. *S. japonicum* occurs in China, Japan, Taiwan, the Philippines, and the Celebes. Concomitant infection with *S. haematobium* and *S. mansoni* is not uncommon, particularly in North Africa. *S. intercalatum* is found only in central and equatorial

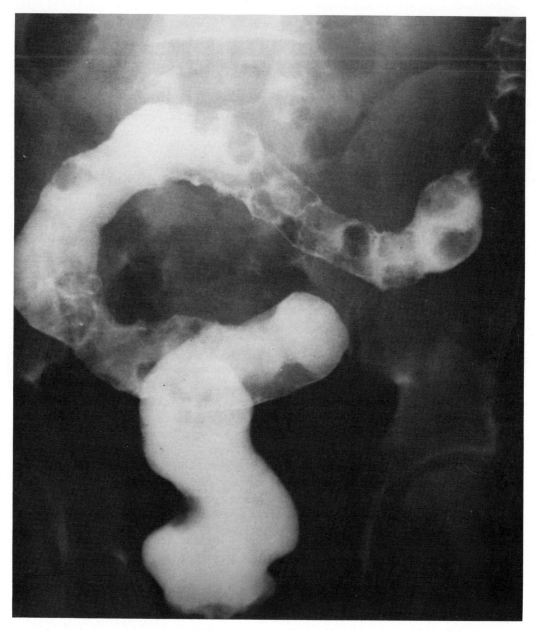

Fig. 62-62 Multiple small filling defects in rectum and sigmoid colon in patient infected with *Schistosoma mansoni.*

Africa. Because there are many different reactions to the different species, parasitologists have been tempted to divide them into separate subcategories, but this is of no importance to radiologists. Infection with schistosomes is so common in many parts of the world that it is part of normal existence, reinfection is usual, and local people disregard many of the symptoms.

The pattern of development is similar in all varieties. The flukes live in pairs and copulate in the portal vein or in its mesenteric tributaries (or the vesical plexus for *S. haematobium*). They are strictly intravenous parasites. Females leave the male after a period of 1 to 20 years and swim upstream to reach the smallest venule possible, where the eggs are deposited. This will be in the wall of the bladder or ureter for *S. haematobium*, the rectum or large intestine for *S. mansoni*, and the small intestine, proximal colon, or rectum for *S. japonicum* and *S. intercalatum*. The division is not absolute: Infection of the intestines with *S. haematobium* can occur. The cycle then depends on the eggs reaching water and the finding of suitable snail hosts, with the subsequent development of cercariae, which penetrate the unbroken skin or buccal mucous membrane to reenter the host. Then, carried through the lymphatics and veins, the larvae eventually reach the portal system and liver, where they mature. The flukes may live for 10 to 15 years and, with variation for each species, may produce an enormous number of eggs. It is the eggs or cercariae that cause most of the clinical problems: Seldom do liver flukes cause any symptoms or radiologic findings unless they embolize during treatment and cause an inflammatory reaction when dead. The clinical disease is much more commonly due to the eggs or miracidia. The characteristic histologic lesion is a severe granuloma with the formation of a nodular scar within which there is usually a calcified egg. There are many factors in the host tissue reaction, but all lead to significant fibrosis, and if this occurs in a vessel, particularly in the lungs, there can be damage to the intima and the wall. Because recanulization of the granuloma can occur, small arteriovenous fistulas or even an aneurysm may develop.

S. mansoni and *S. japonicum* mainly affect the alimentary tract. The discharge of hundreds of eggs through the intestinal mucosa causes a marked fibrotic reaction. If the eggs cannot escape, there is more inflammation around them; this causes the death of the eggs and yet further granuloma formation. This may progress to polyps, strictures, or ulceration. Unfortunately not all the eggs are trapped in the mesenteric venules of the colon or small bowel (or urinary tract). Many are forced back into the portal venous system, penetrate the walls of the small portal veins, and lodge in the periportal connective tissue. There is then the same marked inflammatory re-

action that leads to multiple granulomas of the liver and fibrous tissue formation, followed by obstruction of the small portal veins, before the eggs enter the hepatic sinusoids and cause a presinusoidal block. Portal hypertension therefore occurs long before there is any change in liver function. The vascular changes represent a combination of granulomas, sclerosis, narrowing, and thrombophlebitis, with the development of new capillary networks that form intrahepatic shunts. There may also be extensive portal systemic collaterals outside the liver, with increased pressure in the hepatic artery. Late in the disease fibrosis becomes more generalized, and the liver decreases in size.

The earliest radiographic findings in the colon consist of an edematous mucosa, with mural spicules and tiny ulcers. There is often marked spasm and then loss of haustration, particularly in the descending and sigmoid colon. If there is heavy and chronic infection, multiple polyps may develop, particularly in the rectum and sigmoid and descending colon. They start as submucosal granulomas, lifting the overlying mucosa, and are very friable and liable to bleed. They may become quite large and even cause obstruction or intussusception.[178] The extent of polyp formation varies significantly in different countries, being fairly common in Egypt and Arabia, particularly where there are combined *S. mansoni* and *S. haematobium* infections. Polyps are much less common in the Americas, where stenosing granulomas with pericolic infiltration and strictures are more likely to be found. A pericolic schistosomal abscess (a schistosoma or bilharzioma) may occur in the bowel wall or the mesentery and may simulate carcinoma.[185]

S. japonicum causes similar changes in the small bowel. The flukes live in the superior mesenteric veins and deposit their ova within the small bowel. The changes are very widespread and result from submucosal granulomas (which can be demonstrated by biopsy) and enlarged lymph nodes. As elsewhere, the end result is fibrosis and constriction, and because this affects the mesentery the duodenal loop may be deformed, not only by intrinsic granulomas but also by the adhesions. In the early stages the mucosa is edematous, coarse, and irregular, particularly in the upper jejunum. There is decreased motility because of the thickening, and then relaxation occurs and dilatation results. There is often excess mucus.[187]

The changes in the portal system leading to portal hypertension, marked splenomegaly, and ascites are similar for both *S. mansoni* and *S. japonicum*. Esophageal and gastric varices develop and may be very prominent. They are easily demonstrated by barium swallow studies, splenoportography, or endoscopy.

CT scanning has occasionally demonstrated calcification around the rectum and presacral tissues. It is important to remember that this calcification is within the ova and not in the fibrous tissue or granulomas. Similar calcification has been demonstrated in multiple areas throughout the colon, where it is most easily seen when the colon is distended; and will be laminar in pattern, and will become more amorphous as the bowel collapses. It can be found experimentally about 60 days after infection, but it is not an indicator of severity or the activity of the parasite. It is an incidental finding.

Schistosomiasis is a complex and multifocal disease and is best understood if one realizes that it is primarily a disease of the vascular system that causes a severe granulomatous reaction at various stages in its development. This occurs when the fluke or ova are dead but seldom while either is alive.[182] This is one of the many ways the schistosome is unique and contradictory.

Amebic dysentery (amebiasis)

Amebiasis is infection by a pathogenic protozoan *Entamoeba histolytica*. Many other strains or species of amebas occur in man, but very few are pathogenic. Even *E. histolytica* can be nonpathogenic until combined with bacteria, in which case some amebas produce strong proteolytic enzymes and lysis of the intestinal epithelium occurs. Only then does the patient change from being a carrier to having clinical amebiasis. After invasion, significant antibodies will be found.

Infection occurs when contaminated food or water is swallowed and is usually transmitted by human cyst carriers. In the tropics transmission by water from polluted wells, by food contaminated by human night soil, or by vectors such as cockroaches and flies may also cause human disease. Animals do not appear to be a frequent source of human infection. It has been estimated that more than 20% of the world's population harbor amebas, although only about 6% will develop clinical amebiasis. The infection is found throughout the world, even in nontropical countries. It is not a disease of adults only, and in West Africa more than 60% of all patients are under the age of 10 years (most of these are under the age of 5 years). Even infants in the first year or two of life can be infected. The diagnosis is established by finding amebas in the stools. A single negative examination, even with careful technique, is not sufficient, and even rectal biopsy is necessary. Numerous serologic tests are not all completely reliable, but if both immunosorbent assay and immunoelectrophoresis are performed, there will be no false-negative results. Test results can remain positive for up to 2 years after the disease is eradicated and are therefore less reliable as a therapeutic index.

Clinically the spectrum is very wide, varying from relatively good health to severe illness. The patient's

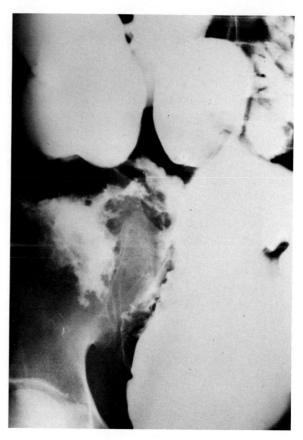

Fig. 62-63 Ameboma adjacent to cecum having cavity connecting with lumen of bowel.

history is quite unreliable, and there may be no episode of dysentery. Symptoms usually develop within 8 to 11 days after invasion, but they sometimes take months or even years to appear. There can be acute dysentery with gripping abdominal pain, tenderness, and fever, but there may be alternating constipation and diarrhea or no bowel symptoms whatsoever. The first attack may subside spontaneously or, alternatively, persist for weeks. Recurrent remission and exacerbation occur in chronic amebic dysentery. Because the amebas spread either directly or by embolism, liver abscesses are common and often spread through the diaphragm and pleura to the lungs. Hematogenous spread may cause pulmonary or brain abscesses. The skin can be infected, particularly when there is a fistula, and abscesses have occurred in the perineum, genitourinary tract, and pelvis.

When there is direct extension through the wall of the large bowel, with associated bacterial infection, a large and sometimes hard tumor (an ameboma) may develop in or adjacent to the bowel (Fig. 62-63). This is common

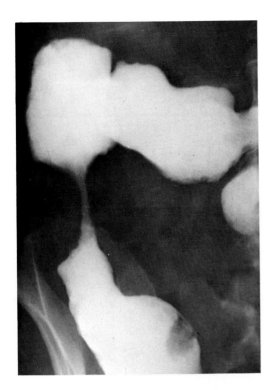

Fig. 62-64 Stricture in ascending colon with severe alteration in mucosal pattern of right half of colon in patient with amebiasis.

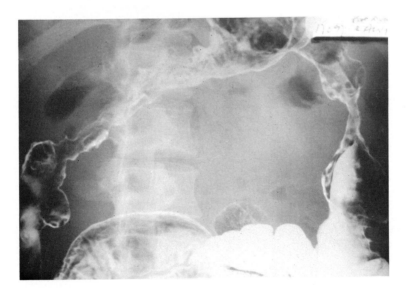

Fig. 62-65 Multiple strictures and complete distortion of mucosal pattern in ascending, transverse, and descending colon in patient with amebiasis.

around the cecum but can occur anywhere in the colon and may strongly resemble a neoplasm with an apple-core lesion.[181] Differentiation may not be possible in some patients, but the smooth tapering edge of the lesion and the presence of amebiasis elsewhere in the colon are the most useful indicators. If there is a reasonable doubt

of an amebic infection, the patient should be treated before surgery: The "malignancy" will often change or even disappear.

The radiologic findings in amebiasis are as numerous and varied as the clinical presentation, and a high index of suspicion is needed.[160] The earliest findings occur around the cecum and ascending colon and are due to the edema and ulceration of the bowel. There will be rigidity and thickening of the bowel wall with an irregular mucosa and multiple tiny ulcers (Figs. 62-64 and 62-65). Normal areas may intervene, and if amebiasis is suspected in any part of the bowel, very careful examination of the bowel elsewhere is indicated. There can be so much spasm and edema that it is difficult to distend any part of the colon. As the ulcers deepen, the edges become undermined and the characteristic flask-shaped ulcer can be demonstrated radiologically. At this stage, the outline of the cecum is often hazy and indistinct, perhaps suggesting inadequate bowel preparation before the examination. The cecum eventually becomes less mobile and rather rigid but usually can be distended with a barium enema (which is not possible with malignancy). The transition from normal to abnormal is very gradual, and, again, this differs from the more abrupt change of a neoplasm. Such areas can occur throughout the bowel, and if the edema is severe, there will be "thumb printing" (Fig. 62-66). The whole colon may be involved, and there may be the appearance of acute ulcerative colitis.[174] Occasionally the terminal ileum becomes infected, because an incompetent ileocecal valve is common and reflux occurs. In very severe and often fatal cases, an

acute toxic megacolon may be seen. In children the symptoms in general are often more acute: one or more amebic ulcers may perforate, and generalized peritonitis or intussusception may occur. Even in children an ameboma may cause obstruction, and transmural peritonitis can also occur.[156]

When the disease is chronic, the picture is that of contraction and rigidity with fixed deformity (Fig. 62-67). The cecum often becomes conical and the terminal ileum rigid and tubular. Multiple fistulas with surrounding abscesses can occur, and late in the disease the bowel wall may be quite smooth, as occurs in the end result of ulcerative colitis.

Abscesses occur anywhere in the liver, although most frequently in the right lobe. They may be solitary or multiple. When close to the diaphragm, there is first loss of movement and then pleural reaction and edema in the nearby lung. Perforation of the abscess through the diaphragm and into the chest may lead to finding of amebas in the sputum. Perforation into the pericardium can be a

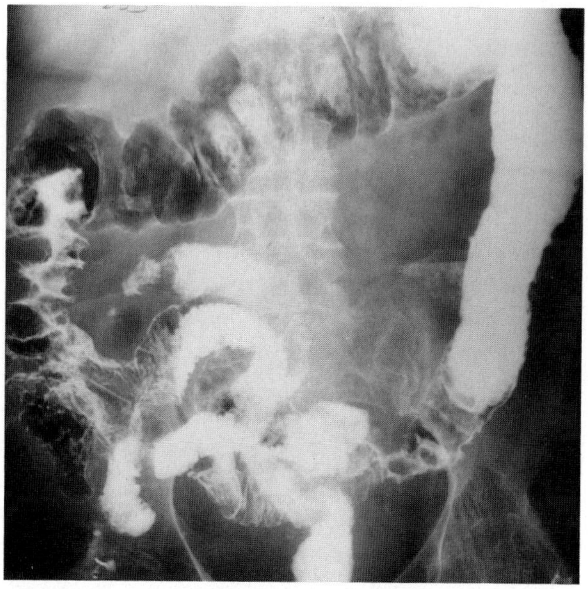

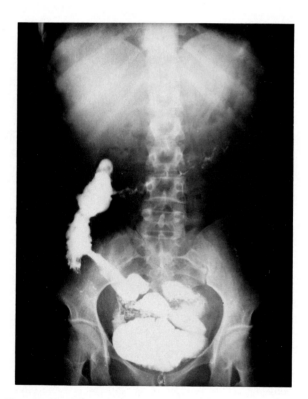

Fig. 62-66 Severe ulcerative colitis in patient with amebiasis with marked "thumb printing" in ascending colon. There are widespread mural spicules and ulceration in descending and sigmoid colon. Terminal ileum is also involved.
(From Reeder, MM, and Palmer, PES: The radiology of tropical diseases, Baltimore, 1981, Williams & Wilkins.) (From Armed Forces Institute of Pathology, No. 67-10134-2 229498-233.)

Fig. 62-67 Fixed, contracted, rigid, and ulcerated cecum caused by chronic amebiasis. Ileocecal valve is fixed and incompetent, and terminal ileum is tubular. There are fistulas from tip of cecum.
(From Reeder, MM, and Palmer, PES: The radiology of tropical diseases, Baltimore, 1981, Williams & Wilkins.)

very dangerous event. The liver abscesses are best demonstrated by CT, ultrasonography (Fig. 62-68) or MRI and are frequently peripheral.[159,175] Angiography will show displacement of the vessels and a ring of increased vascularity around the abscess. Larger abscesses can also be diagnosed by radionuclide scans (Fig. 62-69). With ultrasound it must be remembered that early in the infection some abscesses are isodense and totally or partially hyperechoic.[167] When abscess is suspected clinically and the ultrasound examination is negative, the

examination should be repeated within a day or two, since liquefaction occurs centrally and the sonic findings will change. Alternatively, CT scanning with contrast material may show the hyperemic wall and an otherwise isodense abscess a little earlier. But CT scans or MRI should be used only where ultrasonography produces negative results. In spite of many different descriptions there is no method of imaging that can reliably differentiate an amebic from a pyogenic liver abscess.

A hepatic abscess can rupture into the biliary tract

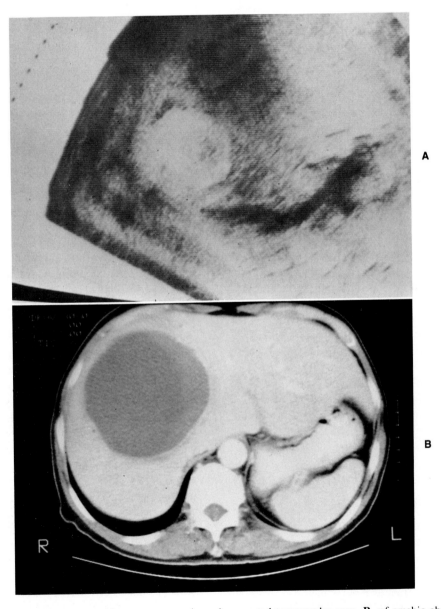

Fig. 62-68 Ultrasonographic appearances, **A,** and computed tomography scan, **B,** of amebic abscesses in liver. Findings are very nonspecific, and amebic abscess cannot be distinguished from any other liver abscess.

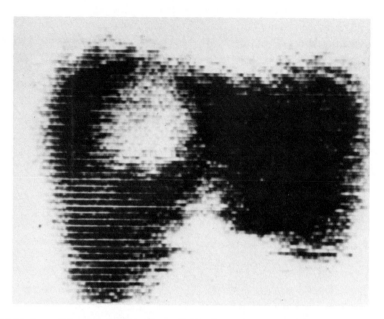

Fig. 62-69 Radionuclide scan (^{99m}Tc-sulfur colloid) shows large amebic abscess in right lobe of liver, spreading upward toward upper surface. Diaphragm was involved, and there was right-sided pleural effusion with edema in right lower lobe.
(From Reeder, MM, and Palmer,PES: The radiology of tropical diseases, Baltimore, 1981, Williams & Wilkins.)

and may cause jaundice. Plain films may show gas within the liver. Perforation can occur into the peritoneum, around the kidneys, or directly into the stomach or gut. Trauma can rupture an abscess either in the liver or elsewhere, and this may be the way in which the abscess is first recognized. After treatment a liver abscess may disappear entirely, may leave some scarring, or occasionally can calcify. Healing may take many months, and the central cavity may persist for years, although it will be sterile.

Amebiasis mimics many diseases, including ulcerative colitis, with or without megacolon; the narrow areas, deep ulcers, fistulas, and skip areas of Crohn's disease; or the tight stricture or mass of malignancy. A serologic check is easy and not only may avoid surgery but may literally be life saving. The radiologist must have a high index of suspicion for amebiasis.

Echinococcosis (hydatid disease)

There are two types of *Echinococcus* infections: *E. granulosus* infection is the most common, and *E. multilocularis* is less common but much more invasive and frequently resembles malignancy. *E. granulosus* infection results in large cysts and is found worldwide but is more common in temperate climates. The life cycle requires two hosts—a dog and a grazing animal, usually sheep, cattle, or pigs. It can also be found in wolves and

some deer. The adult parasite is a tiny tapeworm, usually found by the hundreds or thousands in the small intestine of dogs. Excreted in the feces, the eggs contaminate wide areas of pasture and are subsequently ingested. Man becomes accidentally infected either by contact with infected dogs or by ingesting food, water, or soil containing the eggs. Occasionally uncooked foods, such as salads, may transmit the infection.

In man the external layers of the eggs are digested, and the larvae migrate through the intestinal mucosa into the mesenteric veins and lymphatics and are then carried to many different parts of the body. Because the liver acts as an effective filter, this is the most common site for cysts, exceeding 90% in some series. However, the larvae may lodge anywhere in the body and may be found in the peritoneum, spleen, kidneys, brain, bones, heart, and muscles. Many larvae are overcome by the host reaction, but those that survive develop into tiny cysts containing a small amount of clear fluid. The cyst grows steadily until it becomes clinically evident. The average rate of growth is 1 to 3 cm a year but varies with the type of tissue surrounding it. Thus the cysts grow more rapidly in the lung than in the liver. Each cyst has two walls—a thick outer laminated ectocyst and a more delicate inner membrane, the endocyst. As the cyst grows there is reaction around it in the compressed host tissue, and this forms the third layer, the pericyst. The active

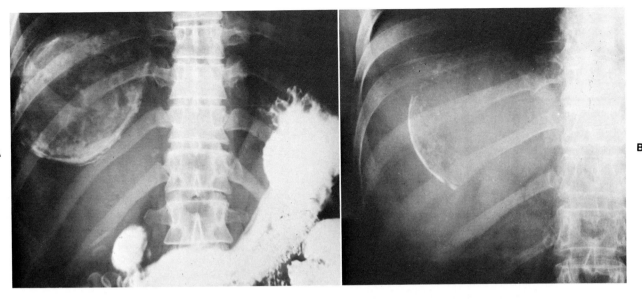

Fig. 62-70 Calcified *Echinococcus* cysts in liver. **A,** Calcified cyst containing multiple daughter cysts in 37-year-old Basque woman. **B,** Segmentally calcified *Echinococcus* cyst in young Greek woman.

part of the cyst is the inner germinal epithelium with its brood capsules and scoleces, from which the new worms develop. The brood capsules usually detach from the germinal layer and may be found as "hydatid sand" at the bottom of the cyst, recognizable on ultrasonograph or CT scans. "Daughter" cysts may develop within the original cyst (Fig. 62-70, *A*), but they are usually thought to be the result of mechanical, chemical, or bacterial insult. CT scanning and ultrasonography have shown multiple septa caused by these daughter cysts within the overall hydatid outline.

Provided the hydatid cyst is contained within the pericyst, there are few local symptoms other than those due to the size of the cyst itself. Once the pericyst is damaged, infection nearly always occurs, and there may be a severe host reaction and sometimes fatal anaphylaxis. About 30% of the cysts die and may become partially or completely calcified, but a partially calcified cyst should not be regarded as harmless (Fig. 62-70).

The clinical symptoms when the cyst is intact are those related to the size of the cyst and the tissue within which it resides. Within the liver most cysts are 10 cm or more in diameter before they are recognized clinically, but eventually there may be pressure on the biliary tract, with indigestion, nausea, or vomiting, and there is sometimes pain. Rupture can be an acute emergency if the cysts break through into the lung or peritoneal cavity, sometimes causing anaphylaxis. On the other hand, hydatid infection can remain latent for many years and be discovered accidentally. Although there are various serologic tests, none is 100% accurate, and multiple methods of detection may be necessary.

On plain radiography these cysts may cause generalized enlargement of the liver or a localized bulge in the hepatic outline, with a hump in the diaphragm in some cases. They are usually spheric and sometimes distorted by the rib cage. In more than 50% of cases partial or crescentic calcification occurs in the cyst wall, or if the cyst has been damaged, the calcification may show that it is collapsed and amorphous.[158] Angiography shows that the cysts are avascular, sometimes with a hypervascular rim in the capillary phase, but the findings are nonspecific, as are the findings on scintigraphy. Ultrasonography, CT scanning, and MRI have made it possible to recognize small cysts and show that they are usually multiple. The ultrasound appearances have been divided into various categories[170,172,180,184]:

1. *Pure fluid.* The cyst is sonolucent with marked enhancement of back wall echoes. The cysts are round and well defined. The smaller cysts are "punched out" and sonolucent, and the actual cyst wall not easily distinguished.

2. *Fluid with a split wall.* The cyst is less well rounded and sags. A floating membrane may be seen internally that is very characteristic of hydatid disease. It suggests lowered intracystic pressure.

3. *Both fluid and septa.* When there are both fluid and septa the cyst is usually well defined but divided into

sections of varying shapes, usually oval or rounded. The back echoes are enhanced, and there is a honeycomb image.

4. *Irregular shape.* Irregular cysts have a variable echo pattern and are usually round but rough in outline. They can be hypoechoic with irregular echoes, hyperechoic and solid without back wall shadows, or of an intermediate phase that may include both of the above, often in clustered nodular groups.

5. *Hyperechoic.* Some cysts are very hyperechoic with a cone-shaped shadow, and only the thick reflecting front wall may be seen.

When there are multiple cysts, there may be considerable overlap. Most hydatid cysts are simple sonolucent cysts that are difficult to distinguish from simple liver cysts, hematoma, or abscess. If the collapsed membrane and septa are recognized, diagnosis is simplified. Sometimes the hydatid sand can be seen at the bottom, and if this moves, it may account for a variation in appearance. Once the cyst is infected, recognition can be very difficult. The differential diagnosis of a hydatid cyst from a hepatoma by ultrasonography is not easy. In countries where hepatomas are common such tumors often show a large irregular echogenic mass with ill-defined and irregular margins and, often, strong echoes within the mass. The European and North American variety of hepatoma is more homogeneous and more closely resembles a metastasis; differentiation from some hydatid cysts can then be difficult.

The CT findings are diagnostically very accurate (Fig. 62-71). The cysts are round, oval, or flattened if they are on the edge of the liver. The attenuation is similar to water. About 80% of the cysts will have marginal calcification, and more than half will have daughter cysts within them. The endocystic membrane can usually be recognized; the contents are not always homogeneous, probably because of hydatid sand. Contrast material seldom enhances the cysts unless there is marked compression of host tissue.

With MRI the cysts are well demonstrated with spin-echo pulse sequences and are equally well seen with either T_1 or T_2 weighting, so it is probably best to use both. A thin, low-intensity rim may be found surrounding the hydatid cysts and can be helpful in the differential diagnosis. This rim is probably caused by the pericyst, which is primarily composed of collagen.

The appearance of a hydatid cyst changes with treatment. After drug therapy the cyst may collapse or slowly shrink, with a decrease in tension within the cyst and a transonic halo. Daughter cysts tend to lose their clarity and even disappear. Change can also happen when there is trauma and the cyst ruptures; numerous daughter cysts may then develop. At surgery cysts may be removed or

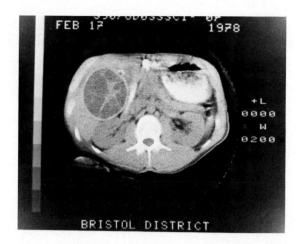

Fig. 62-71 Hydatid cyst demonstrated by computed tomography within liver. Capsule is well seen, and loculations within cyst are well demonstrated.

may be invaginated in the residual space, which may then be filled with omentum. Serial ultrasonography or CT scanning is needed to watch the shrinkage and resulting fibrosis, which may take up to 2 years. Although on ultrasonography a decrease in cyst size, detachment of the cyst membrane, and other signs of regression may occur, the effect of drug therapy is widely variable, and some cysts will continue to grow in spite of treatment. Initial regression may be followed by further progression. Prolonged observation is needed.

Hydatid cysts may occur in the pancreas and show as round, partially calcified cystic lesions. Solitary or even multiple cysts in the spleen or kidney may calcify and have to be differentiated from other cysts, few of which have septa or calcify to the same extent. Cysts elsewhere cause pressure symptoms; some have presented as achalasia resulting from pressure near the cardia, and others have pressed on the rectum or caused symptoms elsewhere in the alimentary tract.

E. multilocularis presents as a very different disease.[182]

It is probably most common in eastern Europe and Turkey but is found in Canada, Alaska, and parts of China and central Asia. It is particularly prevalent in areas of cold and high altitude. The life cycle is much the same as for *E. granulosus,* with dogs, cats, or foxes usually being involved. Although in the beginning it is a benign and afebrile infection, the outcome is usually fatal. Macroscopically it is very difficult to distinguish from malignancy, particularly in liver or kidney (or bone). There are multiple cystic spaces, about 0.5 cm in size, producing a honeycomb or spongy appearance (alveolar echinococcosis). Histologically there is necrosis, a granulomatous inflammatory reaction, and membranes around the multiple small cysts. Clinical signs are those of an enlarging mass within the liver, portal hypertension, splenomegaly, jaundice, and then ascites.

The radiologic appearances of the chronic granulomatous reaction and the multiple small cysts are characteristic. In nearly 70% of infections there will be numerous small calcified spheres with radiolucent centers, ranging from 2 to 4 mm in size. Recognition on ultrasonography is not always easy, since the small cysts are inhomogeneous and may not be easily distinguished from liver tissue. With CT scanning there may be a great variation in the attenuation from +5 to +60 Hounsfield units. Calcification will be demonstrated around the edge of the cysts, but sometimes there is an amorphous, plaquelike, racemose pattern throughout. This combination of clustered microcalcification with necrosis is very suggestive of *E. multilocularis,* but it is not an easy diagnosis. In one series from Turkey 60% of cases were diagnosed as liver malignancy.

Both varieties of hydatid disease can be diagnosed by ERCP, most commonly used when the presenting symptom is jaundice. However, CT scanning and ultrasonography are by far the most satisfactory modalities, unless the plain radiographs show a typical calcified cyst or group of cysts. When found as part of an abdominal examination, it is essential to remember that hydatid disease may occur anywhere in the body. One cyst is unlikely to be the end of the patient's problems.

REFERENCES
Gastrointestinal tuberculosis

1. Abrams, JS, and Holden, WD: Tuberculosis of the gastrointestinal tract, Arch Surg 89:282, 1964.
2. Anscombe, AR, Keddie, NC, and Schofield, PF: Caecal tuberculosis, Gut 8:337, 1967.
3. Ball, PAJ: Abdominal tuberculosis. In Davey, WW, editor: Companion to surgery in Africa, Edinburgh, 1968, E & S Livingstone.
4. Bhansali, SK: Abdominal tuberculosis. Experiences with 300 cases, Am J Gastroenterol 67:324, 1977.
5. Black GA, and Carsky, EW: Duodenal tuberculosis, AJR 131:329, 1978.
6. Brenner, SM, Annes G, and Parker JG: Tuberculous colitis simulating nonspecific granulomatous disease of the colon, Am J Dig Dis 15:85, 1970.
7. Brombart, M, and Massion, J: Radiological differences between ileocecal tuberculosis and Crohn's disease, Am J Dig Dis 6:589, 1961.
8. Burack, WR, and Hollister, RM: Tuberculosis peritonitis: a study of forty-seven proved cases encountered by a general medical unit in twenty-five years, Am J Med 28:510, 1960.
9. Burke, GJ, and Zafar, SA: Problems in distinguishing tuberculosis of bowel from Crohn's disease in Asians, Br Med J 4:395, 1975.
10. Camiel, MR: Ileocecal tuberculosis, Radiology 44:344, 1945.
11. Chazan, BI, and Aitchison, JD: Gastric tuberculosis, Br Med J 2:1288, 1960.
12. El Masri, SH, et al: Abdominal tuberculosis in Sudanese patients, East Afr Med J 54:319, 1977.
13. Gaines, W, Steinbach, HL, and Lowenhaupt, E: Tuberculosis of the stomach, Radiology 58:808, 1952.
14. Gershon-Cohen, J, and Kremens, V: X-ray studies of the ileocecal valve in ileocecal tuberculosis, Radiology 62:251, 1954.
15. Granet, E: Intestinal tuberculosis: a clinical, roentgenological and pathological study of 2086 patients affected with pulmonary tuberculosis, Am J Dig Dis 2:209, 1935.
16. Hancock, DM: Hyperplastic tuberculosis of the distal colon, Br J Surg 46:63, 1958.
17. Herlinger, H: Angiography in the diagnosis of ileocecal tuberculosis, Gastrointest Radiol 2:371, 1978.
18. Hoon, JR, Dockerty, MG, and Pemberton, JdeJ: Collective review: ileocecal tuberculosis including comparision of this disease with nonspecific regional enterocolitis and noncaseous tuberculated enterocolitis, Int Abstr Surg 91:417, 1950.
19. Hughes, HJ, Carr, DT, and Geraci, JE: Tuberculous peritonitis: a review of 34 cases with emphasis on the diagnostic aspects, Dis Chest 38:42, 1960.
20. Kolawole, TM, and Lewis EA: Radiologic study of tuberculosis of the abdomen, Am J Roentgenol 123:348, 1975.
21. Lester, FT, and Tsega, E: Tuberculous peritonitis in Ethiopian patients, J Trop Geogr Med 28:169, 1976.
22. Marshak, RH, and Lindner, AE: Radiology of the small intestine, ed 2, Philadelphia, 1976, W.B. Saunders.
23. McDonald, JB, and Middleton, PJ: Tuberculosis of the colon simulating carcinoma, Radiology 118:293, 1976.
24. Mitchell, RS, and Bristol, LJ: Intestinal tuberculosis: an analysis of 346 cases diagnosed by routine intestinal radiography in 5,529 admissions for pulmonary tuberculosis, 1924-1949, Am J Med Sci 227:241, 1954.
25. Paterson, DE: Tuberculosis of the upper alimentary tract. In Middlemiss, H, editor: Tropical radiology. London, 1961, William Heinemann Medical Books.
26. Pinto, RS, Zausner, J, and Beranbaum, ER: Gastic tuberculosis. Report of a case with discussion of angiographic findings, Am J Roentgenol 110:808, 1970.
27. Reeder, MM, and Palmer, PES: The radiology of tropical diseases, with epidemiological, pathological and clinical correlation, Baltimore, 1981, Williams & Wilkins.
28. Vaidya, MG, and Sodhi, JS: Gastrointestinal tract tuberculosis: a study of 102 cases including 55 hemicolectomies, Clin Radiol 29:189, 1978.
29. Werbeloff, L, et al: The radiology of tuberculosis of the gastrointestinal tract, Br J Radiol 46:329, 1973.

Salmonella Infections and Typhoid Fever

30. Bohrer, SP: Typhoid perforation of the ileum, Br J Radiol 39:37, 1966.
31. Chérigié, E, et al: Aspect radiologique du grêle chez les typhiques, J Radiol Electrol 34:522, 1953.
32. Cockshott, WP: Typhoid. In Schinz, HR, editor: Roentgen diagnosis, ed 2, vol 3, New York, 1969, Grune & Stratton.
33. Elegbeleye, OO: Typhoid fever in Lagos, Nigeria, West Indian Med J 25:39, 1976.
34. Felsenfeld, O: Synopsis of clinical tropical medicine, St. Louis, 1965, C.V. Mosby, pp 43-53.
35. Frimann-Dahl, J: Roentgen examinations in acute abdominal diseases, ed 3, Springfield, Ill., 1974, Charles C Thomas.
36. Golden, R: Radiologic examination of the small intestine, ed 2, Springfield, Ill., 1959, Charles C Thomas.
37. Huckstep, RL: Typhoid fever and other salmonella infections, Edinburgh, 1962, E & S Livingstone.

38. Hunter, GW, III, Swartzwelder, JC, and Clyde, DF: Tropical medicine, ed 5, Philadelphia, 1976, W.B. Saunders.

39. Pontes, JF: Disorders of the small intestine, Ciba Clin Symp 12:107, 1960.

40. Rappaprot, EM, and Rappaport, EO: Typhoid enterocolitis simulating chronic bacillary dysentery: report of a case with cure by chloromycetin, N Engl J Med 242:698, 1950.

41. Reeder, MM, and Palmer, PES: The radiology of tropical diseases, with epidemiological, pathological and clinical correlation, Baltimore, 1981, Williams & Wilkins.

42. Silverman, DN, and Leslie, A: Simulation of chronic bacterial dysentery by paratyphoid B infection, Gastroenterology 4:53, 1945.

43. Slomic, AM, and Rousseau, B: Salmonella colitis: two cases of a milder form, Ann Radiol 19:431, 1976.

44. Wilcocks, C, and Manson-Bahr, PH: Manson's tropical diseases: a manual of diseases of warm climates, ed 17, London, 1976, Baillière Tindall.

Bacillary dysentery

45. Ash, JE, and Spitz, S: Pathology of tropical diseases, Philadelphia, 1945, W.B. Saunders.

46. Christie, AB: Bacillary dysentery, Br Med J 2:285, 1968.

47. Dammin, GJ: Shigellosis. In Binford, CH, and Connor, DH, editors: Pathology of tropical and extraordinary diseases, Washington, D.C., 1976, Armed Forces Institute of Pathology.

48. DeLorimier, AA, et al: Clinical roentgenology, vol 4, Springfield, Ill., 1956, Charles C Thomas.

49. Farman, J, et al: Roentgenology of infectious colitis, Am J Roentgenol 119:375, 1973.

50. Hunter, GW, III, et al: Tropical medicine, ed 5, Philadelphia, 1976, W.B. Saunders.

51. Reeder, MM, and Palmer, PES: The radiology of tropical diseases, with epidemiological, pathological and clinical correlation, Baltimore, 1981, Williams & Wilkins.

52. Schinz, HR, et al: Roentgen-diagnostics, vol 4, New York, 1954, Grune & Stratton.

53. Teplick, JG, and Haskin, ME: Roentgenologic diagnosis, ed 2, Philadelphia, 1974, W.B. Saunders.

Pseudomembranous enterocolitis

54. Benner, EJ, and Tellman, WH: Pseudomembranous colitis as a sequel to oral lincomycin therapy, Am J Gastroenterol 54:55, 1970.

55. Birnbaum, D, Laufer, A, and Freund, M: Pseudomembranous enterocolitis: a clinicopathologic study, Gastroenterology 41:345, 1961.

56. Brown, CH, Ferrante, WA, and Davis, WD Jr: Toxic dilatation of the colon complicating pseudomembranous entercolitis, Am J Dig Dis 13:813, 1968.

57. Ecker, JA, et al: Pseudomembranous enterocolitis—an unwelcome gastrointestinal complication of antibiotic therapy, Am J Gastroenterol 54:214, 1970.

58. Feinberg, SB: The roenten findings in severe pseudomembranous enterocolitis, Radiology 74:778, 1960.

59. Gildenhorn, HL, Springer, EB, and Amromin, GD: Necrotizing enteropathy: roentgenographic features, Am J Roentgenol 88:942, 1962.

60. Goulston, SJ, and McGovern, VJ: Pseudomembranous colitis, Gut 6:207, 1965.

61. Groll, A, et al: Fulminating noninfective pseudomembranous colitis, Gastroenterology 58:88, 1970.

62. Hale, HW, Jr, and Cosgriff, JH, Jr: Pseudomembranous enterocolitis, Am J Surg 94:710, 1957.

63. Pettet, JD, et al: Generalized postoperative pseudomembranous enterocolitis, Proc Staff Meet Mayo Clin 29:342, 1954.

64. Reiner, L, Schlesinger, MJ, and Miller, GM: Pseudomembranous colitis following aureomycin and chloramphenicol AMA Arch Pathol 54:39, 1952.

65. Speare, GS: Staphylococcus pseudomembranous enterocolitis, complication of antibiotic therapy, Am J Surg 88:523, 1954.

Acute gastroenteritis

66. Dodd, K: Gastroenteritis of viral origin, Med Clin North Am 43:1349, 1959.

67. Gorbach, SL: Acute diarrhea—a "toxin" disease? N Engl J Med 283:44, 1970.

Lymphogranuloma venereum

68. Annamunthodo, H: Rectal lymphogranuloma venereum in Jamaica, Dis Colon Rectum 4:17, 1961.

69. Annamunthodo, H, and Marryatt, J: Barium studies in intestinal lymphogranuloma venereum, Br J Radiol 34:53, 1961.

70. Davey, WW: Companion to surgery in Africa, London, 1968, E & S Livingstone.

71. De Lorimier, AA, et al: Clinical roentgenology, vol 4, Springfield, Ill., Charles C Thomas.

72. Helper, M, and Szilagyi, DE: Venereal lymphogranulomatous rectal stricture, Am J Roentgenol 48:179, 1942.

73. Klein, I: Roentgen study of lymphogranuloma venereum: report of 24 cases, Am J Roentgenol 51:70, 1944.

74. Pessel, JF: Lymphogranuloma venereum. In Bockus, HL, editor: Gastroenteology, ed 2, vol 2, Philadelphia, 1964, W.B. Saunders.

75. Reeder, MM, and Palmer, PES: The radiology of tropical diseases, with epidemiological, pathological and clinical correlation, Baltimore, 1981, Williams & Wilkins.

76. Rendich, RA, and Poppel, MH: Lymphogranuloma of the colon, Radiology 33:472, 1939.

77. Spiesman, MG, et al: Lymphogranuloma inguinale: rectal stricture and prestricture, Am J Dig Dis 3:931, 1937.

78. Steinert, R: Stricture of the rectum in lymphopathia venerea and its roentgenologic aspects, Acta Radiol 21:368, 1940.

79. Wright, LT, et al: Lymphogranulomatous strictures of the rectum: résumé of 476 cases, Arch Surg 53:499, 1946.

Tropical sprue

80. Caldwell, WI, et al: The importance and reliability of the radiographic examination of the small bowel in patients with tropical sprue, Radiology 84:227, 1965.

81. Cockshott, WP: Tropical sprue. In Rigler, LG, editor: Textbook of roentgen diagnosis, ed 2, vol 3, New York, 1969, Grune & Stratton.

82. Floch, MH, Caldwell, WL, and Sheehy, TW: Histopathologic interpretation of small bowel roentgenography in tropical sprue, Am J Roentgenol 87:709, 1962.

83. Laws, JW, et al: Correlation of radiological and histological findings in idiopathic steatorrhea, Br Med J 1:1311, 1963.

84. Marshak, RH, and Lindner, AE: Malabsorption syndrome, Semin Roentgenol 1:138, 1966.

85. Marshak, RH, and Lindner, AE: Radiology of the small intestine ed 2, Philadelphia, 1976, W.B. Saunders.

86. Misra, RC, et al: Correlation of clinical, biochemical, radiological, and histological findings in tropical sprue, J Trop Med Hyg 70:6, 1967.

87. Palmer, ED: Functional gastrointestinal disease, Baltimore, 1967, Williams & Wilkins.

88. Paterson, EE, et al: Radiodiagnostic problems in malabsorption, Br J Radiol 38:181, 1965.

89. Reeder, MM, and Palmer, PES: The radiology of tropical diseases, with epidemiological, pathological and clinical correlation, Baltimore, 1981, Williams & Wilkins.

90. Thomas, G, and Clain, DJ: Endemic tropical sprue in Rhodesia, Gut 17:877, 1976.

Gastrointestinal candidiasis

91. Brabander, JO, et al: Intestinal moniliasis in adults, Can Med Assoc J 77:478, 1957.

92. Craig, JM, and Farber, S: The development of disseminated visceral mycosis during therapy for acute leukemia, Am J Pathol 29:601, 1953.

93. Goldberg, HI, and Dodds, WJ: Cobblestone esophagus due to monilial infection, Am J Roentgenol 104:608, 1968.

94. Kaufman, SA, et al: Esophageal moniliasis, Radiology 75:726, 1960.

95. Reeder, MM, and Palmer, PES: The radiology of tropical diseases, with epidemiological, pathological and clinical correlation, Baltimore, 1981, Williams & Wilkins.

96. Rogers, KB: Candida infections in paediatrics. In Winner, HI, and Hurley, R, editors: Symposium on *Candida* infections. London, 1966, E & S Livingstone.

97. Sanders, E, et al: Monilial esophagitis in a patient with hemoglobin SC disease: demonstration of esophageal motor abnormality by cineradiofluorography, Ann Intern Med 57:650, 1962.

98. Smith, JM: Mycoses of the alimentary tract, Gut 10:1035, 1969.

99. Winner, HI, and Hurley, R: *Candida albicans*, London, 1964, J & A Churchill.

Gastrointestinal histoplasmosis

100. Bank, S, et al: Histoplasmosis of the small bowel with "giant" intestinal villi and secondary protein losing enteropathy, Am J Med 39:492, 1965.

101. Dietz, MW: ileocecal histoplasmosis, Radiology 91:285, 1968.

102. Henderson, RG, et al: Histoplasma capsulatum as cause of chronic ulcerative enteritis, JAMA 118:885, 1942.

103. Lee, KR, et al: The radiology corner. Gastrointestinal histoplasmosis, roentgenographic, clinical and pathological correlation, Am J Gastroenterol 63:255, 1975.

104. Negroni, P: Histoplasmosis: diagnosis and treatment (revised ed), Springfield, Ill., 1965, Charles C Thomas.

105. Perez, CA, et al: Some clinical and radiographic features of gastrointestinal histoplasmosis, Radiology 86:482, 1966.

106. Shull, HJ: Human histoplasmosis: disease with protean manifestations often with digestive system involvement, Gastroenterology 25:582, 1953.

107. Silverman, FN, et al: Histoplasmosis, Am J Med 19:410, 1955.

Helminthoma

108. Anthony, PP, and McAdam, IW: Helminthic pseudotumours of the bowel, 34 cases of helminthoma, Gut 13:8, 1972.

109. Ashby, BS, et al: Eosinophil granuloma of the gastrointestinal tract caused by the herring parasite, *Eustoma rotundatum*, Br Med J 1:1141, 1964.

110. Davey, WW: Helminthoma. In Davey, WW, editor: Companion to surgery in Africa, Edinburgh, 1968, E & S Livingstone.

111. Elmes, BGT, and McAdam, IW: Helminthic abscess, a surgical complication of oesophagostomes and hookworms, Ann Trop Med Parasitol 48:1, 1954.

112. Reeder, MM, and Palmer, PES: The radiology of tropical diseases, with epidemiological, pathological and clinical correlation, Baltimore, 1981, Williams & Wilkins.

113. Welchman, JM: Helminthic abscess of the bowel, Br J Radiol 39:372, 1966.

Chagas' disease

114. Anselmi, A, et al: Cardiovascular radiology in acute and chronic Chagas' myocardiopathy. Morphologic and dynamic study of the cardiac contour correlated with the histologic changes observed in myocardiopathies attributed to *Schizotrypanum cruzi*, Am Heart J 73:626, 1967.

115. Atias, A, et al: Megaesophagus, megacolon, and Chagas' disease in Chile, Gastroenterology 44:433, 1963.

116. Brasil, A: Aperistalsis of the esophagus, Rev Bras Gastroenterol 7:21, 1955.

117. Ferreira-Santos, R: Aperistalsis of the esophagus and colon (megaesophagus and megacolon) etiologically related to Chagas' disease, Am J Dig Dis 6:700, 1961.

118. Ferreira-Santos, R, and Carril, CF: Acquired megacolon in Chagas' disease, Dis Colon Rectum 7:353, 1964.

119. Köberle, F: Megaesophagus, Gastroenterology 34:460, 1958.

120. Köberle, F: Enteromegaly and cardiomegaly in Chagas' disease, Gut 4:399, 1963.

121. Reeder, MM, and Hamilton, LC: Tropical diseases of the colon, Semin Roentgenol 3:62, 1968.

122. Reeder, MM, and Hamilton, LC: Radiologic diagnosis of tropical diseases of the gastrointestinal tract, Radiol Clin North Am 7:57, 1969.

123. Reeder, MM, and Palmer, PES: The radiology of tropical diseases, with epidemiological, pathological and clinical correlation, Baltimore, 1981, Williams & Wilkins.

124. Reeder, MM, and Simão, C; Chagas' myocardiopathy, Semin Roentgenol 4:374, 1969.

125. World Health Organization: Chagas' disease: report of a study group, WHO Tech Rep Ser 202:1, 1960.

Trichuriasis

126. Boon, WH, and Hoh, TK: Severe whipworm infestation in children, Singapore Med J 2:34, 1961.

127. Fisher, RM, and Cremin, BJ: Rectal bleeding due to *Trichuris trichiura*, Br J Radiol 43:214, 1970.

128. Getz, L: Massive infection with *Trichuris trichiura* in children: report of four cases with autopsy, Am J Dis Child 70:19, 1945.

129. Hunter, GW, III, Swartzwelder, JC, and Clyde, DF: Tropical medicine, ed 5, Philadelphia, 1976, W.B. Saunders.

130. Jung, RC, and Beaver, PC: Clinical observation on *Trichocephalus trichiurus* (whipworm) infestation in children, Pediatrics 8:548, 1952.

131. Marcial-Rojas, RA: Pathology of protozoal and helminthic diseases, Huntington, New York, 1975, Robert Krieger Publishing.

132. Reeder, MM, Astacio, JE, and Theros, EG: Case of the month from the AFIP: Massive *Trichuris* infestation of the colon, Radiology 90:382, 1968.

133. Reeder, MM, and Hamilton, LC: Tropical diseases of the colon, Semin Roentgenol 3:62, 1968.

134. Reeder, MM, and Palmer, PES: The radiology of tropical diseases, with epidemiological, pathological and clinical correlation, Baltimore, 1981, Williams & Wilkins.

Giardiasis

135. Amini, F: Giardiasis and steatorrhea, J Trop Med Hyg 66:190, 1963.

136. Antia, FP, et al: Giardiasis in adults, Indian J Med Sci 20:471, 1966.

137. Basu, SP: Radiological appearance of duodenal bulb in giardiasis, Bull Calcutta Sch Trop Med 13:64, 1965.

138. Bloch, C, and Tuchman, LR: Diffuse small intestine abnormality due to *Giardia lamblia* with roentgen and clinical reversibility after therapy: case report, J Mt Sinai Hosp 34:116, 1967.

139. Brandborg, LL, et al: Histological demonstration of mucosal invasion by *Giardia lamblia* in man, Gastroenterology 52:143, 1967.

140. Cortner, JA: Giardiasis, a cause of celiac syndrome, Am J Dis Child 98:311, 1959.

141. Gupta, DN, et al: Adult giardiasis. Incidence and absorption studies, J Assoc Physicians India 13:477, 1965.

142. Hermans, PE, et al: Dysgammaglobulinemia associated with nodular lymphoid hyperplasia of the small intestine, Am J Med 40:78, 1966.

143. Hodgson, JR, et al: Roentgenologic features of lymphoid hyperplasia of the small intestine associated with dysgammaglobulinemia, Radiology 88:883, 1967.

144. Hoskins, LC, et al: Clinical giardiasis and intestinal malabsorption, Gastroenterology 53:265, 1967.

145. Marshak, RH, et al: Roentgen manifestations of giardiasis, Am J Roentgenol 104:557, 1968.

146. Marshak, RH, and Lindner, AE: Radiology of the small intestine, ed 2, Philadelphia, 1976, W.B. Saunders.

147. Peterson, GM: Intestinal changes in *Giardia lamblia* infestation, Am J Roentgenol 77:670, 1957.

148. Reeder, MM: RPC of the month from the AFIP, Radiology 93:427, 1969.

149. Reeder, MM, and Hamilton, LC: Radiologic diagnosis of tropical diseases of the gastrointestinal tract, Radiol Clin North Am 7:57, 1969.

150. Reeder, MM, and Palmer, PES: The radiology of tropical diseases, with epidemiological, pathological and clinical correlation, Baltimore, 1981, Williams & Wilkins.

151. Takano, J, and yardley, JH: Jejunal lesions in patients with giardiasis and malabsorption: an electron microscopic study, Bull John Hopkins Hosp 116:413, 1965.

152. Welch, PB: Giardiasis with unusual findings, Gastroenterology 3:98, 1944.

153. Yardley, JH, and Bayless, TM: Giardiasis, Gastroenterology 52:301, 1967.

Parasitic infections

154. Anthony, PP, and McAdam, IW: Helminthic pseudo-tumours of the bowel, 34 cases of helminthoma, Gut 13:8, 1972.

155. Ardran, GM: *Armillifer armillatus*, Br J Radiol 21:342, 1948.

156. Barker, EM: Colonic perforations in amebiasis, S Afr Med J 32:634, 1958.

157. Binford, MC, and Connor, DM: Pathology of tropical and extraordinary diseases, Washington, D.C., 1976, The Armed Forces Institute of Pathology.

158. Bonakdarpour, A: *Echinococcus* disease. Report of 112 cases from Iran and a review of 611 from the United States, AJR 99:660, 1967.

159. Boultbee, JE, et al: Experiences with gray scale ultrasonography in hepatic amoeiasis, Clin Radiol 30:683, 1979.

160. Cardoso, JM, et al: Radiology of invasive amebiasis of the colon, AJR 128:935, 1977.

161. Chartres, JC: Radiological manifestations of parasitism by the tongue worms, Br J Radiol 38:503, 1965.

162. Choi, TK, Wang, KP, and Wong, J: Cholangiographic appearances in clonorchiasis, Br J Radiol 57:681, 1984.

163. Chunge, CN, et al: Other parasitic diseases found in patients with visceral leishmaniasis, E Afr Med J 62:118, 1985.

164. Cremin, BJ: Real time ultrasound in paediatric biliary ascariasis, S Afr Med J 61:914, 1982.

165. Cremin, BJ: Ultrasonic diagnosis in biliary ascariasis, Br J Radiol 55:683, 1985.

166. Dallemand, S, Waxman, M, and Farman J: Radiological manifestations of *Strongyloides stercorealis*, Gastro Radiol 8:45, 1983.

167. Dalrymple, RB, et al: Hyperechoic liver abscesses. Unusual ultrasonic appearances, Clin Radiol 33:541, 1982.

168. Evans, H, et al: Biliary tract changes in the opisthorchiasis, Am J Trop Med Hyg 20:667, 1971.

169. Fisher, RM, and Cremin, BJ: Rectal bleeding due to *Trichuris trichiura*, Br J Radiol 43:214, 1970.

170. Gharbi, HA, et al: Ultrasound examination of the hydatid liver, Radiology 139:459, 1981.

171. Gold, BM, and Meyers, MA: Radiologic manifestations of *Taenia saginata* infestation, Am J Roentgenol 128:493, 1977.

172. Grabbe, HA, et al: Ultrasound examination of the hydatid liver, Ultrasound 139:459, 1981.

173. Iarotski, LS, and Davis, A: The schistosomiasis problem in the world: the results of a WHO questionnaire survey. Bull WHO 59:114, 1981.

174. Juniper, K, Jr: Acute amebic colitis, Am J Med 33:377, 1962.

175. Kern, P, et al: Hepatic amoebic abscess. Ultrasonographic and clinical follow up studies in 20 patients, Ultraschall Med 3:7, 1982.

176. Kuipers, FC: Eosinophilic phlegmonous inflammation of the alimentary canal caused by a parasite from the herring, Pathol Microbiol 27:925, 1964.

177. Manson-Bahr, PH: Manson's tropical diseases, ed 15, London, 1960, Cassell.

177a. Margulis, AR, and Burhenne, HJ: Alimentary tract radiology, ed 3, St. Louis, 1983, The CV Mosby Co.

178. Medina, JT, et al: The roentgen appearance of *Schistosomiasis mansoni* involving the colon, Radiology 85:682, 1965.

179. Okumura, M, et al: Acute intestinal obstruction by ascaris. Analysis of 455 cases, Rev Inst Med Trop Sao Paulo 16:292, 1975.

180. Ralls, WP, et al: Pattern of resolution in successfully treated hepatic amebic abscesses. Sonographic evaluation, Radiology 149:541, 1983.

181. Recio, PM: Ameboma of the colon, Dis Colon Rectum 8:205, 1965.

182. Reeder, MM, and Palmer, PES: The radiology of tropical diseases with epidemiological, pathological and clinical correlation, Baltimore, 1981, Williams & Wilkins.

183. Richman, RH, and Lewicki, AN: Right ileocolitis secondary to anisakiasis, Am J Roentgenol 11:329, 1973.

184. Schulman, A, et al: Pseudo-solid appearance of simple and echinococcal cysts on ultrasonography, S Afr Med J 63:905, 1983.

185. Sobrinho, J, and Kelsch, F: Asbectos tumorais de sequistosomose do colon, Rev Bras Radiol 2:1, 1959.

186. Walsh, JA, and Warren, KS: Selective primary health care: an interim strategy for disease control in developing countries. N Engl J Med 301:967, 1979.

187. Wang, C, et al: Roentgenologic changes of small intestine in *Schistosomiasis japonica*, Chin J Radiol 6:247, 1958.

188. Welchman, JM: Helminthic abscess of the bowel, Br J Radiol 39:372, 1966.

189. World Health Organization: Technical Report Series 666: intestinal protozoan and helminthic infections, 1981.

190. Wynne, JM, and Ellman, BAH: Bolus obstruction by *Ascaris lumbricoides*, S Afr Med J 63:644, 1983.

191. Yokogawa, M, and Yoshimura, H: Clinico-pathologic studies on larval anisakiasis in Japan, Am J Trop Med Hyg 16:723, 1967.

Additional reading

Gupta, SK et al: Duodenal tuberculosis, Clin Radiol 39:159, 1988.

63 *Gastrointestinal Manifestations of AIDS*

SUSAN D. WALL

Since 1981 the acquired immunodeficiency syndrome (AIDS) epidemic has had an unparalled impact on the well being of the people in the United States and the world. As of March, 1988, more than 55,000 persons in the United States alone were diagnosed with this highly morbid epidemic illness, and it had killed more than 31,000 of them. Despite repeated predictions that the rate of newly reported cases may be leveling off, the epidemic has not yet slowed. Indeed, the number of cases reported per year continues to increase in all patient groups. AIDS is concentrated mainly in large metropolitan centers, but it has been reported in communities of all sizes and in all 50 states. Many patients, once diagnosed with AIDS, choose to go home. Hence, their diagnosis may be reported in a large city, but their medical care may be needed in a community that has no large population of homosexual men or IV drug users (the two groups at greatest risk for AIDS in the United States). Consequently, it is appropriate that all radiologists become as informed as possible about the diagnostic clues to AIDS as well as its clinical manifestations, pathophysiology, and mode of transmission. Indeed, radiographic findings may provide the initial suggestion of the diagnosis; radiology often plays a pivotal role in elucidating the early and frequently enigmatic symptomatology of patients with this dreaded syndrome.

AIDS is caused by a retrovirus known as human immunodeficiency virus (HIV). HIV enters the T-helper lymphocytes, where it remains dormant for a variable period of time ranging from weeks to years. Following an as yet unknown stimulus, viral replication occurs, with destruction of those lymphocytes and infection of others. Consequently, there is a profound and unrelenting depression of the immune system that predisposes the patient to opportunistic tumors and opportunistic infections. It is estimated that more than 3.0 million persons in the United States show serological evidence of infection with HIV—most of these people being currently healthy. The virus is transmitted largely by intimate sexual contact but also by exposure to contaminated blood or body secretions. The disease affects mainly homosexual men, IV drug users, and recipients of previously unscreened blood or blood products. Heterosexual contact has had a much smaller impact on the epidemic, and transmission through the delivery of health care is rare. The latency period from the time of viral infection to onset of disease is not yet known, but the mean interval appears to exceed 7 years.[5] However, it is not certain that all persons infected with the virus will develop the disease.

Two laboratory tests currently are used to detect HIV-specific antibodies that indicate prior infection with the virus. These include the enzyme-linked immunosorbent assay (ELISA) as the screening test and the western blot as the confirmatory test. They are not yet optimally effective because of both false positives and false negative results. Currently licensed ELISA tests have a sensitivity between 93% and 99%, and all have specificities greater than 99%. However, reactive tests have a poor positive predictive value when used to screen a general population with a low prevalence of individuals infected with the virus.[14] A positive test result has profound social and medicolegal implications, including the potential for insurability. Laboratory tests that can identify HIF antigen are being developed.

Precautions to prevent the transmission of AIDS in the health care setting should follow the guidelines recommended by the Centers for Disease Control.[6,14] "Universal blood and body-fluid precautions" should be practiced at all times, since medical history, examination, and laboratory testing cannot reliably identify all patients infected with HIV. One should routinely use appropriate barrier precautions to prevent exposure of skin and mucous membrane to blood or other body fluids. Gloves, gowns, masks, and protective eyewear should be used during procedures that are likely to involve contact with blood or other body fluids. Contaminated skin should be washed immediately. Inflamed skin or exudative lesions on a health care worker should be covered at all times. Ventilation devices such as mouthpieces and resuscitation (Ambu) bags should be widely available to minimize the need for emergency mouth-to-mouth resuscitation. Needles should never be recapped, since this is the method by which accidental puncture most often occurs. Puncture-resistant containers should be readily accessible in all rooms for immediate disposal of uncovered needles, scalpel blades, and other sharp items. Reusable instruments can be cleaned with the usual hospital disinfectants, and a simple germicide such as sodium hypochlorite (a 1:10 dilution of household bleach) can be used to clean surfaces upon which blood or body fluids are spilled.[14] The virus is easily killed, and the risk to health-care workers is small. Less than 0.5% of health-care workers have become seropositive for the virus after accidental exposure to HIV-infected blood.[13,14] However, following the precautions that have just been described is prudent.

GASTROINTESTINAL MANIFESTATIONS AND BARIUM RADIOGRAPHY

The GI tract is one of the most frequently involved organ systems in patients with AIDS. Opportunistic tumors (such as Kaposi's sarcoma and lymphoma) and opportunistic pathogens (such as *Candida albicans*, cytomegalovirus, *Cryptosporidium* spp., *Isospora belli*, and atypical *Mycobacterium* spp.) account for most of the recognized gastrointestinal morbidity in AIDS. Their radiographic manifestations are discussed here. Barium radiography can guide endoscopic biopsy and the evaluation of complications, and monitor the progress of therapy. It may be indicated in patients with AIDS who have dysphagia, odynophagia, abdominal pain, diarrhea, symptoms of intermittent obstruction, or gastrointestinal bleeding.

The role of the HIV itself in diarrhea, malabsorption, and other gastrointestinal disorders has not yet been fully elucidated, but its recent recovery from bowel biopsy specimens in patients with AIDS and chronic diarrhea of unknown etiology suggests a direct causative role.[18]

Multifocal gastrointestinal abnormalites (three or more sites) are seen in 65% to 70% of homosexual men with AIDS who are referred for barium examination.[27] Double contrast examination is the preferred technique; it can be directive when diagnosis requires visual inspection by endoscopy or colonoscopy with associated biopsy and/or culture. The cause of multifocal abnor-

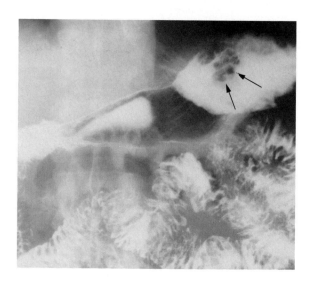

Fig. 63-1 Multifocal abnormalities in 39-year-old man with AIDS and nodular filling defects in gastric fundus due to Kaposi's sarcoma. Also CMV and *Cryptosporidium* organisms both were present in gastric antrum (nondistensible) and in small bowel (thick folds).
(From Wall, SD, Friedman, SL, and Margulis, AR: J Clin Gastroenterol 6:165, 1984.)

malities can be multiple foci of Kaposi's sarcoma, widespread opportunistic infection, multiple opportunistic infections, coexistent tumor and infection (Fig. 63-1), or, less commonly, coexistent Kaposi's sarcoma and lymphoma. With the finding of multifocal gastrointestinal abnormalities on barium radiography, AIDS should be included in the differential diagnosis even in patients not thought to be at high risk for the syndrome.[27]

GASTROINTESTINAL KAPOSI'S SARCOMA

The aggressive clinical course of AIDS-related Kaposi's sarcoma resembles the disseminated lymphadenopathic form seen in young African patients far more than the indolent "classic" form of the disease seen in older men in North America and Europe. Approximately one third of patients with AIDS have Kaposi's sarcoma; the vast majority (95%) of these patients are homosexual or bisexual men. The GI tract is a major target organ of AIDS-related Kaposi's sarcoma, and it is involved at the time of diagnosis or early thereafter in about 50% of patients with cutaneous disease. Occasionally, gastrointestinal lesions precede cutaneous disease. Visceral involvement is considered a manifestation of the multicentric nature of this tumor, not metastatic disease.

Early gastrointestinal Kaposi's sarcoma is not detected on barium radiography because lesions at this stage are macular, and hence they are not evident even with air-contrast technique. However, the appearance on endoscopy is characteristic, and diagnosis is made by visual inspection. Typically there are multiple flat, red-purple, (violaceous) lesions varying in size from a few millimeters to 1-2 cm.[12] Biopsies often are nondiagnostic because the forceps of the flexible fiberoptic endoscope do not reach the submucosa, where the tumor originates.[20] With progression of disease, the lesions become nodular and then are well demonstrated on barium radiography.[15,19,26,27] With air-contrast technique central umbilication may be seen (Fig. 63-2), but "bull's-eye," or "target," lesions are not present in the majority of cases, and this finding should not be required for the radiographic diagnosis of gastrointestinal Kaposi's sarcoma. Advanced disease is demonstrated by the presence of bulky and coalescent nodular lesions[25] (Figs. 63-3 and 63-4). Tumor nodules have been seen in all segments of the GI tract, and their radiographic appearance is similar throughout.

Early gastrointestinal Kaposi's sarcoma generally is asymptomatic. However, even small lesions cause symptoms when they are present in the oropharynx or hypopharynx. Such patients frequently have dysphagia or odynophagia. Pharyngography, which is best performed with an air-contrast technique,[21] will demonstrate well-defined nodular lesions usually without mucosal ulceration.[8] Tumor nodules may be seen at the base of the

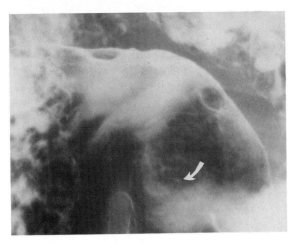

Fig. 63-2 Early Kaposi's sarcoma. Nodular lesions of early Kaposi's sarcoma are present in body and antrum of stomach. Note central umbilication (arrow). (From Wall, SD, et al: AJR 146:1, 1986.)

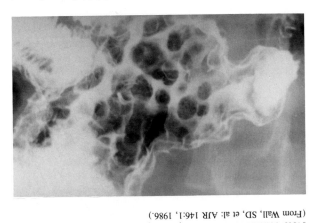

Fig. 63-3 Advanced Kaposi's sarcoma. Multiple, coalescent nodular lesions of advanced Kaposi sarcoma are present throughout stomach in this AIDS patient. (From Wall, SD: Contemp Diag Rad 9(20):1, 1986.)

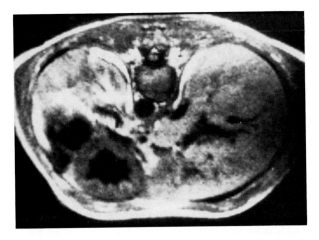

Fig. 63-4 Kaposi's sarcoma. Transaxial magnetic resonance image of stomach in patient with diffuse gastric Kaposi sarcoma demonstrates marked thickening of air-distended stomach. Slight heterogeneity of signal intensity is noted.

the patient, and it is less time consuming. Furthermore, concurrent examination of the remainder of the upper GI tract can be performed readily with pharyngography. Kaposi's sarcoma in the small bowel usually is manifested by focal nodular thickening. With extensive disease, thickening may be diffuse and irregular. Vague abdominal pain and/or diarrhea may be present, but severe complications, such as bleeding, are unusual. Rarely, intussusception (due to a lead mass of Kaposi's sarcoma) or acute appendicitis (due to obstruction of the base of the appendix) has been a presenting manifestation. The barium radiographic findings of gastrointestinal AIDS-related Kaposi sarcoma are not specific, and the differential diagnosis includes lymphoma, metastatic tumor, opportunistic infection, and Crohn's disease.

AIDS-RELATED LYMPHOMA

Gastrointestinal lymphoma seen in patients with AIDS usually is the non-Hodgkins type. The natural history of AIDS-related lymphoma is unusual, since it frequently presents in extranodal sites including abdominal viscera, mucocutaneous surfaces, bone marrow, and brain.[28] Most patients have advanced disease at the time of diagnosis, and the histology usually is a highly malignant subtype. Moreover, the therapeutic response of AIDS-related lymphomas is less than that of non-AIDS lymphomas of similar histology. Hodgkin's disease is seen with less frequency in AIDS patients than is non-Hodgkin's lymphoma, but its natural history also is atypical. In patients with AIDS, Hodgkins disease often presents with non-contiguous sites of involved abdominal, pelvic, and mesenteric lymph nodes, as well as bone marrow disease without splenic involvement.

GASTROINTESTINAL OPPORTUNISTIC INFECTIONS

Candida albicans is the most common opportunistic infection of the GI tract in patients with AIDS.[11] In addition to oral thrush, esophagitis often is seen, and it is diagnostic of AIDS in the proper clinical setting. Early disease causes fold thickening and longitudinal irregular collections of barium among the interstices of mucosal plaques. Advanced disease demonstrates the typical cobblestone appearance seen in non-AIDS patients who are immune compromised for other reasons.[17] Severe disease is manifested additionally by discrete ulceration (Fig. 63-6).

Cytomegalovirus (CMV) esophagitis also occurs frequently in patients with AIDS. It differs radiographically from monilial esophagitis. Early CMV esophagitis is seen on air-contrast radiography as segmental areas of granulation, superficial erosions, and poorly defined, shallow ulcerations.[2] More severe disease typically is manifested by solitary or multiple deep ulcers seen on a background

tongue, posterior oropharynx or hypopharynx, valleculae, and/or pyriform sinuses (Fig. 63-5). Regression has been noted following radiotherapy, but this treatment has limited use because of the severe inflammatory response of the mucosa in patients with AIDS. In selected cases, local radiotherapy has provided palliation for a limited period of time. Pharyngography is a useful screening examination in patients with AIDS and suspected oropharyngeal or hypopharyngeal Kaposi's sarcoma, and for several reasons it may be preferable to laryngoscopy.[8] Barium pharyngography sometimes demonstrates the full extent of disease better than direct visualization at laryngoscopy, because bulky lesions can preclude a complete evaluation, especially of the most caudal extent of tumor. In such a case, radiographic examination can more accurately determine the optimal radiation port when such therapy is indicated. Barium pharyngography requires neither the operating room nor general anesthesia, so it is less expensive than indirect laryngoscopy. Laryngoscopy is a more invasive procedure, and there is more risk to an examiner of exposure to the patient's body fluids. Pharyngography is more easily tolerated by

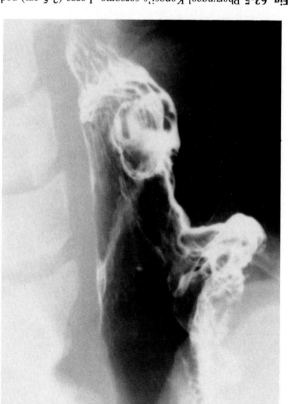

Fig. 63-5 Pharyngeal Kaposi's sarcoma. Large (2.5 cm) nodular lesion of Kaposi's sarcoma is present in pyriform sinus in this man with AIDS. Smaller lesions are present in valleculae and at base of tongue.
(Reprinted from Emeru, CD, et al: AJR 147:919, 1986.)

of normal mucosa (Fig. 63-7). The focal, discretely marginated ulcers of CMV esophagitis may be diamond shaped and frequently has a well-defined peripheral lucency caused by surrounding edema.[2] In patients with AIDS, CMV ulcerations of the esophagus often are seen near the gastroesophageal junction,[2] and there may be extension into the proximal stomach. Another feature characteristic of CMV esophagitis is giant ulceration without abnormality of the surrounding mucosa.[9] Such ulcers are caused by a CMV-induced vasculitis and focal ischemic necrosis.[22] Discrete ulceration of the esophagus also can be caused by herpes simplex or *Mycobacterium avium-intracellulare* in patients with AIDS. Although reported less frequently, the radiographic findings cannot be distinguished from early esophageal ulceration due to CMV.

CMV gastritis also is seen in patients with AIDS, and the radiographic findings are similar to those seen in the esophagus. The most frequent findings are punctate ulceration, thickened folds, and limited distensibility[1] (Fig. 63-8). Similarly, the findings of CMV colitis range from a diffuse pattern of nodular hyperplasia to ischemic necrosis (such as deep ulceration) and very thickened folds due to submucosal hemorrhage.[3] Plain films may reveal signs of toxic megacolon (Fig. 63-9) or perforation. Hemorrhagic CMV colitis may be the cause of death in some patients with AIDS. The diagnosis is confirmed by endoscopic biopsy, and treatment with ganciclovir (DHPG) produces a response in almost 75% of patients.[10] *Cryptosporidium* organisms are protozoa known to cause a self-limiting diarrhea in new-born calves. Before the AIDS epidemic, it rarely caused illness in humans,

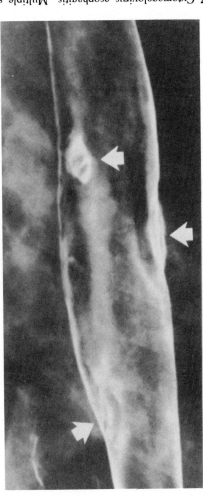

Fig. 63-7 Cytomegalovirus esophagitis. Multiple superficial ulcerations (*arrows*) are present in esophagus of this 27-year-old man with AIDS. Endoscopy and biopsy demonstrated CMV. (From Balthazar, EJ, et al: AJR 149:919, 1987.)

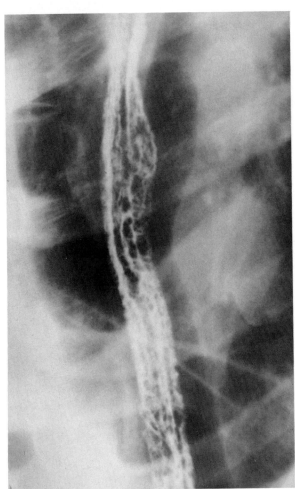

Fig. 63-6 Monilial esophagitis. Severe disease is manifested by focal ulceration (*arrow*) among diffuse nodular irregularity (cobblestoning), with barium collections among interstices of *Candida* plaques.

but it is currently the most frequent cause of enteritis in patients with AIDS. Thickened small bowel folds are most often seen in the duodenum and jejunum. Mild dilatation, fragmentation, and increased secretions may be seen. Cholera-like symptoms may be severe and debilitating, with passage of as much as 10 to 17 L of fluid per day.[4] The diagnosis is confirmed by an examination of stool or duodenal aspirate. *Isospora belli* is a related protozoan that commonly infects the small bowel in association with *Cryptosporidium*. The former can be treated, but rarely is an isolated pathogen. To date, there is no effective treatment for cryptosporidiosis.

Mycobacterium avium-intracellulare (MAI), an atypical bacterium, also can cause enteritis. Barium examination reveals a "pseudo-Whipple" pattern with mild dilation and irregular thickened folds with fine nodularity.[23]

AIDS-RELATED CHOLANGITIS

Acalculous inflammation of the biliary tract in patients with AIDS is thought to be caused by opportunistic infection by *Cryptosporidium* and/or CMV,[7] both of which have been noted in the bile and duodenal contents of such patients. Patients with AIDS-related cholangitis typically present with right upper quadrant and/or epigastric pain, jaundice, or abnormal liver function tests.[7] Nausea, vomiting, and fever also may be present. Computed tomography and ultrasound demonstrate intrahepatic and extrahepatic bile duct dilatation and thickening of the wall of the gallbladder and bile ducts. Endoscopic retrograde

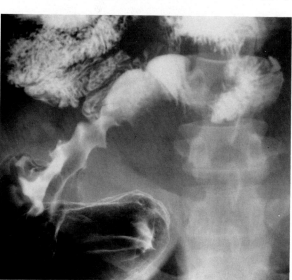

Fig. 63-8 CMV gastritis. Marked thickening of gastric rugal folds and limited distensibility of the body and antrum of stomach was biopsy-proven to be caused by CMV. Multiple superficial ulcerations were seen at endoscopy. (From Balthazar, EJ, Megibow, AJ, and Hulnick, DH: AJR 144:1201, 1985.)

cholangiography demonstrates stricturing and focal dilation like that seen in sclerosing cholangitis.[7,24] (Fig. 63-10). However, papillary stenosis also is seen. The signs and symptoms of AIDS-related cholangitis sometimes are relieved temporarily by endoscopic papillotomy, but this procedure may be complicated by gram-negative bacterial cholangitis.

COMPUTED TOMOGRAPHY

Computed tomography (CT) can sometimes differentiate a patient with AIDS from one with the AIDS-related complex (ARC).[16] CT scans of homosexual men with ARC demonstrates the following triad: (1) splenomegaly (with or without hepatomegaly); (2) increased numbers of small (0.5 to 1.0 cm) lymph nodes in the retroperitoneum and/or mesentery; and (3) rectal thickening with increased attenuation of the perirectal fat. In contrast, large (greater than 1.5 cm) lymph nodes more likely are a manifestation of AIDS because of involvement with lymphoma, MAI (Fig. 63-11), possibly Kaposi's sarcoma. Central low attenuation within the en-

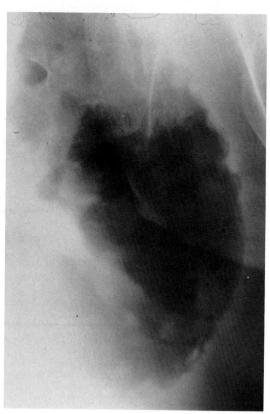

Fig. 63-9 CMV colitis. Plain film of abdomen taken 1 hour before death demonstrates findings of toxic megacolon with diffuse nodular irregularity within air-distended colon. Autopsy confirmed hemorrhagic colitis due to CMV to be cause of death in this patient with AIDS.

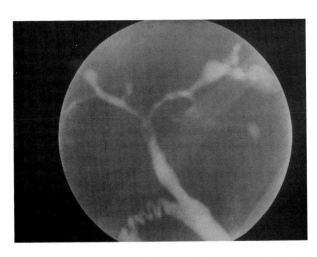

Fig. 63-10 AIDS cholangitis. ERCP demonstrates irregular narrowing of intrahepatic and extrahepatic bile duct as well as focal narrowing of the gallbladder neck *(arrow)*.
(From Dolmatch, BL, et al: Radiology 163:313, 1987.)

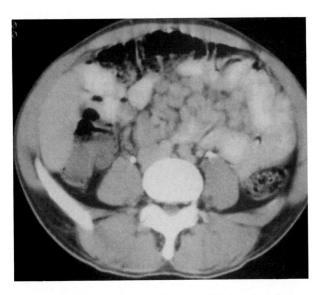

Fig. 63-11 Mesenteric lymphadenopathy. Moderately enlarged lymph nodes are noted throughout mesentery in this patient with AIDS and biopsy-culture proven *Mycobacterium avium-intracellulare*.
(From Wall, SD: Contemp Diag Radiol 9(20)1, 1986.)

larged nodes suggests MAI; very large, bulky nodes suggests lymphoma. The CT attenuation of the liver and spleen is homogeneous throughout in ARC. Focal areas of low attenuation in either organ is not seen with ARC, but is seen with AIDS because of opportunistic tumor (lymphoma more often than Kaposi's sarcoma) or opportunistic infection (most often MAI). A CT-guided biopsy can be diagnostic. All aspirates should be cultured for mycobacterium.

MAGNETIC RESONANCE IMAGING

To date, there is limited experience with magnetic resonance imaging in patients with AIDS. Those with enlarged lymph nodes occasionally have had a central area of low-signal intensity, better seen on T_2-weighted images. It is not yet clear that this finding corresponds with the low attenuation seen on CT scans. Further experience may demonstrate increased sensitivity to focal areas of tumor or infection within the liver or other solid organs; both T_1- and T_2- weighted imaging will be helpful.

REFERENCES

1. Balthazar, EJ, Megibow, AJ, and Hulnick, DH: Cytomegalovirus esophagitis and gastritis in AIDS, AJR 144:1201, 1985.
2. Balthazar, EJ, et al: Cytomegalovirus esophagitis in AIDS: radiographic features in 16 patients, AJR 149:919.
3. Balthazar, EJ, et al: Cytomegalovirus colitis in AIDS: radiographic findings in 11 patients, Radiology 155:585, 1985.
4. Berk, RN, et al: Cryptosporidiosis of the stomach and small intestine in patients with AIDS, AJR 143:549, 1984.
5. Centers for Disease Control: Human immunodeficiency virus infection in the United States, MMWR 36:80, 1987.
6. Centers for Disease Control: Recommendations for prevention of HIV transmission in health-care settings, MMWR 36(25):15, 1987.
7. Dolmatch, BL, et al: AIDS-related cholangitis: radiographic findings in nine patients, Radiology 163:313, 1987.
8. Emery, CD, et al: Pharyngeal Kaposi's sarcoma in patients with AIDS, AJR 147:919, 1986.
9. Farman, DJ, et al: Focal esophageal candidiasis in acquired immunodeficiency syndrome (AIDS), Gastrointest Radiol 11:213, 1986.
10. Federle, MDP: A radiologist looks at AIDS: imaging evaluation based on symptom complexes, Radiology 166:553, 1988.
11. Frager, DH, et al: Gastrointestinal complications of AIDS: radiologic features, Radiology 158:605, 1986.
12. Friedman, SL, Wright, TL, and Altman, DF: Gastrointestinal Kaposi's sarcoma in patients with acquired immunodeficiency syndrome: endoscopic and autopsy finding, Gastroenterology 1:102, 1985.
13. Gerberding, JL, et al: Risk of transmitting the human immunodeficiency virus, cytomegalovirus, and hepatitis B virus to health care workers exposed to patients with AIDS and AIDS-related conditions, J Infect Dis 156:1, 1987.
14. Heller, RM, et al: AIDS awareness in the conduct of radiologic procedures: guidelines to safe practice [editorial], Radiology 166:563, 1988.
15. Hill, CA, Harle, TS, and Mansell, PWA: The prodrome, Kaposi's sarcoma and infections associated with acquired immunodeficiency syndrome: radiologic findings in 39 patients, Radiology 149:393, 1983.
16. Jeffrey, RB, Jr, et al: Abdominal CT in acquired immunodeficiency syndrome, AJR 146:7, 1986.
17. Levine, MS, Macones, PJ, and Laufer, I: *Candida* esophagitis: accuracy of radiographic diagnosis, Radiology 154:581, 1985.
18. Nelson, JA, et al: Human immunodeficiency virus detected in bowel epithelium from patients with gastrointestinal symptoms, Lancet p. 259, 1988.
19. Rose, FHS, et al: Alimentary tract involvement in Kaposi sarcoma: radiographic and endoscopic findings in 25 homosexual men, AJR 139:661, 1982.

20. Safai, B, et al: The natural history of Kaposi's sarcoma in the acquired immunodeficiency syndrome, Ann Intern Med 103:744, 1985.

21. Semenkovich, JW, et al: Barium pharyngography: comparison of single and double contrast, AJR 144:715, 1985.

22. St. Onge, G, and Bezahler, GH: Giant esophageal ulcer associated with cytomegalovirus, Gastroenterology 83:127, 1982.

23. Vincent, ME, and Robbins, AH: Mycobacteium avium-intracellulare complex enteritis: pseudo-Whipple's disease in AIDS, AJR 144:921, 1985.

24. Viteri, AL, Greene, JF, Jr: Bile duct abnormalities in the acquired immune deficiency syndrome. Gastro 92:2014, 1987.

25. Wall, SD: Abdominal radiology of acquired immunodeficiency syndrome, Contemp Diag Radiol 9(20):1, 1986.

26. Wall, SD, Friedman, SL, and Margulis, AR: Gastrointestinal Kaposi's sarcoma in AIDS: radiographic manifestations, J Clin Gastroenterol 6:165, 1984.

27. Wall, SD, et al: Multifocal abnormalities of the gastrointestinal tract in AIDS, AJR 146:1, 1986.

28. Ziegler, JL, et al: Non-Hodgkin lymphoma in 90 homosexual men: relation to generalized lymphadenopathy and the acquired immunodeficiency syndrome, N Engl J Med 311:565, 1984.

PART XIII

POSTOPERATIVE RADIOLOGY

64 *Postoperative Radiology*

H. JOACHIM BURHENNE

GENERAL CONSIDERATIONS

Most surgical procedures on the alimentary tract are successful, but postoperative complications remain a common occurrence. The radiologist must be familiar with a large variety of possible surgical complications, because it is this specialty that is most commonly called on to render a definitive diagnosis. The decision for reoperation, for instance, is usually based on results from radiologic imaging techniques. These now include ultrasonography, CT scanning, needle biopsy, and interventional techniques in addition to contrast studies and nuclear medicine investigation.

Technique

Plain abdominal radiography is helpful in the diagnosis of retained foreign bodies and evaluation of postoperative obstruction and perforation. Barium sulfate remains the most useful diagnostic contrast medium when applied as a biphasic technique. It permits evaluation of postoperative mucosal detail and readily demonstrates obstruction. However, when searching for a postoperative leak or a fistula formation, iodinated contrast material is the agent of choice. We proceed with barium sulfate if there is no evidence of free air on multiple radiographic projections.

1551

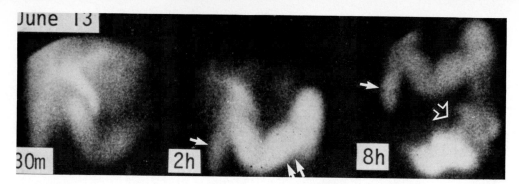

Fig. 64-1 Case 2 demonstrates afferent loop obstruction in patient with subtotal gastrectomy and Billroth II gastroenteroanastomosis for bleeding stomach ulcer. Patient was admitted with epigastric pain that radiated to back and was followed by vomiting. Serial ⁹⁹ᵐTc-IDA images clearly show common duct and afferent loop at 30 minutes. At 2 hours afferent loop contains virtually all the radiopharmaceutical and is markedly dilated *(twin arrows)*. No efferent loop entry was recorded at that time, indicating afferent loop obstruction. This is partial, however, because 8-hour nucleograph depicts distal small bowel activity. Efferent loop is visualized *(open arrow)*. Delayed gallbladder visualization is consistent with chronic cholecystitis *(single solid arrow)*. At surgery afferent loop was dilated to 7 cm, and area of fibrosis and stenosis was found 4 cm proximal to gastroenterostomy.

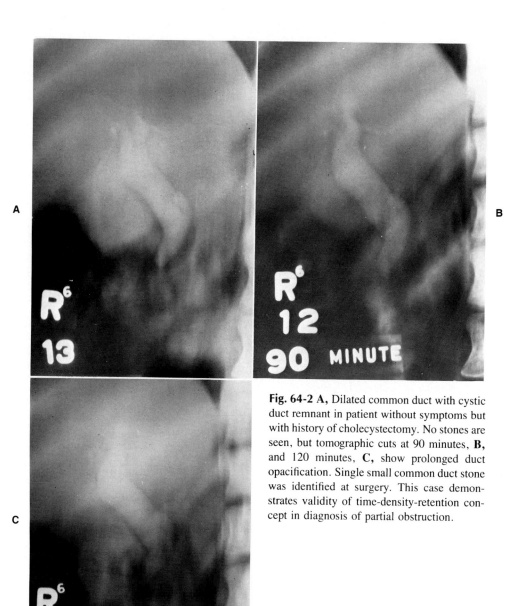

Fig. 64-2 A, Dilated common duct with cystic duct remnant in patient without symptoms but with history of cholecystectomy. No stones are seen, but tomographic cuts at 90 minutes, **B,** and 120 minutes, **C,** show prolonged duct opacification. Single small common duct stone was identified at surgery. This case demonstrates validity of time-density-retention concept in diagnosis of partial obstruction.

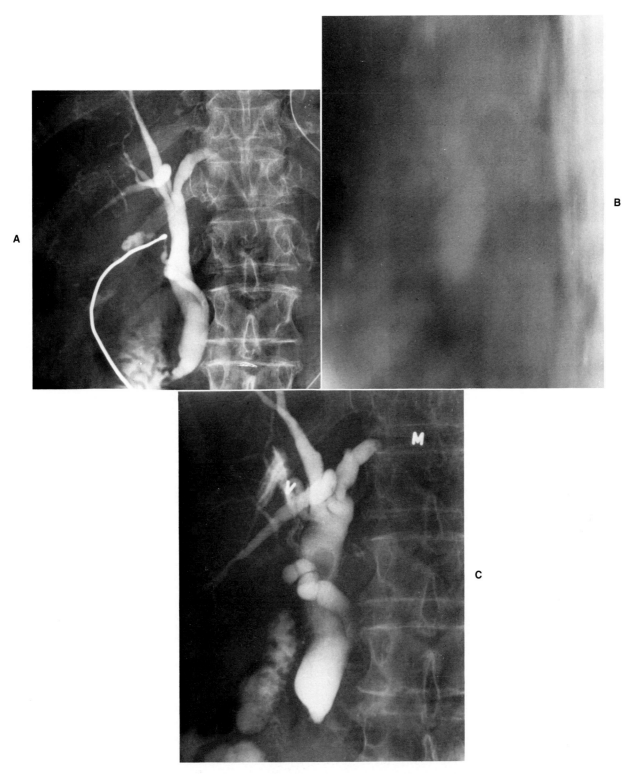

Fig. 64-3 A, Operative cholangiogram in 1977 demonstrates some extrahepatic bile duct dilatation. **B,** Intravenous cholangiography in 1979 demonstrates further dilatation of common hepatic duct in this patient with symptoms. Interval duct dilatation since operative cholangiography indicates partial obstruction. **C,** Transhepatic cholangiogram 1 day after intravenous cholangiography demonstrates common duct stone. Note also long, retained cystic duct remnant.

Isotope studies provide a functional evaluation of the postoperative status by allowing assessment of complications in both upper gastrointestinal and biliary tracts (Fig. 64-1). Intraabdominal bile leaks, for instance, are readily disclosed by serial ^{99m}Tc-IDA imaging.[7]

The technique of intravenous cholangiography has been largely supplanted in recent years with the advent of diagnostic ultrasound and nuclear medicine techniques. The time-density-retention concept of intravenous cholangiography demonstrates partial obstruction in a fashion similar to that of nuclear medicine investigation (Fig. 64-2). Interval increase in the size of the extrahepatic bile ducts after operation is now better identified with ultrasonography, particularly since common duct stones are often not visualized with intravenous cholangiography, even when tomography is an added technique (Fig. 64-3). Intravenous cholangiography with meglumine iotroxate (Biliscopin, Schering AG, Berlin), a new intravenous contrast agent, is still in use in European centers. Recent reports have demonstrated a high diagnostic yield when preoperative infusion cholangiography is compared to routine operative cholangiography.[1]

Reoperation

The importance and frequency of postoperative complications with regard to the alimentary tract are amplified by statistics of reoperation. If one eliminates figures for simple appendectomy, the reoperation rate after surgery on the alimentary tract is approximately 5%. Reoperation is accompanied by an operative mortality significantly higher than that associated with the original surgical procedure. Thus, of 100 patients undergoing surgery, five will require early reoperation and two of these will die in spite of the secondary procedure.[11] The most common indications for reoperation are bleeding, obstruction, fistula, and peritonitis.

Pulmonary complications

In spite of advances in care of the surgical patient, pulmonary problems continue to constitute the most frequent postoperative complications: primarily atelectasis, pneumonia, thromboembolism, and aspiration.[10] These are seen in 10% of patients.

Abscesses

Abscesses continue to be a common occurrence after surgery on the alimentary tract. The most common location is subphrenic, with 52% of abscesses occurring after surgery on the gastric and biliary tracts. The bacterial flora consists of multiple strains of aerobic and anaerobic organisms. The overall mortality is 30% for patients with subphrenic abscesses.[9] In some reports as many as 42% of patients died, but the results are better if the abscess cavity is adequately drained.[2]

The subphrenic space is dependent in position and

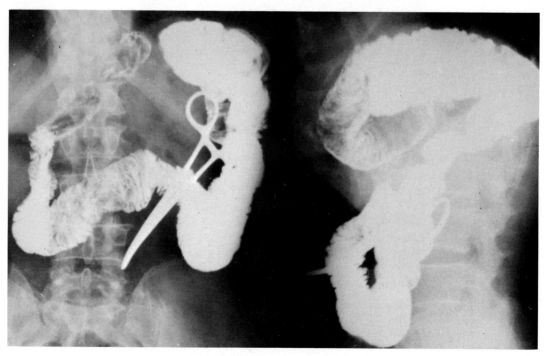

Fig. 64-4 Retained hemostat after gastroduodenostomy, seen in anteroposterior and lateral projections.

potentially large, but the clinical diagnosis is often difficult or impossible. Many subphrenic abscesses exhibit few localizing symptoms. Clinical features may be masked when the patient is receiving antibiotics for presumed sepsis located elsewhere.[8] Patients with pleural effusion or diaphragmatic elevation or both require further examination with more modern imaging modalities, such as ultrasonography[5] or CT scanning. The same imaging techniques are used frequently today by radiologists as a guide for percutaneous abscess drainage.

Retained foreign matter

Surgical instruments or sponges may be retained after surgery on the alimentary tract (Fig. 64-4).[3] Manufacturers use saturated barium sulfate in plastic compounds to prepare sponge indicators in the form of a string or ribbon. Federal specifications call for discernibility under ⅝ inch of aluminum ladder (Fig. 64-5). Retained surgical sponges may result in encapsulated abscesses, chronic sinus tracts, fecal fistulas, and erosion into neighboring viscera.[6] Sponge indicators may change their radiographic appearance after they disintegrate, and the result may be abscess formation, but standardized surgical sponges are usually readily recognized on plain radiographs (Fig. 64-6). CT scanning may be of help in detecting retained sponges, particularly if they do not contain radiopaque markers.[4] Anteroposterior and lateral radiographs are usually sufficient to give an immediate answer to the location of any retained surgical device.[12] Early recognition of retained surgical sponges will prevent possible complications (Figs. 64-7 and 64-8).

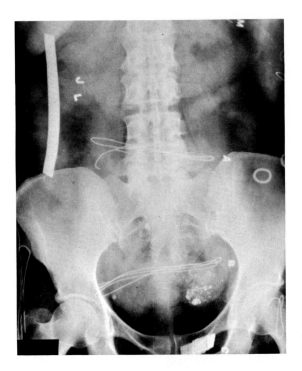

Fig. 64-5 Samples of indicators used for sponges of various sizes made by different manufacturers. Sample radiograph, obtained by draping material over abdomen, is kept in radiology department for reference.

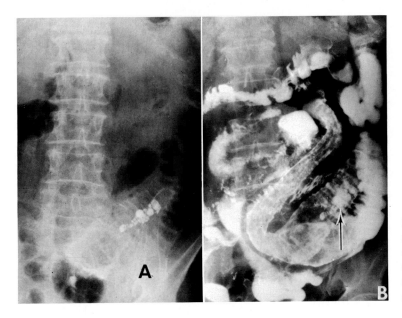

Fig. 64-6 A, Retained sponge 8 weeks after laparotomy, with atypical appearance of opaque indicator seen on plain radiograph. **B,** Sponge indicator is beginning to disintegrate in presence of surrounding small bowel inflammation and abscess formation.

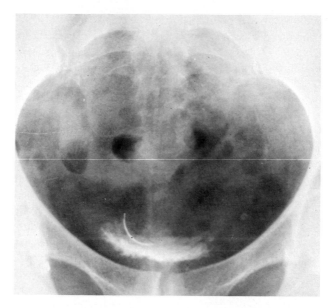

Fig. 64-7 Retained needle beginning to create symptoms 8 years after surgery.

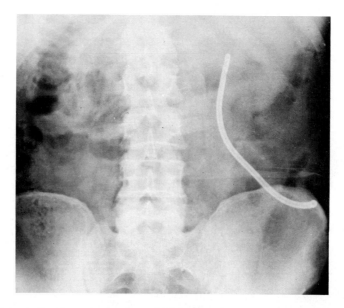

Fig. 64-8 Abdominal radiograph of patient with persistent sinus drainage. Catheter was expected and not reported by radiologist. However, unknown to surgeon, this catheter had slipped completely inside sinus and was responsible for continuous drainage.

ESOPHAGUS[13-47]

A wide variety of esophageal surgical procedures have been devised, primarily for correction of a hiatus hernia and gastroesophageal reflux. It is not surprising that the postoperative complication rate is high when we realize that the operations are destructive in nature and when we consider the uncertainties concerning normal function of the esophagogastric junction.[36]

Instrumentation

Perforation of the esophagus is the most serious possible complication during esophagoscopy, gastroscopy, dilatation of the esophagus, tamponade for esophageal varices, or simple intubation of the esophagus for any reason. The fiberesophagoscopy perforation rate is nearly 0.5%, representing no significant improvement in safety over older semirigid esophagoscopes,[30] and the more fre-

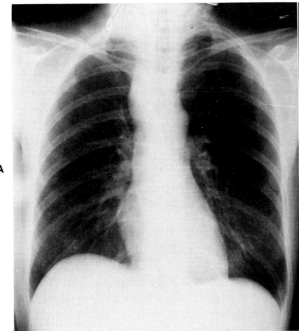

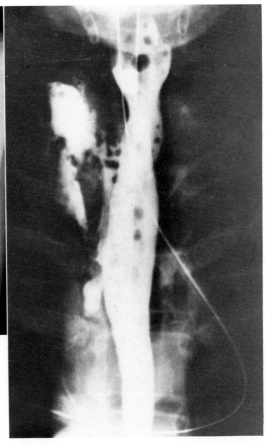

A   B

Fig. 64-9 Esophageal perforation and mediastinal abscess 24 hours after esophagoscopy. **A,** Right superior mediastinal widening. **B,** Gastrografin study demonstrates point of esophageal perforation.

quent use of fiberendoscopes in comparison with previously developed instruments has led to an increase in the number of perforations.[32] Not only the incidence but also the location of perforation with the fiberscope are similar to those with rigid esophagoscope.[35]

Pneumomediastinum and subcutaneous emphysema are the most frequent radiographic findings with esophageal perforation; others are widening of the mediastinum and pleural effusion. Contrast studies with water-soluble media should identify the point of perforation. The early diagnosis of perforation of the esophagus is most important, because this injury represents a surgical emergency demanding immediate treatment in order to decrease mortality[46] (Fig. 64-9).

The incidence of instrumental perforation of the esophagus has been stated as one to five times in every 1000 endoscopic examinations,[36] but perforation after dilatation for achalasia occurs approximately 10 to 15 times in every 1000 procedures.

Esophageal perforation as an iatrogenic injury has also been reported with insertion of nasogastric tubes, upper airway suctioning, passage of feeding tubes, inadvertent placement of endotracheal tubes into the cervical esophagus, and with use of the Sengstaken-Blakemore tube.[25] Endoscopic pneumatic balloon dilatation for achalasia

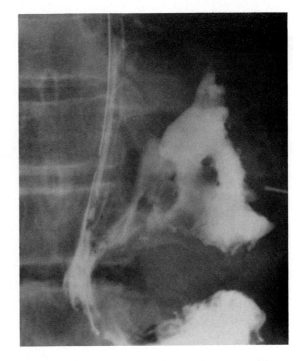

Fig. 64-10 Distal esophageal perforation demonstrated by contrast study after endoscopic pneumatic balloon dilatation for achalasia.

Endoscopic pneumatic balloon dilatation for achalasia may result in perforation of the esophagus (Fig. 64-10).[13]

A thorough review of iatrogenic complications involving the esophagus has been presented by Meyers and Ghahremani.[33]

Correction of hiatus hernia and gastroesophageal reflux

The objectives of surgery for a hiatus hernia or gastroesophageal reflux involve restoration or normal anatomic relationships at the esophagogastric junction, with additional construction of a valve or closing mechanism. Surgical results, postoperative complications, and the radiologic appearance vary for the different operations.

Allison's repair

Allison's hiatus hernia repair[14] is less commonly used today. After the distal esophagus is elevated from the mediastinum and dissected to expose the crura, sutures are placed to approximate the crura, and mattress sutures are placed through the diaphragm. The hiatus should be snug about the esophagus, just permitting the passage of a fingertip. A thoracic approach is used. Recurrence rate of hiatus hernia on radiologic examination is about 30%

of cases for paraesophageal hernias but is larger for sliding hiatus hernias. Not all patients with radiologic recurrence have recurrence of symptoms.

Esophagogastropexy

Esophagogastropexy involves traction of the distal esophagus into the abdominal cavity and fixation of the gastric fundus to its left margin with two rows of sutures. It increases the entrance angle of the esophagus into the stomach at the cardia and elongates the abdominal portion of the esophagus. These changes are apparent on radiographic examination, with the gastric air bubble closely approximating the diaphragmatic hiatus.

Posterior gastropexy (Hill)

According to Hill,[28] the key to the formation of a sliding hiatus hernia is failure or attenuation of the posterior attachment of the esophagus to the preaortic fascia. His corrective surgical procedure involves transabdominal reduction of the hernia, closure of the hiatus posterior to the esophagus, and anchoring of the gastroesophageal junction to the preaortic fascia and median arcuate ligament, resulting in posterior gastropexy. The distortion by the posterior gastropexy of the fundus is best seen radiologically on lateral views (Fig. 64-11).

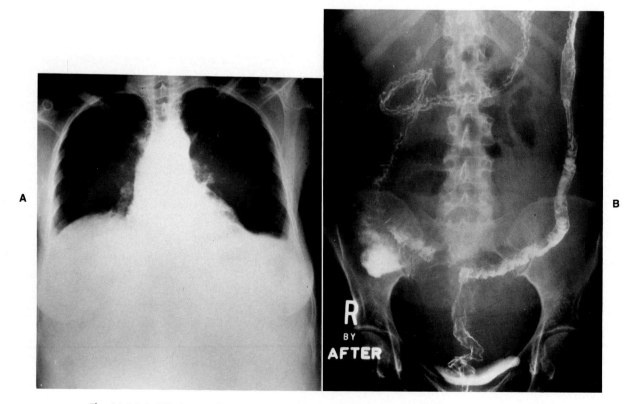

Fig. 64-11 A, Diaphragmatic elevation and left pleural effusion in patient with inadvertent ligature of thoracic duct during posterior gastropexy. **B,** Chylous ascites in same patient.

Anterior gastropexy (Nissen 1)

Nissen's procedure[34] employs a simple anterior gastropexy in which the stomach is sutured to the anterior abdominal wall. The procedure is applicable only when the hernia is reducible. The objections have been that the sutures holding the gastropexy may cut through the stomach, or the abdominal wall may relax, permitting recurrence of the hernia. Early postoperative radiographic investigation with follow-up studies should identify recurrence. Nissen found that a hiatus hernia complicated by reflux esophagitis needed a different surgical approach, and he added fundoplication to gastropexy to

prevent reflux. This combined operation is his procedure of choice today for treating a sliding hiatus hernia.

Fundoplication (Nissen 2)

The abdominal esophagus is usually mobilized through an abdominal approach. The posterior aspect of the fundus is then placed behind the abdominal esophagus from left to right and wrapped around it to form a cuff that is sutured together anteriorly for about 5 cm (Fig. 64-12). A wide-bore esophageal tube is in place throughout the procedure to ensure an adequate esophageal diameter.[34]

The upper gastrointestinal study after Nissen's fundoplication often shows elongation of the abdominal portion of the esophagus, with the gastric air bubble in the fundus adjacent to it. The cuff of the gastric fundus narrows the distal esophagus to prevent reflux, but narrowing may be so pronounced that an inability to belch exists. Permanent gaseous distention of the fundus is present on abdominal radiographs. Other possible complications of fundoplication such as separation of sutures, abscess formation, and fistula formation are also best demonstrated by radiologic investigation. If preliminary films show no evidence of free air, barium is the contrast agent of choice. The radiographic appearance after Nissen's fundoplication has been well described.[42] The mass-like deformity of the fundus must be differentiated from a neoplasm. All types of fundoplication may give the radiographic appearance of a pseudotumor. Pseudotumors that diminished in size during the early postoperative period and then remained constant were seen in 33 of 34 patients in one report.[23] The postoperative appearance may also simulate a paraesophageal hernia.[26] Cineradiography aids in the postoperative detection of re-

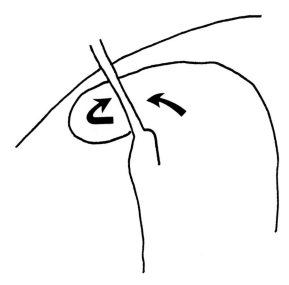

Fig. 64-12 Nissen's fundoplication. Medial portion of gastric fundus is placed behind distal esophagus from left to right and then sutured in front of it to construct fundal cuff around it.

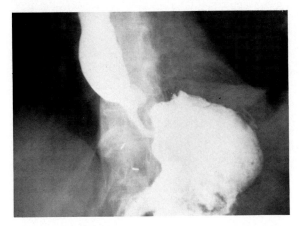

Fig. 64-13 Tight distal esophageal channel after fundoplication with esophageal distention and partial obstruction. Patient also has plication defect on lesser curvature after gastrojejunostomy.

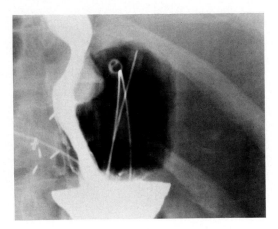

Fig. 64-14 Pseudotumor after fundoplication.

flux even when conventional methods produce normal results.[38] Another complication of fundoplication is postoperative diaphragmatic herniation resulting from disruption of the diaphragmatic incision. The supradiaphragmatic portion of the stomach may incarcerate or present as a volvulus on radiographic studies[15] (Figs. 64-13 and 64-14).

Mark IV procedure (Belsey)

The esophagogastric junction and cardia are mobilized, and the acute esophagogastric angle is restored by plicating the stomach to the esophagus. This restores the abdominal segment of the esophagus. A snug closure of the esophageal hiatus of the diaphragm behind the esophagus is then accomplished by approximation of the separated right crus.[16] The radiologic examination demonstrates the pseudotumor decreasing in size over the first few postoperative weeks. Early esophageal narrowing caused by surgical edema must be differentiated from possible stricture of the elongated abdominal portion of the esophagus.[19]

The characteristic features of the radiologic appearance of common hiatus hernia repairs have also been described by Feigen and associates.[24] Radiologic examination is also helpful in identifying the maintenance of antireflux prosthetic devices inserted into the esophagogastric junction, a more recent technique[31] (Fig. 64-15).

Stricture repair

The procedure by Thal[43] was designed for patients with a fibrous stricture in the distal esophagus caused by reflux esophagitis. A left thoracotomy approach is used. The strictured area is incised, and the incision is extended into the upper portion of the stomach. This defect is covered by the serosal surface of the proximal stomach, which is wrapped over it, enlarging the previous stricture. The procedure may be modified by a fundoplication. The radiographic changes include a large air-filled sac overlying the left cardiac border on the chest radiograph and the barium column in the esophagus separated from the gastric fundus by a radiolucent vertical line.[22] The pseudotumor seen with hiatus hernia may also be present after the Thal procedure[21] (Fig. 64-16).

Other benign lesions

The radiographic appearances after repair of esophageal lesions in the pediatric age group are described in Chapter 69. Radiologic examination is important not only to follow-up of these conditions, including esophageal atresia, chalasia, achalasia, and duplication cysts, but also after correction of symptomatic lower esophageal rings, esophageal webs, and diverticula. Complications of pneumatic dilatations and distal esophageal myotomy are best diagnosed by radiologic techniques. Recurrence, fistula formation, perforation, and disordered motility are

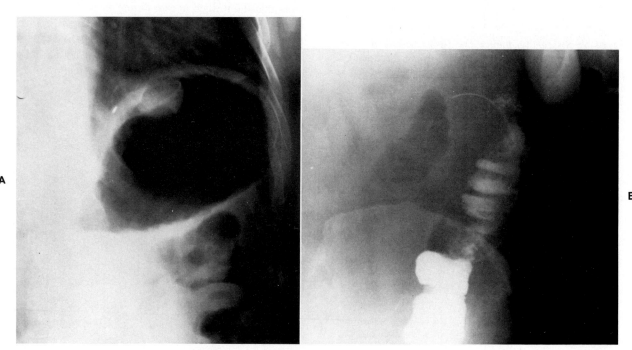

A   **B**

Fig. 64-15 A, Antireflux ring prosthesis placed for correction of esophagogastric reflux. **B,** Prosthetic device separated and migrated into left lower quadrant and was surgically removed.
(Courtesy Dr. L. Warren Burhenne.)

readily detected. The most common complication noted after Heller esophagomyotomy is reflux esophagitis.[11] Eccentric ballooning at the site of myotomy should be recognized as a normal and frequent postoperative finding.[41] Fistula formation and recurrence are the most common complications after surgery for epiphrenic diverticula.

The radiologic appearance of the distal esophagus after sclerotherapy for varices often shows longitudinal tram-like filling defects and eccentric patchy and nodular defects.[40] Radiologic changes seen in the mediastinum and pleural space on CT scanning are other changes described after the use of sclerosing agents.[29]

Esophageal resection and reconstruction

Benign or malignant lesions of the esophagus may require resection or a bypass (Fig. 64-17). Carcinoma and benign strictures are the common indications. Reconstruction with jejunum, colon, stomach, or tubes formed from the stomach are procedures in use (Figs. 64-18 to 64-20). Viscera used for a palliative bypass or reconstruction of the esophagus may be placed subcutaneously, in the retrosternal space, or into the thorax. The indications for preoperative radiologic studies were reviewed by Calenoff and Norfray.[18] Common early postoperative complications include fistula or stricture formation at the cervical anastomosis, transplant gangrene,

and gastric stasis. Late complications include reflux, stricture at the distal anastomosis, gastric stasis, and recurrent carcinoma. Disruption or a stricture at the cervical anastomosis occurs in a third of the patients. Radiologic studies with an iodinated contrast medium are most helpful in investigating postoperative problems (Fig. 64-21).

Permanent esophageal intubation has been used to maintain patency in obstructing benign or malignant lesions. A variety of tubes are in use.[47] Complications from surgical placement of tubes for esophageal cancer are significantly decreased if radiologic balloon dilatation precedes the surgical procedure.[20] Obstruction or displacement of Celestin tubes may be verified by radiologic means (Fig. 64-22).

Reversed gastric tubes fashioned from the stomach may be used for reconstruction,[27] but mobilization of the entire stomach for total esophageal replacement has gained renewed interest. Arteriographic studies have demonstrated that the viability of the fundus is not dependent on anastomotic circulation.[44] The radiographic appearance of the esophagus and stomach after laser treatment for obstructing carcinoma[45] and the radiographic patterns indicative of recurrence of esophageal carcinoma after transhiatal esophagectomy and gastric interposition[17] have recently been described. Fistula formation from the esophagus to the trachea may occur after

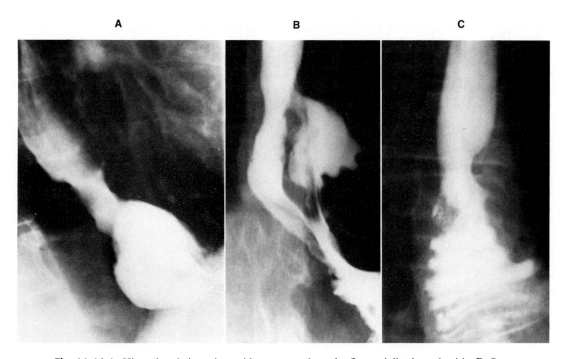

Fig. 64-16 A, Hiatus hernia in patient with gastroesophageal reflux and distal esophagitis. **B,** Same patient after Thal procedure with fistula between esophageal stricture incision and serosal patch of gastric fundus. **C,** Jejunoesophagogastric interposition after revision of previous (Thal) procedure.

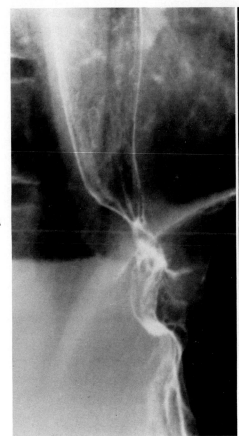

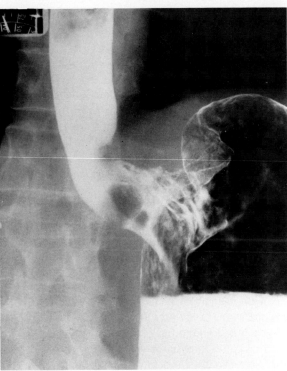

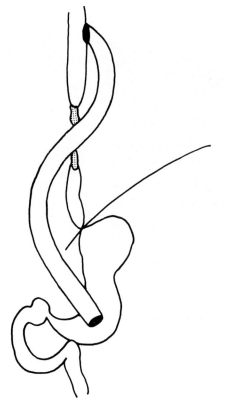

Fig. 64-17 A, Mass and constriction at esophagogastric junction due to villous adenoma. **B,** Malignant recurrence 2 years after resection.
(Courtesy Dr. Morgan Parkes.)

Fig. 64-18 Bypass procedure for esophageal carcinoma with interposed segment of jejunum demonstrating proximal and distal anastomosis.

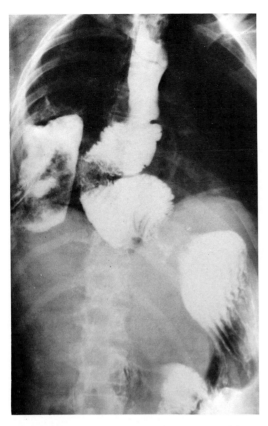

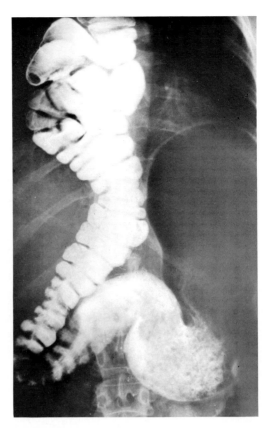

Fig. 64-19 Distal esophageal resection and jejunal interposition. Partial obstruction is caused by fibrosis at jejunogastrostomy; there is also jejunal perforation into right pleural space.

Fig. 64-20 Vagotomy without pyloroplasty, resulting in gastric outlet obstruction in patient with colonic esophagogastric interposition.

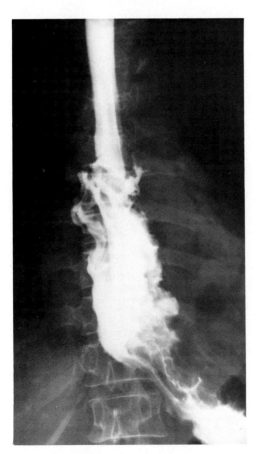

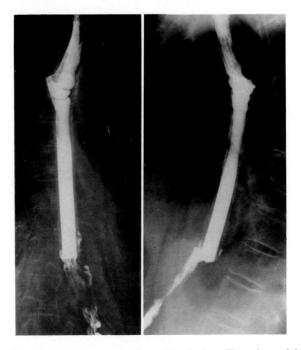

Fig. 64-21 Gastric interposition after resection of small distal esophageal carcinoma.

Fig. 64-22 Permanent esophageal intubation. There is partial obstruction at distal end that is due to relative stiffness of Celestin tube. Mechanical difficulty is not apparent on anteroposterior projection.

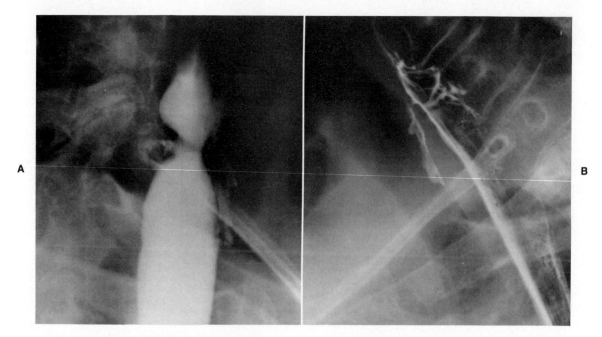

Fig. 64-23 A, Malignant stricture in high esophagus after radiation therapy demonstrates extravasation. **B,** Air contrast study demonstrates esophagotracheal fistula.

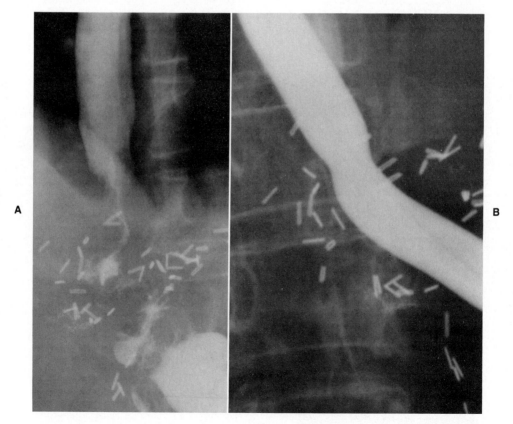

Fig. 64-24 A, Esophagojejunostomy narrowing after total gastric resection for carcinoma. **B,** Radiologic balloon dilatation of the anastomosis was readily accomplished under fluoroscopy, but symptom relief from obstruction could not be obtained. Endoscopic biopsy revealed tumor recurrence at the esophagojejunostomy anastomosis.

radiation therapy for esophageal carcinoma (Fig. 64-23).

Radiologic interventional techniques for esophageal stricture dilatation are described in Chapter 78 (Fig. 64-24).

Vagotomy

Esophageal complications after vagotomy are infrequent but may be serious. They can be classified into three categories: (1) those resulting from operative injury, such as perforation, devascularization, or periesophageal hemorrhage; (2) postoperative dysphagia caused by neurogenic disorder, edema and hematoma formation, periesophageal fibrosis, or esophagitis and (3) the development of a hiatus hernia, which is usually a late complication.[37] Transient postvagotomy dysphagia in the early postoperative period characteristically occurs with the first ingestion of solid foods on the seventh to fourteenth postoperative days. The dysphagia is accompanied by the typical radiographic findings. Persistent tapered narrowing of the terminal 3 to 4 cm of the esophagus may also be present.[39]

STOMACH AND DUODENUM[48-266]
Gastric surgery

The incidence of peptic ulcer disease is decreasing. Estimates in the 1960s that 7.5% of the population in America and England had peptic ulcer disease and that at least 1% of these patients underwent gastric surgery each year are no longer true.[50,67] The decrease had occurred mainly for duodenal ulcer disease and duodenal ulcer surgery and has been estimated to be at least 30% for these.[176,232] Duodenal ulcer, however, remains three or four times more common than gastric ulcer disease clinically. It has become clearer that gastric ulcer is a different entity from duodenal ulcer. One of three gastric ulcers may be related to the use of medication.[83] Alcohol users are also more likely to be subjects of gastric ulcers.

Choice of operative procedure

There is no general agreement as to the proper operation for the patient with intractable duodenal ulcer, or gastric ulcer. The physician must be guided by the surgeon's skill and preferences.[233]

Surgical procedures for peptic disease may be divided into three groups or combinations thereof: gastrectomy, vagotomy, and added drainage operations. The gastrectomy may be distal, pylorus preserving, proximal, or total. Vagotomy may be truncal, total gastric, proximal gastric, or selective. Added drainage operations include pyloroplasty and gastrojejunostomy.[231] The operative mortality is 10% for total gastrectomy, 2% for partial gastrectomy, and 1% or less for vagotomy.

Proximal gastric vagotomy is the safest antiulcer operation with regard to mortality. It has been used more commonly since its description in 1970.[53] The vagal nerves to the gastric fundus and corpus are divided, but those to the gastric antrum, pylorus, and all the other abdominal viscera are left intact. Because the gastric antrum and pylorus are not vagally denervated, an added gastric drainage procedure need not accompany the selective vagotomy. Fistulas, peritonitis, and intraabdominal abscesses are unlikely after proximal gastric vagotomy, but the incidence of recurrent ulcers after this procedure is as yet unknown; the incidence appears to be 5%,[231] which is higher than for partial gastrectomy where the antrum has been removed. A controlled randomized trial of highly selective vagotomy versus selective vagotomy and pyloroplasty in the treatment of patients with duodenal ulcer revealed a 22% persistence or recurrence of ulcers.[154]

As a general rule it seems clear that very different gastric operations for duodenal ulcer give similar functional results.[145] Vagotomy combined with antrectomy is generally considered by most surgeons the operation of choice in good-risk patients, whereas vagotomy with drainage is reserved for elderly and poor-risk patients.[233]

Radiology in postoperative examination of the stomach

Contrast-enhanced radiologic examination remains the most important tool in the diagnosis of both early and late complications of operations on the stomach and duodenum (Fig. 64-25). Obstruction, retention, and fistulas are clearly shown; most benign and malignant recurrences are diagnosed; and functional postgastrectomy abnormalities are successfully investigated.

The radiologist must remember that food ingestion and symptoms of certain postoperative disorders occur primarily with the patient erect. Upright radiographs are therefore taken in patients with retention and dumping. Delayed films at 30 and 60 minutes are used to evaluate retention in the gastric pouch or proximal loop.

It is important to assess the preference of emptying from the gastric pouch in either the proximal or the distal jejunum. Radiographs may be obtained with the patient semierect or recumbent. If this does not clarify the layout of the anastomosis, the patient is turned through a complete circle in the erect position during the drinking of contrast agent in order to separate the two anastomotic loops. This procedure also helps the radiologist determine the length of the proximal loop and whether the jejunum was attached in a retrocolic or antecolic fashion. Cinefluorography is particularly helpful in recording and studying preferential emptying in either jejunal loop and in studying the position of these loops in relation to the stomach and colon.

Radiologic assessment of the amount of stomach remaining may be misleading, since the gastric pouch reduces in size when a large stoma and rapid emptying are present. It may enlarge when the stoma is small.

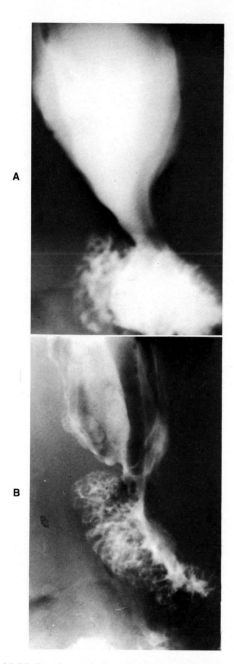

Fig. 64-25 Routine technique for postoperative examination includes full-column films, **A,** and mucosal air contrast studies of gastric pouch, stoma, and anastomotic loop, **B.**

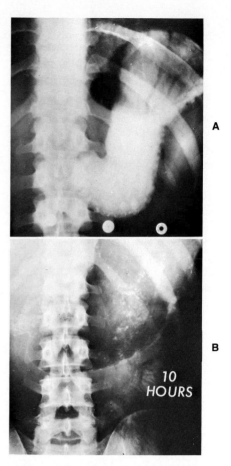

Fig. 64-26 Early postoperative contrast study after vagotomy and pyloroplasty. **A,** With patient in supine position, retention simulates gastric outlet obstruction. **B,** Delayed film of same patient after he was turned to right lateral decubitus position. Emptying occurred by gravity, but gastric atony persists.

Patients with gastric retention after vagotomy or pyloroplasty must be examined in the right lateral decubitus position (Fig. 64-26). Contrast material retained in the aperistaltic stomach with the patient supine may simulate pyloric obstruction. The contrast medium of choice is barium with an added suspending agent, but an iodinated contrast medium is recommended if an anastomotic leak or blowout of the duodenal stump is suspected and if free air is present on routine abdominal radiographs. A more physiologic contrast medium[166] or a mixture of barium

and food may be used.[220] Hiemsche[133] observed hypotonia and widening of the gastric remnant with more functional behavior and with intermittent discharge through the stoma when food was used. Barium solutions pass more rapidly through the anastomosis. A mixture of food and barium will allow more realistic assessment of partial obstruction than will liquid barium[79] (Fig. 64-27).

Accuracy in diagnosing almost all postgastrectomy sequelae increases if postoperative radiologic baseline studies are obtained. They are invaluable for later comparison and represent a necessary part of the surgical record. Unnecessary surgery for suspected tumors in patients with plication defects, for instance, can be avoided if baseline studies are available. Although this postoperative radiologic study has been strongly recommended by surgeons, gastroenterologists, and radiologists alike,[127,165,264] it is usually not done because of the added expense, difficulties in follow-up, and lack of

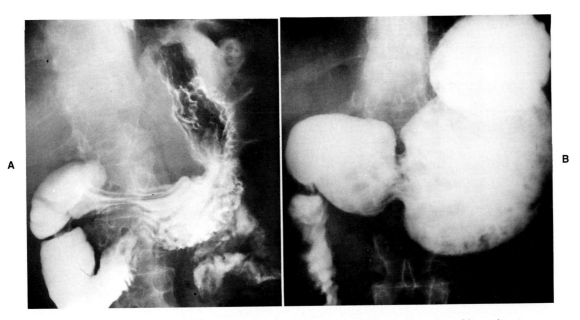

Fig. 64-27 A, Patient with history of previous duodenostomy presenting symptoms of intermittent obstruction. Slight narrowing resulting from scarring, but no obstruction, is seen in descending duodenum. **B,** Partial obstruction is demonstrated with use of mixture of food and barium on same day subsequent to routine upper gastrointestinal contrast investigation.

persistence by the physician. Because edema at the anastomosis usually subsides within 2 weeks,[151,219] the baseline study is best obtained at about 2 or 3 weeks after the gastrectomy.[254]

The complete radiographic evaluation of any patient after gastrectomy includes the identification of 12 basic variants of gastric surgery[78]:

1. Extent of gastric resection
2. End or side anastomosis
3. Anterior or posterior anastomosis
4. Superior or inferior anastomosis
5. Large or small stomal diameter
6. Slow or rapid gastric emptying
7. Antecolic or retrocolic gastrojejunostomy
8. Right-to-left or left-to-right direction of anastomosis
9. Short or long proximal jejunal limb
10. Horizontal or oblique plane of anastomosis
11. Direction of gastric emptying
12. Evidence of previous vagotomy

The identification of these variants is the key to postgastrectomy diagnosis and enables the radiologist to reconstruct the operative procedure performed.

Radiographic anatomy and terminology of gastric surgery

The radiologist must be familiar with all types of gastric operations (Table 64-1). Many varieties of gastroduodenostomy and gastrojejunostomy are performed (Fig. 64-28).

If all variants of gastric surgery are analyzed, 12 basic components become evident (Table 64-1). Different combinations of these variants determine different surgical procedures. The knowledge of these building stones is fundamental to the understanding of postoperative anatomy and disease. Accurate diagnostic interpretation of postgastrectomy radiographs depends on an analysis of these components of surgical anatomy in any patient.

Eponyms and descriptive terminology

The eponyms used to designate various operative procedures on the stomach differ, and no uniformity exists.[78] Eponyms therefore serve a limited purpose in the patient's record. In radiology of the postoperative alimentary tract, descriptive terminology is best for all purposes. It is precise and may be applied to any existing or further operative modification. Examples of descriptive terminology for postoperative radiologic anatomy are given in Fig. 64-29.

The more common eponyms used in North America may be defined as follows:

Billroth I—Any partial gastrectomy (antrectomy) with gastroduodenostomy

Billroth II—All varieties of partial gastrectomy (antrectomy) and gastrojejunostomy

Pólya—Any antrectomy with gastrojejunostomy in which the entire cut end of the stomach is used for the anastomosis

Hofmeister—An antrectomy with gastrojejunostomy with a restricted stoma and partial closure of the cut end of the stomach; at present, the names *Polya* and *Hofmeister* are

☐ **TABLE 64-1**

Systematic arrangement of gastric operations according to their morphologic alterations

No gastric reaction—no anastomosis		Partial gastric resection and enteroanastomosis—cont'd	
Gastrotomy	For exploration	Gastrectomy with gastrojejunostomy	May be end-to-side, side-to-side, or end-to-end, with full or restricted stoma, retrocolic or antecolic, right-to-left or left-to-right anastomosis
Gastrostomy	For feeding or decompression		
Gastropexy or gastrorrhaphy	For ptosis, volvulus, and herniation		
Simple excision	For ulcer	**Total gastrectomy**	
Simple closure	For perforation	Esophagojejunostomy	May be end-to-end or end-to-side
Gastroplasty	For stenosis		
Pylorotomy	For stenosis	Esophagoduodenostomy	May be end-to-end
Pyloroplasty	For drainage		
Vagotomy	For ulcer therapy, complete or selective	Interposition operation	Utilizing small or large bowel or ileocolic segment; may be performed with partial gastrectomy or esophagectomy
Enteroanastomosis—no gastric resection			
Gastroduodenostomy	For pyloric obstruction and drainage	**Combined operations**	
		Vagotomy	
Gastroenterostomy	For ulcer or obstruction and drainage; may be anterior, posterior, antecolic, retrocolic, right-to-left anastomosis, or left-to-right anastomosis	Antrectomy or hemigastrectomy	For ulcer disease
		Total or partial vagotomy with pyloroplasty or gastroenterostomy	For ulcer disease
Partial gastric resection—no enteroanastomosis			
Wedge resection	For ulcer, biopsy, or benign lesion		
Segmental resection	For ulcer or tumor		
Partial gastric resection and enteroanastomosis			
Gastrectomy with gastroduodenostomy	May be end-to-end, end-to-side, side-to-end, or side-to-side with superior, inferior, posterior, or anterior anastomosis		

Modified from Burhenne, HJ: Am J Roentgenol 91:731, 1964. © 1964, American Roentgen Ray Society.

used no matter whether the anastomosis is antecolic, retrocolic, left to right, or right to left

Roux-en-Y—Any end-to-side jejunojejunostomy with or without anastomosis with the esophagus, stomach, duodenum, gallbladder, bile duct, or pancreas

Sequelae of gastric surgery
Pneumoperitoneum

The usual pneumoperitoneum after laparotomy makes difficult the radiographic diagnosis of a postoperative air leak from an insufficient suture, duodenal stump blowout, or other perforation. This is further complicated by the fact that considerable variation exists for the length of time that air persists in the peritoneal cavity in different patients. It is not affected by the presence or absence of peritonitis or by the type of surgical procedure performed. Bryant and coworkers[75] demonstrated that the

body habitus affects the occurrence and duration of trapped air. Wolf and Khilnani[262] concluded that persistence of air for more than 4 days in patients with a sthenic habitus or in children suggests a leak. Bryant and associates have stressed that the time at which pneumoperitoneum disappears depends primarily on the amount of air initially present. Bevan[65] has stated, as a general guideline, that 100 to 500 ml persist for 1 week, 500 to 1000 ml for 10 days, and 1000 ml or more for 2 weeks.

Localized intraperitoneal air in the perihepatic spaces of the right upper quadrant may be present without evidence in general of a pneumoperitoneum.[177] It must also be remembered that as a sign of a pneumoperitoneum, air outlining the inside and outside of the wall of the gut may be simulated when two loops of distended intestine lie in contact with each other.[99] Little diagnostic difficulty arises if serial films demonstrate an increase in the

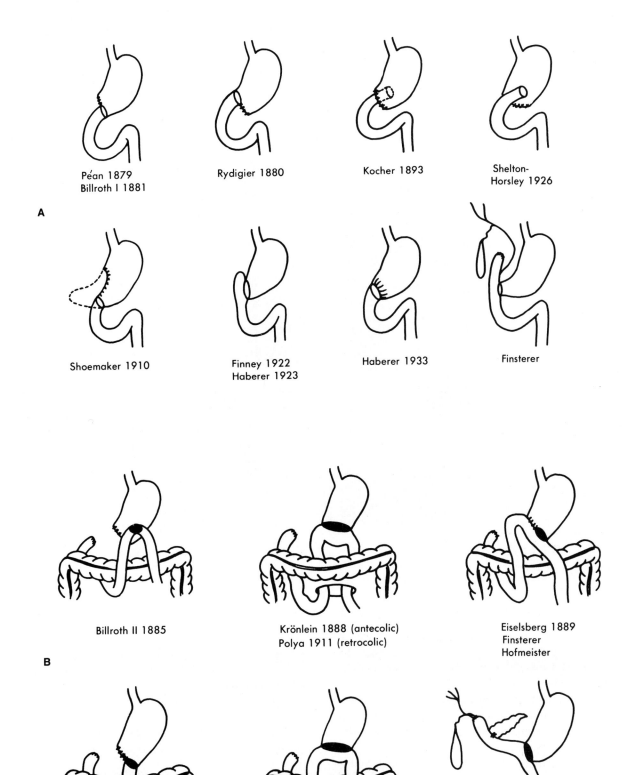

A

Péan 1879
Billroth I 1881

Rydigier 1880

Kocher 1893

Shelton-
Horsley 1926

Shoemaker 1910

Finney 1922
Haberer 1923

Haberer 1933

Finsterer

B

Billroth II 1885

Krönlein 1888 (antecolic)
Polya 1911 (retrocolic)

Eiselsberg 1889
Finsterer
Hofmeister

Roux-en-Y 1893

Moynihan 1923

Whipple 1935-1940

Fig. 64-28 A, Varieties of gastroduodenostomy. **B,** Varieties of gastrojejunostomy.
(From Burhenne, HJ: Am J Roentgenol 91:731, 1964. © 1964, American Roentgen Ray Society.)

Operation   Roentgen-anatomy   Terminology

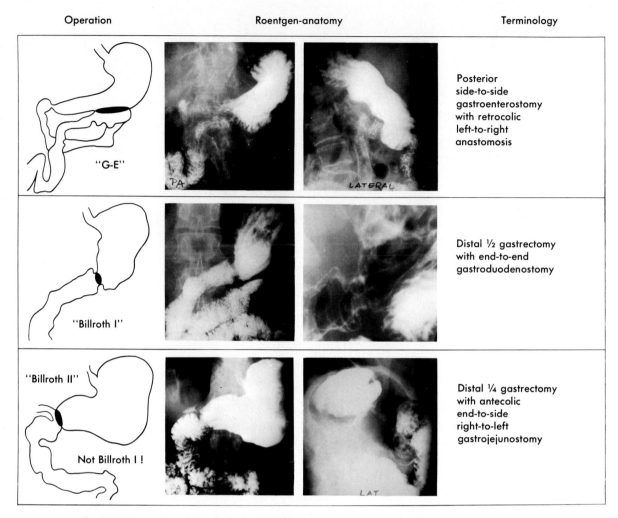

Fig. 64-29 Examples of descriptive terminology as compared with eponyms for operative procedures of stomach.
(From Burhenne, HJ: Am J Roentgenol 91:731, 1964. © 1964, American Roentgen Ray Society.)

amount of peritoneal air. Such progression indicates a leak from the gut except in cases where air continues to enter the abdominal cavity through an indwelling drain.[130]

Gas present in the hepatic portal venous system gives a distinctive radiographic appearance. This sign usually indicates bowel infarction but may be present in cases of ulcerative colitis, intraabdominal abscess, small bowel obstruction, peritoneoscopy with accidental air insufflation into a mesenteric vein, and gastric ulcer.[159]

Paralytic ileus and gastric atony

Gastric atony is present for 24 to 48 hours after most major gastric surgical procedures. Retention of gastric contents may occur without any mechanical obstruction. This motor dysfunction of the stomach is present partic-

ularly if gastric surgery has been combined with vagotomy, and the early postoperative atony may extend to a flaccid duodenum.[195] Preexisting pyloric obstruction[153] and preoperative obstructing duodenal ulcer disease markedly increase the frequency and severity of postvagotomy gastric atony.

Cannon[84] demonstrated as early as 1907 the retardation of discharge through the pylorus after vagotomy. Roth and colleagues[207] found gastric stasis in 12% of cases after vagotomy. Radiologic contrast studies may show marked gastric retention early after surgery. Bezoars may develop.[62] The rate of emptying of the stomach after vagotomy, however, may be increased with added pyloroplasty late after surgery in patients with postvagotomy diarrhea.[93]

Postoperative ileus is not an invariable consequence

Operation	Roentgen-anatomy	Terminology

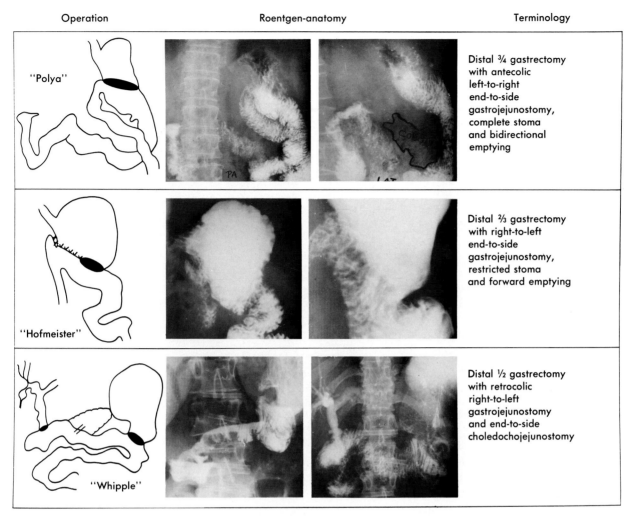

"Polya" — Distal ¾ gastrectomy with antecolic left-to-right end-to-side gastrojejunostomy, complete stoma and bidirectional emptying

"Hofmeister" — Distal ⅔ gastrectomy with right-to-left end-to-side gastrojejunostomy, restricted stoma and forward emptying

"Whipple" — Distal ½ gastrectomy with retrocolic right-to-left gastrojejunostomy and end-to-side choledochojejunostomy

Fig. 64-29, cont'd. Examples of descriptive terminology as compared with eponyms for operative procedures of stomach.

of abdominal surgery.[57] Wells and associates[255] found intestinal contractions to begin 2 to 3 hours after major abdominal operations. The retention appeared to be limited to the stomach and was related to the extent of the operation and duration of anesthesia. Rothnie and coworkers[208] suggested that the early postoperative silent abdomen is caused not by intestinal paralysis but probably by the absence of intestinal contents. They have recommended that fluids be given if they can be made to enter the small bowel. Ross and colleagues[205] used a radiotelemetering capsule to study postoperative motility in the small bowel. Small intestinal movements returned about 10 hours after vagotomy, about 4 hours after various gastric operations, and within 1 hour after those operations not involving handling of the viscera.

Women with long, J-shaped stomachs usually show poor gastric emptying in the erect position after pyloroplasty. Manual gastric emptying by the fluoroscopist is helpful in the radiographic demonstration of the width of the pyloric region to exclude obstruction.

Acute gastric dilatation

Acute gastric dilatation is a serious postoperative complication. It is a sudden and excessive distention of the stomach by fluid and gas and is often accompanied by vomiting, dehydration, and peripheral vascular collapse. It is often associated with immobilization of the patient or extensive postoperative ileus.[59]

Acute gastric dilatation is an equally serious clinical problem when it occurs in a patient without gastrectomy. It has been reported in association with anorexia nervosa, where it may lead to spontaneous rupture of the stomach.[107] The body cast syndrome consists of acute gastric dilatation associated with the application of a plaster hip spica or body jacket. Gastric perforation with peritonitis also may occur in this condition.[63] Rupture of the stomach has been reported in eight cases after the administration of oxygen by nasal catheter.[59]

Rupture, leakage, fistula, and abscess

Rupture of the duodenal stump is one of the gravest complications of gastric surgery and may occur without warning as soon as the first or as late as the nineteenth day after gastrojejunostomy.[210] It causes death in about half of the cases.* It has been reported in as many as 5% of cases after gastrojejunostomy and partial gastrectomy.[192]

Anastomotic leakage often occurs on the lesser curvature angle where the circular and linear suture lines meet (Fig. 64-30). It may lead to peritonitis, sinuses, and abscesses. Leakage after total gastrectomy is often fatal.[61]

A leak of the anastomotic suture line is probably related to an area of ischemia. Rodgers[203] found ischemia and gangrene when the blood supply to the stomach had been jeopardized, particularly when the short gastric arteries had been divided. Infarction of the gastric remnant may occur.

Early intervention in cases of duodenal stump rupture and anastomotic leakage is mandatory. Radiographic examination with an iodinated contrast medium is indicated (Fig. 64-31). Samuel and associates[213] demonstrated nine of 12 postoperative leaks radiographically.

Leakage from the anastomosis usually results in left subdiaphragmatic sinuses and abscess formation, whereas leakage from the duodenal stump causes the same conditions in the right subdiaphragmatic region. In the patients studied by Samuel and coworkers, the left subphrenic and right subphrenic spaces and the area surrounding the anastomosis were the sites of abscess formation in an equal number of cases. Internal fistulas may be formed to the colon, duodenum, small bowel, gallbladder, urinary tract, or pancreas, and external fistulas may be formed to the skin (Fig. 64-32).

Catheter trauma plays an important part in neonatal gastric perforations and was the cause in 11 of 143 cases reported by Inouye and Evans.[136] Prolapsing gastrostomy tubes may obstruct the stomach or duodenum,[97,112] possibly resulting in esophageal rupture. Resultant fatalities have also been reported.[119] Complications from passing long intestinal tubes in patients may occur.[227] Tucker and Izant[244] reported that iatrogenic factors were responsible in four of 26 gastrointestinal perforations that occurred

---

*References 85, 118, 136, 192, 203, 210.

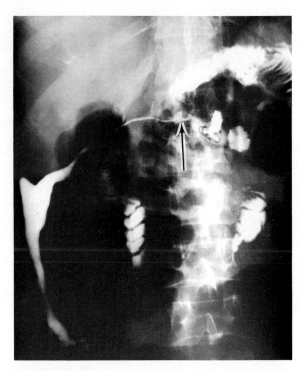

Fig. 64-30 Leakage at line of anastomosis *(arrow)*, with contrast material outlining sinus tract to abscess in right flank of peritoneal cavity.

postoperatively. The Mallory-Weiss syndrome and esophageal or gastric laceration can occur with forceful emesis[265] or with a hiccup while the patient is under anesthesia.[118]

Plain, erect, and decubitus radiographs readily show air-fluid levels below the diaphragm or in the lesser sac. These may be the result of leakage from the anastomosis or duodenal stump. Leakage usually occurs between the third and seventh postoperative days. An iodinated contrast medium is used to demonstrate the site of leakage and the sinuses connecting to abscess cavities.

Fistulas with external skin openings may be studied with the use of an iodinated contrast medium that outlines the tract and the abscess cavities. A vacuum device facilitates the injection of the contrast medium.[73]

Hemorrhage

The incidence of postgastrectomy hemorrhage is 3%[240,247] but may be as high as 12% in emergency surgery[240] or 30% in patients operated on for hemorrhage.[225]

Postoperative hemorrhage may be caused by any of the following:
1. Inflammation or infection
2. Intussusception
3. Gastrojejunal prolapse[158]

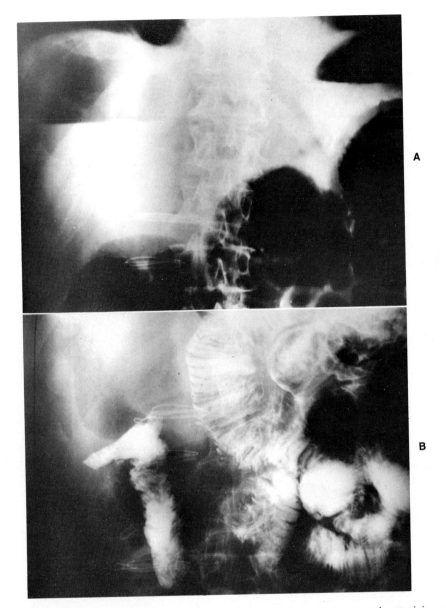

Fig. 64-31 Erect abdominal radiograph taken 5 days after subtotal gastrectomy and gastrojejunostomy for duodenal ulcer. **A,** Large air-fluid cavity is present in right subdiaphragmatic region, consistent with visceral perforation. **B,** Contrast study with iodinated medium demonstrates blowout of duodenal stump with leakage.

4. Misplaced or slipped sutures
5. Artery buttressed to the duodenal stump
6. Thrombocytopenia of extensive replacement transfusions during surgery
7. Erosions on plication defects
8. Neoplasm
9. Second ulcer overlooked at the time of operation
10. Ulcer recurrence or marginal ulcer
11. Hemorrhagic gastritis[252]

Splenic injury during gastrectomy[161] or as a complication of vagotomy[230] is not infrequent and is usually caused by injury of the gastrosplenic or phrenosplenic attachment. It must be considered in the postoperative diagnosis, since splenic injury may not have been diagnosed during surgery. The radiographic signs of splenic hemorrhage are those of a mass in the left upper quadrant with loss of visceral definition, deviation of adjacent hollow viscera, or elevation of the diaphragm.

The site of bleeding is often successfully demonstrated during arteriography and provides important information in a critical situation, particularly with massive bleeding from the duodenal stump.[184,229]

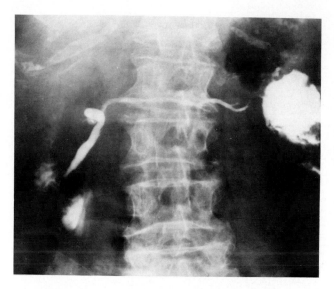

Fig. 64-32 External sinus tract to abscess cavity after attempted gastric drainage of pancreatic cyst shows antegrade drainage and connection with barium pancreatogram.

Obstruction

Stomal obstructions are caused by edema, submucosal hematoma, mechanical fault at the stoma, stricture after anastomotic ulcer, peristomal fat thickening caused by necrosis after anastomotic leakage or ligation of omental vessels, bezoar, intussusception, or internal hernia and are best diagnosed by radiographic examination. Mathieson[172] found stomal or small bowel obstruction after partial gastrectomy in 4.6% of 648 cases. It occurs most often with posterior gastrojejunostomy and least often with gastroduodenostomy.[131] Contrast-enhanced radiologic examination readily distinguishes between obstruction at the stoma and gastric atony with a patent anastomosis.[201] Anastomotic strictures of the upper gastrointestinal tract are amenable to fluoroscopically guided balloon dilatation.[100] Contrast examination is indicated if gastric retention persists for longer than 4 to 5 days after surgery.[234] Vagotomy without pyloroplasty often results in obstruction of the gastric outlet. The radiographic findings after incomplete pyloromyotomy have been well described.[137]

A gastric bezoar has been described after gastroduodenostomy alone[224] (Fig. 64-33), but in most cases the pyloroplasty or partial gastrectomy had been performed in association with vagotomy.[182,238] Also, yeast bezoars have been reported after gastrectomy combined with vagotomy.[138] Yeast bezoar formation is now seen more commonly with the increased use of vagotomy. The bezoar usually appears within 1 year of the operation. It may disappear without any therapy.[193] Other, more recent reports also indicate an increase in yeast overgrowth in gastric surgery after gastrojejunostomy.[237] Clot bezoars in hemorrhage may result in gastric outlet obstruction.

Prolapse of the gastric mucosa into the anastomotic opening may cause partial obstruction. Seaman[223] studied

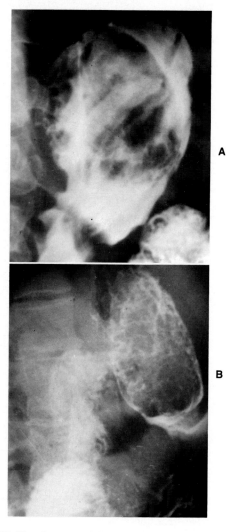

Fig. 64-33 Phytobezoar proximal to gastroduodenostomy, assuming shape of gastric pouch.
(Courtesy Dr. W. Gaines.)

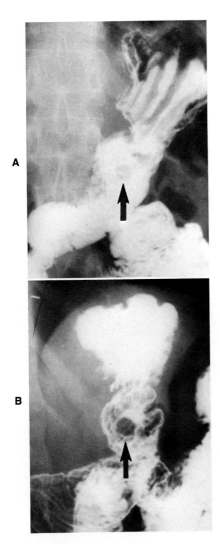

Fig. 64-34 Small smooth filling defect *(arrow)* just distal to point of gastroduodenostomy in patient with occult bleeding. At surgery, prolapse of gastric mucosa with small erosive bleeding point was found.

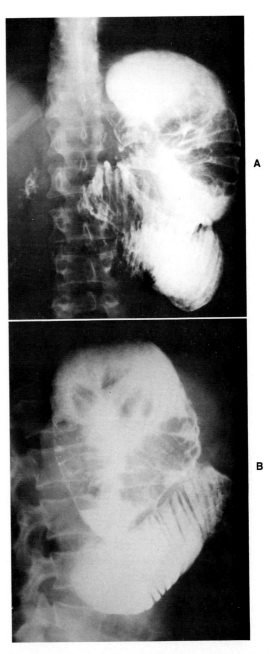

Fig. 64-35 Retrograde jejunogastric intussusception with obstruction, necessitating surgical intervention. Stretched and enlarged valvulae conniventes of intussuscepted jejunum are visualized within dilated gastric pouch and indicate impaired circulation.
(Courtesy Dr. R. Rousseau.)

24 patients with mucosal prolapse through a gastrojejunostomy stoma and found the majority of them to have no symptoms. Stretching of the gastric mucosa and jejunal filling defects are seen radiologically when prolapse is present.[158] Mucosal prolapse can be difficult to differentiate from a neoplasm at the anastomosis (Fig. 64-34). Some degree of postoperative mucosal prolapse through the anastomosis is frequently present and usually causes no delay in emptying.[121]

Intussusceptions must be considered in the differential diagnosis of stomach obstruction. Intussusceptions occur antegrade or retrograde.[114] Jejunum invaginates into the gastric pouch in retrograde jejunogastric intussusception. This type may be either acute or chronic and may occur either early or late after surgery. The acute type presents with a triad of (1) high intestinal obstruction, (2) left hypochondriac mass, and (3) hematemesis.[102] In addition to the obstruction, a striated filling defect in the stomach is seen on radiogrpahic examination and is considered pathognomonic[245] (Fig. 64-35). The valvulae conniventes seen radiographically within the gastric pouch are

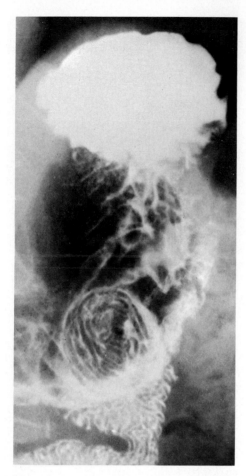

Fig. 64-36 Asymptomatic partial retrograde jejunogastric intussusception of proximal jejunal loop after gastroenterostomy. There is no obstruction.

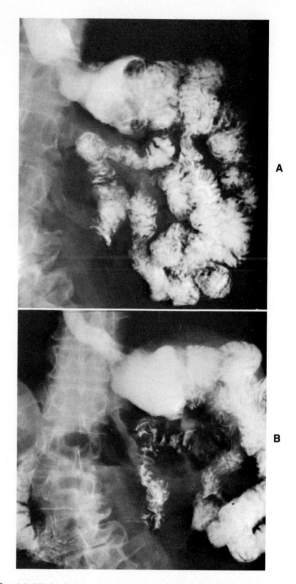

Fig. 64-37 A, Subtotal gastrectomy with retrograde jejunogastric intussusception. **B,** It is self-reducing and asymptomatic.

stretched and enlarged because of pressure edema or strangulation.[196] An outline of the jejunal mucosa by barium is characteristic (Fig. 64-36). Chronic jejunogastric intussusception may be self-reducing[200] and may be intermittent[87] (Fig. 64-37). In the acute form of delayed jejunogastric intussusception, a correct diagnosis and prompt surgical intervention are critical to the patient's survival.[76] The incidence of retrograde jejunogastric intussusception is about three in 2000 gastric operations. It is most often seen after gastrojejunostomy. The intussuscipiens is the distal (efferent) loop in 75% of cases, the proximal (afferent) loop in most other cases, and, rarely, both loops[72] (Fig. 64-38). The radiographic diagnosis of jejunogastric intussusception is important in early postoperative symptomatic cases, since a 100% mortality has been reported in undiagnosed cases.[49,157]

The second form of postgastrectomy intussusception is the antegrade or direct gastrojejunal intussusception (Fig. 64-39). The pouch may intussuscept with the jejunal loop as intussusceptum. A leiomyoma or another tumor may be the leading point.[196] A rare complication described as following total gastric resection is antegrade jejunojejunal intussusception.[113] Retrograde intussusception has also been reported after total gastrectomy combined with Roux-en-Y reconstruction.[237]

Vomiting with upper gastrointestinal obstruction may lead to spontaneous rupture of the esophagus, the so-called Boerhaave's syndrome.[68] Postemetic hemorrhage may be caused by the Mallory-Weiss syndrome. The correct radiologic diagnosis in this condition can be made by arteriography[152] and only rarely with barium contrast studies.

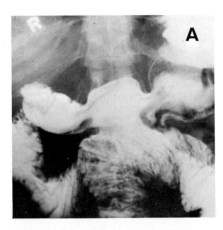
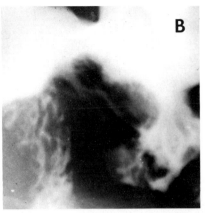

Fig. 64-38 A, Asymptomatic partial retrograde intussusception after gastroenterostomy through large stoma is not unusual with active jejunal peristalsis. **B,** Intussusception involves both jejunal loops.

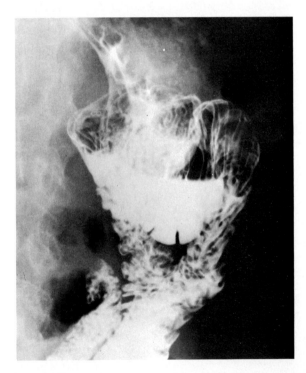

Fig. 64-39 Antegrade gastrojejunal intussusception in patient who had intermittent vomiting.

Plication defects

Local excision and simple closure rarely leave permanent mucosal defects. Norberg[185] failed to see the site of invagination of perforated peptic ulcers in all of 142 cases studied radiographically 5 years after surgery. Defects after surgical closure, when seen radiologically, may be difficult to differentiate from ulcer deformity. Persistence of an overlooked ulcer must also be considered in the differential diagnosis.[190,191]

Temporary or permanent distortion of the mucosal pattern (plication defect, Hofmeister's defect, Shoemaker's defect, mucoma) may occur after gastrostomy, gastrotomy, and any other type of surgical intervention with suturing or inversion (Figs. 64-40 to 64-42). These changes are more pronounced in the early postoperative period. A number of plication defects have been described,[198] and their appearance varies with different techniques of anatomosis and suturing. Granulomas, ischemic necrosis, and separation sometimes accompany plication defects.[74] Associated foreign body granulomas simulating tumors have been described.[104] Although plication defects are seen adjacent to the cardia after vagotomy,[111] they usually occur after partial gastrectomy and are found on the lesser curvature, just above the anastomosis, where partial closure of the cut end of the stomach is performed.[151,189,215,217]

Surgical plication of the mucosa results in a filling defect, as seen on the radiograph (Figs. 64-43 and 64-44). Such filling defects may be as large as 5 cm but may become less prominent or disappear in follow-up studies.[109] Plication defects are readily differentiated from neoplasms if postoperative baseline studies are available. Exploration is indicated if the radiologic defect is in an area where suturing is not customary (Fig. 64-45).

A characteristic pseudodiverticulum deformity sometimes occur after the Heineke-Mikulicz pyloroplasty.[78,260] A longitudinal incision into muscle on the anterior aspect of the pyloric ring is made, and the layers are closed in a transverse direction. The resulting pseudodiverticulum, or beagle-ear sign[81] (Fig. 64-46), with a slight constriction on both its antral and duodenal sides, has been confirmed in cadaver studies.[243] Bloch and Wolf[66] consider cinefluorography to be the method of choice for exami-

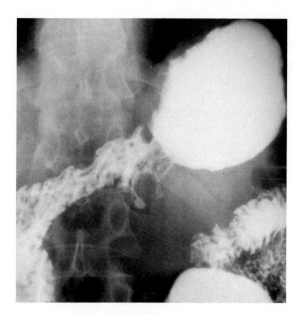

Fig. 64-40 Plication defects at gastroduodenostomy caused by inversion of mucosal margin at anastomosis.

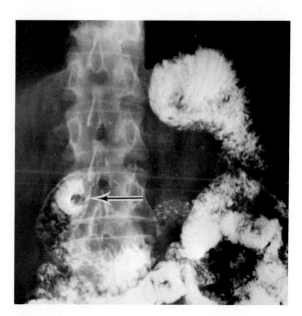

Fig. 64-41 Plication defect in duodenum *(arrow)* after total gastrectomy, resulting from inverted duodenal stump.

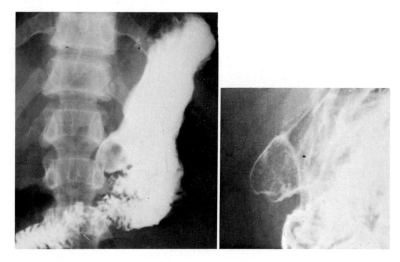

Fig. 64-42 Large plication defect in remaining portion of distal stomach after gastrojejunostomy. Defect, resembling benign tumor, was caused by surgical inversion of gastric antrum. Postoperative baseline studies had not been obtained.
(Courtesy Dr. R. Raphael.)

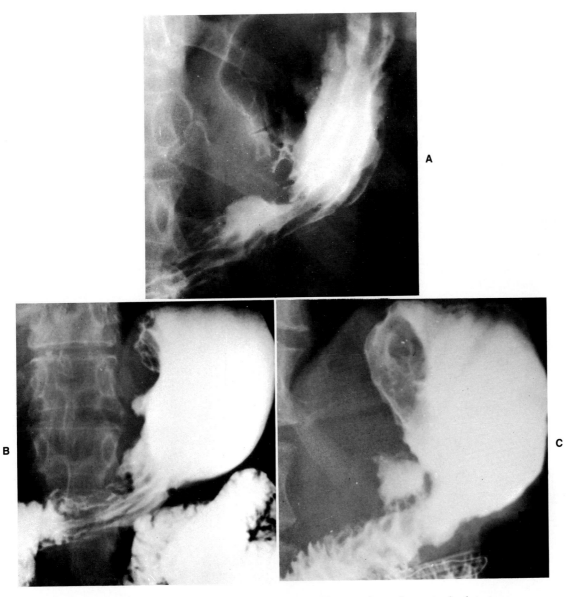

Fig. 64-43 Plication defects in typical location in three different patients after gastroduodenostomy: **A,** with inverted mucosa at point of partial closure on lesser curvature of stomach; **B,** with plication deformity resembling diverticulum; **C,** with preexisting duodenal diverticulum and high plication deformity at cardia, giving appearance of mass.

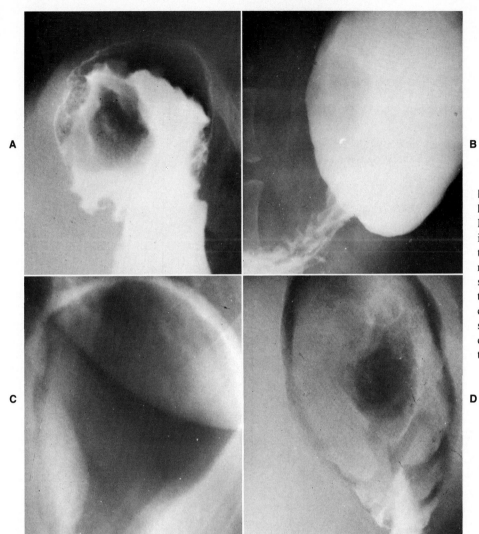

Fig. 64-44 Plication defect on high lesser curvature in typical location just above anastomosis in patient with gastroduodenostomy. **A** and **B,** Plication defect resembling tumor. **C,** Plication stretched and elongated with patient in erect position. **D,** Mucosal conversion resulting from suturing and plication on lesser curvature, seen in lateral projection.

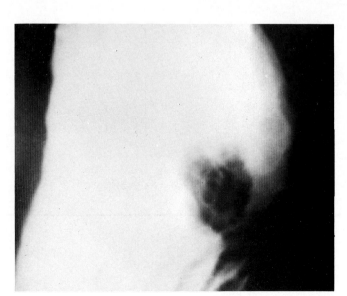

Fig. 64-45 Filling defect seen after gastrojejunostomy in atypical location on greater curvature was histologically shown to be adenomatous polyp.
(Courtesy Dr. O. Klausenstock.)

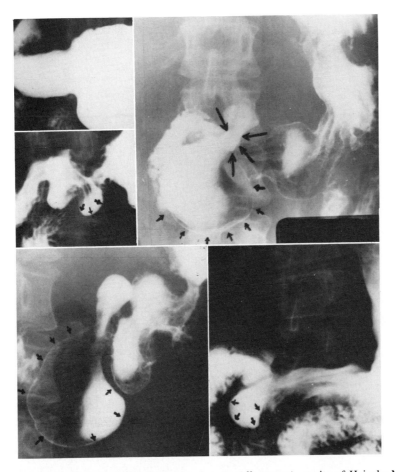

Fig. 64-46 Beagle-ear sign, or pseudodiverticulum *(small arrows)*, at site of Heineke-Mikulicz pyloroplasty, illustrated in four different patients. Normal preoperative greater curvature is demonstrated in first patient. Recurrent duodenal ulcer is present in second patient *(large arrows)*. (Modified from Burhenne, HJ: Semin Radiol 6:182, 1971.)

nation of this postoperative deformity. Recurrent ulcer can be recognized in the presence of pyloroplasty deformity.[258]

A postanastomotic dilatation simulating a duodenal bulb is seen within 6 months of Billroth I procedures in 50% of cases and within 1 year in 75%.[151]

Suture granulomas of the stomach may give a radiographic appearance similar to that of plication deformities. A plea has been made for the use of absorbable suture material in gastric resection surgery.[122] The distal esophagus that has invaginated into the stomach gives a masslike defect in the gastric fundus, which simulates a neoplasm.[91,106]

Retained gastric antrum

Surgical retention of the endocrinologically active gastric antrum gives poor results (Fig. 64-47). Antral exclusion operations, with transection of the stomach, end-to-side gastrojejunostomy, and retention of the gastric antrum in continuity with the pylorus and duodenum, are followed by a incidence of marginal ulcers of 30% to 50%.[148,186] Resection of the retained antrum is mandatory and results in relief of symptoms. The radiographic signs for the retained antrum are described elsewhere.[80] Reflux of barium from the duodenum by way of the pylorus into the antrum is diagnostic.

Five gastrins have now been described,[253] but the relation of ulcer disease to gastrin remains unclear. Hypergastrinemia is associated with pernicious anemia, the Zollinger-Ellison syndrome (or gastrinoma), antral G cell hyperplasia (an entity recently described in which the gastrin-producing cells of the antrum are greatly increased in number), renal disease, and extensive resection of the small intestine. Vagal control of gastrin secretion has been demonstrated.[60]

The syndrome of the retained gastric antrum can also be diagnosed by ^{99m}Tc-pertechnetate scintiphotography.[218] The combination of basic gastric acid secretory studies

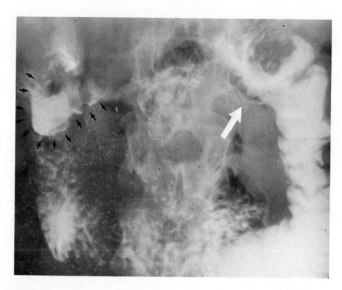

Fig. 64-47 Marginal ulcer *(large arrow)* seen with air contrast in patient after gastrojejunostomy. Reflux occurred by way of pylorus into retained gastric antrum with gastric mucosa *(small arrows)*. (From Burhenne, HJ: Am J Roentgenol 101:459, 1967. © 1967, American Roentgen Ray Society.)

and serum gastrin determinations may identify three causes of recurrent ulcer: incomplete vagotomy, retained antrum, and Zollinger-Ellison tumor.[235]

Postoperative ulcer disease

Esophagitis has been reported to follow gastric surgery[128] and has been related to bile reflux.[179] Clarke and coworkers[90] consider esophageal reflux to be common after abdominal vagotomy for a duodenal ulcer. Reflux was noted radiologically in 50% of cases after gastroduodenostomy and in 27% of cases after gastrojejunostomy and partial gastrectomy.[261] Vestibular spasm may occur after vagotomy.[98] Small, asymptomatic hiatus hernias have been enlarged and symptomatic after vagotomy.[140]

Dysphagia occurring a few weeks after surgery may also be related to a benign stricture of the distal esophagus. Low and Palmer[162] reported six patients with a confirmed postoperative esophageal stricture. Indwelling nasogastric tubes were left in place in these patients from 2 to 21 days. Low and Palmer have suggested that the mucosal trauma by the intubation and persistent regurgitation led to the stricture.

Gastritis commonly occurs early after surgery but usually subsides within a few weeks.[188] Reflux of bile salts has been considered as a cause of gastritis after surgery.[69] Inflammatory changes surrounding the anastomosis may cause hemorrhage or a delay in emptying. Reflux bile gastritis may result in considerable swelling of the gastric mucosa, and large gastric folds can be seen in the gastric remnant on radiologic examination. The radiologist can

play a significant role in alerting the clinician to the presence of this entity.[241]

Jejunitis in the anastomotic loop was found in 38% of cases after partial gastric resection.[129]

A *recurrent ulcer* may be seen on radiographic studies at the original ulcer site after simple excision or wedge resection. Recurrence of gastric ulcer is also seen after gastroenterostomy alone. A vicious circle of secretions and food has been held responsible. Recurrence of duodenal ulcers in the bulb after gastrojejunostomy is rare except with anastomotic obstruction (Figs. 64-48 and 64-49).

The *marginal ulcer* has been known as postoperative ulcer, jejunal ulcer, stomal ulcer, anastomotic ulcer, gastrojejunal ulcer, and recurrent ulcer. It is not a recurrent one but a new ulceration occurring, after gastric surgery, in the jejunum just distal to the anastomosis. Marginal ulcers almost never originate in the gastric mucosa or at the anastomotic margin. Most occur in the first 2 cm of an anastomotic jejunum, most frequently in the distal jejunal loop.[143] Marginal ulcers may encroach on the anastomotic margin secondarily.

Although bleeding can be the presenting symptom of a marginal ulcer, pain is usually felt and is slightly more to the left than was the original duodenal ulcer pain. More pain, bleeding, and perforation than in the original ulcer are typical. Men are affected more often than women in a ratio of 9:1.[199] Bleeding occurs in 50% of marginal ulcers,[248] and 45% have some obstruction at the stoma.[263]

Although marginal ulcers may occur within 1 week

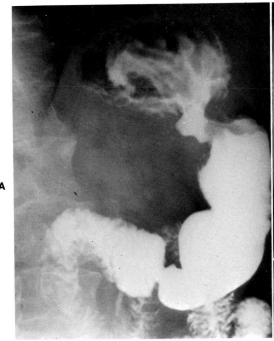

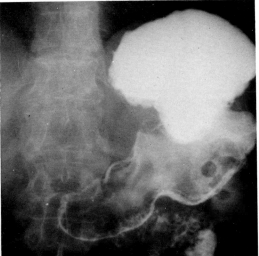

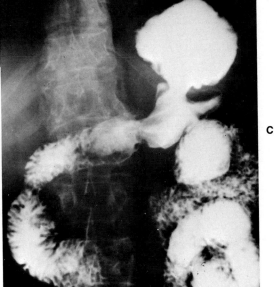

Fig. 64-48 A, Benign gastric ulcer treated with sleeve resection. **B,** Large gastric ulcer recurred at same site. **C,** When, however, large gastric ulcer was left in place and antrum was resected, this gastric ulcer healed and marked scarring occurred.

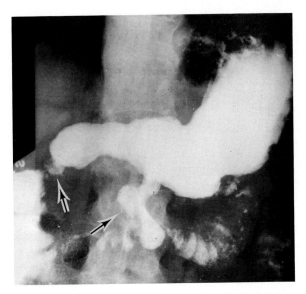

Fig. 64-49 Patient with gastroenterostomy for duodenal ulcer disease. Duodenal ulcer recurred within 1 year *(left arrow),* and marginal ulcer at gastroenterostomy *(right arrow)* is present.

after surgery,[168] most become symptomatic within 2 to 4 years after partial gastrectomy. The length of follow-up influences the incidence of marginal ulcer given in different reports. Working with one group of patients, Welch[252] noted marginal ulcers in 1% of patients 2 years after surgery and in 8% at the end of 5 years. The incidence of marginal ulcer also depends on the type of surgical procedure, the sex of the patient, the location

of the original ulcer, and the history of previous hemorrhage.[146]

The radiographic diagnosis of marginal ulcer is possible in about 50% of cases,[221,263] but some suggestive abnormality is seen in 80% of cases.[174,263] Ellis[105] demonstrated marginal ulcers more readily after partial gastrectomy than after gastroenterostomy. The ulcer crater cannot be demonstrated if it is superficial.[246] Concentrically arranged mucosal folds may be present[236] (Figs. 64-50 and 64-51). Comparison with previous ra-

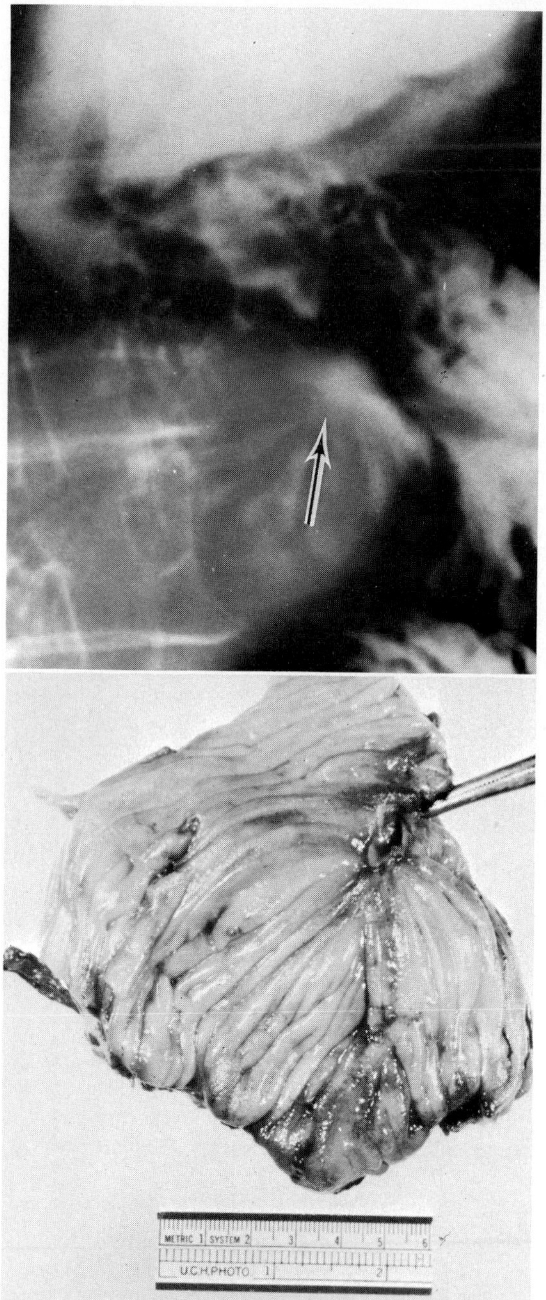

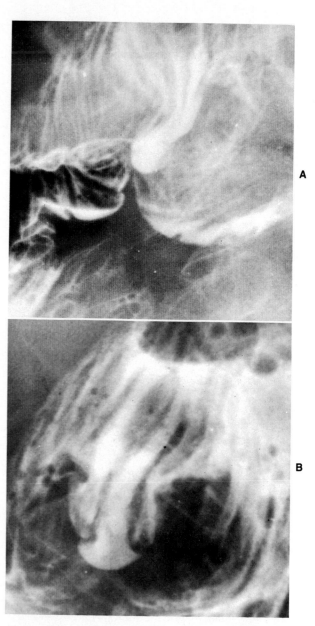

Fig. 64-50 A, Concentrically arranged jejunal folds point to marginal ulcer *(arrow).* **B,** Specimen of resected jejunum.

Fig. 64-51 A, Marginal ulcer simulated by converging folds of small jejunal pouch often seen opposite stoma. **B,** Another view of pouch. It results from foreshortening on inner aspect of anastomotic jejunal loop.

diographic studies is mandatory and most helpful in the diagnosis (Figs. 64-52 and 64-53). Inflammatory changes surrounding the anastomosis are suggestive.[86] Rigidity of the jejunum may at times be the only abnormality found in patients with jejunal ulcers.[216] Another indirect radiographic sign is the inflammatory change sometimes present in the colon in the area adjacent to the anastomosis.[169]

Endoscopic examination is the procedure of choice

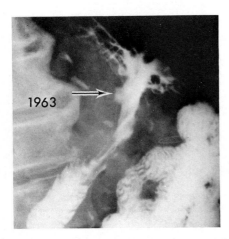

Fig. 64-52 Radiographic appearance consistent with marginal ulcer *(arrow)* after gastroduodenostomy (see Fig. 64-53).

for detection of marginal ulcer disease, but with proper care the double barium contrast examination can provide adequate information.[212] The double barium contrast examination is advocated as the radiologic technique of choice to evaluate mucosal detail in the gastric remnant and in the anastomosis. The use of intravenous glucagon (0.5 to 1 mg) usually further improves the visualization of the anastomosis and the immediate postanastomotic segment of the jejunum.[187]

Gastrojejunocolic fistula

Untreated marginal ulcers have been reported to result in gastrojejunocolic fistulas in 17% of cases.[264] The fistula between the jejunum and the colon represents a grave complication of marginal ulcers and gastric surgery. The patient has diarrhea and weight loss in most cases, with pain and vomiting present in half of the cases and fetor ex ore and bleeding present in about a third. Gastrojejunocolic fistula is attended by a high mortality, especially if recognized late. At the time of surgery the marginal ulcer is usually healed because of the alkaline reflux of colonic contents. Jejunocolic fistulas are unusual in women. Fitzgerald and McMullin[110] found only six such cases in 400 fistulas. The number of marginal ulcers resulting in fistulas is given as 6.6% by Walters[248] and 10% by McBurney and colleagues.[174]

Radiologic techniques provide the most accurate means of diagnosis, and diagnoses are correct in 90% of

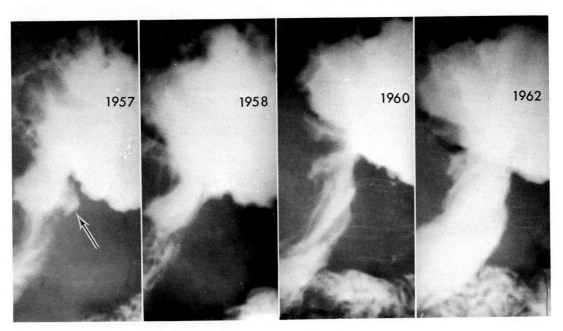

Fig. 64-53 Review of previous radiographic studies in same patient as in Fig. 64-52 shows marginal ulcer in 1957 *(arrow)* on opposite side. Barium collection considered an ulcer in 1963 had been present for 6 years; it contained some mucosal pattern in 1962. Collection apparently represents deformity resulting from either scarring or suturing.

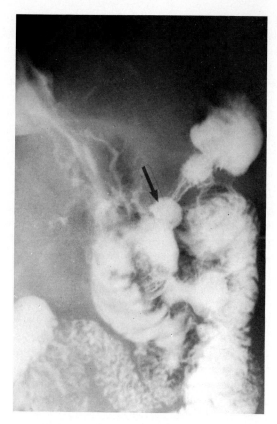

Fig. 64-54 Gastrojejunocolic fistula after gastrojejunostomy. Colon is filling *(arrow)*. No marginal ulcer was seen at time of operation, 4 days after this radiograph was obtained. Barium collection at point of colonic connection apparently represents haustral filling.

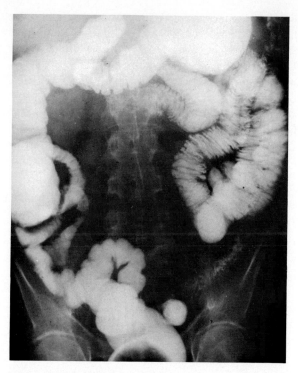

Fig. 64-55 Barium enema in same patient as in Fig. 64-54, with proximal jejunal filling from colon, is more diagnostic for gastrojejunocolic fistula.

gastrojejunocolic fistulas.[171] The barium enema is more diagnostic than the upper gastrointestinal study (Figs. 64-54 and 64-55). In the 31 cases of fistula after marginal ulcers studies by Thoeny and associates,[239] the diagnosis was made in every instance where a barium enema was performed, whereas the fistula was demonstrated by upper gastrointestinal study in only 11% of cases.

Fistulas caused by carcinoma of the colon or stomach[135] and those caused by inadvertent gastroileostomy or gastrocolostomy must be differentiated radiologically from gastrojejunocolic fistulas.

Ulcerogenic tumors

Marginal ulcers associated with ulcerogenic tumors are particularly resistant to medical therapy. Even irradiation, which has given good results for marginal ulcers,[150] characteristically yields no improvement. Total gastrectomy is the most effective treatment for gastric hypersecretion and peptic ulceration.[259] The gastrinlike substance[120] excreted by ulcerogenic tumors of the pancreas (the Zollinger-Ellison syndrome) or polyglandular adenomas provides a mechanism for ulcerogenesis similar to the gastrin produced by a retained gastric antrum after gastrectomy.[80]

The radiographic findings of large or multiple marginal ulcers, with may occur in an unusual position, should alert the radiologist to the diagnostic possibility of ulcerogenic tumors or a retained antrum (Fig. 64-56). The lacy or cobweblike small bowel pattern caused by hypersecretion[251] is an additional radiologic sign to the correct diagnosis.

Postgastrectomy carcinoma

The radiologic diagnosis of malignancy in the postgastrectomy state is difficult, particularly if no postoperative baseline study is available for comparison.[144] Postgastrectomy gastric carcinoma may be recurrent (Fig. 64-57) or primary.

Bachman and Parmer[56] reviewed the radiographic findings in 41 cases of malignant recurrence. The radiologic studies were not revealing in half the cases. When present, mucosal effacement and destruction (Fig. 64-58) or ulceration, narrowing of the stoma, and filling defects were helpful in reaching a diagnosis. However, plication filling defects after suturing may have a similar appearance. The diagnosis is also difficult, because a gastric pouch consisting of the fundus does not exhibit peri-

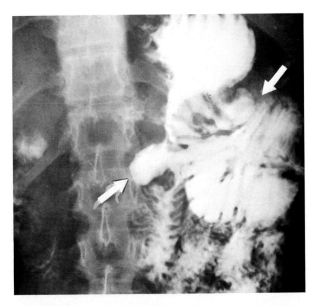

Fig. 64-56 Two large marginal ulcers *(arrows)* occurring early after gastrojejunostomy in patient with ulcerogenic tumor of pancreas.

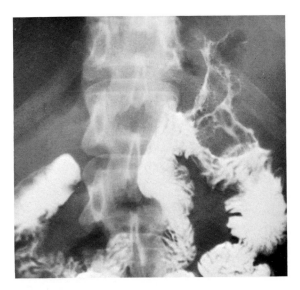

Fig. 64-58 Mucosal effacement in entire gastric pouch caused by recurrence of adenocarcinoma.

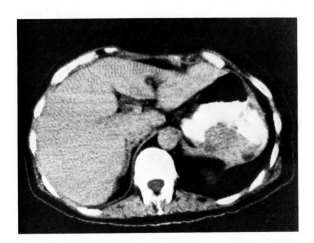

Fig. 64-57 Recurrence of carcinoma of stomach after partial gastrectomy demonstrates large mass in gastric remnant that is infiltrating tail of pancreas when seen on computed tomography.

stalsis. Because of rapid emptying its filling and distention with barium are difficult. Exfoliative cytologic studies are more diagnostic and probably should be done in all cases with narrowing of the stoma or other suggestive radiologic or clinical findings.[116]

Recurring hyperplastic gastric polyps after total gastrectomy may present as another differential diagnostic problem to the radiologist. Polyps may be hyperplastic, adenomatous, or villous. Hyperplastic polyps are more common and are often multiple. They are usually less than 2 cm in size, and the smooth or slightly lobulated

appearance radiologically concurs with their benign character.[139]

Similarly difficult is the radiologic diagnosis of primary gastric carcinoma developing after gastrectomy.[222] Carcinoma of the gastric pouch is more frequent in men than in women and more frequent after surgery for a gastric ulcer.[214] Carcinoma is less common at the anastomosis[55] than within the gastric remnant.[64] Fixation of the anastomosis during breathing maneuvers may be present.[246] The incidence of cancer after surgery for a gastric ulcer exceeds the expected rate, and the incidence appears to be less than that expected after surgery for a duodenal ulcer.[67] Awareness of the increased incidence of carcinoma in the gastric remnant has not been accompanied by improved diagnosis or prolonged survival. The degree of increase has been reported as anywhere from twofold to sixfold.[82] If postoperative deformities make the radiologic differential diagnosis uncertain, direct visualization by fiberendoscopy and biopsy is recommended.

Postgastrectomy syndromes
Dumping

One must differentiate between mechnaical dumping, the early postprandial dumping syndrome, and late postprandial hypoglycemia. The latter occurs 90 to 120 minute after eating and is readily corrected by the ingestion of sugars.

MECHANICAL DUMPING

Mechanical dumping merely refers to rapid emptying of a contrast medium or food from the stomach into the small bowel and is sometimes present with an intact stomach. It may be seen with all types of gastric surgery but is most common after subtotal gastrectomy and gastrojejunostomy. It occurs less frequently after gastroduodenostomy than after gastrojejunostomy, and it is probably less pronounced if the cut end of the stomach has been restricted to a smaller stoma.[48] Liljedahl and coworkers[160] have used cinefluorography to evaluate the motility pattern to the intestinal tract after gastric surgery and have reconfirmed that the patient's status after gastroduodenostomy (Billroth I) is similar to that of healthy subjects, whereas the stomach empties with great rapidity after gastrojejunostomy (Billroth II).

Mechanical dumping of the stomach results in loss of gastric reservoir function, which is easily shown radiographically. A somewhat better reservoir capacity of the gastric pouch is demonstrated with the use of food instead of barium. Stoma size did not appear to be a critical factor in Schlaeger's study,[220] whereas Abbott and collegues[48] believe that the anastomotic opening is decisive. They converted large stomas to a smaller size, with good gastric reservoir capacity resulting in all patients. McCaughand and Bowers,[175] Zollinger and Williams,[266] and Lahey and Marshall[156] have also placed emphasis on a small stoma. Jejunal interposition has also been used to improve reservoir function after gastrectomy.[94] Similar results have been seen with colonic replacement of the stomach.[125]

DUMPING SYNDROME

The dumping syndrome causes early postprandial vascular symptoms of sweating, flushing, palpitation, and feelings of weakness and dizziness. The symptoms are relieved when the patient lies down.

The mechanism of the dumping syndrome is not clearly understood. Machella[164] related it to hypertonic solution entering the jejunum rapidly with mechanical dumping. This osmotically active solution then results in a fluid shift from the blood compartment into the small bowel. Absorption of the contents does not take place until isotonicity is established.[70] The resulting drop in blood plasma volume accompanying the vasomotor symptoms are shown by Roberts and coworkers[202] (Fig. 64-59).

Amdrup and colleagues[52] stated that dumping can be provoked in all subjects when hypertonic solution is introduced into the small intestine in sufficient amounts, but the individual variation in intensity of symptoms has not been explained. An additional factor may be responsible, such as hyperglycemia, postural hypotension,[132] failure of reflex vasoconstriction,[95,134] vascular hypoosmolality,[163] or serotonin release.[141,194] The symptoms are improved by diet.

The incidence of the dumping syndrome varies from 1% to 5% for symptoms considered significant[71,126,149,211,252] and from 10% to 30% for some of the symptoms of dumping.[108,117,129,146,151] Women are affected more than men in a ratio of 2:1.[167]

In the radiographic investigation of the dumping syndrome, food mixtures,[48] a physiologic contrast medium,[166] and a combination of barium and 50% glucose solution[51,54,183] have been used. Symptoms of the dumping syndrome may be provoked by the ingestion of hypertonic contrast mixtures. A dilution effect[77] of the con-

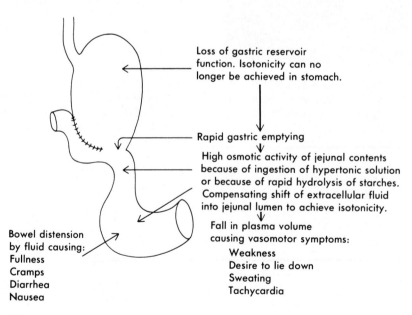

Loss of gastric reservoir function. Isotonicity can no longer be achieved in stomach.

Rapid gastric emptying

High osmotic activity of jejunal contents because of ingestion of hypertonic solution or because of rapid hydrolysis of starches. Compensating shift of extracellular fluid into jejunal lumen to achieve isotonicity.

Fall in plasma volume causing vasomotor symptoms:
Weakness
Desire to lie down
Sweating
Tachycardia

Bowel distension by fluid causing:
Fullness
Cramps
Diarrhea
Nausea

Fig. 64-59 Outline of proposed mechanism in dumping syndrome. Hyperglycemia and release of serotonin have also been implicated.

trast is seen at the time of onset of symptoms[156]; both effects are caused by the shift of fluid into the small bowel.

Sigstad[228] studied 49 patients given hypertonic glucose test meals and found a greater percentage of a fall in plasma volume in "dumpers" than in "nondumpers." The radiologic findings in the dumping syndrome are not diagnostic, since the dilution effect has also been observed in patients without symptoms. The fluid shift appears to represent only a part of the responsible mechanism.

Malabsorption

Malabsorption states after gastric resection may occur with deficient production of extrinsic factors,[142] decreased vitamin B_{12} absorption,[88] increased fat content in the stool,[149,250] or iron deficiency anemia.[96,129]

The calcium metabolism is sometimes altered,[101] with a decrease in calcium levels, particularly after Pólya's gastrectomy in older patients.[181] The radiologic changes resemble osteoporosis or osteomalacia[115] or a combination of the two, with rarefaction, accentuated bony trabeculae, wedging, biconcavity, multiple rib fractures, and Looser's zones in the scapulae and pubic rami.[123] DuBerger and associates[103] described five cases of Milkman's syndrome after gastric surgery, with fractures (Fig. 64-60).

Histologic changes seen in the small bowel can resemble those of the idiopathic malabsorption syndrome,[147] but Sherlock and coworkers[226] found no correlation between the mucosal change and the presence of decreased fat absorption. Ross and colleagues[206] reported gluten enteropathy after partial gastrectomy.

Surgical reconstruction of a food reservoir with interposed jejunal loops[204] or a substitute stomach[173] after total gastrectomy has improved postoperative nutrition. Normal growth and development after gastrectomy in children under the age of 12 years have been reported.[180] In adults, nevertheless, weight loss remains the most common sequela of gastrectomy.[127] The average postoperative weight loss is given as 11.5 kg by Henning and colleagues.[129]

Weight loss and a change in immunity result in reactivation of pulmonary tuberculosis after gastrectomy, with a greater than expected frequency.[127,249] There is no increased incidence when results of preoperative chest films are normal.[242] The routine use of chest films has been stressed by several authors.[58,89,234]

Postvagotomy functional changes

Functional changes after vagotomy are not clearly understood, and some discrepancies are found in the literature.

Diarrhea was reported by Marshall[170] in 32% of cases after gastric surgery if vagotomy was added. This is in contrast to Stammers and Williams'[234] incidence of diarrhea in only four of 28 patients after vagotomy. No conclusive difference of effect was noted between total and selective vagotomy,[257] although more recent reports on selective vagotomy have demonstrated a lower rate of diarrhea.[154]

An increase in the incidence of gallstones after vagotomy has been noted. Rudick and Hutchinson[209] found gallbladder dilatation only after total vagotomy, not after selective vagotomy. No interference with gallbladder emptying after a fatty meal was observed in their radiologic studies.

Gastric operation for morbid obesity

Because of a high complication rate with the small bowel bypass for morbid obesity, the recent surgical approach to this disease has been gastric bypass procedures. Eighty to ninety percent of the stomach, including the antrum, is excluded, and a high gastrojejunostomy is performed (Fig. 64-61). Sufficient acid-secreting cells are present to suppress the production of gastrin. The small proximal stomach limits the amount of food intake and promotes the feeling of satiety. Jejunum and ileum are left in the food stream to permit absorption.[92] In 1980 an entirely new concept in gastric restriction surgery was introduced in Oslo. Instead of stapling, a band is placed around the proximal stomach to create, in one step, a small pouch and stoma. Silicone gastric banding is a simple and effective operation for morbid obesity.[155] It is the least invasive of all gastric restriction procedures,

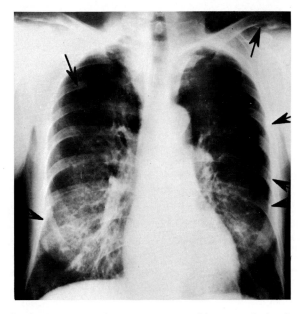

Fig. 64-60 Multiple fractures *(arrows)* with osteomalacia after subtotal gastrectomy.

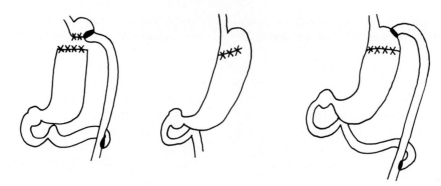

Fig. 64-61 Varieties of gastric operations for morbid obesity with 80% to 95% of stomach excluded in two bypass procedures (*left* and *right*) and with proximal stomach partially closed *(center).*

because the stomach is not cut or stapled. If necessary, this operation can be easily revised or reversed. Complications of gastric bypass surgery, including leakage at the anastomosis, anastomotic stenosis, and abscess formation, can be treated with interventional radiologic procedures.[178]

Immediate complications after a gastric bypass for morbid obesity include leaks at the anastomosis or early obstruction. Delayed symptoms may be due to esophagitis, gastritis, or stomal ulceration or possible enlargement of the gastric pouch. Vomiting and an increase in pouch size may occur with dietary noncompliance.[124] Preoperative gastrointestinal examination should exclude the presence of a hiatus hernia or peptic ulcer disease. Bezoar formation has also been reported.[92] Radiographic examination with Gastrografin has been recommended in the investigation of early postoperative changes.[197] Knowledge of the different gastric exclusion operations for the treatment of morbid obesity is important to the radiologist in evaluating these patients after surgery (Fig. 64-62).

SMALL BOWEL[267-319]

Surgery on the small bowel is well tolerated in general, and anastomoses involving small intestinal segments heal well in the absence of disease at the site. Postoperative leakage is less common than elsewhere in the alimentary tract, and fistula formation indicates ischemia or some other, underlying pathologic condition such as regional enteritis. Because of the microflora in the small intestine, all procedures are potentially septic, particularly if small bowel obstruction occurs.

Intestinal resection, intestinal bypass, interposition procedures, and ileostomy are the most common operations.

Resections are performed for Crohn's disease, intestinal tuberculosis, gangrene, and tumors. The average length of the normal small intestine has been reported as

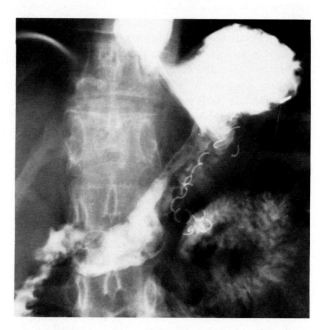

Fig. 64-62 This variation of gastric surgery for morbid obesity shows partial occlusion of stomach on greater curvature side in order to decrease gastric lumen.

450 cm. An assessment of the length of small bowel remaining is one of the indications for radiologic examination. The critical length of residual bowel depends on the site or resection.

There is an increased frequency of bowel action after vagotomy, but the incidence of problematic diarrhea is rare. Patients examined 2 years after pyloroplasty and vagotomy demonstrated an increased diameter of the small bowel segment, prolonged transit time, and increased barium precipitation. These changes were radiologically impossible to differentiate from those seen in sprue.[291]

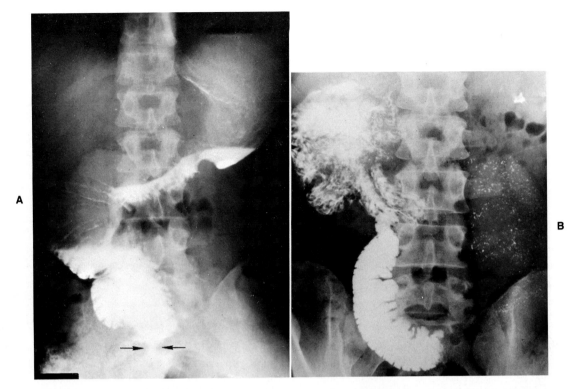

Fig. 64-63 A, High jejunal obstruction caused by scarring *(arrows)* after gastroduodenostomy. Duodenum had been mobilized by Kocher's maneuver. **B,** Same patient returned subsequently with internal hernia through surgical defect in omentum.

Obstruction in the anastomotic jejunal loop

Obstruction in the anastomotic jejunal loop may result from postgastrectomy internal hernia (Fig. 64-63). There are three potential hernial rings after gastrojejunostomy: (1) the postcolic retroanastomotic space, (2) the antecolic retroanastomotic space, and (3) the defect in the transverse mesocolon.[289] The last of these is usually closed after retrocolic gastrojejunostomy, and the omentum is sutured to the stomach pouch. Obstruction may occur if the mesocolon has been sutured to the jejunum.[283] If the proximal loop lies above the mesocolon and the distal loop passes through the mesocolon, posterior herniation behind the anastomosis is impossible.[277] This method of handling the jejunal loop in posterior anastomosis also avoids tension on the omental stitches. These may otherwise pull out and the anastomotic loop may slide up, and torsion and obstruction will result. Internal hernias through the gap in the mesocolon involve either the proximal or the distal loop, or both. Long, proximal (afferent) loops are more prone to herniation and chronic incarceration.[295]

In Carillo's review[271] of immediate complications of gastrectomy, proximal loop obstruction was the second most common cause of postoperative death, the first being duodenal leakage. Kinking, fibrosis, tumor recurrence, or pressure by the mesentery of one anastomotic loop on the other may result in obstruction (Figs. 64-64 and 64-65). Sometimes on films of a barium enema examination a portion of the transverse colon is seen to have been pulled up with the retrocolic anastomosis. The antecolic anastomosis often results in radiographic changes caused by pressure on the transverse colon.[309]

Small bowel obstruction

Obstructions in the small bowel are readily diagnosed by radiographs. The causes of obstruction are adhesions, internal hernias, and intussusceptions.[274] Small bowel obstruction also results from bowel compression by the tautly interposed mesentery.[319] Intestinal obstructions caused by bezoars occur in the jejunum[149] or ileum.[272] After gastrectomy, patients should avoid whole oranges or similar foods containing fibers that may cause phytobezoars.[297,303,304]

The degree of postoperative obstruction in the duodenum or small bowel is sometimes better demonstrated with the use of food and barium than with barium liquid alone.[270]

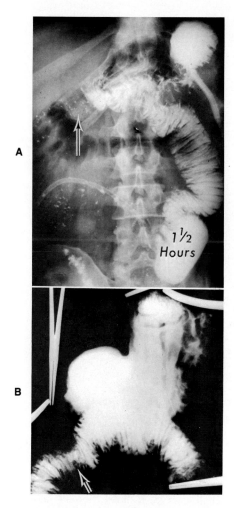

Fig. 64-64 Patient with vomiting after partial distal gastrectomy and side-to-side, left-to-right gastroenterostomy and preferential filling of long proximal jejunal loop. **A,** Delayed film shows proximal loop stasis and partial obstruction at distal jejunal loop *(arrow)*. **B,** Contrast filling of resected specimen with narrowing because of scarring *(arrow)*, extensive enough to cause significant symptoms.

Inadvertent distal gastroenterostomy

Gastroileostomy is a surgical emergency. If the ligament of Treitz is not identified by the surgeon at the time of gastrojejunostomy, an inadvertent anastomosis between the stomach and the ileum is possible.[299,300,307] This results in a rapid loss of weight, hunger after meals, and the passage of undigested food. The patient dies unless the gastroileostomy is revised.[308]

The radiologist must follow the same rule as the surgeon and identify the position of the ligament of Treitz during radiologic examination. Katz and Karp,[287] who found 135 instances of gastroileostomy reported up to 1967, have discussed the radiologic findings and stressed

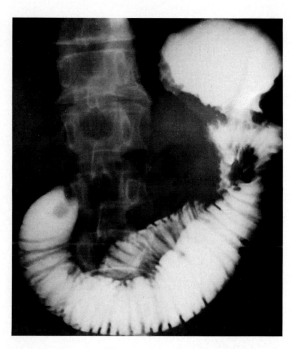

Fig. 64-65 Partial obstruction of both limbs of anastomotic jejunal loop resulting from malignant recurrence in patient who had had partial distal gastrectomy and gastrojejunostomy for carcinoma of antrum. Note plication defect in duodenum caused by inverted stump.

that a preoperative diagnosis of this lesion has never been made without a correctly interpreted radiographic study. The principal radiographic finding is a proximal loop crossing to the right iliac fossa, with rapid appearance of barium in the colon. If the proximal (afferent) jejunal loop does not lead to the ligament of Treitz and if the distal (efferent) jejunal loop can be traced over a relatively short distance to the ileocecal valve, the diagnosis is not difficult (Fig. 64-66).

Gastrojejunocolic fistula, the sequela of marginal ulcers, must be considered in the differential diagnosis of gastroileostomy. With the former condition the patient, however, does not usually have symptoms as early after surgery. The barium enema study is more diagnostic of gastrojejunocolic fistula than is the upper gastrointestinal study.

When an inadvertent gastroileostomy has been formed, the diagnosis is more readily made by upper gastrointestinal study than by a barium enema. However, a barium enema may be used in addition to flood the small bowel and thereby demonstrate the distance from the ileocecal valve to the anastomosis.

Reflux into the stomach after a barium enema and small bowel filling may, however, occur in the intact gastrointestinal tract and is therefore not necessarily indicative of a fistula.[313]

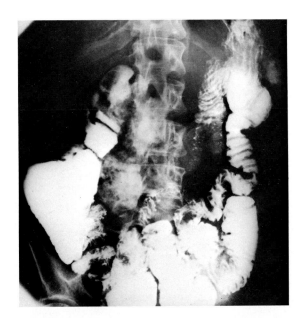

Fig. 64-66 Inadvertent gastroileostomy with relatively short bowel between gastric remnant and ileocecal valve. Proximal jejunal limb of anastomosis is long and leads to right lower quadrant.

Inadvertent *gastrocolostomy* is fatal if not diagnosed. The diagnosis is readily made by both upper gastrointestinal study and a barium enema. No radiographic illustrations previous to the one shown in Fig. 64-67 were found in my study of the literature.

Dysfunction of the proximal jejunal loop

Undue length of the proximal (afferent) loop is considered undesirable.[282,314] If the proximal loop is attached to the greater curvature instead of the lesser curvature, this left-to-right anastomosis results in preferential emptying of the stomach into the proximal loop (Fig. 64-68). It leads to regurgitation and proximal loop stasis and may result in the so-called proximal (afferent) loop syndrome or blind loop syndrome, with vitamin B$_{12}$ deficiency and resulting anemia. I agree with Hafter[282] that this type of left-to-right anastomosis may lead to the afferent loop syndrome. Preferential emptying into the proximal loop and delayed emptying into the distal loop are present with proximal loop stasis, bilious vomiting, and associated anemia in some cases (Fig. 64-69). Surgical conversion into a gastroduodenostomy or revision of the gastrojejunostomy into a conventional right-to-left anastomosis with the proximal loop leading to the lesser curvature results in correction of the symptoms.

Ideally the proximal loop should be short, perhaps no more than 10 cm long.[308] The gastrojejunostomy can be even closer to the duodenojejunal junction in a retrocolic anastomosis.[315]

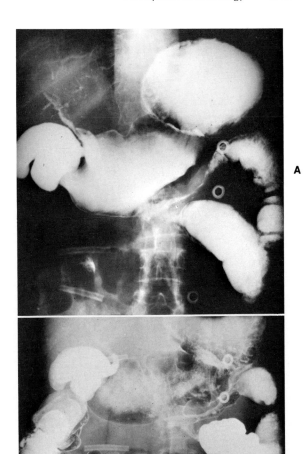

Fig. 64-67 Inadvertent gastrocolostomy in patient who had had cholecystoduodenostomy and gastrojejunostomy scheduled for obstructing carcinoma of pancreas. **A,** Upper gastrointestinal study shows filling of anastomotic colonic loop. **B,** Subsequent barium enema outlines remainder of colon. There is no small bowel filling. Patient lost 20 pounds in 2 weeks after surgery. Anastomosis was revised with good results.

Afferent loop syndrome

The afferent loop syndrome is characterized by postprandial epigastric fullness relieved by bilious vomiting.[281] Stasis in the afferent loop is present, and a high bacterial count may be found on aspiration of the contents of the loop. The predominant organism is a gram-negative bacillus with the flora generally resembling that

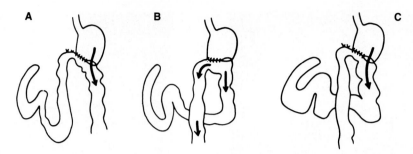

Fig. 64-68 A, Desirable emptying in forward direction in right-to-left anastomosis with oblique cut end of stomach. **B,** Bidirectional emptying with horizontal plane of left-to-right anastomosis. **C,** Undesirable preferential filling of proximal jejunal loop with left-to-right anastomosis and oblique plane of anastomosis resulting in proximal loop stasis.

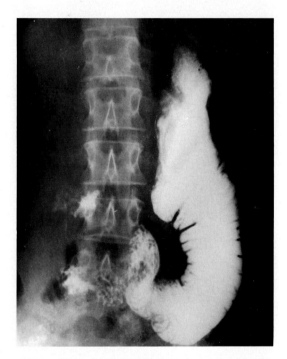

Fig. 64-69 Contrast study demonstrates preferential filling of proximal jejunal loop and duodenum, with stasis. There was no filling of distal jejunal loop on early films. Patient vomited part of barium.

in colon in both quantity and quality. The abnormal bacterial flora[280] and megaloblastic anemia[267] may be corrected by antibiotic therapy.[317] At laparotomy the proximal loop has been found to be hypertrophied. This condition may be classified under the blind loop syndrome.[316] The proximal (afferent) loop syndrome resulting from a left-to-right anastomosis has already been discussed.

Madsen[293] has separated from this chronic form of afferent loop difficulty a more acute afferent loop problem that is characterized by pronounced obstruction. If left untreated, the outcome of this acute form may be death. Four deaths occured in Carillo's five patients[271] with proximal loop obstructions. Causes can be torsion,[273] kinking, or twisted long loops.[282] Also, pressures of one limb of the anastomosis may cause partial obstruction of the other.[316]

Radiologic examination plays an important part in the diagnosis of the afferent loop syndrome. The point of obstruction in either the proximal or distal jejunum can be demonstrated. The direction of gastric emptying is important. Serial films or cinefluorograms may be obtained with the patient in the erect position. Filling of the proximal loop is not in itself considered abnormal. Most of the contrast medium should, however, empty in a forward direction into the distal jejunum. There should be good emptying of the contrast medium from the proximal jejunum.[312,351] If preferential proximal loop filling occurs with the proximal loop distention and if stasis and delayed emptying are recorded on serial films, partial obstruction at or just beyond the anastomosis may be responsible (Fig. 64-70).

Radiologic assessment of the afferent loop by selective intubation methods is able to demonstrate abnormalities such as (1) afferent loop obstruction, (2) duodenal leak, (3) retained antrum, and (4) blind loop syndrome.[284]

Blind pouch syndrome

Stagnant dilated segments of small intestine may be demonstrated radiologically after side-to-side anastomosis of the small intestine. This dilatation usually occurs 5 to 15 years after surgery. It may also be present if a side-to-end or side-to-side anastomosis has been performed between the small intestine and the large intestine. End-to-end anastomosis is now the procedure of choice.

In the classic blind loop syndrome a segment of small intestine has been completely bypassed by enteroanastomosis. The diagnosis of the stagnant loop syndrome is made with demonstration of a structural lesion of the

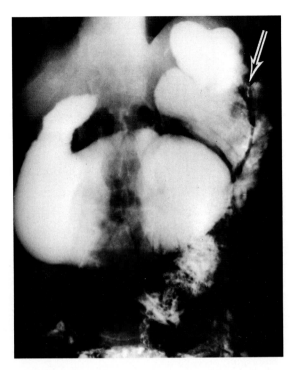

Fig. 64-70 Proximal (afferent) loop distention resulting from partial obstruction with scarring after marginal ulcer at distal jejunal loop *(arrow)*.

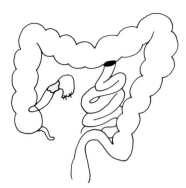

Fig. 64-71 Ileal transverse colostomy with end-to-side anastomosis bypassing distal ileal lesion and right colon.

small bowel that is accompanied by bacterial colonization of the small intestine and evidence of malabsorption. Steatorrhea and macrocytic anemia are the chief clinical features.[269] Radiographic features of the blind pouch syndrome are gas-filled structures on plain radiographs. If filled with fluid, they may resemble soft tissue masses and show air-fluid levels on upright radiographs.[290] Barium studies demonstrate the pouches and the anastomotic site. Blind pouch formation may also be accompanied by gastrointestinal bleeding. Familiarity with the clinical and radiographic features can aid in a prompt and precise preoperative diagnosis. Segmental resection and end-to-end anastomosis are curative.[294]

Intestinal bypass

Most commonly, an intestinal bypass is carried out as a palliative procedure for obstructing nonresectable gastrointestinal cancer (Figs. 64-71 and 64-72). Other indications include radiation injury to the small bowel, hyperlipidemia, and morbid obesity.

End-to-side or end-to-end jejunoileal bypass procedures have been performed. The surgical procedure for intestinal short-circuiting was introduced by Payne and associates[302] in 1963 for the treatment of morbid obesity. With their procedure there is an end-to-side anastomosis of the proximal 14 inches of jejunum with the distal 4 inches of terminal ileum (Fig. 64-73). Scott's

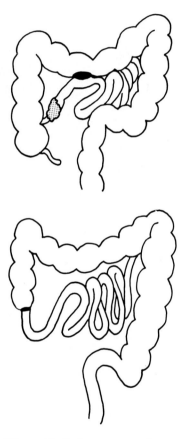

Fig. 64-72 Side-to-side ileal transverse colostomy bypassing unresectable distal ileal lesion *(top);* resection of resectable ileal lesion is followed by end-to-end ileal right colostomy *(bottom).*

procedure[306] uses an end-to-end jejunoileal anastomosis with the bypassed small bowel segment decompressed into the large intestine (Figs. 64-74 and 64-75).

The radiologist should be familiar with the normal and abnormal radiologic changes that occur after a small bowel bypass. The described postoperative complica-

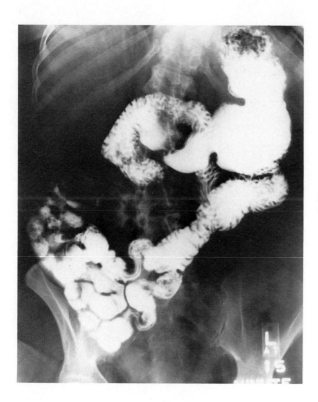

Fig. 64-73 Small bowel bypass procedure for morbid obesity with end-to-side jejunoileostomy (Payne's procedure).

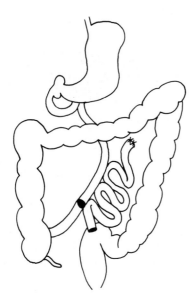

Fig. 64-74 Scott's procedure with end-to-end jejunoileal anastomosis with bypassed small bowel segment anastomosed to large intestine.

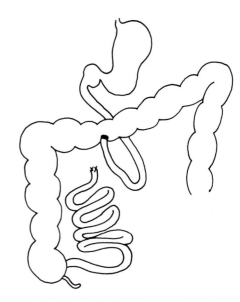

Fig. 64-75 Small bowel bypass with jejunocolonic anastomosis.

tions include bypass enteritis,[301] pneumatosis intestinalis,[296] chronic inflammation of the excluded bowel,[276] liver failure,[268] beriberi,[285] hyperoxaluria,[310] urolithiasis,[318] and cholelithiasis.[318] Complications for Scott's procedure are, in addition, bypass enteritis and the defunctionalized bowel syndrome.[286]

Multiple intestinal air-fluid levels and the distention of the jejunum and ileum are common and expected postoperative sequelae of small bowel bypass procedures for morbid obesity. The radiologist must be familiar with these findings in order to avoid the misdiagnosis of bowel obstruction. If this complication is suspected, contrast studies by rectum and by mouth are indicated.[311]

Intussusception involving the excluded small bowel segment is an infrequent complication after intestinal bypass procedures for morbid obesity.[298] Because the bypassed segment of bowel may not be seen on plain radiographs or contrast studies, ultrasonography[305] or CT scanning may be used to demonstrate the intussuscepted segment of bowel. The tubular-appearing mass void of intestinal content gives a characteristic doughnut appearance.[292]

Because of a high complication rate after a jejunoileal bypass for morbid obesity, gastric exclusion operations are now preferred.

Ileostomy and ileal pouches

Necrosis, ileostomy, ileostomy prolapse, fistula formation, peristomal hernia, ileostomy stenosis, and bleeding are the complications of conventional ileostomies. The ileostomy segment should be examined in an oblique or tangential position during contrast studies to identify abnormalities, particularly hernia and stenosis. This is best done at the end of the reflux examination without a catheter in place.

The continent ileostomy by Kock is now more commonly performed (Fig. 64-76). A small bowel pouch is constructed from a 30 cm segment of ileum just proximal to the distal 10 cm. The distal ileum is brought through the abdominal wall to create a stoma, and the pouch is attached to the anterior abdominal wall. In addition, a nipple valve is created by invaginating the distal segment of ileum back into the pouch for a distance of 2 to 4 cm (Fig. 64-77). The radiologic features of Kock's ileostomy have been described by Diner and Cockrill.[275] Radiologic studies may be of particular value in follow-up by demonstrating postoperative nipple valve extrusion and inflammatory changes in the pouch.[275] About 30% of patients with Kock's ileostomy require revisions for malfunctioning of the valve. The continent ileal reservoir by Kock is considered contraindicated if Crohn's disease is present.

Total colectomy with ileostomy has been a preferred procedure for patients with severe long-standing ulcerative colitis. However, because an ileostomy was not a viable or an acceptable surgical option for many young patients with active life-styles, other surgical procedures were introduced. Most recently, an ileal pouch with ileoanal mucosal anastomosis has been used. This procedure consists of mucosal proctectomy and subtotal colectomy with ileoanal anastomosis and an ileal pelvic pouch immediately above the anastomosis to maintain reservoir function. The reservoir is created from 15 to 20 cm of ileum and may have a side-to-side configuration, a J shape, or an S shape (Figs. 64-78 and 64-79).

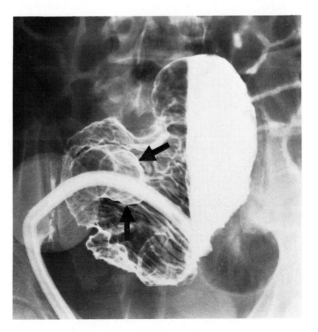

Fig. 64-77 Double contrast study of a normal and intact nipple valve.
(From Stephens, D, Mantell, B, and Kelly, K: AJR 132:717, 1979. © 1979, American Roentgen Ray Society.)

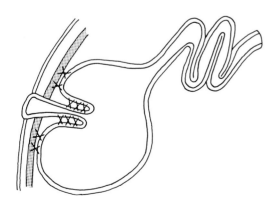

Fig. 64-76 Kock's continent ileostomy with distal ileal pouch and nipple valve.

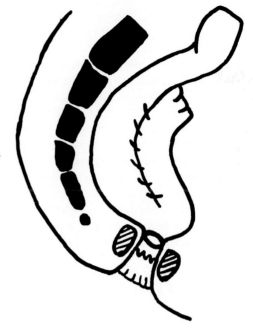

Fig. 64-78 The completed reservoir after ileoanal anastomosis when seen in the lateral projection.

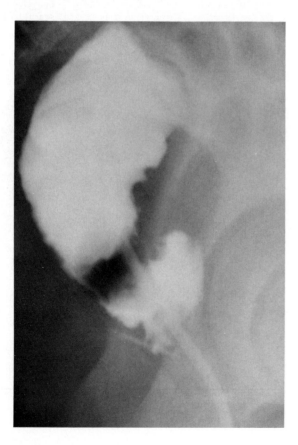

Fig. 64-79 Small leak at the ileoanal anastomosis after subtotal colectomy.

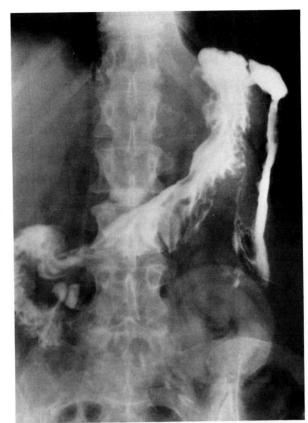

Fig. 64-80 Upper gastrointestinal study outlining fistula from stomach to postoperative bed after resection of splenic flexure.

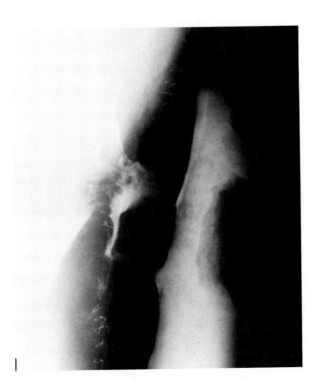

Fig. 64-81 External colonic fistula through incisional dehiscence, with knuckle of colonic wall caught between stitches.

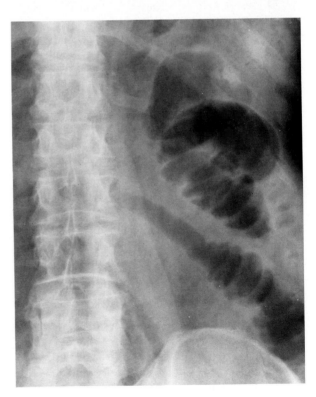

Fig. 64-82 Kinked mesentery with small bowel gangrene after colonic resection.

Small bowel obstruction and leakage at the ileoanal anastomosis are the most commonly detected complications on radiologic examination.[288] Other complications include leaks from the anastomotic reservoir or late anal fistulas.[278]

Another complication associated with pouch ileostomy is bacterial overgrowth and stasis, which may be associated with formation of enteroliths detectable by plain abdominal radiography.[279]

COLON[320-328]

Complications after colonic surgery include anastomotic failure, ileus, fistula, hemorrhage, and sepsis such as wound infection, peritonitis, abscess formation, and enteritis. Radiologic studies are useful in identifying free air or abscess formation on plain films, anastomotic leakage and fistula formation with Gastrografin studies, and bowel obstruction with barium contrast examination (Figs. 64-80 to 64-82).

Obstruction is less common after colonic surgery than it is after small intestine surgery, but the rate of anastomotic breakdown after large bowel surgery is high. If an anastomotic leak is suspected, radiographic enema examination with an iodinated contrast medium is indicated. Contrast studies may demonstrate more than one fistula, or the internal fistula may go to the small bowel or bladder. Radiographic studies will also delineate the size of abscess cavities. Unsuspected loculations can be identified by ultrasonography.

Paralytic ileus and peritonitis may result from anastomotic leakage in the colon. Enema examination will clarify cases of pseudoobstruction of the colon after surgery. Cecal rupture as a result of paralytic ileus is an unusual complication, also called *Ogilvie's syndrome*. The cecal diameter may reach 20 cm.[322]

Tumor recurrence at the colonic anastomosis can be identified by barium enema examination (Figs. 64-83 and 64-84); some narrowing at the colon anastomosis is usually present after surgery. The narrowing is smooth and concentric, and the invagination of the serosal surfaces at the anastomosis usually results in a mucosal collar. Postoperative barium enema examinations as a baseline study of the anastomosis are recommended. This is best done after 2 months and after the postoperative edema has subsided.

Colostomy

A variety of complications may occur at a transverse or sigmoid colostomy site. These include hernia, stricture, bleeding, retraction, prolapse, obstruction, abscess, and perforation. These complications are not uncommon but also are usually not serious (Fig. 64-85).

Colostomy barium examinations can be cumbersome and time-consuming because of the barium spillage. A soft rubber catheter is usually inserted into the colostomy. The patient holds the inflated balloon on the outside against the stoma. The balloon is never inflated inside the patient. A variety of other techniques are in use.[321,323,324] A standard colostomy irrigation bag is easy to use and requires little time for completion.[320] The colostomy should be examined in several projections, including a tangential view to evaluate the colon segment in the abdominal wall.

Radiation effects

Radiation effects on the colon may be seen after treatment of malignant lesions of the female pelvic organs, bladder, and prostate. Earlier changes after radiation include proctocolitis with edematous and sometimes ulcerated mucosa. Rectal bleeding may be present, but most patients demonstrate no specific radiographic findings associated with these clinical signs and symptoms.[326]

A late radiation effect seen radiographically is a chronic large bowel injury, which usually occurs 6 to 24 months after completion of radiation therapy.[328] A segmental stricture is often noted in the distal colon or rectum, along with proximal bowel dilatation. This is caused by chronic postradiation ischemia with mucosal atrophy and fibrosis.

The barium enema study serves the following purposes according to Meyer[325]:
1. A baseline for comparison should symptoms develop at a later date
2. Direct visualization of anatomic relations between the colon and other pelvic structures
3. Screening for intrinsic colon disease such as diverticulitis, ulcerative colitis, or Crohn's disease, which might modify the treatment plan

A lateral view of the rectum is an essential part of the examination. The examination with retention balloons is hazardous because of potential perforation of the stricture.

Local recurrences after resection for carcinoma of the rectum are best studied by CT scanning, which facilitates evaluation of local recurrence, extension of tumor, and possible involvement of the cecum.[327]

RECTUM

Anterior resection of the rectum may be accompanied by hemorrhage. The diagnosis of a hematoma can be made by CT scanning in order to facilitate evacuation. Barium enema examination may be helpful in estimating progress and in determining the time for colostomy closure.

Complications after abdominoperineal resection of the rectum may be at the sigmoid colostomy or at the peri-

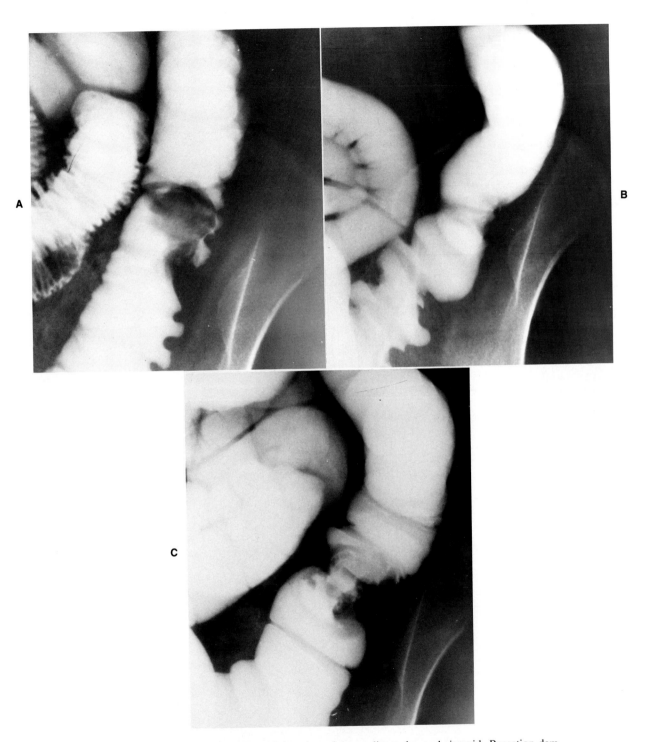

Fig. 64-83 A, Pedunculated polyp at junction of descending colon and sigmoid. Resection demonstrated adenocarcinoma extending into stalk. **B,** Baseline study after local resection, not segmental resection. **C,** Two layers later, recurrence of concentric adenocarcinoma.

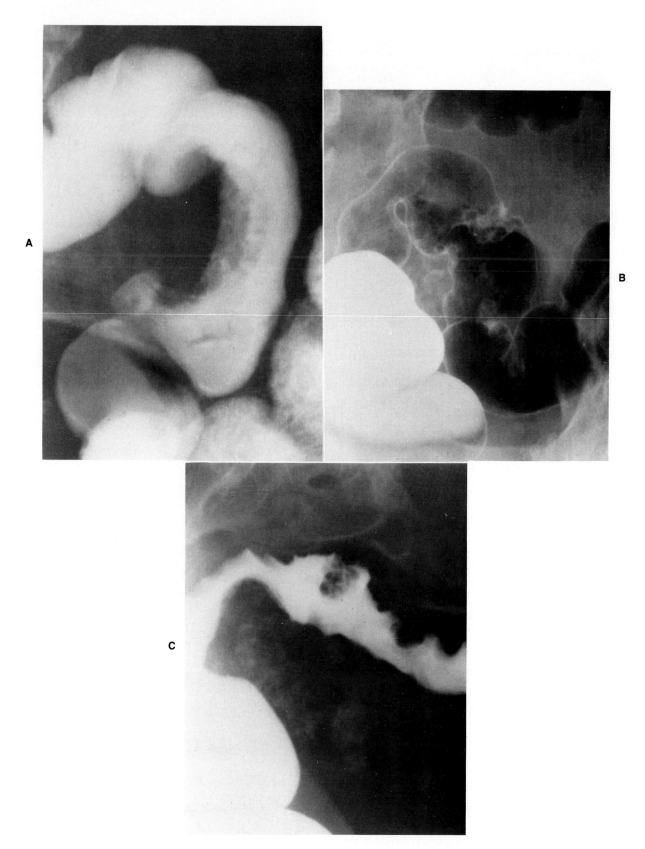

Fig. 64-84 A, Carcinoma of sigmoid colon before segmental resection. **B** and **C,** Polypoid filling defect at anastomotic margin on follow-up study 6 months later. Second operation demonstrated presence of suture granuloma but no recurrence.

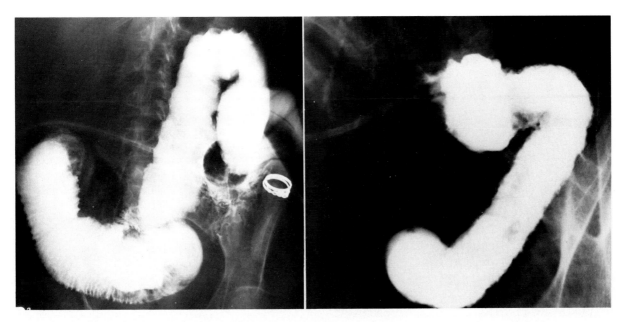

Fig. 64-85 Patient underwent ileal transverse colostomy for regional enteritis of ileum and right colon. Filling of both colostomy segments now shows active granulomatous disease in remaining colon.

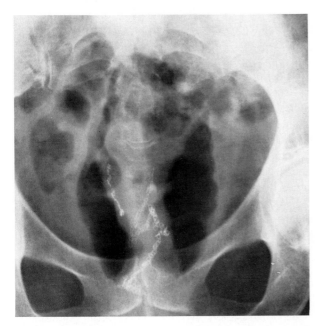

Fig. 64-86 Anastomotic leak at low colonic anastomosis with pelvic perirectal abscess formation.

toneal floor (Fig. 64-86), or the lower urinary tract may be involved. Prolapse of small intestine through a pelvic peritoneal dehiscence may be diagnosed radiographically.

Pull-through operations for cancer of the rectum require postoperative radiographic examination to evaluate possible suture line recurrence. The complication of en-

terocolitis after Swenson's operation for megacolon can be evaluated with the same radiologic technique. In Soave's procedure the outermost layer of the rectum is left in situ. D'Allaine's anterior resection and posterior anastomosis may be followed by early complications involving the urinary tract or the late complication of anal stenosis.

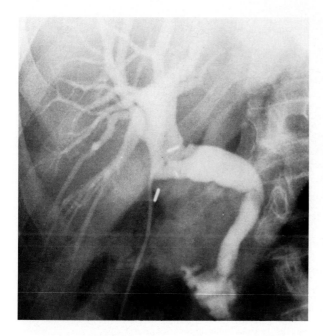

Fig. 64-87 Primary operative cholangiogram with cystic duct cannula shows cystic duct to enter right hepatic duct. No common hepatic duct is present. Cholangiogram shows duct system to be clear. No exploration of common duct was undertaken.

BILIARY TRACT[329-441]

General considerations

The first cholecystectomy for cholelithiasis in 1882 by Langenbuch was a milestone in biliary tract surgery.[361] Choledochotomy by Courvoisier followed in 1890. Radiographic visualization of the bile ducts then became possible by two important techniques: (1) Mirizzi[390] performed direct cholangiography on the operating table in 1932, and (2) transhepatic cholangiography was attempted as early as 1921[338] but did not become accepted and practical until 1952.[344]

We realize the importance of surgical biliary tract radiology when we read that more than half a million patients are hospitalized for gallbladder disease in the United States each year,[423] with two thirds of these patients undergoing surgery.[357] Cholangiography has developed into a major tool for diagnostic evaluation in these patients before, during, and after surgery.

Terminology

Operative or surgical cholangiography consists of two phases with different indications. *Primary cholangiography* is done before the common duct is explored, before the biliary tract is manipulated, and before the decision is made concerning exploration of the biliary duct system (Fig. 64-87). This procedure is also described as diagnostic, preexploratory, or precholedochotomy cholangiography. *Secondary operative cholangiography* is performed after exploration of the common duct, usually through the T-tube, but before closure

of the abdomen. It is the final check on remaining disease and is also described as control, postexploratory, or postcholedochotomy cholangiography. *Postoperative T-tube cholangiography* is usually performed through the indwelling tube within 7 to 10 days after surgery.

Radiomanometry combines pressure readings with contrast injection. It was introduced by Mallet-Guy[387] but was not widely applied. It is primarily used by surgeons interested in dykinesia of the biliary tract.[371] Endoscopic sphincterotomy can provide relief of pain in patients with parallel pain-pressure relationships. Postsphincterotomy manometry showed disappearance of manometric pressure elevation, and results of morphine-Prostigmin tests turned negative.[425]

Dyskinesia of the biliary tract continues to be poorly understood, particularly since most abnormalities of intraductal pressure can be traced to morphologic and mechanical abnormalities in the biliary tract.

Cholescystocholangiography is operative injection into the gallbladder, with opacification of the biliary tree. This technique is of great value in the diagnosis of congenital anomalies of the biliary tract (Figs. 64-88 to 64-90).

Technique

Calculous disease accounts for most surgical procedures on the biliary tract. *Plain films, ultrasonograms, and oral cholecystograms* provide the preoperative diagnosis in almost all cases, whereas transhepatic cholangiograms may be required if jaundice is present (Fig. 64-91).

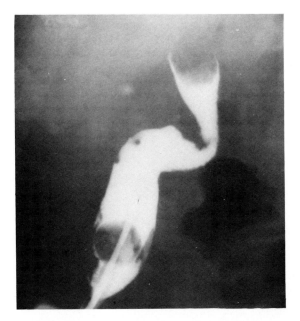

Fig. 64-88 Direct cholecystography without cholangiography shows cystic duct obstruction by large solitary stone.

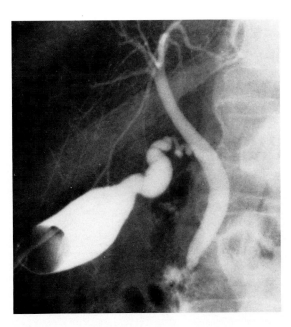

Fig. 64-89 Cholecystocholangiogram demonstrates biliary tract to be normal.

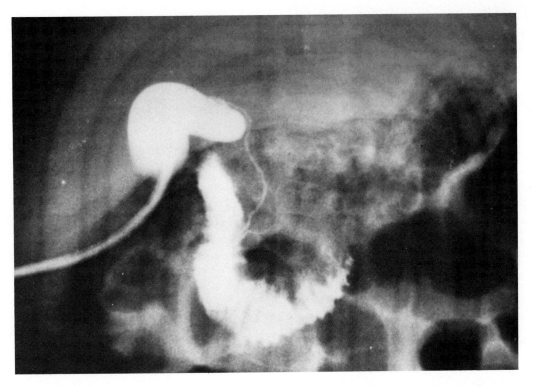

Fig. 64-90 Operative cholecystocholangiography in jaundiced infant with agenesis of hepatic duct. Microcholedochus is apparently caused by disuse.

If elective cholecystectomy has been scheduled for cholelithiasis, a recent radiographic study must be available, because it has been shown that stones up to 1 cm in size and up to 30 in number[368] can be evacuated spontaneously.[389] These so-called disappearing gallstones are often encountered in the postpregnancy state[333] (Fig. 64-92).

The primary operative cholangiogram is the first order of business after laparotomy.[341] The cystic duct is isolated, and either a cannula[330,380] or a bulb-tipped urethral catheter[385] may be used for injection, but the cannulation of the cystic duct with a small polyethylene tube appears to be most satisfactory.[378] The cystic duct remains intubated until usable radiographs are obtained. This interval

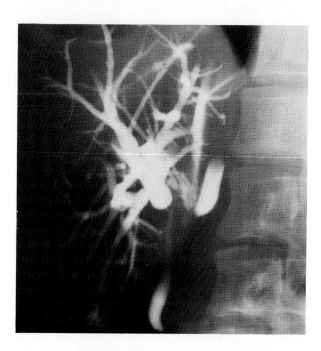

Fig. 64-91 Transhepatic cholangiography in jaundiced patient shows strictures at porta hepatis.

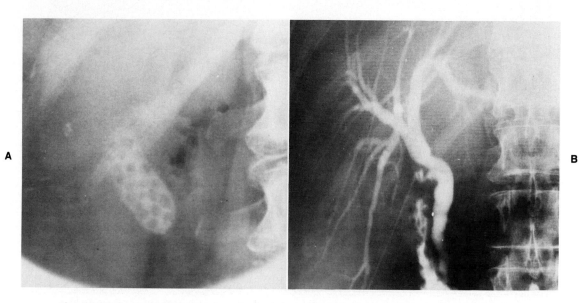

Fig. 64-92 A, Oral cholecystogram obtained 4 months before elective cholecystectomy reveals numerous small gallstones. **B,** At time of surgery, gallbladder contained no stones and primary operative cholangiograms were normal. Surgery could have been avoided in this case of "disappearing gallstones," with repeat oral cholecystogram obtained before surgery. Stones of this size may readily pass through ampulla of Vater.

is used for cholecystectomy so that the duration of anesthesia is shortened. Direct needle puncture of the common duct is also practiced[355,363] (Fig. 64-93).

The operating table is rotated 10 to 15 degrees along the longitudinal axis to the right to project the distal biliary tract away from the lumbar spine. Grid lines must cross the abdomen at a right angle to the longitudinal axis of the body if a movable grid is not available.

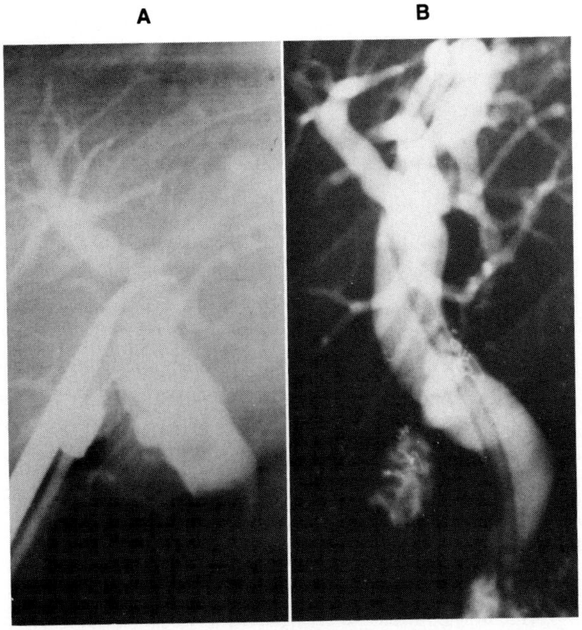

The contrast medium used for direct injection during operative cholangiography must be opaque enough for marginal delineation of the bile duct, yet dilute enough to permit visualization of stones through the contrast medium. A 50% or 60% concentration of the contrast medium (Hypaque or Renografin) diluted half and half with normal saline permits good visualization at 90 kV. Further dilution is required if the extrahepatic bile ducts are dilated beyond 10 mm. At least two films are obtained. The first injection is accomplished with 5 ml or less of the contrast medium injected at low pressure close to gravity. The second radiograph is obtained after injection of less than 10 ml under mild pressure. An increase above normal intraductal pressure usually results in contraction of the sphincter of Oddi with retrograde filling of the intrahepatic radicals (Fig. 64-94).

Television monitors in the surgical suite are convenient[432] but do not match the detail seen on radiographs. I have found routine portable radiography to be quite adequate in the surgical suite. It requires less time than television fluoroscopy.

Serial photofluorography is used when cholangiography presents problems, particularly if delay occurs at the sphincter of Oddi.[393,441] It is useful for evaluation of pharmacoradiologic effects on the biliary tract and its sphincters.[422]

It is not necessary to administer medication to induce spasm of the sphincter of Oddi so that better visualization is obtained, but glucagon may be used to relieve spasm at the choledochoduodenal junction.

Fig. 64-93 A, Primary operative cholangiogram with injection into markedly dilated hepatic duct with stone obstruction. **B,** Secondary operative cholangiogram obtained after relief of obstruction shows decrease in diameter of hepatic duct.

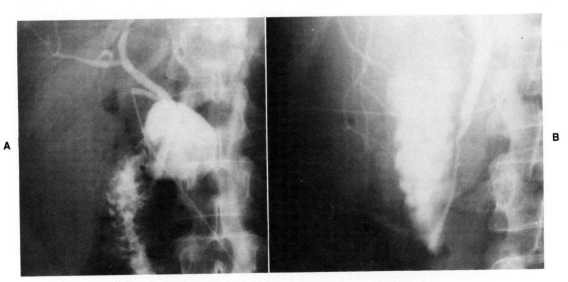

Fig. 64-94 A, First radiograph of primary operative cholangiogram was obtained too late in this patient. Also, too much contrast medium was used. Opaque medium in duodenal bulb is obscuring common duct. Injecting physician, furthermore, should stand on right side of patient. **B,** High injection pressure resulting in sphincter contraction and jet.

Barium cholangiography is practical,[384] particularly if duodenobiliary reflux occurs[345] or if an intestinal anastomosis is present.[436] The absence of air in the biliary ducts after anastomosis to the intestinal tract suggests anastomotic obstruction[366] (Figs. 64-95 to 64-97).

Intraoperative ultrasonography has been used more

recently for the detection of common bile duct calculi. It cannot replace operative cholangiography but is useful in selected cases as an added intraoperative procedure. Its use requires specific training and a prolonged period of learning for the biliary surgeon.[377]

Intraoperative choledochoscopy is another addition to the surgical armamentarium to reduce the rate of retained common duct stones. This technique can detect lesions missed by cholangiography and help in the differential diagnosis of common duct disease. Complications include perforation, fistula formation, pancreatitis, and abscess formation (Fig. 64-98).[347]

Interpretation, pitfalls, and mistakes

With good technique the accuracy of operative cholangiography should be 90% to 95%. Duct stones measuring 3 mm or smaller, however, may be missed in half of the cases.[334] Stones also may be overlooked if their density corresponds to that of the contrast medium.[421]

Attention to details of radiographic technique is the obligation of the radiologist.[426] Good films can be obtained with portable equipment.[409] Custer and Clore[346] analyzed the sources of error in their material on operative cholangiography and found technically unsatisfactory radiographs to be the leading cause.

Air bubbles

Air bubbles must be eliminated by working in a closed system and using aspiration and injection with saline. This applies also to T-tube cholangiograms. The T-tube is best clamped in these patients for at least 12 hours

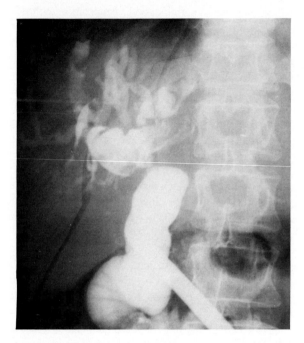

Fig. 64-95 Barium cholangiography permits evaluation of diameter and patency of hepatojejunostomy.

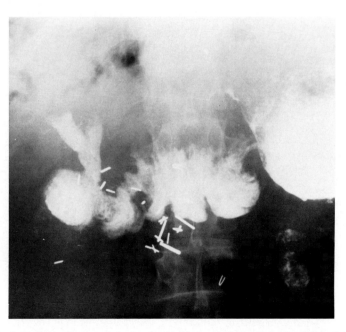

Fig. 64-96 Barium cholangiogram shows patency of hepatojejunostomy after Whipple's procedure for carcinoma of pancreas.

before radiographic examination is undertaken. A needle is then introduced through the wall of the rubber catheter to maintain a closed-fluid system.

The differentiation between air bubbles and stones in the duct system may be made by placing the patient in the Trendelenburg and semierect positions. However, not everything that is round and rises in fluid is an air bubble; gallstones do not have to be faceted, and cholesterol stones may float in contrast medium. Elsey and Jacobs[353] have shown that the specific gravity of the lightest cholesterol stone is 1.04, which is the greatest specific gravity that native bile reaches. This means that stones can hardly float in native bile but may float after the addition of contrast medium. Air bubbles, on the other hand, fortunately are never faceted and never sink in bile or contrast medium.

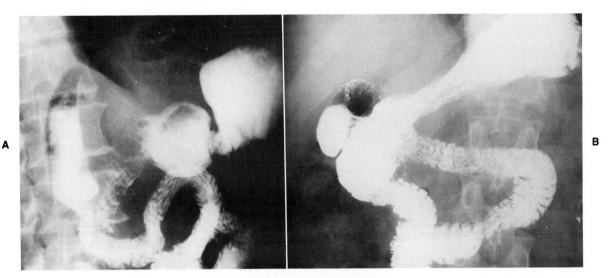

Fig. 64-97 Cholecystoduodenostomy, **A,** and cholecystojejunostomy with Roux-en-Y jejunojejunostomy, **B.** Both cases show barium reflux into gallbladder. Pneumocholangiogram is less frequently present when compared with direct anastomosis of duct system to intestinal tract.

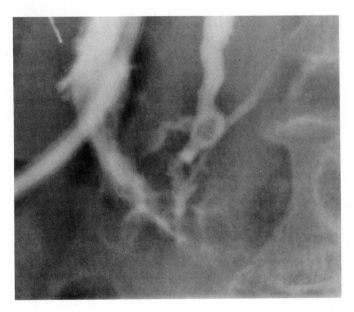

Fig. 64-98 Postoperative T-tube cholangiogram 7 days after common duct exploration and operative choledochoscopy shows a traumatic fistula from the distal common duct to the duodenum. The surgeon was unable to remove the distal common duct stone with the use of the choledochoscope. The stone was removed 4 weeks later by radiologic intervention.

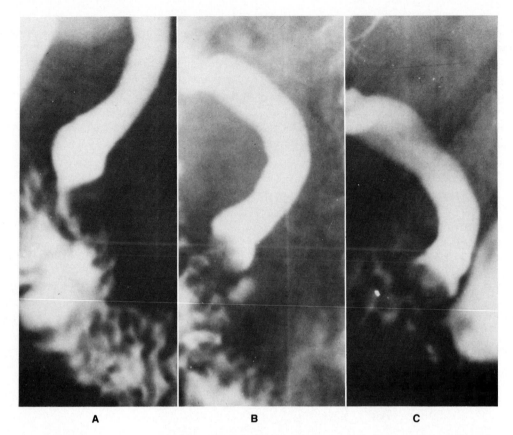

A   B   C

Fig. 64-99 Serial films showing the normal distal duct, **A,** some contraction at sphincter, **B,** and prominent contraction at sphincter simulating common duct stone, **C.** This "pseudocalculus sign" is frequently seen in secondary operative cholangiography following duct instrumentation.

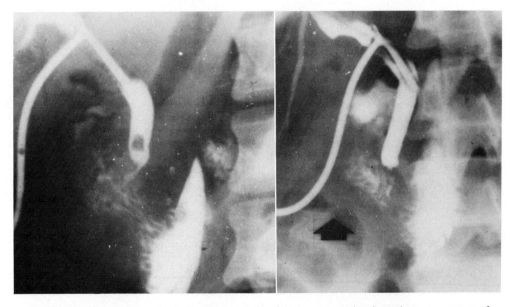

Fig. 64-100 Cinefluorography during T-tube cholangiogram was used to investigate movement of small common duct stone in this patient with no T-tube drainage when supine, but right upper quadrant pain and prominent T-tube drainage when out of bed. **A,** Small stone moved back into common duct with patient supine. **B,** Stone cannot be seen on spot films with patient erect. Cinefluorographic frame analysis showed stone to move into intramural portion of distal common duct, with partial duct obstruction.

Filling defects of the common bile duct may result from external compression, distortion by the needle or catheter used for injection, pressure by the hepatic artery, and other causes. The intramural, or third, portion of the common duct normally may be narrowed where it runs in a groove posteriorly in the head of the pancreas.

Blockage at the sphincter of Oddi may be caused by spasm, particularly after manipulation of the common duct or instrumentation of the sphincter of Oddi. This contraction may even simulate stones in the distal duct. Serial films are necessary for clarification (Figs. 64-99 and 64-100). One must be aware of this possibility, particularly on the second operative cholangiogram, because misinterpretation may lead to unnecessary second exploration.[360] Obstruction of the entrance of the common duct in the duodenum can be expected in half of the cases after instrumentation.[337] If a primary cholangiogram is obtained routinely, the "pseudocalculus" will not be misinterpreted.[414]

Pneumocholangiogram

The presence of gas in the biliary tract may be caused by previous surgical anastomoses, by fistula from a gallstone, by inflammation, by peptic or malignant disease, by gas-forming organisms, or by incompetence of the sphincter of Oddi from medication, tumor, adhesions, or paralytic intestinal ileus.[404] Incompetence of the sphincter of Oddi with reflux of gas and barium has also been seen in newborn infants with duodenal atresia.[359] The pneumocholangiogram caused by gas-forming organisms must be quite unusual, whereas insufficiency of the sphincter with air reflux is more common than was initially thought, particularly if we accept the fact that patients pass gallstones spontaneously. Reflux of gas and barium also occurs in cases where the common duct enters the wall of the duodenal diverticulum[394] (Fig. 64-101). The sphincter musculature is often deficient in these cases. An air cholangiogram is also seen as a sequela of trauma[437] or as a complication of attempted thoracocentesis.[399]

Absence of the pneumocholangiogram sign in patients with other symptoms of a gallstone ileus should raise the suspicion of a second stone in the duct system causing obstruction proximal to a fistula.

Anatomic variations

Cholangiography may demonstrate absence of the cystic duct and gallbladder and duplication of the gallblad-

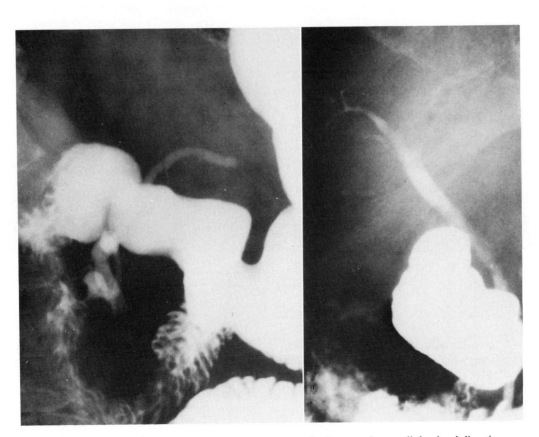

Fig. 64-101 Reflux of barium into bile duct and pancreatic duct entering small duodenal diverticulum.

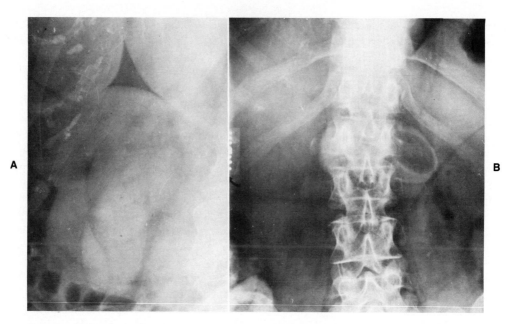

Fig. 64-102 A, Oral cholecystogram shows double gallbladder. **B,** Gallbladder containing large calculus with herniation into lesser sac.

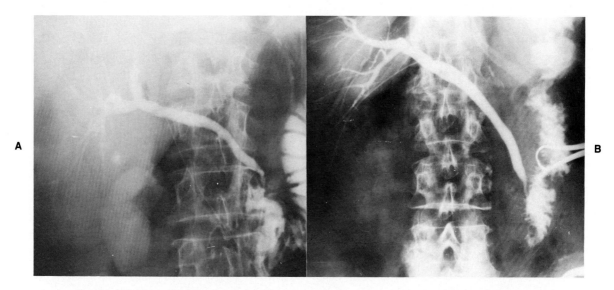

Fig. 64-103 Elongated biliary tract with gastroduodenostomy, **A,** and gastrojejunostomy, **B.** Descending duodenum had been mobilized in both cases.

der, with one[419] or two cystic ducts[397] entering the main duct. Guyer and McLoughlin[365] have concluded that there are not likely to be more than 150 proved cases of a double gallbladder in the world literature and that, of these, only 15 cases have been demonstrated radiologically and subsequently confirmed at surgery (Fig. 64-102). The gallbladder and cystic duct may by positioned anomalously on the left or in the midline. The latter is also seen with herniation of the gallbladder through the foramen of Winslow into the lesser sac.

The common duct elongates and extends to the left of the midline after a surgical procedure with mobilization of the duodenum, the so-called Kocher's maneuver (Fig. 64-103).

Even triplication of the gallbladder has been described in five instances.[408]

The size of the biliary ducts can be measured quite accurately on radiographs. Magnification should amount to 20%.

Compensatory dilatation of the common bile duct after cholecystectomy is not a normal occurrence.[362,391] An increase in diameter after surgery is indicative of biliary tract disease.[352] The common duct in patients without symptoms usually retains its size after surgery, as seen on preoperative films,[374] although normal common bile ducts show a slight but definite increase in both outer and inner circumferences with age in men and women.[386] Most authors therefore feel that in a patient with symptoms after cholecystectomy, cholangiograms that show dilatation on comparison with operative studies indicate an abnormality. I have seen some instances of immediate decrease in common duct diameter when I compared surgical cholangiograms of the same seated patient just before and after relief of common duct obstruction. This difference, which is accompanied by a change in intraductal pressure, is slight and appears to be caused by elastic fibers in the wall of the common duct.

The papilla of Vater is located in the third portion of the duodenum in 8% of patients.[412]

According to one study the ampulla of Vater should be considered abnormally narrow if a 3 mm dilator cannot be passed through it with ease.[340] The largest dilators passed in this study of normal ampullae averaged 6 mm in diameter. It is therefore plausible that common duct stones up to this size may pass spontaneously into the duodenum—an explanation for the entity of so-called disappearing gallstones. Passage of small gallstones into the duodenum is probably more common than is presently accepted.[341]

Also more common than is realized by radiologists and surgeons is the high percentage of anomalies of the major ducts of the biliary tree (Fig. 64-104). Schulenburg[411] found anatomic variations of the biliary tract in 230 of 1093 surgical patients, an incidence of 21%. Anomalies of the cystic duct were present in 13.7% of cases and were most commonly a low insertion into the common duct, with portions of the distal cystic duct running in a common sheet with the major duct. This explains the necessarily high incidence of cystic duct remnant. Hayes[369] found an even higher incidence of biliary duct anomalies. He has pointed out the risk of improperly identifying all structures and doing surgical damage to the biliary drainage. This emphasizes another strength of the primary operative cholangiogram—delineation of duct anomalies before exploration. The high degree of duct visualization after operative cholangiography cannot be achieved with preoperative intravenous cholangiography. Indeed, radiologists rarely identify duct anomalies by the latter method.

A third entity that is more common than is generally

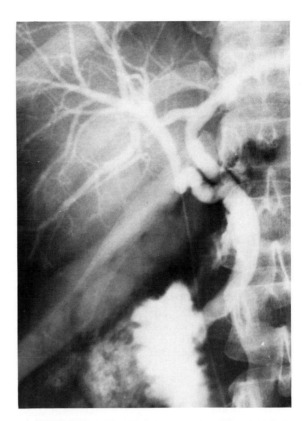

Fig. 64-104 Right hepatic duct joins cystic duct. If this information is available from primary operative cholangiogram, duct transection close to common duct can be avoided.

recognized is the insertion of the common bile duct into duodenal diverticula[394] (Fig. 64-105).

If the distal end of the common duct herniates into the lumen of the duodenum, it may simulate the radiographic appearance of the intraduodenal diverticulum.[354]

Routine versus selective primary operative cholangiography

Routine primary operative cholangiography implies that patients scheduled for cholecystectomy undergo this procedure before common duct exploration. Surgeons advocating *selective* operative cholangiography use this technique only with certain indications. This practice implies that clinical indications for common duct exploration are as accurate as the radiologic assessment. Control studies, however, demonstrate operative cholangiography to be more accurate than any other means of determining need for choledochotomy, including conventional common duct exploration.[329,331,378,383]

Arguments against routine operative cholangiography

Difficulties in operating room technique are responsible for errors, but this problem should be lessened if

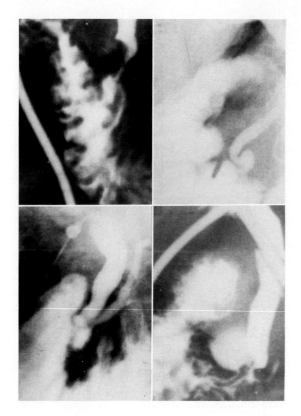

Fig. 64-105 Four different patients with entrance of biliary tract into wall or neck of duodenal diverticulum. Reflux is common.

the surgical team is accustomed to routine cholangiography. Poor technical results are more likely if cholangiography is performed only occasionally.

The time added to the duration of the operation and anesthesia in performing cholangiography has been criticized, but experienced surgeons who use operative cholangiography routinely estimate the added time as 5 to 10 minutes and no more than 10 to 20 minutes.[378,417] Furthermore routine radiographic studies decrease the incidence of exploratory choledochotomy, a procedure that adds at least double that amount of time to the operation. Cholecystectomy is usually begun during the time the radiographs are developed and reviewed.

False-positive and false-negative readings are a factor. The percentage of false-positive readings is given as 4% to 7%. False-negative readings may be as high as 7% to 10%.[403] These figures, however, must be compared with the false-positive and false-negative surgical judgment that relies only on classic clinical criteria for common duct surgery. The higher radiographic accuracy is given as 78%, in comparison with the 54% accuracy for clinical judgment.[379] Most authors who have used routine cholangiography have cut their number of common duct explorations to about half.

Difficulties in cooperation among surgeons, anesthetists, and radiologists may exist. This problem is usually eliminated when all three specialists appreciate the value of routine operative cholangiography and become interested in efficient teamwork. The radiologist must be available to give immediate readings in all cases. He also must be willing to go into the surgical suite in difficult cases in order to discuss the radiographs and help in the performance of repeat contrast injection.

Exposure of physician, personnel, and patient to radiation must be considered. The anesthetist should wear a lead apron during the injection. All other personnel should step at least 10 feet from the table or behind a portable lead screen. Television monitoring in the surgical suite may lengthen the procedure and add to the radiation hazard.

Pancreatic reflux and postoperative pancreatitis are listed as disadvantages. Bardenheier and coworkers[336] checked their records on 840 cases and found a 4% incidence of postoperative pancreatitis. It occurred 10 times as often in patients undergoing common duct exploration (342 cases) as in those patients who had operative cholangiography alone (498 cases). Nine percent of the radiographic studies showed pancreatic reflux. Pancreatic duct filling occurs frequently during operative cholangiography.[435] Beneventano and Schein[337] observed it in 45% of cases but found no evidence of pancreatitis. Even gallstones may enter pancreatic ducts in a retrograde fashion.[332]

Arguments in favor of routine operative cholangiography

Classic clinical indications for common duct exploration are often unreliable. Common duct stones may occur in the absence of duct dilatation and in the absence of jaundice (Fig. 64-106). Even duct palpation is unreliable for determining the presence or absence of common duct stones,[363] particularly in the distal common duct where it may be buried posteriorly in the head of the pancreas.

Information obtained before choledochotomy is essential to determine the presence of duct disease. The surgical procedure can be tailored accordingly, particularly with regard to the large number of anomalies of the biliary tract. Warren[429] reviewed the records on surgical repair of more than 1600 biliary strictures and showed 96% of them to be iatrogenic. Walters and associates' review[428] of their experience with another 429 strictures of the common duct is a further reminder that this is not a rare complication. Warren stressed that the surgeon identify the anatomy of the biliary tract before common duct exploration to avoid this dreaded complication.

Cholangiography aids in the preexploratory identification of calculi, neoplasms (Figs. 64-107 and 64-108),

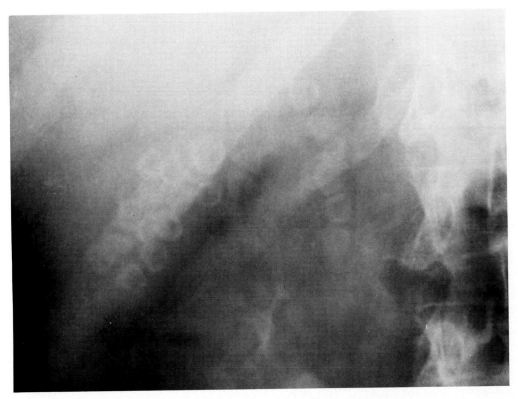

Fig. 64-106 Incidental discovery of multiple gallstones and common duct stones in patient without abdominal symptoms undergoing excretory urography before hysterectomy.

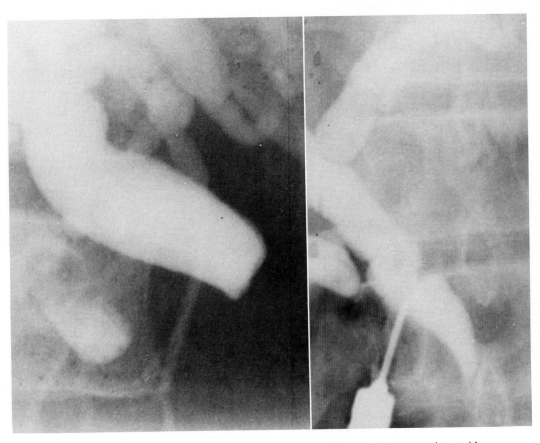

Fig. 64-107 High common duct obstruction with characteristic tapering in two patients with carcinoma of pancreas.

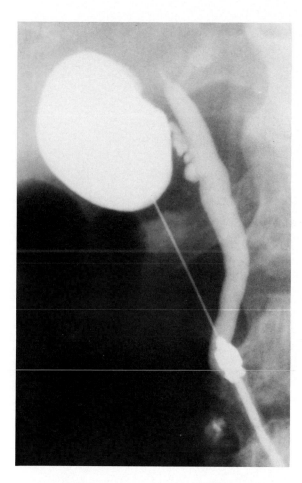

Fig. 64-108 Direct needle cholecystocholangiogram in patient with hepatic duct obstruction caused by ductal carcinoma. Rattail sign is present.

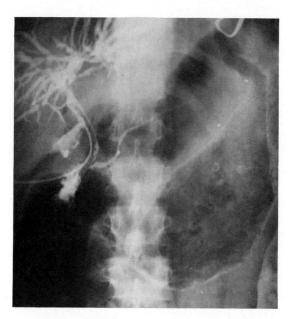

Fig. 64-109 Patient with sclerosing cholangitis of extrahepatic ducts. Surgical cholangiography before common duct exploration and before cholecystectomy is mandatory to preserve gallbladder for anastomosis.

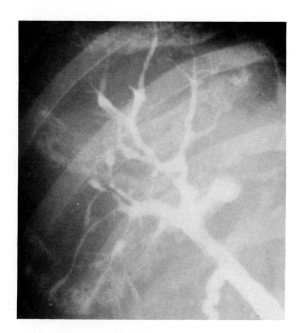

Fig. 64-110 Intrahepatic cholangitis.

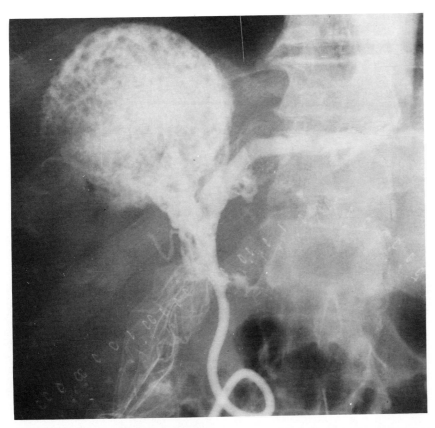

Fig. 64-111 Contrast medium enters large liver abscess cavity during operative cholangiography.

sclerosing cholangitis (Fig. 64-109), metastatic intra-hepatic disease, cholangitis (Fig. 64-110), liver abscess (Fig. 64-111), strictures (Fig. 64-112), fibrosis of the papilla of Vater (Fig. 64-113), and biliary parasites. Car-oli's disease shows bile stasis in the cavernous ectasia of the intrahepatic ducts that predisposes to stone for-mation.[392]

Reduction in the number of choledochotomies was accomplished with the use of routine cholangiography by several authors. When their results with this routine radiographic procedure were compared with those with-out it, the incidence of choledochotomies was cut in half.[331,342,378,410]

A decrease in the number of retained stones and reex-plorations was demonstrated by Hicken and McAllister[372] and Parent and Peloquin.[398] Their comparative analyses showed that twice as many stones were missed when cholangiography was not used (Figs. 64-114 and 64-115).

It must be stressed that the radiographic cholangio-gram is not competing with clinical indications for com-mon duct explorations, since the best results are obtained if clinical judgment is combined with routine operative cholangiography.

Complications

Cholangiovenous reflux may occur with forced injec-tions but requires only a moderate increase above the secretion pressure of the liver in the presence of common duct obstruction. The contrast medium (as well as bac-teria) enters the bloodstream through communications between the bile capillaries and the liver sinusoids[375] and is excreted with opacification of the kidneys. In a recent study examining intraoperative and postoperative bile cultures and the use of antibiotics before cholangiogra-phy, 6.5% of cholangiograms were followed by an ad-verse reaction. Two of these were severe reactions man-ifested by signs of septic shock. The administration of antibiotics, however, was not associated with a reduction in adverse reactions. The cholangiographic technique of gravity infusion of contrast material, however, produced no severe reactions. The avoidance of intraductal pressure above 20 cm of water during postoperative cholangiog-raphy should avoid cholangiovenous reflux.[348]

Bile peritonitis occurs when there is leakage of bile from the liver or the extrahepatic biliary tree into the peritoneal cavity, particularly if injuries to the main ducts or surgical transection of aberrant divisional ducts are not recognized during surgery.[424] Soft tissue masses seen

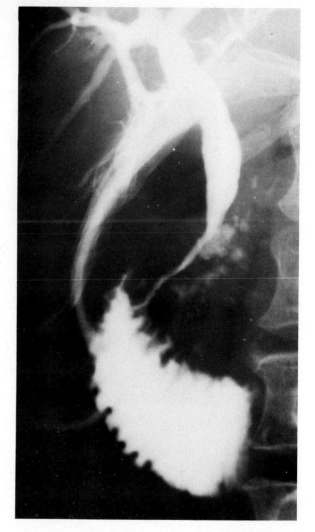

Fig. 64-112 Stricture of distal common duct with chronic pancreatitis. If T-tube is in place, stricture dilatation may be accomplished under fluoroscopic control.

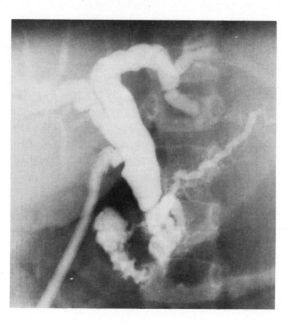

Fig. 64-113 Extensive pancreatic reflux in patient with fibrosis of distal common duct and papilla of Vater.

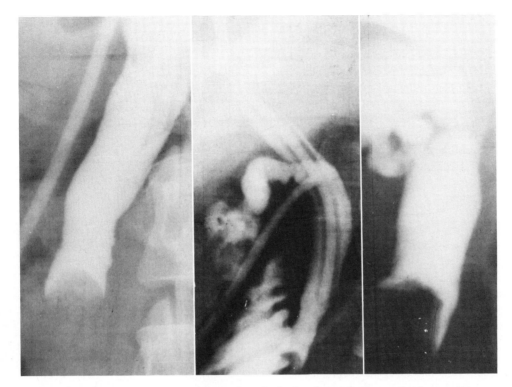

Fig. 64-114 Biliary duct termination at point of calculus obstruction is usually characteristic.

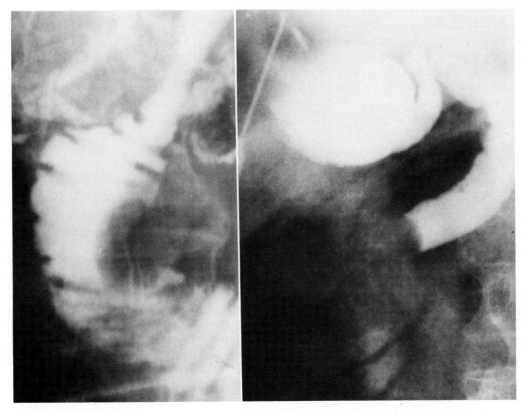

Fig. 64-115 Impacted distal common duct stone with associated surrounding edema may result in prominent filling defect in descending duodenum on barium examination.

on plain abdominal radiographs after surgery, with or without change in the flank stripe, are caused by collections of bile.[431] Delay in diagnosis is common.[407] Preoperative abdominal films must be compared with postoperative studies so that ill-defined masses can be recognized.[335] The bile collections may be loculated, and several masses may be seen because of association peritonitis (Fig. 64-116).

Excessive T-tube drainage after cholecystectomy may be caused by distal common duct obstruction. Testing the bile for the presence of amylase confirms the reflux of pancreatic secretions.

Biliary fistulas

Severance of an unrecognized aberrant bile duct during surgery may lead to persistent postcholecystectomy biliary fistulas. Aberrant bile ducts may be overlooked if primary intraoperative cholangiography is not done. When leakage of bile after cholecystectomy does not resolve, transhepatic cholangiography offers a safe and accurate means of identifying the source of leakage.[405]

Aberrant or accessory bile ducts are not uncommon. Aberrant ducts may enter into the cystic or common duct. This occurs in about 3.5% of cases.[370] Avulsion of the left hepatic duct may also lead to iatrogenic fistula formation.[415]

Most spontaneous internal and external biliary fistulas are caused by cholelithiasis.[349,400] The classic radiographic findings of gallstone ileus are small bowel distention, air in the biliary tract, and an abnormally located gallstone that is usually solitary, large, and laminated. Fistulas to the stomach or duodenum are demonstrated with a contrast medium given by mouth.[406] One series of 819 cases of spontaneous internal biliary fistulas consisted of cholecystoduodenal fistulas in 51%, cholecystocolic fistulas in 21%, and choledochoduodenal fistulas in 19%. Rare types are cholecystogastric, choledochogastric, and cholecystocholedochal fistulas. Gallstones are associated with approximately 90% of fistulas that primarily involve the gallbladder.[401] In another series the fistulas lead to the duodenum in 431 cases, to the colon in 92 cases, and to the duodenum and large bowel in 20 cases.[349] Barium enema studies are diagnostic if the colon is involved, but cholecystograms and cholangiography is sometimes indicated.

If the diagnosis of gallstone ileus is considered, the radiologist should always search for a second stone in the biliary tract. If the fistula is from the gallbladder to the intestinal tract, the common bile duct may not contain gas. Intravenous cholangiography aids in these cases in excluding a second stone in the common bile duct.[416] The diagnosis of choledocholithiasis has been made by barium enema studies in cases of cholecystocolonic fistulas.[364]

Carcinoma of the biliary tract (Fig. 64-117), duode-

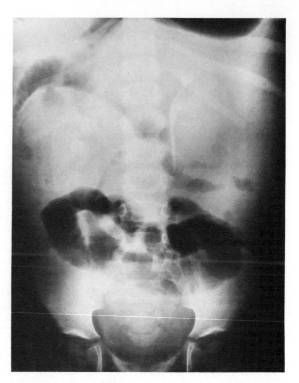

Fig. 64-116 Abdominal masses caused by loculated bile collection with peritonitis after abdominal trauma and bile duct laceration.

num, or colon; diverticulitis; ulcerative colitis; and decubitus erosion from cholecystostomy tubes indwelling for long periods of time[376] make up the small group of noncalculous causes of biliary fistulas. Ascending cholangitis and gastrointestinal bleeding may complicate internal biliary fistulas. Feculent vomiting is often present with fistulas to the colon.[418]

Fistulas have also been reported between the common bile duct and the right renal pelvis,[396] between the biliary tract and the pleural space, and between the biliary and bronchial tracts.[356] The latter two have been observed after trauma, with hepatic abscess, with gonococcal disease, and with biliary tract obstruction.

Postcholecystectomy syndrome

If symptoms occur or persist after cholecystectomy, several of the entities under the heading "postcholecystectomy syndrome" must be considered. These include retained duct stones, cystic duct remnants (Fig. 64-118), duct strictures and injuries, sphincter of Oddi spasm and fibrosis, and neoplastic disease, including neuroma of the cystic duct, pancreatitis, and bile peritonitis. Persistent symptoms also have been ascribed to disorders outside the biliary tract, such as hiatus hernia, peptic ulceration, abdominal angina, coronary artery disease, and spastic colon.[350]

By far the most common cause of postcholecystec-

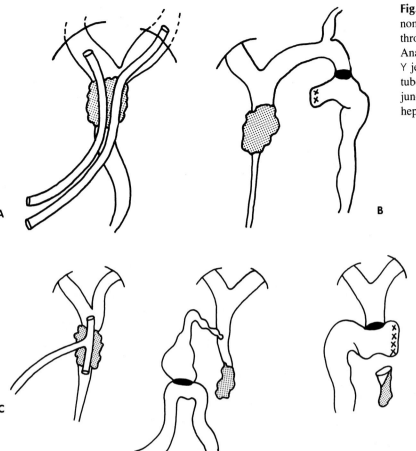

Fig. 64-117 Operations for bile duct carcinoma. **A,** Surgical placement of drainage tubes through common hepatic duct carcinoma. **B,** Anastomosis of left hepatic duct to Roux-en-Y jejunal loop (Longmire's procedure). **C,** T-tube placement through tumor, cholecystojejunostomy for bypass of distal obstruction, and hepatojejunostomy for drainage and bypass.

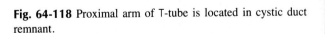

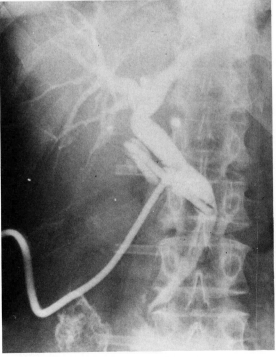

Fig. 64-118 Proximal arm of T-tube is located in cystic duct remnant.

tomy symptoms is retained stones in the biliary tract. Intrahepatic stones overlooked at the time of surgery may have moved distally. Other abnormalities listed under the postcholecystectomy syndrome are indeed rare. Although retained cystic duct stumps are common, it is unlikely that this postoperative finding causes symptoms in the absence of retained stones in the cystic duct. The intramural variant of a cystic duct in apposition to the common duct and covered by a common sheath occurs in 22% of studied cadavers[413] (Fig. 64-119). Bodvall and Overgaard[339] studied 500 cases postoperatively and found cystic duct remnants longer than 1 cm in 40%. When present, the cystic duct remnant occurred in the same number of patients with and without symptoms, so that the remnant per se hardly can be incriminated as producing symptoms. A cystic duct remnant, however, may be associated with tumors or inflammation, or it may contain stones (Fig. 64-120). Resection of cystic duct remnants containing stones has relieved symptoms.[427]

Fibrosis and inflammation of the sphincter of Oddi may give rise to postoperative symptoms. This probably accounts for the majority of cases previously labeled "biliary dyskinesia."

Portorak[402] demonstrated that normal function begins to return about 10 days after sphincterotomy and that return to normal is complete in 95% of cases 6 months after surgery. Barium reflux from the duodenum into the biliary tract is present in only 4% of cases after a 6-month postoperative interval. For permanent drainage, particularly in patients with recurrent and reformed biliary tract stones, choledochoduodenostomy is needed. Barium reflux persists in almost all of the cases.

The initial radiologic imaging procedure for patients with postcholecystectomy symptoms is ultrasonography. The caliber of intrahepatic and extrahepatic bile ducts can be assessed readily. The easiest identification is that of the common hepatic duct above the portal vein. Normally it should measure up to 4 mm in diameter on ultrasonography. Distention may indicate persistence of preoperative distention, or partial obstruction may be present. If baseline measurements are not available in patients without symptoms after cholecystectomy, further investigation, such as transhepatic cholangiography or endoscopic retrograde contrast studies, may be required. New or retained stones, strictures and fistulas, and tumor obstruction can be diagnosed. Intravenous cholangiography still has a place in the investigation of nonjaundiced postcholecystectomy state. It may reveal the presence of stones or strictures (Fig. 64-121). Negative results of ultrasonography or intravenous cholangiography do not

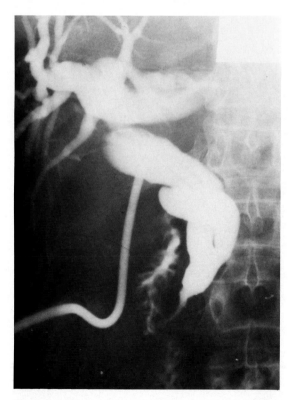

Fig. 64-119 Large cystic duct remnant in patient with fibrosis of sphincter of Oddi. Cystic duct enters low and is in common sheet with major duct. Cystic duct anomaly is common and is responsible for frequently seen cystic duct remnant.

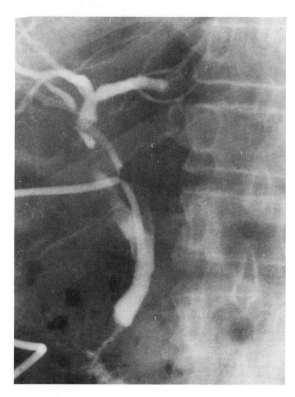

Fig. 64-120 Retained stone in cystic duct remnant.

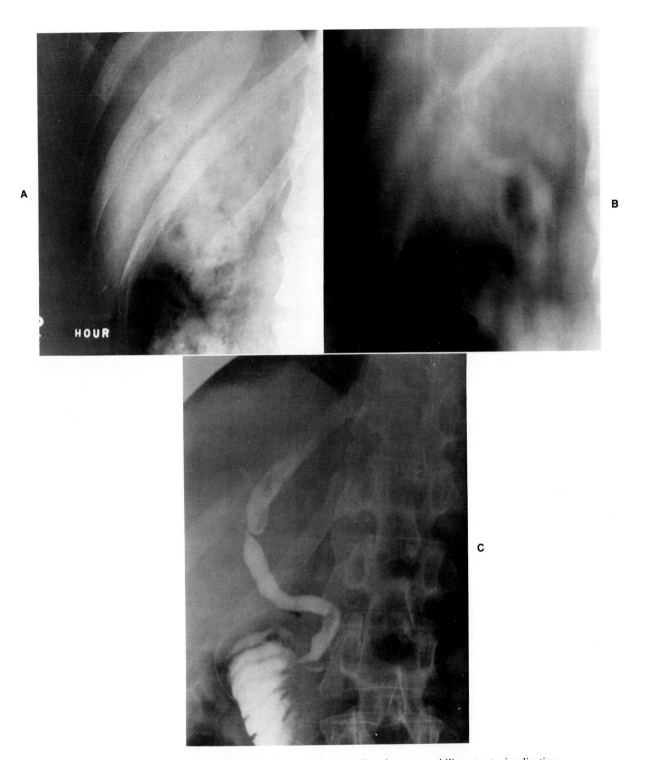

Fig. 64-121 A, Symptomatic patient but without jaundice shows poor biliary tract visualization on right upper quadrant radiograph 30 minutes after injection during intravenous cholangiography. **B,** Tomography now demonstrates high stricture with stone in left hepatic duct proximal to it. **C,** Operative cholangiogram confirms stricture and bile duct stone.

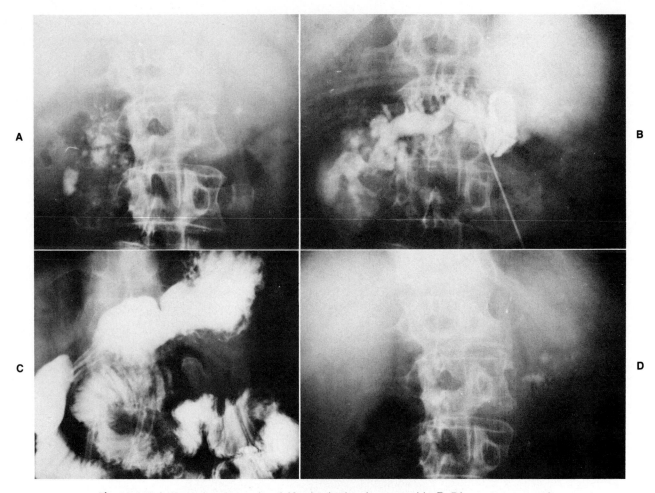

Fig. 64-122 A, Extensive pancreatic calcification in chronic pancreatitis. **B,** Direct pancreatography into dilated duct in same patient. **C,** Puestow's pancreaticojejunostomy was performed. **D,** Radiograph obtained 6 months later shows that most of pancreatic calcification has been passed through anastomosis between pancreatic duct and jejunum.

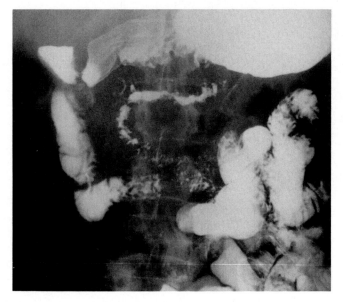

Fig. 64-123 Retrograde barium pancreatogram after longitudinal pancreaticojejunostomy for chronic pancreatitis (Puestow's procedure). Deformity of pancreatic duct remains, but many pancreatic calcifications have passed spontaneously.

exclude the presence of stones in the distal duct. Poor visualization in the distal common duct, caused by inadequate contrast concentration or overlying duodenal gas, is responsible. Early opacification of intrahepatic ducts and delayed emptying from the common duct during intravenous cholangiography may indicate partial obstruction. Transhepatic cholangiography is then the radiologic technique of choice for diagnosis.

LIVER

Complications are not infrequent after partial hepatectomy.[367] Radiologic imaging procedures assist in the diagnosis of subphrenic and subhepatic abscesses, pleural effusion, postoperative bleeding, wound infection, and biliary fistulas. Nuclear medicine HIDA scans are particularly helpful in delineating the anatomy of persistent fistula drainage. Serial abdominal CT studies are useful in monitoring bleeding,[358] whereas low attenuation at the surgical margin after partial hepatectomy is an expected finding on CT examination.[382]

Radiologic techniques are often helpful in patients with an abnormal course after liver transplantation. Direct cholangiography can diagnose biliary obstruction and bile leaks.[438] Stricture at the site of surgical anastomosis in the common bile duct may be associated with bile sludge deposition.[395] Cholangiography will also assist in the evaluation of liver abscesses, stones, and problems associated with internal biliary stents.[440] Because the hepatic artery provides the only blood supply to the biliary tree of the liver allograft, posttransplantation arterial occlusion may result in a biliary complication. Patients with transplants who have nonanastomotic contrast leakage or nonanastomotic strictures on cholangiography should be evaluated for occlusion of the hepatic artery as the probable cause.[439]

A region of low attenuation on CT scan around the peripheral portal tracts, the periportal collar sign, suggests acute liver rejection after liver transplantation. The sign corresponds histopathologically with the lymphocytic portal infiltration but also can be caused by dilated lymphatic vessels as a consequence of total interruption at the time of surgery.[388,430] Angiography is not advocated as a test for transplant rejection. Hematomas, bilomas, and seromas are best localized by CT scanning.[381,433]

PANCREAS

Pancreatic pseudocysts can be anastomosed to stomach and duodenum, or to the small intestine by a Roux-en-Y drainage procedure. Pancreatic fistulas follow external drainage in about 20% to 30% of cases. ERCP is then often indicated to evaluate communication with major pancreatic ducts.[343] Failure of caudal pancreaticojejunostomy to relieve symptoms in patients with multiple points of ductal obstruction lead to the Puestow procedure, which involves longitudinal opening of the pancreatic duct and invagination of the pancreas into the Roux-en-Y jejunal loop (Figs. 64-122 and 64-123). Complications encountered after operation include pancreatic fistula, abscesses, and pneumonia. Percutaneous drainage of pancreatic and peripancreatic fluid collections can be achieved with radiographically guided catheter insertion. This interventional radiographic procedure can help to stabilize patients until surgical intervention is possible. Careful patient selection is important because of a significant associated morbidity and mortality.[420] Pancreaticoduodenectomy (Whipple procedure) is the surgical procedure for cancer in the periampullary area. Although 5-year survival rates are better for ampullary carcinoma, a low 5-year survival rate of 4% for carcinoma of the pancreas has lead surgeons to question whether pancreaticoduodenectomy is so ineffective that resection should not be considered.[434]

REFERENCES
General considerations

1. Alinder, G, et al: Pre-operative infusion cholangiography compared to routine operative cholangiography at elective cholecystectomy, Br J Surg 73:383, 1986.
2. De Cosee, JJ, et al: Subphrenic abscess, Surg Gynecol Obstet 138:841, 1974.
3. Klein, J, et al: The forgotten surgical foreign body, Gastrointest Radiol 13:173, 1988.
4. Kokubo, T, et al: Retained surgical sponges: CT and US appearance, Radiology 165:415, 1987.
5. Kressel, HY, and Filley, RA: Ultrasonographic appearance of gas-containing abscesses in the abdomen, Am J Roentgenol 130:71, 1978.
6. Mason, LB: Migration of surgical sponge into small intestine, JAMA 205:938, 1968.
7. Rosenthall, L, et al: ^{99m}Tc-IDA hepatobiliary imaging following upper abdominal surgery, Radiology 130:735, 1979.
8. Sanders, RC: Post-operative pleural effusion and subphrenic abscess, Clin Radiol 21:308, 1970.
9. Wang, SMS, and Wilson, SE: Subphrenic abscess: the new epidemiology, Arch Surg 112:934, 1977.
10. Welch, CE: Abdominal surgery, N Engl J Med 275:1232, 1966.
11. White, TT, and Harrison, RC: Reoperative gastrointestinal surgery, ed 2, Boston, 1979, Little, Brown.
12. Williams, RG, Bradd, DG, and Nelson, JA: Gossypiboma—the problem of the retained surgical sponge, Radiology 129:323, 1978.

Esophagus

13. Agha, FP, and Lee, HL: The esophagus after endoscopic pneumatic balloon dilatation for achalasia, Am J Roentgenol 146:25, 1986.
14. Allison, PR: Hiatus hernia: a 20-year retrospective study, Ann Surg 178:272, 1973.
15. Balison, JR, Macgregor, AMC, and Woodward, ER: Postoperative diaphragmatic herniation following transthoracic fundoplication, Arch Surg 106:164, 1973.
16. Baue, AE, and Belsey, RH: The treatment of sliding hiatus hernia and reflux esophagitis by the Mark IV technique, Surgery 62:398, 1967.

17. Becker, CD, et al: Patterns of recurrence of esophageal carcinoma after transhiatal esophagectomy and gastric interposition, Am J Roentgenol 148:273, 1987.

18. Calenoff, L, and Norfray, J: The reconstructed esophagus, Am J Roentgenol 125:864, 1975.

19. Childress, MH, and Martel, W: Radiologic appearance of the Collis-Belsey fundoplication, J Can Assoc Radiol 28:282, 1977.

20. Chisholm, RJ, et al: Radiologic dilatation preceding surgical tube placement for esophageal cancer, Am J Surg 151:397, 1986.

21. Cohen, WN: The fundoplication repair of sliding oesophageal hiatus hernia: its roentgenographic appearance, Am J Roentgenol 104:625, 1968.

22. Cooke, GM: Radiographic appearances following the Thal procedure, J Can Assoc Radiol 26:279, 1975.

23. Ettinger, A, Paul, RE, Jr, and Moran, JM: Gastric pseudotumor after fundoplication, Gastroenterology 61:299, 1971.

24. Feigen, DS, et al: The radiological appearance of hiatal hernia repairs, Radiology 110:71, 1974.

25. Ghahremani, GG: Complications of gastrointestinal intubation. In Meyers, MA, and Ghahremani, GG, editors: Iatrogenic gastrointestinal complications, New York, 1981, Springer-Verlag.

26. Gompels, BM, and Harrison, GK: Barium studies following the Niseen-Rossetti operation for oesophageal stricture due to reflux, Br J Radiol 45:137, 1972.

27. Heimlich, HJ: Reconstruction of entire esophagus and restoration of swallowing with reversed gastric tube, NY State J Med 61:2478, 1961.

28. Hill, LD: An effective operation for hiatal hernia: an 8-year appraisal, Ann Surg 166:681, 1967.

29. Ikezoe, J, et al: Computed tomography following endoscopic sclerotherapy of esophageal varices, Acta Radiol 28:415, 1987.

30. Katz, D: Morbidity and mortality in standard and flexible gastrointestinal endoscopy, Gastrointest Endosc 15:134, 1969.

31. Lewis, RA, Angelchik, JP, and Cohen, R: A new surgical prosthesis for hiatal hernia repair, Radiology 135:630, 1980.

32. Meyers, MA, and Ghahremani, GG: Complications of fiberoptic endoscopy. I. Esophagoscopy and gastroscopy, Radiology 115:293, 1975.

33. Meyers, MA, and Ghahremani, GG, editors: Iatrogenic gastrointestinal complications, New York, 1981, Springer-Verlag.

34. Nissen, R: Gastropexy and fundoplication in surgical treatment of hiatal hernia, Am J Dig Dis 6:954, 1961.

35. Nouel, O, et al: Iatrogenic perforations of the esophagus during fiberoptic endoscopy: radiologic signs, J Radiol Electrol 59:113, 1978.

36. Payne, WS, and Ellis, FH, Jr: Complications of esophageal and diaphragmatic surgery. In Artz, CP, and Hardy, JD, editors: Management of surgical complications, ed 3, Philadelphia, 1975, W. B. Saunders.

37. Postlethwait, RW, Kim, SK, and Dillon, ML: Esophageal complications of vagotomy, Surg Gynecol Obstet 128:481, 1969.

38. Punto, L, and Mokka, REM: Roentgencinematography and manometry following Nissen's fundoplication, Fortschr Rontgenstr 128:124, 1978.

39. Rogers, LF: Transient post-vagotomy dysphagia: a distinct clinical and roentgenographic entity, Am J Roentgenol 125:956, 1975.

40. Rose, JD, Roberts, GM, and Smith, PM: The radiological appearances of the oesophagus after sclerotherapy for varices, Clin Radiol 36:355, 1985.

41. Rubesin, SE, et al: Distal esophageal ballooning following Heller myotomy, Radiology 167:345, 1988.

42. Skucas, J, et al: An evaluation of the Nissen fundoplication, Radiology 118:539, 1976.

43. Thal, AP: A unified approach to surgical problems of the oesophagogastric junction, Ann Surg 168:542, 1968.

44. Thomas, DM, et al: The anatomical basis for gastric mobilization in total oesophagectomy, Br J Surg 66:230, 1979.

45. Wolf, EL, et al: Radiographic appearance of the esophagus and stomach after laser treatment of obstructing carcinoma, Am J Roentgenol 146:519, 1986.

46. Wolloch, Y, et al: Iatrogenic perforations of the esophagus: therapeutic considerations, Arch Surg 118:357, 1974.

47. Zaino, C, and Beneventano, TC, editors: Radiologic examination of the orohypopharynx and esophagus, New York, 1977, Springer-Verlag.

Stomach and duodenum

48. Abbott, WE, et al: The etiology and management of the dumping syndrome following a gastroenterostomy or subtotal gastrectomy, Gastroenterology 39:12, 1960.

49. Aleman, S: Jejuno-gastric intussusception, a rare complication of the operated stomach, Acta Radiol [Diagn] (Stockh) 29:383, 1948.

50. Allen, JG: Physiology and treatment of peptic ulcer, Chicago, 1959, University of Chicago Press.

51. Amdrup, E: Postgastrectomy syndromes, Am J Dig Dis 11:432, 1966.

52. Amdrup, E, Hjorth, P, and Jørgensen, JB: Radiological demonstration of variations in the fluid content of the small intestine during dumping attacks, Br J Radiol 31:542, 1958.

53. Amdrup, E, and Jensen, HG: Selective vagotomy of the parietal cell mass preserving innervation of the undrained antrum, Gastroenterology 59:522, 1970.

54. Andreassen, M, Davidsen, HG, and Fenger, HH: The dumping syndrome and its radiologic evaluation, Acta Chir Scand 121:134, 1961.

55. Aronson, AR, and Darling, DR: Carcinoma at the margin of the gastrojejunal stoma: review of the literature and report of a case, Gastroenterology 36:686, 1959.

56. Bachman, AL, and Parmer, EA: Radiographic diagnosis of recurrence following resection for gastric cancer, Radiology 84:913, 1965.

57. Baker, LW, and Dudley, HA: Auscultation of the abdomen in surgical patients, Lancet 2:517, 1961.

58. Balint, JA: Pulmonary tuberculosis and partial gastrectomy, Gastroenterologia (Basel) 90:65, 1958.

59. Barichello, AW, et al: Rupture of the stomach following oxygen therapy by nasal catheter: report of a case and review of the literature, Can Med Assoc J 98:855, 1968.

60. Becker, HD, Reeder, DD, and Thompson, JC: Direct measurement of vagal release of gastrin, Surgery 75:101, 1974.

61. Belding, HH: Mechanical complications of gastrectomy, Surg Gynecol Obstet 117:578, 1963.

62. Benoit, D, et al: Gastric stasis following vagotomy, J Radiol Electrol 52:275, 1971.

63. Berk, RN, and Coulson, DB: Body cast syndrome, Radiology 94:303, 1970.

64. Berkowitz, D, Cooney, P, and Bralow, SP: Carcinoma of stomach appearing after previous gastric surgery for benign ulcer disease, Gastroenterology 36:691, 1959.

65. Bevan, PG: The incidence of postoperative pneumoperitoneum and its significance, Br Med J 2:605, 1961.

66. Bloch, C, and Wolf, BS: The gastroduodenal channel after pyloroplasty and vagotomy: a cineradiographic study, Radiology 84:43, 1965.

67. Bockus, HL: Gastroenterology, ed 2, vol 1, Philadelphia, 1963, W.B. Saunders.

68. Bolooki, H, et al: Spontaneous rupture of esophagus: Boerhaave's syndrome, Ann Surg 174:319, 1971.

69. Borg, I: Gastric flow and acidity before and after Billroth II and Billroth I for gastroduodenal ulcer, Acta Chir Scand [Suppl] 251:1, 1959.

70. Borgström, SE: The efferent loop dumping syndrome and its relation to intestinal absorption studied by an intubation technique, Acta Chir Scand [Suppl] 265:1, 1960.

71. Bowers, RF, and Stockard, CG: Dumping syndrome following pyloroplasty, Arch Surg 92:39, 1966.

72. Bradford, B, Jr, and Boggs, JE: Jejunogastric intussusception—an unusual complication of gastric surgery, Arch Surg 77:201, 1958.

73. Brekkan, A: Fistulography with vacuum suction, Acta Radiol (Stockh) 57:77, 1962.

74. Bret, P, Amiel, M, and Descos, L: Les images lacunaires des moignons de gastrectomie, Ann Radiol (Paris) 7:519, 1964.

75. Bryant, LR, Wiot, JF, and Kloecker, RJ: A study of the factors affecting the incidence and duration of postoperative pneumoperitoneum, Surg Gynecol Obstet 117:145, 1963.

76. Bundrick, TJ, Turner, MA, and Cho, SR: Retrograde jejunogastric intussusception, Rev Interam Radiol 11:21, 1981.

77. Burhenne, HJ: Radiographic confirmation of the hyperosmolar-hypovolemic concept of the dumping syndrome. In Schmid, E, editor: Proceedings of the World Congress of Gastroenterology, 2 vols, Basel, Switzerland, 1963, S. Karger.

78. Burhenne, HJ: Roentgen anatomy and terminology of gastric surgery, Am J Roentgenol 91:731, 1964.

79. Burhenne, HJ: Roentgenologic approach to a physiologic examination of the alimentary tract. In Gamble, JR, and Wilbur, DL, editors: Current concepts of clinical gastroenterology, Boston, 1965, Little, Brown.

80. Burhenne, HJ: The retained gastric antrum, Am J Roentgenol 101:459, 1967.

81. Burhenne, HJ: Postoperative defects of the stomach, Semin Roentgenol 6:182, 1971.

82. Burrell, M, Touloukian, JS, and Curtis, AM: Roentgen manifestations of carcinoma in the gastric remnant, Gastrointest Radiol 5:331, 1980.

83. Cameron, AJ: Aspirin and gastric ulcer, Mayo Clin Proc 50:565, 1975.

84. Cannon, WB: The motor activities of the stomach and small intestine after splanchnic and vagus section, Am J Physiol 17:429, 1907.

85. Cariollo, FX: The immediate complications of gastrectomy: a twelve-year review of early post-operative complications in ulcer surgery, Medical Annals of the District of Columbia 32:159, 1963.

86. Carman, RD, and Balfour, DC: Gastrojejunal ulcers, JAMA 65:227, 1915.

87. Caudell, WS, and Lee, CM, Jr: Acute and chronic jejunogastric intussusception, N Engl J Med 253:635, 1955.

88. Cavassini, GB, et al: L'assorbimento della vitamina B_{12}-CO_{58} nei gastroresecati totali e parziali, Arch Ital Mal Appar Dig 32:11, 1965.

89. Chornas, I, and Love, RW, Jr: Postgastrectomy state and tuberculosis, Arch Surg 92:704, 1966.

90. Clarke, SD, Penry, JB, and Ward, P: Oesophageal reflux after abdominal vagotomy, Lancet 2:824, 1965.

91. Cohen, WN: The fundoplication repair of sliding esophageal hiatus hernia: its roentgenographic appearance, Am J Roentgenol 104:625, 1968.

92. Cohen, WN, Mason, EE, and Blommers, TJ: Gastric bypass for morbid obesity, Radiology 122:609, 1977.

93. Colmer, MR, et al: Pattern of gastric emptying after vagotomy and pyloroplasty, Br Med J 2:448, 1973.

94. Cornell, GN, et al: Use of jejunal interposition with total gastrectomy, Ann Surg 152:430, 1960.

95. Cox, HT, and Allan, WR: The dumping syndrome: an investigation and a cause, Lancet 2:672, 1961.

96. Cueto, J, et al: Vitamin B_{12} and iron deficiency after partial gastrectomy, Arch Surg 91:995, 1965.

97. Currarino, G, and Votteler, T: Prolapse of the gastrostomy catheter in children, Am J Roentgenol 123:1737, 1975.

98. Dagradi, AE, et al: Terminal esophageal (vestibular) spasm after vagotomy, Arch Surg 85:955, 1962.

99. deLacey, G, Bloomberg, T, and Wignall, BK: Pneumoperitoneum: the misleading double wall sign, Clin Radiol 28:445, 1977.

100. de Lange, EE, and Shaffer, HA, Jr: Anastomotic strictures of the upper gastrointestinal tract: results of balloon dilation, Radiology 167:45, 1988.

101. Deller, DJ, and Begley, MD: Bone changes after partial gastrectomy: calcium metabolism and the bones after partial gastrectomy. I. Calcium features and radiology of the bones, Aust Ann Med 12:282, 1963.

102. Devor, D, and Passaro, E, Jr: Jejunogastric intussusception: review of 4 cases—diagnosis and management, Ann Surg 163:93, 1966.

103. DuBerger, L, Masson, G, and Sylvester, J: Milkman's syndrome—five cases of severe osteomalacia following gastric surgery, J Can Assoc Radiol 11:57, 1960.

104. Eklof, O, and Ohlsson, S: Postoperative plication deformity with foreign-body granuloma simulating tumour of the stomach: report of three cases, Acta Chir Scand 123:125, 1961.

105. Ellis, K: Gastrojejunal ulcer, Radiology 71:187, 1958.

106. Ettinger, A, Paul, RE, Jr, and Moran, JM: Gastric pseudotumor after fundoplication, Gastroenterology 61:299, 1971.

107. Evans, DS: Acute dilatation and spontaneous rupture of the stomach, Br J Surg 55:940, 1968.

108. Fisher, JA, Taylor, W, and Cannon, JA: Dumping syndrome: correlation between its experimental production and clinical incidence, Surg Gynecol Obstet 100:559, 1955.

109. Fisher, MS: The Hofmeister defect: a normal change in the postoperative stomach, Am J Roentgenol 84:1082, 1960.

110. Fitzgerald, P, and McMullin, JP: Gastrojejunocolic fistula, Ir J Med Sci 389:230, 1958.

111. Fogen, M: Röntgenoilogische Veränderungen an der kardia nach Osophagofundostomie, Radiol Clin (Basel) 34:254, 1965.

112. Frech, RS, Roper, C, and McAlister, WH: Esophageal rupture secondary to pyloric obstruction by a gastrostomy Foley catheter balloon, J Can Assoc Radiol 21:263, 1970.

113. Frederick, PL, and Sizer, JS: Antegrade jejunojejunal intussusception: a rare complication following total gastric resection, Ann Surg 161:597, 1965.

114. Freeman, FJ, Bernatz, PE, and Brown, PW, Jr: Retrograde intussusception after total gastrectomy: report of a case, Arch Surg 93:586, 1966.

115. Garrick, R, Ireland, AW, and Posen, S: Bone abnormalities after gastric surgery: prospective histological study, Ann Intern Med 75:221, 1971.

116. Gibbs, DD: Carcinoma in gastric remnants after partial gastrectomy for benign ulceration: a study of three cases illustrating the diagnostic contribution of exfoliative cytology, Gut 3:322, 1962.

117. Goligher, JC, and Riley, TR: Incidence and mechanism of early dumping syndrome after gastrectomy; clinical and radiological study, Lancet 1:630, 1952.

118. Goodman, JM: Mallory-Weiss syndrome and hypofibrinogenemia: complications during surgery, JAMA 190:72, 1964.

119. Goodman, LR, Wittenberg, J, and Messer, R: Duodenal obstruction—an unusual complication of a gastrostomy feeding catheter, Br J Radiol 44:883, 1971.

120. Gregory, RA, et al: Extraction of gastrin-like substance from a pancreatic tumour in a case of Zollinger-Ellison syndrome, Lancet 1:1045, 1960.

121. Grimous, M, Moreau, G, and Lemozy, J: Le prolapsus postoperatoire transanastomotique de la muqueuse gastrique, Arch Mal Appar Dig 53:649, 1964.

122. Gueller, R, et al: Suture granulomas simulating tumors: a preventable postgastrectomy complication, Am J Dig Dis 21:223, 1976.

123. Hall, GH, and Neale, G: Bone rarefaction after partial gastrectomy, Ann Intern Med 59:455, 1963.

124. Halverson, JD, and Koehler, RE: Gastric bypass, Surgery 90:446, 1981.

125. Harrison, BB: Colonic replacement of stomach, early results of radiological investigation, Lancet 1:25, 1952.

126. Harvey, HD: A follow-up study of surgically treated peptic ulcer over forty-six years, Md State Med J 12:383, 1963.

127. Haubrich, WS: Sequelae of gastric surgery for peptic ulcer. In Bockus, HL, editor: Gastroenterology, Philadelphia, 1963, W.B. Saunders, vol 1.

128. Helsinger, N, Jr: Esophagitis following total gastrectomy: a clinical and experimental study, Acta Chir Scand [Suppl] 273:1, 1961.

129. Henning, N, et al: Störungen nach Magenresektion, Dtsch Med Wochenschr 91:843, 1966.

130. Heslin, DJ, and Malt, RA: Progressive post-operative pneumoperitoneum: air entering through drain sites, Am J Roentgenol 92:1166, 1964.

131. Hibner, R, and Richard, V: Stomach or small bowel obstruction following partial gastrectomy: report of thirty cases, Am J Surg 96:309, 1958.

132. Hickler, RB, et al: Evaluation of autonomic nervous system response in patients with the dumping syndrome, Surg Forum 11:318, 1960.

133. Hiemsche, W: Zur Methodik de Rontgenologischen Funktionsprufung operierter Magen, Fortschr Rontgenstr 92:395, 1961.

134. Hinshaw, DB, Joergenson, EJ, and Stafford, CE: Preoperative "dumping studies" in peptic ulcer patients, Arch Surg 80:738, 1960.

135. Hoffmann, RN: Gastrocolic fistula and gastric ulcer with prolonged glucocorticoid therapy, JAMA 195:493, 1966.

136. Inouye, WY, and Evans, G: Neonatal gastric perforation: a report of six cases and a review of 143 cases, Arch Surg 88:471, 1964.

137. Jamroz, GA, Blocker, SH, and McAlister, WH: Radiographic findings after incomplete pyloromyotomy, Gastrointest Radiol 11:139, 1986.

138. Jepsen, OL: The presence of yeast fungi in gastric contents after gastrectomy and vagotomy, Fortschr Rontgenstr 109:269, 1968.

139. Joffe, N, Goldman, H, and Antonioli, DA: Recurring hyperplastic gastric polyps following subtotal gastrectomy, Am J Roentgenol 130:301, 1978.

140. Johnson, JR: Esophageal hiatal hernia following vagotomy, Calif Med 103:439, 1965.

141. Johnson, LP, et al: Serotonin antagonists in experimental and clinical "dumping," Ann Surg 156:537, 1962.

142. Jones, CT, et al: Peptic ulceration: some haematological and metabolic consequences of gastric surgery, Lancet 2:425, 1962.

143. Avery Jones, FA, and Gummer, JW: Peptic ulcer. In Clinical gastroenterology, Oxford, 1961, Blackwell Scientific Publications.

144. Joosten F, et al: Röntgenologie des Magenstumpfkarzinoms, ROFO 139:8, 1983.

145. Jordon, PH: Elective operations for duodenal ulcer, N Engl J Med 287:1329, 1972.

146. Jordon, SM: Report of the Committee on Surgical Procedures of the National Committee on Peptic Ulcer of the American Gastroenterological Association, Gastroenterology 22:297, 1952.

147. Joske, RA, and Blackwell, JB: Alimentary histology in the malabsorption syndrome following partial gastrectomy, Lancet 2:379, 1959.

148. Kay, AW: The pyloric antrum and peptic ulceration, Gastroenterologia (Basel) 89:282, 1958.

149. Kiefer, ED: Postgastrectomy syndrome, Am J Gastroenterol 35:352, 1961.

150. Kiefer, ED, and Smedal, MI: Radiation therapy for stomach ulcers occurring after subtotal gastrectomy, JAMA 169:451, 1959.

151. Kim, SY, and Evans, JA: The roentgen appearance of the stomach and duodenum following the Billroth I gastric resection, Am J Roentgenol 81:576, 1959.

152. Koehler, PR: New approaches to the radiological diagnosis of Mallory-Weiss syndrome, Br J Radiol 42:354, 1969.

153. Kraft, RO, Fry, WJ, and DeWeese, MS: Postvagotomy gastric atony, Arch Surg 88:865, 1964.

154. Kronborg, O, and Madsen, P: A controlled, randomized trial of highly selective vagotomy versus selective vagotomy and pyloroplasty in the treatment of duodenal ulcers, Gut 16:268, 1975.

155. Kuzmak, LI: Silicone gastric banding: a simple and effective operation for morbid obesity, Contemp Surg 28:13, 1986.

156. Lahey, FH, and Marshall, SF: The surgical treatment of peptic ulcer, N Engl J Med 246:115, 1952.

157. Lawson, EH, and Whitener, DL: Retrograde jejunogastric intussusception: report of a case, Arch Surg 60:242, 1950.

158. LeVine, M, et al: Gastrojejunal mucosal prolapse, Radiology 80:30, 1963.

159. Liebman, PR, et al: Hepatic-portal venous gas in adults: etiology, pathophysiology and clinical significance, Ann Surg 187:281, 1978.

160. Liljedahl, SO, et al: Cineroentgenographic studies of gastrointestinal motility in healthy subjects and in patients with gastric or duodenal ulcer, Acta Chir Scand 117:206, 1959.

161. Lord, MD, and Gourevitch, A: The peritoneal anatomy of the spleen with special reference to the operation of partial gastrectomy, Br J Surg 52:202, 1965.

162. Low, WC, and Palmer, ED: Esophageal stricture as a complication of gastric surgery, Am J Med Sci 254:342, 1967.

163. Lucas, CE, and Read, RC: Vascular hypertonicity: a mechanism for vasodilatation in the dumping syndrome, Surgery 60:395, 1966.

164. Machella, TE: Mechanism of post-gastrectomy "dumping" syndrome, Ann Surg 130:145, 1949.

165. Machella, TE: Postgastrectomy problems, Am J Dig Dis 6:76, 1961.

166. Madsen, P, and Rasmussen, T: Postgastrectomy roentgenography with a physiologic contrast medium, Acta Radiol [Diagn] (Stockh) 2:153, 1964.

167. Magnuson, FK, Judd, ES, and Dearing, WH: Comparison of postgastrectomy complications in gastric and duodenal ulcer patients, Am Surg 32:375, 1966.

168. Maingot, R: Abdominal operations, ed 3, New York, 1955, Appleton-Century-Crofts.

169. Marshak, RH, and Block, C: Colonic changes secondary to marginal ulcer, Am J Dig Dis 6:1126, 1961.

170. Marshall, RL: Diarrhoea following gastric surgery with partial reference to diarrhoea following vagotomy, J R Coll Surg Edinb 9:307, 1964.

171. Marshall, SF, and Knud-Hansen, J: Gastrojejunocolic and gastrocolic fistulas, Ann Surg 145:770, 1957.

172. Mathieson, AJ: Prolonged delay in gastric emptying after partial gastrectomy: its management with particular reference to stomach dysfunction, Br J Surg 52:657, 1965.

173. Maurer, HJ: Funktionsunterschungen nach totaler Magenresektion, Fortschr Rontgenstr 101:463, 1964.

174. McBurney, RP, Farrar, J, and Sanders, RL: Gastrojejunal ulcer and gastrojejunocolic fistula, Am Surg 24:709, 1958.

175. McCaughan, JJ, Jr, and Bowers, RF: Favorable post-gastrectomy results in Billroth II patients with a small stomach, Arch Surg 77:837, 1958.

176. Mendeloff, AI, and Dunn, JP: Digestive diseases: vital and health statistics monograph, Cambridge, 1971, Harvard University Press.

177. Menuck, L, and Siemers, PT: Pneumoperitoneum: importance of right upper quadrant features, Am J Roentgenol 127:753, 1976.

178. Mishlin, JD, et al: Interventional radiologic treatment of complications following gastric bypass surgery for morbid obesity, Gastrointest Radiol 13:9, 1988.

179. Moffat, RC, and Berkas, EM: Bile esophagitis, Arch Surg 91:963, 1965.

180. Moore, TC: Gastrectomy in infancy and childhood. II. Results of an international survey, Ann Surg 162:91, 1965.

181. Morgan, DB, et al: Osteomalacia after gastrectomy, Lancet 2:1089, 1965.

182. Moseley, RV: Pyloric obstruction by phytobezoar following pyloroplasty and vagotomy, Arch Surg 94:290, 1967.

183. Nägele, E: Klinish-röntgenologische Untersuchunger zum Dupling-Syndrom, Dtsch Arch Klin Med 209:689, 1964.

184. Nathens, MS, and Verna, J: Aortographic demonstration of massive bleeding from duodenal stump, J Can Assoc Radiol 21:194, 1970.

185. Norberg, PB: Results of the original treatment of perforated peptic ulcer: a clinical and roentgenologic study, Acta Chir Scan [Suppl] 1:1, 1959.

186. Oglivie, WH: Approach to gastric surgery, Lancet 2:295, 1938.

187. Ominsky, SH, and Moss, AA: The postoperative stomach: a comparative study of double-contrast barium examination and endoscopy, Gastrointest Radiol 4:17, 1979.

188. Palmer, ED: Further observations on postoperative gastritis: histopathologic aspects, with a note on jejunitis, Gastroenterology 25:405, 1953.

189. Palmer, ED: Mucoma of the postoperative stomach, Bull Gastroenterol Endosc 9:7, 1963.

190. Pastremoli, A: Sul significata dell 'immagine di plus che talvolta si rescontra dopo intervento di sutura per ulcera gastroduodenale perforata, Minerva Radiol 9:357, 1964.

191. Pastremoli, A: Osservasioni radiologiche dopo intervento di sutura per ulcera gastroduodenale perforate, Radiol Med (Torino) 50:593, 1964.

192. Patterson, HC: Morbidity following gastric resection for duodenal ulcer with and without vagotomy, Am Surg 31:175, 1965.

193. Perttala, Y, et al: Yeast bezoar formation following gastric surgery, Am J Roentgenol 125:365, 1975.

194. Peskin, GW, and Miller, LD: The use of serotonin antagonists in postgastrectomy syndromes, Am J Surg 109:7, 1965.

195. Piskorz, A, et al: Badanie radiologiczne czynnosci zoladka i dwunastnicy po wagoantrekotomii z powodu choroby wrzodowej dwynastnicy, Pol Tyg Lek 20:915, 1965.

196. Poppel, MH: Gastric intussusceptions, Radiology 78:602, 1962.

197. Poulos, A, et al: Gastric operation for the morbidly obese, Am J Roentgenol 136:867, 1981.

198. Prevot, R: Uber Beutel, Taschen, und Burzel am operierten Magen, Roentgenpraxis 5:101, 1933.

199. Raterman, L, and Buckwalter, JA: The treatment of marginal ulcer, Arch Surg 85:114, 1962.

200. Reyelt, WP, Jr, and Anderson, AA: Retrograde jejunogastric intussusception, Surg Gynecol Obstet 119:1305, 1964.

201. Rimer, DG: Gastric retention without mechanical obstruction: a review, Arch Intern Med 117:287, 1966.

202. Roberts, KE, et al: Cardiovascular and blood volume alterations resulting from intrajejunal administration of hypertonic solutions to gastrectomized patients: relationship of these changes to dumping syndrome, Ann Surg 140:631, 1954.

203. Rodgers, JB: Infarction of the gastric remnant following subtotal gastrectomy, Arch Surg 92:917, 1966.

204. Rosi, PA, and Cahill, WJ: Is total gastrectomy compatible with normal living? Q Bull NW Univ Med School 35:326, 1961.

205. Ross, B, Watson, BW, and Kay, AW: Studies on the effect of vagotomy on small intestinal motility using the radiotelemetering capsule, Gut 4:77, 1963.

206. Ross, JR, Mekhjian, HS, and Gibb, SP: Gluten enteropathy following partial gastrectomy, Lahey Clin Found Bull 15:59, 1966.

207. Roth, JL, Vilardell, F, and Affolter, H: Post-vagotomy gastric stasis, Ann NY Acad Sci 99:203, 1962.

208. Rothnie, NG, Harper, RA, and Catchpole, BN: Early postoperative gastrointestinal activity, Lancet 2:64, 1963.

209. Rudick, J, and Hutchinson, JS: Evaluation of vagotomy and biliary function by combined oral cholecystography and intravenous cholangiography, Ann Surg 162:234, 1965.

210. Rudko, M, and Price, WE: Duodenal stump perforation, J Okla Med Assoc 58:337, 1965.

211. Saikku, LA, and Halonen, V: Dumping syndrome: evaluation of severity of dumping syndrome by clinical and roentgenological methods, Acta Chir Scan 109:339, 1955.

212. Salter, RH, et al: Endoscopic and radiologic assessment of recurrent ulceration after peptic ulcer surgery, Br J Radiol 51:257, 1978.

213. Samuel, E, et al: Radiology of the post-operative abdomen, Clin Radiol 14:133, 1963.

214. Sarasin, R, and Franco, R: Les cancers de l'estomac chex es malades operes pour ulcere benin, Radiol Clin (Basel) 32:243, 1963.

215. Sasson, L: Tumor-simulating deformities after subtotal gastrectomy: a study of the problems of the deformities of the postoperative stomach produced by operative distortions which give the appearance of tumor growth, JAMA 174:280, 1960.

216. Schatzki, R: The significance of rigidity of the jejunum in the diagnosis of postoperative jejunal ulcers, Am J Roentgenol 103:330, 1968.

217. Schautz, R: Zur Differentialdiagnose und Variabilität von Fremdkörpergranulomen, Z Artztl Wochenschr 9:630, 1954.

218. Schiarretta, G, et al: Retained gastric antrum syndrome diagnosed by (^{99m}Tc) pertechnetate scintiphotography in man: hormonal and radioisotopic study of two cases, J Nucl Med 19:377, 1978.

219. Schinz, HS, et al: Roentgen diagnosis, New York, 1954, Grune & Stratton, vol 4.

220. Schlaeger, R: Radiologic observations with barium and food in the postgastrectomy state, NY J Med 60:1780, 1960.

221. Schulman, A: Anastomotic, gastrojejunal ulcer: accuracy of radiological diagnosis in surgically proven cases, Br J Radiol 44:422, 1971.

222. Schulz, HG: Zur Röntgendiagnostik der primären Magenstumpfkarzinome, Fortschr Rontgenstr 103:399, 1966.

223. Seaman, WB: Prolapsed gastric mucosa through a gastrojejunostomy, Am J Roentgenol 110:304, 1970.

224. Segal, AW, et al: Bezoars occurring in the gastric remnant after gastrectomy, S Afr Med J 44:1176, 1970.

225. Serebro, HA, and Mendeloff, AI: Late results of medical and surgical treatment of bleeding peptic ulcer, Lancet 2:505, 1966.

226. Sherlock, P, Glass, GB, and McNeer, G: Histological alternations in the jejunum after total gastrectomy, Am J Med Sci 252:442, 1966.

227. Schulman, H: Passing the Cantor tube in a patient with a gastroenterostomy: an unusual complication, Am J Roentgenol 110:332, 1970.

228. Sigstad, H: Post-gastrectomy radiology with a physiologic contrast medium: comparison between dumpers and nondumpers, Radiology 101:233, 1971.

229. Silverberg, PW: The arteriographic demonstration of bleeding in the duodenal stump, Radiology 100:315, 1971.

230. Simmons, RL, et al: Technical complications of transabdominal vagotomy, Arch Surg 92:922, 1966.

231. Sircus, W, and Smith, AN, editors: Scientific foundations of gastroenterology, London, 1980, William Heinemann Medical Books.

232. Smith, MP: Decline in duodenal ulcer surgery, JAMA 237:987, 1977.

233. Spiro, HM: Clinical gastroenterology, ed 2, New York, 1977, MacMillan Publishing.

234. Stammers, FA, and Williams, JA: Partial gastrectomy: complications and metabolic consequences, London, 1963, Butterworth.

235. Stremple, JF, and Elliott, DW: Gastrin determinations in symptomatic patients before and after standard ulcer operations, Arch Surg 110:875, 1975.

236. Strittmatter, WC, and Wise, RE: Roentgenologic diagnosis of jejunal or marginal ulcer, Cleve Clin Q 20:286, 1953.

237. Strom, BG, Beaudry, R, and Morin, F: Yeast overgrowth in operated stomach, J Can Assoc Radiol 29:161, 1978.

238. Szemes, G, and Amberg, JR: Gastric bezoars after partial gastrectomy: report of five cases, Radiology 90:765, 1968.

239. Thoeny RH, Hodgson, JR, and Scudamore, HH: The roentgenologic diagnosis of gastrocolic and gastrojejunocolic fistulas, Am J Roentgenol 83:876, 1960.

240. Thompson, JE, and Rodgers, JB: The management and prevention of abdominal complications associated with gastric and duodenal surgery, Am Surg 30:553, 1964.

241. Thorfinnson, PC, and Brow, JR: Reflux bile gastritis, J Can Assoc Radiol 25:263, 1974.

242. Thorn, PA, Brookes, VS, and Waterhouse, JA: Peptic ulcer, partial gastrectomy, and pulmonary tuberculosis, Br Med J 1:603, 1956.

243. Toye, DK, Hutton, JF, and Williams, JA: Radiological anatomy after pyloroplasty, Gut 11:358, 1970.

244. Tucker, AS, and Izant, RJ, Jr: How serious are gastrointestinal perforations in infancy? Radiology 81:112, 1963.

245. Tuschka, O: Jejunogastric intussusception, JAMA 186:1092, 1963.

246. Vargha, J: Funktionelle Röntgenuntersuchungen der Anastomose bei Anastomosenkarzinomen, Radiol Diagn (Berl) 3:215:, 1962.

247. Wallensten, S: Results of surgical therapy of peptic ulcer by partial gastrectomy according to Billroth I and Billroth II methods, Acta Chir Scand [Suppl] 191:1, 1954.

248. Walters, W: Six to ten-year follow-up of the surgical treatment of duodenal, gastric and gastrojejunal ulcer, Gastroenterologia (Basel) 93:15, 1960.

249. Warthin, TA: Reactivation of pulmonary tuberculosis in relation to subtotal gastrectomy for peptic ulcer, Am J Med Sci 225:421, 1953.

250. Wastell, C, and Ellis, H: Faecal fat excretion and stool colour after vagotomy and pyloroplasty, Br Med J 1:1194, 1966.

251. Weber, JM, Lewis, S, and Heasley, KH: Observations on the small bowel pattern associated with the Zollinger-Ellison syndrome, Am J Roentgenol 82:973, 1959.

252. Welch, CE: Abdominal surgery, N Engl J Med 275:1232, 1966.

253. Welch, CE: Abdominal surgery (first of three parts), N Engl J Med 293:858, 1975.

254. Wellauer, J: Der operierte Magen: Rontgentaktik und-Technik, Bibl Gastroenterol 6:137, 1964.

255. Wells, C, et al: Postoperative gastrointestinal motility, Lancet 1:4, 1964.

256. Whitehouse, GH, and Temple, JG: The evaluation of dumping and diarrhoea after gastric surgery using a physiological test meal, Clin Radiol 28:143, 1977.

257. Williams, EJ, and Irvine, WT: Effects of total and selective vagotomy, Lancet 1:1053, 1966.

258. Williams, JA, and Toye, DK: Recurrent ulcer after vagotomy and pyloroplasty: the x-ray appearances and their value in diagnosis, Gut 11:405, 1970.

259. Wilson, SD, and Ellison, EH: Survival in patients with the Zollinger-Ellison syndrome treated by total gastrectomy, Am J Surg 111:787, 1966.

260. Wilson, WJ, and Weintraub, HD: The post-pyloroplasty antrum, Am J Roentgenol 96:408, 1966.

261. Windsor, CW: Gastro-oesophageal reflux after partial gastrectomy, Br Med J 2:1233, 1964.

262. Wolf, BS, and Khilnami, MT: Progress in gastrotenterological radiology, Gastroenterology 51:542, 1966.

263. Wychulis, AR, Priestley, JT, and Foulk, WT: A study of 360 patients with gastrojejunal ulceration, Surg Gynecol Obstet 122:89, 1966.

264. Zatzkin, HR, and Riera, A: Upper gastro-intestinal examination after gastric surgery, Radiology 55:193, 1950.

265. Zikria, BA, et al: Mallory-Weiss syndrome and emetogenic (spontaneous) rupture of the esophagus, Ann Surg 162:151, 1965.

266. Zollinger, RM, and Williams, RD: Consideration in surgical treatment for duodenal ulcer, JAMA 160:367, 1956.

Small bowel

267. Adams, JF: Postgastrectomy megaloblastic anaemia and the loop syndrome, Gastroenterologia (Basel) 89:326, 1958.

268. Andreassy, MRJ, Haff, RC, and Lobritz, RW: Liver failure after jejunoileal shunt, Arch Surg 110:332, 1975.

269. Botsford, TW, and Gazzaniga, AB: Blind pouch syndrome: a complication of side-to-side intestinal anastomosis, Am J Surg 113:486, 1967.

270. Burhenne, HJ: Roentgenologic approach to a physiologic examination of the alimentary tract. In Gamble, JR, and Wilbur, DL, editors: Current concepts of clinical gastroenterology, Boston, 1965, Little, Brown.

271. Carillo, FX: The immediate complications of gastrectomy: a twelve-year review of early postoperative complication in ulcer surgery, Medical Annals of the District of Columbia 32:159:1963.

272. Chun, JJ, and Dinan, JJ: Small bowel obstruction due to phytobezoar in gastric subjects, Can J Surg 8:272, 1965.

273. Coffey, RR: Afferent loop syndrome after Billroth II gastrectomy, Am J Surg 108:610, 1964.

274. Coletti, L, and Bossart, PA: Intestinal obstruction during the early postoperative period, Arch Surg 88:774, 1964.

275. Diner, WC, and Cockrill, HH: The continent ileostomy (Kock pouch): roentgenologic features, Gastrointest Radiol 4:65, 1979.

276. Drenick, EJ, et al: Bypass enteropathy: intestinal and systemic manifestations following small-bowel bypass, JAMA 236:269, 1976.

277. Dunphy, JE: A method of handling the jejunal loop in gastrectomy with a posterior anastomosis, Surg Gynecol Obstet 110:109, 1960.

278. Fleshman, JW, et al: The ileal reservoir and ileoanal anastomosis procedure: factors affecting technical and functional outcome, Dis Colon Rectum 31:10, 1988.

279. Fox, ER, Chung, T, and Laufer, I: Enteroliths in a continent iliostomy, Am J Roentgenol 150:105, 1988.

280. Goldstein, F, Wirtz, CW, and Kramer, S: The relationship of afferent limb stasis and bacterial flora to the production of postgastrectomy steatorrhea, Gastroenterology 40:47, 1961.

281. Gribovsky, E: The dietary and medical treatment of postgastrectomy symptoms, Am J Gastroenterol 36:645, 1961.

282. Hafter, E: Praktische Gastroenterologie, ed 2, Stuttgart, 1962, Georg Thieme Varlag.

283. Hardy, JD: Gastric resection: pathophysiology and management of certain complications, Am J Gastroenterol 32:136, 1959.

284. Ho, CS, and Lipinsky, JK: Selective intubation of the afferent loop, Am J Roentgenol 130:481, 1978.

285. Jewell, WR, Hermreck, AS, and Hardin, CA: Complications of jejunoileal bypass for morbid obesity, Arch Surg 110:1039, 1975.

286. Karasick, D, and Karasick, S: Obstructive and enteropathic syndromes after jejonoileal bypass surgery, Gastrointest Radiol 6:129, 1981.

287. Katz, I, and Karp, FL: Inadvertent gastroileostomy, Am J Roentgenol 99:162, 1967.

288. Kremers, PW, et al: Radiology of the ileoanal reservoir, Am J Roentgenol 145:559, 1985.

289. Larsen, RR, Saliba, NS, and Sawyer, KC: Postgastrectomy internal hernia, Arch Surg 89:725, 1964.

290. Levine, M, Katz, I, and Lampros, PJ: Blind pouch formation secondary to side-to-side intestinal anastomosis, Am J Roentgenol 89:706, 1963.

291. Lewicki, AM, et al: The small bowel following pyloroplasty and vagotomy, Radiology 109:539, 1973.

292. Lo, G, Fisch, AE, and Brodey, PA: CT of the intussuscepted excluded loop after intestinal bypass, Am J Roentgenol 137:157, 1981.

293. Madsen, P: The afferent loop syndrome: a roentgen and cineroentgenographic study, Acta Chir Scand 129:417, 1965.

294. Maglinte, DDT: "Bline pouch" syndrome: a cause of gastrointestinal bleeding, Radiology 132:314, 1979.

295. Mallet-Guy, P, Paillet, P, and Rochet, Y: Y incarceration chronique de l'anse anastomotique dans la beche mesocolique apres gastrectomie, Lyon Chir 54:12, 1958.

296. Martyak, SN, and Curtis, LE: Pneumatosis intestinalis: a complication of jejunoileal bypass, JAMA 235:1038, 1976.

297. McCabe, R, and Knox, WG: Phytobezoar in gastrectomized patients: a cause of small bowel obstruction, Arch Surg 86:264, 1963.

298. Miller, DR: Intussusception of the by-passed segment after jejunoileal by-pass for obesity: a cryptic problem, Am J Gastroenterol 72:434, 1979.

299. Moretz, WH: Inadvertent gastro-ileostomy, Ann Surg 130:124, 1949.

300. Palumbo, PJ, et al: Inadvertent gastroileostomy, Gastroenterology 45:505, 1963.

301. Passaro, E, Jr, Dreneck, E, and Wilson, SE: Bypass enteritis: a new complication of jejunoileal bypass for obesity, Am J Surg 131:169, 1976.

302. Payne, JH, DeWind, LT, and Commons, RR: Metabolic observations in patients with jejunocolic shunts, Am J Surg 106:273, 1963.

303. Riegel, N: Intestinal obstruction due to orange pulp in a patient with partial gastrectomy, vagotomy, and gastrojejunostomy, Am Surg 32:407, 1966.

304. Rogers, LF, Davis, EK, and Harle, TS: Phytobezoar formation and food boli following gastric surgery, Am J Roentgenol 119:280, 1973.

305. Sarti, DA, and Zablen, MA: The ultrasonic findings in intussusception of the blind loop in jejunoileal bypass for obesity, J Clin Ultrasound 7:50, 1979.

306. Scott, HW: The surgical management of patients with morbid obesity, J R Coll Surg 22:241, 1977.

307. Sherwin, B, and Messe, AA: Inadvertent gastroileostomy, Gastroenterology 21:382, 1952.

308. Stammers, FA, and Williams, JA: Partial gastrectomy: complications and metabolic consequences, London, 1963, Butterworth.

309. Stiris, G, and Traetteberg, K: Changes in the transverse colon following partial gastric resection, Acta Radiol [Diagn] (Stockh) 1:1100, 1963.

310. Vainder, M, and Kelly, J: Renal tubular dysfunction secondary to jejunoileal bypass, JAMA 235:1257, 1976.

311. Wade, DH, Richards, V, and Burhenne, HJ: Radiographic changes after small bowel bypass for morbid obesity, Radiol Clin North Am 14:493, 1976.

312. Waugh, JM, and Hood, RT, Jr: Gastric operations: a historic review, I. Q Rev Surg Obstet Gynecol 10:201, 1953.

313. Weissman, I: Enterogastric regurgitation during barium enema examination, Am J Roentgenol 88:637, 1962.

314. Welch, CE: Abdominal surgery, N Engl J Med 275:1232, 1966.

315. Welch, CE, and Ellis, DS: Physiology of the surgically altered stomach, Ann Rev Med 12:19, 1961.

316. Williams, JA, and Stammer, FA: Criteria for reoperation tightened up after analysis of the results in thirty-nine cases, Acta Gastroenterol Belg 27:610, 1965.

317. Wirts, CW, et al: The correction of postgastrectomy malabsorption following a jejunal interposition operation, Gastroenterology 49:141, 1965.

318. Wise, LW, and Stein, T: Biliary and urinary calculi: pathogenesis following small bowel bypass for obesity, Arch Surg 110:1043, 1975.

319. Witt, CB, Jr, and Averbrook, BD: Intestinal obstruction following jejunal interposition operation, Arch Surg 93:498, 1966.

Colon

320. Bartow, JH, and Rao, BR: Simplified barium enema examination via colostomy, Am J Roentgenol 135:1302, 1980.

321. Burhenne, HJ: Technique of colostomy examination, Radiology 97:183, 1970.

322. Gierson, ED, et al: Caecal rupture due to colonic ileus, Br J Surg 62:383, 1975.

323. Goldstein, HM, and Miller, MH: Air contrast colon examination in patients with colostomies, Am J Roentgenol 127:607, 1976.

324. Lane, RE: Colostomy enema, Radiology 100:36, 1977.

325. Meyer, JE: Radiography of the distal colon and rectum after irradiation of carcinoma of the cervix, Am J Roentgenol 136:691, 1981.

326. Moss, WT, Brand, WN, and Battifora, H: Radiation oncology: rationale, technique, results, ed 5, St. Louis, 1979, C.V. Mosby.

327. Steinbrich, W, et al: Computed tomography in the diagnosis of local recurrences after resection for carcinoma of the rectum, ROFO 131:499, 1979.

328. Strockbine, MD, Hancock, JE, and Fletcher, GH: Complications in 831 patients with squamous cell carcinoma of the intact uterine cervix treated with 3000 rad or more whole pelvic irradiation, Am J Roentgenol 108:293, 1970.

Biliary tract, liver, and pancreas

329. Acosta, JM, et al: Operative cholangiography, Arch Surg 99:29, 1969.
330. Aldrete, JS, and Judd, ES: Metallic cannula as an aid to cystic duct operative cholangiography, Mayo Clin Proc 41:839, 1966.
331. Allen, KL: Routine operative cholangiography, Am J Surg 118:573, 1969.
332. Andersson, A, et al: Concretions in the pancreatic duct diagnosed by cholangiography, Acta Radiol (Stockh) 8:183, 1969.
333. Arcomano, JP, Schwinger, HN, and DeAngelis, J: The spontaneous disappearance of gallstones, Am J Roentgenol 99:637, 1967.
334. Ashmore, JD, et al: Experimental evaluation of operative cholangiography in relation to calculus size, Surgery 40:191, 1956.
335. Babbitt, DP, and Thatcher, DS: Radiographic findings in postoperative bile collections, Radiology 84:471, 1965.
336. Bardenheier, JA, Kaminski, DL, and Willman, VL: Pancreatitis after biliary tract surgery, Am J Surg 116:773, 1968.
337. Beneventono, TC, and Schein, CJ: Pseudocalculus sign seen in cholangiography, Arch Surg 98:731, 1969.
338. Bockhart, H, and Moller, W: Versuche ueber die Funktion der Gallenblase und ihre Roentgendarstellung, Dtsch Chir 161:168, 1921.
339. Bodvall, B, and Overgaard, B: Cystic duct remnant after cholecystostomy, Ann Surg 163:382, 1966.
340. Braasch, JW, and McCann, JC, Jr: Choledochoduodenal junction size, Surgery 62:258, 1967.
341. Burhenne, HJ: Problem areas in the biliary tract, Curr Probl Radiol 5:3, 1975.
342. Burnett, WE, et al: Operative cholangiography, Ann Surg 168:551, 1968.
343. Carey, LC, and Ellison, EC: Pancreas, In Fromme, D, editor: Gastrointestinal surgery, New York, 1985, Churchhill-Livingstone.
344. Carter, RF, and Saypol, GM: Transabdominal cholangiography, JAMA 148:253, 1952.
345. Cugini, A, and Sosso, A: Retrograde cholangiography from transpapillary duodenobiliary reflux, Ann Radiol Diagn (Bologna) 35:163, 1962.
346. Custer, MD, Jr, and Clore, JN, Jr: Source of error in operative cholangiography, Arch Surg 100:664, 1970.
347. Dayton, MR, Conter, R, and Tompkins, RK: Incidence of complications with operative choledochoscopy, Am J Surg 147:139, 1984.
348. Dellinger, EP, et al: Determinants of adverse reaction following postoperative T-tube cholangiogram, Ann Surg 191:397, 1980.
349. Dowse, JL: Cholecysto-duodenocolic fistulae due to gallstone, Br J Surg 50:776, 1963.
350. Dreiling, DA: The post-cholecystectomy syndrome, Am J Dig Dis 7:603, 1962.
351. Edmunds, R, Rucker, C, and Finby, N: Intravenous cholangiography, Arch Surg 90:73, 1965.
352. Edmunds, R, et al: The common duct after cholecystectomy, Arch Surg 103:79, 1971.
353. Elsey, EC, and Jacobs, DL: Floating gallbladder stones, Am J Roentgenol 65:73, 1951.
354. Engelholm, L, et al: Die intraduodenal Choledochocele, Fortschr Rontgenstr 108:403, 1968.
355. Ferguson, HL, and Sampliner, JE: Operative needle cholangiography: a clinical evaluation, Am Surg 35:476, 1969.
356. Ferguson, TB, and Burford, TH: Pleurobiliary and bronchobiliary fistulas, Arch Surg 95:380, 1967.
357. Ferris, DO, and Sterling, WA: Surgery of the billiary tract, Surg Clin North Am 47:861, 1967.
358. Foley, WD, et al: Treatment of blunt hepatic injuries: role of CT, Radiology 164:635, 1987.
359. Frates, RE: Incompetence of the sphincter of Oddi in the newborn, Radiology 85:875, 1965.
360. Ginzburg, L, Gefen, A, and Friedman, IH: Pseudo-obstruction after choledochotomy, Ann Surg 166:83, 1967.
361. Glenn, F, and Grafe, W, Jr: Historical events in biliary tract surgery, Arch Surg 93:848, 1966.
362. Graham, MF, et al: The size of the normal common hepatic duct following cholecystectomy: an ultrasonographic study, Radiology 135:137, 1980.
363. Griffin, TF, and Wild, AA: The case for preoperative cholangiography, Br J Surg 54:609, 1967.
364. Gudas, PP, Haberman, GC, and Belcher, HV: Cholecystocolonic fistula, Arch Surg 95:228, 1967.
365. Guyer, PB, and McLoughlin, M: Congenital double gallbladder, Br J Radiol 40:214, 1967.
366. Hafner, HM: Examinations following choledochoduodenostomy, Helv Chir Acta 26:334, 1959.
367. Hanks, JB, et al: Surgical resection for benign and malignant liver disease, Ann Surg 191:584, 1980.
368. Hansson, K, and Ramberg, L: A case of spontaneous and complete disappearance of gallstones, Radiologe 1:97, 1961.
369. Hayes, MA: Biliary duct anomalies, unexpected high rate, JAMA 197:30, 1966.
370. Hayes, MA, Goldenberg, IS, and Bishop, CC: The developmental basis for bile duct anomalies, Surg Gynecol Obstet 107:447, 1958.
371. Hess, W: Surgery of the biliary passages and the pancreas, New York, 1965, W. Van Nostrand.
372. Hicken, NF, and McAllister, AJ: Operative cholangiography as an aid in reducing the incidence of "overlooked" common bile duct stones, Surgery 55:753, 1964.
373. Howard, JM, and Short, WF: An evaluation of pancreatography in suspected pancreatic disease, Surg Gynecol Obstet 129:319, 1969.
374. Hughes, J, et al: The common duct after cholecystectomy: initial report of a ten-year-study, JAMA 197:89, 1966.
375. Hultborn, A, Jacobsson, B, and Rosengren, B: Cholangio-venous reflux: a clinical and experimental study, Acta Chir Scand 123:111, 1962.
376. Hutchin, P, Harrison, TS and Halasz, NA: Postoperative cholecystocolic fistula, Ann Surg 157:587, 1963.
377. Jakimowicz, JJ, et al: Comparison of operative ultrasonography and radiography in screening of the common bile duct for calculi, World J Surg 11:628, 1987.
378. Jolly, PC, et al: Operative cholangiography, Ann Surg 168:551, 1968.
379. Jolly, PC, et al: Operative cholangiography, Northwest Medicine 68:639, 1969.
380. Kramer, SG: Technical aid to operative cholangiography, Surgery 64:403, 1968.
381. Letourneau, JG, et al: Liver allograft transplantation: postoperative CT findings, AJR 148:1099, 1987.
382. Letourneau, JG, et al: Upper abdomen: CT findings following partial hepatectomy, Radiology 166:139, 1988.
383. Letton, AH, and Wilson, JP: Routine cholangiography during biliary tract operation, Ann Surg 163:937, 1966.
384. Lucas, CE, and Read, RC: Barium cholangiography, Radiology 87:1043, 1966.
385. Luttwak, EM: A simple method of operative cholangiography, Surg Gynecol Obstet 128:603, 1969.
386. Mahour, GH, Wakim, KG, and Ferris, DO: Common bile duct in man: its diameter and circumference, Ann Surg 165:415, 1967.

387. Mallet-Guy, P: L'intervention biliaire sous controle radiomano-métrique, Lyon Chir 39:50, 1944.

388. Marincek, B, et al: CT appearance of impaired lymphatic drainage in liver transplants, Am J Roentgenol 147:519, 1986.

389. Marguis, JR, and Densler, J: The disappearing limy bile syndrome, Radiology 94:311, 1970.

390. Mirizzi, PL: La colangiografia durante las operaciones de las vias biliares, Bol Trabv Soc Buenos Aires 16:1133, 1932.

391. Mueller, PR, et al: Postcholecystectomy bile duct dilation: myth or reality, Am J Roentgenol 136:355, 1981.

392. Mujahed, Z, Glenn, F, and Evans, J: Communicating cavernous ectasia of the intrahepatic ducts (Carolis' disease), Am J Roentgenol 113:21, 1971.

393. Myers, RN, et al: Cinecholangiography as an aid in the interpretation of T-tube cholangiogram deformities, Surg Gynecol Obstet 119:47, 1964.

394. Nelson, JA, and Burhenne, HJ: Anomalous biliary and pancreatic duct insertion into duodenal diverticula, Radiology 120:49, 1976.

395. Olutola, PS, Hutton, L, and Wall, WJ: Radiologic assessment of bile duct complications in liver transplantation: initial experience, J Can Assoc Radiol 37:276, 1986.

396. Op den Orth, JO: A radiologically demonstrated fistula between the common bile duct and the right renal pelvis, Radiol Clin Biol 38:402, 1969.

397. Palmisano, DJ: Double gallbladder, Am J Surg 118:463, 1969.

398. Parent, M, and Peloguin, A: Preoperative cholangiography, Can J Surg 6:129, 1963.

399. Perlin, E, et al: The air cholangiogram as an unusal sequela to thoracocentesis, JAMA 210:2280, 1969.

400. Piedad, OH, and Well, PB: Spontaneous internal biliary fistula: obstructive and nonobstructive types: 20-year review of 55 cases, Ann Surg 175:75, 1972.

401. Pitman, RG, and Davies, A: The clinical and radiological features of spontaneous internal biliary fistulae, Br J Surg 50:414, 1963.

402. Portorak, JL: An attempt to evaluate the function of the sphincter of Oddi after sphincterotomy, Pol Tyg Lek 21:137, 1966.

403. Pyrtek, LJ, and Bartus, SH: Critical evaluation of routine and selective operating room cholangiography, Am J Surg 103:761, 1962.

404. Raknerud, N: Gas in the biliary ducts, Tidsskr Nor Laegeforen 89:1024, 1969.

405. Rappoport, AS, and Diamond, AB: Cholangiographic demonstration of postoperative bile leakage from aberrant biliary ducts, Gastrointest Radiol 6:273, 1981.

406. Rominger, CJ, and Canino, CW: Internal biliary tract fistulae, Am J Roentgenol 90:835, 1963.

407. Rosato, EF, Berkowitz, HD, and Roberts, B: Bile ascites, Surg Gynecol Obstet 130:494, 1970.

408. Ross, RJ, and Sachs, MD: Triplication of the gallbladder, Am J Roentgenol 104:656, 1968.

409. Schulenburg, CA: Operative cholangiography, London, 1966, Butterworth.

410. Schulenburg, CA: Postoperative cholangiography, London, 1966, Butterworth.

411. Schulenburg, CA: Anomalies of the biliary tract as demonstrated by operative cholangiography, Med Proc 16:351, 1970.

412. Schwartz, A, and Birnbaum, D: Roentgenologic study of the topography of the choledocho-duodenal junction, Am J Roentgenol 87:772, 1962.

413. Schwarz, E: The intramural cystic duct remnant, Am J Roentgenol 86:930, 1961.

414. Senter, KL, and Berne, CJ: Significance of non-passage of radiopaque media through the ampulla of Vater during cholangiography, Am J Surg 112:7, 1966.

415. Sewell, JA: Avulsion of left hepatic duct, Ann Surg 165:628, 1967.

416. Shehadi, WH: Roentgen observation in cases of fistulae of the biliary tract, JAMA 174:2204, 1960.

417. Shehadi, WH: Clinical radiology of the biliary tract, New York, 1963, McGraw-Hill.

418. Shocket, E, Evans, J, and Jonas, S: Cholecystoduodenocolic fistula with gallstone ileus, Arch Surg 101:523, 1970.

419. Simendinger, EA, Krutky, TA, and Reodica, RE: Double gallbladder with double cholelithiasis, JAMA 215:1823, 1971.

420. Stanley, JH, et al: Percutaneous drainage of pancreatic and peripancreatic fluid collections, Cardiovasc Intervent Radiol 1:21, 1988.

421. Staple, TW, and McAlister, WH: In vitro and in vivo visualization of biliary calculi, Am J Roentgenol 94:495, 1965.

422. Stassa, G, and Grafe, WR: The cineradiographic evaluation of the biliary tract after drug therapy following cholecystectomy, sphincterotomy, and vagotomy, Radiology 91:297, 1968.

423. Statistical bulletin, Metropolitan Life Insurance 46:9, 1965.

424. Tabrisky, J, and Pollack, EL: The aberrant division bile duct, Radiology 99:537, 1971.

425. Tanaka, M, et al: Manometric diagnosis of spincter of Oddi spasm as a cause of postcholecystectomy pain and the treatment by endoscopic sphincterotomy, Ann Surg 202:712, 1985.

426. Turner, MA, Cho, S-R, and Messmer, JM: Pitfalls in cholangiographic interpretation, RadioGraphics 7:1067, 1987.

427. Viost, JC: Cystic duct remnants [thesis], University of Minnesota, 1957.

428. Walters, W, Nixon, JW, Jr, and Hodgins, TE: Strictures of the common duct: five to 25-year follow-up of 217 operations, Ann Surg 149:781, 1959.

429. Warren, KW: Pitfalls of gallbladder surgery, Hosp Prac 2:29, 1967.

430. Wechsler, RJ, et al: The periportal collar: a CT sign of liver transplant rejection, Radiology 165:57, 1987.

431. Weston, WJ: Post-operative bile peritonitis: its radiological diagnosis, Aust Radiol 11:34, 1967.

432. Whitaker, PH, Parkinson, EG, and Hughes, JH: Television fluoroscopy for operative cholangiography: an analysis of 150 cases, Clin Radiol 19:368, 1968.

433. White, RM, et al: Liver transplant rejection: angiographic findings in 35 patients, Am J Roentgenol 148:1095, 1987.

434. Wise, L, Pizzimbono, C, and Dehner, LP: Periampullary cancer, Am J Surg 131:141, 1976.

435. Wise, RE: Cholangiography and duct pancreatography in the diagnosis of pancreatic disease, Semin Roentgenol 3:288, 1968.

436. Wise, RE, and Keefe, JP: Radiological evaluation of hepaticojejunal anastomosis, Surg Clin North Am 48:579, 1968.

437. Wolfel, DA, and Brogdon, BG: Intrahepatic air—a sign of trauma, Radiology 91:952, 1968.

438. Zajko, AB, et al: Cholangiography and interventional biliary radiology in adult liver transplantation, Am J Roentgenol 144:127, 1985.

439. Zajko, AB, et al: Cholangiographic findings in hepatic artery occlusion after liver transplantation, Am J Roentgenol 149:485, 1987.

440. Zajko, AB, et al: Percutaneous transhepatic cholangiography and biliary drainage after liver transplantation: a five-year experience, Gastrointest Radiol 12:137, 1987.

441. Zakl, KS: Cineradiographical examination of the common bile duct, Pol Przegl Radiol (Warszawa) 28:353, 1964.

PART XIV

RETROPERITONEAL SPACE

65 *Radiology*

MORTON A. MEYERS

Disease processes originating within the alimentary tract may extend through the extraperitoneal spaces, and abnormalities primarily arising within other extraperitoneal sites may significantly affect the bowel.[37] In uncovering extraperitoneal origins and complications in a spectrum of diseases involving the alimentary tract, however,"the clinician is often left with only his flair and his diagnostic first principles to guide him."[10] Symptoms and signs may be obscure, delayed, or nonspecific,[1,58] and the area is generally not accessible to auscultation, palpation, or percussion. Radiologic evaluation thus plays a critical role.

ETIOLOGY OF EXTRAPERITONEAL EFFUSIONS

Extraperitoneal infection is usually a complication of infection, injury, or malignancy in adjacent retroperitoneal or intraperitoneal organs. Unless diagnosed early and treated adequately, extraperitoneal abscess is associated with prolonged morbidity and high mortality. Spread may involve the anterior abdominal wall, subcutaneous tissues of the back or flank, subdiaphragmatic space, mediastinum, thoracic cavity, psoas muscle, thigh, or hip.

Extraperitoneal blood is usually caused by trauma, ruptured aneurysm, malignancy, bleeding diathesis, or overanticoagulation.

Extraperitoneal gas is most often the result of bowel perforation from inflammation of ulcerative disease, blunt or penetrating trauma, a foreign body, iatrogenic manipulation, or a gas-producing infection originating in extraperitoneal organs. Often it is not until the gas is recognized radiologically that attention is directed to or confirms the presence of an acute process in the abdomen.

NORMAL AND PATHOLOGIC ANATOMY

Basic to an understanding of the pathogenesis of spread of diseases and their radiologic criteria is a precise knowledge of the anatomy of the extraperitoneal fascial planes, compartments, and relationships.[37,41] These features can be applied diagnostically in conventional radiologic modalities and have been further confirmed and readily documented by ultrasonography and particularly computed tomography (CT).[27,37]

Radiologically loss of visualization of the lateral margin of the psoas muscle had classically been considered the hallmark of extraperitoneal effusions. This sign, however, is unreliable, since 25% to 44% of normal individuals show unequal visualization of the psoas borders.[11,63] Furthermore, the psoas outline may disappear with only very minimal rotation or scoliosis of the lumbar spine,[57] and extraperitoneal fat may be scanty in emaciated pa-

tients or in those who have lost weight. A reliable sign, however, is *segmental* loss of visualization of the psoas border. Such asymmetry in properly centered films immediately localizes a collection to a specific extraperitoneal compartment.[37]

The retroperitoneal space is bounded anteriorly by the posterior parietal peritoneum and posteriorly by the transversalis fascia and extends from the pelvic brim inferiorly to the diaphragm superiorly. Central to the division of the extraperitoneal region are the conspicuous anterior and posterior layers of renal fascia (Gerota's fascia) (Fig.

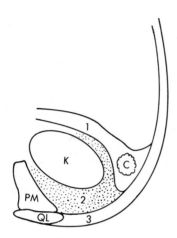

Fig. 65-1 Fascial definitions of three extraperitoneal spaces. Transverse diagram of left flank. *1,* Anterior pararenal space; *2,* perirenal space; *3,* posterior pararenal space. Note their relationships to kidney *(K),* descending colon *(C),* psoas muscle *(PM),* and quadratus lumborum muscle *(QL).*
(Modified from Meyers, MA: Semin Roentgenol 8:445, 1973.)

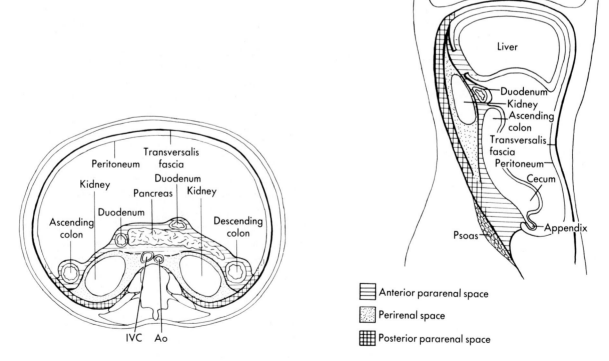

Fig. 65-2 Contents and relationships of three extraperitoneal compartments.
(Modified from Meyers, MA: Semin Roentgenol 8:445, 1973.)

65-1); these two layers fuse behind the ascending or descending colon to form the single lateroconal fascia, which then continues around the flank to blend with the peritoneal reflection. These fascial relationships are readily confirmed by CT.[27,37] Three distinct extraperitoneal compartments are thus demarcated (Figs. 65-1 and 65-2):

1. *Anterior pararenal space.* Lying between the posterior parietal peritoneum and anterior renal fascia, this space contains the pancreas and retroperitoneal portions of the alimentary tract. Ventrally the anterior pararenal space is anatomically continuous with the roots of the small bowel mesentery and transverse colon.[45]

2. *Perirenal space.* Lying within the cone of renal fascia, this space contains the kidney and renal vessels, the adrenal gland, the proximal ureter, and a variable amount of fat.

3. *Posterior pararenal space.* Lying between the posterior renal fascia and the transversalis fascia, this space contains no organs; its fat continues laterally as the properitoneal flank stripe.

Table 65-1 summarizes the major radiologic criteria of collections localized specifically to each of these three compartments.[37,44]

The normal thickness of the fascial planes is 1 to 2 mm. A fascia that is focally thickened or greater than 2 to 3 mm in width is usually abnormal.[48,49] Renal fascial thickening may be caused by edema, hyperemia fibrosis, or lipolysis.[47] It has been reported in a large variety of pathologic conditions,[5,19,48] including inflammatory, malignant, and traumatic processes, and is further nonspecific in not allowing diagnostic localization to a primary extraperitoneal site, since it may be related to disease in the kidney, perirenal space, or pararenal compartments.[27,33,49]

Rarely the appearance of thickened fascia may be simulated on CT supine scans by intraperitoneal fluid within posterior peritoneal recesses, particularly on the left[14,15,53] (Fig. 65-3). The posterior renal fascia has been shown by dissection studies to be divided into two laminae at a variable point from the kidney.[51] The thinner anterior leaf extends anteriorly to be continuous with the anterior renal fascia. The thicker posterior lamina becomes the lateroconal fascia. Fig. 65-4 clearly displays these laminae in two different patients. A potential space between the two laminae is thus anatomically continuous with the anterior pararenal space.[51]

Variations in the origin of the lateroconal fascia may explain the uncommon occurrence of retrorenal colon or extension of ascitic fluid.[21,26,55] Kunin [24] has identified three groups of bridging connective tissue septa that may divide the perirenal space into relatively discrete compartments. These include fibrous lamellae that connect the renal capsule to the perirenal fascia and some that connect the anterior and posterior renal fasciae, but the most commonly visible in well-fatted patients is the posterior renorenal bridging septum.[24,30] This is attached only to the renal capsule and runs parallel to the surface of the kidney. The septa may thicken in response to the

☐ **TABLE 65-1**

Radiologic criteria for localizing extraperitoneal fluid and gas collections

Radiologic features	Anterior pararenal space	Perirenal space	Posterior pararenal space
Perirenal fat and renal outline	Preserved	Obliterated	Preserved
Axis of density	Vertical	Vertical (acute)	Inferolateral (parallel to psoas margin)
		Inferomedial (chronic)	
Kidney displacement	Lateral and superior	Anterior, medial, and superior	Anterior, lateral, and superior
Psoas muscle outline	Preserved	Upper half obliterated	Obliterated in lower half or throughout
Flank stripe	Preserved	Preserved	Obliterated
Hepatic and splenic angles	Obliterated	Obliterated	Preserved or obliterated
Displacement of ascending or descending colon	Anterior and lateral	Lateral	Anterior and medial
Displacement of descending duodenum or duodenojejunal junction	Anterior	Anterior	Anterior

From Meyers, MA: Dynamic radiology of the abdomen: normal and pathologic anatomy, New York, 1982, Springer-Verlag.

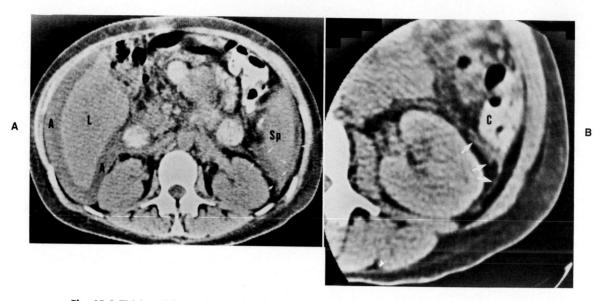

Fig. 65-3 Thickened fascia simulated by intraperitoneal fluid. **A,** CT scan and **B,** magnified view at lower level. Ascitic fluid *(A)* surrounds liver *(L)*. Small amount of ascites around spleen *(Sp)* in splenorenal recess *(arrows)* results in appearance of thickened left anterior renal fascia. *C,* Descending colon.

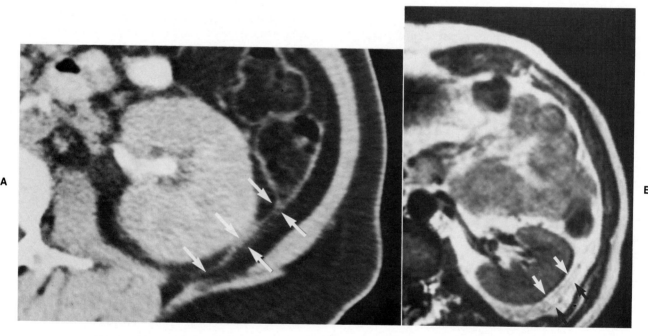

Fig. 65-4 In vivo identification of two layers of posterior renal fascia. **A,** CT demonstrates enlarged left kidney, caused by acute pyelonephritis, abutting posterior renal fascia and presence of double line of posterior renal fascia *(arrows)*. Inner line adjacent to kidney is thickened, and potential space between two leaves of posterior renal fascia is now seen. **B,** Magnetic resonance imaging discretely shows two layers of posterior renal fascia *(arrows)*.

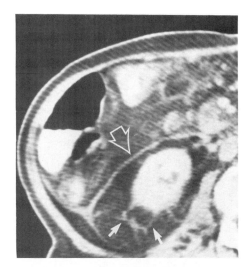

Fig. 65-5 Bridging renal septa. Among multiple bridging septa, most conspicuous is dorsal renorenal septum *(arrows)*. These are associated with thickened anterior renal fascia *(open arrow)*.

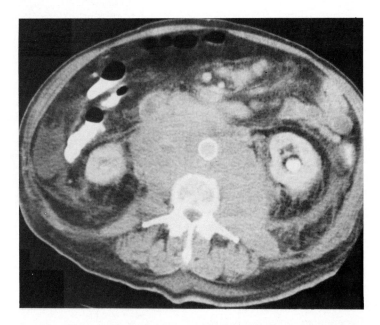

Fig. 65-6 Lymphatic stranding through the extraperitoneal spaces. In patient with non-Hodgkin's lymphoma with gross paraaortic-paracaval adenopathy, CT demonstrates extraperitoneal lymphedema with thickening of fasciae and septa.

same stimuli that cause thickening and increased visibility of the anterior and posterior renal fasciae[16,30] (Figs. 65-5 and 65-6).

ANTERIOR PARARENAL SPACE

The anterior pararenal compartment is the most common site of extraperitoneal infection.[1] Most arise from primary lesions of the alimentary tract, especially the colon, extraperitoneal appendix, pancreas, and duodenum. The exudates originate from perforating malignan-

cies, inflammatory conditions, penetrating peptic ulcers, and accidental or iatrogenic trauma.[1,29] Collections are generally bounded unilaterally on the side of origin (Fig. 65-7).

Extraperitoneal perforation of the colon and appendix

Fig. 65-8 illustrates that extraperitoneal perforations of the colon can be identified as clearly localized to the anterior pararenal space. The extraperitoneal collection

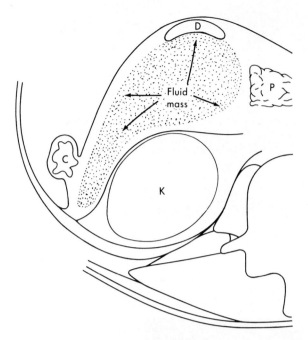

Fig. 65-7 Fluid collection in anterior pararenal space on right, with viscus displacement. *P,* Pancreas; *D,* duodenum; *C,* colon; *K,* kidney.
(Modified from Meyers, MA, et al: Radiology 104:249, 1972.)

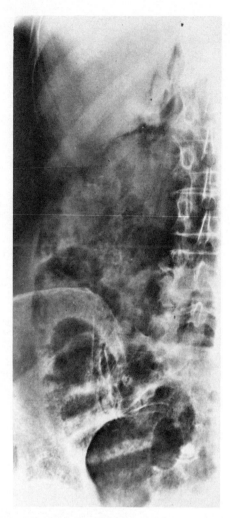

Fig. 65-8 Perforation of hepatic flexure. Mottled lucent areas on right represent collections of gas that extend medially over psoas muscle and approach spine. Flank stripe is intact. These changes localize extraperitoneal gas to anterior pararenal space.
(From Meyers, MA and Ghahremani, G: Radiology 115:301, 1975.)

of mottled gaseous lucencies is oriented with a general vertical axis, medially overlaps the psoas muscle and approaches the spine, and does not obscure the flank stripe laterally. In this patient, who developed fever after numerous scattered polyps were removed by colonoscopic cautery, the characteristic findings localize the site of perforation to the ascending colon.

The severe inflammatory changes or true abscess that may be associated with regional enteritis or ganulomatous enterocolitis resides within the anterior pararenal space. This explains anatomically the urologic complications of this disease.[37] The process commonly produces obstructive pressure on the ureter after it has emerged from the cone of renal fascia, typically at the L5 or lumbosacral level, producing hydronephrosis (Fig. 65-9). In adults similar changes may be caused by perforated carcinoma or diverticulitis of the colon (Fig. 65-10). In children, particularly, extraperitoneal appendicitis and its associated abscess within the anterior pararenal space may produce similar consequences.[37]

An ascending retrocecal position of the appendix is surprisingly common; its incidence ranges from 26% in surgical cases[5,6] to 65% in an autopsy series.[62] In this position the appendix may be intraperitoneal but is frequently extraperitoneal within the anterior pararenal space (Fig. 65-11). Many complications of appendicitis are related to anatomic variations in the position of the appendix, reflected clinically in the problem of differential diagnosis of acute appendiceal disease and lesions of the gallbladder, liver, right kidney, and base of the right lung or pleura. The radiologic features, however, constitute a characteristic pattern that permits precise localization and diagnosis.[37,40,42,43] Inflammation associated with an intraperitoneal ascending retrocecal appendix occurs in the right paracolic gutter and involves the lateral haustral row of the ascending colon (Fig. 65-12). In contrast, inflammation associated with an *extraperitoneal* ascending retrocecal appendix affects primarily the posterior haustral row (Fig. 65-13). The appendix itself may show definite abnormalities, including mass displacement, sinus tracts, and opacification of the abscess cavity.

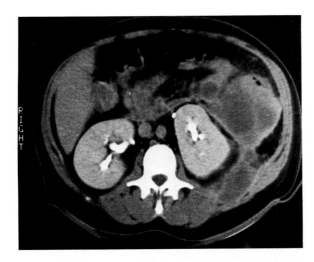

Fig. 65-21 Fluid collection arising from tail of pancreas within left anterior pararenal space continues to widen space between two leaves of posterior renal fascia. Perirenal space is grossly uninvolved.

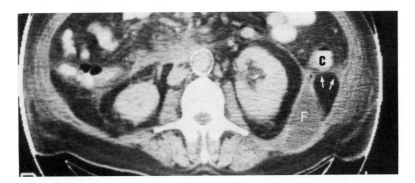

Fig. 65-22 Extension of pancreatitis to posterior abdominal wall. Accompanying thickening of renal fasciae and lateroconal fascia *(arrows)*, is a loculation of fluid *(F)* between leaves of posterior renal fascia immediately behind descending colon *(C)*.

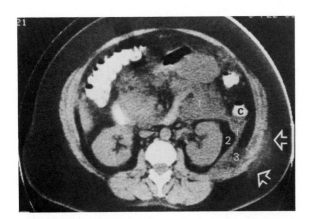

Fig. 65-23 Grey Turner's sign caused by pancreatitis. Extravasated pancreatic fluid in left anterior pararenal space *(1)* dissects between leaves of posterior renal fascia with loculated fluid collection *(f)* near descending colon *(c)*. Perirenal space *(2)* is maintained. Inflammatory changes have reached adjacent portion of posterior pararenal space *(3)* and subcutaneous tissues in left flank *(arrow)* at clinical site of discoloration.

topoulos and co-workers[51] have emphasized the typical appearance of this posterior extension of pancreatitis as a widening of the posterior renal fascia that tapers posteriorly, I have observed that variability in the origin of the division into two leaves accounts for the varied appearances of fluid accumulation in this plane (Fig. 65-22).

Posteriorly these collections at some axial level generally become contiguous with the lateral edge of the quadratus lumborum muscle. In the flank communication may be established to the posterior pararenal space and to the structures of the abdominal wall (Figs. 65-22 and 65-23). I have shown[41] that these pathways provide an anatomic-radiologic explanation for the classic clinical sign of subcutaneous discoloration in the costovertebral angle (Grey Turner's sign), which may be associated with acute pancreatitis.[8,61]

The liberated digestive enzymes of severe pancreatitis may dissect within fascial planes to result in an interesting extension to the posterior pararenal space from the an-

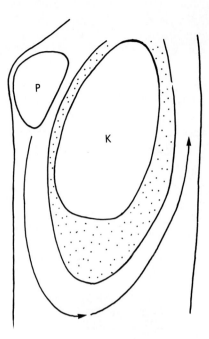

Fig. 65-24 One route of extension from anterior to posterior pararenal space. Parasagittal diagram illustrates spread from pancreas *(P)* around inferior border of perirenal space *(stippled area surrounding kidney, K)* into posterior pararenal compartment.
(From Meyers, MA: Semin Roentgenol 8:445, 1973.)

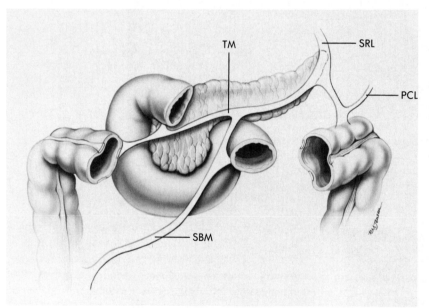

Fig. 65-25 Relationships of pancreas to transverse mesocolon *(TM)* and small bowel mesentery *(SBM)*. Splenorenal *(SRL)* and phrenicocolic *(PCL)* ligaments are shown.
(Modified from Meyers, MA, and Evans, JA: Am J Roentgenol 119:151, 1973.)

terior pararenal space without the contamination of the intervening perirenal compartment. This may be a consequence either of violation of the lateroconal fascia[27,37] or the process spreading from the pancreas down the anterior pararenal space and then rising posterior to the cone of renal fascia within the posterior pararenal space[33,41] (Fig. 65-24). The kidney and colon are pushed forward, and the psoas muscle and flank stripe are obliterated.

Despite the digestive effects of pancreatic fluid, the renal facia almost invariably is not transgressed, so that the perirenal fat and kidney retain their integrity. Indeed,

in acute pancreatitis, CT documentation of extrapancreatic fluid collections with perirenal spread and without renal involvement is rare.[4,15]

Many pancreatic processes may have a variety of effects on other segments of the alimentary tract, but it is their extension through the anterior extraperitoneal compartments that brings them into relationship with specific segments of the bowel. It has been established, for example, that localized changes on characteristic portions of the small intestine and colon are produced by the extravasated enzymes of pancreatitis, which follow definite anatomic planes.[37,38] The lesions range from tran-

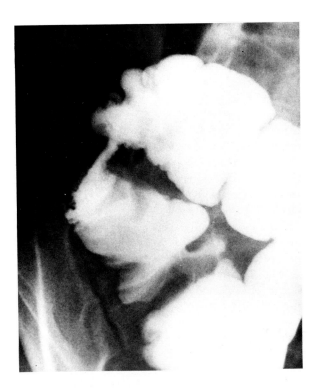

Fig. 65-26 Extrinsic stricture of distal ascending colon caused by acute suppurative pancreatitis. Barium enema demonstrates annular constricting lesion caused by fat necrosis from pancreatitis.
(From Meyers, MA, and Evans, JA: AJR 119:151, 1973. © 1973, American Roentgen Ray Society.)

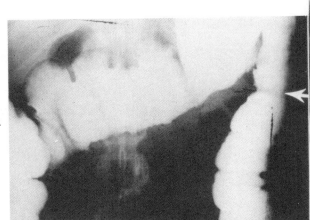

A

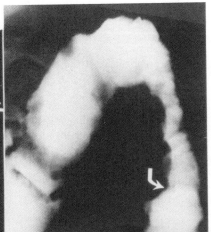

B

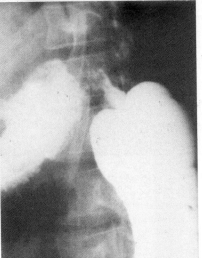

C

Fig. 65-27 Traumatic pancreatitis. **A,** Flattening of inferior haustal contour of transverse colon is typical evidence of extension from pancreas across anterior pararenal space and through leaves of transverse mesocolon. Pseudosacculations result on uninvolved superior border. Process ends abruptly at level of phrenicocolic ligament at anatomic splenic flexure of colon *(arrows).* **B,** Spot film documents scalloped narrowing of splenic flexure. Intramural lesions end precisely at level of phrenicocolic ligament *(arrow).* **C,** Three months later there is marked fibrotic stenosis of splenic flexure, reducing its lumen to diameter of less than 3 mm. Surgical resection of stricture, induced by fat necrosis, was required.
(From Meyers, MA, and Evans, JA: AJR 119:151, 1973.)

sient spasm to ischemic atrophy and, particularly with the effects of fat necrosis, the development of obstructive structures and remote exudative abscesses.

The mesenteric pathways that are most often involved and that direct the spread of pancreatic enzymes from the anterior pararenal space to remote sites in the intestinal tract are the transverse mesocolon and the small bowel mesentery[22,37] (Fig. 65-25). In this way spread reaches the transverse colon, duodenum, jejunal loops, and ileocecal region.

Although involvement of the hepatic flexure, as originally reported by Price[50] when he coined the term *colon cut-off sign,* is rare (Fig. 65-26), the anatomic splenic flexure is the single most common colonic site involved.[37] This is caused by the natural drainage from the tail of the pancreas into the phrenicocolic ligament.[12,32,37] Barium enema study may show narrowing with irregular nodular or serrated margins and distorted mucosal folds from the extramural inflammatory infiltrate. The process characteristically stops abruptly at the level of the anatomic splenic flexure.[37,38] Occasionally a significant degree of retrograde obstruction may be met. A granulomatous and fibrotic reaction may then result in a stricture of the splenic flexure (Fig. 65-27). If the inflammatory

process erodes through the wall of the colon at this site, extraperitoneal sinus tracts or fistulas to adherent small bowel loops may be demonstrated (Fig. 65-28). Extraperitoneal dissection inferiorly may result in pseudocyst formation within the anterior pararenal space and occasionally may progress inferiorly to the pelvis or even as far as the groin[33,34,54] (Fig. 65-29).

In a similar manner the inflammatory process associated with extravasated pancreatic enzymes may disseminate along the root of the small bowel mesentery, either for a portion or for its entire length. Compression of the third portion of the duodenum may result from an indurated mesenteric root. This typically occurs in its mid portion, which may appear sharply cut off (Fig. 65-30) with dilatation and stasis proximally. Such a mechanical process undoubtedly accounts for many instances of the duodenal "ileus" seen in acute pancreatitis. As the enzymes progress farther down the root of the mesentery, jejunitis may be evident (Fig. 65-31). Chronic recurrent pancreatitis may be the cause of some cases of malabsorption by virtue of ischemic effects with mucosal atrophy.[37,38] If the process extends the full length of the root of the small bowel mesentery, an exudative abscess or a type of pseudocyst may develop in the ileocecal

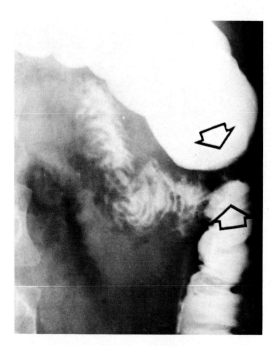

Fig. 65-28 Acute suppurative pancreatitis. Extravasated enzymes within phrenicocolic ligament have resulted in fistulization from narrowed anatomic splenic flexure *(arrows)* to small bowel loop and long extraperitoneal sinus tract.
(From Meyers, MA: Radiology 95:539, 1970.)

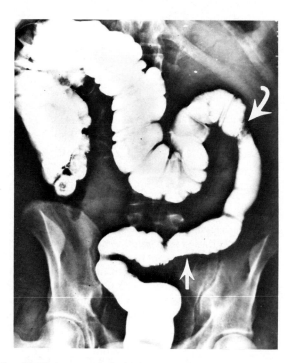

Fig. 65-29 Acute pancreatitis. Pseudocyst formation in tail of pancreas depresses distal transverse colon. In addition, extravasated enzymes within phrenicocolic ligament result in localized narrowing of anatomic splenic flexure *(curved arrow).* Inferior extension extraperitoneally on left is revealed by compression of sigmoid colon *(arrow).*
(Courtesy Dr. Jack Farman.)

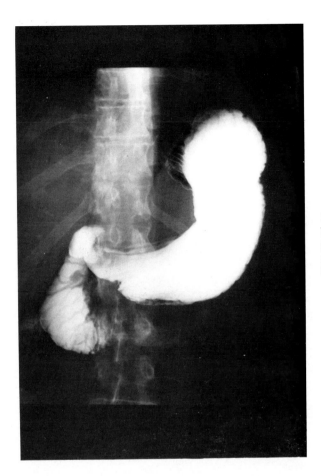

Fig. 65-30 Obstruction of mid portion of transverse duodenum by pancreatitis extending down mesenteric root. Associated finding is enlargement of Vater's ampulla.
(From Meyers, MA, and Evans, JA: AJR 119:151, 1973. © 1973, American Roentgen Ray Society.)

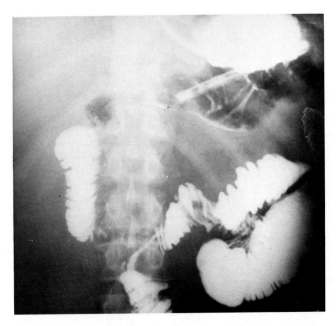

Fig. 65-31 Jejunitis caused by acute pancreatitis. Besides displacement and mucosal changes in duodenal loop, evidence of extension of pancreatic enzymes into small bowel mesentery is shown by their effects on proximal jejunal loops. These demonstrate mucosal edema and sites of spastic narrowing with proximal dilatation.

area.[37,38] This process explains the misleading presentation of acute appendicitis with peritoneal signs localized predominantly in the right lower quadrant in some cases of fulminating acute pancreatitis.

PERIRENAL SPACE

Many patients with renal disease have symptoms that seem to arise from the digestive tract. Clinical investigation is thus often initiated with barium contrast studies. Characteristic effects on specific portions of the bowel may uncover the primary site, redirect the course of evaluation, or document the extent of disease.*

Renointestinal anatomic relationships
Right kidney

The right kidney is in intimate relationship to two segments of the GI tract—the descending duodenum and the hepatic flexure of the colon (Figs. 65-32 and 65-33):

---

*References 34, 36, 37, 39, 42, 43, 44.

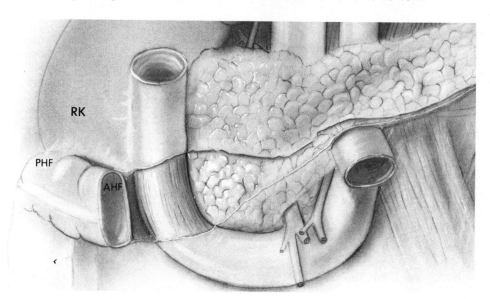

Fig. 65-32 Anatomic relationships of right kidney *(RK)* to descending duodenum and to colon, including posterior *(PHF)* and anterior *(AHF)* hepatic flexures. Root of transverse mesocolon begins at anterior hepatic flexure and extends across descending duodenum and pancreas.
(Modified from Meyers, MA, and Whalen, JP: AJR 117:263, 1973. © 1973, American Roentgen Ray Society.)

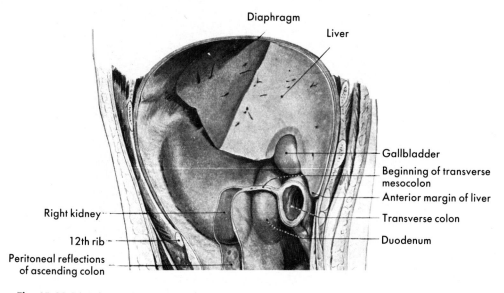

Fig. 65-33 Right parasagittal drawing showing anatomic relationships of right kidney.
(From Meyers, MA: AJR 123:386, 1975. © 1975, American Roentgen Ray Society.)

1. Beyond its postapical segment, the second portion of the duodenum descends immediately in front of the right kidney.

2. The colon courses obliquely over the lower pole of the kidney, precisely at its level between the posterior hepatic flexure, which is related superiorly to the deep inferior visceral surface of the liver, and the anterior hepatic flexure, which is related superiorly to the gallbladder. The lower renal pole is inframesocolic and related laterally and anteriorly to the distal ascending colon.

Left kidney

The relationships of the left kidney to the bowel are most intimate to the distal transverse and proximal descending colon (Fig. 65-34). The former is related to the anterior surface of the lower half of the kidney at variable distances, depending on the length of the transverse mesocolon. The lower pole is fully inframesocolic. The extraperitoneal descending colon passes downward along the lateral border of the left kidney, turning somewhat medially toward the psoas muscle.

Radiologic features

Characteristic mass displacements

Right renal masses typically cause medial and anterior displacement of the descending duodenum, whereas the immediate postapical segment tends to be unaffected (Fig. 65-35). In right lateral projections the anterior displacement may result in a gentle axis inferiorly and anteriorly or in a more striking ventral bowing (Fig. 65-36). The right colon segment most typically involved is that extending between the posterior and anterior flexures. This demonstrates displacement inferiorly, medially, and anteriorly (Fig. 65-37). A mass originating in

the lower pole, however, characteristically elevates the colon between the two hepatic flexures (Fig. 65-38).

Left renal masses arising in the upper half may displace the distal transverse colon inferiorly and anteriorly. Those originating in the lower half are often first revealed by typical compression and lateral and anterior displacement of the descending limb of the distal transverse colon (Fig. 65-39). Masses projecting from the lower pole displace the descending colon laterally and anteriorly (Fig. 65-40). The anatomic splenic flexure tends to be unaffected.

Invasive hypernephroma

Renal neoplasms may invade adjacent segments of bowel directly, occasionally as recurrences many years after resection of the primary tumor. They tend to produce bulky intraluminal masses without significant obstruction, because they generally elicit no desmoplastic response.[37-39] Recognition of the usual sites of involvement and identification of any extraluminal soft tissue mass leads to the correct diagnosis. On the right the descending duodenum (Fig. 65-41) and on the left the distal transverse colon or proximal descending colon (Fig. 65-42) are most often involved. Even on other sides, the characteristic findings remain evident (Fig. 65-43).

Perinephritis and renointestinal fistulas

Advanced perirenal infection may break through fascial boundaries to involve overlying bowel.[34-37] The pathogenesis involves a site of renal infection that breaks through the capsule of the kidney to contaminate the perirenal space, either diffusely or as a localized abscess, which most commonly coalesces dorsolateral to the lower renal pole.[33,37,41] Fulminating infection may then reach

Text continued on p. 1658.

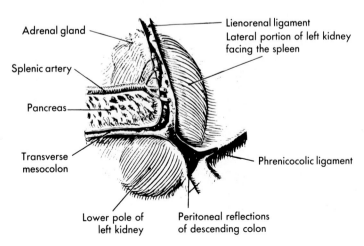

Adrenal gland

Splenic artery

Pancreas

Transverse mesocolon

Lower pole of left kidney

Lienorenal ligament
Lateral portion of left kidney facing the spleen

Phrenicocolic ligament

Peritoneal reflections of descending colon

Fig. 65-34 Frontal drawing emphasizing relationship of left kidney to colon by virtue of their peritoneal reflections.
(From Meyers, MA: AJR 123:386, 1975. © 1975, American Roentgen Ray Society.)

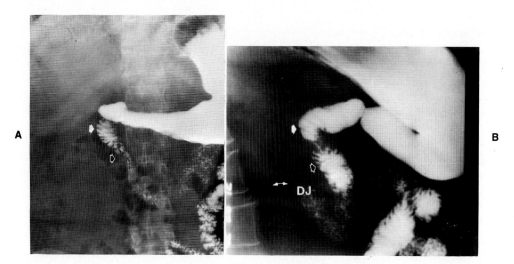

Fig. 65-35 Displacement of descending duodenum by right renal cyst. Frontal, **A,** and right lateral, **B,** views. Postapical portion of duodenum descends normally *(closed arrows),* but there is medial and anterior deflection of distal two thirds *(open arrows).* Descending duodenum projects anterior to duodenojejunal junction *(DJ, double arrow).* In **A,** note that renal mass also causes elevation of hepatic flexure of colon.

(From Meyers, MA: AJR 123:386, 1975. © 1975, American Roentgen Ray Society.)

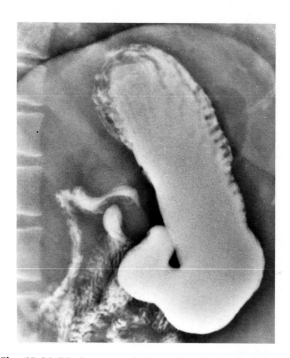

Fig. 65-36 Displacement of descending duodenum by right renal cyst. Bowed anterior displacement of second portion of duodenum.

(From Meyers, MA: AJR 123:386, 1975. © 1975, American Roentgen Ray Society.)

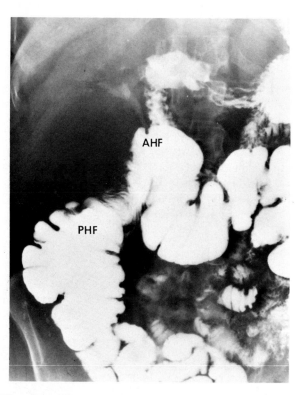

Fig. 65-37 Displacement of right colon by right renal cyst. Large intestine between posterior *(PHF)* and anterior *(AHF)* hepatic flexures is displaced inferiorly and medially, with extrinsic compression on its superior haustral row. Posterior flexure is mildly displaced downward as mass, originating in middle third of kidney, extends laterally into flank. Note that there is no displacement of descending duodenum.

(From Meyers, MA: AJR 123:386, 1975. © 1975, American Roentgen Ray Society.)

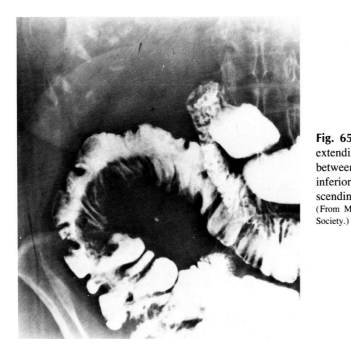

Fig. 65-38 Displacement of right colon by right renal cyst extending from lower pole. Superior displacement of segment between two hepatic flexures, with extrinsic compression of its inferior haustral row. Mass also affects ascending colon. Descending duodenum is uninvolved.
(From Meyers, MA: AJR 123:386, 1975. © 1975, American Roentgen Ray Society.)

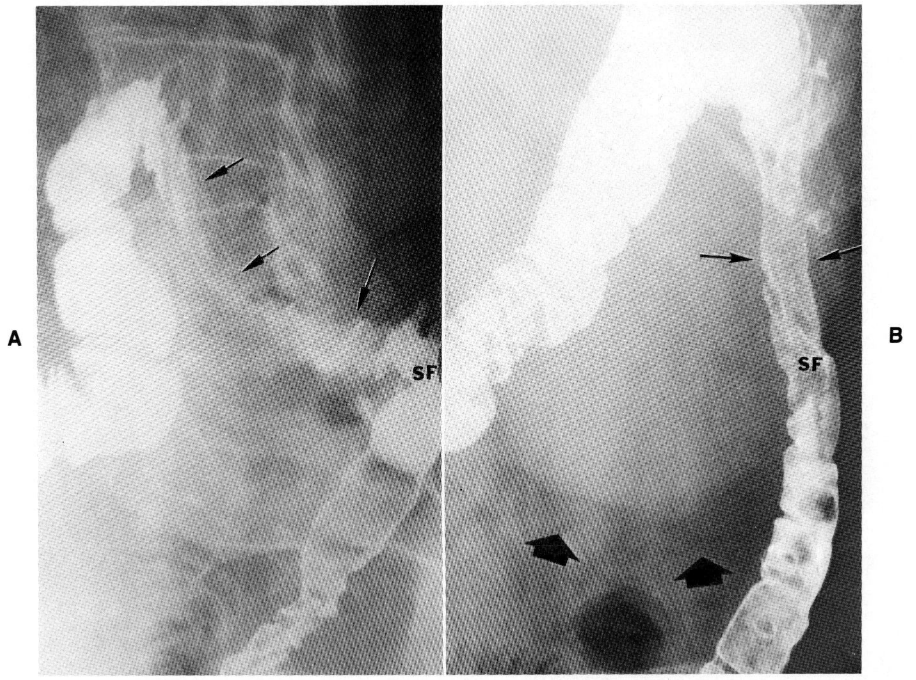

Fig. 65-39 Displacement of left colon by left renal cyst. **A,** Anatomic splenic flexure *(SF)* is maintained, but there is lateral and anterior displacement of descending limb of distal transverse colon *(arrows)*. **B,** Anteroposterior compression of its lumen is indicated also on frontal view. Mass enlargement of lower pole of kidney is identifiable *(large arrows)*.
(From Meyers, MA: AJR 123:386, 1975. © 1975, American Roentgen Ray Society.)

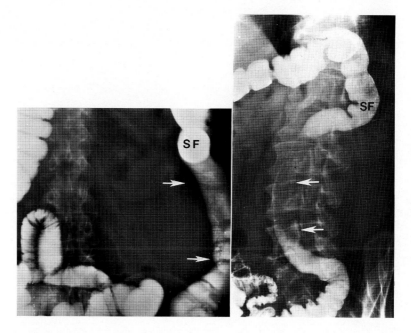

Fig. 65-40 Displacement of left colon by left renal cyst. Descending colon is displaced laterally and anteriorly *(arrows)* by large cyst originating from lower renal pole. Anatomic splenic flexure *(SF)* is unaffected.
(From Meyers, MA: AJR 123:386, 1975. © 1975, American Roentgen Ray Society.)

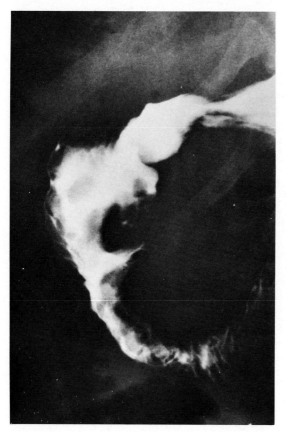

Fig. 65-41 Direct invasion of descending duodenum by right hypernephroma. There are multiple bulky intraluminal masses without fibrotic angulation of duodenum.
(Courtesy Dr. Emil Balthazar.)

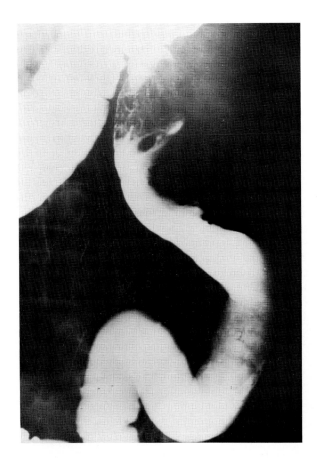

Fig. 65-42 Direct invasion of colon by left renal carcinoma. This produces extrinsic and intramural masses of distal transverse and proximal descending colon with bulky polypoid intraluminal extensions.
(From Meyers, MA, and McSweeney, J: Radiology 105:1, 1972.)

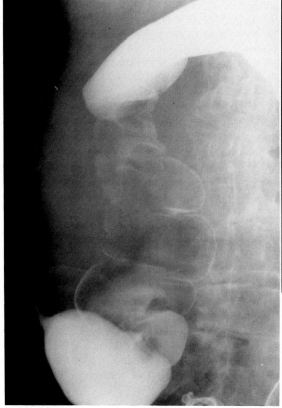

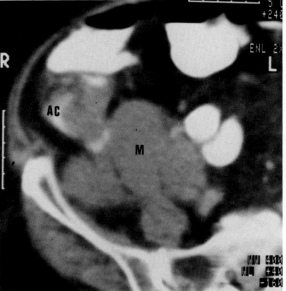

Fig. 65-43 Right hypernephroma invading ascending colon. Barium enema **(A)** and CT scan **(B)** show large lobulated tumor mass *(M)* extending inferiorly from region of right kidney, where it displaces and invades ascending colon *(AC)*.
(Courtesy Dr. Michiel Feldberg, Utrecht, Netherlands.)

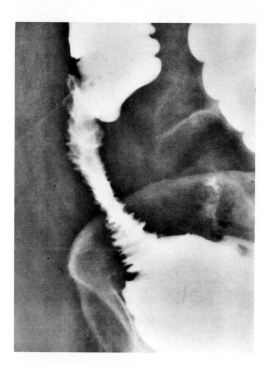

Fig. 65-44 Colonic changes caused by right perinephritis. Barium enema study shows mass displacement and inflammatory mucosal thickening of ascending colon. These changes are caused by perirenal abscess complicating xanthogranulomatous pyelonephritis.
(From Meyers, MA: Dynamic radiology of the abdomen: normal and pathologic anatomy, New York, 1976, Springer-Verlag.)

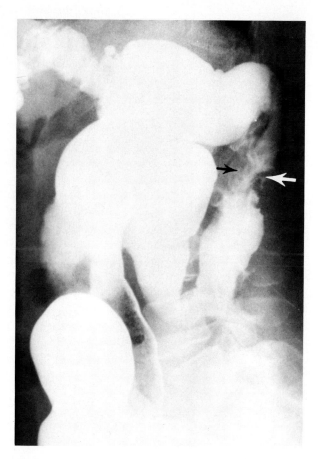

Fig. 65-45 Colonic changes caused by left perinephritis. Lateral radiograph of barium enema study demonstrates persistent irregular narrowing *(arrows)* with intact mucosal folds just distal to splenic flexure. These changes are caused by perirenal abscesses that are adherent to descending colon.
(From Meyers, MA: Radiology 111:525, 1974.)

typical segments of the large intestine. Changes reflecting at least inflammatory adherence may affect principally the medial or posterior contour of the colon or may be circumferential. They are manifested primarily by spastic narrowing, scalloped induration, and inflammatory mucosal thickening (Fig. 65-44 and 65-45).

A gross extraperitoneal sinus collection represents advanced transmural erosion. Most renointestinal fistulas are caused by an underlying chronic pyelonephritis and stone disease that establishes communication usually with the descending duodenum or left colon.[3]

Renal agenesis and ectopia

Agenesis or ectopia of the kidney is frequently accompanied by characteristic malposition of specific portions of the bowel.[31,44] Particular segments of the intestine may occupy the area of the renal fossa on the side of agenesis or ectopia or show characteristic displacement and extrinsic mass effect by an ectopic kidney in as many as 75% of the cases.[44] Identification of the characteristic changes on plain films or on an initial barium contrast study uncovers the renal anomaly, which may have multiple clinical implications. The incidence of renal disease

in a congenitally solitary kidney as a cause of death is high.[2,9] In an ectopic kidney the incidence of complications such as lithiasis, infection, and hydronephrosis approaches 50%.[13] Furthermore, anomalies of structures arising from the urogenital ridge are associated with these renal conditions in as many as 18.5% of cases.[2,9,13]

On the right side the descending duodenum may be abnormally positioned posteriorly, projecting well over the lumbar spine in the lateral view. Proximal jejunal loops may also occupy a similar position, filling in the renal fossa and coursing abnormally posteriorly (Fig. 65-46). These bowel changes can be easily distinguished from a right paraduodenal hernia.[31]

On the left side there may be striking posteromedial malposition of the distal transverse colon and anatomic splenic flexure into the "empty" renal fossa area (Fig. 65-47). In these instances the descending colon is normally positioned, a distinguishing feature from a de-

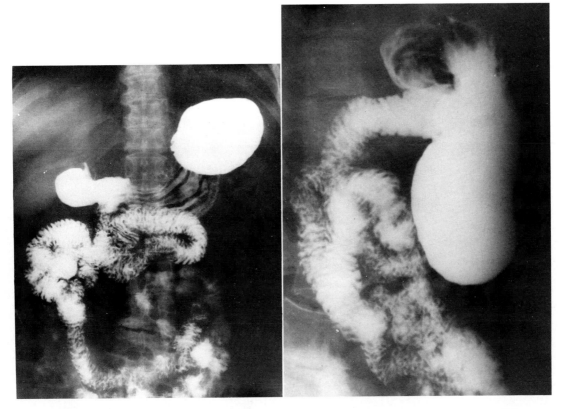

Fig. 65-46 Right renal agenesis with intestinal malposition. Upper GI series demonstrates striking posterior malposition of descending duodenum and proximal jejunal loops in right flank region, simulating some features of right paraduodenal hernia.
(From Meyers, MA, et al: AJR 117:323, 1973. © 1973, American Roentgen Ray Society.)

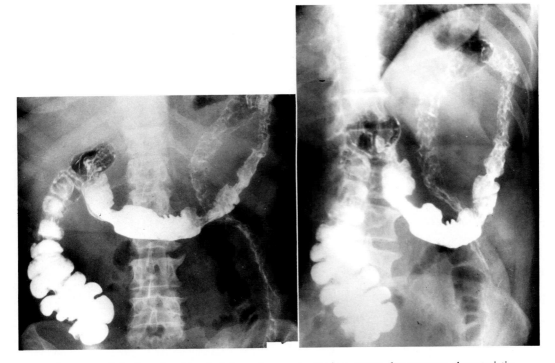

Fig. 65-47 Colonic malposition in left renal agenesis. Barium enema demonstrates characteristic medial and posterior malposition of distal transverse colon and anatomic splenic flexure into area of left renal bed.
(From Meyers, MA, et al: AJR 117:323, 1973. © 1973, American Roentgen Ray Society.)

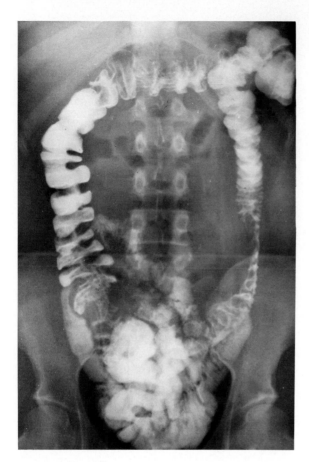

Fig. 65-48 Ectopic kidney in 24-year-old woman with left lower quadrant mass. Barium enema examination demonstrates extrinsic mass impression on medial aspect of lower descending colon, produced by ectopic left kidney. Note also that anatomic splenic flexure is sharply angulated into "empty" renal fossa, further confirming that LLQ mass is ectopic kidney.
(From Meyers, MA, et al: AJR 117:323, 1973. © 1973, American Roentgen Ray Society.)

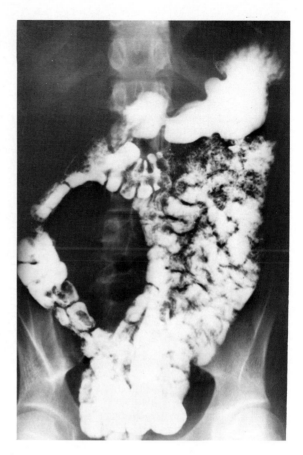

Fig. 65-49 Ectopic kidney. Small bowel series. Inframesocolic mass displacement of small bowel and colon in right lower quadrant. Note reniform contour of mass displacement.
(From Meyers, MA, et al: AJR 117:323, 1973. © 1973, American Roentgen Ray Society.)

scending colon on a mesentery and other normal variants.

These changes in intestinal position have not been seen after acquired atrophy of the kidney. However, similar angulated malposition of the hepatic or splenic flexure of the colon may be noted after anterior nephrectomies.[37]

In renal ectopia not only may the "empty" renal fossa occur, but there is often direct mass effect by the ectopic kidney itself—most typically the medial borders of the ascending or descending colon (Fig. 65-48) and small bowel loop (Fig. 65-49).[37,39]

POSTERIOR PARARENAL SPACE

Because the posterior pararenal space contains no major organs from which disease processes may directly arise, collections solely limited to this compartment originate by other mechanisms.[7] It is a common site of spontaneous retroperitoneal hemorrhage in conditions such as bleeding diathesis, overanticoagulation, and hemorrhage from trauma (including stab wounds and fractures of the ribs or vertebrae).[37]

Ruptured abdominal aorta or infected graft

Bleeding from a ruptured abdominal aortic aneurysm or infection complicating an aortic graft frequently extends to this compartment.[23,28,37] The distinctive complex of findings is evaluated easily (Fig. 65-50). Although these conditions may be strongly suspected on plain films (Fig. 65-51),[25,46] their presence and extent are clearly demonstrable by CT (Figs. 65-52 and 65-53). Aneurysms also rupture first into the psoas muscle and then into the posterior pararenal space.[20] Infection localized to this space is also encountered occasionally as a complication of bowel surgery with fascial transgression.[37]

Perforation of the rectum or sigmoid colon

Extravasates originating in the pelvis, as in perforation of the rectum or sigmoid colon, may spread upward into this compartment. Because the rectum is subperitoneal

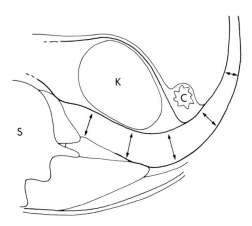

Fig. 65-50 Fluid collection in posterior pararenal space on left, with viscus displacement. There is direct extension into properitoneal fat. *K,* Kidney; *C,* colon; *S,* spine.
(From Meyers, MA, et al: Radiology 104:249, 1972.)

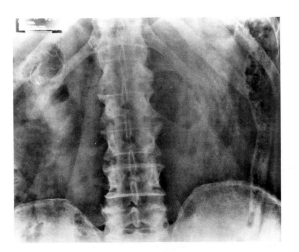

Fig. 65-51 Ruptured aneurysm of abdominal aorta. Plain film demonstrates streaky radiolucent lines on left in area of ill-defined mass that also causes loss of visualization of psoas muscle border. These changes are caused by blood dissecting, often in sheets, through posterior pararenal fat.
(Courtesy Dr. John Williams.)

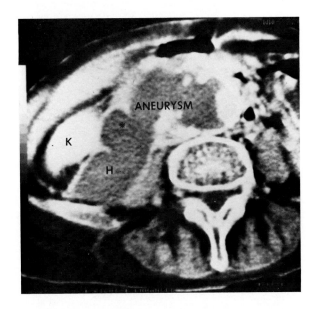

Fig. 65-52 Posterior pararenal hemorrhage from ruptured aneurysm of abdominal aorta. CT demonstrates hemorrhage *(H)* localizing in posterior pararenal space behind kidney *(K).* Slice level shows precisely the site of leakage *(asterisk)* from large calcified aneurysm.
(Courtesy Dr. Michael Oliphant.)

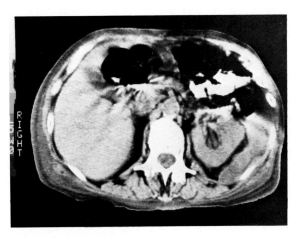

Fig. 65-53 Left posterior pararenal abscess caused by infected aortic graft. Perirenal space is spared.
(Courtesy Dr. Patrick Freeny.)

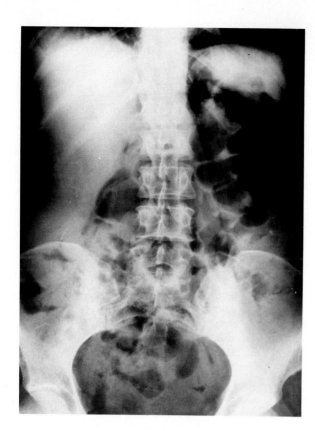

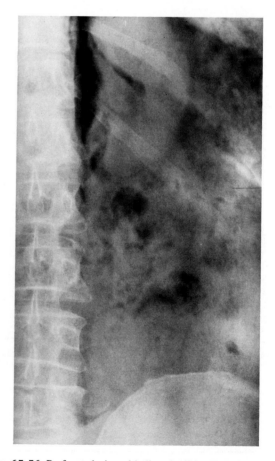

Fig. 65-54 Rectal perforation. Extraperitoneal gas parallels lateral borders of psoas muscles and outlines upper pole of left kidney, adrenal gland, medial border of spleen, medial crus of diaphragm, and immediate subphrenic tissues. These findings localize gas to posterior pararenal compartment.
(From Myers, MA: Radiology 111:17, 1974.)

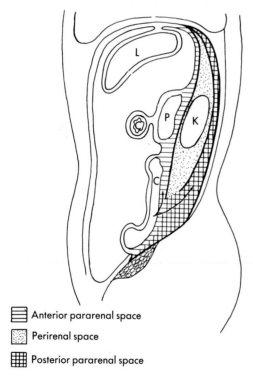

▤ Anterior pararenal space

▦ Perirenal space

▩ Posterior pararenal space

Fig. 65-55 Relationships and structures of three extraperitoneal spaces on left. Sigmoid colon is in continuity with anterior and posterior pararenal compartments. *L,* Liver; *P,* pancreas; *K,* kidney; *C,* colon.
(Modified from Meyers, MA: Semin Roentgenol 8:445, 1973.)

Fig. 65-56 Perforated sigmoid diverticulitis. Extraperitoneal gas extends anterior to psoas muscle toward spine within anterior pararenal space. Superiorly gas extends within posterior pararenal space outlining adrenal gland, posteromedial border of spleen, and medial crus of diaphragm.
(From Meyers, MA: Radiology 111:17, 1974.)

and lies in the midline, gas that escapes from its lumen rises up both sides within the extraperitoneal tissues, with preferential spread into the posterior compartments.[35,37] The gas may then parallel the lateral contour of the psoas muscles, outlining the suprarenal and subdiaphragmatic tissues (Fig. 65-54).

Since the sigmoid colon lies below the limits of the cone of renal fascia and is in anatomic continuity with both the anterior and posterior pararenal spaces (Fig. 65-55), gas from a perforation may enter one or both compartments. The gas may extend medially over the psoas muscle in the form of mottled radiolucencies, but extension into the posterior compartment often dominates the radiologic findings (Fig. 65-56).

The gas may enter the properitoneal flank fat directly but superiorly is characterized by its outlining of the adrenal gland and upper renal pole, the medial crus of the diaphram, and the extraperitoneal subdiaphragmatic plane. Only if the sigmoid perforation occurs between the leaves of the mesocolon does the extraperitoneal gas rise bilaterally within the anterior pararenal spaces.[35,37]

REFERENCES

1. Altemeier, WA, and Alexander, JW: Retroperitoneal abscess, Arch Surg 83:512, 1961.
2. Ashley, DJ, and Mostofi, FK: Renal agenesis and dysgenesis, J Urol 83:211, 1960.
3. Bissada, NK, Cole, AT, and Fried, FA: Renoalimentary fistula: unusual urological problem, J Urol 110:273, 1973.
4. Casolo, F, Bianco, R, and Franceschelli, N: Perirenal fluid collection complicating chronic pancreatitis: CT demonstration, Gastrointest Radiol 12:117, 1987.
5. Chintapalli, K, et al: Renal fascial thickening in pancreatitis, J Comput Assist Tomogr 6:983, 1982.
6. Collins, DC: 71,000 human appendix specimens: a final report summarizing forty years' study, Am J Proctol 14:365, 1963.
7. Cullen, TS: A new sign in ruptured extrauterine pregnancy, Am J Obstet 78:457, 1918.
8. Dickson, AP, and Imrie, CW: The incidence and prognosis of body wall ecchymosis in acute pancreatitis, Surg Gynecol Obstet 159:343, 1984.
9. Doroshow, L, and Abeshouse, BS: Congenital unilateral solitary kidney: report of 37 cases and review of the literature, Urol Surg 11:219, 1961.
10. Editorial: Periureteric fibrosis, Lancet 2:780, 1957.
11. Elkin, M, and Cohen, G: Diagnostic value of the psoas shadow, Clin Radiol 13:210, 1962.
12. Fallis, LS: Cullen's sign in acute pancreatitis, Ann Surg 106:54, 1937.
13. Farman, F: Anomalies of the kidneys. In Alken, CE, editor: Handbuch der Urology, vol 7, Malformations, Berlin, 1968, Springer-Verlag.
14. Feldberg, MAM: Computed tomography of the retroperitoneum: an anatomical and pathological atlas with emphasis on the fascial planes, Boston, 1983, Martinus Nijhoff Publishers.
15. Feldberg, MAM, et al: Pancreatic lesions and transfascial perirenal spread: computed tomographic demonstration, Gastrointest Radiol 12:121, 1987.
16. Feurstein, IM, et al: Perirenal cobwebs: the expanding CT differential diagnosis, J Comput Assist Tomogr 8:1128, 1984.
17. Glazer, GM, et al: CT detection of duodenal perforation, AJR 137:333, 1981.
18. Griffin, JF, Sekiya, T, and Isherwood, I: Computed tomography of pararenal fluid collections in acute pancreatitis, Clin Radiol 35:181, 1984.
19. Hadar, H, and Meiraz, D: Thickened renal fascia: a sign of retroperitoneal pathology, J Comput Assist Tomogr 5:193, 1981.
20. Hopper, KD, Sherman, JL, and Ghaed, N: Aortic rupture into retroperitoneum (letter), AJR 145:435, 1985.
21. Hopper, KD, et al: The retrorenal colon in the supine and prone patient, Radiology 162:443, 1987.
22. Jeffrey, RB, Federle, MP, and Laing, FC: Computed tomography of mesenteric involvement of fulminant pancreatitis, Radiology 147:185, 1983.
23. Kam, J, Patel, S, and Ward, RE: Computed tomography of aortic and aortoiliofemoral grafts, J Comput Assist Tomogr 6:298, 1982.
24. Kunin, M: Bridging septa of the perinephric space: anatomic, pathologic and diagnostic considerations, Radiology 158:361, 1986.
25. Loughran, CF: A review of the plain abdominal radiography in acute rupture of abdominal aortic aneurysms, Clin Radiol 37:383, 1986.
26. Love, L, Demos, TC, and Posniak, H: CT of retrorenal fluid collections, AJR 145:87, 1985.
27. Love, L, et al: Computed tomography of the extraperitoneal spaces, AJR 136:781, 1981.
28. Mark, A, et al: CT evaluation of complications of abdominal aortic surgery, Radiology 145:409, 1982.
29. McCort, J: Anterior pararenal-space infection, Mt Sinai J Med 51:482, 1984.
30. McLennan, BL, Lee, JKT, and Peterson, RR: Anatomy of the perirenal area, Radiology 158:555, 1986.
31. Meyers, MA: Paraduodenal hernias: radiologic and arteriographic diagnosis, Radiology 95:29, 1970.
32. Meyers, MA: Roentgen significance of the phrenicocolic ligament, Radiology 95:539, 1970.
33. Meyers, MA: Acute extraperitoneal infection, Semin Roentgenol 8:445, 1973.
34. Meyers, MA: Colonic changes secondary to left perinephritis: new observations, Radiology 111:525, 1974.
35. Meyers, MA: Radiologic features of the spread and localization of extraperitoneal gas and their relationship to its source: an anatomical approach, Radiology 111:17, 1974.
36. Meyers, MA: The reno-alimentary relationships: anatomic-reontgen study of their clinical significance, AJR 123:386, 1975.
37. Meyers, MA: Dynamic radiology of the abdomen: normal and pathologic anatomy, ed 2, New York, 1982, Springer-Verlag.
38. Meyers, MA, and Evans, JA: Effects of pancreatitis on the small bowel and colon: spread along mesenteric planes, AJR 119:151, 1973.
39. Meyers, MA, and McSweeney, J: Secondary neoplasms of bowel, Radiology 105:1, 1972.
40. Meyers, MA, and Oliphant, M: Ascending retrocecal appendicitis, Radiology 110:293, 1974.
41. Meyers, MA, et al: Radiologic features of extraperitoneal effusions: an anatomic approach, Radiology 104:249, 1972.
42. Meyers, MA, et al: Haustral anatomy and pathology: a new look. I. Roentgen identification of normal patterns and relationships, Radiology 108:497, 1973.
43. Meyers, MA, et al: Haustral anatomy and pathology: a new look. II. Roentgen interpretation of pathologic alterations, Radiology 108:505, 1973.
44. Meyers, MA, et al: Malposition and displacement of bowel in renal agenesis and ectopia: new observations, AJR 117:323, 1973.
45. Meyers, MA, et al: The peritoneal ligaments and mesenteries: pathways of intra-abdominal spread of disease, Radiology 163:593, 1987.

46. Nichols, GB, and Schilling, PJ: Pseudo-retroperitoneal gas in rupture of aneurysm of abdominal aorta, AJR 125:134, 1975.

47. Nicholson, RL: Abnormalities of the perinephric fascia and fat in pancreatitis, Radiology 139:125, 1981.

48. Parienty, RA, and Pradel, J: Radiological evaluation of the peri- and pararenal spaces by computed tomography, Crit Rev Diagn Imaging 20:1, 1983.

49. Parienty, RA, et al: Visibility and thickening of the renal fascia on computed tomograms, Radiology 139:119, 1981.

50. Price, CWR: "Colon cut-off sign" in acute pancreatitis, Med J Aust 1:313, 1956.

51. Raptopoulos, V, et al: Renal fascial pathway: posterior extension of pancreatic effusions within the anterior pararenal space, Radiology 158:367, 1986.

52. Roman, E, Silva, Y, and Lucas, C: Management of blunt duodenal injury, Surg Gynecol Obstet 132:7, 1971.

53. Rubenstein, WA, et al: Posterior peritoneal recesses: assessment using CT, Radiology 156:461, 1985.

54. Salvo, AF, and Nematolahi, H: Distant dissection of a pancreatic pseudocyst into the right groin, Am J Surg 126:430, 1973.

55. Sherman, JL, et al: The retrorenal colon on computed tomography: a normal variant, J Comput Assist Tomogr 9:339, 1985.

56. Siegelman, SS, et al: CT on fluid collections associated with pancreatitis, AJR 134:1121, 1980.

57. Skarby, HG: Beitrage 2ur Diagnostic der Paranephritiden mit Besonderer Berucksichtigung des Rontgenver Fahrens, Acta Radiol Suppl 62:1, 1946.

58. Stevenson, EO, and Ozeran, RS: Retroperitoneal space abscesses, Surg Gynecol Obstet 128:1202, 1969.

59. Susman, N, Hammerman, AM, and Cohen, E: The renal halo sign in pancreatitis, Radiology 142:323, 1982.

60. Toxopeus, MD, Lucas, CE, and Krabbenhoft, KL: Roentgenographic diagnosis in blunt retroperitoneal duodenal rupture, AJR 115:281, 1972.

61. Turner, GG: Local discoloration of the abdominal wall as a sign of acute pancreatitis, Br J Surg 7:394, 1919.

62. Wakely, CPG: The position of the vermiform appendix as ascertained by an analysis of 10,000 cases, J Anat 67:277, 1933.

63. Williams, SM, et al: The psoas sign: a reevaluation, Radiography 5:525, 1985.

66 *Ultrasonography*

SERGIO A. AJZEN
GREGORY J. ALLEN
PETER L. COOPERBERG

GENERAL CONSIDERATIONS

Before the advent of the newer imaging techniques, the retroperitoneum was one of the most difficult areas of the body to evaluate. Moreover, signs and symptoms of retroperitoneal diseases are frequently vague and poorly localized.[47] Whalen[88] and Meyers[65] added considerably to our understanding of retroperitoneal abnormalities as they appear on plain and contrast opacified gastrointestinal (GI) and genitourinary tract radiographs. Nonetheless, these concepts are difficult to appreciate, and the ability to produce cross-sectional images with ultrasound and computed tomography (CT) has facilitated the demonstration of retroperitoneal anatomy and pathologic conditions. Although ultrasound has proved particularly useful in the evaluation of the retroperitoneal spaces, the scattering effect of peritoneal fat and the inability to penetrate bowel gas and bone are major drawbacks. If the patient is relatively large, small masses may be difficult to visualize with ultrasound. Whereas larger masses or fluid collections may be identified, one cannot confidently exclude small retroperitoneal masses. It is not helpful to direct ultrasound through the posterior aspect of the patient, since well-developed paraspinal muscles, ribs, spine, and bony pelvis prevent penetration of the ultrasound beam. These problems do not affect visualization of the retroperitoneum by CT, which therefore has a higher success rate in visualizing the retroperitoneal structures. Nonetheless, retroperitoneal abnormalities frequently attain a large enough volume that they may be demonstrated by the more economical and less invasive ultrasound approach. CT can then be reserved for patients in whom ultrasound cannot provide adequate images or for the exclusion of small masses when the ultrasound study has demonstrated no abnormality.

Normal anatomy

The retroperitoneum is an intraabdominal compartment dorsal to the parietal peritoneum that extends from the diaphragm to the pelvis. It is bounded anteriorly by the liver and spleen, the luminal GI tract, and the bladder in the pelvis. It is bounded posteriorly by the spine, ribs, bony pelvis, and erector spinae and quadratus lumborum muscles. The normal organs contained in the retroperitoneal space include the kidneys, adrenal glands, pancreas, great vessels of the abdomen, and portions of the duodenum and colon. The sympathetic chain, autonomic plexus, somatic nerves, and lymph nodes are also present in variable amounts of fat in the retroperitoneum.

The retroperitoneal space can be further subdivided by the perirenal (Gerota's) fascia into the anterior pararenal space, the perirenal space, and the posterior pararenal space. The anterior pararenal space contains the aorta, vena cava, and pancreas. This space is also continuous through the mesentery with the alimentary tract. The perirenal space includes the kidneys and adrenal glands. The posterior pararenal space contains no organs.

A common misconception is that the retroperitoneum is a deep posterior space. However, the retroperitoneum passes over the spine anteriorly and in thin individuals may be just deep to the anterior abdominal wall. The lower pole of either kidney may be easily palpated in a thin patient, despite its retroperitoneal location. Most important, masses arising from the retroperitoneum may initially be easily palpable structures, even in large patients, thus confusing clinicians about their origin.

Generally, when abdominal retroperitoneal masses are large, it can be difficult to identify their retroperitoneal origin by ultrasound or even by CT. Usually the only ultrasonographic evidence to indicate that a lesion arises in the retroperitoneum is anterior displacement of known retroperitoneal structures. With CT scanning the fascial planes of the retroperitoneum may be well delineated by fat, and lesions, especially smaller ones, may then be clearly seen to lie behind the parietal peritoneum. Not infrequently one can even specify which of the three retroperitoneal compartments is involved.

Since Chapter 42 is devoted to the pancreas, and since the adrenal glands and kidney are considered beyond the scope of this book, this chapter considers the ultrasonographic evaluation of the abdominal aorta and its branches, the inferior vena cava, and abnormal fluid collections and masses that can arise in the retroperitoneum.

ABDOMINAL AORTA
Technique

The abdominal aorta is usually easily visualized by longitudinal scanning just to the left of the midline (Fig. 66-1, A). Generally the origins of the celiac and superior mesenteric arteries can be demonstrated on both longitudinal (Fig. 66-1, B) and transverse scans. The aorta usually courses parallel to the spine just to the left of the midline. In elderly patients it is commonly tortuous and may cause clinical confusion with an abdominal aortic aneurysm. Only the lateral aspect of the tortuous aorta

may be palpated, or a plain abdominal film may show a curvilinear calcification. A tortuous aorta used to be difficult to evaluate with static articulated arm B scanning. However, the real-time transducers make it particularly easy to follow the course of a tortuous aorta and pick the appropriate plane of section for the best longitudinal axis. In addition, one can use the real-time transducer array as a compression device to judiciously compress the overlying bowel gas out of the way, achieving visualization of the more deeply situated abdominal aorta. In larger patients the aorta can be seen by moving the transducer laterally toward either side of the abdomen and angling back toward where one expects to see the abdominal aorta. One can generally find a "window," unobscured by bowel gas, through which the aorta can be visualized. Persistence with these techniques makes the "nonvisualized" aorta exceedingly rare. After scanning longitudinally through the long axis of the aorta to its bifurcation, the transducer is angled obliquely to follow the aorta into the common iliac arteries. One can even produce a pseudocoronal view of the distal abdominal aorta and origin of the iliac arteries by putting the patient into a left side–down decubitus position and aiming the transducer medially from the right side of the abdomen. Sometimes this works better in the opposite direction, with the patient right side down and the transducer aimed from the left side.[67] Transverse images of the aorta and iliac arteries are obtained by carefully scanning through the short axis of the vessels. It is important to appreciate that if the aorta is tortuous, the short axis of the aorta is not necessarily the true transverse section of the abdomen (Fig. 66-1, C). This distinction is important to avoid sectioning the aorta obliquely and thereby elongating its apparent transverse diameter. It is also important to appreciate this distinction to avoid elongating the anteroposterior diameter. Occasionally, the abdominal aorta and its bifurcation into the common iliac arteries can be visualized by a coronal scan through the right lobe of the liver and/or right kidney (Fig. 66-1, D).

We do not measure the caliber of the normal abdominal aorta. If the aorta is ectatic or aneurysmal, the depth, width, and length of the aneurysm are measured. Diameter measurements are from outside edges of the aortic wall, as this compares to what is seen at surgery.[40]

Ninety-five percent of abdominal aortic aneurysms do not involve the renal arteries. Most commonly the aneurysmal portion involves only the distal third of the abdominal aorta, and one can confidently exclude renal artery involvement. If the aneurysm is noted to extend more proximally, one can attempt to search for the origin of the renal arteries (Fig. 66-2).[45] This is commonly very difficult. Even if one can identify the right renal artery passing behind the inferior vena cava, this can be at a

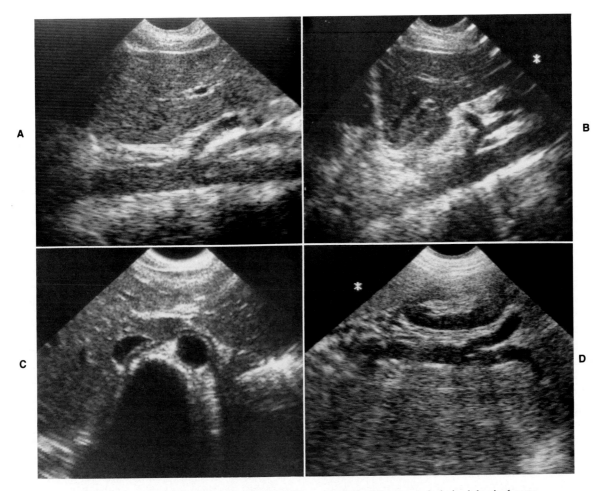

Fig. 66-1 A, Sagittal scan showing left lobe of liver anteriorly. More posteriorly is abdominal aorta with celiac and superior mesenteric artery branches arising anteriorly toward right side of image. Inferiorly and just deep to left lobe of liver lies cross-section of body of pancreas. Anterior to more superior portion of aorta is crus of diaphragm and gastroesophageal junction. **B,** Sagittal scan showing congenital abnormality of common trunk arising from aorta and giving off celiac axis anteriorly and superiorly and superior mesenteric artery directed inferiorly. **C,** Transverse scan high in abdomen showing abdominal aorta to left, IVC to right, and crus of diaphragm passing over abdominal aorta and posterior to IVC. **D,** Coronal scan through right lobe of liver and right kidney showing distal abdominal aorta and its bifurcation into common iliac arteries.

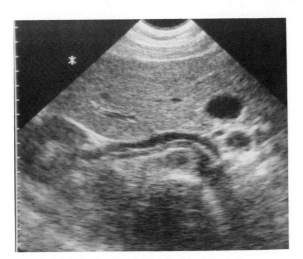

Fig. 66-2 Transverse scan aimed from right anterior axillary line showing right renal artery arising from aorta posterior to right renal vein coursing to IVC. Right kidney can be seen toward left side of image, and gallbladder and portal vein are noted toward right side of image.

significantly lower level than its origin from the aorta. Therefore the portion of the renal artery may be seen at the level of the aneurysm but arises from the normal aorta above that level. Furthermore, the renal arteries are best seen when there is no aneurysm, since the large bulk of the aneurysm tends to displace bowel gas superiorly and obscures visualization. If an aneurysm is noted to originate in the region of the mid-abdominal aorta, an aortogram is suggested to evaluate the origin of its branches.

Normal anatomy

The normal abdominal aorta is situated anterolateral to the spine at the level of the diaphragm and, coursing anteriorly and medially, becomes anterior to the spine at the lower lumbar level. Therefore, on supine longitudinal scanning, the abdominal aorta will go in a posterior-to-anterior direction as one scans inferiorly. The normal aorta tapers gradually from superior to inferior and normally measures less than 3 cm in diameter superiorly.

Deep to the abdominal aorta, one should see the undulating echo of the anterior border of the lumbar spine, and there should be no space or mass between the spine and the abdominal aorta. Anteriorly one can generally see the gastroesophageal junction as a small target appearance just anterior to the most superior portion of the abdominal aorta (see Fig. 66-1, A). More superiorly the aorta is frequently obscured by overlying lung. The right crus of the diaphragm lies anterior to the proximal abdominal aorta and is seen on ultrasound as a thin, echo-free line (see Fig. 66-1, C). In most patients one can see the origin of the celiac and superior mesenteric arteries. Most frequently these arteries arise from the left side of the anterior aspect of the abdominal aorta. In exceptionally thin patients one may not be able to show the origin of these branches in the same longitudinal plane that shows the widest diameter of the abdominal aorta. If the plane of section is moved toward the left and angled back toward the midline, one can then line up the branches to show their origin from the aorta. The left gastric branch of the celiac courses superiorly for a short segment, and this can be seen on a longitudinal scan. On a transverse scan one can see the splenic artery continuing to the left from the celiac axis, and the hepatic branch generally arises to the left of the abdominal aorta and crosses back over the aorta as it courses to the right, anterior to the portal vein, into the porta hepatis. Occasionally, the main hepatic artery or an accessory hepatic artery arises from the superior mesenteric artery. This can be seen posterior to the portal vein. Inferior to the origin of the superior mesenteric artery, one can frequently see the left renal vein traversing anterior to the abdominal aorta. Inferior to that, the third portion of the duodenum crosses the aorta deep to the superior mesenteric artery, but this is

very rarely identified. The superior mesenteric vein may be situated in a position anterior to the abdominal aorta rather than toward the right. This should not be confused with the superior mesenteric artery, which can be traced to its origin from the aorta. Furthermore, the superior mesenteric vein generally is completely echo free, whereas the superior mesenteric artery generally contains some fine echoes. These are probably artifact echoes arising either from the lateral walls, which are always included within the ultrasound beam, or perhaps reverberation artifacts from the anterior wall of the vessel. Furthermore, the superior mesenteric artery is generally encased by very echogenic fat in the root of the small bowel mesentery. The neck of the pancreas is situated anterior to the superior mesenteric vein, and the uncinate process is posterior to it. These are frequently seen in the plane of section that shows the long axis of the abdominal aorta. Inferior to the level of the pancreas, there is normally only bowel interposed between the anterior abdominal wall and the aorta. Usually the contained gas can be easily displaced so that the aorta can be visualized down to its bifurcation at the level of the umbilicus.

Abnormalities

Although it would be useful to demonstrate arteriosclerotic narrowing and obliteration of the abdominal aorta and its major branches, this is generally not feasible by ultrasound techniques. Irregularities of the posterior and lateral walls of the abdominal aorta may be demonstrated, but this is generally not clinically useful. There are too many artifacts of the anterior wall of the aorta, because of reverberation, to accurately demonstrate irregularities in this location. Calcified arteriosclerotic plaques may cause acoustic shadowing (and resultant signal loss) similar to that seen deep to gallbladder calculi. Most commonly stenosis or complete occlusion involves the iliac arteries. Since gas interferes with the identification of these vessels, arteriography is necessary to evaluate these lesions. Doppler ultrasound has been used to help identify stenoses at the origin of the celiac, superior mesenteric, and renal arteries.[2,25,48,58] However, these techniques are exceedingly difficult technically.

Abdominal aortic aneurysm

Ultrasonography of the abdominal aorta is most important clinically in detection and measurement of abdominal aortic aneurysms.[56,79,90] Although clinical evaluation by palpation will detect many aneurysms, it is not accurate in quantitating their diameters. Also, aneurysms can be missed on physical examination in large patients, and in thin patients or those with considerable lumbar lordosis an aneurysm may be simulated by palpating the relatively superficial, pulsatile aorta together with the

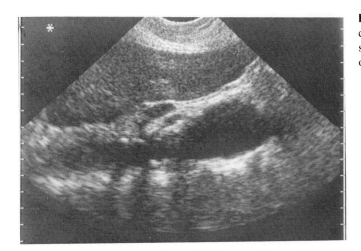

Fig. 66-3 Longitudinal scan showing aneurysmal ectasia of distal abdominal aorta just distal to origin of celiac and superior mesenteric arteries (and presumably distal to level of renal arteries as well).

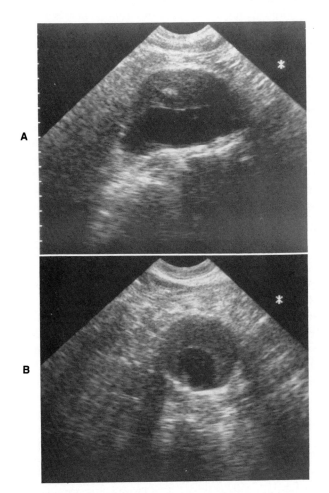

Fig. 66-4 A, Longitudinal and, **B,** transverse views showing abdominal aortic aneurysm with considerable thrombus in anterior portion.

lumbar spine. Before the use of ultrasound to confirm abdominal aortic aneurysms, many patients were operated on with the expectation of having an abdominal aneurysm and were found to have normal aortas. Perhaps the most useful role of ultrasound is to confirm the presence of a clinically suspected abdominal aneurysm in all cases before surgery.

When the distal aorta is aneurysmally dilated, the overlying bowel will usually be displaced, allowing excellent ultrasonographic visualization of the aneurysm. As described, it is important to obtain images through the long axis of the aorta, showing the longitudinal extent of the aneurysm (Figs. 66-3 and 66-4).

On transverse scans the size of the aneurysm is measured from its outer walls, which correlates with the findings at surgery. Since it is impossible to assess the depth of an aneurysm clinically or even at operation, the diameter measurement most appropriate for clinical and surgical evaluation is the transverse diameter. This measurement, however, is less accurate by ultrasound than anteroposterior diameter for three reasons. First, the ultrasound beam is tangential to the lateral aortic wall, so that strong discrete echoes are not produced, and choice of measurement points is thus more subjective. Also, whereas measurements along the axis of the ultrasound beam are highly accurate, measurements perpendicular to the sound beam are less accurate; that is, axial resolution is much higher than lateral resolution. Furthermore, axial measurments depend only on the speed of sound in tissue. Lateral measurements are based on mechanical and electronic calibration, and without frequent evaluation and adjustment they may become inaccurate. It is important to give the anteroposterior diameter, the transverse diameter, and the length of the aneurysm, because the usual surgical determinant for operation is that the greatest diameter exceed 5 cm. If the diameter of an aneurysm is less than 5 cm, the ultrasound examination should be repeated at yearly or half-yearly intervals to assess growth. The reported annual growth rate of a 3 to 5.9 cm abdominal aortic aneurysm is 0.23 to 0.28 cm per year.[28] An aneurysm of 4 to 5 cm may require surgery if it is symptomatic or increases in diameter by more than 1 cm in one year.[28] Other authors consider 6 cm as the cutoff for operation in asymptomatic individuals.[85] If the aneurysm is less than 6 cm, patients rarely die from rupture and have a 75% 1-year survival rate.[85] If the diameter is greater than 6 cm, there is a 50% survival at one year.[85] If the aneurysm is greater than 7 cm, there is a greater than 75% risk of fatal rupture; if it is less than 5 cm, there is less than a 1% rupture rate.[60,85] The operative mortality before rupture is 5%, but with emergency surgery for rupture the mortality increases to 50%.[76]

In studies comparing CT with ultrasound for aneurysm measurment, CT has been slightly more accurate[29,74]; however, there appears to be no significant benefit of CT over ultrasound. Also, ultrasound has the advantage of showing the long axis of the aorta, which is not seen on CT unless reformations are done. Since abdominal aortic aneurysms were detectable with the earliest ultrasound equipment, most of the studies comparing aneurysm size by ultrasound with findings at surgery or radiography used early real-time or static B-scan techniques and presumably measured inner to inner diameter; nonetheless, reasonable accuracy was achieved. Considerable improvement in instrumentation has occurred since then. Ultrasound was within 0.5 cm in 75% of cases and within 1 cm in 92% of patients in a study done in 1978.[42]

Ultrasonography can detect not only the size of the aneurysm but also the presence of thrombus within the aneurysm. Although this is not really clinically important, generally the soft echoes of the thrombus are clearly differentiated from the smaller lumen within the aneurysm (Fig. 66-4).[41] The nonthrombosed lumen follows the course of the normal proximal aorta, as might be expected. This explains why an aortogram may appear almost normal in patients with considerable circumferential thrombus. If the aorta is completely clotted and therefore obstructed, it can be difficult to differentiate noise echoes within the lumen from true clot echoes.[1] It is the differentiation of nonthrombosed lumen with flowing blood from surrounding thrombus that allows one to visualize the thrombus. Doppler may also be of help.

Aside from proving that a palpable, pulsatile mass in the mid abdomen is not a normal aorta, it is also important to differentiate an aneurysm from a preaortic or paraaortic mass that is transmitting the pulsation. Numerous cases of these masses mimicking aneurysms have been documented in the literature.[23,61,82] The "silhouette sign" of the inability to visualize the abdominal aorta within per-

iaortic lymph node masses, popularized with earlier ultrasound technology, is no longer a problem with modern real-time techniques. There is generally no difficulty in differentiating periaortic masses from an abdominal aortic aneurysm. Retroperitoneal fibrosis can occasionally cause confusion with an aneurysm.

To evaluate extension of an abdominal aneurysm into the iliac arteries, it is necessary to identify two dilated tubular structures below the level of the aorta on transverse scanning.[7,31] Although the abdominal aorta generally bifurcates at about the level of the umbilicus, and it is assumed that any extent to the umbilicus would be into the iliac arteries, it is common for the abdominal aorta to elongate and become tortuous, especially in patients who are prone to develop aortic aneurysms. The course of the common iliac arteries in arteriosclerotic disease is frequently very tortuous and may extend in a horizontal plane or even curve slightly anteriorly. It is therefore virtually impossible to determine where an aortic aneurysm commences, unless one can show both iliac arteries side by side in a transverse scan. Occasionally, a double lumen will be seen within the thrombus in the abdominal aorta proximal to the bifurcation of the aorta. Performing transverse scans inferior to that level will confirm two separate structures representing the iliac aneurysms. Occasionally, on transverse scans at the level of the umbilicus the inferior vena cava will be distended and situated to the right of and posterior to the aneurysm. It is important not to mistake the vena cava for a normal right iliac artery and assume that the aneurysm is extending into the left iliac artery.

Aortic dissection

Another useful role of ultrasonography is in the detection and evaluation of the patient with a dissection involving the abdominal aorta (Fig. 66-5).[7,15] Originally called *dissecting aneurysm*, the aorta is rarely aneurysmal although often enlarged, and *aortic dissection* has become the favored term.[19] In this case a hematoma dissects along the aortic media, weakened usually by degenerative changes, and begins in either the aortic root or aortic arch. Currently the most popular classification of aortic dissection recognizes two types. Type A involves the ascending aorta or the ascending and descending aorta. It is the most common and most lethal type. Type B does not involve the ascending aorta and usually begins at or just distal to the left subclavian artery, extending down into the descending and abdominal aorta.[19] Ultrasound is not useful to diagnose an intrathoracic dissection. Occasionally, involvement of the aortic root may be demonstrated by M-mode or two-dimensional echocardiography.[38,52] CT or aortography is necessary for the accurate diagnosis of an intrathoracic aneurysm. In the abdomen ultrasound may demonstrate the abnormal echo from the

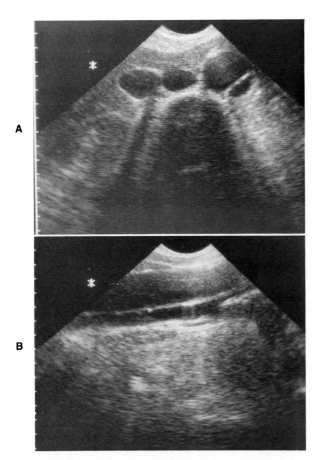

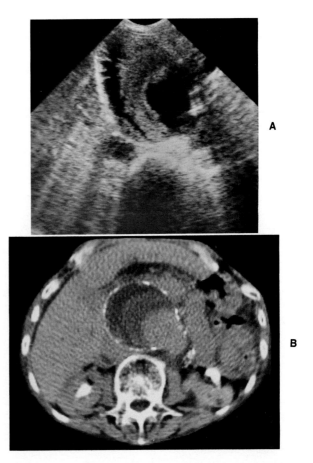

Fig. 66-5 Abdominal aortic dissection. **A,** Transverse scan showing, from right ot left, gallbladder, IVC, and abdominal aorta with intimal flap posteriorly and to left. **B,** Longitudinal scan between sagittal and coronal showing intimal flap separating false lumen (toward top of image) from true lumen extending into both right and left iliac arteries (toward right of image).

Fig. 66-6 A, Transverse sonogram and, **B,** CT scan showing reliquefaction of peripheral portion of thrombus in aortic aneurysm. Note peripherally situated calcification of intima clearly differentiating this from dissection.

intimal flap within the aorta.[15,19,28,52] Sometimes a dramatic back-and-forth motion of the intimal flap can be seen with each cardiac pulsation.[17]

The thoracic extent of the aneurysm cannot be evaluated by ultrasonography, but occasionally the involvement of the aortic root may be demonstrated by M-mode two-dimensional echocardiography.[38,52]

Occasionally, reliquefaction of the peripheral portion of the clot can take place in an abdominal aortic aneurysm (Fig. 66-6).[46] This appearance can cause confusion and suggest a dissection or even a leak to the unwary radiologist.

Ruptured aortic aneurysm

In addition to the patient who has a palpable pulsatile abdominal mass, ultrasound can be useful in the patient with unexplained abdominal back pain. Approximately 55% of patients with ruptured aortic aneurysm who come to the emergency room are not diagnosed until surgery

or postmortem. Most frequently they are misdiagnosed as renal colic. However, ultrasonography frequently cannot identify the hematoma because of the paralytic ileus that obscures the deeper structures. Also, the hematoma need not have considerable volume but may be more platelike. CT is superior in displaying the site and extent of a retroperitoneal hematoma (Fig. 66-7). However, in that clinical setting the demonstration by ultrasonography of an abdominal aortic aneurysm should be sufficient to alert the clinician to the likely diagnosis. We have seen several cases in which an aneurysm was found in a patient with unexplained abdominal pain, and the correct diagnosis of a slow leak was made at surgery. Despite the inconvenience, it might be useful to perform ultrasound examinations of those patients with unexplained abdominal pain who come to the emergency room.

Aneurysms of the branches of the abdominal aorta may be demonstrated by ultrasound. These are generally mycotic aneurysms but also can be seen particularly in

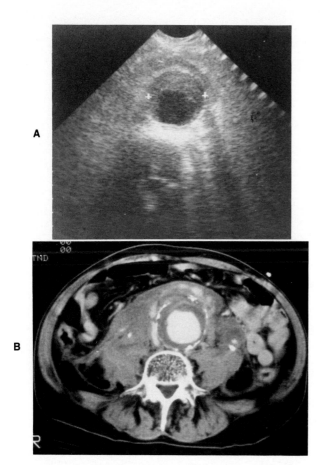

Fig. 66-7 A, Transverse sonogram showing abdominal aortic aneurysm with virtually unappreciated pancake of leaking hematoma. **B,** CT scan at approximately same level showing thin rim of hematoma anteriorly and large collections to both sides.

the renal arteries of patients with fasculitis. It can be exceedingly difficult to make a specific diagnosis of such an aneurysm by ultrasound, and arteriography is generally necessary.

Postoperative evaluation

Ultrasound can be used in an attempt to identify a hematoma[32] or false aneurysm following end-to-side or end-to-end grafts for aortoiliac stenosis or aortic aneurysmectomy.[33,91] Ultrasound can delineate the proximal anastomosis in 84% of patients and the iliac graft in 88% to 90% of patients,[34] but sometimes visualization of the graft following aneurysmectomy can be difficult, since the original aneurysm is not completely excised. Generally a small hematoma persists for a variable period following aneurysmectomy or aortoiliac grafting. An extensive paraaortic hematoma may be a normal finding after repair of an abdominal aortic aneurysm if it had ruptured.[60] Such a postoperative hematoma would other-

wise indicate a complication such as anastomotic leak. It is impossible to differentiate a bland hematoma from an infected hematoma by ultrasound. In fact, if there is gas within the infected hematoma, the hematoma may be completely obscured. CT is the preferred method to assess an infected postoperative hematoma related to aortic surgery. Fine-needle aspiration of a recognized hematoma with either CT or ultrasound guidance may be helpful in the appropriate clinical setting.

Pulsed Doppler, duplex scanning and more recently color flow Doppler can be particularly helpful in identifying flow in false aneurysms. This can differentiate the false aneurysm from a simple perigraft hematoma or other fluid collection.

INFERIOR VENA CAVA
Technique

Scanning of the inferior vena cava (IVC) can be performed in the supine or left lateral decubitus position.[4] Longitudinal scans 2 to 4 cm to the right of the midline generally show the long axis of the IVC. Starting at the level of the diaphragm, the IVC is evaluated in longitudinal and transverse views at least to the level of the uncinate process of the pancreas. Since the degree of distention of the vena cava dramatically depends on both cardiac and intrathoracic pressure, real-time imaging is particularly useful.[39] There is great variability in the degree to which the IVC distends. Many young women will show a greatly distended IVC almost throughout the respiratory cycle. The IVC should increase in caliber with held breath or expiration and decrease with inspiration or the Valsalva maneuver. However, commonly the IVC will be collapsed throughout most of the respiratory cycle and distended maximally only at the right combination of held inspiration and the appropriate phase of the cardiac cycle.

Normal anatomy

The IVC is seen at a higher level in the abdomen than the abdominal aorta, since it enters the liver just after leaving the right atrium. (There is generally air-containing lung anterior to the abdominal aorta at that level.) At the superior aspect of the liver the three hepatic veins (right, middle, and left) can be seen to enter the vena cava. The IVC in this region is surrounded by liver on three sides—on the left, anteriorly, and on the right.

More inferiorly the caudate lobe is anterior to the IVC. Medial and posterior to the IVC is the right crus of the diaphragm. The main portal vein in the region of the porta hepatis is intimately related to the anterior aspect of the IVC. Inferior to that level, the common bile duct is directly anterior to the IVC. The right renal artery courses obliquely behind (dorsal to) the IVC and frequently causes a sharp indentation in the posterior wall of the IVC. Occasionally, the right renal vein can be visualized on a transverse scan running toward the right kidney (see Fig. 66-2). The left renal vein can be consistently visualized posterior to the superior mesenteric artery and anterior to the abdominal aorta. The left renal vein can be best seen during a Valsalva maneuver when it, like the IVC, is distended. The portion of the left renal vein to the left of the abdominal aorta may appear larger than expected and most frequently is more distended than the portion crossing the aorta.[8] It is important not to mistake this portion of the left renal vein for an abnormal fluid collection or mass. The head of the pancreas may cause an indentation on the anterior aspect of the IVC. Distal to the level of the head of the pancreas, the IVC is generally not adequately visualized, because it is either collapsed or obscured by overlying bowel gas.

Occasionally, especially in thin individuals, small echoes can be seen moving in the direction of blood flow within the IVC or in the hepatic and portal veins. These are clearly not artifacts, since they move with the flow pattern within these veins and slow down during the Valsalva maneuver. They are not indicative of any specific disease process. Several explanations have been proposed for this effect,[3,16,92] but it appears to be best explained by the rouleaux formation that occurs in slow flow rates or in large caliber vessels, both conditions providing low shear rates[70,80] that allow red blood cell aggregation.

Congenital anomalies

The congenital anomalies involving the IVC are duplication,[44,75,77] transposition,[77] left renal vein anomalies[77] (Fig. 66-8), and hemiazygos continuation.[23,83] Left-sided or hemiazygos continuation of the IVC has a confusing appearance on ultrasound, suggesting an abnormal structure posterior and to the left of the abdominal aorta (Fig. 66-9).[23,83]

Congestive failure

Whereas there is considerable variation among normal subjects in the ability of the IVC to distend during the Valsalva maneuver and the degree of collapse on inspiration, patients who have right-sided congestive failure characteristically demonstrate a very large IVC and large hepatic veins that do not collapse during inspiration.[86] This is usually not a major indication for ultrasound, since the jugular veins can be evaluated clinically. However, in cases of unexplained hepatomegaly, especially in large patients in whom the jugular veins cannot be well visualized, the demonstration of these large turgid veins can give an indication as to the cause of the hepatomegaly. Also, the IVC and hepatic veins may reflect

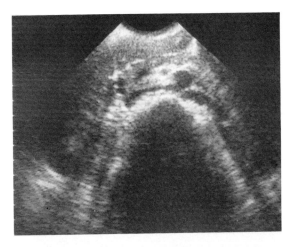

Fig. 66-8 Transverse scan showing retroaortic left renal vein.

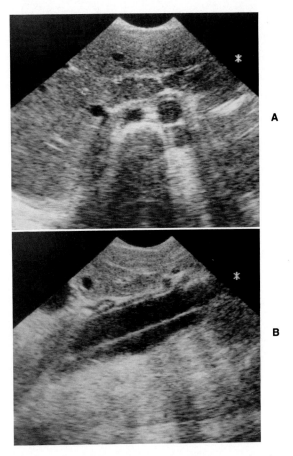

Fig. 66-9 A, Transverse and, **B,** longitudinal scans showing vascular structure posterior to abdominal aorta toward left side, which is large hemiazygos vein. Structure resembling IVC to right of aorta is actually azygos vein, situated behind right crus of diaphragm. Note crus of diaphragm and gastroesophageal junction anterior to abdominal aorta on sagittal scan.

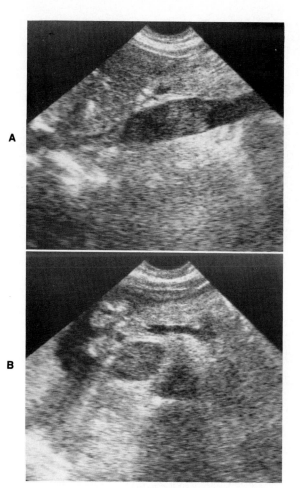

Fig. 66-10 Tumor thrombus in IVC from right renal carcinoma. **A,** Longitudinal and, **B,** transverse scans showing distention of vena cava with tumor thrombus.

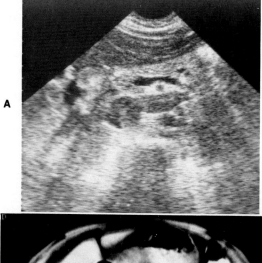

Fig. 66-11 Tumor thrombus in left renal vein and IVC on sonogram **(A)** and CT scan **(B).**

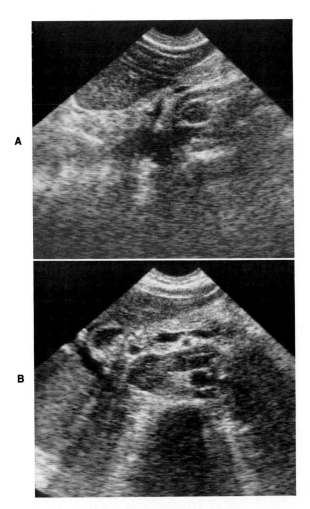

Fig. 66-12 A, Longitudinal and, **B,** transverse sonograms showing tumor extending into circumaortic left renal vein. Note on longitudinal scan oval structure between superior mesenteric artery and aorta. On transverse scan tumor can be seen distending left renal vein between superior mesenteric artery and aorta. Note also tumor distention of retroaortic left renal vein between abdominal aorta and anterior border of vertebral body.

large ventricular pulsations in patients with tricuspid insufficiency.

Thrombosis

Rarely thrombosis of the IVC may occur in the Budd-Chiari syndrome.[59,63] More commonly thrombosis occurs more inferiorly at the level of the renal veins.[26,68] These are caused by renal cell carcinomas that frequently invade the renal vein, and they may extend up the IVC even as far as the right atrium (Figs. 66-10 to 66-12).[27,36] IVC involvement most commonly arises from large tumors of the right kidney[30] because of the close proximity to the

IVC.[27,36] One should specifically search for IVC involvement in any patient with hypernephroma.[62] Tumors of adrenal, hepatic, and neurogenic origin can invade as well as displace the IVC.[4,81] Other less common tumors that involve the IVC are retroperitoneal liposarcoma, leiomyosarcoma, pheochromocytoma, osteosarcoma, and rhabdomyosarcoma.[43,73] IVC involvement by a benign renal angiomyolipoma has been detected ultrasonographically.[54]

If the IVC can be seen, tumor involvement is not difficult to diagnose. The question that usually arises is whether the tumor is compressing the cava or invading it. It is most helpful to visualize echo-free blood both anterior and posterior to the thrombus to indicate its intraluminal nature. Occasionally, the mass within the IVC may be noted first on the ultrasound examination. In this case both kidneys and adrenal glands should be examined carefully for the primary lesion.

External compression

Unlike the abdominal aorta, the contour of which appears normally tapering from superior to inferior, the caliber of the IVC reflects the normal and abnormal structures that are apposed to it. Both the caudate lobe and the head of the pancreas may cause mild indentation of the anterior surface of the IVC. The normal upper pole of the right kidney may mildly indent the posterolateral aspect of the IVC. The right renal artery can cause a sharply marginated indentation. However, tumors in the liver, head of the pancreas, right adrenal gland, upper pole of the right kidney, and enlarged lymph nodes (Fig. 66-13) may cause more irregular and significant indentation of a well-distended IVC.[4,53] These should not be used as the only sign of an abnormality; the remainder of the lesion should be carefully identified.

Inferior vena cava filters

Stainless steel wire cages, such as the Kimray-Greenfield filter, may be placed in the IVC to prevent thromboemboli from reaching the lungs in patients in whom anticoagulation is contraindicated or ineffective. These are subject to a variety of complications, such as thrombosis and occlusion of the IVC in 3% to 5% of cases, caudad migration in 30% to 50%, and cephalad migration in 5% to 10%.[64] Prong penetration of the IVC and retroperitoneal hematomas have been reported.[57] Ultrasound has been recommended as a means of routine follow-up of uncomplicated filters[57] and can accurately identify the filter in 89% of cases (Fig. 66-14).[69] With the addition of pulsed Doppler, 100% accuracy has been reported in identifying normal blood flow in patient venae cavae and in determining thrombosis, except for a few technically inadequate studies.[69]

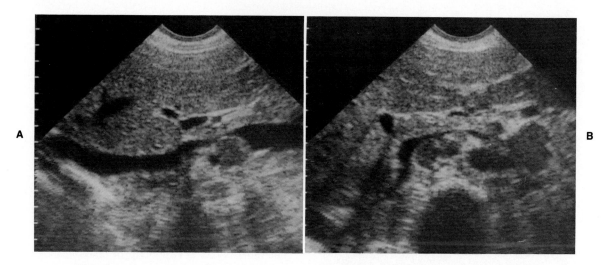

Fig. 66-13 A, Longitudinal and, **B,** transverse scans showing enlarged lymph node indenting posterior aspect of IVC.

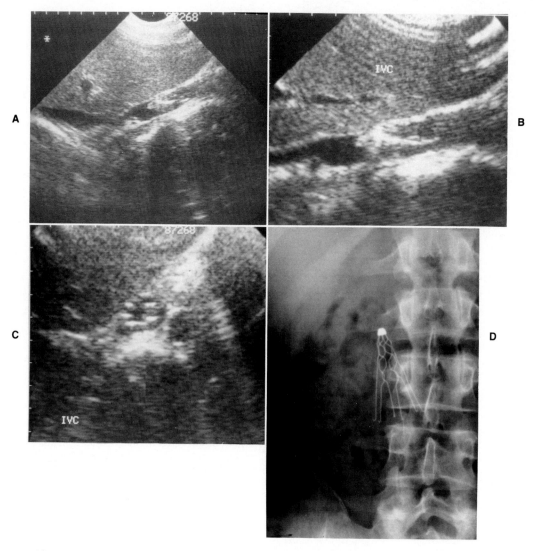

Fig. 66-14 A and **B,** Sagittal scan through IVC showing a Kimray-Greenfield filter with clot. **C,** Transverse scan showing individual six limbs of filter. **D,** Radiograph showing radiopaque filter.

RETROPERITONEAL MASSES

Masses in the retroperitoneum may displace a kidney anteriorly or laterally or may displace the aorta or IVC anteriorly. If there is no displacement of one of these structures, it can be difficult to decide whether a mass is retroperitoneal or intraperitoneal by ultrasound alone. Thus one might be able to specifically diagnose an abscess or lymphoma as being retroperitoneal if it extends posterior to the aorta. However, if the mass is situated more anteriorly, one cannot specify whether the mass is solely intraperitoneal or retroperitoneal. Right upper quadrant retroperitoneal fat is displaced in a characteristic manner by masses originating in the retroperitoneum, and this pattern of displacement may help to localize the origin of the mass.[35,37] Fortunately, there is generally not much clinical benefit in knowing specifically whether a mass of this type is strictly intraperitoneal or retroperitoneal; this knowledge will not usually alter therapy.

It is easiest to divide abnormalities that arise in the retroperitoneum into those that are cystic and those that are solid. Cystic abnormalities include abscesses, hematomas, seromas, lymphoceles, and urinomas. Basically these can all have an identical appearance on ultrasound and cannot be distinguished on the basis of ultrasound alone.[61] Fortunately, ultrasonographically guided fine-needle aspiration can easily allow the differentiation. Solid masses are almost always malignant and are usually primary sarcomas, lymphomas, or metastatic involvement of the retrocrural and paraaortic lymph nodes. Fine-needle aspiration biopsy can easily be guided ultrasonographically if the lesion is detected by ultrasound. Retroperitoneal fibrosis is another condition that can have a similar ultrasonographic appearance to paraaortic lymph node enlargement.

Abnormal fluid collections: abscesses

Despite advances in antibiotics and surgical technique, retroperitoneal abscesses remain a significant clinical problem. These are usually caused by infection (Crohn's disease, appendicitis, pyelonephritis, perinephric abscess, tuberculous or pyogenic spondylitis), trauma, bowel perforation, surgery, or malignancy in adjacent retroperitoneal or intraperitoneal structures.[51,55,89] A pancreatic abscess may arise as an infection in a pancreatic pseudocyst or may be a complication of pancreatitis. Although these latter fluid collections can occur anywhere, there is a predilection for the fluid to extend into the posterior pararenal space on the left side (Fig. 66-15). A perirenal abscess can arise from an infection in the kidney. The most common presentations are pain in the lower abdomen or flank with fever of unknown source or postoperatively. Generally there are no localizing signs. If there are localizing features, the

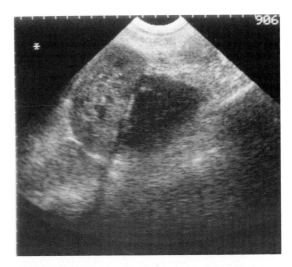

Fig. 66-15 Longitudinal scan in left flank showing left kidney elevated by abscess in left posterior pararenal space.

ultrasound examination should be concentrated in that area, but in any case a complete examination of the upper, mid, and lower abdomen and pelvis should be performed.

Although it is possible to miss an abscess on ultrasound examination because of overlying bowel gas and the inability to penetrate bone or thick muscles from other approaches, the most common cause for missing an abscess is failure to recognize the abscess because of the presence of gas in the abscess cavity. A large amount of gas in an abscess is indistinguishable from gas within a bowel loop. If the gas is in the form of microbubbles and if the abscess is in a location remote from bowel loops, it is possible to demonstrate an echogenic mass that can have the appearance of a solid lesion.[49] On the other hand, the presence of gas within an abscess allows its demonstration by plain film radiography and CT (Fig. 66-16).

Although an abscess on ultrasound may contain debris echoes or demonstrate a thickened wall, the spectrum of findings in abscesses ranges from a completely echo-free fluid collection to a very densely echogenic mass if microbubbles are present.[20] If clinical findings indicate that the fluid collection is an abscess, confirmation by ^{67}Ga or indium-labeled leukocyte isotope scan may help to prove the infectious nature, or the demonstration of microbubbles on CT may be confirmatory. A simpler and more direct approach for the definite diagnosis is fine-needle percutaneous aspiration.[89] Since the localization of the abnormal fluid collection can easily be identified in relation to the external landmarks, the angle of approach and depth of penetration may easily be determined from the ultrasound image. With the use of a 22-gauge spinal needle, even thick, purulent material may be as-

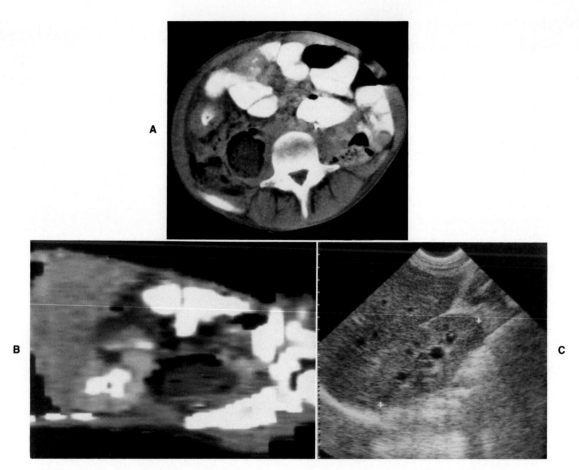

Fig. 66-16 A, CT scan and, **B,** sagittal reconstruction showing gas-containing right psoas abscess. Note on sagittal reconstruction that lower pole of mildly hydronephrotic right kidney is elevated by abscess. **C,** Sonogram in same case showing lower pole of mildly hydronephrotic right kidney elevated by gas-containing abscess. Intraluminal bowel gas should not be present in that location.

pirated. The applications of fine-needle aspiration are twofold. First, it can confirm that the abnormal fluid collection is in fact an abscess and not a seroma or other fluid collection. As part of this, the aspirated material can be sent for bacteriologic tests, including antibiotic susceptibility studies. Second, many abscess cavities are easily accessible by a percutaneous approach for therapeutic drainage under ultrasonographic or CT control.[23] Surgical and anesthetic morbidity, mortality, and excessive cost can accordingly be avoided in a significant number of patients.

Hemorrhage

Retroperitoneal bleeding may occur spontaneously but more commonly occurs in association with hemophilia,[50] anticoagulant therapy, or trauma.[22] There is essentially no difference in the ultrasonographic appearance of a hematoma from that of an abscess. It may be completely echo-free and exhibit all the characteristics of a cystic structure, including a smooth deep border, and be enhanced through transmission of the ultrasound. On the other hand, the hematoma may appear as an inhomogeneously solid structure when there is considerable clot of varying stages within it. It may have relatively poorly defined margins and may appear identical to a solid lesion. If the clinical story is not clear, one can again use fine-needle percutaneous aspiration to confirm the diagnosis. The dark appearance of the blood or the lack of clotting can differentiate a hematoma from a traumatic tap. Generally the history of trauma or interference with the clotting mechanism, combined with a drop in hemoglobin, should suffice in the presence of a large retroperitoneal mass to diagnose a hematoma.

Most commonly, ultrasonography can detect an abscess or hematoma. However, if there is strong clinical suspicion, CT scanning should be performed, especially on relatively large individuals.

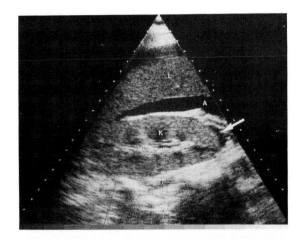

Fig. 66-17 Longitudinal scan showing ascites *(A)* in Morison's pouch separating liver *(L)* from Gerota's fascia around kidney *(K)*. Note small fluid collection in perirenal space *(arrow)*.

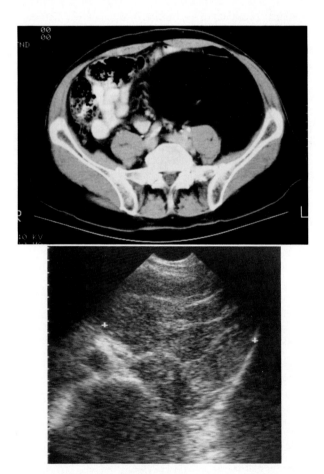

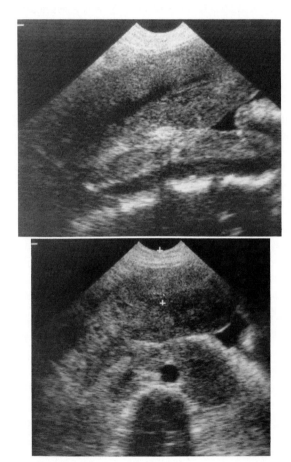

Fig. 66-18 A, CT scan showing large left-sided liposarcoma. **B,** Sonogram showing nondescript mass displacing bowel gass from left flank.

Fig. 66-19 Intraperitoneal and retroperitoneal tumor. **A,** Longitudinal and, **B,** transverse scans showing retroperitoneal tumor around aorta separated from intraperitoneal tumor more anteriorly by small amount of ascites and clear-cut plane of cleavage.

Other masses

Urinomas may be seen in association with renal trauma, surgery, or obstruction from a ureteral calculus (Fig. 66-17). Localization to the perirenal space is suggestive of the diagnosis, but confident distinction from abscess cannot usually be made without fine-needle aspiration or surgical confirmation. Lymphoceles usually result from surgery—renal transplants, radical gynecologic procedures, and extensive urologic operations. They appear ultrasonographically simply as abnormal fluid collections in the abdomen, and there is nothing about the images to allow specific diagnosis. Again, a fine-needle percutaneous aspiration should provide a definitive diagnosis.[82]

Primary neoplasm

Both benign[84,87] and malignant[10-12] primary tumors can arise in the retroperitoneal area. These are most commonly malignancies but may be relatively low grade and frequently are completely resectable. The most common type is a liposarcoma[47] (Fig. 66-18), but virtually any type of sarcomatous lesion can arise in the retroperitoneum, including those arising from muscle, blood vessel, and connective or neurogenic tissue. These tumors may be large, displacing other retroperitoneal structures, such as the kidney, vena cava, and aorta, and even intraperitoneal structures, such as the bowel, liver, and spleen. Since they frequently attain large dimensions, they are often palpable through the anterior abdominal wall and are easily seen ultrasonographically (Fig. 66-19). There is nothing specific about the ultrasonographic appearance of these lesions. They may be homogeneously solid. They may exhibit enhancement through transmission. Or there may be discrete cystic areas within the lesion caused by necrosis and/or hemorrhage into the tumor, a finding particularly seen in leiomyosarcomas.

Again, fine-needle aspiration biopsy can help make a preoperative diagnosis.

LYMPHOMA AND METASTASES

CT and lymphangiography are the principal techniques for staging and identifying retroperitoneal involvement in Hodgkin's disease, non-Hodgkin's lymphoma, and retroperitoneal metastatic disease.* Early studies[20] showed only a slight advantage of CT over ultrasound; however, if the patient is at all large, CT is far superior. It is important to be able to recognize retroperitoneal involvement in lymphoma and metastatic disease, since ultrasound examinations are frequently performed in patients with lymphoma and known primary malignancies. Furthermore, patients with these condi-

---

*References 6, 13, 66, 71, 72, 78.

tions may initially have generalized symptoms, such as abdominal pain, weight loss, or fever. The finding, for example, of an enlarged spleen on an ultrasound examination should direct one to the retroperitoneal area, specifically to the paraaortic region, to assess the possibility of lymph node enlargement (Figs. 66-20 to 66-22).

The crura of the diaphragm are easily identified on CT, since they are outlined on both sides by fat. Ultrasound can frequently identify the right crus of the diaphragm, especially in thin individuals (see Fig. 66-1, C).[9] This is an important area to examine, since relatively small involved lymph nodes can be detected in this region and identified as abnormal (Fig. 66-23). Massive enlargement of lymph nodes in the paraaortic region can easily be identified by demonstrating displacement of the abdominal aorta away from the spine with large masses surrounding the aorta on all sides. There is generally a lobular appearance to the outline of the masses. This can be differentiated from circumferential thrombus in an aneurysm, since thrombus has a softer echo texture with a clearly defined lumen and yet no strong specular echo separating the lumen from the thrombus as there would be between the abdominal aorta and periaortic nodes. It can be difficult, however, to assess whether the enlarged lymph nodes are completely retroperitoneal or involve the intraperitoneal region as well or vice versa (see Fig. 66-19). Only when one can demonstrate elevation of the aorta away from the spine can one be sure that the process involves the retroperitoneal compartment. Intraperitoneal lymph nodes, extending along the course of the superior mesenteric artery, can be easily identified, as well as

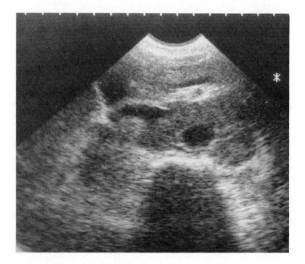

Fig. 66-20 Transverse sonogram showing lobulated lymph node masses around abdominal aorta and elevating IVC.

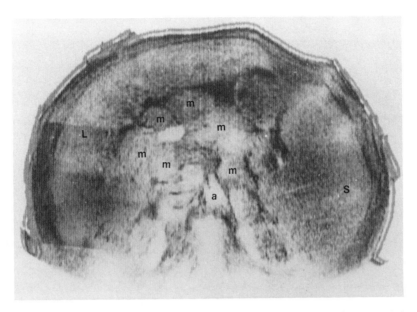

Fig. 66-21 Old static scan showing enlarged spleen *(S)* and multiple lymph node masses *(m)* around aorta *(a)*, IVC, and portal vein. Stomach can be seen between left lobe of liver *(L)* and spleen.

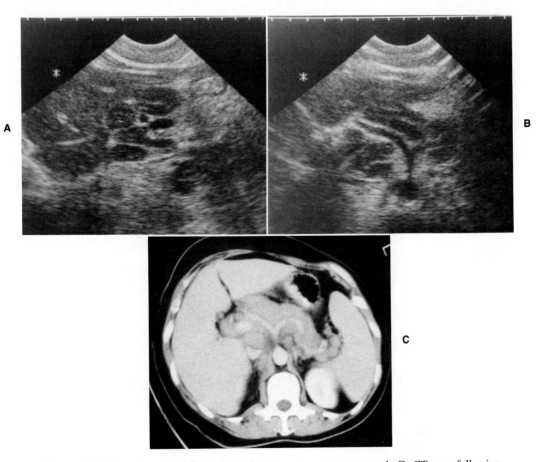

Fig. 66-22 Celiac axis nodes. **A,** Sagittal, **B,** transverse sonograms, and, **C,** CT scan following bolus of intravenous contrast medium showing multiple enlarged lymph nodes around celiac axis.

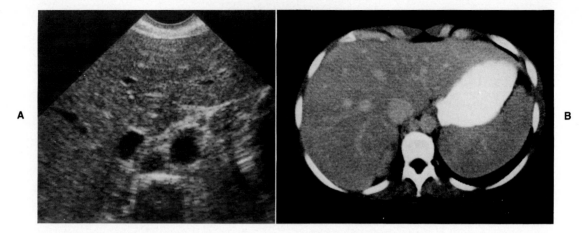

Fig. 66-23 Retrocrural node. **A,** Transverse sonogram and, **B,** CT scan showing small but definitely abnormal retrocrural lymph node.

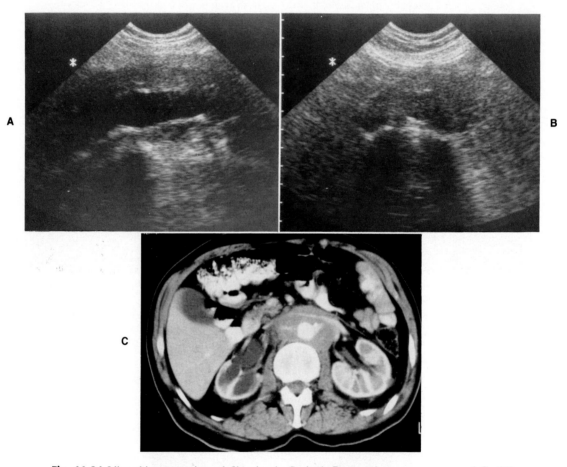

Fig. 66-24 Idiopathic retroperitoneal fibrosis. **A,** Sagittal, **B,** transverse sonograms, and **C,** CT scan following bolus injection of intravenous contrast medium showing relatively large mass of fibrous tissue around abdominal aorta. There is also right hydronephrosis. This degree of involvement is more exuberant than usually seen with retroperitoneal fibrosis.

nodes at the root of the mesentery and in the sites mentioned.

Although lymph nodes involved with lymphomatous processes generally achieve a larger size than those from secondary tumors, many of the latter can appear virtually indistinguishable from lymphomatous masses. This is particularly true of periaortic retroperitoneal metastases from carcinoma of the prostate and carcinoma of the testis. Retroperitoneal tumors may also invade as well as displace the head of the pancreas. Lesions in the region of the head of the pancreas, the porta hepatis, and the celiac artery are particularly prone to occur with chronic lymphocytic leukemia.

The characteristic features of lymph node enlargement vary from an echo-poor to echo-free lesion with a smooth deep wall and fairly good through transmission. Lymph nodes thus can occasionally be mistaken for abnormal fluid collections. One characteristic feature of lymph node involvement is the lobulated contour. Even if the lesion looks entirely "cystic" on ultrasound, if it has a lobulated contour, one should consider lymph node enlargement most likely.

Here again the best method of confirmation would be fine-needle percutaneous aspiration biopsy.[93,94] If the patient has a history of lymphoma, this would not be necessary. However, if there is no antecedent history, it is important to differentiate lymphoma from adenocarcinoma metastases and especially to differentiate loculated fluid collections from abnormal lymph node masses. Unless the cytology can be specific for a lymphosarcoma, especially histocytic, a histologic biopsy rather than fine-needle aspiration biopsy is necessary to diagnose the specific type of lymphoma and to assess prognosis and therapy. In these situations the architecture and growth pattern of the abnormal cells is more important than the appearance of the individual cells. Cytologic confirmation of adenocarcinoma averts the need for laparotomy. Even if a known primary tumor was treated previously, fine-needle percutaneous aspiration biopsy is of value to prove that the new lesion is a metastasis from the original tumor. This is especially true if further therapy is required, since pathologic proof is generally needed by oncologists before radiotherapy or further chemotherapy.

Although ultrasound has been reportedly used for radiotherapy planning, CT has been the preferred modality for identification, staging, and follow-up of lymphoma.[66]

RETROPERITONEAL FIBROSIS

Retroperitoneal fibrosis is for the most part an idiopathic condition that may be primary or, rarely, secondary to drugs or retroperitoneal tumors. It can appear similar to paraaortic lymphadenopathy, the isthmus of a horseshoe kidney, and retroperitoneal hematomas[5,14,21] on ultrasonographic examination. Generally lymphomas tend to be more lobulated and, if they are confluent, larger. In retroperitoneal fibrosis the periaortic involvement is smoother and does not achieve the large dimensions of periaortic nodal masses (Fig. 66-24). A helpful finding on CT or ultrasound is elevation of the aorta off the spine by nodal enlargement, which does not occur in retroperitoneal fibrosis.[18] Although hydronephrosis can occur with both lymphoma and retroperitoneal fibrosis, it more commonly occurs with the latter. It is interesting that the hydronephrosis is less severe than would be expected for the degree of uremia. Ultrasound or CT can be used for following response to steroid treatment for retroperitoneal fibrosis, including the frequently found hydronephrosis.

REFERENCES

1. Anderson, JC, Baltaxe, HA, and Wolf, GL: Inability to show clot: one limitation of ultrasonography of the abdominal aorta, Radiology 132:693, 1979.
2. Atkinson, T, and Wells, PNT: Pulsed Doppler ultrasound and its clinical application, Yale J Biol Med 50:367, 1977.
3. Beitler, JC, et al: The effects of temperature on blood flow ultrasonic echogenicity in vitro, J Ultrasound Med 2:259, 1983.
4. Bernardino, ME, et al: Ultrasonic demonstration of inferior vena caval involvement with right adrenal gland masses, J Clin Ultrasound 6:167, 1978.
5. Bowie, JD, and Bernstein, JR: Retroperitoneal fibrosis: ultrasound findings and case report, J Clin Ultrasound 4:435, 1976.
6. Bragg, DG, et al: New concepts in the non-Hodgkin lymphomas: radiologic implications, Radiology 159:289, 1986.
7. Bresnihan, ER, and Keates, PG: Ultrasound and dissection of the abdominal aorta, Clin Radiol 31:105, 1980.
8. Buschi, AJ, et al: Distended left renal vein: CT/sonographic normal variants, AJR 135:339, 1980.
9. Callen, PW, et al: Ultrasonography of the diaphragmatic crura, Radiology 130:712, 1979.
10. Carroll, BA: Lymphoma, Clin Diagn Ultrasound: Ultrasound Cancer 6:52, 1981.
11. Carroll, BA: Ultrasound of lymphoma, Semin Ultrasound 3:114, 1982.
12. Carroll, BA, and Ta, HN: The ultrasound appearance of extranodal abdominal lymphoma, Radiology 136:419, 1980.
13. Castellino, RA: Hodgkin disease: practical concepts for the diagnostic radiologist, Radiology 159:305, 1986.
14. Center, S, Schwab, R, and Goldberg, BB: The value of ultrasonography as an aid in the treatment of idiopathic retroperitoneal fibrosis, J Ultrasound Med 1:87, 1982.
15. Conrad, MR, et al: Real-time ultrasound in the diagnosis of acute dissecting aneurysm of the abdominal aorta, AJR 132:115, 1979.
16. Cosgrove, DO, and Arger, PH: Intravenous echoes due to laminar flow: experimental observation, AJR 139:953, 1982.
17. Curiati, WL, et al: Echographic demonstration of mobility of the dissecting flap of an aortic aneurysm, Radiology 123:173, 1977.
18. Degesys, GE, et al: Retroperitoneal fibrosis: use of CT in distinguishing among possible causes, AJR 146:57, 1986.
19. DeSanctis, RW, et al: Medical progress: aortic dissection, N Engl J Med 317:1060, 1987.
20. Doust, BD, Quiroz, F, and Stewart, JM: Ultrasonic distinction of abscesses from other intra-abdominal fluid collections, Radiology 125:213, 1977.

21. Fagan, CJ, et al: Retroperitoneal fibrosis: ultrasound and CT features, AJR 133:239, 1979.

22. Foley, LC, and Teele, RL: Ultrasound of epigastric injuries after blunt trauma, AJR 132:583, 1978.

23. Garris, JB, Kangarloo, H, and Sample, WF: Ultrasonic diagnosis of intrahepatic interruption of the inferior vena cava with azygos (hemiazygos) continuation, Radiology 134:179, 1980.

24. Gerzof, SG, and Gale, ME: Computed tomography and ultrasonography for diagnosis and treatment of renal and retroperitoneal abscess, Urol Clin North Am 9:185, 1982.

25. Gill, RW: Pulsed Doppler with B-mode imaging for quantitative blood flow measurement, Ultrasound Med Biol 5:223, 1979.

26. Goiney, R: Ultrasound imaging of inferior vena cava thrombosis, J Ultrasound Med 4:387, 1985.

27. Goldstein, HM, et al: Ultrasonic detection of renal tumor extension into the inferior vena cava, AJR 130:1083, 1978.

28. Gomes, MN: Clinical and surgical aspects of abdominal aortic aneurysms, Semin Ultrasound 3:156, 1982.

29. Gomes, MN, Hakkai, HG, and Schellinger, D: Ultrasonography and CT scanning: a comparative study of abdominal aortic aneurysms, Comput Tomogr 2:99, 1978.

30. Goncharenko, V, et al: Incidence and distribution of venous extension in 70 hypernephromas, AJR 133:263, 1979.

31. Gooding, GAW: Ultrasonography of the iliac arteries, Radiology 135:161, 1980.

32. Gooding, GAW: Ruptured abdominal aorta: postoperative ultrasound appearance, Radiology 145:781, 1982.

33. Gooding, GAW, et al: B-mode ultrasonography of prosthetic vascular grafts, Radiology 127:763, 1978.

34. Gooding, GAW, et al: The aortofemoral graft: detection and identification of healing complications by ultrasonography, Surgery 89:94, 1981.

35. Gore, RM, Callen, PW, and Filly, RA: Displaced retroperitoneal fat: sonographic guide to right upper quadrant mass localization, Radiology 142:701, 1982.

36. Gosink, BB: The inferior vena cava: mass effects, AJR 130:533, 1978.

37. Graif, M, Manor, A, and Itzchak, Y: Sonographic differentiation of extra- and intrahepatic masses, AJR 147:553, 1983.

38. Granato, JE, et al: Utility of two-dimensional echocardiography in suspected ascending aortic dissection, Am J Cardiol 56:123, 1985.

39. Grant, E, et al: Normal inferior vena cava: caliber changes observed by dynamic ultrasound, AJR 135:335, 1980.

40. Hardy, DC, et al: Measurements of the abdominal aortic aneurysms: plain radiograph and ultrasonographic correlation, Radiology 141:821, 1981.

41. Harter, LP, Gross, BH, and Callen, PW: Ultrasonic evaluation of abdominal aortic thrombus, J Ultrasound Med 1:315, 1982.

42. Hertzer, NR, and Beven, EG: Ultrasound aortic measurement and selective aneurysmectomy, JAMA 240:1966, 1978.

43. Hoffman, JC, et al: Pheochromocytoma invasion of the inferior vena cava: sonographic evaluation, Radiology 149:793, 1983.

44. Hoffman, JC, et al: Sonographic demonstration of an anatomic variant of the inferior vena cava, J Ultrasound Med 2:421, 1983.

45. Isikoff, MB, and Hill, MC: Sonography of the renal arteries: left lateral decubitus position, AJR 134:1177, 1980.

46. King, PS, Cooperberg, PL, and Madigan, SM: The anechoic crescent in abdominal aortic aneurysms: not a sign of dissection, AJR 146:345, 1986.

47. Koenigsberg, M, Hoffman, JC, and Schnur, MJ: Sonographic evaluation of the retroperitoneum. In Raymond, HW, and Zwiebel, WJ, editors: Seminars in ultrasound, vol 3, New York, 1982, Grune & Stratton.

48. Kossoff, G: Doppler: its use in the abdomen and pelvis—the leading edge in diagnostic ultrasound [lecture], Atlantic City, NJ, 1987.

49. Kressel, HY, and Filly, RA: Ultrasonographic appearance of gas-containing abscesses in the abdomen, AJR 130:71, 1978.

50. Kumari, S, et al: Gray scale ultrasound evaluation of iliopsoas hematomas in hemophiliacs, AJR 133:103, 1979.

51. Kumari, S, et al: Fluid collections of the psoas in children, Semin Ultrasound 3:139, 1982.

52. Kumari, SS, et al: Occult aortic dissection and diagnosis by ultrasound, Br J Radiol 53:1093, 1980.

53. Kurtz, AB, et al: Ultrasound diagnosis of masses elevating the inferior vena cava, AJR 132:401, 1979.

54. Kutcher, R, et al: Renal angiomyolipoma with sonographic demonstration of extension into the inferior vena cava, Radiology 143:755, 1982.

55. Laing, FC, and Jacobs, RP: Value of ultrasonography in detection of retroperitoneal inflammatory masses, Radiology 123:169, 1977.

56. Lee, TG, and Henderson, SC: Ultrasonic aortography: unexpected findings, AJR 128:273, 1977.

57. Liu, GC, et al: Inferior vena caval filters: noninvasive evaluation, Radiology 160:521, 1986.

58. Loh, C, Atkinson, T, and Halliwell, M: The differentiation of bile ducts and blood vessels using a pulsed Doppler system, Ultrasound Med Biol 4:37, 1978.

59. Makuuchi, M, et al: Primary Budd-Chiari syndrome: ultrasonic demonstration, Radiology 152:775, 1984.

60. Marcus, R, and Edell, SL: Sonographic evaluation of iliac artery aneurysms, Am J Surg 140:666, 1980.

61. McCullough, DL, and Leopold, GR: Diagnosis of retroperitoneal fluid collections by ultrasonography: a series of surgically proved cases, J Urol 115:656, 1976.

62. McDonald, DG: The complete echographic evaluation of solid renal masses, J Clin Ultrasound 6:402, 1978.

63. Menu, Y, et al: Budd-Chiari syndrome: US evaluation, Radiology 157:761, 1985.

64. Messmer, JM, et al: Greenfield caval filters: long-term radiographic follow-up study, Radiology 156:613, 1985.

65. Meyers, MA: Dynamic radiology of the abdomen, New York, 1976, Springer-Verlag.

66. Newman, CH, et al: Clinical value of ultrasonography for the management of non-Hodgkin's lymphoma patients as compared with abdominal computed tomography, J Comput Assist Tomogr 7:666, 1983.

67. Pardes, JG, et al: The oblique coronal view in sonography of the retroperitoneum, AJR 144:1241, 1985.

68. Park, JH, et al: Sonographic evaluation of inferior vena caval obstruction: correlative study with vena cavography, AJR 145:757, 1985.

69. Pasto, ME, et al: The Kimray-Greenfield filter: evaluation by duplex real-time pulsed Doppler ultrasound, Radiology 148:223, 1983.

70. Pavivansalo, MJ, et al: Direct visualization of laminar blood flow in abdominal aorta using real-time ultrasound, J Clin Ultrasound 14:135, 1986.

71. Pera, A, et al: Lymphangiography and CT in the followup of patients with lymphoma, Radiology 164:631, 1987.

72. Poskitt, KJ, et al: Sonography and CT in staging nonseminomatous testicular tumors, AJR 144:939, 1985.

73. Pussel, SJ, and Cosgrove, DO: Ultrasound features of tumor thrombus in the inferior vena cava in retroperitoneal tumor, Br J Radiol 54:866, 1987.

74. Raskin, MM, and Cunningham, JB: Comparison of computed tomography and ultrasound for abdominal aortic aneurysms: a preliminary study, J Comput Assist Tomogr 2:27, 1978.

67 *Computed Tomography and Magnetic Resonance Imaging*

BARBARA E. DEMAS
HEDVIG HRICAK

Computed tomography and magnetic resonance imaging have advanced our knowledge of retroperitoneal anatomy, facilitated diagnosis of retroperitoneal pathology, guided attempts at therapeutic intervention, and allowed evaluation of therapeutic response. These imaging modalities, which combine sensitive soft tissue contrast resolution with sectional morphologic display, are widely available and in routine clinical application. Their importance is such that they have beome procedures of first choice in the evaluation of abdominal and pelvic pathology. The role of these modalities in the evaluation of pancreatic, duodenal, and colonic diseases has been discussed in earlier chapters of this text. Renal and adrenal diseases are outside this chapter's intended area of concentration. Instead we will concentrate attention on the assessment of vascular, lymphatic, and miscellaneous mesenchymal diseases of the retroperitoneal space.

TECHNIQUES OF EXAMINATION
Computed tomography

The details of CT examination technique for evaluation of the retroperitoneum vary slightly with use of different commercial models of scanners, but certain basic principles are common to all units. Generous bowel opacification is critical if misdiagnosis of pseudotumors caused by fluid-filled intestinal loops is to be avoided. Adequate bowel opacification can be achieved by oral administration of 16 to 24 oz of a 2% iodinated contrast solution 30 to 45 minutes before scanning, supplemented by administration of an additional 6 to 8 oz 5 to 10 minutes before scan initiation. Nonenhanced scans may be useful in the assessment of calcific renal and adrenal lesions, ureteral calculi, and suspected hemorrhagic retroperitoneal fluid collections.[19] However, for routine scanning, intravenous contrast enhancement is of tremendous value. It is standard in most radiology departments. For evaluation of an adult patient with normal renal function, intravenous administration of 100 to 150 ml of 60% iodinated contrast material is typical. Use of an automated injection device allows consistent, controlled injection rates. Generally rates of 1.0 to 2.0 ml/

second produce excellent vascular opacification when scanning is performed within the first 1 to 5 minutes after initiation of contrast injection. Incremental dynamic scanning—that is, rapid-sequence scanning with sequential table movement—has become increasingly popular in recent years because it can be performed during the intravenous administration of iodinated contrast material by bolus technique. This combination of scan timing and contrast delivery allows production of images during the period when intravenous concentration of contrast material is maximal, facilitating the demonstration of vascular and perivascular anatomy, delineation of intrarenal anatomy, depiction of pancreatic parenchymal boundaries, and visualization of interfaces between relatively hypervascular inflammatory and neoplastic masses and adjacent normal structures (Fig. 67-1). Modern CT scanners allow selection of individual section scan durations of 5 seconds or less with interscan delay intervals shorter than 10 seconds. To avoid motion artifact when scan times at the upper end of the available range are chosen, it may be necessary to require the patient to suspend respiration during the radiographic exposure. Interscan delays may be lengthened accordingly to allow breathing. For screening purposes sequential sections through the retroperitoneum may be 10 mm in thickness. Detailed evaluation of the pancreas, kidneys or adrenals, or individual vascular structures may require use of 3-

to 5-mm sections. The retroperitoneum is generally examined as a part of a complete abdominal and pelvic CT study, and sequential sections are usually contiguous, a situation mandated by the need for complete evaluation of abdominal and pelvic viscera. However, when the primary reason for examination is to search for retroperitoneal adenopathy, published data indicate that the use of 5- to 10-mm interslice gaps does not greatly degrade information content.

Magnetic resonance imaging

Routine clinical examination of the retroperitoneum with MR techniques involves use of spin echo pulse sequences with both short and long recovery times (TR) and echo delay times (TE) to generate images with tissue contrast dependent on differences in either T_1 and T_2 values. Selection of TR and TE values to produce T_1- and T_2-weighted images (T_1WI, T_2WI) varies depending on the magnetic field strength employed and the options offered by different manufacturer's equipment. For units with moderate field strengths (0.3 to 1.0 Tesla), T_1WI can be generated with TR values of less than 1000 msec and TE values of less than 40 msec. Typically TR/TE combinations of 500 to 600 msec/20 to 30 msec are chosen. T_2WI can be acquired using TR values of 1500 to 2000 msec and TE values of 60 msec or more. When high–field strength imagers are used (1.5 to 2.0 tesla),

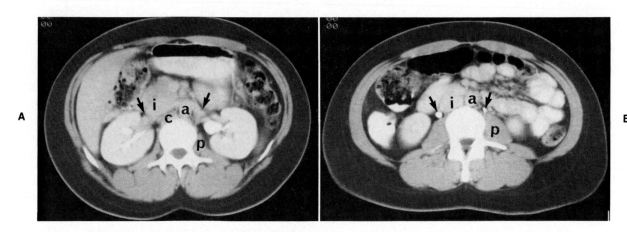

Fig. 67-1 A, Normal anatomy of retroperitoneum at level of kidneys is demonstrated in this CT image obtained at level of hila during administration of iodinated contrast material. Renal parenchyma is fairly densely enhanced, and contrast material has been excreted into collecting structures. Both left and right renal veins *(arrows)* are clearly delineated as they course medially to enter inferior vena cava(i). Left renal vein crosses midline anterior to aorta *(a)*. Kidneys are surrounded by low-density fat, and intrinsic soft tissue contrast is high. Psoas muscles *(p)* and diaphragmatic crura *(c)* are clearly delineated. **B,** Normal retroperitoneal anatomy at slightly more caudal level. Ureters *(arrows)* are imaged as circular structures containing very densely opacified urine. They lie lateral to inferior vena cava *(i)* and aorta *(a)* and anteromedial to psoas muscles *(p)*. Their normal caliber varies with peristaltic motion but is usually symmetric.

T_1 values are prolonged. T_1WI may be produced with TR/TE combinations similar to those employed with low to moderate field systems, but the generation of T_2WI will require additional TR and TE prolongation. TR values of 2000 to 2500 msec and TE values of 70 to 80 msec are preferred.

Initial evaluation of retroperitoneal anatomy is best made with transverse plane images. However, supplemental sagittal or coronal plane scans may be helpful when it is necessary to clarify the spatial relationships of retroperitoneal tumors to intraperitoneal or retroperitoneal viscera, to delineate the cephalad extent of intravenous thrombi or aortic aneurysms, or to confirm subtle structural abnormalities detected in transverse plane im-

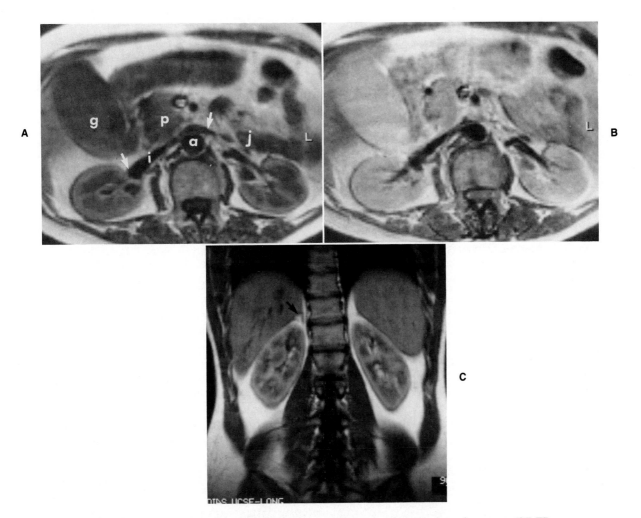

Fig. 67-2 A, Transverse plane MR image demonstrating normal retroperitoneal anatomy (SE TR is 500 msec; TE is 30 msec). Kidneys demonstrate high-intensity peripheral cortex and low-intensity medulla in this T_1-weighted scan. Perinephric fat is of high intensity. Renal veins *(arrows),* IVC *(i),* and aorta *(a)* are free of internal signal. Psoas muscles, quadratus lumborum muscles, and deep musculature of back produce signal of low intensity. Also labeled are pancreatic head *(p),* gallbladder *(g),* and jejeunum *(j).* **B,** T_2-weighted MR image of same patient (SE TR is 2000 msec; TE is 60 msec). Signal intensity of renal medulla and cortex have increased, and contrast between these two areas has decreased; however, visual contrast between kidney, liver, and skeletal muscle has been accentuated. Dark rim adjacent to right kidney's lateral margin and bright rim along left kidney's lateral aspect are chemical shift artifacts in direction of frequency-encoding gradient. **C,** Coronal plane T_1-weighted MR image of normal retroperitoneal viscera (SE TR is 500 msec; TE is 30 msec). Corticomedullary boundaries are well defined. Anatomic relationships between upper poles of kidneys and liver and spleen are demonstrated. Pyramidal shape of right adrenal gland *(arrow)* can be readily appreciated.

ages. T_1WI, which maximize contrast between retroperitoneal organs, lymph nodes, and surrounding fat, are the most useful in the delineation of intrarenal anatomy, detection of adenopathy, and demonstration of retroperitoneal fluid collections. However, T_2WI are valuable for visualization of interfaces between inflammatory and neoplastic masses and viscera, skeletal muscle, and bone cortex. Evaluation of both T_1WI and T_2WI is essential in any attempt at tissue characterization using MRI criteria (Fig. 67-2).

Assessment of vascular anatomy and luminal pathology may require the addition of special techniques to the routine spin echo pulse sequences. For example, synchronization of image acquisition with the systolic phase of the cardiac cycle can minimize signal artifacts caused by slow blood flow. Use of gradient reversal rather than 180-degree refocussing pulses can confirm the presence of flowing blood within a vessel lumen. Evaluation of images designed to demonstrate phase shifts may distinguish a signal caused by stationary thrombus from that caused by slow blood flow.

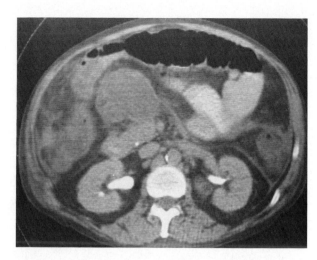

Fig. 67-3 This CT scan, obtained at level of renal hila, shows thickening of perirenal fascia and fluid in anterior pararenal space caused by acute pancreatitis. Pseudocyst is evident in region of pancreatic head.

COMPARTMENTAL ANATOMY OF THE RETROPERITONEAL SPACE

The work of Myers and Whalen, which includes cadaver anatomic studies with detailed anatomic and radiologic correlation, has shown that the retroperitoneum is divided by fascial planes into three major compartments.[59,60,86] These are (1) the anterior pararenal space bounded anteriorly by the parietal peritoneum and posteriorly by Zuckerkandl's fascia, (2) the perirenal space bounded anteriorly by Zuckerkandl's fascia and posteriorly by Gerota's fascia, and (3) the posterior pararenal space limited anteriorly by Gerota's fascia and posteriorly by transversalis fascia. The anterior pararenal space contains the pancreas, second and third portions of the duodenum, and ascending and descending portions of the colon. The perirenal space contains the kidneys, adrenal glands, associated vascular and lymphatic structures, and perinephric fat. The posterior pararenal space contains only fat. The anterior and posterior perirenal fascial layers fuse laterally to form the lateroconal fascia, which then blends with the transversalis fascia. The anterior and posterior pararenal spaces communicate near the iliac fossa below the lower cone of renal fascia, and the right and left perinephric spaces may communicate across the midline.[39] The midline vascular structures, including the aorta and inferior vena cava, provide branches to and receive tributaries from the retroperitoneal and intraperitoneal viscera and may be considered to lie in the perinephric space. The site and completeness of fusion of the perinephric fascial layers is variable, and the location of the lateroconal fascia may be opposite the mid-

portion of the kidney or in a retrorenal location.[48,71] Knowledge of this compartmental fascial anatomy is important in the interpretation of CT and MR images—chiefly in the determination of location, extent, and probable source of retroperitoneal fluid collections[13,40,41,49,65] (Fig. 67-3). Pancreatic effusions, for example, originate in and occupy the anterior pararenal space but may enter the posterior pararenal space at the level of the iliac fossa. If the lateroconal fascia is quite dorsally positioned, anterior pararenal fluid collections may, in cross-sectional images, be seen to extend dorsal to the kidney.[48,71,72] Posterior pararenal fluid collections will alter the CT attenuation and the MR signal intensity of the fat within the anatomic compartment. Perirenal hematomas or urinomas may be limited by fibrous septa running from the renal capsule to the perinephric fascia. Inflammatory and neoplastic processes may thicken fascial sheets and render them more conspicuous in cross-sectional images.[54,64]

ABDOMINAL AORTA
Anatomy

The aorta enters the abdomen through the diaphragmatic aortic hiatus at the level of the lower border of the twelfth thoracic vertebral body. The aortic hiatus, which is formed by the right and left crura connected by the median arcuate ligament, also transmits the thoracic duct and the azygous and hemiazygous veins. The abdominal aorta runs caudally in a left prevertebral position to its point of bifurcation into the common iliac arteries anterior to the fourth lumbar vertebral body. The aorta is in close contact with the right sided inferior vena cava.

Proceeding caudally, the aorta lies immediately dorsal to the aortic and celiac plexi, the pancreas and splenic vein, the left renal vein, the third portion of the duodenum, and the mesenteric root.[87] The origins of its major branches, the celiac, superior mesenteric, renal, inferior mesenteric, and lumbar arteries, are usually visible in transverse plane images. However, the distal portions of these arteries are often tortuous and are seen only segmentally in tomographic sections. The aorta of the normal adult does not exceed 3 cm in diameter in the suprarenal portion. The lumen normally tapers distally.

In CT images the aorta is seen as a round structure which is, in nonenhanced scans, of soft tissue density. In such scans it is impossible to distinguish the boundary of the aortic wall from the adjacent unopacified intraluminal blood. Contrast-enhanced scans increase the visibility of this interface. The aortic wall is normally symmetrically thin and smoothly contoured.

In multiplanar MR images the aorta and its branches are demonstrated as tubular structures free of intraluminal signals. The signal void within vascular lumina is caused by a variety of physical phenomena that are related to the presence of flowing blood and are described as time of flight and phase shift effects. The result of these phenomena is that vascular anatomy is very clearly delineated without a need for administration of exogenous contrast agents. The aortic wall is shown as a thin symmetric structure of low signal intensity. The surrounding retroperitoneal fat is of very high intensity, further accentuating the aortic contour. The origins of the aorta's major branches are visible in transverse-plane MR images. The renal artery origins are well delineated in the coronal plane, whereas those of the celiac, superior mesenteric, and inferior mesenteric arteries are demonstrated in the sagittal plane.

Arteriosclerotic disease

Arteriosclerosis, an idiopathic, progressive disease of arterial walls, is characterized by the deposition of intimal plaques made up of fibroblasts, smooth muscle cells, and lipid material. It causes adventitial fibrosis and degeneration of the internal elastic lamina and media. The clinical effects of these abnormalities are reflected in local arterial occlusions and aneurysm formation.

CT scans demonstrate the presence of arteriosclerosis in the aorta and its major branches chiefly by revealing arterial wall calcification and vascular tortuosity. Contrast-enhanced scans show luminal narrowing caused by wall thickening and may reveal low-density fatty plaques projecting into the column of opacified blood.

MR images in the presence of atherosclerosis show increases in the width of the aortic wall, diminution of luminal caliber, and intimal plaques (Fig. 67-4). The

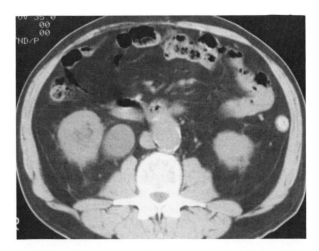

Fig. 67-4 Atherosclerotic disease and abdominal aortic aneurysm. This CT scan shows calcification in aortic wall, dilatation of aortic lumen, and mild compression and deformity of adjacent IVC. Dilated right extrarenal pelvis and proximal ureter are incidentally noted.

plaques themselves are more often visible in MR images than in CT scans, but signal artifacts from abnormally slow or turbulent blood flow may obscure or be confused with mural plaques or thrombi. Synchronization of scan generation with the systolic phase of the cardiac cycle may assist in image interpretation by decreasing flow-related artifacts.

Aortic aneurysms

Aneurysmal dilatation of the abdominal aorta occurs most frequently as a complication of arteriosclerosis, but may be caused as well by antecedent injury or syphilitic or bacterial infection. The abdominal aorta is the most common site of atherosclerotic aneurysm formation. Degeneration of the internal elastic lamina, fragmentation of the elastic tissue of the media, and smooth muscle degeneration decrease the tensile strength of the aortic wall and cause fusiform dilatation and tortuosity. Progressive widening of the aortic lumen may cause a more saccular configuration often associated with deposition of intraluminal thrombus. Abdominal aortic aneurysms are most frequently infrarenal in location. Determination of the presence or absence of dilatation at the origins of the renal and iliac arteries is important for surgical treatment planning. Quantitative measurement of the aortic diameter is essential for diagnosis and can be used to predict prognosis when surgical repair is under debate.

CT images demonstrate the external boundaries of the aortic wall and the fusiform or saccular nature of progressive distal aortic dilatation (Fig. 67-4). Contrast-enhanced scans often reveal peripheral luminal thrombi which are crescent shaped and low in density.[50] The diameter of the patent portion of the vascular lumen can be easily appreciated. The distinction of aortic aneurysm from aortic dissection is usually simple.[32] An aortic aneurysm is characterized by the presence of a dilated, thin-walled vessel with a single, round, residual lumen. Transverse diameter and wall thickness are proportionally increased, and heavy wall calcification may be present. An aortic dissection produces the appearance of two opacified lumina, the native lumen being deformed in contour with one flat wall. Differential enhancement rates are observed between the true and false lumena. High-density clotting may be seen at multiple levels. Wall thickness is disporportionately increased as compared with luminal diameter, and central calcification may be present.

CT scans are more sensitive than arteriograms in the detection of aortic aneurysms, because arteriograms, showing only the patent part of the lumen, may underestimate dilatation.[3,11,17,20,44] CT images reliably document the relationships of the cephalic and caudal limits of aneurysms to the renal and iliac arteries. However, CT is less likely than arteriography to demonstrate the presence of multiple renal arteries.[63] Although CT can be employed for diagnosis, arteriography remains important for surgical treatment planning.[20,63]

The ability of MRI to define aneurysmal dimensions and renal artery origins in the transverse plane is comparable with that of CT.[1,2,25,44] MRI allows direct acquisition of coronal and sagittal plane images, which may provide better delineation of multiple renal arteries. Use of cardiac gating or phase images may be helpful in separating flow artifacts from intraluminal thrombus. Crescentic mural thrombi will be of low to medium signal intensity on T_1WI, contrasting with the signal void of the patent portion of the lumen. Lee et al. compared measurements of MR-imaged aneurysm diameter in 20 patients and found that aneurysmal dimensions in MRI fell within 5 mm of those obtained sonographically.[44] Wall thickening and atheromatous plaques are generally present, but wall calcification may be difficult to detect unless it is massive.

PROSTHETIC AORTIC GRAFTS
Normal anatomy

When incorporated into the retroperitoneum, prosthetic aortic grafts appear in CT scans as well-defined tubular structures with very–high density walls. Their position and that of the native aorta vary with the chosen route of surgical anastomosis. End-to-side prosthesis to native aorta anastamoses are common. In this situation transverse-plane images show that the native aorta remains intact and in normal position. The graft lies ventral to the native aorta, and its proximal terminus blends into the anterior aortic wall below the renal arteries. End-to-end anastomoses require that the native aorta be transected, the aneurysm resected, and the distal portion of the native aorta oversewn. The native aorta then appears as a discrete, rounded density dorsal to the graft. The cephalad portion of the graft is continuous with the proximal native aorta. When vessel size and surrounding fibrosis prevent aneurysm resection, the prosthetic graft may be placed within the native aneurysmal lumen. In this case the calcified aortic wall and mural thrombus will surround the dense margins of the prosthesis.[51]

Vascular prosthesis infection may occur early or late in the postoperative period. Reilly et al. have reported a series of 92 patients who developed graft infections at intervals ranging from 3 days to 17 years after surgery.[67] CT manifestations of graft infections include perigraft fluid collections and gas in the surrounding soft tissue (Fig. 67-5). Diagnosis in the early postoperative period is difficult; hematoma and edema may normally persist for several weeks. Mark et al. stated that detection of perigraft fluid more than 6 weeks postoperatively or gas collections more than 2 weeks postoperatively should suggest infection.[51,52]

Aortic prosthetic grafts appear in MRI as tubular structures with low-intensity walls free of intraluminal signals (Fig. 67-6). Anatomic relationships of grafts to native vessels are familiar from knowledge of CT findings. Graft infections are signalled by the presence of surrounding fluid collections.[38] However, fluid may normally be present for several weeks postoperatively, and clinical data must be coordinated with imaging findings. MRI does not routinely detect perigraft gas collections, since it cannot distinguish such gas collections from mural calcification.

INFERIOR VENA CAVA

The inferior vena cava (IVC) begins at the junction of the common iliac veins anterior to the fifth lumbar vertebral body and ascends in a right prevertebral location in close contact with the aorta. It passes between the right and caudate lobes of the liver and traverses the caval diaphragmatic hiatus at the level of the eighth thoracic vertebral body. Just above the diaphragm it drains into the right atrium. The inferior vena cava receives venous drainage from the lower extremities, abdominal wall, pelvic, abdominal, and retroperitoneal viscera. It lies ventral to the right renal and adrenal arteries and the right adrenal gland; medial to the right kidney and ureter; and dorsal to the pancreatic head, second and third portions of the duodenum, portal vein, small bowel mesentery, and right common iliac artery.[12,82]

In CT images the IVC is evident as a tubular structure (circular in cross section) in a right paramedian location

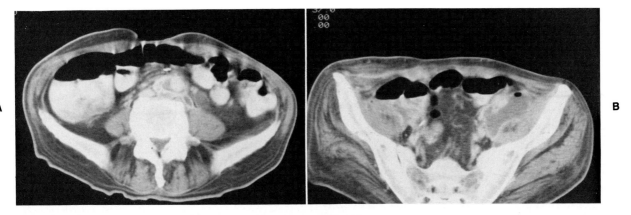

Fig. 67-5 A, Lumen of prosthetic aortic graft is opacified, and low-density fluid collection surrounds graft in this scan demonstrating graft infection. Inflammatory tissue infiltrating region of graft enhances fairly densely. **B,** Fluid collection surrounding left iliac limb of graft contains pocket of gas—a sign of abscess formation if present more than 2 weeks after surgery.

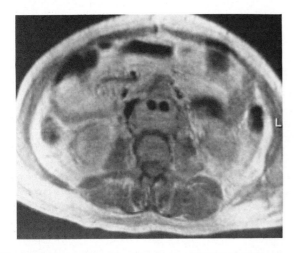

Fig. 67-6 Transverse plane MR image (SE TR is 2000 msec; TE is 30 msec) of aortic prosthesis. Graft limbs are tubular and free of internal signal. Fluid- or thrombus-filled native aorta surrounds prosthetic graft.

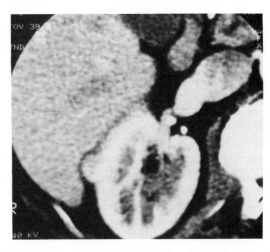

Fig. 67-7 CT scan obtained with first minute of intravenous contrast injection shows dense enhancement of renal cortex with dramatic demonstration of corticomedullary boundary. Small mass arises from lateral cortex of kidney. This tumor is stage 1 renal cell carcinoma. Laminar flow of opacified blood from renal veins causes peripheral high and central low density in IVC. This is an artifact commonly seen during incremental dynamic scanning and should not be mistaken for tumor thrombus.

anterior to the spine. Sites of iliac vessel and renal vein entry are routinely well delineated. The diameter of the IVC is extremely variable with phase of inspiration and may be markedly dilated during a Valsalva maneuver. IVC opacification is easily accomplished during contrast-enhanced dynamic scanning. However, care must be taken to avoid confusion of central low-density defects caused by laminar flow of contrast-opacified blood from the renal veins with true intraluminal thrombi (Fig. 67-7). Such artifacts may be encountered following either arm or foot vein contrast injections and may be eliminated by combining dynamic scanning with delayed images in the region of the suprarenal IVC.[4,81]

Congenital anomalies of the IVC

The embryologic development of the inferior vena cava occurs by means of appearance and regression of three paired venous systems, the posterior cardinal, subcardinal, and supracardinal veins. The posterior cardinal veins develop first, followed by the subcardinal veins, which gradually take over their drainage. The right hepatic vein anastamoses with the right subcardinal vein. The supracardinal veins located dorsal to the subcardinal veins anastamose with the subcardinal veins to form the renal segment of the IVC. The caudal portion of the right supracardinal vein becomes the prerenal segment of the IVC. The cranial portions of the supracardinal veins become the azygous system. The posterior cardinal veins and caudal portion of the left supracardinal vein disappear during the course of normal embryonic development.

Failure of the hepatic-subcardinal anastomosis results in absence of the intrahepatic portion of the IVC with continuation of venous drainage to the heart via the azygous-hemizygous system. Failure of resorption of the left supracardinal vein results in IVC duplication. Persistence of the left supracardinal vein with resorption of the right supracardinal vein causes IVC transposition.

These congenital variants of IVC anatomy are visible in both CT and MR images.[28,35,55,70] With interruption of the hepatic portion of the IVC and azygous continuation of venous drainage the lumen of the IVC is not visible between the caudate and right lobes of the liver and the lumina of the azygous and hemizygous veins are grossly dilated (Fig. 67-8). These vessels are best seen in their retrocrural locations. In IVC duplication tubular venous structures are visible on either side of the aorta. The left-sided IVC is often the larger of the two. It crosses the midline at the level of the renal vessels and enters the right IVC, which ascends as a single vessel into the liver. In IVC transposition a single left-sided IVC crosses the midline at the renal hilar level and ascends into the liver to the right of the spine. These anomalies are best appreciated in contrast-enhanced CT images. In nonenhanced scans a left-sided IVC imaged in cross section may resemble a paraaortic lymph node. Scrutiny of sequential sections clarifies the tubular rather than nodular configuration of the aberrant vessel. The anatomic abnormalities evident in contrast-enhanced CT images are readily seen in MR images in which vessels are conspicuous by their absence of internal signal.

Venous thrombosis

Thrombosis within the IVC prevents luminal opacification and may partially or totally occlude blood flow (Fig. 67-9). If the IVC lumen is severely compromised, dilated retroperitoneal collateral vessels will be apparent.[62] It is not generally possible to distinguish tumor thrombus from blood clot in CT images in the absence of clinical history.[53] Both types of thrombus are of heterogeneous density in nonenhanced scans.[31] Tumor thrombus is more likely than blood clot to cause IVC widening. Intravascular tumors may be enhanced by contrast.

MRI shows both tumor thrombus and blood clot as focal sites of intraluminal signal in the IVC. Both tend to emit a low-intensity signal in T_1WI and a high-intensity

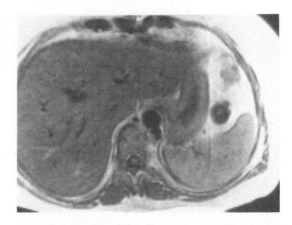

Fig. 67-8 Transverse plane MR image (SE, T_1-weighted cardiac gated) of upper abdomen in patient with interruption of inferior vena cava in its intrahepatic portion and continuation of venous drainage from infrarenal portion of IVC through azygous and hemizygous veins. Note absence of intrahepatic IVC lumen and dilatation of retrocrural portions of azygous and hemiazygous veins.

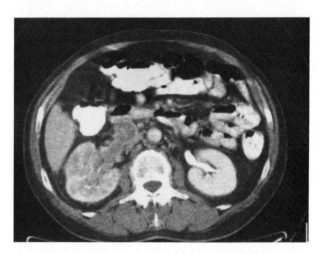

Fig. 67-9 Thrombotic occlusion of IVC and right renal vein. Lumina of these vessels are occupied by clot of variable—but predominantly low—density. Right kidney is swollen, and parenchymal enhancement is patchy. Excretion of contrast material is delayed in right kidney.

signal in T_2WI. Tumor thrombus may resemble primary tumor in its signal-intensity pattern with TR/TE variation and may be heterogeneous in appearance. If occlusion is only partial, it may be possible to identify normal patterns of blood flow in the patent portion of the IVC lumen (Fig. 67-10). The advantages of MRI in the assessment of venous thrombosis are its lack of need for exogenous contrast and its multiplanar capability, which facilitates delineation of the cephalad extent of thrombus.

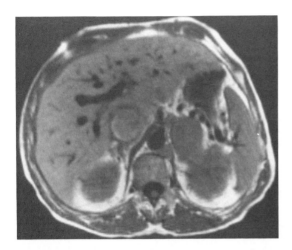

Fig. 67-10 Transverse plane MR image (SE TR is 500 msec; TE is 30 msec) of patient with stage 3A renal cell carcinoma. Large mass arises from left kidney. Tumor thrombus produces signal within lumen of left renal vein and IVC. High-intensity signal in IVC periphery is caused by slowly flowing blood in patent part of lumen.

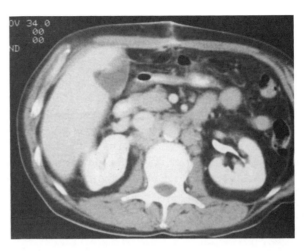

Fig. 67-11 Lobulated soft tissue masses surround the aorta and elevate IVC in this patient with non-Hodgkin's lymphoma involving retroperitoneal lymph nodes.

LYMPHATIC SYSTEM

The lymphatic structures of the retroperitoneum include the lumbar trunks that receive drainage from the lower extremities, lower abdominal wall, genitourinary structures of the pelvis, distal small bowel and colon, superficial and deep efferent lymph vessels, and associated lymph nodes. The lumbar trunks are paraaortic in location. They empty into the cisterna chyli, which lies at the level of the first two lumbar vertebral bodies between the aorta and the azygous vein. The superficial and deep lymphatic vessels are not visible in either CT or MR images. The lymph nodes that lie along the courses of and receive drainage from the lymph vessels are often visible even if not enlarged—and particularly if they are surrounded by retroperitoneal fat. In the pelvis lymph nodes are found anterior, lateral, and medial to the external iliac artery, and caudal to the external iliac vein adjacent to the pelvic side wall. External iliac nodes drain the inguinal nodes, the anterior abdominal wall, and the pelvic viscera. Internal iliac nodes receive lymphatic drainage from the pelvic viscera, perineum, and deep gluteal region. Obturator nodes, which lie adjacent to the obturator vessels, receive efferent drainage from the genitourinary organs of the pelvis.[57] Progressive drainage from these nodal groups is into the common iliac and paraaortic chains. Lymphatic drainage from the testes parallels venous drainage. The right testicular nodal drainage is to right paraaortic nodes at the level of the renal hilum. The left testis's lymphatic drainage is to a nodal group at the level of the left renal vein. Normal lymph nodes are ovoid and normally vary in size from about 1 mm to 25 mm in diameter, the larger nodes being found in the inguinal regions.[87]

Before the introduction of CT, radiographic evaluation of retroperitoneal lymph node abnormalities required performance of bipedal lymphangiography. This procedure remains valuable in the assessment of internal morphology of retroperitoneal nodes. However, mesenteric, peripancreatic, obturator, hepatic and splenic hilar, and retrocrural lymph nodes are not opacified by bipedal lymphangiographic techniques. Both CT and MRI can demonstrate the presence of normal-sized and enlarged lymph nodes in the pelvic, paraaortic, retrocrural, and intraabdominal locations. CT has assumed an important role in the detection of abdominal and pelvic lymph node enlargement. MRI has been of value in the detection of lymph node enlargement for the staging of genitourinary tumors.

In CT images lymph nodes are visible as rounded structures of soft tissue attenuation lying in perivascular locations. Nodes are more conspicuous if they are surrounded by fat, and detection of retroperitoneal adenopathy can be difficult in emaciated patients. Delineation of pelvic lymph nodes and distinction of nodes from tortuous vessels are facilitated by vascular opacification. CT criteria for lymph node abnormality are based on size. Retrocrural lymph nodes are said to be abnormal when they exceed 6 mm in diameter. Abdominal and paraaortic nodes are believed to be enlarged when their diameters are greater than 15 mm (Fig. 67-11). Deep pelvic nodes are enlarged if they exceed 12 mm in diameter. Radiologists using these size criteria have reported accuracies of 70% to 90% in the detection of lymph node metastases from prostatic, cervical, and bladder carcinomas, and abdominal lymphomas.* CT cannot reliably distinguish benign from malignant causes of lymph node enlargement, although clinical data and the detection of characteristic abnormalities in other organs may increase diagnostic accuracy.[10,37,46,58] CT images may reveal changes in lymph node size and attenuation during response to chemotherapy, and CT is routinely employed in posttreatment examination of patients with lymphomas and testicular neoplasms. Although decreases in the density and homogeneity of lymph node masses may accompany tumor necrosis, a decrease in size remains the most reliable evidence of therapeutic response.[61]

In T_1-weighted MR images lymph nodes appear as rounded structures of medium signal intensity surrounded by high-intensity fat or adjacent to the signal and void of retroperitoneal or pelvic vessels. Lymph nodes increase in signal intensity in T_2WI, and contrast between nodes and skeletal muscle is optimal in such scans. MRI is similar to CT in its ability to delineate lymph nodes, although with its lesser spatial resolution, it may overestimate the sizes of nodes lying in conglomerate masses. MRI criteria for nodal disease rest in size measurements (Fig. 67-12). Differences in T_2 values between normal and pathologic nodes have been reported, but overlap between T_2 values of normal, hyperplastic, and neoplastic nodes has been great.[14] MRI accuracy has been comparable to that reported for CT in the evaluation of nodal metastases from prostatic, cervical, endometrial, bladder, and renal malignancies.[17,33,34,36,88]

Retroperitoneal hemorrhage

Hemorrhage into the retroperitoneal space may occur as a result of relatively minor trauma in patients receiving anticoagulant therapy, or it may be caused by surgery, translumbar aortography, renal biopsy, major blunt or penetrating trauma, or aortic aneurysmal rupture.** CT features of retroperitoneal hematoma include a fairly dense mass lesion which infiltrates retroperitoneal fat, displaces retroperitoneal viscera, enlarges psoas or iliacus muscles or obscures aortic outlines.[6,27,74] Nonenhanced scans are helpful in distinguishing hemorrhagic collections of high density from urinomas of water density (Figs. 67-13 and 67-14).

Hemorrhage caused by excessive anticoagulation or by aortic rupture most often occupies the posterior para-

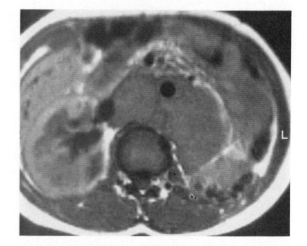

Fig. 67-12 Transverse plane MR image (SE TR is 500 msec; TE is 30 msec) reveals bulky adenopathy surrounding aorta and elevating it from spine. IVC is displaced. Left kidney is absent; patient had undergone radical left nephrectomy for renal cell carcinoma. Adenopathy represents recurrent retroperitoneal tumor.

renal space. However, if hematoma volume is large, any or all of the retroperitoneal compartments may be affected. Localized hematoma in the perirenal space has been reported in cases of aneurysmal rupture.[7] Retroperitoneal hematomas initially appear more dense than skeletal muscle, but their CT attenuation decreases, as does their size, during the several-day period of resolution.[6]

The MRI appearance of hemorrhage into the retroperitoneal space varies with TR/TE and with hematoma age. Hemorrhagic collection less than 4 to 7 days old will be of an intensity similar to skeletal muscle in T_1WI. Progressive T_1 shortening causes an increase in signal intensity after that period, although central portions of blood collections may remain of low intensity. In T_2WI both subacute and chronic hematomas emit a high-intensity signal near the intensity of fat.

Retroperitoneal fibrosis

Retroperitoneal fibrosis may be idiopathic or associated with primary or metastatic malignant retroperitoneal neoplasms. It produces clinical effects by causing ureteral obstruction or, more rarely, by causing compression of mesenteric vessels, aorta, IVC, duodenum, or bile ducts. CT images reveal either a bulky retroperitoneal mass (similar in appearance to retroperitoneal adenopathy, hemorrhage, or mesenchymal neoplasm) or a plaque-like sheet of tissue that encases the ureters, IVC, and aorta.[5,8,9,23,73] Fibrotic tissue within the retroperitoneal

---

*References 15, 16, 30, 42, 43, 45, 47, 56, 66, 78, 83.
**References 7, 21, 22, 27, 69, 75-77.

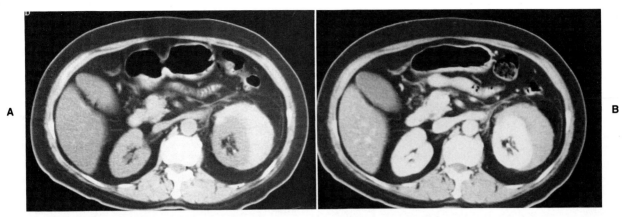

Fig. 67-13 A, Left-sided subcapsular hematoma appears of relatively high density as compared with renal tissue in this nonenhanced CT scan. Density of subcapsular collection suggests hematoma rather than urinoma as appropriate diagnosis, since unopacified urine would be intermediate in density between renal tissue and surrounding fat. Clear confinement of collection and compression rather than displacement of kidney are signs that hematoma is subcapsular and not perinephric in location. **B,** After administration of intravenous contrast material, enhancement of renal parenchyma causes reversal of relative densities of kidney and subcapsular blood.

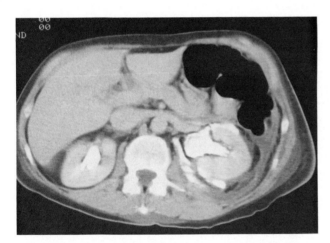

Fig. 67-14 Urinoma caused by intraoperative ureteral injury. Unopacified urine infiltrates both anterior and posterior pararenal spaces, and opacified urine extravasated during time of CT scanning surrounds renal pelvis and enters perinephric space.

mass may enhance dramatically during administration of iodinated contrast material.[73,80] Displacement of the aorta and IVC is unusual, but vascular encasement is typical. A definitive diagnosis may require a biopsy because radiographic features overlap with those of a variety of retroperitoneal tumors and because fibrosis and neoplasms may coexist.

The MRI appearance of retroperitoneal fibrosis varies with the proportions of fibrotic tissue and associated inflammatory reaction. If the proportion of fibrous tissue is high, the characteristically short T_2 value of such tissue will cause the emitted signal to be of low intensity. Bulky masses and dense plaques have been reported. Vascular encasement may be appreciated without the use of ex-

ogenous contrast agents. MRI cannot distinguish idiopathic retroperitoneal fibrosis from that associated with a metastatic neoplasm.

Retroperitoneal sarcomas

A variety of mesenchymal tumors may arise from tissues of the retroperitoneum. The majority are malignant. The most common of these tumors are liposarcomas, leiomyosarcomas, malignant fibrous histiocytomas, rhabdomyosarcomas, and malignant teratomas. Liposarcomas are the most frequently encountered of these neoplasms. Their CT features vary with histologic characteristics.[26,82] Poorly differentiated tumors contain little or no visible fatty tissue, and CT scans show a solid mass

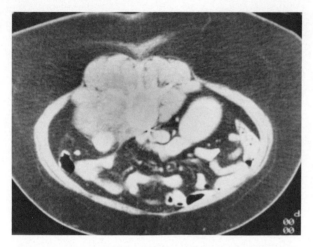

Fig. 67-15 Primary retroperitoneal liposarcoma. Mass of heterogeneous density involves left psoas and quadrants lumborum muscles and invades deep musculature of back. It abuts vertebral body and (at different level) was noted to invade spine. It encases and obstructs left ureter. Although this is most frequently detected of retroperitoneal sarcoma tissue types, one cannot distinguish it on basis of CT criteria from other primary and metastatic soft tissue neoplasms.

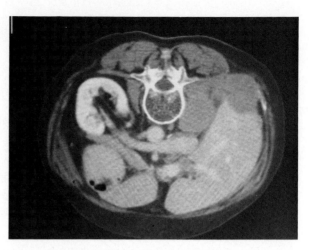

Fig. 67-16 Melanoma metastatic to right renal fossa. Lobulated mass of attenuation similar to that of adjacent psoas muscle invades posterior abdominal wall and indents right lobe of liver. This is a locally recurrent lesion in patient who had undergone right nephrectomy 2 years earlier for metastatic melanoma.

of soft tissue density (Fig. 67-15). Tissue necrosis, cyst formation, or minimal fatty content will cause heterogeneity of density with focal sites of low attenuation. Calcification may be present. Tumor boundaries are generally indistinct, and invasion of skeletal muscle, retroperitoneal organs, and major vessels is common. Use of dynamic scanning techniques with rapid infusion of contrast material may accentuate tumor interfaces with skeletal muscle or viscera and will delineate vascular anatomy. Retroperitoneal sarcomas are often greater than 10 cm in diameter at the time of diagnosis, so determination of the site of tumor origin can be difficult. Signs of retroperitoneal origin include anterior displacement of the IVC, portal vein, kidney, or duodenum.[18] Although diagnostic probabilities can be estimated on the basis of tumor prevalence, it is generally impossible to distinguish poorly differentiated or mixed liposarcomas from other types of sarcomas or from certain metastatic tumors on the basis of radiographic findings (Fig. 67-16). CT is appropriately performed for preoperative staging, while a biopsy is required for histologic diagnosis.

Although only a small number of retroperitoneal sarcomas have been described in the MRI literature, experience gained with truncal and extremity sarcomas indicates that sensitive soft tissue contrast resolution and multiplanar display will facilitate tumor staging.[9a] MRI provides clear delineation of tumor boundaries with skeletal muscle, liver, kidney, and spleen (Fig. 67-17). It demonstrates tumor vascularity and documents major

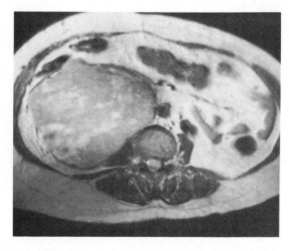

Fig. 67-17 Transverse plane MR image (TR is 2000 msec; TE is 80 msec) of primary retroperitoneal liposarcoma. Large mass lies on right paraspinal location. It emits signal of high but heterogeneous intensity. It displaces and occludes in IVC. Collateral venous drainage from pelvis occurs through dilated gonadal vein.

vessel encasement. It does not delineate peritoneal, mesenteric, or bowel implants reliably or clearly.

PSOAS MUSCLES

The paired psoas muscles originate at the transverse processes of the twelfth thoracic vertebral bodies and insert on the lesser trochanters of the femurs. Because they pass behind the arcuate ligament of the diaphragm, the psoas muscles provide a route of communication between the thorax, retroperitoneum, pelvis, and thigh. These muscles are covered by dense fascia and so constitute discrete anatomic compartments. Psoas abscesses may occur as a result of infection in the vertebral column, as a result of aortic graft infection, as a complication of renal transplantation, or as a consequence of duodenal or colonic disease. Psoas abscesses cause enlargement in muscular contour and a decrease in the muscle's density. In the absence of obvious fluid and air collections it is not possible to distinguish an abscess from a phlegmon within the psoas muscle. A psoas hematoma can simulate abscess or tumor.[24,68] Extension of retroperitoneal primary or metastatic neoplasms may distort psoas contour and alter psoas attenuation.

The normal psoas muscles emit low-intensity signals on both T_1 and T_2-weighted images. They are clearly distinguished from high-intensity retroperitoneal fat and from the vertebral column. Fat planes between the psoas, quadrants lumborum, and iliacus muscles are readily discriminated. Contrast between the psoas and the adjacent kidney is maximal on T_2-weighted images.

Psoas abscess formation raises the intensity and enlarges the contour of the muscle.[85] Adjacent inflammatory disease, such as that seen in rejection of a renal allograft in the iliac fossa or in an appendiceal abscess, also raises psoas signal intensity. These abnormalities are conspicuous on T_2-weighted images. A psoas hematoma causes contour abnormality but is similar in intensity to normal muscle in T_1-weighted images obtained immediately after injury. Progressive T_1 shortening during hematoma resolution will lead to production of a strong signal on T_1- and T_2-weighted images after several days.

GENERAL CONSIDERATIONS

The excellent soft tissue contrast resolution and tomographic image production offered by CT and MRI have simplified noninvasive evaluation of retroperitoneal anatomy and pathology. CT at the current state of technology offers rapid, convenient, reliable production of high-quality images and can be used to evaluate anatomy in all parts of the body. These practical features are of great advantage, particularly when the retroperitoneum is to be evaluated as a part of a total body screening (as for metastatic disease from a known malignancy). MRI provides direct multiplanar imaging, which may resolve anatomic questions raised by transverse plane CT images. MRI does not require the use of exogenous contrast agents for assessment of arterial and venous anatomy. The dramatic tissue contrast provided in T_1- and T_2-weighted MR images may allow discrimination of tissue interfaces that are indistinct in CT scans. The two mo-

dalities are equivalent in their ability to detect and characterize lymphadenopathy. Because MRI is more time consuming and more costly, it must be used in a more carefully targeted fashion than CT would require. MRI remains in a state of rapid technical development, and comparison of the values of CT and MRI may be premature.

REFERENCES

1. Amparo, EG, et al: Magnetic resonance imaging of aortic disease: preliminary results, AJR 143:1203, 1984.
2. Amparo, EG, et al: Comparison of magnetic resonance imaging and ultrasonography in the evaluation of abdominal aortic aneurysms, Radiology 154:451, 1985.
3. Axelbaum, SP, et al: Computed tomography evaluation of aortic aneurysms, AJR 127:75, 1976.
4. Barnes, PA, Bernardino, ME, and Thomas, JL: Flow phenomenon mimicking thrombus: a possible pitfall of the pedal infusion technique, J Comput Assist Tomogr 6:304, 1982.
5. Breen, B, et al: CT in retroperitoneal fibrosis, AJR 137:535-538, 1981.
6. Cisternino, SJ, Neiman, HL, and Malave, SR, Jr: Diagnosis of retroperitoneal hemorrhage by serial computed tomography, J Comput Assist Tomogr 3:686, 1979.
7. Clayton, MJ, Walsh, JW, and Brewer, WH. Contained rupture of abdominal aortic aneurysms: sonographic and CT diagnosis, AJR 138:154, 1982.
8. Dalla-Palma, L, et al: Computed tomography in the diagnosis of retroperitoneal fibrosis, Urol Radiol 3:77, 1981.
9. Degesys, GE, et al: Retroperitoneal fibrosis: use of CT in distinguishing among possible causes, AJR 146:57, 1986.
9a. Demas, BE, et al: Soft tissue sarcomas of the extremities: comparison of MR and CT in determining the extent of disease, AJR 150:615g, 1988.
10. Deutch, SJ, Sandler, MA, and Alpern, MB: Abdominal lymphadenopathy in benign diseases: CT detection, Radiology 163:335, 1987.
11. Dixon, AK, et al: Computed tomography (CT) of abdominal aortic aneurysms determination of longitudinal extent, Br J Surg 68:47, 1981.
12. Dlugy, RC, and Gittes, RF: The adrenals. In Walsh, PC, et al, editors: Campbell's urology, Philadelphia, 1986, WB Saunders.
13. Dodds, WJ, et al: The retroperitoneal spaces revisited, AJR 147:1155, 1986.
14. Dooms, GC, et al: Characterization of lymphadenopathy by magnetic resonance relaxation times: preliminary results, Radiology 155:691, 1985.
15. Dunnick, NR, and Javaslpour, N: Value of CT and lymphography: distinguishing retroperitoneal metastases from nonseminomatous testicular tumors, AJR 136:1093, 1981.
16. Ehrlichman, RJ, et al: Computerized tomography and lymphangiography in staging testis tumors, J Urol 126:179, 1980.
17. Ellis, HH, et al: Comparison of NMR and CT imaging in the evaluation of metastatic retroperitoneal lymphadenopathy from testicular carcinoma, J Comput Assist Tomogr 8:709, 1985.
18. Engel, IA, et al: Large posterior abdominal masses: computed tomographic localization, Radiology 149:203, 1984.
19. Englestad, B, McClennan, BL, and Levitt, RG: The role of precontrast images in CT of the kidney, Radiology 136:153, 1980.
20. Eriksson, I, et al: Preoperative evaluation of abdominal aortic aneurysms: is there a need for aortography? Acta Chir Scand 147:533, 1981.

21. Federle, MP, et al: Evaluation of abdominal trauma by computed tomography, Radiology 138:637, 1981.

22. Federle, MP, et al: Computed tomography in blunt abdominal trauma, Arch Surg 117:654, 1982.

23. Feinstein, RS, et al: Computerized tomography in the diagnosis of retroperitoneal fibrosis, J Urol 126:255, 1981.

24. Feldberg, MA, Koehler, PR, and Van Waes, PFGM: Psoas compartment disease studied by computed tomography, Radiology 148:505, 1983.

25. Flak, B, et al: Magnetic resonance imaging of the abdominal aorta, AJR 144:991, 1985.

26. Friedman, AC, et al: Computed tomography of abdominal fatty masses, Radiology 139:415, 1981.

27. Gavant, ML, Salazar, JE, and Ellis, J: Intrarenal rupture of the abdominal aorta: CT features, J Comput Assist Tomogr 10:516, 1986.

28. Ginaldi, S, Chuang, VP, and Wallace, S: Absence of hepatic segment of the inferior vena cava with azygous continuation, J Comput Assist Tomogr 4:112, 1980.

29. Glazer, GM, Callen, PW, and Parker, JI: CT diagnosis of tumor thrombus in the inferior vena cava: avoiding the false positive diagnosis, AJR 137:1265, 1981.

30. Glazer, GM, et al: Computed tomographic detection of retroperitoneal adenopathy, Radiology 143:147, 1982.

31. Glazer, GM, et al: Computed tomography of renal vein thrombosis, J Comput Assist Tomogr 8:288, 1984.

32. Heiberg, E, et al: CT characteristics of aortic atherosclerotic aneurysm versus aortic dissection, J Comput Assist Tomogr 9:78, 1985.

33. Hricak, H, and Sandles, LG: Invasive cervical carcinoma: comparison of MR imaging and surgical findings, Radiology 166:623, 1988.

34. Hricak, H, Stern, J, and Fisher, MR: MRI in the evaluation of endometrial carcinoma and its staging, Radiology 162:297, 1987.

35. Hricak, H, et al: Abdominal venous system: assessment using MR, Radiology 156:415, 1985.

36. Hricak, H, et al: Prostatic carcinoma: staging by clinical assessment, CT, and MR imaging, Radiology 162:231, 1987.

37. Jones, B, et al: Lymphadenopathy in celiac disease computed tomographic observations, AJR 142:1127, 1984.

38. Justich, E, et al: Infected aortoiliofemoral grafts: magnetic resonance imaging, Radiology 154:133, 1985.

39. Kneeland, JB, et al: Perirenal spaces: CT evidence for communication across the midline, Radiology 164:657, 1987.

40. Kunin, M: Bridging septa of the paranephric space: anatomic, pathologic, and diagnostic considerations, Radiology 158:361, 1986.

41. Laor, E, et al: On percutaneous drainage of retroperitoneal fluid collections: when is primary surgical drainage preferable? Urology 26:114, 1985.

42. Lee, JKT, et al: Accuracy of computed tomography in detecting abdominal and pelvic adenopathy in lymphoma, AJR 131:311, 1978.

43. Lee, JKT, et al: Accuracy of CT in detecting intraabdominal and pelvic lymph node metastases from pelvic cancers, AJR 131:675, 1978.

44. Lee, JKT, et al: Magnetic resonance imaging of abdominal aortic aneurysms, AJR 143:1197, 1984.

45. Levine, MS, et al: Detecting lymphatic metastases from prostatic carcinoma: superiority of CT, AJR 137:207, 1981.

46. Li, DKB, and Rennie, CS: Abdominal computed tomography in Whipple's disease, J Comput Assist Tomogr 5:249, 1981.

47. Lien, HH, et al: Comparison of computed tomography, lymphography, and phlebography in 200 consecutive patients with regard to retroperitoneal metastases from testicular tumor, Radiology 146:129, 1983.

48. Love, L, Demos, TC, and Pasniak, H: CT of retrorenal fluid collections, AJR 145:87, 1986.

49. Love, L, et al: Computed tomography of extraperitoneal spaces, AJR 136:781, 1981.

50. Machida, K, and Tasaka, A: CT patterns of mural thrombus in aortic aneurysms, J Comput Assist Tomogr 4:840, 1980.

51. Mark, A, et al: CT evaluation of complications of abdominal aortic surgery, Radiology 145:409, 1982.

52. Mark, AS, et al: Detection of abdominal aortic graft infection: comparison of CT and in-labeled white blood cell scans, AJR 144:315, 1985.

53. Marks, WM, et al: CT diagnosis of tumor thrombosis of the renal vein and inferior vena cava, AJR 131:843, 1978.

54. Marx, WJ, and Patel, SK: Renal fascia: its radiographic importance, Urology 13:1, 1979.

55. Mayo, J, et al: Anomalies of the inferior vena cava, AJR 140:339, 1983.

56. McCullough, DL, Prout, GR, and Daly, JS: Carcinoma of the prostate and lymphatic metastases, J Urol 111:65, 1974.

57. McLaughlin, AP, et al: Prostatic carcinoma: incidence and location of unsuspected lymphatic metastases, J Urol 115:89, 1976.

58. Meranze, S, et al: Sarcoidosis on computed tomography, J Comput Assist Tomogr 9:50, 1985.

59. Meyers, MA: Dynamic radiology of the abdomen: normal and pathologic anatomy, Berlin, 1976, Springer-Verlag.

60. Meyers, MA, et al: Radiologic features of extraperitoneal effusions: an anatomic approach, Radiology 104:249, 1972.

61. Oliver, TW, Bernardino, ME, and Sones, PJ: Monitoring the response of lymphoma patients to therapy: correlation of abdominal CT findings with clinical course histologic reel type, Radiology 149:219, 1983.

62. Pagani, JJ, Thomas, JL, and Bernardino, ME: Computed tomographic manifestations of abdominal and pelvic venous collaterals, Radiology 142:415, 1982.

63. Papanicolaou, N, et al: Preoperative evaluation of abdominal aortic aneurysms by computed tomography, AJR 146:711, 1986.

64. Parienty, RA, et al: Visibility and thickening of the renal fascia on computed tomograms, Radiology 139:119.

65. Raptopoulos, V, et al: Renal facial pathways: posterior extension of pancreatic effusions within the pararenal space, Radiology 158:367, 1986.

66. Redman, HC, et al: Computed tomography as an adjunct in the staging of Hodgkin's disease and non-Hodgkin's lymphomas, Radiology 124:381, 1977.

67. Reilly, LM, et al: Late results following surgical management of vascular graft infections, J Vasc Surg 1:36, 1984.

68. Rolls, PW, et al: CT of inflammatory disease of the psoas muscle, AJR 134:767, 1980.

69. Rosen, A, et al: CT diagnosis of ruptured abdominal aortic aneurysm, AJR 143:265, 1984.

70. Royal, SA, and Callen, PW: CT evaluation of anomalies of the inferior vena cava and left renal vein, AJR 132:759, 1979.

71. Rubenstein, WA, and Whalen, JP: Commentary: extraperitoneal spaces, AJR 147:1162, 1986.

72. Rubenstein, WA, et al: Posterior peritoneal recesses: assessment using CT, Radiology 156:461, 1985.

73. Rubenstein, WA, et al: CT of fibrous tissues and tumors with sonographic correlation, AJR 147:1067, 1986.

74. Sagel, SS, et al: Detection of retroperitoneal hemorrhage by computed tomography, AJR 129:403, 1977.

75. Sandler, CM, Jackson, H, and Kaminsky, R: Right perirenal hematoma secondary to a leaking abdominal aortic aneurysm, J Comput Assist Tomogr 5:264, 1981.

76. Schaner, EG, Balow, JE, and Doppman, JL: Computed tomography in the diagnosis of subcapsular and perirenal hematoma, AJR 129:83, 1977.

77. Sclafani, S, et al: Lumbar arterial injury: radiologic diagnosis and management, Radiology 165:709, 1987.

78. Thomas, JL, Bernardino, ME, and Bracken, RB: Staging of testicular carcinoma: comparison of CT and lymphangiography, AJR 137:991, 1981.

79. Deleted in proofs.

80. Vint, VC, et al: Aortic perianeurysmal fibrosis: CT density enhancement and ureteral obstruction, AJR 134:577, 1980.

81. Vogelzang, RL, et al: Inferior vena cava CT pseudothrombus produced by rapid arm vein contrast infusion, AJR 144:843, 1985.

82. Waligore, MP, et al: Lipomatous tumors of the abdominal cavity: CT appearance and pathologic conditions, AJR 137:539, 1981.

83. Walsh, JW, et al: Computed tomographic detection of pelvic and inguinal lymph node metastases from primary and recurrent pelvic malignant disease, Radiology 137:157, 1980.

84. Weinerman, PM, et al: Pelvic adenopathy from bladder and prostate carcinoma: detection by rapid sequence computed tomography, AJR 140:95, 1983.

85. Weinreb, JC, Cohen, JM, and Maravilla, KR: Illiopsoas muscles: MR study of normal anatomy and disease, Radiology 156:435, 1985.

86. Whalen, JP: Radiology of the abdomen: anatomic basis, Philadelphia, 1976, Lea & Febiger.

87. Williams, PL, and Warwick, R, editors: Gray's anatomy, ed 26, Philadelphia, 1980, WB Saunders.

88. Zirinsky, K, et al: The portacaval space: CT with MR correlation, Radiology 156:453, 1985.

68 Lymphography

RONALD A. CASTELLINO

TECHNIQUE

COMPLICATIONS

INDICATIONS
  Detection of subdiaphragmatic lymph node metastases
  Surgical guidance
  Radiotherapy port planning and evaluating the
    response to therapy
  Detection of a relapse by surveillance abdominal films
  Repeat lymphography
  Percutaneous fine-needle aspiration biopsy

INTERPRETATION

ACCURACY

CONCLUSION

With all radiologic imaging techniques, with the important exception of lymphography (and certain types of radionuclide studies), one must await an increase in lymph node size before one is able to detect evidence of lymph node abnormality. A distinct advantage of lymphography is that, in addition to demonstrating lymph node size, it displays the internal architecture of the opacified lymph node. Lymphography thus is capable of depicting abnormalities within normal-size lymph nodes (Figs. 68-1, 68-2, 68-4, 68-10, and 68-12).

Since the introduction of lymphography as a clinical tool in the mid 1950s,[21] it has become an accepted diagnostic modality for evaluating patients with a variety of malignant diseases.[10,41] Lymphography perhaps finds its most frequent and accepted use in evaluating patients with malignant lymphoma, including Hodgkin's disease. It is also used in patients with solid tumors of the pelvis (uterine cervix and corpus, ovary, testis, prostate, external genitalia, and bladder), soft tissue and bone tumors of the lower trunk and lower extremity, and malignant melanoma. The most commonly performed lymphographic study—the bipedal or lower extremity lymphogram—opacifies many lymph nodes of the pelvis and retroperitoneum and is discussed in this chapter.

TECHNIQUE

The basic technique of lymphography remains similar to that originally described by Kinmonth[21] and consists of:

1. Identification of a lymphatic channel (usually aided by its absorption of vital blue dye)
2. Cannulation of the surgically exposed lymphatic channel
3. Infusion of an oily radiopaque contrast medium (Ethiodol*)
4. Radiographic documentation of the opacified lymphatic channels (initial films) and lymph nodes (delayed or 24-hour films)

With experience, bilateral cannulation of the lymphatics on the dorsum of the feet can be accomplished in almost all patients. At times only one side can be cannulated; nevertheless, this often produces a clinically diagnostic study, since the ipsilateral iliac and paralumbar (paraaortic and paracaval) lymph nodes are opacified, as

---

*Savage Laboratories, Melville, N.Y.

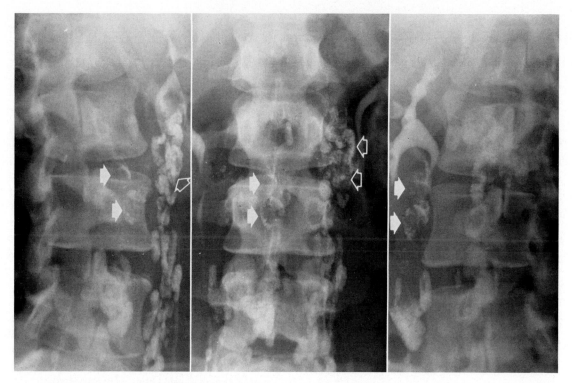

Fig. 68-1 Focal abnormalities of internal architecture in normal-size lymph nodes. This 16-year-old girl with Hodgkin's disease had lymphogram performed for staging. Lymphogram showed several normal-size or minimally enlarged lymph nodes containing filling defects *(closed arrows)* and foaminess *(open arrows)*, interpreted as being involved with tumor (biopsy proved). Such lymph nodes may appear normal to surgeon at laparotomy, so lymphogram can play important role in guiding surgical biopsy. Note normal excretory urogram.
(From Castellino, RA, et al: Lymphology 8:74, 1975.)

well as the contralateral paralumbar lymph nodes by crossover channels. Thus only the contralateral iliac nodes are not demonstrated. Bilateral failure of lymphatic cannulation is rare, except in the very young child[5] (less than 3 years of age) or in patients with leg edema in whom identification of lymphatic channels with infusion of sufficient contrast to permit a diagnostic study is impaired.

Although lymphography is more commonly performed on adults, in the vast majority of cases this study can be technically performed on children with an acceptably low complication rate and high diagnostic accuracy. The same surgical instrument tray is used for children and adults. The major differences between performing lymphograms on adults and children is the frequent use of general anesthesia for the younger child and the infusion of small volumes of contrast medium in children. A detailed discussion of lymphography in childhood can be found elsewhere.[5]

It is often desirable to perform a repeat lymphogram. The technical approach is similar, and there are no added difficulties in performing the repeat study. A similar rate for successful repeat lymphatic cannulation can be obtained both in adults and in children.[7,12]

Serious complications related to lymphography are rare,[5,38] particularly over the past 20 years, owing to a decrease in the volume of Ethiodol that is infused. It is important to carefully monitor the ascent of Ethiodol to infuse enough contrast medium to provide an adequate study with a minimum of spillover into the pulmonary vascular bed. I terminate the infusion when lymphatic channels are opacified at the level of L4 or L5, since at that time there is sufficient contrast medium within the lymphatic channels of the leg to ascend and opacify the more cephalad paralumbar lymphatics and lymph nodes. Most adults require no more than 10 to 12 ml total for a diagnostic study, and 1 to 3 ml total is often sufficient in children up to the age of 4 years. The important point is to tailor the volume of contrast to be infused in each patient by careful radiographic monitoring, rather than rely on any predictive dose schedule.

Since the internal architectural patterns of the opaci-

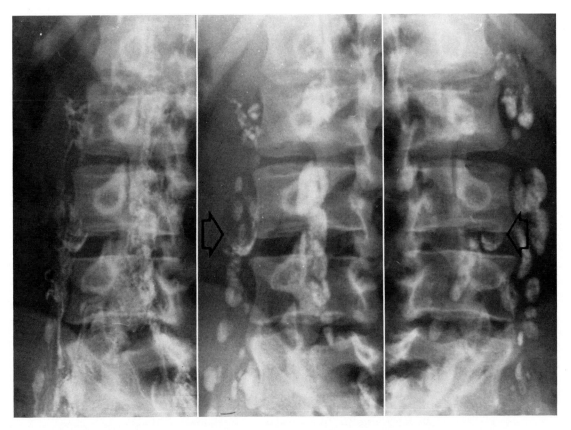

Fig. 68-2 Focal defect in moderately enlarged lymph nodes *(arrows)*. This 21-year-old man had right testicular tumor. Lymphogram performed for staging demonstrated moderately enlarged lymph node whose architecture was extensively replaced, interpreted as representing metastatic tumor (biopsy proved).

fied lymph nodes must be carefully evaluated, it is critical to obtain as sharp a radiographic image as possible. Careful attention must be paid to patient positioning, coning of the roentgen beam, use of a fine-focal spot tube, and radiographic factors that will minimize the exposure time and keep the kilovoltage low to enhance the radiographic contrast. Films are usually performed immediately following the infusion of contrast material; these document the opacified lymphatic channels (initial films) and are followed by radiographs in multiple projections of the opacified lymph nodes the next day (24-hour films). The oblique projections are particularly helpful views, since they displace the paraaortic-paracaval lymph nodes from the underlying lumbar spine and open for better display the posteroanterior sweep of the iliac lymph nodes (Figs. 68-1 to 68-3). At times tomography may display a suspicious finding to better advantage and thus provide a more confident interpretation (Figs. 68-4 and 68-5). Although some advocate the frequent or routine use of tomography, routine tomography is not currently used in most medical centers.

COMPLICATIONS

The complications associated with lymphography are related to the pulmonary (and at times systemic) embolization of Ethiodol; allergic (or idiosyncratic) reactions to the injected local anesthetic, vital blue dye, or Ethiodol; and the surgical cutdown.[16,22] Minor complaints such as transient mild fever or cough, limited wound infections, or urticaria are little cause for concern. However, occasional reports of death related to the lymphographic procedure have appeared in the literature, including anaphylactic reactions (which can be caused by the local anesthetic, the Ethiodol, or, most commonly, the vital blue dye) or Ethiodol embolization to the central nervous system. Lymphography should not be performed on patients with right-to-left cardiovascular shunts because of the increased risk of systemic Ethiodol embolization. Lymphography should also not be performed on patients with significant preexisting pulmonary disease, since the Ethiodol pulmonary embolization that occurs in virtually all cases may precipitate respiratory decompensation in patients with marginal respiratory function.

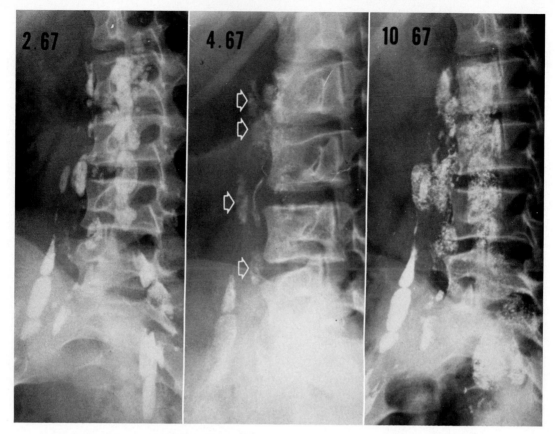

Fig. 68-3 Surveillance abdominal radiographs detecting disease activity. This young girl with non-Hodgkin's lymphoma had staging lymphogram interpreted as being normal. However, surveillance film 2 months later showed interval increase in size of some lymph nodes *(arrows),* suggesting active disease. Repeat lymphogram performed 6 months later to confirm these findings showed further increase in lymph node size and development of foamy internal architecture, confirming development of disease relapse.

(From Castellino, RA, et al: Lymphology 8:74, 1975.)

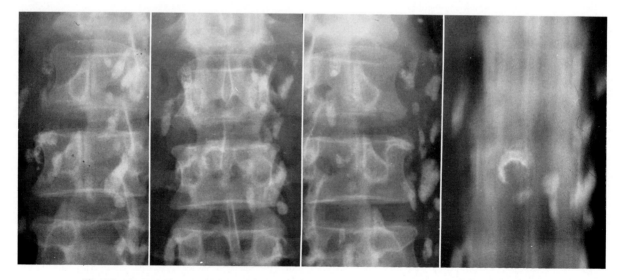

Fig. 68-4 Value of tomography to delineate focal lesions. This 38-year-old man had seminoma of right testicle. Lymphogram demonstrated lymph nodes of normal size. However, analysis of internal architecture on oblique and frontal views demonstrated at least one node to contain what appeared to be discrete filling defect. Should lymphographic appearances not be convincing on standard projections, then tomography at times will clearly demonstrate abnormality. Note that it is evaluation of internal architecture of lymph nodes and not lymph node size, shape, or position that provides information leading to diagnosis of lymph node metastases.

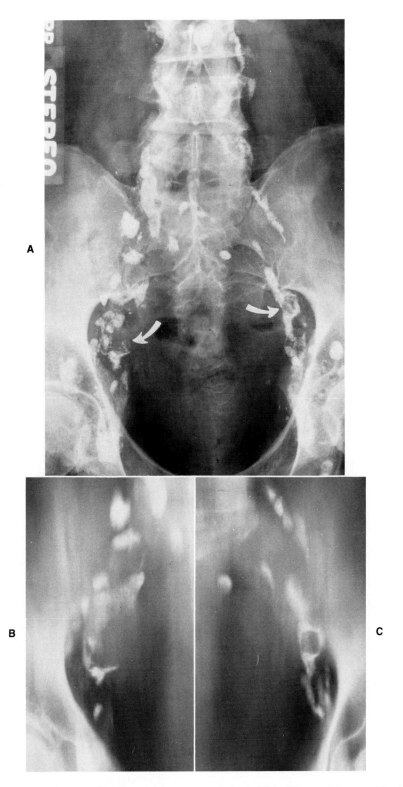

Fig. 68-5 Focal defects (well delineated by tomography). **A,** This 60-year-old man with adeno-carcinoma of prostate had staging lymphogram. Discrete filling defect was noted in left iliac lymph node, but less well-defined lymph node abnormality was present in right pelvis *(arrows).* **B** and **C,** Frontal tomograms clearly demonstrated focal defect in left pelvic lymph node and more definitely outlined extent of lymph node replacement on right.

The incidence of complications related to lymphography before 1968 was determined by a questionnaire.[22] In more than 32,000 examinations there were 81 cases of pulmonary infarction, 10 cases of pulmonary edema, 6 cases of hypotensive crises, 97 cases of hypersensitivity reactions ranging from hives to vasomotor collapse, and 9 cases of severe cerebral disorders, which resulted in 3 of the 18 deaths. The applicability of this data to lymphography as practiced today is questionable, since currently much smaller volumes of Ethiodol are infused and an improved understanding of risk factors has provided better screening of patients for this procedure.

A comprehensive retrospective review of all lymphograms performed on children less than 16 years of age at three medical centers revealed no instance of permanent adverse sequelae or death in 1079 consecutive cases.[5] There were 6 (0.5%) complications, of which 4 were urticaria (0.37%), 1 an acute cardiovascular collapse (0.09%) successfully treated medically, and 1 a transient upper extremity monoplegia (0.09%). Although lymphography has an acceptably low complication rate, it is an invasive procedure and is not entirely without potential risk.

INDICATIONS
Detection of subdiaphragmatic lymph node metastases

In patients with biopsy-proved malignant disease, the lymphogram can provide information on whether the opacified subdiaphragmatic lymph nodes are involved with tumor and, if so, the anatomic extent of this tumor involvement. This information is of obvious value for accurate staging in previously untreated patients so that optimal therapy can be undertaken (Figs. 68-1, 68-2, 68-4, to 68-6, and 68-8). In patients who have been previously treated, lymphography provides similar infor-

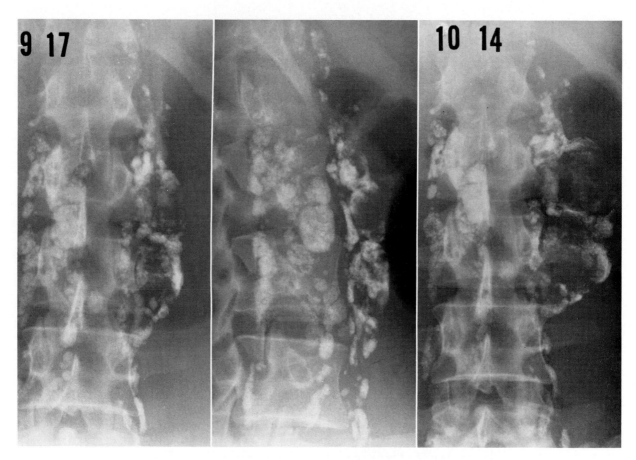

Fig. 68-6 Focal defects in moderately enlarged lymph nodes with marked progression of disease noted on surveillance films. This 22-year-old women with Hodgkin's disease had staging lymphogram that demonstrated abnormal lymph nodes in left mid paraaortic region. These lymph nodes demonstrated focal filling defects and were moderately enlarged and interpreted as representing Hodgkin's disease. Surveillance abdominal film 1 month later showed marked increase in size in previously abnormal lymph nodes, indicating rapid progression of disease.

mation; however, detailed knowledge of the patient's prior treatment is necessary, since radiotherapy, chemotherapy, and surgery can modify the appearance of the opacified lymph nodes and can lead to interpretive difficulties unless this is taken into account.[24,28,29]

Surgical guidance

In patients undergoing a staging laparotomy procedure, the information derived from the lymphogram will guide the surgeon to sample those nodes that are of most concern on the lymphogram, thus maximizing the possibility of documenting subdiaphragmatic metastases. Intraoperative radiographs can be taken to ensure that the abnormal node or nodes have been sampled and to monitor the adequacy of a therapeutic lymph node dissection.

Radiotherapy port planning and evaluating the response to therapy

The opacified lymph nodes can be used to determine radiotherapy fields, and as the tumor is seen to regress during treatment, the ports can be altered to reduce the dose to the surrounding normal tissue. The overall efficacy of radiotherapy or chemotherapy can be readily monitored by observing the response to abnormal opacified lymph nodes on abdominal films. At times evaluation of the residually opacified lymph nodes will be the only available objective means of judging a treatment response.

Detection of a relapse by surveillance abdominal films

The lymph nodes retain sufficient residual radiographic contrast material to permit continued surveillance for an average of 12 months in 70% of patients undergoing lymphography.[15] By simply obtaining an abdominal radiograph following treatment, the size of the lymph nodes can be monitored. An interval increase in lymph node size usually signifies recurrent tumor (Figs. 68-3 and 68-6 to 68-8). Such radiographic findings may be the first and only evidence of relapse in an otherwise asymptomatic and apparently tumor-free patient.[6,15] Such changes may also provide confirmatory evidence of a suspected relapse in a patient with equivocal findings of disease recurrence, or they may more precisely evaluate the extent of disease in a patient with a known relapse.

Repeat lymphography

If necessary, the lymphogram can be repeated when there is insufficient residual contrast material to permit critical analysis for adequate lymph node surveillance.[2,7,12] As noted previously, repeat lymphography can be performed with no added technical difficulties and

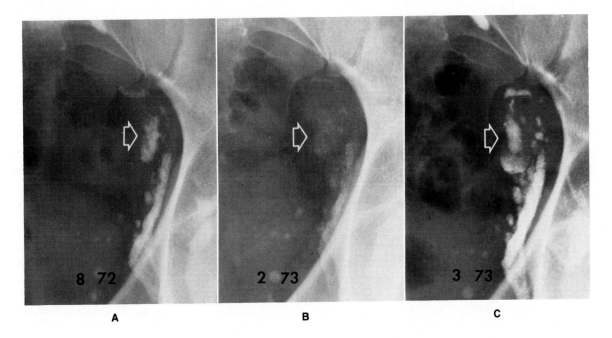

Fig. 68-7 Detection of relapse on routine surveillance abdominal films. This 38-year-old man had right testicular seminoma that was treated by right orchiectomy and radiation to ipsilateral pelvic and bilateral paraaortic lymph nodes. **A,** Initial staging lymphogram was interpreted as being normal. Routine surveillance films were periodically obtained, and radiograph, **B,** taken 6 months later demonstrated interval increase in size of residually opacified lymph node *(arrows)*. To confirm this observation, a repeat lymphogram, **C,** was performed 1 month later and clearly demonstrated interval enlargement of lymph nodes, interpreted as representing metastases (biopsy proved).

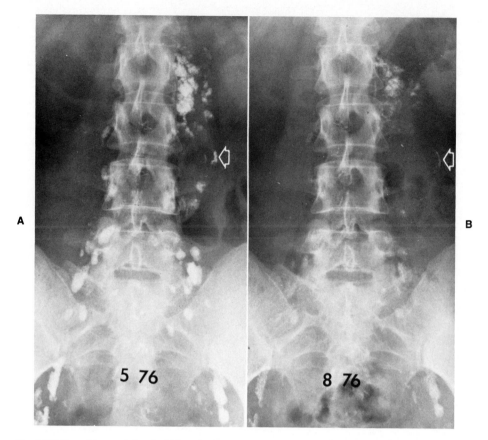

Fig. 68-8 Surveillance abdominal films demonstrating progressive disease. This 51-year-old woman had rectal carcinoma. **A,** Staging lymphogram was interpreted as demonstrating evidence of metastases to left paraaortic region, where lymph nodes were seen to be markedly replaced as well as displaced laterally *(arrows).* **B,** Follow-up film 3 months later demonstrated further lateral displacement of markedly replaced lymph nodes, indicating increasing lymphadenopathy in this region.

with a similar success rate of lymphatic cannulation. Once these lymph nodes are reopacified, they can be compared with their appearances on the prior lymphogram and on the intervening surveillance abdominal films to allow early detection of tumor relapse or to document a suspected tumor recurrence (Figs. 68-3, 68-7, 68-9, and 68-10).

Percutaneous fine-needle aspiration biopsy

Fluoroscopically guided percutaneous needle aspiration of opacified lymph nodes is technically feasible with minimal attendant complications.[18,41] The opacified lymph node is readily localized at fluoroscopy, and the site of maximal abnormality can be identified and sampled with a fine-gauge (22- to 23-gauge) needle (Fig. 68-12). Diagnostic accuracy is high with carcinomas but not as good with lymphomas, since only enough material is recovered for cytologic—and not histologic—study.

INTERPRETATION

Lymph nodes are ovoid structures surrounded by a fibrous capsule. The parenchymal portion of the lymph node consists of two important components: (1) the lymphoid follicles and medullary cords, which are dense aggregations of cells scattered throughout the lymph nodes in the cortex and medulla, respectively, and (2) the sinuses, which consist of an interconnecting network of relatively acellular spaces through which the lymph fluid is conducted. The lymph, carried to the lymph node via afferent lymphatics that pierce the periphery of the lymph node, traverses the lymph node in the sinusoidal network and exits at the hilus in one or more efferent channels. The injected Ethiodol follows the same pathway and, because of its oily particulate nature, is trapped within the sinusoidal system but does not enter the lymphatic follicles or medullary cords. The oily droplets provoke a nonspecific inflammatory response, become

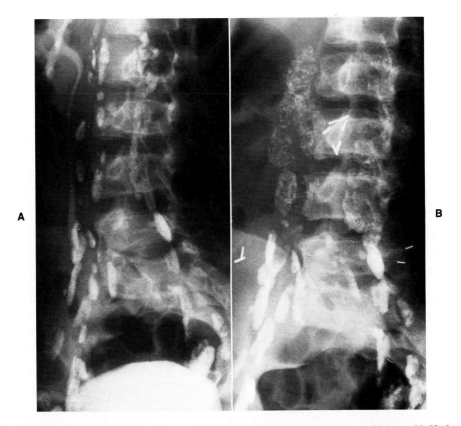

Fig. 68-9 Repeat lymphography documenting relapse of disease. This 11-year-old boy with Hodgkin's disease had staging lymphogram, **A,** which was interpreted as being normal (confirmed at subsequent staging laparotomy). He was treated with supradiaphragmatic irradiation. Three years later, because of suspected relapse based on development of splenomegaly, repeat lymphogram was performed, **B,** which demonstrated development of markedly enlarged and foamy paraaortic lymph nodes, interpreted as represeting tumor (biopsy proved).

surrounded by foreign body giant cells, and are retained within the lymph node for many months.

The lymphographic image of a normal lymph node consists of an ovoid structure that contains a fine, homogeneous stippling of the droplets of contrast material (corresponding to the opacified lymphatic sinuses) intermixed with the radiolucent areas of the node (which correspond to the nonopacified lymphatic follicles). Any process that disturbs this normal relationship between the opacified sinuses and the nonopacified follicles will cause a similar distortion on the radiograph.[40] Thus the lymphadenogram is a very accurate image of the "macroscopic" appearance of the lymph node. However, the nature of an entity causing distortion of the nodal architecture is often determined only by careful microscopic evaluation of the lymph node. These considerations lead to the following conclusions:

1. The lymphadenogram is an excellent method of evaluating the "macroscopic" internal architectural characteristics of lymph nodes. Thus the lymphadenogram can display significant abnormalities in normal-size lymph nodes (Figs. 68-1, 68-2, 68-4, 68-10, and 68-12). An increase in node size is not required to detect abnormalities, which is needed in cross-sectional imaging techniques. Further, the lymphogram can identify lymph nodes that are enlarged as being intrinsically free of significant disease (Figs. 68-11 and 68-12).

2. The histologic nature of the process distorting the internal architecture of the lymph node, although it cannot be determined from the lymphadenogram per se, can often be accurately predicted when correlated with the patient's clinical presentation.

3. Knowledge of patterns of lymphatic spread of various tumors is essential. False-positive lymphographic diagnoses will usually have a benign pro-

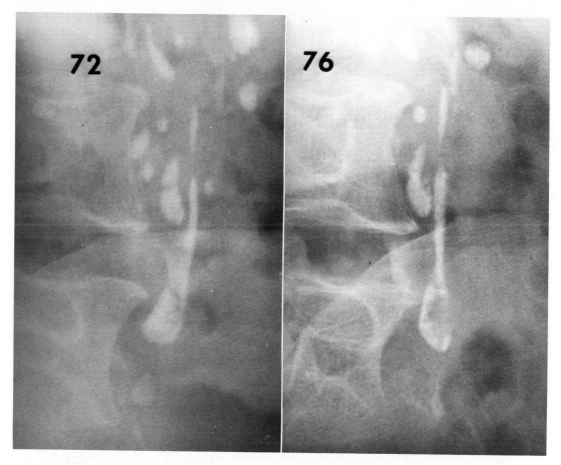

Fig. 68-10 Detection of unsuspected relapse by repeat lymphography. This 70-year-old man with carcinoma of prostate first diagnosed in 1972 had staging lymphogram, **A,** which was interpreted as being normal. He was treated with pelvic radiotherapy. **B,** Repeat lymphogram performed in 1976 demonstrated interval development of prominent filling defect in single lymph node that had not increased in size. However, this lymph node previously had been evenly opacified, so a diagnosis of metastases was made. Biopsy of this lymph node demonstrated metastatic adenocarcinoma of prostate. This convincing evidence of interval development of metastases is based on development of internal architecture abnormalites *without* concomitant lymph node enlargement.

cess as the cause of the structural abnormality that is noted on the lymphadenogram, such as fatty or fibrous infiltration or nonspecific reactive hyperplasia.[3,36]

4. Disease processes that do not sufficiently distort the relationship between the opacified sinuses and the nonopacified follicles, because of their small size, will not be detected on the lymphadenogram. False-negative lymphographic diagnosis will usually be the result of tumor metastases that are less than 2 to 5 mm in size.

A consideration of the size and shape of the individual lymph nodes and their position in their relationship to fixed anatomic points, such as the spine, is helpful in lymphographic interpretation. However, there are great variations in the size and shape of lymph nodes, normal nodes ranging from several millimeters to 3 or 4 cm in largest dimension. It is not unusual to encounter large lymph nodes that are quite normal and normal-size or small lymph nodes that contain focal areas of metastases readily recognizable on the lymphogram. Lymph nodes also vary in their relationship to bony landmarks, since the nodes are closely applied to vessels and tend to be displaced as vessels increase in tortuosity with age. *Thus it is the analysis of the internal architecture of each individual lymph node that is the most critical aspect of accurate lymphographic interpretation.*

Before lymphographic films can be interpreted, pertinent clinical details must be correlated with the lymphographic observations. In patients being evaluated for

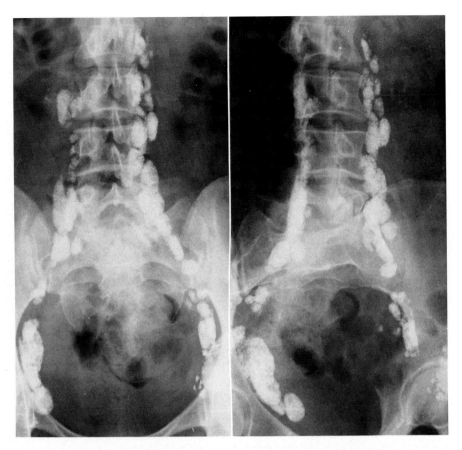

Fig. 68-11 Enlarged lymph nodes caused by reactive (follicular) hyperplasia. This 38-year-old woman was first seen with fever of unknown origin, splenomegaly, and abnormal liver function studies. Lymphogram showed bulky, enlarged, opacified lymph nodes with coarse, granular architecture, characteristic of nonspecific hyperplasia. Lymphographic interpretation was confirmed at exploratory laparotomy when reactive follicular hyperplasia was found in excised paraaortic and splenic hilar lymph nodes and in spleen. Note that although lymph nodes are enlarged, generalized symmetric increase in size and homogeneous granularity is quite suggestive of hyperplasia rather than involvement by tumor.
(From Dunnick, NR, and Castellino, RA: Radiology 125:107, 1977.)

malignant tumors, knowledge of the site or sites of known tumor involvement as well as the histology of the tumor is necessary to evaluate the study, since this provides information on the preferred routes of lymphatic dissemination of the tumor. Since prior radiotherapy, chemotherapy, or surgical excision can affect the appearance of the lymphogram, details of prior treatment are of value in interpreting the films.[28,29]

Every effort should be made to arrive at a definitive radiographic impression, since an "equivocal" diagnosis serves little purpose in patient management and is an all too readily available diagnostic category in which to place the difficult lymphogram. I do not use an "equivocal" diagnostic category but report all lymphograms on patients with known malignant tumors as being either positive or negative for lymph node metastases.

ACCURACY

A large body of literature on the accuracy of lymphography has developed in the past 15 years.[4] These studies are based on a correlation of the radiographic diagnosis with the histologic findings in lymph nodes biopsied at the time of surgical staging in treatment. The best studies are those in which the patients are evaluated in a consecutive and nonselective fashion, the lymph nodes are biopsied within several weeks of the lymphogram, and careful notice is taken that the lymph nodes of radiographic concern have been biopsied by an evaluation of postoperative or intraoperative radiographs. Based on such studies, the following observations about accuracy can be made:

1. The overall diagnostic accuracy, sensitivity, and specificity of lymphography in the initial staging

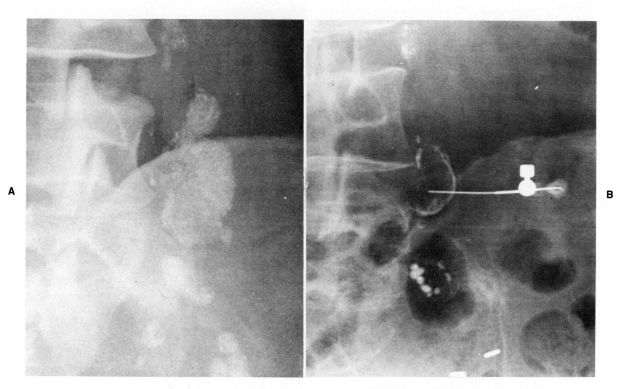

Fig. 68-12 A, Large lymph node at junction between aorta and left common iliac artery. However, internal architecture is normal, indicating that large size of this node is not related to replacement by tumor. This lymph node was biopsied and found to be normal histologically. **B,** Large lymph node at junction between aorta and left common iliac artery has large filling defect with "rim sign," interpreted as being positive for metastases from this patient's known prostatic carcinoma. Percutaneous needle aspiration produced malignant cells.

(**B** from Castellino, RA: Lymphography. In Moss, AA, and Goldberg, HI, editors: CT, ultrasound and x-ray: an integrated approach, © 1979, Masson Publishing USA, Inc, New York.)

of patients with Hodgkin's disease and non-Hodgkin's lymphoma is 90% or greater.[3,20,27] The majority of lymphographic diagnostic errors in this group of patients appears to be false-positive lymphographic diagnoses.[3] The role of lymphography in patients with mycosis fungoides is still unclear,[8,14] but it is probably of limited clinical usefulness.

2. The overall lymphographic accuracy in patients with carcinomas of the pelvic organs, such as uterine cervix,[11,17,23,37] ovary,[35] testicle,[13,25,31,32] and prostate,[1,26,39] is lower, ranging between 75% and 90%. In this group of malignant tumors by far the greatest cause of erroneous lymphographic interpretation is a false-negative lymphogram caused by the presence of small foci of metastasis that are not detected within the opacified lymph nodes—that is, a low sensitivity.

3. The diagnostic accuracy in patients with soft tissue and bone sarcomas, malignant melanomas,[34] and some of the less frequently studied carcinomas (such as bladder, uterine corpus, external genitalia, and rectosigmoid) is not as well established.[11,19,30,33] However, a diagnostic accuracy similar to that obtained in other solid tumors seems likely.

4. Lymphography in childhood tumors appears to be accompanied by a diagnostic accuracy of 95% or more.[5] This is perhaps related to the much smaller incidence of fibrolipomatous changes within pelvic lymph nodes in children as compared with that in adults and to the technically superior radiographs obtainable in small children as compared with those obtainable in many muscular or obese adults.

Table 68-1 summarizes the results of several larger studies on the accuracy of lymphography (and at times of CT) in evaluating the paraaortic-paracaval and pelvic lymph nodes. Data is based on histologic correlation of lymph nodes obtained by biopsy. The original articles should be read to determine variables in the clinical designs of these studies. Direct comparison of the results from one study with those of another may not be valid

☐ **TABLE 68-1**
Radiologic-histologic correlation of retroperitoneal and pelvic lymph nodes

Study	Tumor	Number of cases	Radio- graphic study	Accuracy (%)				
				Sensitivity	Specificity	Overall	Positive report	Negative report
Marglin and Castellino[27]	Hodgkin's	416		93	92	92	80	98
	Non-Hodgkin's	216	LAG	89	86	88	88	87
	Total	632		91	91	91	84	95
Castellino et al[9]	Hodgkin's	107	LAG	85	98	95	89	97
			CT	65	92	87	65	92
Kademian and Wirtamen[20]	Hodgkin's	131	LAG	90	96	95	87	97
Castellino[1]	Prostate	89	LAG	53	93	79	81	78
Liebner et al[26]	Prostate	149	LAG	56	95	81	86	79
Kolbenstvedt[23]*	Cervix	30	LAG	29	96	79	71	80
Wallace et al[41]	Cervix	103	LAG	77	98	87	98	80
Musumeci et al[31]	Testis	287	LAG	86	88	87	85	89
Lackner et al[25]	Testis	64	LAG	73	79	75	89	56
			CT	80	79	80	90	63
Dunnick and Javodpour[13]	Testis	56	LAG	77	100	82	100	55
		50	CT*	66	100	74	100	48
Musumeci et al[35]	Ovary	77	LAG	79	100	92	100	89
Musumeci et al[34]	Melanoma	118	LAG	94	90	92	92	92

*Equivocal diagnoses assigned to negative interpretation category.

because of different materials and methods. For example, the marked differences in sensitivity reported by the two studies with lymphography in cervical cancer is explained by the larger series being composed almost entirely of patients with earlier stage (stage IB) of disease.

Accuracy is defined in the following terms:

1. Sensitivity—the percentage of patients with histologically positive nodes whose radiographic studies were correctly interpreted as positive
2. Specificity—the percentage of patients with histologically normal nodes whose radiographic studies were correctly interpreted as negative
3. Overall accuracy—the percentage of patients whose radiographic studies were correctly interpreted as positive or negative
4. Accuracy of positive radiographic interpretation—the percentage of patients with radiographic studies interpreted as positive who had histologically abnormal lymph nodes
5. Accuracy of negative radiographic interpretation—the percentage of patients with radiographic studies interpreted as negative whose lymph nodes were histologically free of tumor

CONCLUSION

Lymphography is the only currently available imaging modality that permits an evaluation not only of the size and shape of individual lymph nodes, but also of the details of their internal architecture. Based on a careful scrutiny of the internal architecture of each lymph node in multiple projections, a confident conclusion can be reached on whether there are any alterations within the lymph node of sufficient size to be noted on a "macroscopic" level. Although the cytologic nature of the lymph node alteration cannot be determined from the radiograph, by combining the clinical information on the patient's problem with the appearance on the radiograph, one can render an interpretation that carries a high level of accuracy when compared with many other imaging tests.

Lymphography is an established and widely used imaging procedure in patients with Hodgkin's disease and non-Hodgkin's lymphoma. It is also frequently used in the evaluation of patients with pelvic carcinomas, such as uterine cervix and body, prostate, ovary, and testis. It is a convenient method to serially evaluate response to therapy and relapse by surveillance abdominal films.

REFERENCES

1. Castellino, RA: Lymphography in clinically localized prostate cancer, JNCI. (In press.)
2. Castellino, RA, Bergiron, C, and Markovits, P: Repeat lymphography in children with Hodgkin's disease, Cancer 38:90, 1976.
3. Castellino, RA, Billingham, M, and Dorfman, RF: Lymphographic accuracy in Hodgkin's disease and malignant lymphoma with a

note on the reactive lymph node as a cause of most false-positive lymphograms, Invest Radiol 9:155, 1974.

4. Castellino, RA, and Marglin, SI: Imaging of abdominal and pelvic lymph nodes: lymphography or computed tomography? Invest Radiol 17:433, 1982.

5. Castellino, RA, Musumeci, R, and Markovits, P: Lymphography. In Parker, BR, and Castellino, RA, editors: Pediatric oncologic radiology, St Louis, 1977, The CV Mosby Co.

6. Castellino, RA, et al: Roentgenologic aspects of Hodgkin's disease. II. Role of routine radiographs in detecting initial relapse, Cancer 31:316, 1973.

7. Castellino, RA, et al: Roentgenologic aspects of Hodgkin's disease: repeat lymphangiography, Radiology 109:53, 1973.

8. Castellino, RA, et al: Experience with lymphography in patients with mycosis fungoides, Cancer Treat Rep 63:581, 1979.

9. Castellino, RA, et al: Computed tomography, lymphography, and staging laparotomy: correlations in initial staging of Hodgkin disease, AJR 143:37, 1984.

10. Clouse, ME: Clinical lymphography, Baltimore, 1977, Williams & Wilkins.

11. Douglas, B, MacDonald, JS, and Baker, JW: Lymphography in carcinoma of the uterus, Clin Radiol 23:286, 1972.

12. Dunnick, NR, Fuks, Z, and Castellino, RA: Repeat lymphography in non-Hodgkin's lymphoma, Radiology 115:349, 1975.

13. Dunnick, NR, and Javodpour, N: Value of CT and lymphography: distinguishing retroperitoneal metastases from nonseminomatous testicular tumors, AJR 136:1093, 1981.

14. Escovitz, ES, et al: Mycosis fungoides: a lymphographic assessment, Radiology 112:23, 1974.

15. Fabian, CE, Nudelman, EJ, and Abrams, HL: Postlymphangiogram films as an indication of tumor activity in lymphoma, Invest Radiol 1:386, 1966.

16. Fischer, HW: Complications in lymphography. In Fuchs, WA, Davidson, JW, and Fischer, HW, editors: Recent results in cancer research: lymphography in cancer, Berlin, 1969, Springer-Verlag.

17. Fuchs, WA, and Seiler-Rosenberg, G: Lymphography in carcinoma of the uterine cervix, Acta Radiol [Diagn] (Stockh) 16:353, 1975.

18. Gothlin, JH: Percutaneous transperitoneal fluoroscopy-guided fine-needle biopsy of lymph nodes, Acta Radiol [Diagn] (Stockh) 20:660, 1979.

19. Kademian, MT, Buchler, DA, and Wirtanen, GW: Bipedal lymphangiography in malignancies of the uterine corpus, AJR 129:903, 1977.

20. Kademian, M, and Wirtanen, G: Accuracy of bipedal lymphography in Hodgkin's disease, AJR 129:1041, 1977.

21. Kinmonth, JB: Lymphangiography in clinical surgery and particularly in the treatment of lymphoedema, Ann R Coll Surg Engl 15:300, 1954.

22. Koehler, PR: Current status of lymphography, Lymphology 1:116, 1968.

23. Kolbenstvedt, A: Lymphography in the diagnosis of metastases from carcinoma of the uterine cervix stages I and II, Acta Radiol (Stockh) 16:81, 1975.

24. Kuhn, E, Molnar, Z, and Bohm, K: Postirradiation changes on the lymphatics studied by lymphography, Fortschr Roentgenstr 131:92, 1979.

25. Lackner, K, et al: Computed tomographic demonstration of lymph node metastases from malignant testicular tumors: a comparison of lymphography in computer tomography, Forschr Roentgenstr 130:636, 1979.

26. Liebner, EJ, Stefani, S, and Uro-Oncology Research Group: An evaluation of lymphography with nodal biopsy in localized carcinoma of the prostate, Cancer 45:728, 1980.

27. Marglin, S, and Castellino, R: Lymphographic accuracy in 632 consecutive, previously untreated cases of Hodgkin's disease and non-Hodgkin lymphoma, Radiology 140:351, 1981.

28. Markovits, P, Blanche, R, and Charbit, A: Radiologic aspects of lymphangiography after chemotherapy for malignant lymphomas: anatomic-radiologic correlations, Ann Radiol 13:539, 1970.

29. Markovits, P, et al: Radiological appearances of lymphograms performed after radiotherapy, Ann Radiol 12:835, 1969.

30. Merrin, C, et al: The clinical value of lymphangiography: are the nodes surrounding the obturator nerve visualized? J Urol 117:762, 1977.

31. Musumeci, R, et al: Tumors of the testis: lymphography and other imaging techniques, Ettore Majorana Int Sci Sr Life Sci 18:99, 1985.

32. Musumeci, R, et al: Lymphographic evaluation of 285 testicular tumors, Tumori 60:365, 1974.

33. Musumeci, R, et al: Reliability and value of diagnostic lymphography in carcinoma of the sigmoid, rectum and anus, Tumori 61:465, 1975.

34. Musumeci, R, et al: Lymphographic evaluation of 250 patients with malignant melanoma, Cancer 38:1568, 1976.

35. Musumeci, R, et al: Retroperitoneal metastases from ovarian cancer, AJR 134:499, 1980.

36. Parker, BR, Blank, N, and Castellino, RA: Lymphographic appearance of benign conditions stimulating lymphoma, Radiology 111:267, 1974.

37. Piver, MS, Wallace, S, and Castro, JR: The accuracy of lymphangiography in carcinoma of the uterine cervix, AJR 111:278, 1971.

38. Sokol, GH, et al: Complications of lymphangiography in patients of advanced age, AJR 128:43, 1977.

39. Spellman, MC, et al: An evaluation of lymphography in localized carcinoma of the prostate, Radiology 125:637, 1977.

40. Tjernberg, B: Lymphography: an animal study of the diagnosis of Vx2 carcinoma and inflammation, Acta Radiol (Suppl) (Stockh) 214:1, 1962.

41. Wallace, S, Jing, B, and Zornoza, J: Lymphangiography in the determination of the extent of metastatic carcinoma: the potential value of percutaneous lymph node biopsy, Cancer 39:706, 1977.

PART XV

PEDIATRIC RADIOLOGY

69 *Gastrointestinal Tract*

EDWARD B. SINGLETON

SYMPTOMS REQUIRING RADIOLOGIC EXAMINATION
Abdominal pain
Vomiting
Constipation or diarrhea
Bleeding
Malabsorption and abnormal motility

METHOD OF RADIOLOGIC INVESTIGATION
Contrast media
Preparation of patients
Examination

CONGENITAL LESIONS OF THE ESOPHAGUS
Pharyngeal incoordination
Esophageal atresia and fistula
Solitary tracheoesophageal fistula
Stenosis or congenital stricture
Neurenteric cysts
Gastroesophagel reflux
Achalasia

ACQUIRED LESIONS OF THE ESOPHAGUS
Caustic strictures
Foreign bodies
Esophageal varices

DIAPHRAGMATIC HERNIAS
CONGENITAL INTESTINAL OBSTRUCTION
Obstruction in the duodenum
Obstruction in the jejunum or ileum
Lower obstruction
Meconium ileus
Obstruction of the colon
Small left colon syndrome
Imperforate anus

MISCELLANEOUS ABNORMALITIES OF THE ALIMENTARY TRACT
Necrotizing enterocolitis
Bowel obstruction caused by hernias
Duplication of the ileum
Neonatal pseudoobstruction
Duplication of the colon
Hypertrophic pyloric stenosis
Intussusception

Inflammatory lesions
Peptic ulcer
Traumatic lesions
Benign polyps
Neoplasms
Malabsorption
Chiliaditis syndrome
Functional constipation

The radiologic investigation of the alimentary tract of the pediatric patient requires a knowledge of many conditions found only in this age group and an appreciation of technical differences in the method of examination as compared with that of the adult patient. Careful fluoroscopic examination and adequate radiographic studies are as essential with children as with adults. The inconvenience of examining an uncooperative infant or child should never serve as an excuse for foregoing a complete radiographic study. The gonadal areas of the patient should be protected, the field size should be made as small as possible consistent with adequate visualization, and image amplification should be used. Equipment capable of a rapid exposure time, using a generator capacity of at least 300 mA, is essential for high-quality radiographs of children.

A detailed radiologic description of all pediatric alimentary tract abnormalities is beyond the scope of this chapter. Other publications provide this information.[16,38,43] The purpose of this chapter is to provide the radiologist with information on some of the differences between pediatric and adult radiology, particularly in the methods of patient preparation and in the technique of examination, and to discuss the radiologic findings in the more common diseases affecting the alimentary tract of infants and children.

SYMPTOMS REQUIRING RADIOLOGIC EXAMINATION

Because routine upper gastrointestinal (GI) tract and colon examinations are neither advisable nor necessary in the pediatric patient, the order in which the various portions of the alimentary tract are to be examined depends on careful clinical evaluation, particularly with infants, who are unable to describe their condition in terms of localization of pain or other symptoms. The major symptoms and signs of alimentary tract disease that require radiologic investigation are abdominal pain, vomiting, constipation or diarrhea, blood in the stools, and abdominal distention. The presence of one of these signs or symptoms indicates the logical site of disease and directs the radiologist to that portion of the alimentary tract to the studied.

Abdominal pain

Abdominal pain in infants is difficult to evaluate, but intermittent crying accompanied by flexion of the thighs and defecation suggests pain of bowel origin. A preliminary scout radiograph of the abdomen is mandatory in such cases to determine whether intestinal obstruction is present. This may be followed by barium enema studies if there is evidence of a low bowel obstruction. An upper GI tract examination is seldom of value in determining the cause of this symptom.

Abdominal pain in the older child is the most common symptom requiring radiologic evaluation of the intestinal tract. The symptom is variable in location, time of appearance, and severity. The child usually points to the periumbilical or epigastric regions when asked where the pain is. The upper GI tract examination is usually performed first, and a 24-hour delayed radiograph may be made to evaluate the colon without subjecting the patient to an unnecessary and usually uninformative separate colon examination. Intravenous pyelograms are frequently more rewarding than upper GI and colon studies. Peptic ulcers are an uncommonly demonstrable lesion in this age group.[41]

Vomiting

Vomiting is the most common sign requiring radiologic study of the infant's GI tract. With the newborn, one must consider the various types of congenital obstructions. A preliminary abdominal scout film is mandatory for the proper evaluation of such cases and should always precede any studies using contrast media. If there is radiographic evidence of a high small bowel obstruction, the use of an ingested contrast medium is unnecessary, because a sufficient amount of air is usually present to identify the location of the obstruction. If the obstruction is obviously in the colon, or if it is impossible to differentiate the level of the obstruction, barium enema

studies are commonly required. An oral contrast medium should not be given if there is a colonic obstruction and is usually unnecessary in the radiologic evaluation of small bowel obstructions. In the young infant physiologic disturbances of deglutition and of the gastroesophageal region, as well as pyloric obstructions, are of foremost consideration.

In older infants and young children vomiting may be due to esophageal stricture or reflux esophagitis. A foreign body in the esophagus is a common cause of unexplained vomiting in this age group.

Constipation or diarrhea

Either constipation or diarrhea should direct attention to the colon or anorectal area, and a barium enema should be the initial examination. If the patient is an infant, aganglionosis and inflammatory diseases of the colon are major considerations. Habitual or functional constipation is more common in the postinfantile age group.

Bleeding

Melena in the infant or child usually is the result of bleeding in the upper GI tract; therefore, an examination of this area should preced colon studies. Hemtaochezia usually indicates bleeding from the colon or from a Meckel's diverticulum.

There are many causes of gastrointestinal bleeding (Table 69-1), and the site may be impossible to determine by radiologic methods. A scout film of the abdomen is indicated with all infants before studies of the upper GI tract or colon.

Malabsorption and abnormal motility

Malabsorption syndromes and disorders of bowel motility are difficult to evaluate radiographically and commonly are impossible to determine in the infant, but such evaluations are more informative with the ambulatory child.

In all instances a logical approach to identifying the suspected disease is required, avoiding unnecessary examinations and preparatory procedures, particularly in the critically ill or dehydrated infant. Although malabsorption disorders may be suspected on the basis of radiographic studies alone, stool analysis, laboratory studies, and an endoscopic bowel biopsy are more informative in arriving at a specific diagnosis.

METHOD OF RADIOLOGIC INVESTIGATION
Contrast media

Barium is the contrast medium of choice in the examination of the upper GI tract and esophagus and in the evaluation of swallowing disorders. Oily preparations of iodide materials have no place in the examination of the alimentary tract; because of their high viscosity, they are

☐ **TABLE 69-1**
Etiology of gastrointestinal bleeding

Chart I—dark blood	Chart II—dark or bright blood	Chart III—bright blood
Swallowed blood	*Hepatobiliary disease*	*Tumors*
Maternal	Hematobilia	Colonic polyps
Bleeding in utero	Hepatitis	Inflammatory
Bleeding nipples	Posttraumatic	Adenomatous
Oral blood	Cholelithiasis	Familial
Respiratory bleeding	Hypoprothrombinemia	Intestinal polyps
Mucosal ulceration	*Aberrant gastric and pancreatic tissue*	Peutz-Jeghers syndrome (melanin spots)
Stress	Duplications	Carcinoma
Anoxia	Meckel's diverticulum	Lymphosarcoma
Trauma	*Volvulus*	Neuroblastoma
Head Injury	Mesenteric thrombosis	Teratomas
Burns	*Intussusception*	Sacrococcygeal
Endocrine lesions	Acute	Ovarian
Adrenal	Chronic	Gastric
Pheochromocytoma	Postoperative	Rhabdomyosarcoma
Corticoma	Rectal	*Enterocolitis*
Cushing tumor	*Systemic disease*	Infectious
Aldosteroma	Allergy	Specific
Parathyroidoma	Milk	Pseudomembranous
Pancreatic	Schönlein-Henoch purpura	Granulomatous
Hypothalamic—pituitary	Glomerulonephritis (purpuras)	Ulcerative
Peptic ulcers	*Trauma*	Idiopathic
Esophagitis	External	Amebic
Gastroduodenal	Blunt	Renal insufficiency
Marginal	Penetrating	*Anorectal*
Obstructive	Internal	Proctitis
Esophageal	Gastrointestinal suction	Fissures
Pyloric	Swallow—foreign body	Fistula
Intestinal	Suppositories	Hemorrhoids
Drugs	Anal—foreign body	Impactions
Aspirin	*Tumors*	Stercorium ulcers
Antibiotics	Hemangioma	
Steroids	Telangiectasia	
Nitrogen mustard		
Numerous poisons		
Varices		
Gastric		
Esophageal		
Intestinal		

Chart I: Peptic ulcers (Esophagitis, Gastroduodenal, Marginal) — Pain

Chart II: Duplications through Rectal (Aberrant gastric and pancreatic tissue, Volvulus, Intussusception) — Pain

Chart III: Carcinoma through Rhabdomyosarcoma — Pain at some stage of disease; Enterocolitis and Anorectal — Pain

extremely difficult for an infant to swallow without aspirating. The use of water-soluble iodide materials is also unnecessary. If aspirated, these may cause a chemical pneumonitis, and if given in sufficient amounts may lead to severe hypovolemia or even death.[22,28] However, nonionic iodide medium is a safe and useful contrast agent, especially in evaluating the low-birth-weight infant and in demonstrating esophageal atresia and tracheoesophageal fistula. Barium-water mixtures and flavored barium mixtures remain the preferred contrast media in most situations.

Preparation of patients

The method of preparation for an examination of the upper alimentary tract depends on the age of the patient. Most infants undergoing examination of the upper GI tract should not be fed for 3 to 4 hours before the fluoroscopic examination. This is also advisable in the evaluation of swallowing difficulties and of questionable abnormalities of the esophagus. One of the hazards of the examination of a young infant who is vomiting is aspiration. This danger is considerably lessened if the infant is examined when the stomach is empty. Older infants and childrens who are not on a night feeding schedule may be prepared in a manner similar to that for adults: they are not permitted to eat or drink after going to sleep the evening before the examination. Needless to say, with this preparation the earlier the fluoroscopic procedure is carried out, the easier it is on the patient and the more appreciative are the parents.

Infants should be given barium from a nursing bottle with an adequate hole in the nipple to allow a sufficient amount to be swallowed. At this age the patient hungrily takes the contrast medium, particularly if a flavoring agent has been added. This is preferable to the administration of barium through a nasogastric tube. In addition, the fluoroscopist has the advantage of studying the infant's ability to suck and to swallow—important physiologic observations in this age group. Esophageal movements are also more easily studied with this method, and the hazard of the infant's gagging and aspirating the contrast medium is less than when the medium is administered by a tube.

Examination

The radiologic examination of the upper GI tract in ambulatory children is similar to that of the adult patient. In the infant contrast material is observed passing down the esophagus with the patient in a supine right anterior oblique position. When this method is used, the esophagus is clear of the spine and can be carefully studied, with particular attention to deglutition and the gastroesophageal junction (Fig. 69-1). This position also allows the contrast medium to pool in the fundus and prevents it from filling the antrum and the pyloric canal before these areas can be studied. The patient is then turned slowly to the right into a left posterior oblique position while the contour of the stomach and the filling of the duodenum are observed fluoroscopically.

In the examination of the infant's and child's colon, the use of Foley or other types of balloon catheters is unnecessary, uncomfortable, and may obscure the rectal area or perforate the rectum (Fig. 69-2). Disposable infant's and children's enema tips are preferable. The small tip is necessary with neonates to prevent injury to the rectal mucosa. Adult tips are suitable for children. In each case the tip is secured by taping the buttocks together (Fig. 69-3).

Adequate cleansing of the colon is not as necessary with the pediatric patient as with the adult. Barium is the contrast medium of choice even in the evaluation of functional constipation or Hirschsprung's disease, provided one is careful to examine only the lower portion of the colon and avoids filling the dilated segment with contrast material. The use of isotonic saline as the vehicle is unnecessary in such cases if one carefully avoids filling the distended portion of the bowel. No preparation is necessary if the examination is for the evaluation of chronic constipation or intussusception.

Only in the examination of the colon for suspected

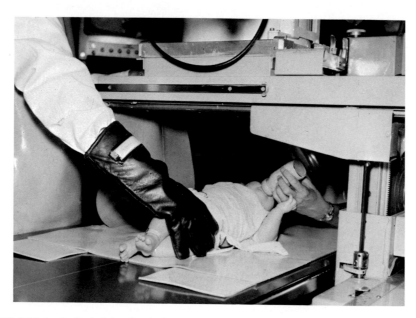

Fig. 69-1 Method of administering barium to young infant undergoing examination of upper GI tract.

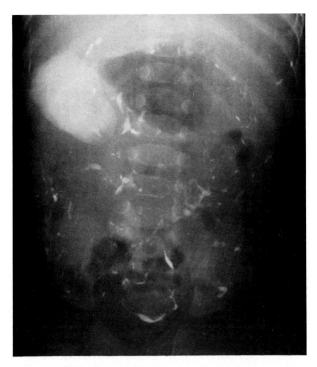

Fig. 69-2 Tear of rectosigmoid by overinflated balloon catheter in 1-week-old infant. Radiograph of abdomen made several weeks later following colostomy for treatment of rectosigmoid perforation shows residual barium scattered throughout peritoneal cavity.
(From Singleton, E.B., Wagner, M.L., and Dutton, R.V.: Radiology of the alimentary tract in infants and children, Philadelphia, 1977, W.B. Saunders.)

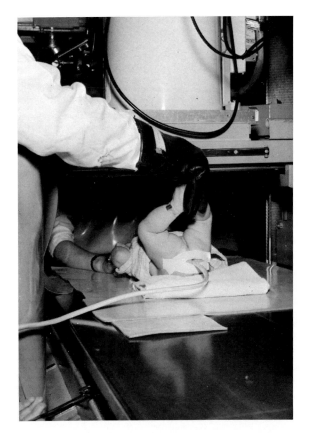

Fig. 69-3 Technique of barium enema examination.

☐ **TABLE 69-2**
Preparations used at Texas Children's Hospital

Procedure	Preparation	Special notes
Esophagus	No preparation if it is the only examination	Infants accustomed to scheduled feedings may have a bottle as late as 5 hours before the study.
Upper GI	Nothing by mouth after midnight	

Colon or barium enema	Under 5 years of age: cleansing saline enemas at 6:00 A.M. (not to exceed four enemas)
	5 to 10 years of age: 1 ounce of senna syrup (or other comparable cathartic) at 4:00 P.M. day preceding examination and enemas preceding examination; milk-free liquid supper and milk-free breakfast may be given
	10 to 15 years of age: 1½ ounces of senna syrup (or other comparable cathartic) at 4:00 P.M. day preceding examination and enemas preceding examination; milk-free liquid supper and milk-free breakfast may be given
		Colon and IVP may be done same day.
		Colon and UGI may *never* be done same day.
		No preparation for:
		  Constipation (obstipation)
		  Suspected megacolon (Hirschsprung's disease)
		  Suspected intussusception, appendicitis, or any other acute condition
		For ulcerative colitis: clear liquids only the day before the examination and NPO for 4 hours before examination time

polyps is thorough cleansing necessary. In such cases a cathartic may be given the evening before and cleansing enemas before the examination. In addition, one may use preliminary barium filling of the colon as a cleansing enema if fecal material is encountered.

Air contrast studies may be of value in demonstrating polyps. Table 69-2 presents the types of preparation that have been used successfully in the Department of Radiology at Texas Children's Hospital.

CONGENITAL LESIONS OF THE ESOPHAGUS
Pharyngeal incoordination

Pharyngeal incoordination occurs most commonly in premature infants and infants who have brain damage, but it may also be seen in normal infants, presumably resulting from an incoordination or immaturity of the swallowing mechanism. Careful fluoroscopic observations of swallowing should be made in infants with dysphagia and those with chronic pneumonitis, particularly if the pneumonia involves the right lobe. Frequently these infants show an inability to suck normally, and once the contrast medium passes into their mouths, their swallowing movements are unsuccessful in propelling the bolus into the esophagus. Instead, the medium may pass into the nasopharynx or be aspirated into the trachea (Fig. 69-4). Pharyngonasal reflux may extend into the eustachian tubes and cause recurrent otitis media. Occasion-

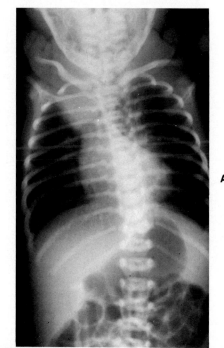

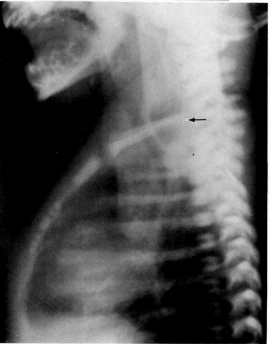

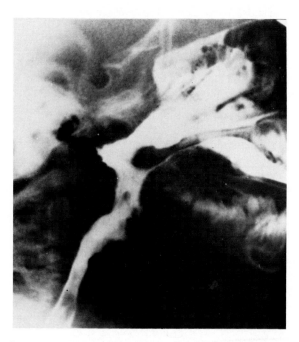

Fig. 69-4 Pharyngonasal reflux in infant with congenital short velum. During deglutition contrast medium passed into nasopharynx because of failure of short palate to occlude nasopharyngeal passage.
(From Singleton, E.B., Wagner, M.L., and Dutton, R.V.: Radiology of the alimentary tract in infants and children, Philadelphia, 1977, W.B. Saunders.)

Fig. 69-5 Esophageal atresia with tracheoesophageal fistula. **A,** Anteroposterior radiograph of chest shows atelectasis and pneumonia of right upper lobe, the most common site for aspiration pneumonia. **B,** Lateral chest radiograph shows air within blind upper esophageal pouch *(arrow).*

ally a deficient gag reflex appears to be present, as determined by the accumulation of the contrast medium in the hypopharynx. Incoordinated movements of the esophagus may also be observed in these infants, with secondary peristaltic waves beginning in the mid or lower portion of the esophagus and passing cephalad. Pharyngeal and esophageal incoordination may be so severe that feeding by gastrostomy is necessary. As the infant grows older, the condition usually improves, and after several weeks or a few months, deglutition may occur normally.

Esophageal atresia and fistula

Esophageal atresia with or without a tracheoesophageal fistula or a tracheoesophageal fistula alone should be suspected in an infant who has an increased amount of mucus and salivation or who strangles during attempted feedings. If esophageal atresia is suspected, preliminary radiographs of the chest and abdomen in both frontal and lateral projections are necessary. If atresia is present, the blind upper esophageal pouch may be distended with air (Fig. 69-5).

The most common form of esophageal atresia combined with a tracheoesophageal fistula is that in which the lower esophageal segment communicates with the tracheobronchial tree. Consequently there is air, usually

in large amounts, in the GI tract. If esophageal atresia alone is present, there is an absence of gas in the stomach.

After the preliminary radiograph of the chest and abdomen has been made, an opaque catheter should be passed under fluoroscopic observation through the infant's nose, and the point at which the passage of the catheter is obstructed should be observed. Unless this is performed under fluoroscopy, the catheter may coil up on itself and give the erroneous impression that it is passing into the stomach. Once the catheter has met an obstruction in the upper blind esophageal pouch, a small amount of barium (1 ml or less) may be injected to delineate more accurately the lower limit of the obstruction (Fig. 69-5) and to determine if an upper tracheoesophageal fistula is present. Then the contrast medium should be aspirated and the nasal tube removed. The examination should be performed with the infant in a prone position (Fig. 69-6).

Many surgeons prefer to perform a gastrostomy on an infant with esophageal atresia before repairing the defect. If this is done, barium may be instilled into the stomach to identify the lower esophageal segment and provide a clearer picture of the length of the atresia (Fig. 69-7). If reflux into the lower esophageal segment does not occur, making the infant gag usually accomplishes this.

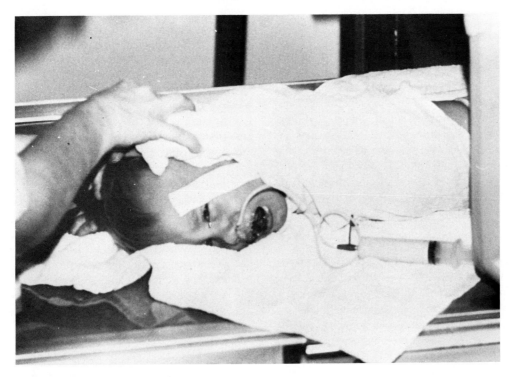

Fig. 69-6 Examination for tracheoesophageal fistula. Tip of catheter is placed in upper esophagus, and infant is in semiprone Trendelenburg position.

(From Singleton, E.B., Wagner, M.L., and Dutton, R.V.: Radiology of the alimentary tract in infants and children, Philadelphia, 1977, W.B. Saunders.)

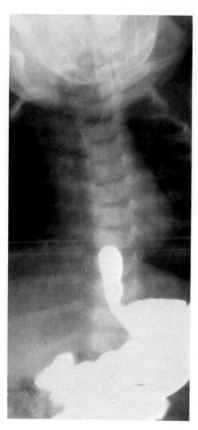

Fig. 69-7 Esophageal atresia. Barium has been introduced through gastrostomy, and reflux into lower esophageal segment outlines length of this segment.

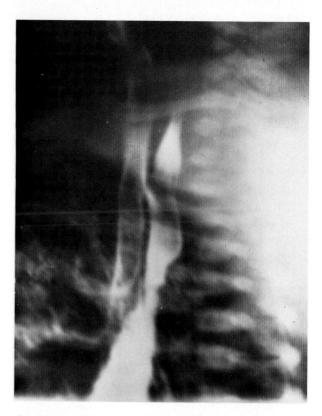

Fig. 69-8 Tracheoesophageal fistula without esophageal atresia. Fistula may be extremely short, making differentiation between this and aspiration of contrast medium into trachea difficult without careful fluoroscopic and videotape recordings.
(From Singleton, E.B., Wagner, M.L., and Dutton, R.V.: Radiology of the alimentary tract in infants and children, Philadelphia, 1977, W.B. Saunders.)

Postoperative fluoroscopic and radiographic examination of the esophagus following the repair of esophageal atresia is of value in determining the patency of the anastomosis and in determining whether dilatations are necessary. Alteration in the physiologic activity of the esophagus below the anastomosis is invariably present. Segmental contractions may occur, but a progressive peristaltic wave from the upper segment through the area of anastomosis into the lower esophagus does not occur.[14]

Solitary tracheoesophageal fistula

The identification of a solitary tracheoesophageal fistula occurring in the absence of esophageal atresia may be very difficult, especially if the communication between the two structures is small. Infants with this condition commonly show chronic pneumonia and atelectasis involving the right upper lobe, but any infant with chronic recurring pneumonia should be investigated for the possibility of a tracheoesophageal fistula. The presence of air distending the esophagus and stomach is a common finding. The use of videotape recordings is of particular value in these cases to determine whether the

contrast medium reaches the tracheobronchial tree through a fistula or is aspirated over the larynx.

After the swallowing mechanism has been studied, a catheter is passed through the nose into the upper portion of the esophagus, and with the patient in a prone position, contrast medium is injected. Forceful distention of the esophagus is often necessary to force contrast medium through the fistula into the trachea. However, this must be performed carefully to avoid overfilling the esophagus and causing aspiration into the trachea.

A tracheoesophageal fistula, if present, may be identified, but more commonly contrast material can be seen extending cephalad in the trachea from the site of the communication (Fig. 69-8). A small fistula may be extremely difficult to identify; frequently several attempts are necessary. Positioning the infant in the prone position with the head down is preferable, because the fistula is directed cephalad from the esophagus. This is presumably the result of the esophagus growing at a greater rate

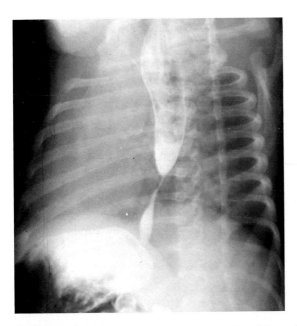

Fig. 69-9 Congenital esophageal stricture. There is stricture of lower third of esophagus with dilatation proximal to this. Gastroesophageal junction is normal, and there was no evidence of gastroesophageal reflux at fluoroscopy.

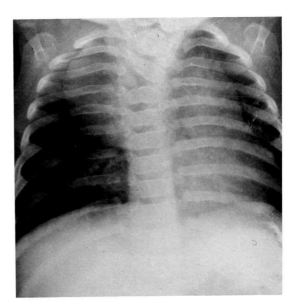

Fig. 69-10 Mediastinal neurenteric cyst in 1-year-old infant. Large mass was seen in right posterior mediastinum. Associated anomalies of upper dorsal spine are present.

than the trachea during intrauterine life, thereby putting the esophageal end of the fistula at a slightly lower level than the tracheal opening.

Stenosis or congenital stricture

Stenosis or congenital stricture of the esophagus probably results from unrecognized intrauterine anoxia with subsequent capillary damage, focal necrosis, cicatricial changes, and stricture formation. Although this process is hypothetical, it offers a better explanation than the hypothesis of a failure of recanalization of the esophagus after the solid stage of embryonic development. Esophageal stenosis of this type is usually located in the mid portion of the esophagus; the lower portion, including the gastroesophageal area, is normal (Fig. 69-9). The possibility that ectopic gastric mucosa in the esophagus produces the stricture is also to be considered but is unlikely. A congenital stenosis of this type is usually not recognized until the infant begins taking solid food, at which time a bolus of meat or a swallowed foreign body becomes lodged at the stricture.

Neurenteric cysts

Neurenteric cysts (esophageal duplications or gastroenteric cysts) represent remnants of one of the accessory Kovalevskys canals that embryologically connects the primitive alimentary tube with the notochord.[29] Pressure of these lesions on the esophagus produces vomiting,

and chest radiographs show a posterior mediastinal mass commonly associated with anomalies of the spine (Fig. 69-10).

Gastroesophagel reflux

Abnormalities of the gastroesophageal junction of young infants are of particular interest. In spite of many theories on the valvular mechanism in this area, it is obvious that the gastroesophageal area is in a tonic or closed state except when forced open by the weight of ingested material, by an esophageal peristaltic wave, or by reflex action following deglutition (Fig. 69-11). If this normal tonicity is not present, gastroesophageal reflux or chalasia (Fig. 69-12) occurs. This is apparently normal to a small degree in many infants, but when severe and persistent it may lead to esophagitis and cicatricial changes with resulting retraction of the cardia into the thorax. In addition, recurrent or chronic pneumonia and even asphyxia and death may occur.[24]

The most common reason for a GI tract examination of the young infant is a complaint by the parents that the infant regurgitates most or part of the feedings. In many cases this is exaggerated by the parent, who confuses normal spitting up with an abnormal condition. Negative results on the fluoroscopic examination in such cases usually indicate that mild but insignificant chalasia is present. Some form of milk allergy or milk incompatibility may be responsible, however, and improvement in

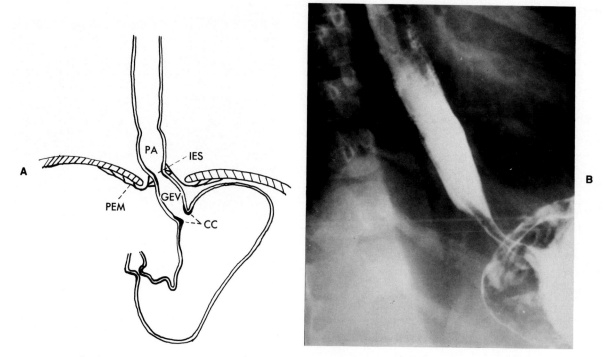

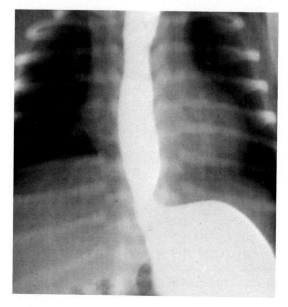

Fig. 69-11 A, Anatomy of lower esophagus. *PA,* Phrenic ampulla; *IES,* inferior esophageal sphincter; *PEM,* phrenoesophageal membrane; *CC,* constrictor cardiae; *GEV,* gastroesophageal vestibule. **B,** Normal gastroesophageal vestibule. Spot film shows tonic constriction of gastroesophageal vestibule during resting phase.
(**A** from Singleton, E.B.: X-ray diagnosis of the alimentary tract in infants and children, Chicago, 1959, Year Book Medical Publishers.)

Fig. 69-12 Chalasia in 3-month-old infant. Pressure was applied to abdomen, resulting in reflux of barium from stomach into esophagus.

such cases will occur if the infant is placed on a diet of milk substitutes.

Chalasia in a severe form may occur in premature infants or infants with brain damage and is occasionally seen in normal infants. Keeping the infant in an upright position after feeding, keeping him or her in a prone position, or thickening the feedings leads to improvement in most cases. In those patients who do not respond to conservative therapy, fundoplication is necessary. The neglect of persistent reflux results in shortened esophagus and hiatus hernia (Fig. 69-13). Once this occurs, persistent reflux is common,[10] and eventual surgical correction, often by colon substitutes, is necessary. Although fundoplication as a treatment for reflux in infants with chronic pneumonia is becoming increasingly popular, conservative therapy should be tried first.

Achalasia

Achalasia is the condition opposite of chalasia. It is characterized by an unusually tonic gastroesophageal vestibule and by a failure of the normal esophageal peristaltic waves or the weight of the ingested food to open it (Fig. 69-14). In time dilatation of the esophagus develops, and surgical correction may be necessary. This

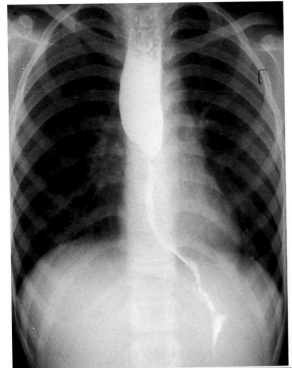

A

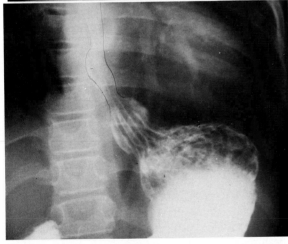

B

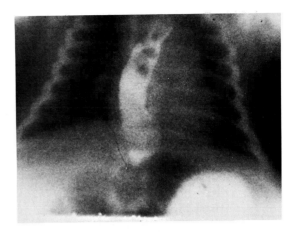

Fig. 69-14 Achalasia in 2-week-old infant (cine study). Gastroesophageal vestibule was abnormally tonic and esophagus dilated, but showed adequate peristaltic movement. Reexamination in 2 months showed no abnormality.

Fig. 69-13 Acquired esophageal stricture caused by gastroesophageal reflux. Patient had history of vomiting from birth. **A,** Esophagram shows constriction of lower half of esophagus. Gastroesophageal reflux was demonstrated at time of fluoroscopy. **B,** Two years later, marked shortening of esophagus has occurred with resulting hiatus hernia.

condition may also be transient and may improve as the infant becomes older.

ACQUIRED LESIONS OF THE ESOPHAGUS
Caustic strictures

Acquired inflammatory lesions of the esophagus are uncommon in older children, but the ingestion of caustic

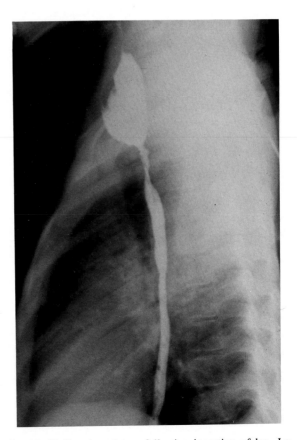

Fig. 69-15 Caustic stricture following ingestion of lye. Localized stricture is identified in proximal portion of thoracic esophagus.

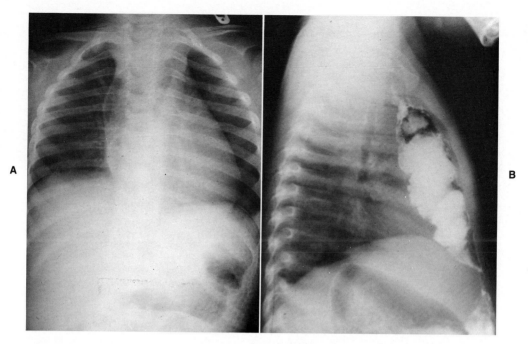

Fig. 69-16 Colon substitute for esophageal stricture in 6-year-old child. **A,** Chest radiograph shows air and fluid level in colon transplant. **B,** Barium outlines transplant and shows characteristic colonic haustrations.

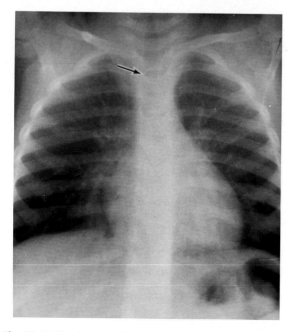

Fig. 69-17 Foreign body in 3-year-old child. Wire segment of Christmas tree ornament can be faintly identified in upper portion of esophagus *(arrow).*

material is a common cause of acute esophagitis and esophageal strictures in younger children (Fig. 69-15). Such strictures usually occur in the upper half of the esophagus and may produce severe dysphagia. If the ingested material is an acid rather than a base, cicatricial changes of the stomach may also develop. One cannot predict the severity of the cicatricial changes that will occur in cases of caustic strictures, but careful radiologic studies during the healing phase and afterward are of value in evaluating the treatment with either dilatation or surgical correction using a colon conduit. In most children who have had this type of esophageal bypass, the overall clinical result is good. The radiographic findings are unusual. Actual peristaltic waves such as are associated with a normal esophagus are not seen (Fig. 69-16). Although segmental contractions do occur, most of the ingested food reaches the stomach as a result of gravity.

Foreign bodies

Foreign bodies tend to become lodged at the thoracic inlet but may also stop at the gastroesophageal vestibule or, less likely, in the upper third of the esophagus, where they pass behind the left main bronchus. Foreign bodies thus found include any objects that the infant can put in his mouth. The presence of a foreign body commonly is unsuspected until a radiologic examination of the esophagus is performed because of the infant's failure to eat

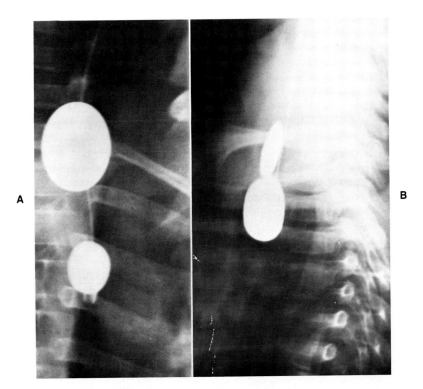

Fig. 69-18 Extraction of metallic coin from esophagus with Foley catheter. **A,** Foley catheter is passed distal to metallic coin and partially inflated with opaque contrast medium. **B,** Catheter has been withdrawn and has made contact with inferior surface of coin before complete extraction. (From Singleton, E.B., Wagner, M.L., and Dutton, R.V.: Radiology of the alimentary tract in infants and children, Philadelphia, 1977, W.B. Saunders.)

and because of excess salivation (Fig. 69-17). Coins lodged at the thoracic inlet frequently can be removed by passing a Foley catheter beyond the object, inflating the catheter balloon with opaque contrast medium, and retracting the catheter and the coin up to the pharynx under fluoroscopic control (Fig. 69-18).[9]

Esophageal varices

Esophageal varices are rare in infants but are not uncommon in children with portal hypertension. The radiographic appearance is similar to that seen in adults. Splenoportograms are of value in determining the extent of the varices and the location of the venous obstruction. Excretory pyelography is advised to exclude renal tubular ectasia, which may accompany congenital cirrhosis.[20] Surgical treatment is continually changing and being reappraised.[23]

DIAPHRAGMATIC HERNIAS

Diaphragmatic hernias are not rare in infants. An acquired esophageal hiatus hernia as the result of gastroesophageal reflux and esophagitis is the most common form. Herniation of bowel through Bochdalek's foramen, the pleuroperitoneal hiatus, is the most common form of congenital diaphragmatic hernias. The hernia is usually on the left, and the left hemithorax is filled with multiple radiolucent blebs, some of which may show fluid levels. Although the radiographic appearance may suggest cystic disease of the lung, the absence of a normal bowel pattern in the abdomen indicates that a hernia is present (Fig. 69-19). Although the condition is usually diagnosed in young infants, it may not be discovered until the child is older (Fig. 69-20). Unusual forms of hernias through Bochdalek's foramen may occur, in which only the spleen or a portion of the stomach may be herniated (Fig. 69-21). Paraesophageal hernias and hernias through Morgani's foramen are less common (Fig. 69-22).

CONGENITAL INTESTINAL OBSTRUCTION

Obstructive lesions of the GI tract in newborn infants are common anomalies, and early recognition is necessary for survival. Prenatal ultrasonography will frequently identify the obstruction (Fig. 69-23). The clinical findings consist of vomiting, abdominal distention, and obstipation. The higher the level of the obstruction, the earlier is the onset of vomiting. If the obstruction is in the lower part of the alimentary tract, abdominal distention and obstipation are the initial signs. In cases of a

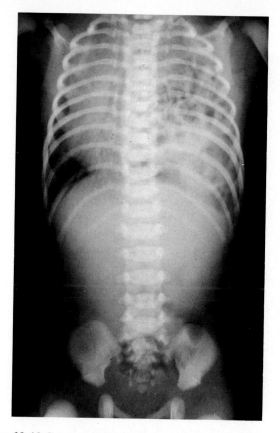

Fig. 69-19 Congenital pleuroperitoneal hiatus hernia. There is absence of gas within abdomen, and multiple gas-filled loops of bowel are seen in left hemithorax with displacement of mediastinum to right.

suspected GI tract obstruction the radiologist is faced with three questions: Is obstruction present? What is the location of the obstruction? What is its cause?

Determining an accurate diagnosis of an intestinal obstruction in the newborn may be difficult if one is not familiar with the many variations of normal gas patterns in this age group.[39] The cardinal signs of an intestinal obstruction in the adult, such as dilated loops of small bowel, air-fluid levels, continuity of loops, and hairpin turns, may be normal variations in the infant. In infants before the ambulatory age one expects to see gas within the stomach, small bowel, and colon. The honeycomb appearance of gas scattered throughout loops of small bowel in a young infant is a normal finding (Fig. 69-24) and is very reassuring in an infant who may be clinically suspected of having an obstructive lesion. However, a large amount of air can be swallowed by a crying infant, and the Mueller effect of sobbing against a closed glottis may force great quantities of air into the stomach (Fig. 69-25). Also, any infant with a disturbance in respiration commonly shows an abundance of gas in the stomach and scattered through the intestinal tract. Distention of loops of small bowel commonly occurs in such conditions, and if films are made with the infant in the upright position, air-fluid levels may be identified. These are

Fig. 69-20 Pleuroperitoneal hiatus hernia in 7-year-old boy. **A,** Radiograph of chest suggests empyema, but patient was asymptomatic. **B,** Fluoroscopic examination demonstrated all of small bowel and most of colon in left hemithorax.

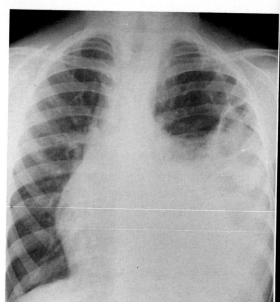

A

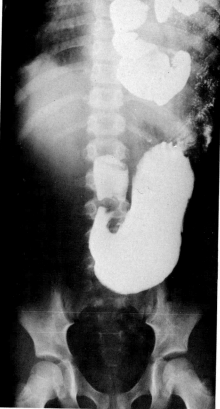

B

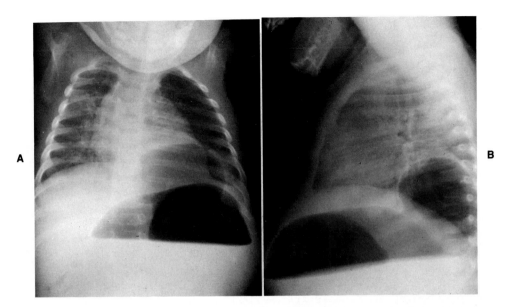

Fig. 69-21 Unusual form of Bochdalek's foramen hernia in young infant. **A,** Chest radiograph shows air-fluid level in stomach as well as collection of air above left hemidiaphragm. **B,** Lateral view shows herniated segment of fundus through pleuroperitoneal foraman to better advantage.

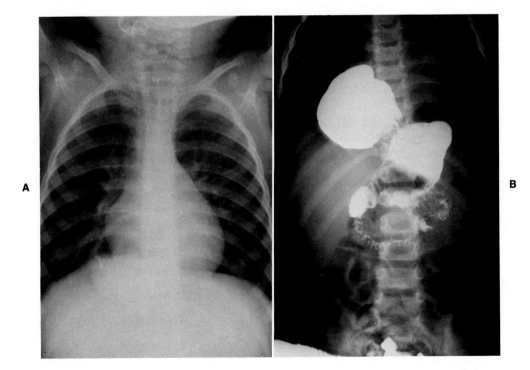

Fig. 69-22 Paraesophageal hiatus hernia in 2-year-old infant. **A,** Air-fluid level is seen in lower medial hemithorax. **B,** GI tract examination shows herniation of proximal half of stomach in paraesophageal region.

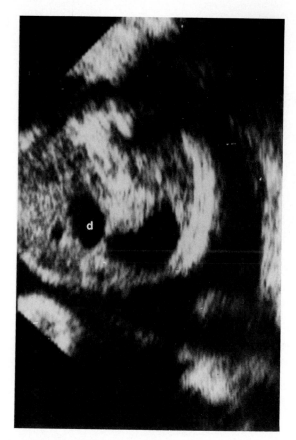

Fig. 69-23 Obstetrical ultrasonographic study of fetus with annular pancreas. Duodenal bulb *(d)* is dilated. Larger echofree fluid-filled stomach is seen to right.

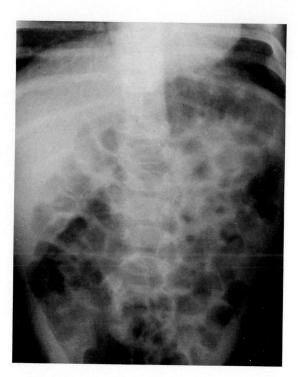

Fig. 69-24 Normal intestinal gas pattern of infant.

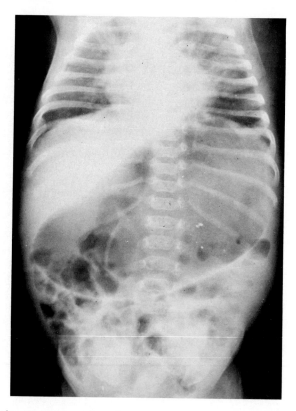

Fig. 69-25 Distention of stomach in young infant caused by prolonged crying.

variations of the normal condition (Fig. 69-26) and are also identical to the radiographic findings of acute enteritis. Consequently it is extremely important that the radiographic findings be carefully correlated with the clinical findings to avoid a misdiagnosis of intestinal obstruction in patients in this age group.

Most cases of small intestinal obstructions in the newborn are characterized by a deficiency in the intestinal gas pattern rather than by the accumulation of a large amount of gas. Air usually enters the stomach during the first few minutes of life, and as a rule an abdominal scout film of a newborn infant shows gas within the stomach. After approximately 30 minutes, air can be identified in the proximal small bowel, and after 3 to 4 hours, air usually has reached the colon. At 6 to 7 hours as a rule gas has reached the distal colon and rectum. A delay in this progression of gas within the intestinal tract may occur in infants who have brain damage (Fig. 69-27), in infants who are born of overly sedated mothers, or in infants who for other reasons do not cry and respond vigorously during the neonatal period. Consequently a delay in the extension of gas into the distal portions of

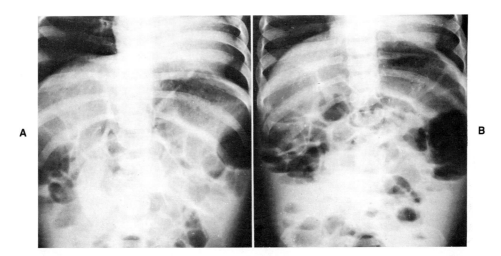

Fig. 69-26 A, Variation of normal gas pattern in infant. **B,** Supine radiograph shows normal honeycombed appearance. Upright film shows multiple air-fluid levels.
(From Singleton, E.B.: X-ray diagnosis of alimentary tract in infants and children, Chicago, 1959, Year Book Medical Publishers.)

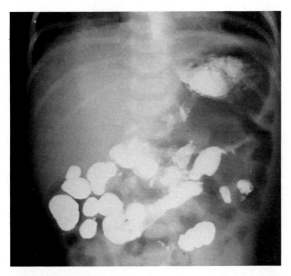

Fig. 69-27 Delay in transient time of contrast medium through small bowel in infant with brain damage. Abdominal radiograph made 10 hours after ingestion of medium shows barium within proximal small bowel.

the small bowel and colon is frequently more informative in the evaluation of a suspected obstruction than is the amount of intestinal gas.

Obstruction in the duodenum

The radiologic identification of a duodenal or proximal small bowel obstruction is relatively easy. Air is present in the bowel proximal to the obstruction, and there is a deficiency of gas distal to the obstructed area. There are several forms of duodenal obstructions, including atresia, stenosis,[32] annular pancreas, and volvulus. The frequent occurrence of duodenal obstructions together with mongolism should alert the radiologist to look for the osseous changes of mongolism in all infants with congenital duodenal obstructions.

The contrast medium of choice for the identification of these lesions is air. If there is insufficient air in the stomach and duodenum for the obstruction to be accurately located, a small catheter may be passed into the stomach and fluid removed and replaced with air. There is no need to use a liquid contrast medium in such cases. The danger of aspiration is a considerable hazard with infants with a proximal bowel obstruction; consequently the use of air as a contrast medium is preferable.

Abdominal radiographs of infants with a duodenal obstruction usually show the so-called double-bubble sign, representing air within the duodenal bulb and the gastric fundus and a deficiency of gas distal to the duodenum. If there is dilatation of the duodenal bulb, the most likely diagnosis is duodenal atresia, duodenal diaphragm, or annular pancreas (Fig. 69-28). A smaller duodenum is more often associated with a volvulus or peritoneal band (Fig. 69-29). Presumably in the former conditions the obstruction has been present for a longer time, with a resulting greater dilatation of the duodenum.

Fluid-aided ultrasonographic examination is advocated by some to diagnose neonatal duodenal obstruction.[11] Vascular injury to an area of the fetal or embryonic gut with resulting necrosis and cicatrization may account for many forms of atresia.[7,42] This condition may be similar to that of necrotizing entercolitis in newborn infants, only having occurred at an earlier stage of intrauterine development.[34] This explanation of bowel atresia

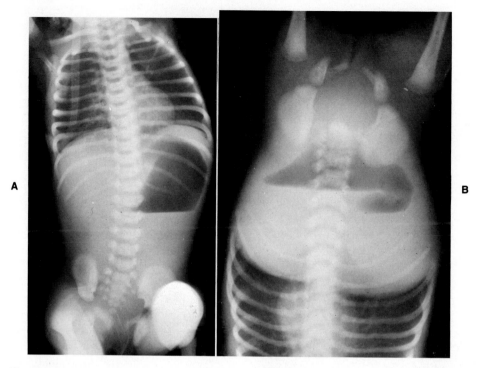

Fig. 69-28 Duodenal atresia. **A,** Upright film shows air within fundus of stomach, but duodenum is not visualized. **B,** Abdominal radiograph made with infant inverted outlines duodenal bulb and pyloric canal.

is especially attractive when one considers the number of cases of atresia in which meconium containing bile and epithelial cells is distal to the obstruction. Because the canalization of the alimentary tract occurs before the formation of bile, the presence of this substance within the colon distal to the obstruction would not be possible on this basis; consequently the obstruction must develop at a later period of intrauterine life.

Obstruction in the jejunum or ileum

Obstructions of the jejunum or proximal ileum cause distention of the proximal small bowel. In these cases, as in duodenal obstructions, air is the only contrast medium necessary. Etiologic considerations include peritoneal bands, atresia and stenosis, herniation of bowel through mesenteric defects (Fig. 69-30), and volvulus. A Z-shaped duodenojejunal loop suggests congenital bands and abnormal mesenteric fixation with potential

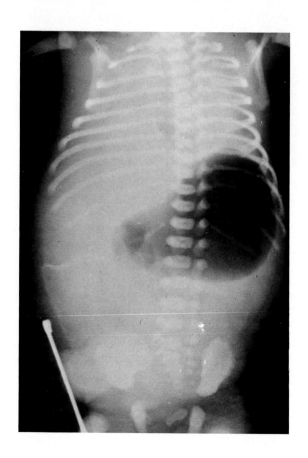

Fig. 69-29 Volvulus obstructing duodenum. Duodenal bulb is identified within air-filled antrum and is not appreciably dilated. Absence of gas distal to duodenum indicates complete obstruction. There is associated meconium peritonitis as determined by calcification within peritoneal cavity.

volvulus.[1] Extrinsic masses may also obstruct the bowel (Fig. 69-31).

Even though scout films in such cases show an obvious high intestinal obstruction, barium enema studies are frequently helpful in alerting the surgeon to the probability that a lower small bowel obstruction may also be present. The identification of an abnormally small colon associated with a high small bowel obstruction usually indicates that additional bowel obstructions are present. The intrauterine development of the colon depends to some extent on the succus entericus produced by the intestinal tract and passed into the colon during its development. Consequently in low small bowel obstructions there is less succus entericus entering the colon. Therefore, if the scout film shows a high small bowel obstruction along with microcolon, there is a high probability that an additional lower obstructive lesion is present. If the intrauterine ischemic insult to the bowel also includes the mesentery, twisting may result and form the so-called apple core or Christmas tree mesentery as well as bowel atresia.

Lower obstruction

Localization of an obstruction is more difficult when it is lower. It may be impossible to determine on abdominal scout films whether the obstruction is in the small bowel or colon. In such cases barium enema studies are informative. If the colon fills completely and appears normal, or if the entire colon is patent but has an unusually small lumen (microcolon), the obstruction is obviously in the terminal portion of the small bowel. The differential diagnoses include ileal atresia, volvulus, peritoneal bands, meconium ileus, and agangliosis (Fig. 69-32). If the cecum is in an abnormal position, one may assume that malrotation and volvulus are present (Fig. 69-33). The embryonic development of the bowel and its relationship to a variety of anomalies, including omphalocele, nonrotation of the foregut, and peritoneal bands, are extremely interesting. Frequently such an obstruction does not develop until later in life (Fig. 69-34).

Because of the variety of complications resulting from a failure of normal rotation and fixation of the fetal intestinal tract, an understanding of the embryology of nor-

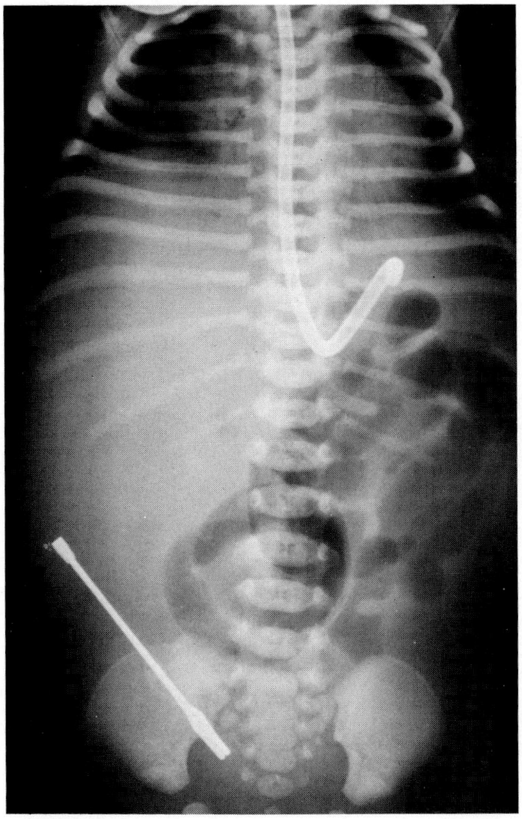

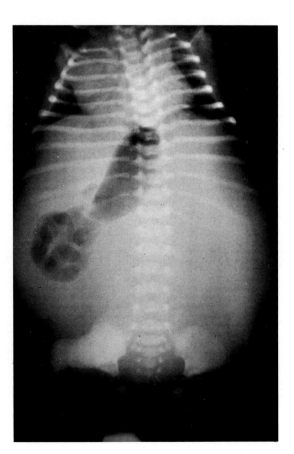

Fig. 69-30 Congenital obstruction caused by volvulus of bowel, which was found at surgery to be incarcerated within mesenteric defect.

Fig. 69-31 Obstruction of proximal jejunum in newborn infant with large solitary left renal cyst.

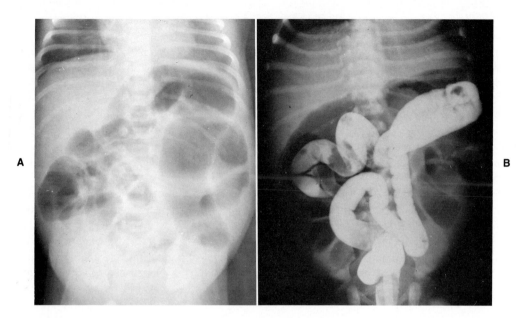

Fig. 69-32 Ileal atresia. **A,** Dilated loops of small bowel are present but without definite gas in colon. **B,** Barium enema shows small colon with obstruction in terminal ileum.

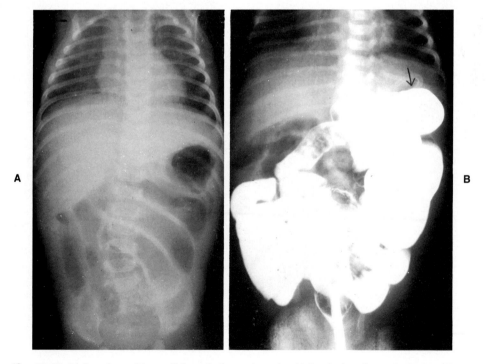

Fig. 69-33 Malrotation with small bowel obstruction. **A,** Abdominal radiograph shows dilated loops of small bowel. **B,** Barium enema study shows cecum in left upper quadrant *(arrow).*

mal midgut rotation is necessary. Beginning at approximately the sixth week of intrauterine life, the alimentary tube undergoes a rapid increase in length and protrudes into the umbilical cord as a single loop, having the superior mesenteric artery as its axis. With further elongation of the loop, possibly initiated by the growth of the liver and by an unequal growth of the duodenal wall associated with development of the pancreas, an initial 90-degree rotation occurs in a counterclockwise direction around the axis of the superior mesenteric artery. Following this there is a continued counterclockwise rotation of the mid intestine with a return of the prearterial segment to the left upper quadrant of the abdomen beneath the axis of the superior mesenteric artery. The subsequent complete 270-degree rotation and packing of the bowel into the coelomic cavity with the last of the midintestine, including the ascending colon and cecum, returning to the right side of the abdomen, completes the rotation process. The third and final stage, which occurs from approximately the eleventh or twelfth week of intrauterine life, is characterized by the fixation of the normal retroperitoneal structures (the duodenum, cecum, and ascending colon) and the fusion of the mid gut and the

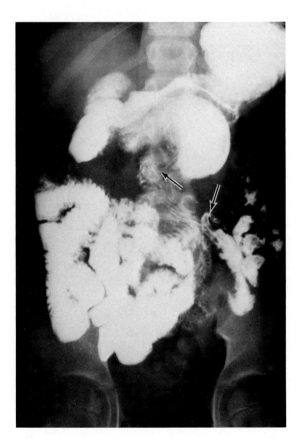

Fig. 69-34 Peritoneal band obstructing proximal jejunum in 6-year-old boy. Cecum and appendix are identified in left mid abdomen *(arrows)*.

mesentery to the posterior parietal peritoneum on a broad base extending from the duodenojejunal junction to the ileocecal junction.

If the normal herniation of the mid gut into the umbilical cord occurs without a return to the abdominal cavity, an omphalocele results. If the return of the intestine occurs after the initial 90-degree stage of rotation, the jejunum returns to the right upper portion of the abdomen and the cecum usually lies in the midline or to the left lower quadrant. There are many additional variations of the rotation process, but in all instances the major complication is an obstruction, which if not present at birth may develop later in life. This is caused by the fact that in all of these situations there is a narrow mesenteric pedicle rather than the normal broad pedicle, and volvulus with a resulting obstruction may easily occur. In addition to this, peritoneal bands, usually extending from the cecum to the posterior portion of the upper peritoneum, are frequently formed and pass across the duodenum, obstructing it.

Volvulus is a common cause of intestinal obstructions during the first few weeks of life. As mentioned previously, it should be suspected if there are plain film indications of a bowel obstruction associated with an abnormally positioned or abnormally movable cecum. In milder forms in which the peritoneal bands (Ladd's bands) produce a duodenal obstruction, upper GI tract studies may be informative by showing the duodenal dilatation, malpositioned Treitz' ligament, and active peristalsis of the duodenum associated with the obstruction near the duodenojejunal obstruction.[1]

Meconium ileus

Meconium ileus deserves special consideration. This is the earliest clinical and radiographic manifestation of fibrocystic disease. Any newborn infant with evidence of an intestinal obstruction should have upright films taken of the abdomen.

If an intestinal obstruction is present, the absence of air-fluid levels within the colon and distal small bowel suggests the presence of meconium ileus[46] (Fig. 69-35). In this condition the meconium is so tenacious and thick that air-fluid levels are usually absent or less prominent than in other forms of mechanical obstructions. The soap bubble appearance of gas and meconium within the small bowel is seen in conditions other than meconium ileus. It is not uncommonly seen in cases of ileal atresia or total colonic aganglionosis.

Obstruction of the colon

With obstructions of the colon one expects to find distention of the entire small bowel as well as distention of the colon proximal to the obstruction. Barium enema studies are of value in confirming this. Colonic atresias

(Fig. 69-36) and stenoses may be identified with such a procedure, but more common causes of obstructions are the meconium plug syndrome and aganglionosis.

Meconium plug syndrome

Meconium plug syndrome may be responsible for obstipation occurring during the neonatal period. The majority of cases respond to digital examination or cleansing enemas. Barium enema studies identify the site of the obstruction. Differentiation of this condition from Hirschsprung's disease may be difficult, but if the plug

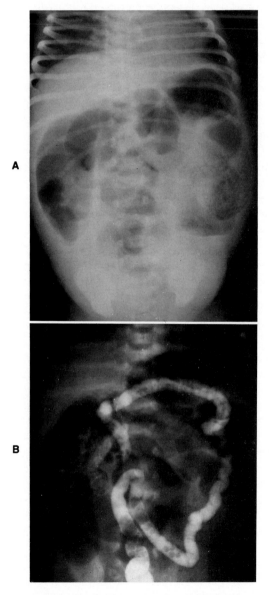

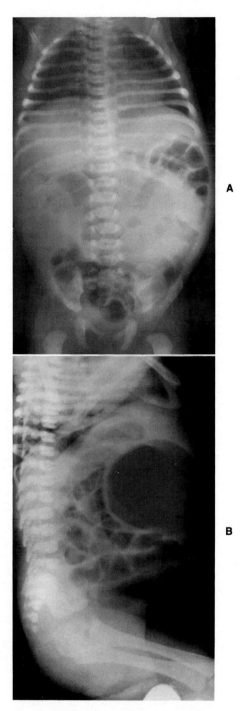

Fig. 69-35 Meconium ileus. **A,** Upright film of abdomen shows soap-bubble appearance of meconium and air within small bowel. There is absence of usual air-fluid level within small bowel, suggestive of meconium ileus. **B,** Barium enema study shows very small colon with obstruction in proximal portion.

Fig. 69-36 Atresia of colon. **A,** Adominal scout film shows ill-defined area of radiolucency in mid abdomen, representing distention of colon proximal to site of atresia. **B,** Lateral view shows dilated transverse portion of colon to better advantage.

can be expelled as a result of the barium enema or hypertonic water-soluble enema with iodine contrast,[47] the resulting clinical course is usually that of a healthy infant. Obstructions produced by a meconium plug may also be present in Hirschsprung's disease.

In any condition in which there has been an obstruction to the passage of meconium into and through the colon during intrauterine life, regardless of whether the cause is ileal atresia, atresia of the proximal portion of the colon, or meconium ileus, barium enema studies show an abnormally small colonic lumen, the so-called microcolon. This should not be misinterpreted as a primary defect of the colon; it simply represents an underdevelopment of the colon because of its failure to serve as a conduit for the movement of meconium into the distal bowel during intrauterine life. The colonic lumen is usually normal in patients with the meconium plug syndrome or Hirschsprung's disease.

Aganglionosis

Aganglionosis or Hirschsprung's disease of the colon may be difficult to diagnose during the neonatal period or early infancy because there has not been sufficient time for megacolon to develop. Constipation is usually the initial complaint, although later in infancy recurrent episodes of diarrhea and constipation may occur because of associated colitis. In the absence of large bowel di-

latation the transition area between the normal rectum and megacolon cannot be identified, and one must rely on the infant's failure to evacuate the enema after 24 to 48 hours.[43] Retention of the enema after this period is presumptive evidence of aganglionosis, but a biopsy of the rectal mucosa and muscularis is necessary for confirmation. If associated colitis is present, however, evacuation may occur quickly (Fig. 69-37).

The bowel proximal to the aganglionic area is distended with air to an extent depending on the severity of the obstruction. In cases of total colonic aganglionosis the small bowel may be markedly distended, far exceeding the diameter of the colon. In the older infant and occasionally in the neonate the transition zone between a small rectum and dilated sigmoid can be identified and the diagnosis readily made during fluoroscopy (Fig. 69-38). In such cases no attempt should be made to fill the entire colon with barium. The examination should be discontinued after the transition zone has been identified. Carrying the examination beyond this point may cause water intoxication and may add to the obstruction.

Small left colon syndrome

The small left colon syndrome produces symptoms similar to those of other colonic obstructions: obstipation, abdominal distention, and occasionally vomiting. Approximately one half of these infants have diabetic moth-

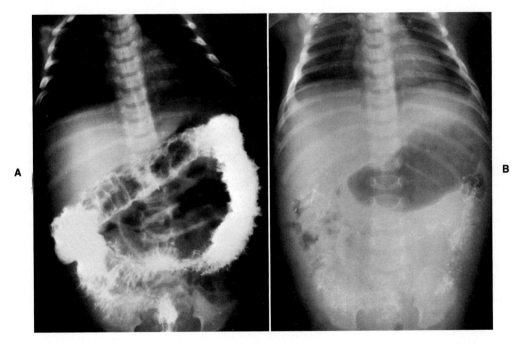

Fig. 69-37 Hirschsprung's disease in 3-week-old infant who had recurrent episodes of diarrhea. **A,** There is marked irregularity of rectosigmoid and descending portions of colon with evidence of extensive ulceration. **B,** Postevacuation film made after barium enema study shows nearly complete evacuation. Biopsy confirmed presence of aganglionosis of rectum.

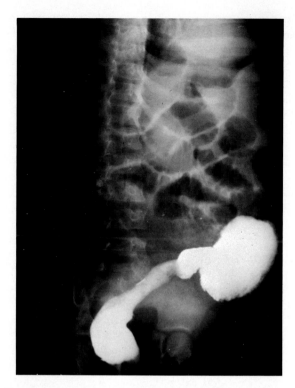

Fig. 69-38 Hirschsprung's disease in 5-year-old child. Rectum is small, and transition zone to dilated sigmoid is identified.

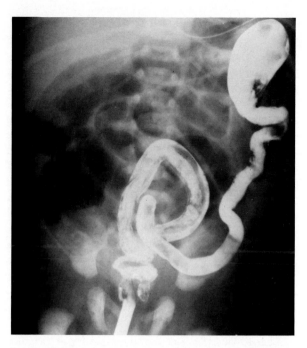

Fig. 69-39 Small left colon in 2-day-old infant. Barium enema examination shows small left colon with transitional dilatation at splenic flexure. Wall of colon is smooth without segmental areas of contraction seen in cases of Hirschsprung's disease. Recovery followed barium enema.

ers. Abdominal scout films show distention of the ascending and transverse portions of the colon and small bowel. The barium enema examination shows the left side of the colon distal to the splenic flexure to be small along with dilation of the colon proximal to this. An acceptable explanation is that the myenteric plexus in the distal portion of the colon is immature.[25] The enema is usually curative (Fig. 69-39). If symptoms persist, aganglionosis is probably present, and a rectal biopsy should be performed.

Microcolon of prematurity is probably a more advanced form of functional obstruction similar to the small left colon syndrome of more mature infants. Maternal therapy of magnesium sulfate for toxemia may be etiologically related in both conditions.[3]

Imperforate anus

Imperforate anus and rectal atresia are common causes of low alimentary tract obstructions in newborns and may be very complex anomalies. The diagnosis of an imperforate anus is readily made with an inspection of the infant, and in both conditions there is, of course, an absence of meconium stools.

The determination of whether the rectal atresia is high or low, that is, above or below the levator ani muscle, can usually be made clinically.[8] If there is a perineal fistula, one can assume the obstruction is low, whereas in patients with a high obstruction a perirenal fistula is not present. Consequently radiographic studies are considered unnecessary in some centers. However, I believe that radiographic studies are helpful, and I routinely obtain a lateral inverted radiograph with a metallic marker placed at the anal dimple (Fig. 69-40). This provides a more accurate evaluation of the level of the obstruction in relation to the pubococcygeal line or levator ani muscle (Fig. 69-41). Because at least 6 hours are usually necessary for swallowed air to reach the rectum of a newborn infant, an examination before this time is usually uninformative. It is important to remember that the apparent distance between the gas in the colon and the anocutaneous region is subject to inaccurate measurements depending on the length of time the infant has been kept in an inverted position before filming and on the amount of meconium that may be packed into the distal rectal segment. If the level is low, a direct needle puncture of the rectal pouch with a small amount of water-soluble iodine contrast medium under fluoroscopic guidance is helpful in more accurately determining the distance to the cutaneous anal region and in demonstrating rectovesical or urethral fistulas.[45]

Because of the combination of anomalies of the vertebrae *(V)*, anus *(A)*, trachea *(T)*, esophagus *(E)*, and

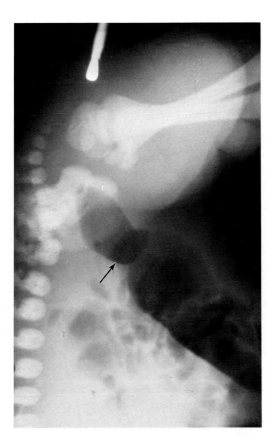

Fig. 69-40 Imperforate anus. Inverted film shows distance between gas in distal rectal segment and anal dimple marked by thermometer. Descending and sigmoid portions of colon are dilated compared with size of rectum, suggesting Hirschsprung's disease, which was later confirmed. *Arrow,* transitional zone.

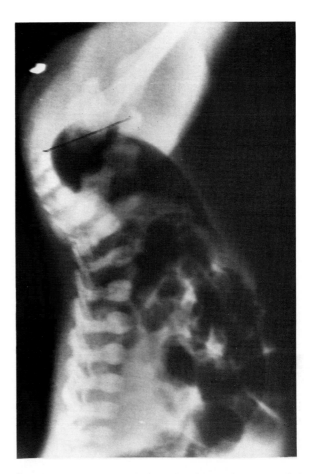

Fig. 69-41 Inverted lateral view of abdomen shows extended rectum extending below pubococcygeal line.

renal structures *(R),* the term *VATER's syndrome* has become popular. Genitourinary tract anomalies are extremely common in patients with anorectal malformations, and excretory urograms are advised. Approximately 70% of male infants with rectal atresia have an associated rectovesical fistula. Consequently the radiologist should carefully observe the vesical area for the presence of air. In female infants rectovaginal communication may be present. The anomaly may be visualized by filling the vagina with contrast material (Fig. 69-42). A dilated air- and fluid-filled vagina may be associated with rectovaginal vesical fistulas.

MISCELLANEOUS ABNORMALITIES OF THE ALIMENTARY TRACT
Necrotizing enterocolitis

A miscellaneous group of alimentary tract abnormalities occur in the neonate. One of these is necrotizing enterocolitis,[7,42] a common complication of prematurity.

The clinical findings are failure to feed, temperature instability, vomiting, distention, and bloody diarrhea. Although there are a variety of theories explaining this condition, the most acceptable is that in infants under stress or in a state of hypoxia, a reflex constriction of mesenteric vessels occurs in an effort to provide the brain and heart with a greater blood flow. Ischemic changes of the bowel develop, and gas passes into the ulcerated mucosa, producing pneumatosis cystoides intestinalis, a pathognomonic finding of necrotizing enterocolitis (Fig. 69-43).[35] If a bowel perforation occurs, pneumoperitoneum is radiographically evident (Fig. 69-44), and immediate surgical intervention is imperative. Before these complications of ischemic bowel disease, the only radiographic change is an alteration of the normal honeycombed bowel pattern. There may be an increase of bowel gas, but in our experience a deficient gas pattern is more common. Gas within the portal circulation is an ominous complication.[6] Colonic and small bowel stric-

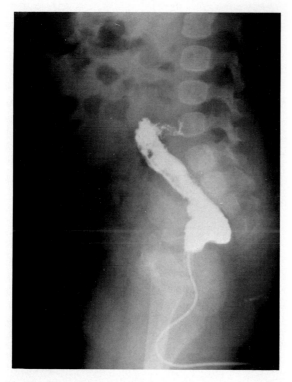

Fig. 69-42 Rectovaginal fistula with imperforate anus. Catheter has been passed into vagina, and contrast medium fills rectum through rectovaginal fistula.

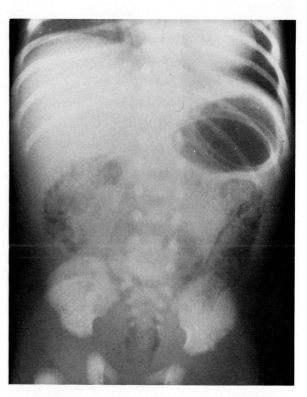

Fig. 69-43 Necrotizing enterocolitis and pneumatosis intestinalis in 1-week-old infant. Gas outlines wall of rectum, sigmoid, and descending portions of colon.

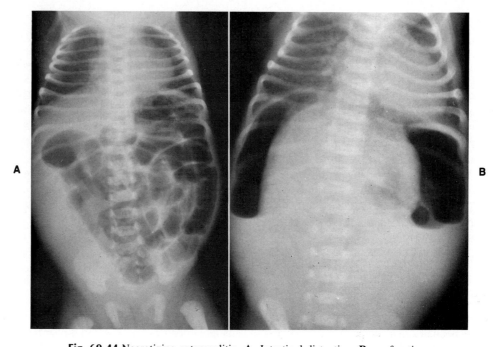

Fig. 69-44 Necrotizing enterocolitis. **A,** Intestinal distention; **B,** perforation.

tures may develop after recovery of necrotizing enterocolitis.[12] The use of nonionic contrast medium provides an excellent method of identifying these obstructions.[15]

Bowel obstruction caused by hernias

An obstruction of the bowel caused by umbilical and inguinal hernias may develop suddenly. Radiographic studies are of value in demonstrating the degree of bowel distention and the location of the obstruction (Fig. 69-45). Although gas in herniated bowel may often be seen, a fullness of the soft tissues of the inguinal area may be the only radiographic clue of an obstruction caused by inguinal hernia. The injection of water-soluble iodine contrast material into the peritoneal cavity may identify unsuspected inguinal hernias.[30] If reduction can be accomplished, the bowel pattern quickly returns to normal. The persistence of abdominal distention suggests the possibility of nonviable bowel.

Duplication of the ileum

Duplication of the ileum and Meckel's diverticulum may present identical radiologic findings. Gastrointestinal bleeding and abdominal pain may be the clinical findings in either case. Radiographic demonstration is frequently impossible unless barium enters the duplication sac and careful small bowel studies are obtained

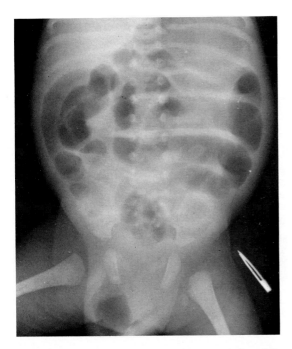

Fig. 69-45 Incarcerated inguinal hernia in young infant. Dilated loops of small bowel are identified, as well as gas in right side of scrotum.

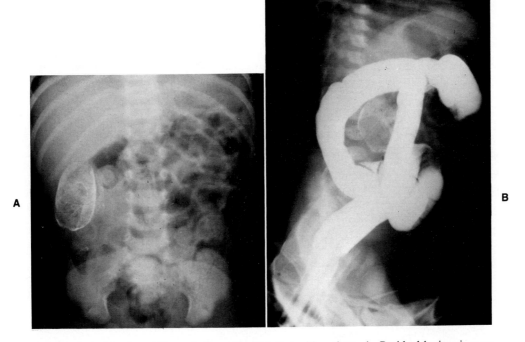

Fig. 69-46 Duplication of ileum in 2-month-old infant with melena. **A,** Residual barium is seen in cystic structure in right side of abdomen following upper GI examination. **B,** Colon examination shows filling of terminal ileum, which is obstructed by extraluminal cyst. Laparotomy disclosed duplication of ileum.

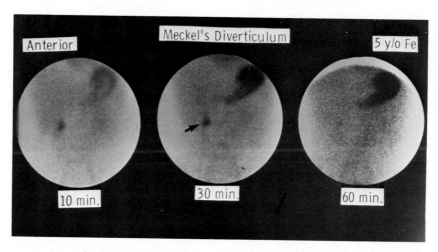

Fig. 69-47 Technetium-99m—pertechnetate nuclide studies.

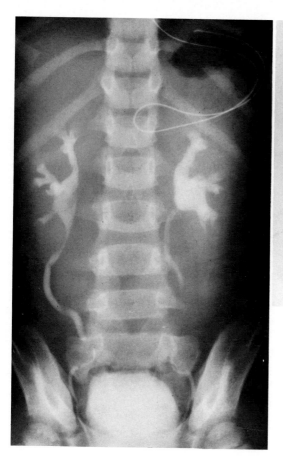

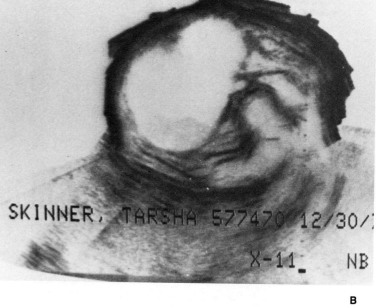

Fig. 69-48 Small bowel duplication. **A,** Intravenous pyelogram studies show displacement of ureters by large abdominal mass. **B,** Ultrasonographic examination shows cystic quality of mass, which contains some debris in its lower portion.

(Fig. 69-46). Positive differentiation is made at the time of laparotomy. Meckel's diverticulum occurs on the antimesenteric side of the ileum, and the duplication is within the mesentery.

Technetium nuclide studies provide a more accurate diagnosis because most cases of Meckel's diverticulum and duplications of the ileum contain gastric mucosa (Fig. 69-47). Ultrasound studies are of help in determining the cystic character of both duplications and large diverticula (Fig. 69-48).

The dilatation of a segment of small bowel following an end-to-side anastomosis for the treatment of an obstructive lesion may produce a marked dilatation of the blind segment and lead to signs of a malabsorption syndrome or chronic macrocytic anemia. The latter is the result of chronic enteritis (Fig. 69-49) and bacterial overgrowth.

Neonatal pseudoobstruction

Neonatal intestinal pseudoobstruction is a form of functional obstruction seen in neonates in whom surgical investigation has shown no evidence of obstruction.[37] Radiologic studies show prolonged intestinal transit and ineffective peristalsis. Some of the patients reported have had microcolon and megacystis. Treatment consists of long-term nutritional support.[4]

Duplication of the colon

Duplication of the colon is a rare anomaly that may be accompanied by the duplication of other pelvic structures (Fig. 69-50).

Hypertrophic pyloric stenosis

Hypertrophic pyloric stenosis is the most common form of acquired alimentary tract obstructions in infants. Although the clinical picture of a palpable olive-size mass in the epigastrium of a 3- to 6-week-old male infant who has projectile vomiting is usually diagnostic of this condition, all too frequently the clinical findings are atypical.

Ultrasound diagnosis of hypertrophic pyloric stenosis has replaced many of the radiologic examinations. In such cases a doughnut configuration is identified in cross-sectional views. The length of the hypertrophied muscle should be at least 16 mm; the cross-sectional diameter, 14 mm; and the muscle thickness, 4 mm or more (Fig. 69-51).[44] If the ultrasound examination is equivocal, the radiologic examination is confirmatory.

The condition was once thought to be congenital, but the development of pyloric stenosis in many infants who have previously had normal GI tract examinations indicates that it is an acquired lesion of unknown cause.

A presumptive diagnosis of hypertrophic pyloric stenosis may be made with a preliminary scout film of the

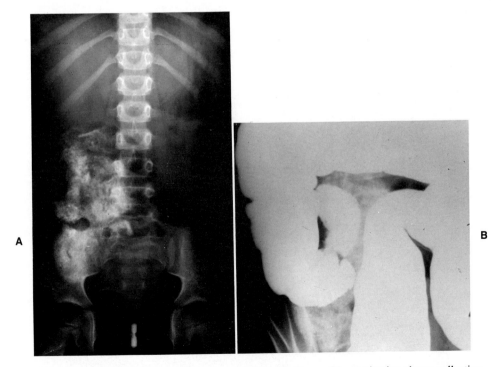

A   **B**

Fig. 69-49 Blind loop syndrome in 4-year-old child. **A,** Upper GI examination shows collection of contrast medium in structure having appearance of ascending colon and cecum. **B,** Barium enema study shows no abnormality of cecum or terminal ileum. At surgery blind ileal loop was discovered resulting from end-to-side anastomosis for treatment of ileal atresia at birth.

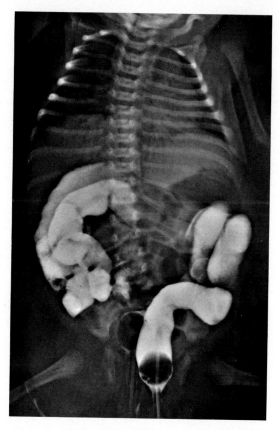

Fig. 69-50 Duplication of entire colon in newborn infant. There were also two vaginal openings and two anal orifices.

abdomen, which shows distention of the stomach with a decrease in the amount of gas distal to the pyloric area. Fluoroscopy is mandatory to determine the true length of the pyloric canal, because a contraction of the gastric antrum on radiographs frequently simulates an abnormally elongated pyloric canal. Only by observing where the gastric waves stop can the radiologist identify the proximal portion of the pyloric canal.

Besides the well-known "string sign" there are other pathognomonic signs of hypertrophic pyloric stenosis. The most common of these is the pyloric beak, which is the extension of the contrast medium into the compressed portion of the distal antrum. In severe cases of hypertrophic pyloric stenosis the contrast medium does not enter the pyloric canal. If the beak can be observed, there is no necessity for prolonging the fluoroscopic observation for the sake of identifying the pyloric canal. The "shoulder sign"[13] and pyloric tit[36] are additional features of hypertrophic pyloric stenosis (Fig. 69-52).

Chalasia occurs in approximately 10% of infants with pyloric stenosis; when present it is of value in explaining the postoperative vomiting of some of these infants. Delayed gastric emptying is invariably present, and although the postoperative examination may show a persistence of the defect of the pyloric canal for a period of weeks or months, the emptying time after surgical correction is normal.

Intussusception

Intussusception offers the radiologist the opportunity of treatment as well as diagnosis. The hydrostatic re-

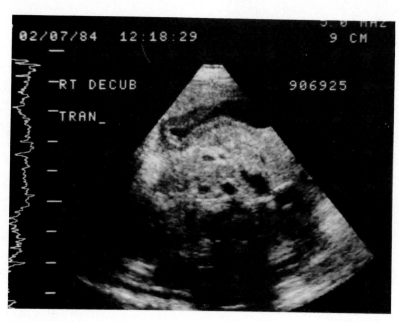

Fig. 69-51 Ultrasonographic examination of hypertrophic pyloric stenosis. Longitudinal scan shows elongated pyloric canal.

duction of an ileocolic or colocolic intussusception should not be considered competitive with surgical reduction, however, for there are indications for both forms of treatment.

The feasibility of hydrostatic reduction can be accurately predicted with an abdominal scout film of infants with this condition (Fig. 69-53). If there is no evidence or only minimal evidence of an intestinal obstruction determined with abdominal radiographs, hydrostatic reduction may be accomplished with ease. If there is radiographic evidence of a moderate obstruction, with distention of the terminal ileum and with a relative decrease in the amount of gas in the colon, reduction may be attempted but is frequently unsuccessful. Even so, a partial reduction facilitates surgical reduction. If there is evidence of a significant obstruction with dilatation of the terminal ileum, hydrostatic reduction is not feasible and prolonged attempts to reduce the intussusception should be avoided. If the patient has evidence of peritonitis, including leukocytosis, abdominal tenderness, and rigidity, even a diagnostic barium enema is contraindicated, because a perforation of the bowel has probably occurred.

The age of the patient is also a factor in selecting patients for hydrostatic reduction. The cause of an intussusception in infancy is usually unknown, and direct causes such as Meckel's diverticulum or a hypertrophied Peyer's patch are rare in this age group, occurring in only 2%.[18] Direct causes are much more common after infancy, and consequently these older patients are not candidates for hydrostatic reduction.

Technique of hydrostatic reduction

The technique of hydrostatic reduction is somewhat different from that required in a routine barium enema study. This is the only examination in which a catheter with an inflated bag can be used to good advantage. It is preferable to begin the study after the infant has been sedated. A barbiturate given in an intravenous infusion allows the infant to rest during the examination and makes hydrostatic reduction much easier than if the infant were awake and struggling. Once the catheter is inserted and inflated, the buttocks should be taped together. Then with the level of the barium in the container kept no more than 3 feet above the table top, contrast material is allowed to flow into the rectum.

The advancing column of barium should be observed carefully. If intussusception is present, a convex meniscus defect is observed. This is usually encountered in the splenic or transverse portion of the colon but may be identified wherever the intussusception is located.

With sustained hydrostatic pressure the contrast medium is seen to flow around the intussusception and gradually to displace it proximally. The retrograde displace-

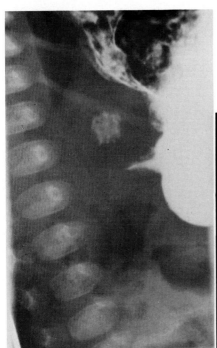

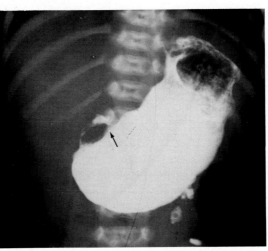

A   **B**

Fig. 69-52 Hypertrophic pyloric stenosis. **A,** Pyloric beak is identified and represents extension of contrast medium into compressed distal antrum and narrowed pyloric canal. **B,** Elongated and angulated pyloric canal is opacified, and "shoulder sign" is demonstrated *(arrow).*

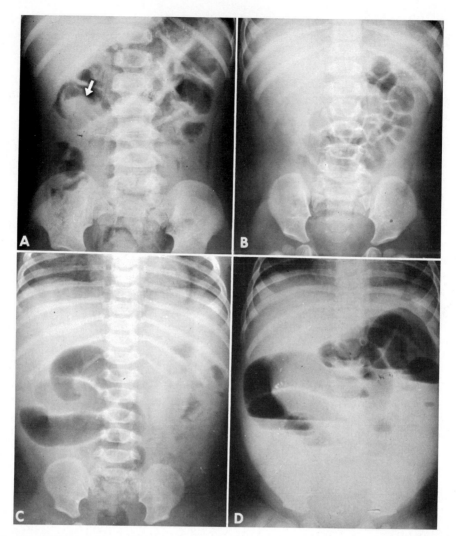

Fig. 69-53 Variations in gas patterns of infants with ileocolic intussusception. **A,** Normal gas pattern with gas in colon and small intestine in normal amounts (*arrow,* location of intussusception). **B,** Nearly complete absence of gas in colon with beginning distention of small bowel. Reduction by hydrostatic pressure should be anticipated but with more difficulty than in patient in **A. C,** Complete absence of colonic gas with distention of terminal ileum. Reduction by hydrostatic method is doubtful. **D,** Marked obstruction with free peritoneal fluid. Attempts at hydrostatic reduction were contraindicated.
(From Singleton, E.B.: Pediatr Clin North Am 10:571, 1963.)

ment of the intussusception is occasionally delayed at the hepatic flexure and invariably in the region of the cecum. It may be necessary on occasion to lessen the hydrostatic pressure by lowering the enema reservoir and allowing the colon to evacuate. Resumption of the hydrostatic pressure in such instances is usually successful in producing further reduction. The appendix often fills with barium as reduction into the ileocecal region occurs. With persistent and sustained hydrostatic pressure, however, complete reduction may be anticipated, and it may be confirmed when contrast medium is seen entering the

terminal ileum (Fig. 69-54). It is necessary to fill several inches of the terminal ileum to be certain that ileoileal intussusception is not also present.

Even if a complete reduction cannot be obtained by hydrostatic means, a partial reduction invariably occurs, and this in turn facilitates surgical reduction. One should keep in mind that intussusception in children past the age of infancy is commonly associated with a direct cause, such as Meckel's diverticulum, a hypertrophied Peyer's patch, aberrant pancreatic tissue, or ileal duplication. Consequently surgical reduction is preferable with these

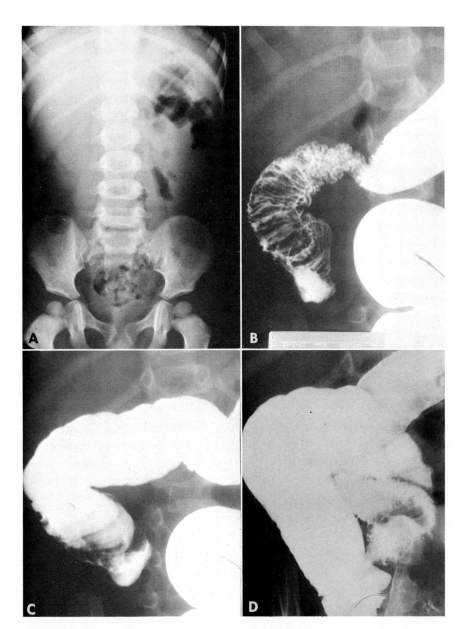

Fig. 69-54 Steps in hydrostatic reduction of intussusception. **A,** Rather common appearance on scout film shows no evidence of significant obstruction. **B,** Intussusception has been reduced to hepatic flexure. **C,** Reduction has been accomplished to region of cecum. **D,** Extensive filling of terminal ileum has occurred, indicating complete reduction.
(From Singleton, E.B.: Pediatr Clin North Am 10:571, 1963.)

older patients. Recurrence of the intussusception after hydrostatic reduction should be considered the result of a definite etiologic lead point, and no attempt should be made to repeat the hydrostatic reduction.

The advantages of hydrostatic reduction are obvious. Laparotomy is avoided, and the hazards of a general anesthetic, even though they are remote, are obviated. Consequently, if the patient is an infant and if the abdominal scout film shows a slight or only a moderate degree of mechanical obstruction, an attempt at hydrostatic reduction should be made. If this attempt is unsuccessful, a partial reduction will at least have been accomplished.

Although ultrasound detection of intussusception is frequently reliable, it must be followed by contrast or air enema if reduction is to be achieved. The use of air under controlled pressure for reduction of intussusception is gaining popularity in many pediatric hospitals.[21]

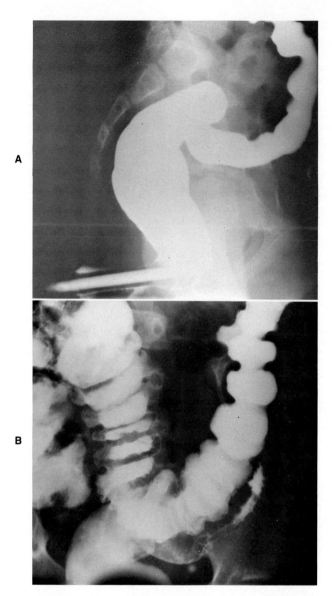

Fig. 69-55 Bacterial colitis in 8-year-old child. **A,** Lateral view of rectosigmoid shows minute areas of ulceration involving rectum and sigmoid. **B,** Postevacuation film shows area of spasm and ulceration in sigmoid.

Inflammatory lesions

Inflammatory lesions of the GI tract are rare in infants. The infectious diarrhea of gastroenteritis in a young infant or child is commonly seen, and the radiographic findings are similar to those seen in a severe adynamic ileus. Air is present in all portions of the intestinal tract, and upright films show multiple fluid levels in the small bowel and colon.

Acute ulcerative colitis

Acute ulcerative colitis as the result of *Shigella, Salmonella,* or another virulent organism is occasionally

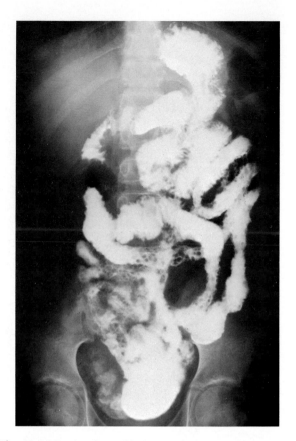

Fig. 69-56 Regional enteritis in 8-year-old boy. There is loss of normal small bowel mucosa as well as multiple granulomatous polyps.

seen in an infant or young child and may mimic the early changes of chronic ulcerative colitis. The radiologic examination shows areas of ulceration in the rectosigmoid region and evidence of distinct irritability of the bowel (Fig. 69-55). Appropriate bacteriologic studies and follow-up radiologic examinations serve to establish this condition as acute colitis rather than a chronic ulcerative form.

Regional enteritis and chronic ulcerative colitis

More chronic forms of enteritis are occasionally encountered in young children. Regional enteritis, granulomatous colitis,[33] and chronic ulcerative colitis are conditions that may affect the pediatric patient. The radiographic features are similar to those seen in the adult (Fig. 69-56). Chronic ulcerative colitis may make its appearance in infancy but occurs more commonly in young children. The onset is frequently acute, and the progression of the condition may be rapid, with radiographic evidence of denudation of the mucous membrane, multiple areas of ulceration, cicatricial changes, and a resulting shortening of the colon. This disease in a young child presents many problems in the type of treatment,

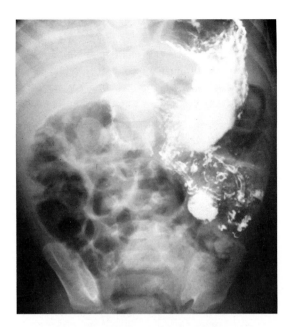

Fig. 69-57 *Ascaris lumbricoides*. Linear filling defects in proximal jejunum represents *Ascaris* worm.

and all too frequently an extensive resection of the colon and permanent colostomy are necessary.

Ascariasis

Chronic bacterial and parasitic infections of the bowel are very rare in the United States and when present are similar to the same conditions seen in the adult. The radiologic identification of *Ascaris* species in the bowel is common in many indigent children, and the radiographic findings are typical. *Ascaris* worms may appear as radiolucent filling defects in the bowel or may be coated by the barium meal; the barium may even outline the linear alimentary tube of the *Ascaris* worm (Fig. 69-57).

Acute appendicitis

Acute appendicitis commonly results in rather specific radiographic findings. This is particularly true if perforation of the appendix has occurred. In such instances one may expect to see on abdominal scout films a distention of the terminal ileum similar to that seen in cases of a mechanical obstruction of this structure. Whether this is the result of localized paralytic ileus adjacent to a periappendiceal abscess or there is an actual mechanical obstruction of the terminal ileum by the pericecal infection is difficult to determine. Free gas within the peritoneal cavity may be identified, particularly in the form of scattered areas of radiolucency in the pericecal region. The peritoneal fat line in such instances is usually obliterated adjacent to the infection.

Commonly an appendicolith, with its characteristic

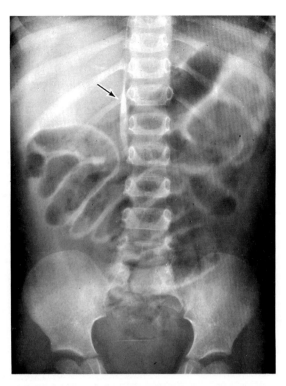

Fig. 69-58 Pneumoperitoneum in child. General radiolucency represents air in peritoneal cavity (*arrow,* falciform ligament). At operation perforated duodenal ulcer was identified.

laminated appearance, can be seen. When present, this is pathognomonic evidence of appendicitis. The identification of an appendicolith before the clinical onset of appendicitis is considered by most authorities to justify a prophylactic appendectomy. In any event the identification of an appendiceal stone should serve as a warning that acute appendicitis with perforation may occur. Filling of the appendix with barium in an attempt to exclude appendicitis in uncertain clinical circumstances is advocated by some but in my experience has occasionally been misleading. The ultrasound identification of a pericecal or pelvic abscess is often helpful.

Peptic ulcer

A peptic ulcer involving the stomach or duodenum is uncommon in children. Anoxic ulcers of the stomach or duodenum may be the cause of severe bleeding or even bowel perforation in the newborn; however, these lesions, because of their small size, are extremely difficult to identify with fluoroscopy. In spite of numerous reports suggesting that peptic ulcers are a common finding in children, the experience of most pediatric radiologists indicates that they are rare.[40] When a peptic ulcer is present, the radiographic features are similar to those seen in adults.

Pneumoperitoneum as a result of a perforating peptic

ulcer in older children or as a result from any cause leading to perforation of the intestinal tract is easily identified in upright films. If films are made with the patient supine, the radiolucency produced by the air about the falciform ligament produces a sign that has been compared to the appearance of a football[27] (Fig. 69-58).

Traumatic lesions

Traumatic lesions of the GI tract should be suspected in any ambulatory infant or child if an obstruction of the small bowel develops. This is particularly true in cases of obstructive lesions of the third portion of the duodenum. Trauma in this area commonly leads to a duodenal hematoma along with distention of the duodenum proximal to the lesion. Hemorrhage in the intestinal tract may also occur in patients with Schönlein-Henoch purpura with or without a history of trauma. The radiographic findings in these patients are highly suggestive because of the thumbprint deformity involving the wall of the affected bowel.[19]

Benign polyps

Benign polyps of the colon are common in young infants and are usually identified at the time of proctoscopy or with radiologic studies of the colon following the appearance of blood in the stool. These juvenile polyps of the colon are benign lesions, and their radiographic identification is not as important as with adult patients (Fig. 69-59). In most instances the polyp after outgrow-

ing its blood supply is passed spontaneously; the only indication for surgical removal is severe bleeding.

Familial polyposis is a more serious condition in which there is potential malignancy. Consequently the accurate identification of the polyps in this condition is very important so that surgical removal can be accomplished.

The Peutz-Jeghers syndrome is another form of polyposis involving the small bowel and occasionally the stomach and colon. Children with this syndrome show characteristic melanin deposits on their lips as well as

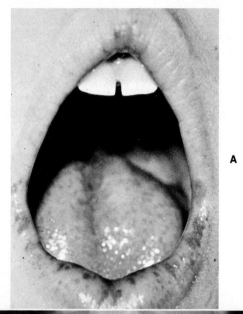

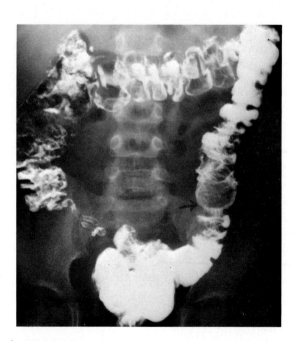

Fig. 69-59 Solitary juvenile polyp in lower descending colon of 5-year-old child.

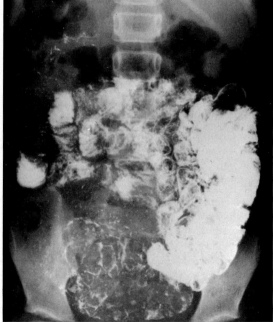

Fig. 69-60 Peutz-Jeghers syndrome. **A,** Pigmentation of lips. **B,** Multiple polyps scattered throughout small intestine with massive collection of tumors in terminal ileum.

on the buccal mucosa (Fig. 69-60). These polyps may produce an intestinal obstruction either as a result of their mass or because of the resulting intussusception. Their localization by radiologic methods is important for surgical removal. Although most of these lesions are hamartomas, there are reports of malignant change occurring.[2]

Neoplasms

Malignant neoplasms of the GI tract are extremely rare in infants but become more common during the later years of childhood. Lymphomas of various forms are the most common malignant neoplasms in this age group, and these show changes similar to identical lesions in the adult patient (Fig. 69-61). The lesion, however, is usually localized and obstructive.

Tumors of the pancreas are extremely rare in children but may occur. Consequently the radiologist should not discount the possibility of an "adult type" of lesions even in a child (Fig. 69-62). Ultrasound studies and CT are valuable complementary studies in patients past infancy.

Malabsorption

The numerous malabsorption syndromes include celiac disease, fibrocystic disease (Fig. 69-63), colla-

gen diseases, agammaglobulinemia, parasitic diseases, chronic enteritis, intestinal lymphangiectasis (Fig. 69-64), hereditary fructose intolerance, disturbance of intestinal hydrolysis of lactose or maltose, and exudative enteropathy, to mention only a few.[26] The radiographic findings are similar in all these. There is coarsening of the mucosal folds of the small bowel along with segmentation and puddling of the barium columns. In the evaluation of the small bowel pattern, one must appreciate the fact that in infants segmentation and irregularity of the small bowel pattern are commonly a normal finding. The mucosal pattern of the colon may be altered in a child with fibrocystic disease. There is coarsening of the mucosal folds as well as multiple cobblestone-like filling defects, seen most commonly in the descending and sigmoid portions.

Chiliaditis syndrome

Chiliaditis syndrome consists of the interposition of the hepatic flexure between the liver and diaphragm. Clinically it is characterized by abdominal pain that becomes increasingly worse during the day and is often accentuated by deep breathing. Radiographic studies show gas within the hepatic flexure interposed between the liver and diaphragm[5] (Fig. 69-65). The validity of this condition as a true clinical syndrome is openly questioned, because an interposition of the bowel between liver and diaphragm is occasionally seen in normal and asymptomatic individuals.

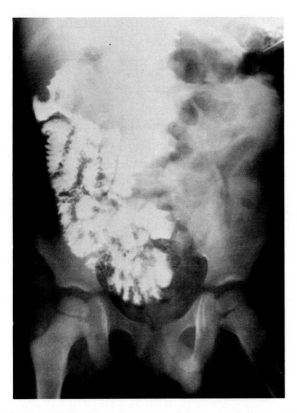

Fig. 69-61 Reticulum cell sarcoma of duodenum is 4-year-old boy. There is loss of normal mucosal pattern. Location of jejunum on right indicates associated nonrotation of bowel.

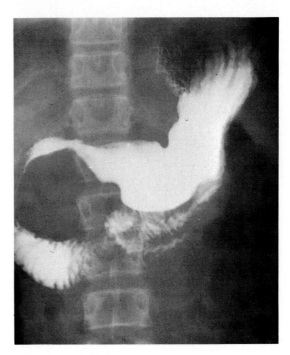

Fig. 69-62 Pancreatic adenoma in 14-year-old boy. There is compression of duodenal loop.

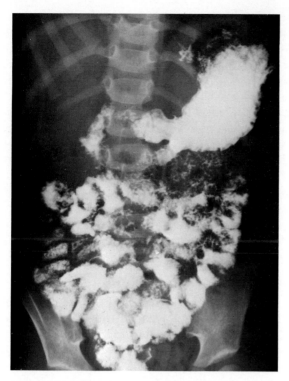

Fig. 69-63 Malabsorption syndrome caused by fibrocystic disease. There is puddling and segmentation of barium within small bowel as well as coarsening of mucosal pattern.

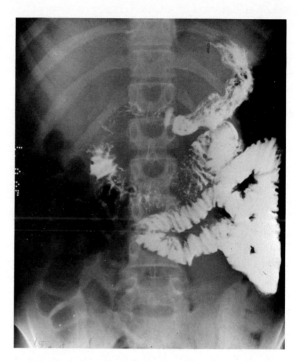

Fig. 69-64 Malabsorption syndrome caused by intestinal lymphangiectasia (exudative enteropathy). There is thickening of mucosal folds.
(Courtesy Dr. J. Dorst and Dr. W. Schubert.)

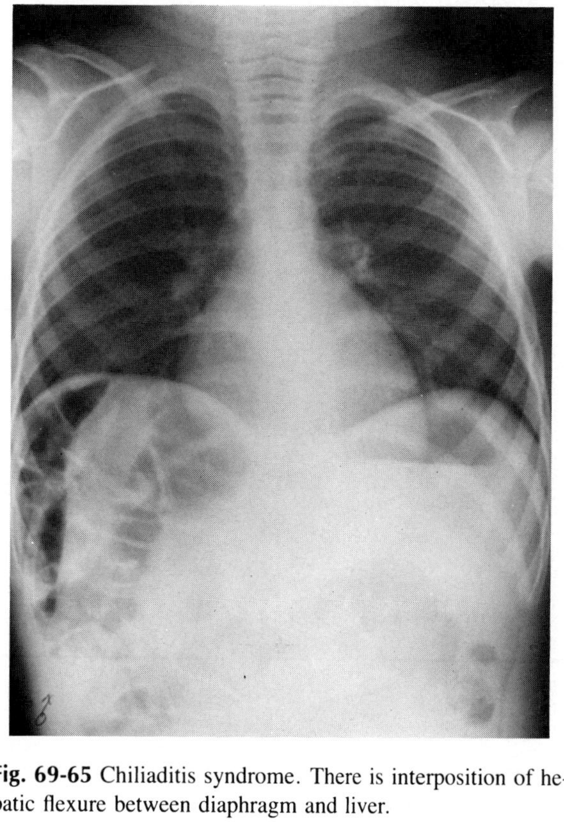

Fig. 69-65 Chiliaditis syndrome. There is interposition of hepatic flexure between diaphragm and liver.

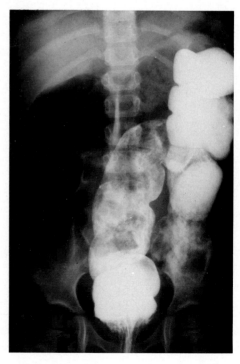

Fig. 69-66 Functional constipation with associated dilatation of rectosigmoid and descending portions of colon.

Functional constipation

Functional constipation in the young infant is a common complaint, and it is the most common reason for colon examinations in this age group. The clinical history is usually diagnostic, and differentiation from Hirschsprung's disease can frequently be made on the basis of clinical information alone. Children with functional constipation are well until late infancy or until toilet training begins, when for an unexplained reason their bowel difficulty begins. This is a result in some cases of an anal fissure and the resulting pain on defecation. In contrast, patients with Hirschsprung's disease have a history of constipation from birth. Children with functional constipation usually constantly soils their underclothes, and when bowel movements occur they are frequently of enormous size. On the other hand, the child with Hirschsprung's disease does not as a rule have a history of soiling, and bowel movements are small.

Radiographic studies are helpful in differentiating these conditions.[43] The child with functional constipation has a very large rectum, and the dilated colon is accompanied by marked elongation and redundancy of the rectosigmoid area (Fig. 69-66). It is difficult to determine whether this increased length of the colon is caused by chronic constipation or present initially and plays an important factor in the patient's symptoms. In all probability children with functional constipation have an excessively long colon initially. In the radiologic examination one should not attempt to fill the colon completely but should simply allow enough barium to enter the distal colon to establish the diagnosis.

REFERENCES

1. Ablow, RC, et al: Z-shaped duodenojejunal loop: sign of mesenteric fixation anomaly and congenital bands, AJR 141:461, 1983.
2. Achord, JJ, and Proctor, HD: Malignant degeneration and metastasis in Peutz-Jeghers syndrome, Arch Intern Med 111:498, 1963.
3. Amodio, J, et al: Microcolon of prematurity: a form of intestinal obstruction, AJR 146:239, 1986.
4. Bagwell, CE, et al: Neonatal intestinal pseudo-obstruction, J Pediatr Surg 19:732, 1984.
5. Behlke, RM: Hepatodiaphragmatic interposition in children, AJR 91:669, 1964.
6. Berdon, WE, and Baker, DH: Roentgenographic diagnosis of Hirschsprung's disease in infancy, AJR 93:432, 1965.
7. Berdon, WE, et al: Necrotizing enterocolitis in the premature infant, Radiology 83:879, 1964.
8. Berdon, WE, et al: The radiologic evaluation of imperforate anus: an approach correlated with current surgical concepts, Radiology 90:466, 1968.
9. Campbell, JB, Quattromani, FL, and Foley, LC: Foley catheter removal of blunt esophageal foreign bodies: experience with 100 consecutive children, Pediatr Radiol 13:116, 1983.
10. Carre, IJ, and Astley, R: Fate of partial thoracic stomach (hiatus hernia) in children, Arch Dis Child 35:484, 1960.
11. Cohen, HL, et al: Neonatal duodenum: fluid-aided ultrasound examination, Radiology 164:805, 1987.
12. Costin, BS, and Singleton, EB: Bowel stenosis as a late complication of acute necrotizing enterocolitis, Radiology 128:435, 1978.
13. Currarino, G: The value of double contrast examination of the stomach with pressure spots in the diagnosis of infantile hypertrophic pyloric stenosis, Radiology 83:873, 1964.
14. Desjardins, JG, Stephens, CA, and Moes, CAF: Results of surgical treatment of congenital tracheoesophageal fistula with note on cinefluorographic findings, Ann Surg 160:141, 1964.
15. Dutton, RV, and Singleton, EB: Use of low osmolar contrast for gastrointestinal studies in low-birth-weight infants, Am J Dis Child 141:635, 1987.
16. Franken, EA, Jr: Gastrointestinal imaging in pediatrics, ed 2, New York 1982, Harper & Row, Publishers.
17. Gillis, DA, and Grantmyre, EB: Meconium plug syndrome and Hirschsprung's disease, Can Med Assoc J 92:225, 1965.
18. Gross, RE: The surgery of infancy and childhood, Philadelphia, 1953, WB Saunders Co.
19. Grossman, H, Berdon, WE, and Baker, DH: Reversible gastrointestinal signs of hemorrhage and edema in the pediatric age group, Radiology 84:33, 1965.
20. Grossman, H, Winchester, PH, and Chisari, FV: Roentgenographic classification of renal cystic disease, AJR 104:319, 1968.
21. Gu, L, et al: Intussusception reduction by rectal insufflation of air, Paper presented at the International Pediatric Radiology Meeting, Toronto, June 1, 1987.
22. Harris, PD, Neuhauser, EBD, and Gerth, R: The osmotic effect of water soluble contrast media on circulating plasma volume, AJR 91:694, 1964.
23. Koop, CE, and Kavianian, A: Reappraisal of colonic replacement of distal esophagus and proximal stomach in management of bleeding varies in children, Surgery 57:454, 1965.
24. Leonidas, JC: Gastroesophageal reflux in infants: role of the upper gastrointestinal series, AJR 143:1350, 1984.
25. LeQuesne, GW, and Reilly, BJ: Functional immaturity of the large bowel in the newborn infant, Radiol Clin North Am 13:331, 1975.
26. Marshak, RH, and Lindner, AE: Malabsorption syndrome, Semin Roentgenol 1:138, 1966.
27. Miller, RE: Perforated viscus in infants: a new roentgen sign, Radiology 74:65, 1960.
28. Nelson, SW, Christoforidis, AJ, and Roenigk, WJ: Dangers and fallibilities of iodinated radiopaque mediums in obstruction of small bowel, Am J Surg 109:546, 1965.
29. Neuhauser, EBD, Harris, GD, and Berrett, A: Roentgenographic features of neurenteric cysts, AJR 79:235, 1958.
30. Oh, KS, et al: Peritoneographic demonstration of femoral hernia, Radiology 127:209, 1978.
31. Ravitch, M: Nonoperative treatment of intussusception: hydrostatic pressure reduction by barium enema, Surg Clin North Am 36:1495, 1956.
32. Rescorla, FJ, and Grosfeld, JL: Intestinal atresia and stenosis: analysis of survival in 120 cases, Surgery 98:668, 1985.
33. Rudhe, U, and Keats, TE: Granulomatous colitis in children, Radiology 84:24, 1965.
34. Santulli, TV, and Blanc, WA: Congenital atresia of the intestine, pathogenesis and treatment, Ann Surg 154:939, 1961.
35. Seaman, WB, Fleming, RJ, and Baker, DH: Pneumatosis intestinalis of the small bowel, Semin Roentgenol 1:234, 1966.
36. Shopfner, CE: The pyloric tit in hypertrophic pyloric stenosis, AJR 91:674, 1964.
37. Sieber, WK, and Girdany, B: Functional intestinal obstruction in the newborn infant with morphologically normal gastrointestinal tract, Surgery 53:357, 1963.
38. Silverman, FN: Caffey's pediatric x-ray diagnosis, ed 8, Chicago, 1985, Year Book Medical Publishers.

39. Singleton, EB: Radiologic evaluation of intestinal obstruction in the newborn, Radiol Clin North Am 1:571, 1963.
40. Singleton, EB: The radiologic incidence of peptic ulcer in infants and children, Radiology 84:956, 1965.
41. Singleton, EB, and Favkus, MH: Incidence of peptic ulcer as determined by radiologic examinations in the pediatric age group, J Pediatr 65:858, 1964.
42. Singleton, EB, Rosenburg, HM, and Samper, L: Radiologic considerations of the perinatal distress syndrome, Radiology 76:200, 1961.
43. Singleton, EB, Wagner, ML, and Dutton, RV: Radiology of the alimentary tract in infants and children, Philadelphia, 1977, WB Saunders.

44. Stunden, RJ, Le Quesne, GW, and Little, KET: The improved ultrasound diagnosis of hypertrophic pyloric stenosis, Pediatr Radiol 16:200, 1986.
45. Wagner, ML, et al: The evaluation of imperforate anus utilizing percutaneous injection of water-soluble iodide contrast material, Pediatr Radiol 1:34, 1973.
46. White, H: Meconium ileus: new roentgen sign, Radiology 66:567, 1956.
47. Wood, BP, and Katzberg, RW: Tween 80/diatrizoate enemas in bowel obstruction, AJR 130:747, 1978.

70 *Systemic Diseases*

J.S. DUNBAR

CYSTIC FIBROSIS OF THE PANCREAS

Cystic fibrosis (CF), a genetic disorder that is transmitted as an autosomal recessive trait, is one of the most important causes of morbidity in children. Though chronic illness and eventual death are largely attributable to pulmonary disease and resultant cor pulmonale, numerous gastrointestinal and hepatic abnormalities result from the pancreatic exocrine dysfunction and generalized mucous obstruction of organ passages that are the hallmarks of the disease.

A candidate gene for locus of CF has been reported[23] and is useful for 97.5% of families at risk of the disease in offspring.

Neonatal manifestations
Meconium ileus

Meconium ileus (MI) occurs in 10% to 15% of neonates with CF.[57,58] In addition to pancreatic insufficiency, these infants have large amounts of abnormally tenacious mucus in the gut. The mucus seems to be important in the pathogenesis of MI.[61] The inspissated meconium causes obstruction, usually at the level of the distal ileum but occasionally proximal or distal to this level.

Failure to pass meconium in the first days of life, progressive abdominal distention and possible vomiting suggest the diagnosis of bowel obstruction. If there is a positive history of CF, the diagnosis of MI must immediately be entertained. Radiographic examination at this stage is important. As with other causes of suspected obstruction, an anteroposterior supine view of the abdomen is the basic film and should include the chest. (The infant may already have intrathoracic disease caused by the CF or by aspiration of vomited material.) A horizontal-beam abdominal film should be added in supine

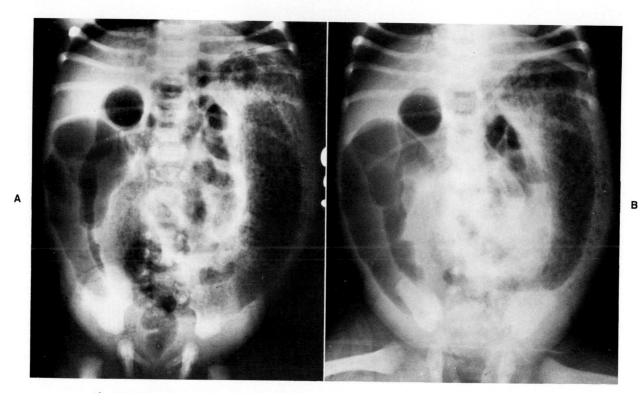

Fig. 70-1 Meconium ileus. Supine, **A,** and upright, **B,** radiographs of abdomen of newborn. There is marked bowel distention, with small amount of gas in rectum. There is granular, salt-and-pepper appearance in some of distended segments of small bowel, which is characteristic of meconium ileus. In upright view, **B,** there is paucity of gas-fluid levels in comparison with severe gut distention.

("cross-table lateral"), upright, or lateral decubitus position to demonstrate or exclude fluid levels and/or free gas in the peritoneal cavity.

The changes shown on the plain films are classically those of a bubbly appearance in the gut[170] in the right lower quadrant and distended bowel proximally, with paucity of fluid levels (Fig. 70-1). However, these changes are not always present, even in cases of uncomplicated meconium ileus[143] (Fig. 70-2), and it is usually difficult to distinguish large from small bowel on plain films in newborns. Thus absence of the classical appearance does not exclude the diagnosis of MI. When there is doubt about the diagnosis, contrast examination of the colon should be done. I use water-soluble contrast for this purpose, because I believe it is safer than barium, and it has no comparative disadvantages. The contrast medium should be at an osmolality level close to that of body fluids; this can be achieved by, for example, meglumine diatrizoate in 15% to 20% solution. The solution is gently instilled into the colon by means of a syringe and small rectal tube or allowed to flow from an elevated enema bag, provided that the flow is carefully controlled.

The finding of microcolon, in which the large bowel is of diminished caliber but normal length, indicates the presence of a distal small bowel obstruction. the finding does not identify the cause, unless the contrast flows by reflux into the terminal ileum and there outlines the accumulation of obstructing meconium. When this occurs, an attempt may be made to relieve the obstruction by using water-soluble contrast material to loosen the impacted meconium and promote its expulsion. Gastrografin, a solution of diatrizoate with a wetting agent (Tween 80) added, has been one of the most recommended contrast media for this therapeutic purpose ever since its effectiveness in relieving meconium ileus was reported by Noblett.[173,234] However, in undiluted form, Gastrografin is hyperosmolar, and therefore poses a danger of causing intravascular to extravascular fluid shift. In addition, the effect of Tween 80 is incompletely understood. Therefore if Gastrografin is used, great caution must be exercised in maintaining the child's fluid and electrolyte balance. An intravenous infusion should be initiated before the procedure is begun and expertly monitored. One of the ordinary water-soluble contrast agents may be used and may be effective, because the success of the enema method appears to rely at least partly on the flushing. There appears to have been no prospective study of the comparative efficacy of the various agents. The limited ability to achieve reflux into the terminal ileum when desired and the possibility of unrecognized

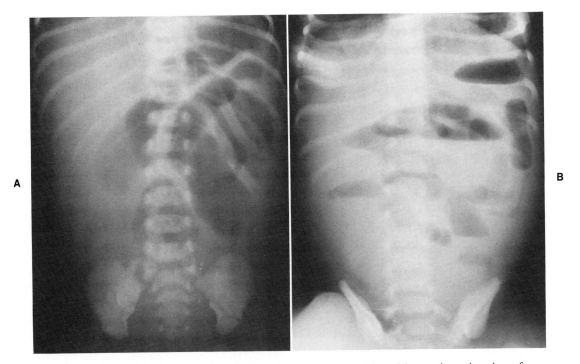

Fig. 70-2 Newborn infant with neconium ileus. **A,** Dilatation of bowel is seen in supine view of abdomen. **B,** Erect view shows number of gas-fluid levels. Note variation in caliber of gas-containing bowel. There is no evidence of classic soap bubble appearance. No atresia or other complication of meconium ileus was found at surgery.

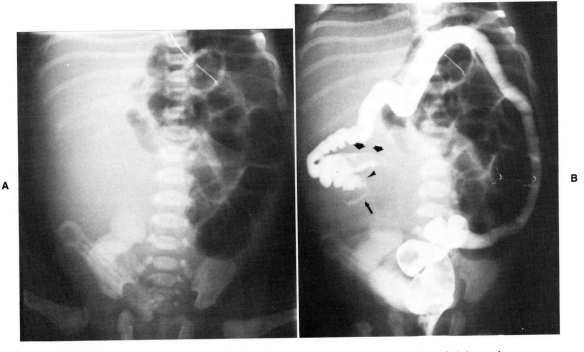

Fig. 70-3 Meconium ileus with pseudocyst formation. **A,** In supine plain film of abdomen large mass occupies right lower abdomen, and proximal to it there is markedly dilated small bowel, with no gas or meconium in large bowel, indicating complete obstruction. **B,** Contrast enema film shows entire colon, cecum *(arrowhead)*, and appendix *(arrow)*. Relux has occurred into terminal ileum, which tapers proximally to pointed termination *(short arrows)*, indicating volvulus of distal ileum with pseudocyst formation, which was confirmed at surgery.

complications of MI or of its treatment indicate the need for caution. Perforations of the colon are reported to occur easily in these infants.[61]

Other complications of meconium ileus include secondary atresia of the small intestine, volvulus, meconium cyst (or pseudocyst—the terms are used almost interchangeably [Fig. 70-3]) and meconium peritonitis. Except for meconium peritonitis, these complications may be difficult to recognize radiographically.[144] Grantmyer and co-workers reported necrotizing enterocolitis after treatment of MI with hyperosmolar Renografin enema containing no Tween 80, and warned that hyperosmolarity of the contrast medium in combination with bowel distention and ischemia may be responsible when perforation or necrotizing enteritis occurs.[98]

Wood and co-workers[244] used Tween 80 in 1% to 2% solution with isotonic sodium diatrizoate in a variety of infants and children with fecal mass obstruction with good results. They suggested that Tween 80 is effective in liquefaction and evacuation of tenacious stool, including that encountered in MI. Leonidas and co-workers reported the deaths of two newborn infants with MI who were treated with Gastrografin, which the authors felt may have contributed substantially to bowel necrosis.[144]

The balance of evidence appears to suggest that the greatest danger to the newborn infant with MI is the use of hyperosmolar contrast media, particularly when the fluid and electrolyte balance are not rigorously monitored and controlled.

Intestinal atresia

Secondary atresia (obliteration of the lumen prenatally of the distal ileum) may complicate CF, presumably because of compromise of the vascularity of the gut in utero.[29,101] Discontinuity of the gut may also result from adhesions associated with meconium peritonitis or from antenatal volvulus.[28] Atresia can also occur in the absence of MI.[150,198] The presence of prominent intestinal gas-fluid levels is unusual in uncomplicated MI[143]

Volvulus

The most common early intestinal complication of MI is prenatal volvulus of the small bowel, usually in the middle or distal ileum. The twisted loop may retain its viability or undergo necrosis. With necrosis, resorption of intestinal loops may occur, resulting in a meconium cyst or pseudocyst[150,198] (Fig. 70-3). Part of the pseudocyst may undergo calcification, demonstrable radiographically before or after birth.

Gastric emptying

Abnormally accelerated gastric emptying during the first hours after milk or formula meal was found in three or four infants with CF by Cavell, who felt that this might be a factor in growth retardation and maldigestion in such patients.[47]

Meconium peritonitis

Calcification outlining parts of the peritoneum of the fetus or neonate signify meconium peritonitis, and about 50% of cases of meconium peritonitis are the result of meconium ileus.[59] The presence of meconium peritonitis in a patient with cystic fibrosis is a grave prognostic sign.[117]

Meconium plug syndrome

The meconium plug syndrome is a common cause of low-grade intestinal obstruction in newborns. The obstruction usually is relieved spontaneously or by means of a diagnostic/therapeutic contrast enema.[66] For reasons that are not clear, a horizontal beam film of the abdomen may show a paucity of fluid levels, as occurs in meconium ileus.[187] This benign condition may be closely simulated by meconium ileus (Fig. 70-4). Therefore any newborn who appears to suffer from meconium plug syndrome, even if there is passage of a typical meconium plug there appears to be complete and recovery, should be checked for CF; in about 15% of cases, CF is the cause.[109,196]

Later manifestations
Meconium ileus equivalent

Some patients with CF, whether or not they had meconium ileus as neonates, have episodes of low-grade obstruction later in life—this is called meconium ileus equivalent[26] (Fig. 70-5). Abdominal radiographs usually show generalized gut dilatation, with bubbly appearing semisolid material in the distal small bowel and ascending colon. A fecal bolus in the distal ileum is almost pathognomonic.[26] Infants, older children, and even occasional adults with CF can be affected. The severity of the meconium ileus equivalent syndrome is not related to the severity of the pulmonary or hepatic disease.[160,185] Numerous factors, including abnormal mucus secretion, dehydration, and inadequate therapy with pancreatic enzymes have been implicated. The symptoms usually respond to medical therapy.[18] Diagnostic barium enema may have a therapeutic effect (Fig. 70-6). In less responsive instances, a water enema containing Mucomyst (acetylcysteine) has occasionally been helpful, in our hands and those of others,[219] but no prospective studies have been done, so it is not known whether the addition of acetylcysteine is truly useful.

Upper gastrointestinal tract

Gastroesophageal Reflux (GER) has been shown to be more common in patients with CF than in their normal

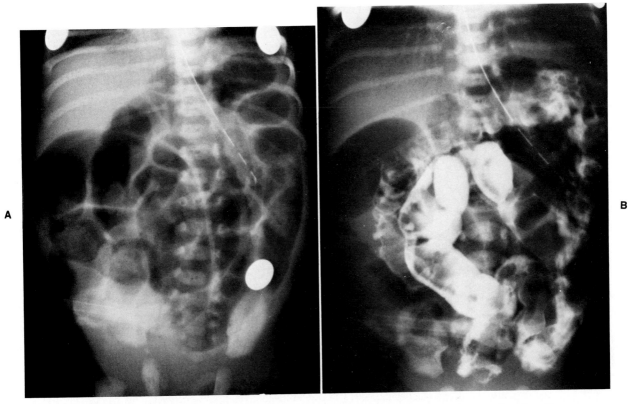

Fig. 70-4 Meconium plug syndrome in patients with cystic fibrosis. **A,** Preliminary supine film of abdomen shows marked distention of gut and empty rectum. **B,** Contrast enema film with water-soluble medium shows colon to be of normal caliber and to contain many long filling defects, characteristic of meconium plugs. After this diagnostic enema, child passed series of meconium plugs, and abdominal distention disapppeared. However, sweat testing subsequently proved cystic fibrosis.

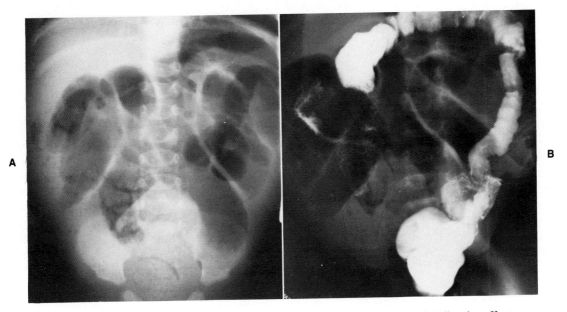

Fig. 70-5 Meconium ileus equivalent in 3-month-old infant with cystic fibrosis. **A,** Dilatation affects mainly small bowel. **B,** There was some difficulty in filling cecum with barium.

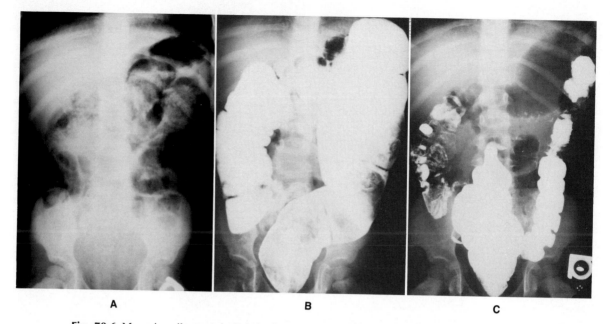

A   B   C

Fig. 70-6 Meconium ileus equivalent in 4-year-old cystic fibrosis patient with mild respiratory involvement and recent onset of crampy abdominal pain. Abdominal radiograph, **A,** shows large collection of fecal material, which was thought to be in colon. Barium enema was performed, **B,** which confirmed that large mass of fecal material was present in colon. After evacuation of barium and fecal material, **C,** no other abnormality was demonstrated. Symptoms were relieved by barium enema.

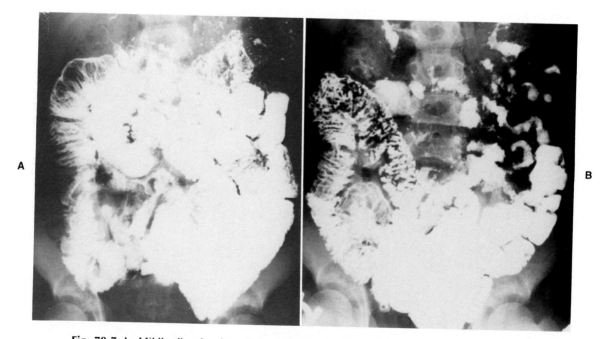

Fig. 70-7 A, Mildly disordered small bowel pattern in 10-year-old girl with cystic fibrosis and abdominal pain of unknown origin. **B,** After further transit of barium, nodular mucosal defects of small bowel are seen, probably as a result of dilated intestinal mucosal glands.

siblings and more common than in controls, though nighttime nasogastric feedings for CF patients appear to be safe.[203] Bendig and co-workers[25] reviewed seven children with CF who had GER. Their signs and symptoms included abdominal pain, peptic esophagitis, upper GI hemorrhage, and esophageal stricture. The mechanical influence of a depressed diaphragm caused by pulmonary hyperinflation, along with increased abdominal pressure and chronic coughing, appeared to contribute to GER. The authors suggested that early diagnosis and treatment are important.

SMALL BOWEL

Duodenal ulcer is occasionally found in older children and adults with CF.[16,179]

On barium study, the small bowel in patients with CF tends to appear abnormal. The duodenal folds are thickened and nodular. Similarly, the loops of jejunum and ileum are dilated, and their mucosal folds thickened, nodular, and distorted (Fig. 70-7). This finding, while characteristic, is not specific to CF. It is similar to that found in celiac disease. True celiac disease in CF patients, however, is extremely rare.[114] Another common finding is that of marginal small bowel filling defects (Fig. 70-7 *B*) that are probably caused by mucous distention of mucosal glands.[21]

Pneumatosis intestinalis

Hernanz-Schulman and co-workers[113] reviewed the clinical and radiographic findings with PI identified among 441 patients with CF. Pneumomediastinum, pneumothorax, or pulmonary interstitial emphysema was found in 95% of the patients with PI, compared with 62% of patients without PI. Dissection of air into the gut wall was often clinically silent, and tended to be self-perpetuating.

Colonic abnormalities

The colonic manifestations of CF include a redundant, velvety appearance of the colon on postevacuation barium enema films. This appearance, first described by Glazer,[90] is characteristic (Fig. 70-8). It may result in part from distended crypt goblet cells,[238] particularly in the older CF patient. I suspect that it is also caused by chronic distention of the colon, which, when relieved by diagnostic barium enema, causes the mucosal redundancy of the empty colon to be displayed. The striking radiographic change so produced has occasionally led to the diagnosis of previously unrecognized CF.

The viscid, tenacious fecal material in the colon of a CF patient may form a mass in the cecum or occasionally elsewhere in the colon. The mass may be perceived radiographically as a fecalith and may be palpable. It may

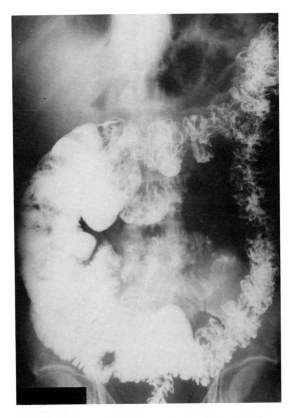

Fig. 70-8 Redundant, hyperplastic mucosal folds of colon are demonstrated on postevacuation barium enema film of adult patient with cystic fibrosis.

cause the signs and symptoms of a colonic neoplasm or suggest appendicitis when there is associated tenderness.[26]

Rectal prolapse is not uncommon in children between the ages of 6 months and 3 years who have untreated CF. Indeed, any young child who has repeated episodes of rectal prolapse should be suspected of having CF.[139]

Intussusception

Partients with CF are abnormally liable to suffer from ileocolic or colocolic intussusception.[101] The chief predisposing factor is likely the adherent fecal material that acts as a lead point for the intussusceptum. It is possible that the redundant mucosa in the small bowel or colon, or both, also acts as a lead point.

The incidence of intussusception in patients with CF has been estimated at 0.2% to 1.0%.[118] It has occurred as the first clinical evidence of CF. Hydrostatic reduction by a barium or water-soluble contrast enema has been reported to be successful in about 75% of such patients, but in some patients so treated, the intussusception recurs. Cecectomy has been performed successfully to prevent further recurrence.[231]

Pancreatic abnormalities

Diabetes is uncommon in CF, but with improved survival rates, its incidence is increasing. When it does develop, it is usually mild in degree.[216a] Radiographically demonstrable pancreatic calcification is uncommon but no longer considered rare (Fig. 70-9). Iannaccone and Antonelli found 5 cases of pancreatic calcification in 60 patients with CF. All were over 5 years of age. Four showed diabetic curves on glucose tolerance testing, and two developed frank diabetes.[122]

The pancreas in CF becomes increasingly abnormal with age. Spehl-Robberecht and co-workers reported that progressive pancreatic abnormalities may be noted by ultrasound in children who have CF. The pattern is normal in infants, but becomes progressively abnormal in patients older than 6 years, with increasing echogenicity and decreased width.[216] Willi and co-workers,[239] in reviewing ultrasound examinations of 24 patients with CF aged 8 to 30 years, also found that the number and severity of organs involved tended to increase with age. When the pancreas was identified, it was usually echogenic and small. The increased echogenicity is caused by fat replacement of pancreatic tissue (Fig. 70-10), and thus can be demonstrated clearly by ultrasound, CT, and magnetic resonance imaging (Fig. 70-11). Daneman and co-workers[52] showed that in some children in whom the pancreas is almost or completely replaced by fat it becomes enlarged. Rarely, the pancreas is virtually completely replaced by large cysts, which are demonstrable by ultrasound. Histologically, they are lined by a single layer of epithelial cells. These cysts have been termed *pancreatic cystosis*.[112]

Liver abnormalities

Textural changes in the liver, reflecting underlying parenchymal disease, are recognizable by ultrasound[239] and also by CT (Fig. 70-11). Cystic fibrosis of the liver accounts for one third of all cases of cirrhosis of the liver in pediatric patients.[59] However, only a small number of patients with CF have symptomatic cirrhosis. At autopsy, focal biliary cirrhosis with concretions in the cholangioles and bile ducts caused by inspissation of bile is a constant finding. These changes may be encountered in postmortem studies of infants, but they increase in frequency and severity with longer survival.[177] As such changes progress, portal hypertension with hepatosplenomegaly, hypersplenism, gastrointestinal bleeding with esophageal varices, and ascites may appear.[26,58,177,179] Fig. 70-12 shows the radiographic changes in a child with CF and exceptionally severe liver cirrhosis—an abnormally small liver, massively enlarged spleen, and esophageal varices.

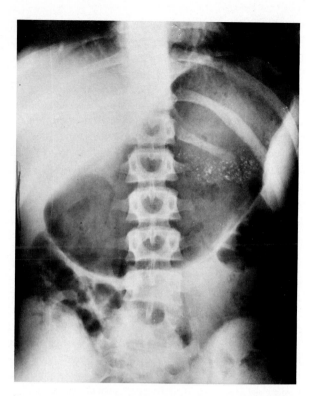

Fig. 70-9 Pancreatic calcification in patient with fibrocystic disease with diabetes. Gas-distended stomach permits clear visualization of pancreatic calcification.
(From Iannaccone, G, and Antonelli, M: Pediatr Radiol 9:85, 1980.)

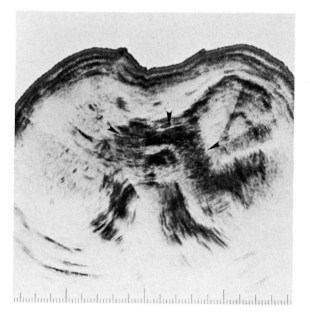

Fig. 70-10 Fat replacement of pancreas in cystic fibrosis. Pancreas is normal in size and shape but is highly echogenic and typical of fat replacement.

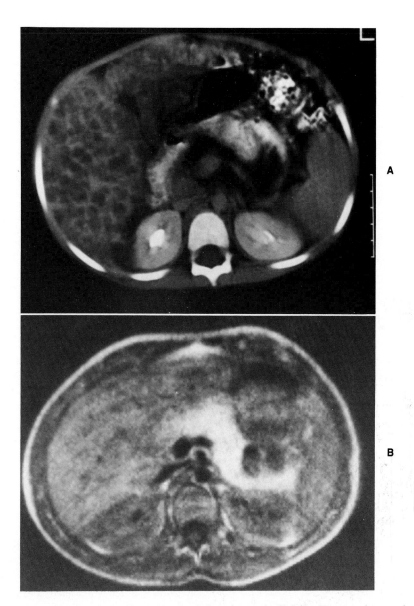

Fig. 70-11 A, Fat replacement of pancreas and liver in cystic fibrosis. Pancreas is completely replaced by low-density fat. There is also extensive fat replacement of the liver in pseudocystic configuration. **B,** Fat replacement of pancreas in cystic fibrosis shown by magnetic resonance imaging.

(Courtesy John C. Egelhoff, DO.)

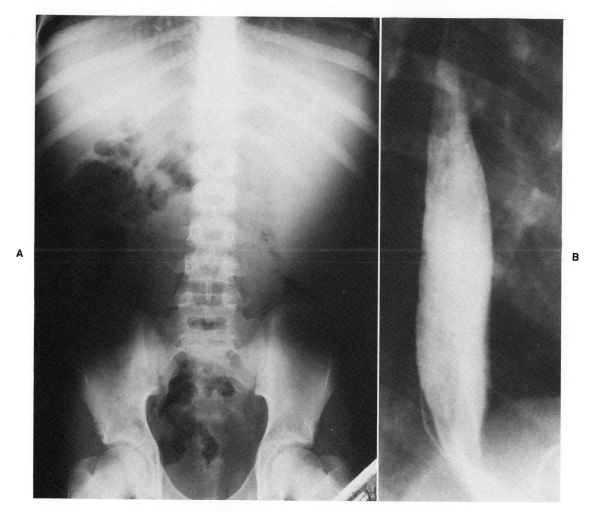

Fig. 70-12 A, Film of 12-year-old cystic fibrosis patient with small liver and splenic enlargement caused by portal hypertension and biliary cirrhosis. **B,** Varix is present in lower esophagus.

Fatty infiltration of the liver is found in 15% of CF patients at autopsy.[51] It cause is not fully understood, but it likely results from a nutrititional deficiency of protein. Of the infants showing fat infiltration of the liver, a significant number have been fed soybean-based formula, indicating that soybean is not an adequate protein source for these children.[85] In addition, there is evidence of a soybean trypsin inhibitor in the formula.[123] Fat replacement of liver parenchyma may be massive in some infants and is recognizable by radiolucency on abdominal films (Fig. 70-13), ultrasound, or CT[202](Fig. 11).

Willi and co-workers[239] reported that half of the CF patients whose abdomens they examined by ultrasound had abnormal hepatic patterns. Regularly increased echogenicity was the most common finding and was unrelated to liver size. Phillips and co-workers[183] found similar sonographic changes.

Gallbladder abnormalities

The gallbladder is usually small in patients with CF.[239] Sometimes, it is so small as to be almost indiscernible.[2] It may contain calculi and/or sludge, and the small gallbladder is most likely to contain calculi.[239] Changes of chronic cholecystitis have occasionally been noted.[29] However, demonstration of biliary disease in patients with CF does not correlate closely with symptoms; many such patients have few or no abdominal symptoms, and surgical treatment should only be recommended when correlation of radiographic and significant clinical findings has been convincingly established.[147]

The appendix in CF

The appendix may fail to fill on barium enema examination of patients with CF. Although filling indicated absence of appendicitis in CF patients, as it usually does

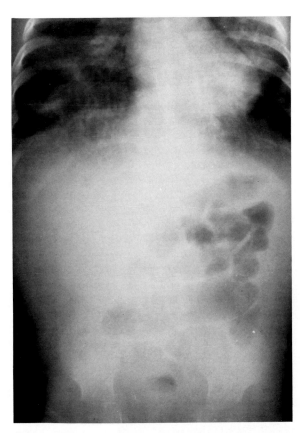

Fig. 70-13 Uncommon finding of fatty, hyperlucent liver in infant with cystic fibrosis. This may have resulted from inability to use dietary protein.

in otherwise normal individuals, lack of filling is not a reliable sign of appendicitis in those with CF. Histologic studies indicate that nonfilling is frequently related to mucus plugging of the appendiceal lumen.[76]

When the appendix is removed from a patient with CF, histologic features enable the diagnosis to be made by the pathologist, even if it has not been suspected clinically.[176,208] Increased activity of mucus-secreting cells with wide, gaping crypts filled with mucus are histologically characteristic and diagnostic.

ENDOCRINE DISORDERS
Hypothyroidism

Neonatal hypothyroidism is difficult to diagnose at birth; the signs are usually not sufficiently developed to be readily recognized.[56] Because delay in diagnosis can cause irreversible mental retardation, it is important that all physicians dealing with young infants be aware of the early clinical (and radiologic, in the case of radiologists) findings of congenital hypothryroidism, even though the majority of cases are discovered by neonatal laboratory screening tests. Constipation that is unresponsive to treatment, is one of these early findings. The radiologist asked to perform a barium enema for constipation in an infant should be aware of hypothyroidism as a possible cause. Delayed ossification of the femoral capital epiphyses can be identified on the abdominal films and/or with fluoroscopy in the course of a barium enema. Because the distal femoral epiphysis is almost always ossified in normal newborn infants, its absence in a possible case of hypothyroidism is highly significant. A glance at the knee with the fluoroscope entails negligible radiation and may help to confirm or eliminate suspected hypothyroidism, or even to first draw attention to this possible diagnosis.

The finding of a small rectum and dilatation of the remainder of the colon in a hypothyroid child have been demonstrated to closely mimic the barium enema changes of Hirschsprung's disease.[8]

IMMUNE DEFICIENCIES
Acquired immune deficiency syndrome

Acquired immune deficiency syndrome (AIDS) appears to be caused by infection with a retrovirus, which has been labeled human immunodeficiency virus (HIV). The infection produces disruption of the four major components of the normal immune system,[8] with the consequences of opportunistic infections, particularly in the lungs, and lymphoma, especially Kaposi's sarcoma. In children with AIDS, Kaposi's sarcoma is less common and less malignant than in adults. Most infants and children with AIDS are born to mothers who are infected with the virus, though the mother may not have the disease clinically. A high proportion of hemophiliac children who receive transfusions and/or factor VIII concentrate develop antibodies to AIDS-associated viruses. Symptoms usually occur within the first 3 to 6 months of age, but may not appear for up to 5 years. Hepatosplenomegaly, lymphadenopathy, failure to thrive, and chronic interstitial pneumonia are the most common clinical manifestations.

The alimentary tract is not as frequently involved in pediatric AIDS as is the respiratory tract, but chronic diarrhea is common. Other gastrointestinal symptoms include oral candidiasis, lymphadenopathy, and parotitis. Children may have HIV infection and show some of the clinical or laboratory abnormalities without meeting the criteria for AIDS diagnosis of the Centers for Disease Control.[54] Radiographically the most common manifestation of pediatric gastrointestinal AIDS is lymphadenopathy; hepatosplenomegaly is second.[10] Histologically, follicular hyperplasia, large lymphocytes and rare multinuceated giant cells are found in the nodes.[54] Typically, the aortic, caval, mesenteric, and porta hepatis lymph nodes are enlarged, usually forming large, bulky masses.

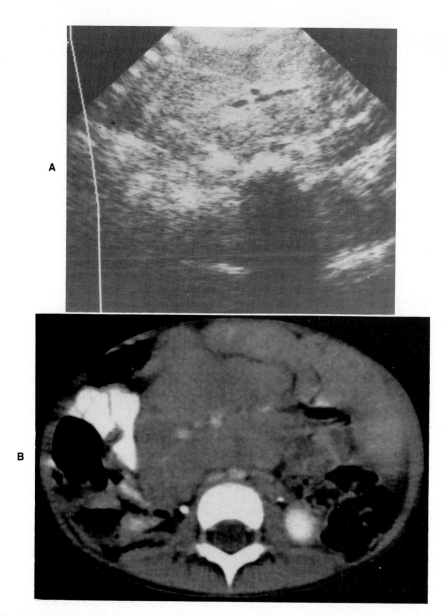

Fig. 70-14 Abdominal ultrasound image of child with AIDS. **A,** Transverse scan shows mesenteric vessels between hyperechoic lymph nodes. **B,** Enhanced CT scan at same level, demonstrating "sandwich sign"—compression of mesenteric vessels between enlarged lymph nodes. Biopsy of nodes revealed Mycobacterium avium intracellulare, and radio findings were confirmed at autopsy. (From Amodio, JB, Abramson, S, and Berdon, WE: Roentgenol 22:66, 1987.)

When these are located around mesenteric vessels, pancaking of the celiac axis or superior mesenteric artery may occur, producing the "sandwich sign,"[10] which may be imaged by ultrasound and/or CT (Fig. 70-14). The nodes, as shown by ultrasound, are usually hypoechoic, but may be variable in appearance. Ascites may also be seen, as may a thick-walled gallbladder.

Pediatric patients with AIDS not uncommonly have oral thrush, and this may be associated with candida esophagitis. Mucosal abnormalities may be seen on barium examination of the esophagus. These abnormalities consist of thickening of the mucosal folds, mucosal plaques, and ulceration. The changes are not specific for the particular opportunistic infection; diagnosis requires endoscopic visualization, biopsy, and culture.

As with other immunocompromised states, cryptosporidiosis may occur in patients with AIDS, causing intractable diarrhea and voluminous stools.[27] Pneumatosis

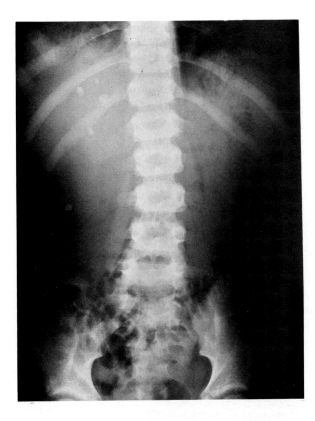

Fig. 70-15 Multiple liver calcifications in patient with chronic granulomatous disease. Liver is enlarged and contains several irregular calcified nodules, presumably representing necrotic residua from hepatic abscesses.
(Courtesy Frank Johnson, MD and David Cavanaugh, MD.)

intestinalis has also been shown radiographically in children with AIDS.[10]

Chronic granulomatomous disease

Chronic granulomatous disease (CGD) is a syndrome of recurrent bacterial or fungal infections associated with defective microbiocidal capacity of phagocytic cells and abnormal oxidative metabolic responses during phagocytosis. About 80% of cases occur in boys, in whom the inheritance is x-linked. In girls, there appears to be an autosomal recessive inheritance pattern.[190] In this disease, recognition and phagocytosis of bacteria occur normally in phagocytic cells, but the ingested microorganisms are not killed. Bacterial multiplication is inhibited, but intracelluar organisms survive and infections persist. The defect is in the oxidative metabolism and production of reacitve oxygen radicals during phagocytosis.

Clinically and radiographically, hepatosplenomegaly is found in most children with the disease but is nonspecific. Similarly, hepatic or perihepatic abscesses have been found. The most common organs in which frank infections appear, and reappear, are the liver, lungs, and bones; the most common bacteria are *Staphylococcus aureus, Seratia marcescens, Klebsiella* spp., and *Pseudomonas cepacia.* The commonest fungus is *Aspergillus fumigatus;* this organism may disseminate and cause serious, even fatal disease, particularly if not recognized and treated early in the infectious episode.

Liver and perihepatic abscesses are common in CGD, but the radiographic findings are usually nonspecific, even with arteriography.[22] However, radionuclide studies using gallium-67 have been shown to help in localizing infection in the liver, and may, particularly when complemented by technetium-99m, ultrasound, and CT, indicate liver suppuration and may succeed in localizing abscesses.[178,221] Calcifications may occur in liver granulomas (FIg. 70-15), and their presence on abdominal films should suggest the diagnosis. Splenic calcification, sometimes speckled, has also been seen.[43] The abdominal lymph nodes may calcify.[92]

Marked motility disturbance of the esophagus may be a manifestation of CGD. In a severe case, a boy with esophageal absent peristalsis and tight lower sphincter and hiatal hernia required a feeding gastrostomy for nutrition after pharmacologic and dilatation treatment failed.[155] Sutcliffe[224] reported dilatation of the esophagus and aquired coarctation of the descending thoracic aorta in CGD.

The most common, relatively specific and radiographically identifiable gut lesion occurring in this disease has

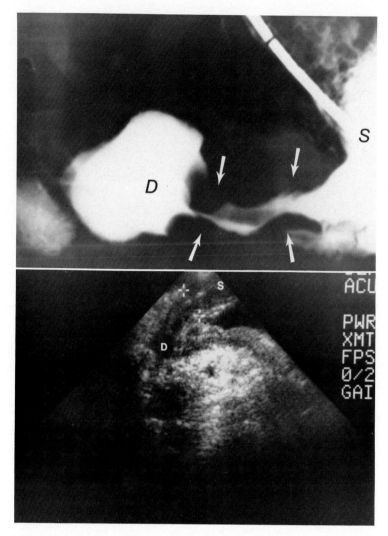

Fig. 70-16 Chronic granulomatous disease—gastric outlet obstruction *(arrows)*. **A,** Fluoroscopic spot film showing marked compression of gastric antrum with irregular mucosa. **B,** Transverse ultrasound image at level of antrum, showing hyperechoic mass causing antral compression. *S,* stomach; *D,* duodenum.

(From Dickerman, JD, Am J Dis Child 140:567, 1986. Copyright 1986, American Medical Association.)

The most common, relatively specific and radiographically identifiable gut lesion occurring in this disease has been antral narrowing. This may be demonstrated by barium studies and/or sonography (Fig. 70-16). The antral changes can resolve quickly, with or without antibiotic therapy.[55,99,136]

The small bowel can become involved and even obstructed. In all eight patients with CGD biopsied by Ament and Ochs,[9] the small bowel and rectum contained either granulomas or pigment-laden histiocytes, typical though not diagnostic of the disease. A patient reported by Harris and Boles developed a partial intestinal obstruction; the distal ileum, right colon, and proximal transverse colon were inflamed, thickened, and narrowed and contained granulomas in their muscular coats.[106] Sty

and co-workers[223] reported a 14-year-old with chronic granulomatous disease who had striking changes and marked nodularity of the entire colon, associated with a paracolic abscess (Fig. 70-17).

Graft-versus-host disease

When a child receives an allogeneic bone marrow transplant (BMT) the lymphoid tissue in the transplanted material may react against the tissues of the host. The most common host tissues attacked are those of the skin, liver, and gastrointestinal tract. The principal clinical findings are skin rash, hepatocellular dysfunction, and secretory diarrhea. Graft-versus-host disease (GVHD) occurs in 50% to 70% of allogeneic transplants, and is lethal in about 15% of afflicted marrow transplant recip-

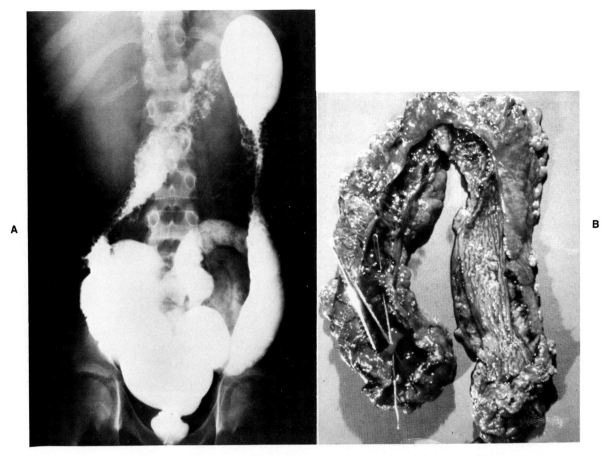

Fig. 70-17 Inflammation of colon in child with chronic granulomatous disease. **A,** Barium enema film shows marked nodularity of entire colon. **B,** Resected specimen of colon showing greatly thickened and nodular wall (**A** from Sty, JR, et al: Radiology 132:618, 1979, **B** courtesy JR Sty, MD.)

ients. Treatment includes immunosuppressive drugs and bowel rest and results in remission of the disease in about 75% of cases.

Efforts to suppress the reaction have included pretreatment of bone marrow to remove T cells responsible for GVHD before engraftment. While this pretreatment may reduce the risk of GVHD, it may increase risk of infection, particularly invasive fungal infection.[186]

The essential element of the intestinal GVHD is granular necrosis of crypt epithelium in the presence of infiltrating lymphocytes.[246]

The main radiographic findings are demonstrable by barium examination of the upper and lower intestinal tract. They consist of severe and rather characteristic changes in the entire intestinal tract, including the stomach, small bowel, and colon. However, the changes are most marked in the small bowel, which shows thickening and flattening of mucosal folds, thickening of the bowel wall, rapid transit of barium, and excess luminal fluid[74]

(Fig. 70-18). The radiographic findings may revert to normal in successfully treated cases. However, Jones and co-workers[125] reviewed the records of 28 patients whose barium studies suggested gastrointestinal inflammation after bone marrow transplantation and either acute GVHD, viral infection, or both. The authors concluded that differentiation between acute GVHD and viral enteritis is not possible on the basis of radiographic findings alone. Fig. 70-19 illustrates one of their cases—an 8-year-old girl whose barium study appears at least consistent with GVHD, but who had clinical evidence of viral enteritis, not GVHD. They advised that both entities be considered when gastrointestinal inflammation occurs after BMT.

Pneumatosis intestinalis (PI) may complicate the course of a child who has had BMT. Yeager and co-workers[248] reported the findings in four children aged 3 to 8 years who developed PI after BMT for acute leukemia or severe aplastic anemia. PI was detected at 48

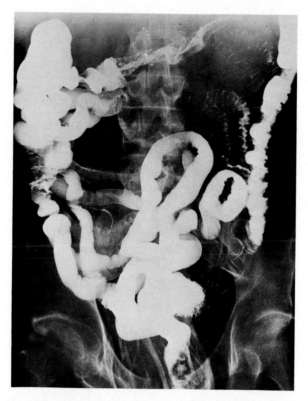

Fig. 70-18 Graft-vs.-host reaction. Barium enema film shows narrowed edematous colon with reflux into narrowed, tubular, separated ileal loops without mucosa and into jejunal loops with thickened folds.
(From Rosenberg, HK, et al: Radiology 138:371, 1981.)

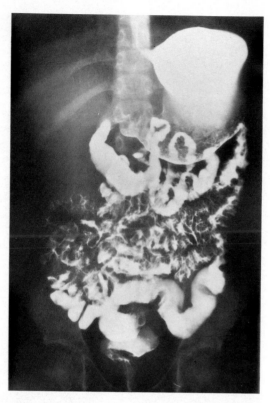

Fig. 70-19 Barium study in 8-year-old girl. Small bowel disorder was felt to be consistent with graft-versus-host disease, but clinical evidence favored viral enteritis.
(From Jones, B, and Kramer, SS: Gastrointestinal inflammation after bone marrow transplantation: graft-versus-host disease or opportunistic infection? AJR 150:277-281, © by American Roentgen Ray Society 1988.)

days (median) after BMT, and was associated with abdominal symptoms and clinical signs. All had severe systemic and/or high-grade cutaneous acute GVHD at some time after BMT and were receiving corticosteroids when PI developed. However, the PI was associated with concomitant severe, acute GVHD in only one patient. The overall survival depended on the frequency and severity of other conditions, such as GVHD and opportunistic infection.

Lymphoid hyperplasia of the gut

Lymphoid follicles may be radiographically visible in the gut of the normal child. In the terminal ileum, the follicles are aggregated into larger masses (Peyer's patches). These masses are easily visualized in standard or compression films. In the normal colon, nodular filling defects up to 2 mm in diameter are frequently seen, with or without umbilication.[45,142] These represent normal lymph follicles. The term *lymphoid hyperplasia* should be reserved for abnormally large follicles, although it is admittedly difficult to be sure in many cases whether the nodules are only unusually large and visible or abnormally so. True lymphoid hyperplasia is found in some patients with immune deficiencies. It may be visualized in the small bowel in and proximal to the terminal ileum[116] (Fig. 70-20) and in the colon.[243] Laufer[142] suggested that, in the colon, the term *lymphoid hyperplasia* be reserved for cases in which the lymph follicles are greater than 2 mm in diameter. I have seen, in a child with an immunologic deficiency, lymph follicles so large in the small and large bowel that they were mistaken for polyposis. In patients with Crohn's disease, lymphoid hyperplasia may also occur and may be indistinguishable from that observed in immune deficiencies.

Sauerbrei and Castelli[199] reported an adult with hypogammaglobulinemia with radiographically demonstrated nodular lymphoid hyperplasia of the small bowel and colon, and they found lymphoid hyperplasia of the gallbladder and appendix pathologically.

Lymphoid hyperplasia of the stomach is rare. The case of a 12-year-old girl in whom the diagnosis was confirmed by endoscopy and endoscopic biopsy was reported by Odes.[175] She was treated with antacids, and her abdominal pain, which was the presenting complaint, disappeared.

In a patient with hypogammaglobulinemia who un-

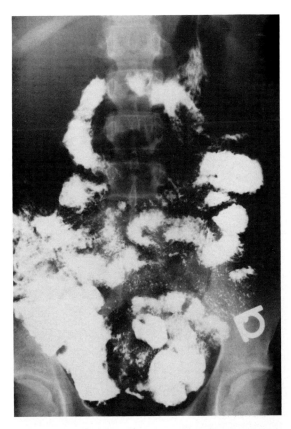

Fig. 70-20 Small bowel examination of patient with severe hypogammaglobulinemia. Radiographs show innumerable small nodules scattered throughout small bowel and moderate disordering of small bowel pattern consistent with malabsorption. Autopsy confirmed that nodular lesions were caused by lymphoid hyperplasia.

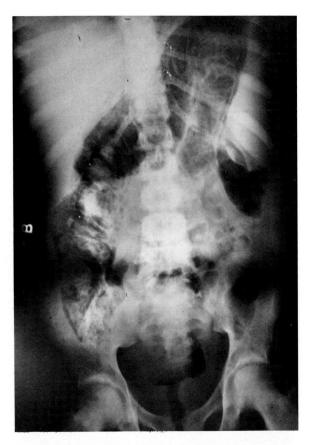

Fig. 70-21 Pneumatosis coli in patient with immune deficiency. Extensive pneumatosis intestinalis is present in right colon, and there is retroperitoneal air in right suprarenal region and along left psoas margin.
(From Kleinman, PK, Brill, PW, and Winchester, P: Am J Dis Child 134:1149, 1980. Copyright 1980, American Medical Association.)

derwent surgical exploration and jejunal biopsy, pathologic examination of the small bowel showed the tiny nodules to be hyperplastic lymph follicles in the lamina propria.[116] The enlarged follicles caused effacement of the villous pattern of the overlying mucosa, producing a polypoid appearance. There was a heavy perifollicular lymphocyte infiltration; the germinal centers within the follicles were large, and there was conspicuous mytotic activity.

Pneumatosis intestinalis

Gas may appear in the wall of the bowel, usually the colon, of children with a variety of conditions, most notable of which are immuune deficencies[135] and steroid therapy. Three mechanisms for this phenomenon have been postulated. First, steroid treatment may shrink the lymph follicles in the gut and thus make its mucosa more permeable. Second, a patient with an immune deficiency is susceptible to pulmonary interstitial emphysema, mediastinal emphysema, retroperitoneal emphysema, and pneumatosis of the gut wall. Third, a severe infection in an immunologically compromised child may lead to necrosis of the bowel wall and permeation by gas from the lumen, by gas-forming organisms, or by both, Fig. 70-21 demonstrates pneumatosis intestinalis (PI) in a child with immune deficiency.

The prognosis of PI in such patients is not necessarily poor; if the respiratory or gut disease can be treated and controlled, PI generally subsides. If there is no identifiable primary lesion, PI may be asymptomatic, and may disappear after lasting some days or weeks.[32,135] PI has been seen following BMT, without notably affecting the prognosis or treatment.[248]

There are two conditions in which gas in the gut wall may signal severe or dangerous disease—typhlitis and necrotizing enterocolitis. These should not be confused with the more benign and indolent pneumatosis intestinalis. Typhlitis (from the Greek *typhlon*, cecum) has come to mean necrotizing inflammation of the cecum. Typhlitis is usually seen in children receiving chemo-

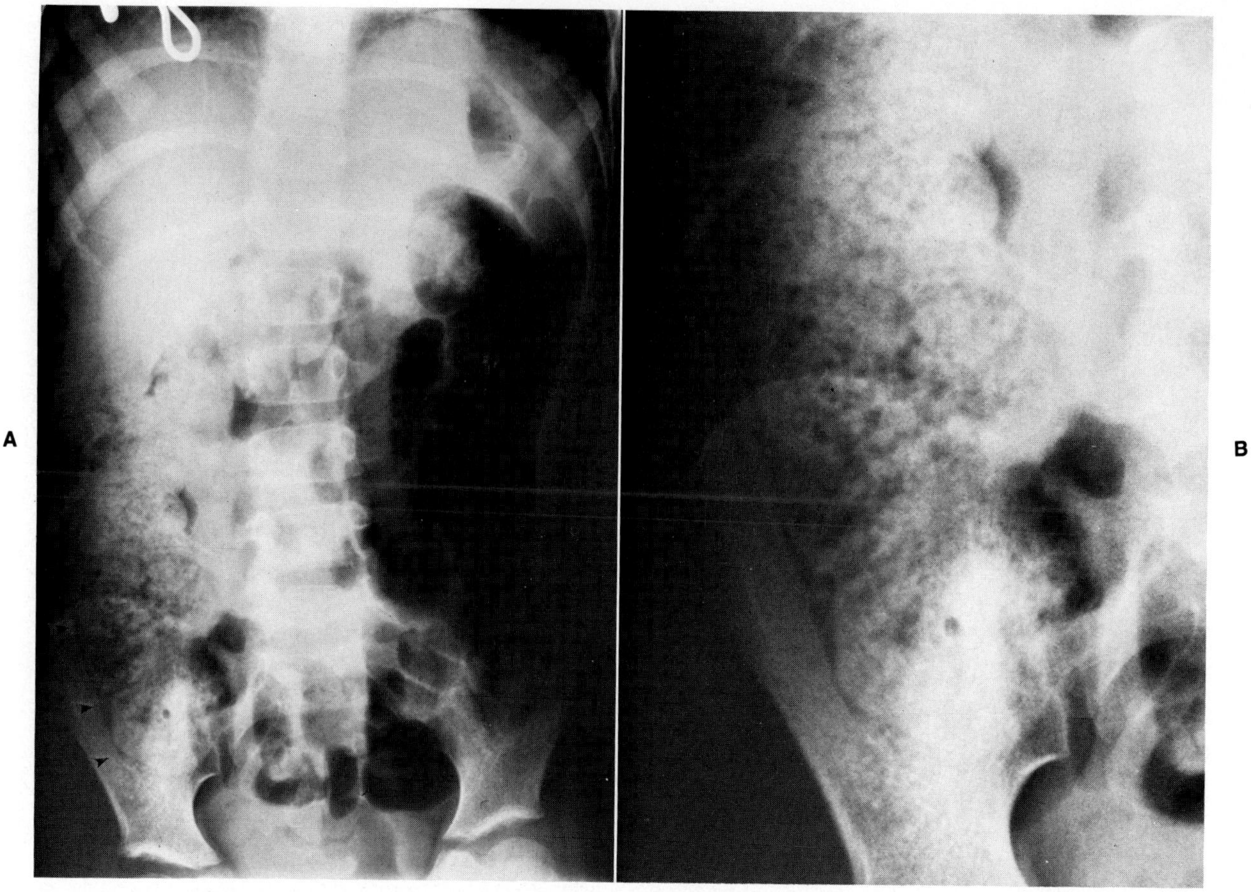

Fig. 70-22 A, Typhlitis complicating leukemia. Plain film of abdomen shows gas in wall of cecum and proximal ascending colon *(arrowheads).* This was considered to be characteristic of leukemic typhlitis and to signify poor prognosis. Child died short time after this complication developed. **B,** Close-up view of cecum and proximal ascending colon.

therapy in late or terminal stages of illness. It is seen in adults, but less commonly, and may occur early in the disease.[1] Surgery is thought to be needed immediately on diagnosis, but is not always successful or essential.[1] The diagnosis has most frequently been made by radiographic recognition of gas in the wall of the cecum and, variably, the ascending colon (Fig. 70-22), together with mass effect and inflammatory changes in the involved bowel. The same findings can be identified by ultrasound.[226]

Esophagitis

Esophagitis may occur in patients with any debilitating condition, including prolonged illness, diabetes, malignancy and impaired immune competence. The latter usually results from the primary disease or its treatment by steroids, chemotherapy, or antibiotics. Primary immune deficiencies are not as likely to predispose to esophagitis, as are secondary deficiencies.

The most common esophageal infection in children

with impaired immune response is candidiasis (formerly called moniliasis and, when clinically recognized in and around the mouth, thrush). Oral and pharyngeal lesions clinically appear as white or gray-white plaques surrounded by erythematous halos. In some patients, however, no oral or pharyngeal lesion is present. Odynophagia and dysphagia, with or without the oral and pharyngeal lesions of thrush, lead to the radiographic examination of the esophagus. The clinical and radiographic abnormalities usually subside rapidly with oral antifungal treatment.

The radiographic appearance of candidiasis in adults is said to be most typically characterized by plaques in the esophageal mucosal.[36] This cannot usually be done in children, partly because the number of cases for study is smaller in the pediatric age group, and partly because it is more difficult to perform a superb double-contrast examination of the esophagus in infants and children than in adults.[232] Fig. 70-23 demonstrates the findings in a child with immune defiency and esophageal candidiasis.

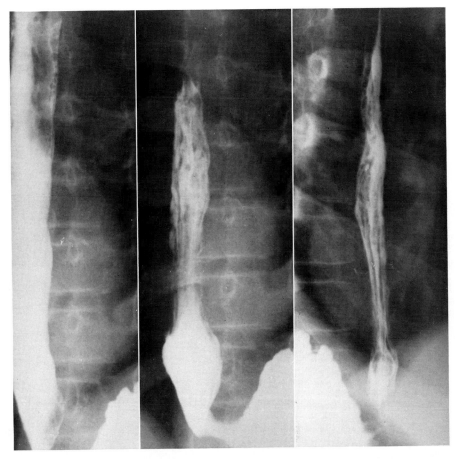

Fig. 70-23 Candida esophagitis in patient with immune deficiency. This child has been treated for leukemia and was therefore presumably more susceptible to opportunistic infection than normal. Radiologic investigation of dysphagia demonstrated coarsening and irregularity of mucosal folds and of esophageal margin. Findings were consistent with esophageal candidiasis, which was successfully treated.

Herpes esophagitis also occurs in immunocompromised patients. The clinically recognizable lesions sometimes begin in the central portion of the face. Small papulovesicular eruptions become necrotic and slowly enlarge peripherally for several weeks before healing commences.[167]

The radiographic findings closely resemble those of candidiasis, though discrete ulcers or discrete plaques on an otherwise normal esophageal background are said to be characteristic.[146] Esophagoscopy viral cultures, or both may be necessary to identify herpes infection. The distinction from other forms of infection is important, because antiviral agents are available that appear to shorten or mitigate viral infections.[110]

A chronic esophageal stricture can result from candidal infection of the esophagus.[129]

In the differential diagnosis of esophagitis complicating an immune deficiency, the effects of medication must be considered. However, though medication-induced esophagitis is reported in adults,[5,33] it appears to be very uncommon in children.[172] Esophagitis and esophageal stricture complicating radiation therapy, reported in adults,[30,93] is almost unknown in infants and children. The same is true of bacterial esophagitis.[235]

Cytomegalovirus infection of the esophagus has been observed radiographically in four homosexual men with AIDS; there was localized ulceration or more diffuse esophagitis, affecting predominantly the distal esophagus.[19] No similar observations in children have yet been published.

HEMATOLOGIC AND ONCOLOGIC DISEASE
Leukemia

Leukemia may involve any portion of the alimentary tract.[189] PI is one of the most commn complications, PI is often asymptomatic, and if symptoms are present, they may not be severe. Jaffe and co-workers[130] reported finding PI unexpectedly in six children with advanced leu-

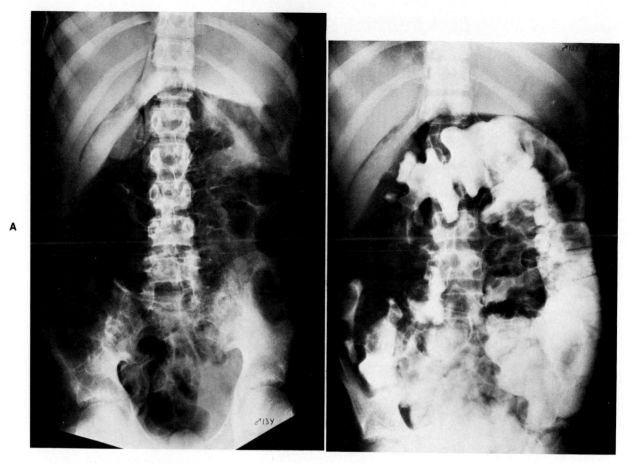

Fig. 70-24 Pneumatosis coli in child with leukemia. While under treatment for leukemia and essentially asymptomatic, this child had routine chest radiograph that showed gas in bowel wall in upper abdomen. Abdominal films demonstrated extensive pneumatosis cystoides coli. He continued to be asymptomatic, and gas spontaneously disappeared from bowel wall and from retroperitoneal space in right adrenal area. **A,** Plain film showing gas in bowel wall and extraperitoneal space. **B,** Confirmation by barium enema examination.

kemia. In one child, spontaneous resolution occurred; in the other five, the PI was confirmed at autopsy, however, death was not attributable to PI in any of the patients. They advised that the condition is probably best treated with antibiotics in the leukemic child with specific attention to any intrinsic abdominal disease and to the leukemic process. Fig. 70-24 shows PI in a leukemic child.

Hunter and Bjelland[120] described 13 patients, including four children, who came to autopsy after dying of leukemia. The complications found included typhlitis, leukemic infiltration of the bowel, ureterocolonic fistula, abscess secondary to typhlitis, and pseudomembranous colitis with *Candida* overgrowth. Of the 13 patients, 8 survived their gastrointestinal complications, and those who died had nonetheless experienced significant palliation. The authors stated that the gastrointestinal compli-

cations of leukemia should not be considered rare, untreatable, or preterminal. Their review included the case of a 16-year-old girl with acute myelogenous leukemia and intussusception. The cause of the intussusception was not established. Fig. 70-23 illustrates typhlitis occurring shortly before death in a leukemic child.

Esophagitis caused by opportunistic organisms is not uncommon in leukemia (Fig. 70-23). Lower esophageal filling defects caused by leukemia have been reported in a child who had dysphagia; the clinical and radiographic findings resolved with radiation therapy.[7]

Although contrast enemas are sometimes needed to better define a colonic or cecal abnormality that may need specific treatment, any kind of anorectal manipulation, including cleansing enemas and diagnostic enemas, may be a danger to the leukemic patient. The child is highly susceptible to infection, and the colonic mucosa may be

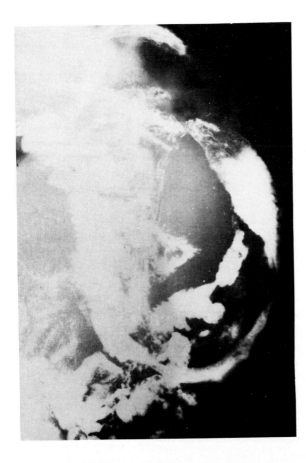

Fig. 70-25 Massive involvement of stomach and small bowel by Burkitt's lymphoma in African child. Note incidental infestation with *Ascaris*.
(Courtesy P Cockshott, M.D.)

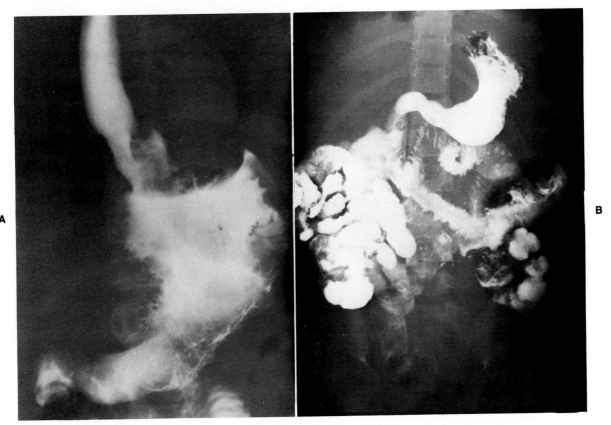

A

B

Fig. 70-26 **A,** Burkitt's lymphoma involving stomach in African child. (Courtesy P Cockshott, M.D.)
B, Burkitt's lymphoma, American type, in African child. Upper gastrointestinal series shows enlarged spleen; rigid, ulcerated, and encased segment of jejunum separated from other segments; and mass in left lower quadrant.

abnormally permeable. Colonic organisms may therefore enter the bloodstream and cause septicemia.[140] If a diagnostic contrast enema is deemed essential, and if there is any likelihood of perforation of the gut, a water-soluble contrast medium should be used in preference to barium.

Lymphoma

Hodgkin's lymphoma does not involve the pediatric gastrointestinal tract sufficiently frequently or severely to be dealt with separately here.

Non-Hodgkin's lymphoma, to the degree that it involves the gastrointestinal tract in children, is mostly Burkitt's lymphoma (BL), a neoplasm related to African lymphoma, that has distinctive histologic, cytologic, and cytochemical criteria.[38] The tumor consists primarily of large, immature lymphoid cells of B-lymphocyte origin.[40] BL deposits are more often extranodal than nodal. Though BL is endemic in tropical Africa and frequently makes its first appearance in the jaw, American BL is uncommon, usually occurs in childhood, and tends to involve the abdominal organs more than the jaw. The abdominal mass or masses that appear in BL sometimes enlarge very rapidly—more so than in any other pediatric malignancy. Indeed, abdominal BL has occasionally had such a fulminant course that it was mistaken clinically for acute appendicitis.

African children are of course not exempt from abdominal Burkitt's lymphoma (Figs. 70-25 and 70-26).

Enlarging submucosal ileal masses in non-Hodgkin's lymphoma occasionally cause ileocolic intussusception (Fig. 70-27). In fact, occurring in a child with intussusception who is older than the usual age for "idiopathic" ileocolic intussusception should be suspected of having cystic fibrosis of the pancreas or non-Hodgkin's lymphoma, for these are the two most common causes of such an event.

The initial assessment of BL previously depended on standard radiographic methods—chest and abdominal films, excretory urography, and barium studies of the gut as specifically indicated. Newer imaging methods have shown their superiority, however, and should form the basis of at least the initial assessment. Glass and coworkers,[89] in reviewing their use of gallium-67 scintigraphy, found that this method demonstrated more sites of tumor involvement than any other method. Pretreatment abdominal CT and ultrasonography were useful for evaluating ascites, density and size of the liver and spleen, renal involvement, and the presence of lymphomatous soft-tissue masses. Sonography was less accurate in localizing tumor deposits but more sensitive to small amounts of ascites. Any of these methods, the authors reported, is effective in following response to chemo-

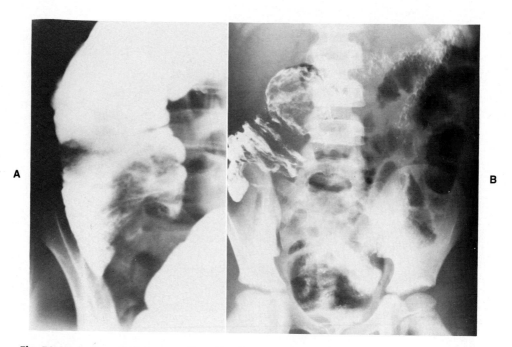

Fig. 70-27 A, Ileocolic intussusception caused by localized non-Hodgkin's lymphoma in 6-year-old boy. **B,** Postevacuation barium enema film shows intraluminal tumor mass remaining in area of hepatic flexure.

therapy, but sequential ^{67}Ga scintigraphy also had prognostic value, as those children whose scintigrams reverted to normal within 6 months survived.

Hemophilia and Christmas disease

Hemophilia is a cause of intramural intestinal bleeding that can be spontaneous or the result of minor trauma. Although numerous cases of intramural hematoma have been reported since the radiographic description by Felson and Levin in 1954,[70] surprisingly few have been described in patients with hemophilia.[88,96] In the duodenum, the resultant intramural mass is sharply marginated, and the valvulae conniventes are spread into a coil-spring pattern similar to that seen in cases of intussusception.[70] The hematoma may result in intestinal obstruction[164] (Fig. 70-28). Khilnani[132] described characteristic thickening of folds of the small intestine with a parallel spiked appearance of their margins that resembles stacked coins. This is particularly noticeable in the jejunum. Multiple lucent filling defects (thumbprinting), caused by mucosal hemorrhage, have also been seen in this disease.[132] Wiot[241] suggested that spontaneous intramural hemorrhage is more infiltrative and less likely to cause a mass than is hemorrhage caused by trauma. Intussusception is also a possible complication of hemorrhage in children with hemophilia.[166] Besides the duo-

denum, intramural bleeding caused by hemophilia has been demonstrated radiographically in the stomach,[96] jejunum,[60] distal ileum and ileocecal valve area,[242] and distal descending colon.[60] When this phenomenon occurs in the stomach, large obstructing hemorrhagic masses may result.[96,100,247]

Christmas disease (Factor IX deficiency, accounting for about 15% of all hemophiliac patients) causes findings similar to those of hemophilia.[166] An early case of a duodenal hematoma was reported in an infant with an undetermined type of hemorrhagic disease, possibly hemophilia.[100]

Because surgery is hazardous in patients with coagulation defects, the radiographic recognition of the effects of hemophilia on the gut is important. Eventual spontaneous disappearance of the clinical and radiographic abnormalities is to be expected.[60]

Henoch-Schönlein purpura

Henoch-Schönlein purpura (nonthrombocytopenic purpura) is a frequently encountered childhood disorder that is included in the differential diagnosis of spontaneous intramural hemorrhage.[241] Abdominal pain may be associated with the finding of dilated, separated loops of small bowel with marginal defects or thumbprinting caused by submucosal hemorrhage.[100] These findings, as

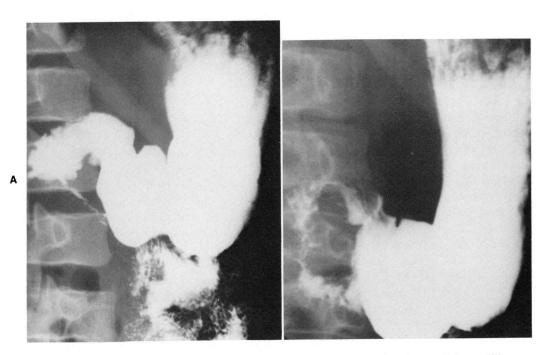

Fig. 70-28 A, Duodenal obstruction caused by intramural hematoma in 15-year-old hemophiliac patient involved in automobile accident. **B,** Nine days later duodenum is normal with exception of slight thickening of mucosal folds.

well as the clinical manifestations of purpura, abdominal pain, and arthralgia, are reversible. Occasionally, intussusception results and may require surgical relief. Matsumoto and co-workers[214] reported a patient who had an ileocolic intussusception and 7 days later a jejunojejunal intussusception. Both required surgical intervention, the second with resection of 30 cm of jejunum. Tsunado[230] reviewed 79 cases, of which 7 (9%) required surgery.

Bryn and co-workers[37] had a patient with Henoch-Schönlein purpura in whom abdominal symptoms antedated the appearance of cutaneous lesions by 3 months. The characteristic radiographic changes of submucosal small bowel hemorrhage contributed to the correct diagnosis (Fig. 70-29). Glasier and co-workers[87] pointed out that small bowel changes in this disorder may be identical to those of Crohn's disease; the colon may be involved in submucosal hemorrhage, and intussusception or even small bowel obstruction may occur. Lombard reported ileal stricture as a late complication.[149]

Sickle cell disease

An autosomal recessive gene for homozygous (SS) disease is carried by approximately 8% of American blacks, and it is estimated that 1 of 500 black neonates has homozygous sickle cell disease. Abdominal crises, caused by occlusion of small blood vessels by spontaneously sickled red cells and manifested by pain, jaundice, elevated liver enzymes, and often leukocytosis, are said to occur in 10% of all patients with sickle cell anemia.

Radiographic investigation infrequently adds substantially to the evaluation of the pediatric sickle cell anemia patient having an acute abdominal crisis. Plain films tend to show a small or invisible spleen, presumably because of progressive autoinfarction, although McCall et al. reported an incidence of 31% splenic calcification.[160] Seldom is any intestinal or other abnormality found that helps to explain the abdominal crisis or identify other abdominal abnormalities that may simulate a sickle cell crisis in a child.

An important exception is biliary calculi. A prospective study has shown gallstones to be present in 17% of sickle cell patients from 10-19 years of age; the incidence rises to 71% at age 30 or older, with an overall incidence after age 10 of 49%.[184] These figures were for calculi demonstrated by plain films and oral cholecystography and would likely be considerably higher if ultrasound were included in a prospective study. Karayalcin and co-workers examined 47 patients with SS disease, aged 2 to 28 years, to determine the prevalence of gallstones. Eight children (17%) had stones demonstrated by oral cholecystography; in seven of these cases ultrasound also demonstrated stones. All eight had been admitted on several occasions for sickle cell crises and four for acute

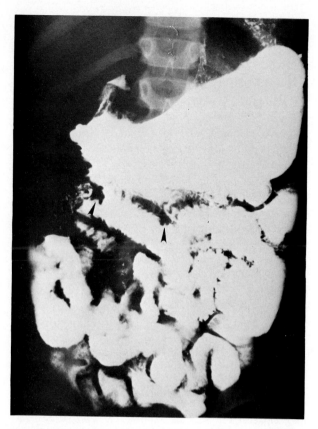

Fig. 70-29 Henoch-Schönlein purpura involving small bowel. Upper gastrointestinal barium examination 6 days before appearance of skin lesions shows separation of bowel loops and thumbprinting *(arrowheads)*, characteristic of submucosal hemorrhage.
(From Byrn, JR, et al: Am J Dis Child 130:1335, 1976. Copyright 1976, American Medical Association.)

hepatic crises. All eight underwent elective cholecystectomy, and gallstones were found in each. They were followed up from 7 to 17 months after cholecystectomy, and none had abdominal symptoms.[126]

Magid and co-workers[153] studied 30 patients with sickle cell disease, all with unusual abdominal pain and/or fever of uncertain cause. They found acute liver, spleen, and appendiceal abnormalities in several patients in or near the pediatric age; a 15-year-old boy had a ruptured spleen, a 19-year-old man had a liver infarct, and a 17-year-old boy had appendiceal fecaliths with periappendiceal abscess. Thus, though most abdominal crises have not appeared to result from any lesion whose treatment can be altered or improved by radiographic investigation, any atypical or persistent signs or symptoms should be taken seriously and submitted to appropriate studies. CT and ultrasound are the methods with the highest yield in such cases. Indeed, if the experience of Karayalcin and co-workers[126] and of Ariyan and co-

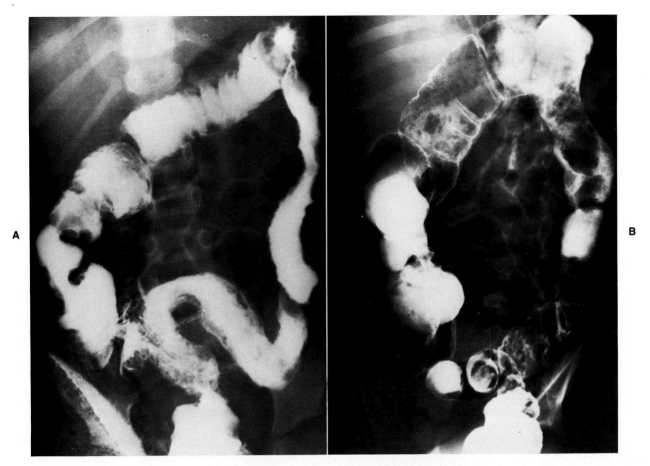

Fig. 70-30 Hemolytic uremic syndrome in 5-year-old boy with bloody diarrhea. Barium enema examination. **A,** showed severe changes of inflammatory disease. Sigmoidoscopy showed superficial mucosal ulceration. Within a few days he had developed typical laboratory and clinical findings of hemolytic uremic syndrome, from which he recovered. Two weeks later, repeat barium enema, **B,** Demonstrated relatively normal mucosal pattern. Area of persistent narrowing in descending colon represents stricture formation.
(From Peterson, RB, et al: Radiology 118:667, 1976.)

workers[13] is confirmed by others, routine ultrasound scanning of the biliary tract of sickle cell patients would appear to be justified.

Hemolytic-uremic syndrome

The hemolytic-uremic syndrome (HUS) is the most common cause of acute renal failure in young children. HUS is a triad of acute renal failure, microangiopathic hemolytic anemia, and thrombocytopenia, most common in children under the age of 4 years there is a prodromal period of 3 to 10 days in which gastrointestinal symptoms occur in 80% or more of patients, followed by pallor, irritability, weakness, lethargy, oliguria, and thrombocytopenia.[95a,127]

If a barium enema examination is performed to investigate the bloody diarrhea, which clinically may appear to be caused by acute colitis, the characteristic changes of transverse ridging and thumbprinting may be shown, indicating hemorrhage or edema or both of the bowel wall[20,134,182] (Fig. 70-30, *A*). Therefore in any young child who develops bloody diarrhea and in whom a barium enema examination shows evidence of edema, hemorrhage, or colitis that is otherwise unexplained, the possibility of HUS should be considered.

A stricture may occur in the colon as a complication of the colitis in HUS[134,182,200] (Fig. 70-30, *B*).

Shwachman syndrome

Shwachman syndrome (exocrine pancreatic insufficiency, blood disorders and metaphyseal dysostosis) is a hereditary disease with exocrine pancreatic insufficiency, cyclic neutropenia, anemia, and thrombocytopenia.[209]

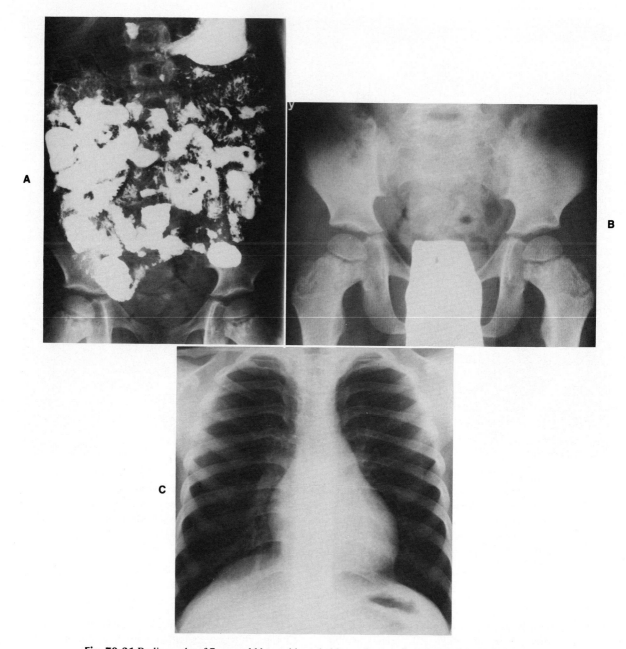

Fig. 70-31 Radiographs of 7-year-old boy with probable syndrome of pancreatic insufficiency, bone marrow dysfunction, and metaphyseal dysostosis. **A,** Small bowel study shows disordered pattern consistent with malabsorption. **B,** There is minimal irregularity of physes and metaphyses of proximal femora. Distal femoral metaphyses were similar in appearance but showed less marked abnormalities. **C,** Chest radiograph taken at age of 10 years showed none of chronic pulmonary disease usually associated with cystic fibrosis.

The patients fail to grow and/or thrive during infancy and have diarrhea, but not gross steatorrhea; they are sometimes thought to have cystic fibrosis initially. There may be a disordered small bowel pattern radiographically (Fig. 70-31, A). The pancreatic acinar tissue is atrophic and may even be replaced by fat[194] in manner similar to that seen in cystic fibrosis. Sweat electrolytes are normal however, and pulmonary abnormalties, though present by respiratory function tests, are not prominent (Fig. 70-31, C). Metaphyseal dystosis may be visible radiographically, but is variable and may be subtle (Fig. 70-31, B) or equivocal.[163] Leukemia has been reported.[245]

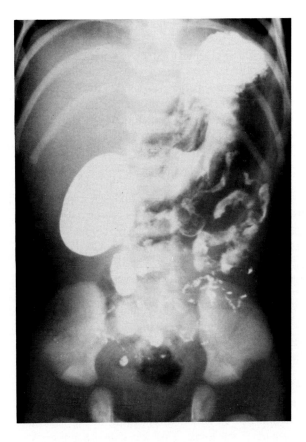

Fig. 70-32 Partial duodenal obstruction is present in this newborn infant with trisomy 21. Pelvis shows widening of iliac wings and horizontally disposed acetabular roofs, characteristic of Down's syndrome.

CHROMOSOMAL DISORDERS
Trisomy 21 (Down's syndrome)

In patients with Down's syndrome, there is a high incidence of clinically significant anomalies of the intestine.[31] Duodenal stenosis and duodenal atresia are most frequently encountered, and their demonstration or suspicion in a newborn infant should alert the radiologist to the possibility that the patient has Down's syndrome.[69,105] Esophageal atresia and Hirschsprung's disease[67] also have a disproportionately high incidence in patients with trisomy 21, but are not as frequent in this syndrome as duodenal anomalies. The characteristic contours of the pelvis in cases of Down's syndrome have been well established since the work of Caffey and Ross.[42] It is thus often possible to recognize that the patient is suffering from this malformation at the time of an investigation for an intestinal obstruction (Fig. 70-32). The gastrointestinal derangements caused by the intestinal anomalies occurring in patients with Down's syndrome do not differ from those discovered in otherwise normal children or in association with other syndromes. The diagnostic radiographic manuevers for detecting and assessing the obstruction and its cause are likewise similar to those used in otherwise normal patients. In view of the known high association of congenital heart disease with trisomy 21, however, the heart and lungs on chest films of such patients should be examined with particular attention. Similarily, when a patient with Down's syndrome is found to have one gastrointestinal anomaly such as esophageal atresia, other anomalies should be anticipated and sought. Smith and Teele[215] have pointed out that occasionally the duodenal obstruction is so mild that it is not recognized in early life, but may come to attention in childhood. In the four cases they reported, all had retained foreign bodies proximal to the duodenal obstruction, and one had symptoms of esophagitis. All had histories of recurrent or intermittent vomiting that was mostly ignored, perhaps because of the associated mental retardation.

Trisomy 13 and 18 syndromes

In trisomy 13 (Patau) syndrome there is an increased incidence of incomplete rotation of the colon and Meckel's diverticulum. Trisomy 18 syndrome is also associated wtih increased incidence of Meckel's diverticulum as well as biliary atresia, absent gallbladder, and esophageal atresia.[191] However, such anomalies are not commonly the presenting or predominating findings in terms of the infant's signs and symptoms. Rather, infants with these syndromes tend to be feeble and fail to thrive.[83]

Aggressive investigations to discover and treat gastrointestinal anomalies are not appropriate for such patients, because the prognosis is poor and the incidence of brain malformations, particularly in trisomy 13, is very high.[214]

Turner syndrome (ovarian agenesis)

Turner syndrome is defined as an abnormality of the x chromosome. The major clinical features are short stature and ovarian dysgenesis with failure of secondary sexual development. There are many associated morphologic abnormalities. The structural abnormalities of internal organ systems may include aortic coarctation, pulmonic stenosis, and renal anomalies. Reported inflammatory changes include giant cell hepatitis and Hashimoto's thyroiditis, as well as recurrent upper respiratory and middle ear infections. An increased incidence of inflammatory bowel disease in patients with Turner syndrome has been reported.[14,188,237] The inflammatory bowel disease may take the form of ulcerative colitis or Crohn's disease.

DISORDERS ASSOCIATED WTIH PHARYNGEAL AND ESOPHAGEAL ABNORMALITIES
Familial dysautonomia (Riley-Day syndrome)

The Riley-Day syndrome (RDS) is a familial autosomal recessive disturbance in autonomic and peripheral sensory functions. It is most common in Ashkenazi Jews, among whom the frequency of the carrier state is estimated to be about 1%.[121] The peripheral nerves have a deficit in the number of small unmyelinated fibers, which normally carry pain, temperature, and taste sensation, and of the large myelinated fibers, which carry afferent impulses from muscle spindles. Clinical findings include labile hypertension, peripheral sensory dysfunction, diminished pain sense, mental retardation, dysarthria, swallowing incordination, and absent or hypoactive tendon and corneal reflexes.

The gastrointestinal tract is regularly involved in patients with RDS; there is almost always impaired pharyngeal and esophageal coordination, which leads to chronic aspiration of ingested liquid and can be demonstrated by barium swallow.[103] This chronic or repeated aspiration of swallowed fluid may be the cause of chronic, recurrent, or resistant pneumonia. Disturbance of motility throughout the esophagus and improper relaxation of the lower esophageal sphincter are also often present; they probably account for the frequent finding of feeding difficulty in early infancy and the symptom of dysphagia in childhood. Scoliosis is common; thus a chest radiograph may show evidence of aspiration pneumonia and scoliosis (Fig. 70-33).

Sandifer syndrome

Kinsbourne[133] in 1964 described five patients with hiatus hernia and an abnormal posturing of the neck and upper part of the trunk. This was called Sandifer syndrome by Sutcliff[224] when he reported an additional seven cases in 1969. In Sutcliffe's cases, all the children had

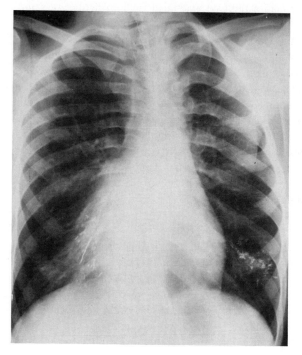

Fig. 70-33 Characteristic findings in patient with familial dysautonomia. Chronic pneumonia is shown in lower lungs, and there is barium in bronchi bilaterally following its aspiration in course of recent contrast examination of pharynx and esophagus. Scoliosis of moderate degree is present and is also characteristic of this disorder.

hiatus hernia. More recently, the emphasis in reported cases of Sandifer syndrome has been on gastroesophageal reflux rather than hiatus hernia.[104,169]

Vomiting is a common symptom, and hemoptysis occasionally occurs. Thus the combination of the rather bizarre head hyperextension and lateral flexion movements in a child who is vomiting should evoke the possibility of Sandifer syndrome. Not all such children vomit, however, and Murphy and Gellis[169] emphasized that in any child with hyperextension of the neck and twisting motions of the head, a radiographic investigation should be carefully performed to search for both reflux and hiatus hernia.

It was originally thought that surgery was curative,[210] but not all patients respond to surgery.[211] Moreover, Murphy and Gellis[169] reported two cases of infants in the first year of life who were successfully treated without surgery by positioning in chalasia chairs.

Because hyperextension and twisting of the head and neck seem not only not to prevent the reflux, but in fact to produce or enhance it, one wonders whether Sandifer syndrome may be a variant of rumination.

Rumination

Rumination (merycism) has long been regarded as a manifestation or complication of emotional deprivation. It is seen primarily in infants from poor, underprivileged, or broken homes. When it develops into a regular pattern, it leads to weight loss, growth failure, severe malnutrition, dehydration, electrolyte imblance, and even death.

Rumination usually begins between the ages of 3 to 6 months, but has been reported to start as early as 5 weeks and as late as 1 year of age.

The infant who ruminates induces vomiting by any one or a combination of movements: extension or twisting of the head, protrusion of the tongue, forward projection of the mandible, arching of the back with contraction of abdominal muscles, and rhythmic chewing movements. There may be mouthing of fingers, sometimes to the point of gagging. The stomach contents are brought up into the mouth and dribble out or are vomited. The remainder is rechewed and reswallowed. The clinical picture thus produced is called rumination because of the strong resemblance to the behavior of ruminant animals, in which recycling of the gastric contents is part of normal digestion. The management of such infants and young children usually consists of loving care. Each time the child begins to ruminate, his or her attention is engaged by an attentive parent or surrogate. This is said to be the most successful method of treatment.[175]

It has been suggested that the vomiting of ruminators is not so much self-induced as spontaneous, caused by hiatus hernia or laxity of the gastroesophageal sphincter mechanism, together with gastroesophageal reflux.[111] Because of this possibility, an infant ruminator should undergo a radiographic examination of the esophagus and stomach, in search of hiatus hernia or reflux, which, if found, may be amenable to surgical treatment.

There has been a report of rumination as a complication of neonatal intensive care.[207]

Epidermolysis bullosa (EB)

Epidermolysis bullosa is a rare hereditary skin disease in which slight trauma disrupts the cohesion between the epidermis and dermis, resulting in the formation of vesicles, bullae, and ulcers. Of the six types that have been described,[180] hypoplastic dystrophic type is an autosomal recessive trait, with its onset at or shortly after birth. Widespread bullae follow minor trauma, affecting both the skin and mucosa, and heal with excessive scarring; the other types do not tend to scar much, if at all. These changes also occur in the esophagus, and may result in esophageal stenosis or webs.[115] Becker and Swinyard[24] reported four cases in infants and children. Segmental areas of the esophagus are involved with stenotic changes. The upper third is more frequently affected than the lower third (Fig. 70-34). Ulcers, vesicles, and bullae may be demonstrated endoscopically, and esophageal stenosis and its complications are recognized radiographically.[64] The complications include retention or impaction of swallowed food, osteoporosis, distal soft tissue atrophy, and acquired webbing between fingers and toes. Fonkalsrud and Ament[78] reported successful surgical treatment of esophageal stenoses by colonic interposition between the pharynx and stomach. Feurle and co-workers,[72] however, stated that conservative methods, including phenytoin to reduce epithelial detachment and strict avoidance of all possible causes of even minor trauma to the esophagus, gave satisfactory results. Balloon diatation was used instead of bougienage for treatment of stenosis.[72]

Tishler and co-workers reported the radiographic findings in the esophagus in four patients wtih epidermolysis bullosa dystrophica, ages 5 to 67 years. The most impressive radiographic finding was bullae formation in virtually any part of the esophagus, often with subsequent scar formation.[227]

Pyloric atresia associated with epidermolysis bullosa has been reported by several observers.[3,38,137] This combination has been called the "letalis" type, because the infant does not usually survive, although one of Korber and Glasson's two patients underwent successful surgery and was well at the age of 11 months.[137] Acquired pyloric obstruction has also occurred in this condition.[119]

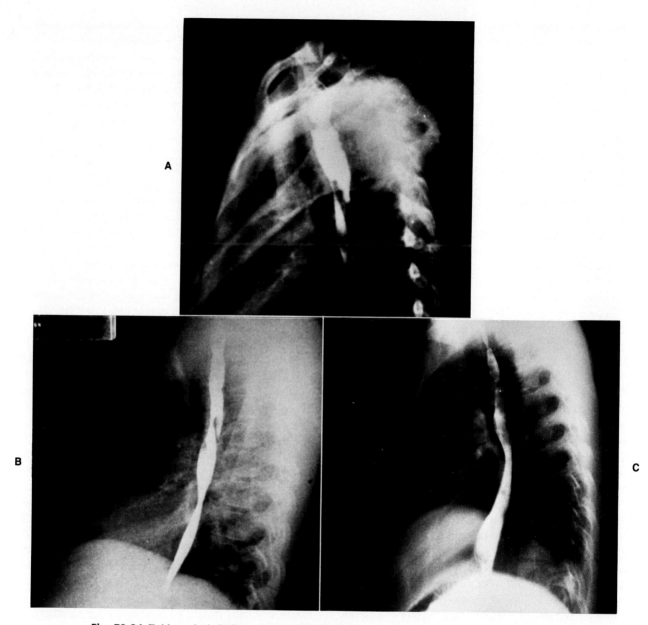

Fig. 70-34 Epidermolysis bullosa dystrophica. **A,** Area of annular stenosis is present, and just below it barium-filled pocket representing ulcer and/or abscess. **B,** One month later there is improvement. **C,** Fourteen months later two stenotic areas are present in upper esophagus. (From Becker, MH, and Swinyard, CA: Radiology 90:124, 1968.)

COLLAGEN VASCULAR DISEASE
Polyarteritis nodosa

Medium and small arteries are the sites of inflammation in polyarteritis nodosa (PN).[201] It is rare in childhood, and males are affected more frequently than females. The cause is unknown, but the disease has been reported to follow drug exposure. Hepatitis B antigen has been associated with a few cases, as have strepto-coccal infections and serous otitis media. The clinical signs and symptoms are those of a systemic illness and include fever, lethargy, weakness, weight loss, arthralgia, arthritis, and skin changes. Abdominal pain, bleeding ulcerations, and infarction can follow involvement of gastrointestinal vessels. The prognosis is poor, with some improvement from treatment with steroids and/or chemotherapeutic agents such as cyclophosphamide.

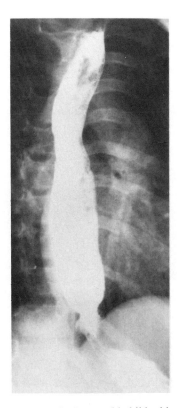

Fig. 70-35 Esophagram in 8-year-old child with scleroderma. Persistent dilatation with abnormal motility.
(From Shanks, MJ, and Blane, CE: Radiographic findings of scleroderma in childhood, AJR 141:657-660, © by American Roentgen Ray Society 1983.)

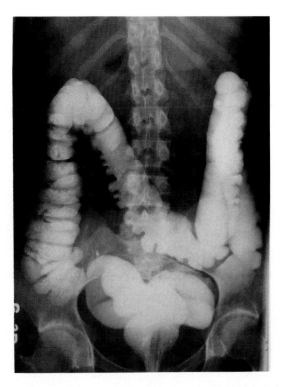

Fig. 70-36 Barium enema of child with scleroderma. Colon shows marked loss of haustration, which is characteristic of scleroderma.

Fujioka and co-workers[82] reported that two of their patients with PN were suspected of having intussusception, and small bowel intussusception was documented by surgery in a third child. The incidence of renal compared to intestinal involvement was the same as in adults. Angiography, especially when demonstrating microaneurysms, ws helpful but not specific. Angiography can be of some help in selecting a biopsy site. Small bowel disease, shown by barium examination, included thickening of mucosal folds, mild segmental dilatation, and prolonged barium transit time—all nonspecific changes.

Scleroderma (progressive systemic sclerosis)

Scleroderma is rare in children, and usually has a patchy, focal distribution.[201] Gut disturbances are less common than in adults with the disease. Shanks and co-workers found in a review of 12 children with scleroderma that dilatation and decreased motility of the esophagus were present in a few, but that the changes were nonspecific[206] (Fig. 70-35). Loss of haustration in the colon (Fig. 70-36) is a characteristic finding in children as in adults,[156] although it may simulate ulcerative colitis and "laxative colon."

Dilatation of the duodenum to the point of crossing of the superior mesenteric artery occurs in pediatric scleroderma, but the dilatation results not from obstruction by the crossing artery, but from loss of intrinsic muscle tone[95] and likely from weight loss in afflicted children. The duodenal dilatation may come and go.

Dermatomyositis

Dermatomyositis is a multisystem disease of unknown cause. The cardinal abnormality is nonsuppurative inflammation of striated muscle, usually with typical associated cutaneous lesions.[201] Affected muscles tend to become stiff, sore, swollen, edematous, and brawny. The proximal limb muscles are most typically and usually most severely involved. Diminished or lost function is the result. There may be demonstrable abnormalities throughout the gastrointestinal tract, but the pharynx, esophagus, and duodenum are most often shown to be abnormal in function and structure by radiographic studies. Swallowing disorders,[102] duodenal perforation[154] extensive bowel necrosis with multiple perforations,[73] pneumatosis intestinalis with a benign course,[35] and gas-

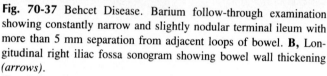

Fig. 70-37 Behcet Disease. Barium follow-through examination showing constantly narrow and slightly nodular terminal ileum with more than 5 mm separation from adjacent loops of bowel. **B,** Longitudinal right iliac fossa sonogram showing bowel wall thickening *(arrows)*.
(From Stringer, DA, Pediat Radiol 16:131, 1968.)

tric and duodenal ulcers[219] have been reported; all are uncommon in this uncommon disease, which affects girls more than boys.

Behçet's disease.

Behçet's disease is of unknown cause. It involves multiple organs and is characterized by ulcerations of the buccal and genital mucosa, skin lesions, and ocular changes. The optic changes include chronic uneitis with hypopyon and optic neuritis.[12] The histologic changes are those of inflammation and fibrinoid necrosis. Involvement of the gut is common, the terminal ileum and colon being the most common sites.[17] The rectum is almost never involved; this is important, because the ulcerative changes shown radiographically are prone to be misdiagnosed as those os ulcerative colitis, which very rarely spares the rectum. Perforation of the gut may occur; Ketch and co-workers[131] reported the recovery of an adult after extensive surgery.

Behçet's disease in children is particularly uncommon. Vlymen and Moskowitz[233] reported Behçet disease in two teenage girls in whom esophageal ulceration or stricture or both led to dysphagia. Ileocolitis with fistula formation occurred in one patient and ileal inflammation without perforation or colitis in the other. They pointed out that the findings may simulate those of Crohn's disease in children. Stringer and co-workers[222] published the

findings in four cases with barium and ultrasound studies (Fig. 70-37). They too emphasized the difficulty in distinguishing this entity from other chronic inflammatory gut disorders, especially Crohn's disease. They recommended that three major clinical criteria be met before the diagnosis is established.

Kawasaki's disease (mucocutaneous lymph node syndrome)

This entity, long known in Japan, was first described in English by Kawasaki and co-workers[128] in 1974, and is now frequently recognized in North America. Most patients are younger than 5 years old. The main features are fever, conjunctivitis, reddening of the lips and oral mucosa, swelling of cervical lymph nodes, and a typical skin rash, followed by desquamation. Most patients recover, but some develop complications affecting the heart, coronary arteries, and systemic arteries.[49] Many patients develop hydrops of the gallbladder, but it usually subsides spontaneously.

Gastrointestinal manifestations are much less common; the chief of these is, or is caused by, vascular insufficiency, producing small bowel obstruction.[168,240] Intestinal pseudo-obstruction has also been seen with a favorable outcome, but it also has caused death.[79] Vascular distribution is diffuse,[141] so occasional gut involvement would appear to be inevitable.

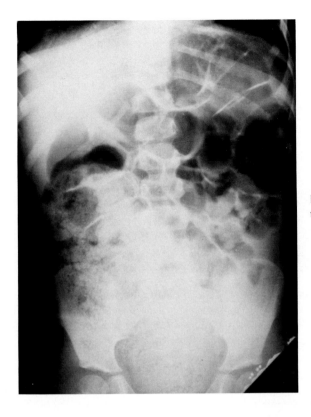

Fig. 70-38 Typical functional megacolon with large amount of retained feces shown in plain film of abdomen of 4-year-old boy.

PSYCHOGENIC DISORDERS AND CHILD ABUSE
Functional megacolon (chronic constipation)

Chronic constipation is common in children and often difficult to manage. It is thought to be frequently psychogenic. Radiographic examinations are often performed to assess the degree of fecal retention and to exclude an organic cause.

The severity of fecal retention can be evaluated by a plain film of the abdomen (Fig. 70-38). This must be done without preparation, because laxatives and cleansing enemas remove the stool, which is the sole criterion for assessing retention. There are no agreed-on criteria for chronic constipation as seen on plain films, however, and surgeons, pediatricians, and radiologists tend to diagnose as constipation findings that are in no way different from the fecal content of the normal child's abdomen. The clinician is looking for an explanation of the child's symptoms, and may be predisposed to overdiagnosis. Radiologists become accustomed to looking at scout films after colonic cleansing and before gastrointestinal and urologic studies, and the normally feces-filled colon may come to look "bad."

In the radiographic search for a cause of childhood chronic constipation, the emphasis should be on the diagnosis or exclusion of Hirschsprung's disease. In the otherwise healthy child, organic causes of fecal retention other than Hirschsprung's disease are rare. If the rectum is clinically or radiographically found to be filled or distended with feces, Hirschsprung's disease is highly unlikely. In many such cases, no further radiographic evaluation is necessary. The impression of a feces-filled or distended rectum can sometimes be confirmed by a lateral projection of the pelvis, thus obviating barium enema.

If it is decided that a barium enema should be performed, however, the colon should be examined in the unprepared state. Then the radiographic findings faithfully represent the clinical situation, not the empty colon after "good preparation." More importantly, if Hirschsprung's disease is present, it may be missed if the colon has been emptied. The empty colon then fails to show the diagnostic findings of a transition zone between dilatation proximally and collapse distally.

Only enough barium should be used to exclude findings of colorectal stenosis or Hirschsprung's disease. As soon as the contrast enters dilated colon, the flow should be stopped. Thus the problem of possible temporary aggravation of constipation, caused by inspissated barium, is averted. In addition, it is wise to use a dilute suspension of barium and to suspend the barium in normal saline instead of plain tap water to avoid the possibility of water intoxication, which can come about through excessive absorption from the large mucosal surface of a distended colon.[249]

A lateral projection of the rectum, taken after barium

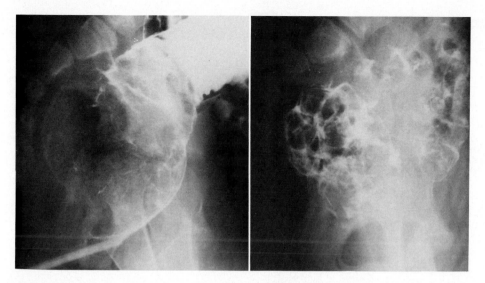

Fig. 70-39 Lateral radiographs of distal sigmoid and rectum in child with chronic constipation. **A,** Before evacuation rectum is distended with large fecal mass. **B,** After evacuation rectum is almost completely evacuated. Mucosa appears moderately redundant after discharge of large rectal fecal mass.

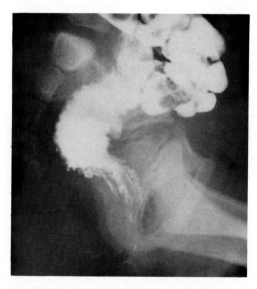

Fig. 70-40 Lateral film of sigmoid, rectum, and anal canal following cleansing of bowel in patient with chronic constipation. Previously distended rectum is now almost completely empty, and redundant mucosa and wide retrorectal space simulate inflammatory change.

evacuation and preferably before as well, is essential in the evaluation of all such problems (Fig. 70-39). If the chronically distended rectum is completely emptied, the postevacuation film may show a pattern of large, redundant mucosal folds that resemble those found in fibrocystic disease of the pancreas or may even suggest hypertrophic or inflamed mucosa (Fig. 70-40).

Notwithstanding the possibility of overdiagnosis, constipation sometimes does cause abdominal pain. Pediatric surgeons and pediatric radiologists are aware of this, because they are not infrequently confronted with a patient who has acute mild or severe abdominal pain and the only finding, clinically and radiographically, is a distended abdomen. Most of the distention is evidently caused by a large amount of feces in the colon and rectum (Fig. 70-41). The diagnosis of pain caused by constipation is suggested by these findings, and confirmed by relief of the pain following a successful cleansing enema. Indeed, one experienced pediatric surgeon states that constipation is the most common cause of acute abdominal pain in childhood.[173]

Anorexia nervosa

Anorexia nervosa (AN) is a common condition with marked female predominance, characterized by decreased food intake and sometimes vomiting. Its causes are widely accepted as psychogenic.

There are no characteristic radiographic findings in AN, but such patients not infrequently develop dilatation of the duodenum, with narrowing and compression of its distal portion as it crosses the vertebral column. The condition may therefore come to be labeled as superior mesenteric artery syndrome. Because the syndrome may indeed occur as a complication of weight loss from any cause, it may be found by barium study in patients with AN, but should not be mistaken for the primary cause

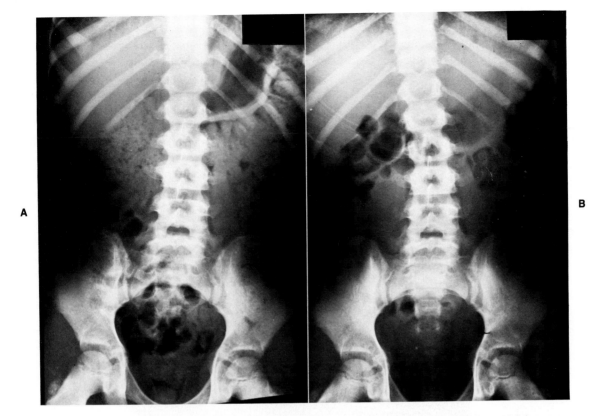

Fig. 70-41 Constipation causing abdominal pain. **A,** Plain film of abdomen in child complaining of abdominal pain shows no abnormality except considerable amounts of feces throughout colon. **B,** After cleansing enemas repeat abdominal film shows colon to be nearly empty; pain was relieved.

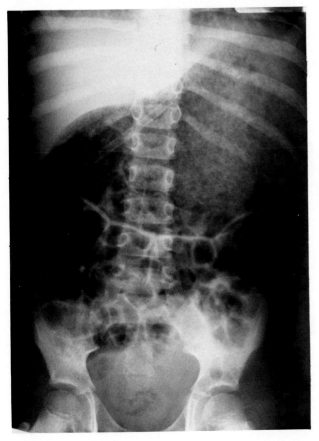

Fig. 70-42 Neglect and/or deprivation in child with history of abdominal distention. Plain film of abdomen showed stomach distended with irregular, bubbly material. History of eating large amounts of toilet paper was elicited. It was thought that child was in environment of neglect.

of the child's weight loss and vomiting.[205] AN usually disappears with the successful treatment of the primary condition.

Child abuse

Acute gastric dilatation with a large amount of food (or other material) in the stomach may be a sign of child abuse or deprivation.[79] Fig. 70-42 illustrates such a case.

This child was admitted to hospital with recent onset of abdominal distention, abdominal pain, and vomiting. Abdominal films showed marked distention of the stomach by a mass of soft material interspersed with gas. The history then obtained from the father revealed that the child had been found eating large amounts of toilet paper. It is presumed that he was emotionally or physically deprived.

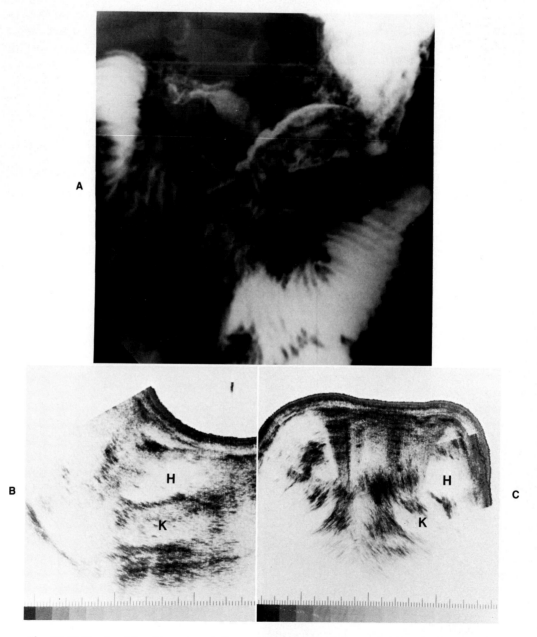

Fig. 70-43 Duodenojejunal hematoma in battered infant. **A,** Barium examination of upper gastrointestinal tract shows long segment of duodenum and proximal jejunum widened, with separation of plicae conniventes, characteristic of duodenojejunal hematoma. **B** and **C,** Ultrasound confirms hematoma *(H)* anterior to left kidney *(K).*

Battered infants may sustain trauma to many organs, including those of the gastrointestinal tract. Rupture of the liver, pneumoperitoneum, chylous ascites,[34] mesenteric tear, and pancreatic disruption[48,213] have all been described as being caused by trauma, as has secondary celiac syndrome. One of the most common lesions found in children with abdominal trauma, including those in whom the trauma is part of abuse, is a duodenal or duodenojejunal hematoma (Fig. 70-43). Plain films of the abdomen may show pneumoperitoneum or ascites and may provide the first clues to the diagnosis of abuse by demonstrating rib fractures (Fig. 70-44). Ultrasound is of great value in demonstrating an abdominal mass that may be unclear or invisible on radiographs. It shows the pancreas well and thus can demonstrate or help to exclude pancreatic traumatic lesions, including swelling and pseudocysts. It is essential to consider the battered-baby syndrome in any case in which a traumatic intraabdominal lesion is shown or suspected. The skeletal findings in the battered child have been well described.[65,212] Slovis and co-workers[213] pointed out that traumatic pancreatitis in the abused child may cause secondary inflammatory bone lesions, presumably caused by intramedullary fat necrosis. They also noted that bile peritonitis may result

from childhood abdominal trauma. Cohen and co-workers[48] also reported bone lesions developing as complications of child abuse, including pancreatic trauma. Boysen[34] showed that abdominal distention caused by chylous ascites may be the presenting abnormality in cases of child abuse.

MISCELLANEOUS DISORDERS
Neurofibromatosis

The protean manifestations of neurofibromatosis occasionally include intrabdominal masses and gastrointestinal abnormalities,[84] but pediatric gut lesions caused by this disease are very uncommon. Buntin and Fitzgerald[39] pointed out that before the stigmata of neurofibromatosis appear, or while they are so subtle as to be missed, a patient may suffer severe anemia because of an ulcerative neurofibromatous polyp in the jejunum. Though gastrointestinal neurofibromas occur at all ages, they are most common at ages 40 to 60 and are usually benign. The most common symptoms are abdominal pain, gastrointestinal bleeding, a palpable mass, and manifestations of bowel obstruction.[53] Perforation caused by an intestinal neurofibroma has been reported.[236]

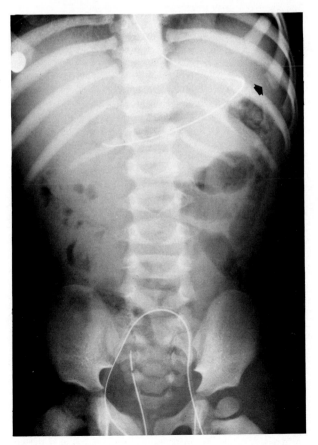

Fig. 70-44 Battered infant. Child was admitted with symptoms and signs of shock and acute abdomen. Plain radiograph showed nonspecific changes of slightly and irregularly distended gut, but fractuures of rib ends (most obvious indicated by arrow) indicated abuse and severe and likely repeated trauma. At laparotomy long segment of distal ileum was seen to have traumatically separated from its mesentery and undergone necrosis.

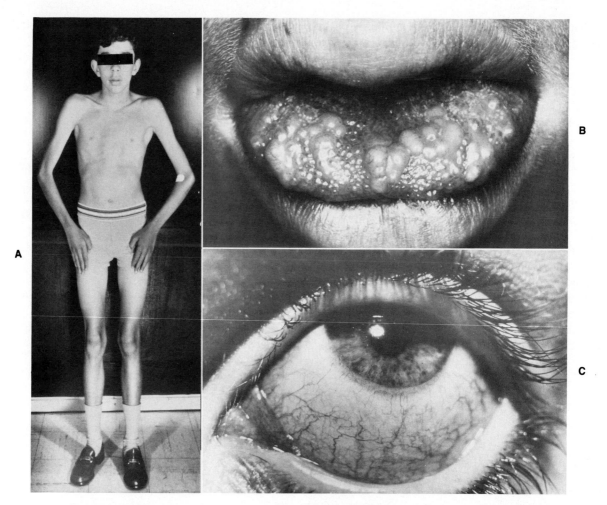

Fig. 70-45 Mucosal neuroma syndrome. **A,** Marfanoid changes. Patient also has high palate, slight kyphosis, and pes cavus, which are not seen. **B,** Close-up view demonstrates prominent lips and fleshy neuromas on anterior third of tongue. **C,** Whitish neuromatous tissue can be seen heaped up along limbus of cornea.
(From Anderson, TE, Spackman, TJ, and Schwartz, SS: Radiology 101:93, 1971.)

Multiple endocrine neoplasia IIB syndrome (mucosal neuroma syndrome)

Multiple endocrine neoplasia (MEN) IIB is now recognized as a clinically characteristic constellation of findings. It had been reported earlier as "plexiform neurofibromatosis of the colon simulating Hirschsprung's disease,"[218] and may cause clinical signs and symptoms that mimic Hirschsprung's disease—chronic constipation and abdominal distention—before typical clinical features (Fig. 70-45) become apparent. The clinical changes include long, slender extremities and other features similar to Marfan's syndrome, prominent lips with nodules on the vermilion border, nodular deformity of the tongue, and corneal limbus thickening.[11] Barium enema (Fig. 70-46) shows a nodular, mucosal redundancy of the colon, without ulceration or exudate. All of these clinical and radiographic nodular lesions are caused by mucosal neuromas, and they usually precede the thyroid and adrenal neoplasms that are characteristic of this class of multiple endocrine neoplasia. Carney[46] found in a review of 17 patients that oral lesions were present at birth in seven children, and appeared before age 6 years in another six. Lucaya et al[151] reported an 8-year-old boy with multiple mucosal neuromas and a medullary thyroid carcinoma whose diagnosis was first suggested by the findings of a barium enema.

This syndrome, now classified as MEN IIB, has also been called mucosal neuroma syndrome, MEN type II, sipple syndrome, and MEN type III syndrome.[62]

For the radiologist confronted with a child who is suspected of having chronic constipation or Hirschsprung's disease, the important message is that if the co-

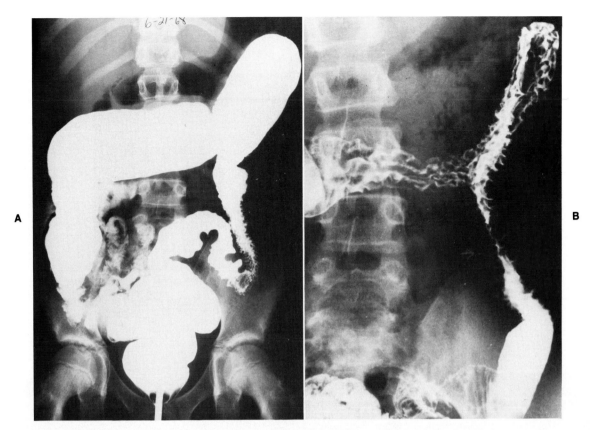

Fig. 70-46 A, Barium-filled colon has unusual haustral markings and segmental area of spasm. **B,** Evacuation film demonstrated thick mucosal folds without ulceration or exudate. Diverticulum may be seen in descending colon.

(From Anderson, TE, Spackman, TJ, and Schwartz, SS: Radiology 101:93, 1971.)

lonic mucosa appears unduly rich, nodular, and redundant, as shown in Fig. 70-46, the possibility of the MEN IIB syndrome should be raised and clinical and histologic evidence sought.

Alagille syndrome (arterial hepatic dysplasia)

Alagille syndrome has a familial tendency and possibly autosomal dominant inheritance with variable expressivity.[67] The major manifestations include neonatal intrahepatic cholestasis, hypoplasia and stenosis of pulmonary arteries, distinctive facies, and skeletal anomalies. The course may be benign,[193] or progressive and fatal.[97]

The radiographically important gastrointestinal findings are limited to the liver and biliary system. Cholangiography shows both a decrease in the number of intrahepatic ducts and focal areas of duct dysplasia in extrahepatic ducts.[97,195]

Blue rubber bleb nevus syndrome

Also known as gastrointestinal cutaneous angiomatosis, blue rubber bleb nevus syndrome is uncommon, though more than 40 cases have now been reported. It consists of rubbery blue cutaneous nevi and hemangiomatoses, frequently hemorrhagic, in the bowel. The skin lesions, usually present at birth, vary in number from 1 to 100. They have a characteristic color and appearance (Fig. 70-47, *A*). They empty when pressed and refill when released.[162] The gastrointestinal lesions, which can be shown as polypoid by barium studies (Fig. 70-47, *B* and *C*), may require surgery, sometimes repeatedly for blood loss, or even for secondary intussusception.[36,228]

Rarely, the musculoskeletal system may be involved.[161]

Pseudomembranous colitis

A dangerous and fulminating disease, pseudomembranous colitis may be caused by recent surgery,[181] debilitation,[44] or broad-spectrum antibiotic therapy. The latter is most prone to occur after administration of clindamycin,[20] with overgrowth of *Clostridium difficile*, which produces a powerful toxin.[4] For this reason clindamycin is now infrequently used, although occasionally other antibiotics can have the same effect. The radio-

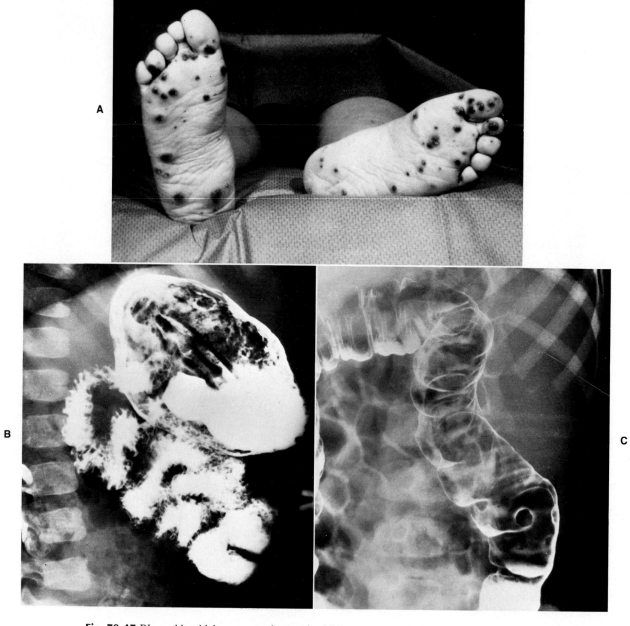

Fig. 70-47 Blue rubber bleb nevus syndrome. **A,** Clinical photograph shows multiple blue rubber blebs on soles of feet. There were numerous similar lesions elsewhere. **B,** In fundus and body of stomach are numerous polypoid filling defects. **C,** Barium enema film shows several polyps in transverse and sigmoid colon.
(From McCauley, RGK, Leonidas, JC, and Bartoshesky, LE: Radiology 133:375, 1979.)

graphic findings on barium enema have been well described, and appear to be at least suggestive of the diagnosis.[217] They consist of edema, inflammation, and discrete or confluent plaques. It is widely agreed, however, that in most cases where this diagnosis in entertained, the child's condition is so grave that radiographic procedures are contraindicated. Endoscopy, with membrane and culture material obtained for laboratory examination, is the procedure of choice.[80,217]

Cowden (multiple hamartoma) syndrome

Cowden syndrome is a rare condition named after the first patient who was described. The clinical findings are diagnostic, with distinctive facies and multiple mucocutaneous papular lesions of characteristic morphology on the face, extremities and oral mucosa. There are abnormalities of multiple organs, particularly the breast and thyroid, with predisposition to malignancies at these sites, the skin, and colon. The radiographic findings, which may be demonstrated in children or adults, are striking, with innumerable polypoid lesions throughout the gastrointestinal tract, especially vividly demonstrable in the esophagus and stomach.[81,91,107]

Degos syndrome (malignant atrophic papulosis)

Degos disease is a progressive, frequently fatal, arterial occlusive vasculitis. It is manifested especially by skin (atrophic papulosis) lesions and lesions in the gastrointestinal tract and complicated by infarction, perforation, and peritonitis. The nervous system may also be affected. Degos and co-workers described a 5-month-old infant with biopsy-proved lesions who died of complications of neocrotic small bowel.[148] Another fatal case was that of an infant who died of small bowel perforations secondary to endarteritis obliterans.[229] The radiographic signs are nonspecific and include edema of the mucosal folds of the gut and punctate ulcerations during episodes of abdominal pain.

Fabry's disease

Fabry's disease is an x-linked disorder caused by the accumulation of ceramide trihexoside in many organs resulting from a specific enzyme deficiency. Its clinical features may include rash, limb pain, corneal haze, renal failure, hypertension, and cerebral vascular disease. The major clinical problems are usually those of renal insufficiency. Gastrointestinal disorders are known but uncommon in adults and rare in children. Rowe and co-workers[197] reported four adult patients with intestinal involvement. The small bowel changes consisted of thickening of folds and mild dilatation throughout, and the ileum had and unusual granular appearance. Colonic haustral markings were diminished. Flynn and co-

workers[77] reported nonspecific small bowel abnormalities in 14-year-old twins.

Familial Mediterranean fever

Familial Mediterranean fever (familial recurring polyserositis), is a form of amyloidosis, affecting people of mediterranean origin, mainly Sephardic Jews. The disease is apparently independently inherited.[108] It is characterized by recurrent episodes of fever and inflammation of one or more serosal membranes and/or joints—the latter typically being the proximal limb joints. The joint findings are not specific radiographically, but sometimes sclerosis or even fusion of sacroiliac joints occurs. Thus in any child of Mediterranean origin suffering from acute abdominal symptoms, sclerosis of sacroiliac joints noted on plain films of the abdomen may be a valuable clue to the diagnosis, which is otherwise easily overlooked.

During acute attacks of pain, plain films show adynamic ileus of the small gut,[204] and barium examination shows discontinuity of the small bowel column, with dilatation and delayed transit. All these findings disappear when the pain subsides,[68] but there have been instances of small bowel obstruction later, caused by peritoneal bands.[225]

A C5a inhibitor deficiency in peritoneal fluids from patients with the disease has been reported.[159]

REFERENCES

1. Abramson, SJ, et al: Childhood typhlitis: its increasing association with acute myelogenous leukemia, Radiology 146:61, 1983.
2. Abramson, SJ, et al: Gastrointestinal manifestations of cystic fibrosis, Semin Roentgenol 22:97, 1987.
3. Adashi, EY, Louis, FJ, and Vasquez, M: An unusual case of epidermolysis bullosa hereditaria letalis with cutaneous scarring and pyloric atresia, J Pediatr 96:443, 1980.
4. Adler, SP, Tattamangalam, C, and Berman, WF: *Clostridium difficile* associated with pseudomembranous colitis, Am J Dis Child 135:820, 1981.
5. Agha, FP, Wilson, JAP, Nostrand, TT, Medication-induced esophagitis, Gastrointes Radiol 11:7, 1986.
6. Deleted in proofs.
7. Al-Rashid, RA, and Harned, RK: Dysphagia due to leukemic involvement of the esophagus, Am J Dis Child 121:75, 1971.
8. Amman, AJ: In Behrman, RE, Vaughan, VC, Nelson, WE, editors: Nelson textbook of pediatrics, ed 13, Philadelphia, 1987, WB Saunders.
9. Ament, ME, and Ochs, HD: Gastrointestinal complications of chronic granulomatous disease, N Engl J Med 288:282, 1973.
10. Amodio, JB, et al: Pediatric AIDS, Semin Roentgenol 22:66, 1987.
11. Anderson, TE, Spackman, TJ, and Schwartz, SS: Roentgen findings in intestinal ganglioneuromatosis, Radiology 101:93, 1971.
12. Apt, L, and Gaffney, WL: Behçet's disease. In Rudolph, AM, editor: Pediatrics, ed 16, New York, 1977, Appleton-Century-Crofts.
13. Ariyan, S, Shessel, FS, and Pickett, LK: Cholecystitis and cholelithiasis masking as abdominal crises in sickle cell disease, Pediatrics 58:252, 1976.

14. Arulanantham, K, Kramer, MS, and Gryboski, JD: The association of inflammatory bowel disease and x chromosomal abnormality, Pediatrics 66:63, 1980.
15. Deleted in proofs.
16. Aterman, K: Duodenal ulceration and fibrocystic pancreas disease, Am J Dis Child 101:210, 1961.
17. Baba, S, et al: Intestinal Behçet's disease: report of 5 cases, Dis Colon Rectum 19:428, 1976.
18. Baghdassarian, OM, Koehler, PR, and Schultze, C: Massive neonatal ascites, Radiology 76:586, 1961.
19. Balthazer, EJ, Megibow, AJ, and Hulnick, DH: Cytomegalovirus esophagitis and gastritis in AIDS, AJR 144:1201, 1985.
20. Bartlett, JG, et al: Role of *Clostridium difficile* in antibiotic associated pseudomembranous colitis, Gastroenterology 75:778, 1978.
21. Bartram, CI, and Small, E: The intestinal radiological changes in older people with pancreatic cystic fibrosis, Br J Radiol 44:195, 1976.
22. Bassani, F, et al: Chronic granulomatous disease, Pediatr Radiol 11:105, 1981.
23. Beaudet, AL, Experience with new DNA markers for the diagnosis of cystic fibrosis, N Engl J Med 318:50, 1988.
24. Becker, MH, and Swinyard, CA: Epidermolysis bullosa dystrophica in children: radiologic manifestations, Radiology 90:124, 1968.
25. Bendig, DW, et al: Complicatios of gastroesophaeal reflux in patients with cystic fibrosis, J Pediatr 100:536, 1982.
26. Berk, RN, and Lee FA: The late gastrointestinal manifestations of cystic fibrosis of the pancreas, Radiology 106:377, 1973.
27. Berkowitz, CD, and Seidel, JS: Spontaneous resolution of crytosporidiosis in children with acquired immunodeficiency syndrome, Am J Dis Child 139:967, 1985.
28. Bernstein, J, et al: The occurrence of intestinal atresia in newborns with meconium ileus, Am J Dis Child 99:804, 1960.
29. Blanc, WA, Santulli, TV, and Anderson, DH: Pathogenesis of jejunoileal atresia, Am J Dis Child 98:564, 1959.
30. Boal, DKB, Newburger, PE, and Teele, RL: Esophagitis induced by combined radiation and adriamycin, AJR 132:567, 1979.
31. Bodian, M, et al: Congenital duodenal obstruction and mongolism, Br Med J 1:77, 1952.
32. Borns, PF, and Johnston, TA: Indolent pneumatosis of the bowel wall associated with immune suppressive therapy, Ann Radiol 16:163, 1973.
33. Bova, JG, et al: Medication-induced esophagitis: diagnosis by double-contrast esophagography, AJR, 148:731, 1987.
34. Boysen, BE: Chylous ascites: manifestation of the battered child syndrome, Am J Dis Child 129:1338, 1975.
35. Braunstein, EM, and White, SJ: Pneumatosis intestinalis in dermatomyositis, Br J Radiol 53:1011, 1980.
36. Browne, AF, Katz, S, and Miser, J: Blue rubber bleb nevi as a cause of intussusception, J Pediatr Surg 18:7, 1983.
37. Bryn, JR, et al: Unusual manifestations of Henoch-Schonlein syndrome, Am J Dis Child 130:1335, 1976.
38. Bull, MJ, et al: Epidermolysis bullosa—pyloric atresia: an autosomal recessive syndrome, Am J Dis Child 137:449, 1983.
39. Buntin, PT, and Fitzgerald, JF: Gastrointestinal neurofibromatosis, Am J Dis Child 119:521, 1970.
40. Burkitt, D: A sarcoma involving the jaws of African children, Br J Surg 46:218, 1958.
41. Burkitt, D, and O'Connor, GT: Malignant lymphoma in African children: clinical syndrome, Cancer 14:258, 1961.
42. Caffey, J, and Ross, S: Mongolism (mongoloid deficiency) during early infancy: some newly recognized diagnostic changes in the pelvis bones, Pediatrics 17:642, 1956.
43. Caldicott, WJH, and Baehner, RL: Chronic granulomatous disease in childhood, AJR 103:133, 1968.
44. Cammerer, RC, et al: Clinical spectrum of pseudomembranous colitis, JAMA 235:2502, 1976.
45. Capitanio, MA, and Kirkpatrick, JA: Lymphoid hyperplasia of the colon in children: roentgen observations, Radiology, 94:323, 1970.
46. Carney, JA, and Hayles, AB: Alimentary tract manifestations of multiple endocrine neoplasia type IIB, Mayo Clin Proc 52:543, 1977.
47. Cavell, B: Gastric emptying in infants with cystic fibrosis, Acta Paediatr Scand 70:635, 1981.
48. Cohen, H, Haller, JO, and Friedman, AP: Pancreatitis, child abuse, and skeletal lesions, Pediatr Radiol 10:175, 1981.
49. Cook, A, and L'Heureux, P: Radiographic findings in the mucocutaneous lymph node syndrome, AJR 132:107, 1979.
50. Cordonnier, JK, and Izant, RJ, JR: Meconium ileus equivalent, Surgery 54:667, 1962.
51. Craig, JM, Haddad, H, and Shwachman, H: The pathological changes in the liver in cystic fibrosi of the pancresa. Am J Dis Child 93:357, 1957.
52. Daneman A, et al: Pancreatic changes in cystic fibrosis: CT and sonographic appearances, AJR 141:653, 1983.
53. Davis, GB, and Berk, RN: Intestinal neurofibromas in von-Recklinghausen's disease, Am J Gastroenterol 60:410, 1973.
54. DeVita, VT, JR, Hillman, S, and Rosenberg, SA: AIDS: etiology, diagnosis treatment and prevention, JB Lippincott, Philadelphia, 1985.
55. Dickerman, JD, Colletti RB, and Tampas, JP: Gastric outlet obstruction in chronic granulomatous disease of childhood, Am J Dis Child 140:567, 1986.
56. diGeorge, AM: In Behrman, RE, Vaughan, VC, and Nelson, WE, editors: Nelson Textbook of Pediatrics ed 13 Philadelphia, 1987, WB Saunders.
57. di Sant'Agnese, PA: Cystic fibrosis of the pancreas, Am J Med 21:406, 1956.
58. di Sant'Agnese, PA, and Blanc, WA: A distinctive type of biliary cirrhosis of the liver associated with cystic fibrosis of the pancreas: recognition through signs of portal hypertension, Pediatrics 18:387, 1956.
59. di Sant'Agnese, PA, and Lepore, MJ: Involvement of abdominal organs in cystic fibrosis of the pancreas, Gastroenterology 40:64, 1961.
60. Dodds, WJ, Spitzer, RM, and Friedland, GW: Gastrointestinal roentgenographic manifestations of hemophilia, AJR 110:413, 1970.
61. Donnison, AB, Shwachman, H, and Gross, RE: A review of 164 children with meconium ileus seen at Children's Hospital Medical Center, Boston, Pediatrics 37:833, 1966.
62. Doppman, JL: Multiple endocrine syndromes—a nightmare for the endocrinologic radiologist, Semin Roentgeno 20:7, 1985.
63. Deleted in proofs.
64. DuPree, E, Hodges, F, Jr, and Simon J: Epidermolysis of the esophagus, Am J Dis Child 117:349, 1969.
65. Ellerstein, NS, and Norris, KJ: Value of radiologic skeletal survey in assessment of abused children, Pediatrics 74:1075, 1984.
66. Ellis, DG, and Clatworthy, HW, JR: The meconium plug syndrome revisited, J Pediatr Surg 1:54, 1966.
67. Emanuel, B, Padorr, MP, and Swenson, O: Mongolism associated with Hirschsprung's disease, J Pediatr 66:437, 1965.
68. Eyler, WR, Nixon RK, and Priest, RJ: Familial recurring polyserositis, AJR 84:262, 1960.
69. Federman, DD: Down's syndrome, Clin Pediatr 4:331, 1965.
70. Felson, B, and Levin, EJ: Intramural hematoma of the duodenum: a diagnostic roentgen sign, Radiology 63:823, 1954.

71. Ferriero, DM, Wolfsdorf, JI: Hemolytic uremic syndrome associated with Kawasaki disease, Pediatrics 68:405, 1981.

72. Feurle, GE, et al: Management of esophageal stenosis in recessive dystrophic epidermolysis bullosa, Gastroenterology 87:1376, 1984.

73. Fischer, TJ, Cipel, L, and Stiehm, ER: Pneumatosis intestinalis associated with fatal childhood dermatomyositis, Pediatrics 6:127, 1978.

74. Fisk, JD, et al: Gastrointestinal radiographic features of human graft-vs.-host disease, AJR 136:329, 1981.

75. Fleisher, DR: Infant rumination syndrome, Am J Dis Child 133:266, 1979.

76. Fletcher, BD, and Abramowsky, CR: Contrast enemas in cystic fibrosis: implications of appendiceal nonfilling, AJR 137:323, 1981.

77. Flynn, DM, et al: Gut lesions in Fabry's disease without a rash, Arch Dis Child 47:26, 1972.

78. Fonkalsrud, EW, and Ament, ME: Surgical management of esophageal stricture due to recessive dystrophic epidermolysis bullosa, J Pediatr Surg 12:221, 1977.

79. Franken, EA, et al: Intestinal pseudo-obstruction in mucocutaneous lymph-node syndrome, Radiology 130:649, 1979.

80. Franken, DA, and Smith, WL: Gastrointestinal imaging in pediatrics, Philadelphia, 1982, Harper & Row.

81. Fritsch, P, et al: The multiple hamartoma (Cowden) syndrome, Hautarzt 32:285, 1981.

82. Fujioka, M, et al: Polyarteritis nodosa in children: radiological aspects and diagnostic correlation, Radiology 136:359, 1980.

83. Gellis, SS, and Feingold, M: Atlas of mental retardation syndromes: visual diagnosis of facies and physical findings, Washington, DC, 1968, U.S. Government Printing Office.

84. Ghrist, TD: Gatrointestinal involvement in neurofibromatosis, Arch Intern Med 112:357, 1963.

85. Gibson, B, et al: Roentgenographically visible fatty liver in cystic fibrosis, Pediatrics 59:778, 1977.

86. Girdany, BR. In Silverman, FN, editor: Caffey's pediatric x-ray diagnosis: an integrated imaging approach, ed 8, Chicago, 1985, Year Book.

87. Glasier, CM, et al: Henoch-Schonlein syndrome in children: gastrointestinal manifestations, AJR 136:1081, 1981.

88. Glass, GC: Hemorrhage in a newly born infant, causing intestinal and biliary obstruction: report of a case with necropsy, Am J Dis Child, 54:1052, 1937.

89. Glass, RB, et al: Gallium scintigraphy in American Burkitt lymphoma: accurate assessment of tumor load and prognosis, AJR 145:671, 1985.

90. Glazer, J: Personal communication. Cited in White, H, and Rowley WF: Cystic fibrosis of the pancreas: clinical and roentgenographic manifestations, Radiol Clin North Am 1:539, 1961.

91. Gold, BM, and Zarrani, MH: Radiologic manifestations of Cowen disease, AJR 135:385, 1980.

92. Gold, RH et al: Roentgenographic features of the neutrophil dysfunction syndromes, Radiology 102:1045, 1969.

93. Goldstein, HLM, et al: Radiological manifestations of radiation induced injury to the normal upper gastrointestinal tract, Radiology 117:135, 1975.

94. Goldstein, SJ, and Crooks, DJM: Colitis in Behçet's syndrome, Radiology 128:321, 1978.

95. Gondos, B: Duodenal compression defect and the "superior mesenteric artery syndrome," Radiology 123:575, 1977.

95a. Gonzalez, R, and Michael, A: In Behrman RE, Vaughan, VC, and Nelson WE, editors: Nelson textbook of pediatrics, ed 13, Philadelphia, 1987, WB Saunders.

96. Gordon, RA, et al: Intramural gastric hematoma in a hemophiliac with an inhibitor, Pediatrics 67:417, 1981.

97. Gorelick, FS, et al: Biliary tract anomalies in patients with arteriohepatic dysplasia, Dig Dis Sci 27:815, 1982.

98. Grantmyer, EB, Butler, GJ, and Gillis, DA: Necrotizing enterocolitis after renografin-76 treatment of meconium ileus, AJR 136:990, 1981.

99. Griscom, NT, et al: Gastric antral narrowing in chronic granulomatous disease of childhood, Pediatrics 54:456, 1974.

100. Grossman, H, Berdon, WE, and Baker, DH: Reversible gastrointestinal signs of hemorrhage and edema in the pediatric age group, Radiology 84:33, 1965.

101. Grossman, H, Berdon, WE, and Baker, DH: Gastrointestinal findings in cystic fibrosis. AJR 97:227, 1966.

102. Grünebaum M, and Salinger, H: Radiological findings in polymyositis-dermatomyositis involving the pharynx and upper esophagus, Clin Radiol 22:97, 1971.

103. Gyepes, MT, and Linde, LM: Familial dysautonomia: the mechanism of aspiration, Radiology 91:471, 1968.

104. Hadari, A, et al: Sandifer's syndrome: a rare complication of hiatal hernia. A case report. Z Kinderchir 39:202, 1984.

105. Hall, B: Mongolism in newborn infants, Clin Pediatr 5:4, 1966.

106. Harris, CH, and Boles, ET: Intestinal lesions in chronic granulomatous disease in childhood, J Pediatr Surg 8:955, 1973.

107. Hauser, H, et al: Radiological findings in multiple hamartoma syndrome (Cowden disease), Radiology 137:317, 1980.

108. Heller, H, Sohar, E, and Grafni, J: Amyloidosis in familial Mediterranean fever: an independent, genetically determined character, Arch Intern Med 107:539, 1961.

109. Hen, J, Jr, Dolan, TF, Jr, and Touloukian, RJ: Meconium plug syndrome associated with cystic fibrosis and Hirschsprung's disease, Pediatrics 66:466, 1980.

110. Herbst, JJ: In Behrman, RE, Vaughan, VC, and Nelson, WE, editors: Nelson textbook of pediatrics, ed 13, Philadelphia, 1987, WB Saunders.

111. Herbst, J, Friedland, GW, and Zboralske, FF: Hiatal hernia and "rumination" in infants and children. J Pediatr 78:261, 1971.

112. Hernanz-Schulman, M, et al: Pancreatic cystosis in cystic fibrosis, Radiology 158:629, 1986.

113. Hernanz-Schulman, M, et al: Pneumatosis intestinalis in cystic fibrosis, Radiology 160:497, 1986.

114. Hide, DW, and Burman, D: An infant with both cystic fibrosis and coeliac disease, Arch Dis Child 44:533, 1969.

115. Hillemeier, C, et al: Esophageal web: a previously unrecognized complication of epidermolysis bullosa, Pediatrics 67:678, 1981.

116. Hodgson, JR, Hoffman, HN, and Huizenga, DA: Roentgenologic features of lymphoid hyperplasia of the small intestine associated with dysgammaglobulinemia, Radiology 88:883, 1967.

117. Holsclaw, DS, Eckstein, HB, and Nixon, HH: Meconium ileus: a 20-year review of 109 cases, Am J Dis Child 109:101, 1965.

118. Holsclaw, DS, Rocmans, C, and Shwachman, H: Intussusception in patients with cystic fibrosis, Pediatrics 48:51, 1971.

119. Honig, PJ, Yoder, M, and Ziegler, M: Acquired pyloric obstruction in a patient with epidermolysis bullosa letalis, J Pediatr 102:598, 1983.

120. Hunter, TB, Bjelland, JC: Gastrointestinal complications of leukemia and its treatment, AJR 142:513, 1984.

121. Huttenlocher, PR: In Behrman, RE, Vaughan, VC, and Nelson, WE, editors: Nelson textbook of pediatrics, ed 13, Philadelphia, 1987, WB Saunders.

122. Iannaccone, G, and Antonelli, M: Calcification of the pancreas in cystic fibrosis, Pediatr Radiol 9:85, 1980.

123. Issenman, RB: Personal communication, 1987.

124. Jaffe, N, Carlson, DH, and Vawter, GF: Pneumatosis cystoides intestinalis in acute leukemia, Cancer 30:239, 1972.

125. Jones, B, et al: Gastrointestinal inflammation after bone marrow transplanation: graft-versus-host disease or opportunistic infection?, AJR 150:277, 1988.

126. Karayalcin, G, et al: Cholelithiasis in children with sickle cell disease, Am J Dis Child 133:306, 1979.

127. Kawanami, T, Bowen, A, and Girdany, BR: Enterocolitis: prodrome of the hemolytic-uremic syndrome, Radiology 151:91, 1984.

128. Kawasaki, T, et al: A new infantile acute febrile mucocutaneous lymph node syndrome (MLNS) prevailing in Japan, Pediatrics 54:271, 1974.

129. Kelvin, FM, et al: Chronic oesophageal stricture due to moniliasis, Br J Radiol 51:826, 1978.

130. Deleted in proofs.

131. Ketch, LL, Buerk, CA, and Liechty, RD: Surgical implications of Behçet's disease, Arch Surg 115:759, 1980.

132. Khilnani, MT, et al: Intramural intestinal hemorrhage, Am J Roentgenol 92:1061, 1964.

133. Kinsbourne, M: Hiatus hernia with contortions of the neck, Lancet 1:1058, 1964.

134. Kirks, DR: The radiology of enteritis due to hemolytic-uremic syndrome, Pediatr Radiol 12:179, 1982.

135. Kleinman, PK, Brill, PW, and Winchester, P: Pneumatosis intestinalis, Am J Dis Child 134:1149, 1980.

136. Kopen, PA, and McAlister, WH: Upper gastrointestinal and ultrasound examinations of gastric antral involvement in chronic granulomatous disease, Pediatr Radiol 14:91, 1984.

137. Korber, JS, and Glasson, MJ: Pyloric atresia associated with epidermolysis bullosa, J Pediatr 90:600, 1977.

138. Kramer, NR, Karasic, D, and Karasick, S: "Micro-gallbladder": a clue to cystic fibrosis, JCAR 34:271, 1983.

139. Kulczycki, LL, and Shwachman, H: Studies in cystic fibrosis of the pancreas: occurrence of rectal prolapse, N Engl J Med 259:409, 1985.

140. Lampkin, BC: Personal communication.

141. Landing, BH, and Larson, AJ: Are infantile periarteritis nodosa with coronary artery involvement and fatal mucocutaneous lymph node the same? comparison of 20 patients from North America, with patients from Hawaii and Japan, Pediatrics 59:651, 1977.

142. Laufer, I, and deSa, D: Lymphoid follicular pattern: a normal feature of the pediatric colon, AJR 130:51, 1978.

143. Leonidas, JC, et al: Meconium ileus and its complications: a reappraisal of plain film roentgen diagnostic criteria, AJR 108:598, 1970.

144. Leonidas, JC, et al: Possible adverse effects of methylglucamine diatrizoate compounds on the bowel of newborn infants with meconium ileus, Radiology 121:693, 1976.

145. Levine, MS, Macones, AJ, and Laufer, I: Candida esophagitis: accuracy of radiographic diagnosis, Radiology 154:581, 1985.

146. Levine, MS, et al: Opportunistic esophagitis in AIDS: radiographic diagnosis, Radiology 165:815, 1987.

147. L'Heureux, PR, et al: Gallbladder disease in cystic fibrosis, AJR 128:953, 1977.

148. Llop, FAM, et al: Degos malignant atrophic papulosis, Ann Esp Pediatr 13:437, 1980.

149. Lombard, KA, et al: Ileal stricture as a late complication of Henoch-Schönlein purpura, Pediatrics 77:396, 1986.

150. Louw, JH, and Barnard, CN: Congenital intestinal atresia: observations of its origin, Lancet 2:1065, 1955.

151. Lucaya, J, et al: Syndrome of multiple mucosal neuromas, medullary thyroid carcinoma, and pheocromocytoma: cause of colon diverticula in children, AJR 133:1186, 1979.

152. Deleted in proofs.

153. Magid, D, et al: Abdominal pain in sickle cell disease: the role of CT, Radiology 163:325, 1987.

154. Magill, HL, et al: Duodenal perforation in childhood dermatomyositis, Pediatr Radiol 14:28, 1984.

155. Markowitz, JF, et al: Progressive esophageal dysfunction in chronic granulomatous disease, J Pediatr Gastroenterol Nutr 1:145, 1982.

156. Martel, W, Chang, SF, and Abell, MR: Loss of colonic huastration in progressive systemic sclerosis, AJRRT, 126:704, 1976.

157. Martin, LW: Personal communication, 1988.

158. Matsumoto, S, et al: Recurrent intussusception combined with Scholein-Henoch's purpura, J Jpn Soc Pediatr Surg 14:909, 1978.

159. Matzner, Y, and Brzezinski, A: C5a inhibitor deficiency in peritoneal fluids from patients with familial mediteranean fever, N Engl J Med 311:287, 1984.

160. McCall, IW, Vaidya, S, and Serjeant, GR: Splenic opacification in homozygous sickle disease, Clin Radiol 32:611, 1981.

161. McCarthy, JC, Goldberg, MJ, and Zimbler, S: Orthopaedic dysfunction in the blue rubber-bleb nevus syndrome, J Bone Joint Surg 64A:280, 1982.

162. McCauley, RGK, Leonidas, JC, and Bartoshesky, LE: Blue rubber bleb nevus syndrome, Radiology 133:375, 1979.

163. McLennan, TW, and Steinbach, HL: Shwachman's syndrome: the broad spectrum of bony abnormalities, Radiology 112:167, 1974.

164. Mestel, AL: Lymphosarcoma of the small intestine in infancy and childhood, Ann Surg 149:87, 1959.

165. Metheny, JA: Dermatomyositis: a vocal and swallowing disease entity, Laryngoscope 88:147, 1978.

166. Middlemiss, JH: Hemophilia and Christmas disease, Clin Radiol 11:40, 1960.

167. Muller, SA, Herrmann, AC, Jr, and Winkelmann, RK: Herpes simplex infections in hematologic malignancies, Am J Med 52:102, 1972.

168. Murphy, DJ, Jr, et al: Small bowel obstruction as a complication of Kawasaki disease, Clin Pediatr 26:193, 1987.

169. Murphy, WJ, Jr, and Gellis SS: Torticollis with hiatus hernia in infancy: Sandifer syndrome, Am J Dis Child 131:564, 1977.

170. Neuhauser, EBD: Roentgen rays associated with pancreatic insufficiency in early life, Radiology 46:319, 1946.

171. Deleted in proofs.

172. Newburger, PE, Cassady, JR, and Jaffe, N: Esophagitis due to adriamycin and radiation therapy for childhood malignancy, Cancer 42:417, 1978.

173. Noblett, HR: Treatment of uncomplicated meconium ileus by Gastrografin enema: a preliminary report, J Pediatr Surg 4:190, 1969.

174. Deleted in proofs.

175. Odes, HS, et al: Benign lymphoid hyperplasia of the stomach, Pediatr Radiol 10:244, 1981.

176. Oestreich, AE, and Adelstein, EH: Appendicitis as the presenting complaint in cystic fibrosis, Pediatr Surg, 17:191, 1982.

177. Oppenheimer, EH, and Esterly, JR: Hepatic changes in young infants with cystic fibrosis: possible relation to focal biliary cirrhosis, J Pediatr 86:683, 1975.

178. Papanicolaou, N, Curnette, JT, and Nathan, DG: Gallium-67 scintigraphy in children with chronic granulomatous disease, Pediatr Radiol 13:137, 1983.

179. Park, RW, and Grand, RJ: Gastrointestinal manifestations of cystic fibrosis: a review, Gastroenterology 81:1143, 1981.

180. Pearson, RW: Epidermolysis bullosa. In Rudolph, AM, editor: Pediatrics, ed 16, New York, 1977, Appleton-Century-Crofts.

181. Perelman, R, et al: Pseudomembranous colitis following obstruction in a neonate, Clin Pediatr 20:212, 1981.

182. Peterson, RB, et al: Radiographic features of colitis associated with the hemolytic-uremic syndrome, Radiology 118:667, 1976.

183. Phillips, HE, et al: Pancreatic sonography in cystic fibrosis, AJR 137:69, 1981.

184. Phillips, JC, and Gerald, BE: The incidence of cholelithiasis in sickle cell disease, AJR 113:27, 1971.

185. Pilling, DW, and Steiner, GM: The radiology of meconium ileus equivalent, Br J Radiol 54:562, 1981.

186. Pirsch, JD, and Make, DG: Infectious complications in adults with bone marrow transplantation and T-cell depletion of donor marrow: increased susceptibility to fungal infections, Ann Intern Med 104:619, 1986.

187. Pochaczevsky, R, and Leonidas, JC: The meconium plug syndrome, Am J Roentgenol 120:342, 1974.

188. Price, WH: A high incidence of chronic inflammatory bowel disease in patients with Turner's syndrome, J Med Genet 16;263, 1979.

189. Prolla, JD, and Kirsner, JB: The gastrointestinal lesions and complications of the leukemias, Ann Intern Med 61:1084, 1964.

190. Quie, PG: In Behrman, RE, Vaughan, VC, and Nelson, WE, editors: Nelson textbook of pediatrics, ed 13, Philadelphia, 1987, WB Saunders.

191. Rabinowitz, JG, et al: Trisomy 18, esophageal atresia, anomalies of the radius and congenital hypoplstic thrombocytopenia, Radiology 89:488, 1967.

192. Reilly, BJ, and Neuhauser, EBD: Renal tubular ectasia in cystic disease of the kidneys and liver, AJR 84:546, 1960.

193. Riely, CA, et al: Arteriohepatic dysplasia: a benign syndrome of intrahepatic cholestasis with multiple organ involvement, Ann Intern Med 91:520, 1979.

194. Robberecht, E, et al: Pancreatic lipomatosis in the Shwachman-Diamond syndrome: identification by sonography and CT scan, Pediatr Radiol 15:348, 1985.

195. Rosenfield, NS, et al: Arteriohepatic dysplasia: radiologic features of a new syndrome, AJR 135:1217, 1980.

196. Rosenstein, BJ, and Langbaum, TS: Incidence of meconium abnormalities in newborn children with cystic fibrosis, Am J Dis Child 134:72, 1980.

197. Rowe, JW, Gilliam, JI, and Warthin, TA: Intestinal manifestations of Fabry's disease, Ann Intern Med 81:628, 1974.

198. Santulli, TV, and Blanc, WA: Congenital atresia of intestine: pathogenesis and treatment, Ann Surg 154:939, 1961.

199. Sauerbrei, E, and Castelli, M: Hypogammaglobulinemia and nodular lymphoid hyperplasia of the gut, J Can Assoc Radiol 30:62, 1979.

200. Sawaf, H, et al: Ischemic colitis and stricture after hemolytic-uremic syndrome, Pediatrics 61:315, 1978.

201. Schaller, JG, and Wedgwood, RJ: Behrman, RE, Vaughn, VC, and Nelson, WE, editors: In Nelson Textbook of pediatrics, ed 13, Philadelphia, 1987, WB Saunders.

202. Schwartz, A, Dorkin, H, Carter, B: CT appearance of the liver in a patient with biliary cirrhosis and cystic fibrosis, J Comput Assist Tomogr 7:530, 1983.

203. Scott, RB, O'Loughlin, EV, Gall, DG: Gastroesophageal reflux in patients with cystic fibrosis, J Pediatr 106:223, 1985.

204. Shahin, N, Sohar, E, and Dalith, F: Roentgenologic findings in familial Mediterranean fever. AJR 84:269, 1960.

205. Shandling, B: The so-called superior mesenteric artery syndrome, Am J Dis Child 130:1371, 1976.

206. Shanks, MJ, et al: Radiographic findings of scleroderma in childhood, AJR 141:657, 1983.

207. Sheagren, TG, et al: Rumination: a new complication of neonatal intensive care, Pediatrics 66:551, 1980.

208. Shwachman, H, and Holsclaw, D: Examination of the appendix at laparotomy as a diagnostic clue in cystic fibrosis, N Engl J Med 286:1300, 1972.

209. Shwachman, H, et al: The syndrome of pancreatic insufficiency and bone marrow dysfunction, J Pediatr 65:645, 1964.

210. Sidaway, MD: Torsion spasm and hiatus hernia, Ann Radiol 8:15, 1965.

211. Siegel, NJ, et al: Syndrome of hiatus hernia with torsion spasms and abnormal posturing (Sandifer's syndrome). Am J Dis Child 121:53, 1971.

212. Silverman, FN: Unrecognized trauma in infants, the battered child syndrome, and the syndrome of ambroise Tardieu: the Rigler Lecture, Radiology 104:337, 1972.

213. Slovis, TL, et al: Pancreatitis and the battered child syndrome, AJR 125:456, 1975.

214. Smith, DW, Jones, KLJ: Recognizable patterns of human malformation: Genetic, embryologic and clinical aspects. In Major Problems in Clinical Pediatrics, vol VII, Philadelphia, 1982, WB Saunders.

215. Smith, GV, and Teele, RL: Delayed diagnosis of duodenal obstruction in Down syndrome, AJR 134:937, 1980.

216. Spehl-Robbrecht, M, et al: Ultrasonic study of pancreas in cystic fibrosis, Ann Radiol 24:49, 1981.

216a. Sperling, MA: In Behrman, RE, Vaughn, VC, and Nelson, WE: Nelson textbook of pediatrics, ed 13, Philadelphia, 1987, WB Saunders.

217. Stanley, RJ, Melson, GL, and Tedesco, FJ: The spectrum of radiographic findings in antibiotic-related pseudomembranous colitis, Radiology 111:519, 1974.

218. Staple, TW, McAlister, WH, and Anderson, MS: Plexiform neurofibromatosis of the colon simulating Hirschsprung's disease, AJR 91:840, 1964.

219. Steiner, RM, et al: The radiologic findings in dermatomyositis of childhood, Radiol. 111:385, 1974.

220. Deleted in proofs.

221. Stricof, DD, Glazer, GM, and Amendola, MA: Chronic granulomatous disease: value of the newer imaging modalities, Pediatr Radiol 14:328, 1984.

222. Stringer, DA, et al: Behçet syndrome involving the gastrointestinal tract: a diagnostic dilemma in childhood, Pediatr Radiol 16:131, 1986.

223. Sty, JR, et al: Involvement of colon in chronic granulomatous disease of childhood, Radiology 132:618, 1979.

224. Sutcliffe, J: Torsion spasms and abnormal postures in children with hiatus hernia: Sandifer's syndrome, Progr Pediatr Radiol 2:190, 1969.

225. Tal, Y, et al: Intestinal obstruction caused by primary adhesions due to familial Mediterranean Fever, J Pediatr Surg 15:186, 1980.

226. Teefey, SN, et al: Sonographic diagnosis in neutropenic typhlitis, AJR 149:731, 1987.

227. Tishler, JM, Han, SY, Helman, CA: Esophageal involvement in epidermolysis bullosa dystrophica, AJR 141:1283, 1983.

228. Travis, RC: Case of the month: an unusual cause of gastrointestinal haemorrhage, Br J Radiol 60:933, 1987.

229. Tschumi, A, et al: Meligne atrophisierende Papulose (Degos-Syndrom) im Sauglingsalter, eine polytope Vasculitis, Helv Paediatr Acta 36(Suppl.):13, 1976.

230. Tsunado, A, and Ishida, M: Surgical complications of Schonlein-Henoch purpura, Z Kinderchir 8:63, 1970.

231. Tucker, AS, et al: Intussusception in older children: a complication of cystic fibrosis, Ann Radiol 16:173, 1973.

232. Vahey, TN, Maglinte, DT, and Chernish, SM: State-of-the-art barium examination in opportunistic esophagitis, Dig Dis Sci 31:1192, 1986.

233. Vlymen, WJ, and Moskowitz, PS: Roentgenographic manifestations of esophageal and intestinal involvement in Behçet's disease in children, Pediatr Radiol 10:193, 1981.

234. Wagget, J, et al: The nonoperative treatment of meconium ileus by gastrografin enema, J Pediatr 77:407, 1970.

235. Walsh, TJ, Belitsos, NJ, and Hamilton, SR: Bacterial esophagitis in immunocompromised patients, Arch Intern Med 146:1345, 1986.

236. Warshauer, F, and Nelson, RE: Neurofibroma of jejunum with perforation, Am Surg 19:467, 1953.

237. Weinrieb, IJ, Fineman, RM, and Spiro, HM: Turner syndrome and inflammatroy bowel disease, N Engl J Med 294:1221, 1976.

238. Weinstein, LD, Clemett, AR, and Herskovic, T: Morphologic and radiologic findings in the intestines in cystic fibrosis, Gastroenterology 54:1282, 1968.

239. Willi, UV, Reddish, JM, and Teele, RL: Cystic fibrosis: its characteristic appearance on abdominal sonography, AJR 134:1005, 1980.

240. Williams, JR, Jr: Vascular insufficiency of the intestines, Gastroenterology 61:757, 1971.

241. Wiot, JF: Intramural small intestinal hemorrhage: a differential diagnosis, Semin Roentgenol 1:219, 1966.

242. Wolf, BS: Case #29: intramural hematoma of terminal ileum and ileocecal valve due to hemophilia, J Mt Sinai Hosp 25:89, 1958.

243. Wolfson, JJ, et al: Lymphoid hyperplasia of the large intestine associated with dysgammaglobulinemia: report of a case, AJR 108:610, 1970.

244. Wood, BP, and Katzberg, RW: Tween 80/diatrizoate enemas in bowel obstruction, AJR 130:747, 1978.

245. Woods, WG, Roloff, JS, and Lukens, JN: The occurrence of leukemia in patients with the Shwachman syndrome, J Pediatr 99:425, 1981.

246. Woofruff, JM, et al: The pathology of graft-vs-host reaction (GVHR) in adults receiving bone marrow transplants, Transplant Proc 8:675, 1976.

247. Wright, FW, and Matthews, JM: Hemophilic pseudotumor of the stomach, Radiology 98:547, 1971.

248. Yeager, AM, et al: Pneumatosis Intestinalis in children after allogeneic bone marrow transplantation, Pediatr Radiol 17:18, 1987.

249. Ziskind, A, and Gellis, SS: Water intoxication following tap water enemas, Am J Dis Child 96:699, 1958.

71 *Biliary System*

RONALD A. COHEN
HOOSHANG TAYBI

GENERAL CONSIDERATIONS

Advances in imaging techniques have improved our diagnostic capabilities for evaluating the liver, biliary system, and pancreas. Ultrasound is frequently the first imaging examination, and computed tomography (CT) and magnetic resonance imaging (MRI) are used in selected cases.[54,107] Most of the interventional radiologic techniques used in adults can be adapted for use in children.[31,104] Hepatobiliary scintigraphy remains a useful tool for assessing anatomy and function in biliary disease.[59] Others, such as sulfur colloid liver-spleen scans, are used much less often because of the availability of more sensitive imaging modalities. Angiography is now used in selected cases, primarily for evaluation of portal hypertension or identification of blood supply in hepatic tumors.[102]

LIVER

The liver is relatively large in newborns. As the child grows, the liver size becomes less prominent.[29] Scintigraphy and sonographic measurements of liver size have shown a high correlation. Plain film evaluation of liver size is difficult, particularly if there is a prominent Riedel's lobe. Standards for sonographic size have been developed.[32,50,69]

Congenital anomalies

The major liver malformations include anomalous lobation, hypoplasia or absence of a lobe, accessory lobe, attached by a pedicle, and ectopic tissue without a connection (Fig. 71-1). A horizontal, symmetric liver is associated with abdominal heterotaxy (asplenia and polysplenia syndromes).

Herniation of the liver through a diaphragmatic hernia usually is present at birth but may be delayed. Group B streptococcal pneumonia has been associated with late onset right-sided diaphragmatic hernia. Ultrasound and scintigraphic studies aid in diagnosis.

Congenital hepatic fibrosis is characterized by the proliferation of fibrous tissue, cystic dilatation of the small bile ducts, and hypoplasia of the smaller portal vein radicles. Tubular ectasia of the kidneys resembling medullary sponge kidney has been commonly reported.[28] Por-

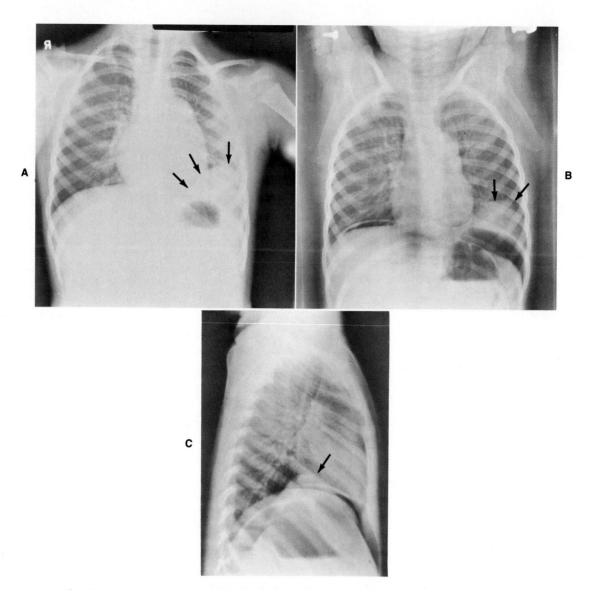

Fig 71-1 Intrathoracic ectopia of liver. **A,** Radiograph of 3-year-old boy with congenital heart disease (partial absence of pericardium on left side of heart and pulmonary stenosis) shows mass *(arrows)* above left leaf of diaphragm. Posteroanterior, **B,** and lateral, **C,** pneumoperitoneograms disclose extraperitoneal-intrathoracic position of mass *(arrows)*. Surgery showed mass to be located on diaphragm with vascular communication through diaphragm. Resected mass proved to be accessory lobe of liver with normal architecture and preservation of liver cells.
(Courtesy James Vaudgna, MD; from Taybi, H: Med Radiogr Photogr 54:19, 1978.)

tal hypertension develops in these patients, and hemorrhage caused by varices is often the initial clinical manifestation. The disease may be sporadic or autosomal recessive. It is sometimes referred to as juvenile polycystic disease. Caroli's disease has also been associated with hepatic fibrosis.[28,60,65]

Infantile polycystic kidney disease is an autosomal recessive disorder that is most often fatal. Some patients develop hepatic fibrosis and portal hypertension.[79] In others multiple hepatic cysts have been noted at autopsy. In adult-type (autosomal dominant) polycystic kidney disease, hepatic cysts develop in about one third of patients.

Many inherited metabolic diseases may affect the liver in children. These include glycogen storage diseases, mucopolysaccaridoses, Gaucher's disease, other storage diseases, cystic fibrosis, Wilson's disease, α_1-antitrypsin deficiency, galactosemia, fructose intolerance, tyrosi-

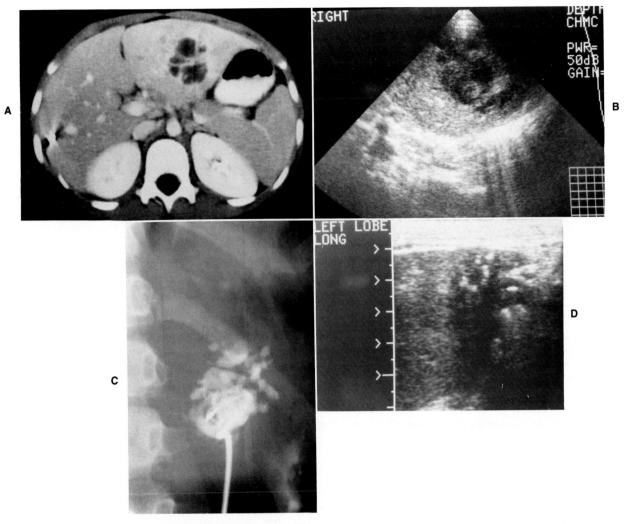

Fig. 71-2 Pyogenic liver abscess in 11-year-old boy with chronic granulomatous disease. **A,** Surgical clip in right lobe is from surgical drainage of abscess several years earlier. CT scan demonstrates septated low-attenuation mass in left lobe. **B,** Transverse ultrasonogram shows complex hypoechoic mass. **C,** Percutaneous drain was placed with ultrasound guidance. Contrast injection shows complex abscess cavity. **D,** Longitudinal ultrasonogram 14 months later shows calcification where abscess had been. Patient recovered completely from this episode.

nemia, and others. Variable degrees of hepatic enlargement or cirrhosis occur in these disorders.[35] Some conditions are associated with development of hepatic tumors, such as glycogen storage disease type 1 (von Gierke's disease), tyrosinemia, galactosemia, and anabolic steroid therapy.

Acquired diseases

Infectious hepatitis is usually caused by the type A hepatitis virus. Type B hepatitis also occurs in infants and children, particularly those at risk because of blood transfusions, infected mothers, or drug abuse. Other causes of hepatitis include cytomegalovirus, Epstein-Barr virus, varicella, and leptospirosis. Ultrasound findings are variable. Hepatic enlargement, increased periportal echoes, poor definition of vascular structures, and gallbladder wall thickening have been reported.[43,91]

Pyogenic liver abscesses in children often occur when there is a compromise in immune defense mechanisms, as in chronic granulomatous disease or childhood malignancies (Fig. 71-2)[18,23,53] Umbilical venous catheterization and sepsis are factors in some newborn infants. The organisms most commonly found are *Staphylococcus* species, *Streptococcus* species, coliforms, or mixed

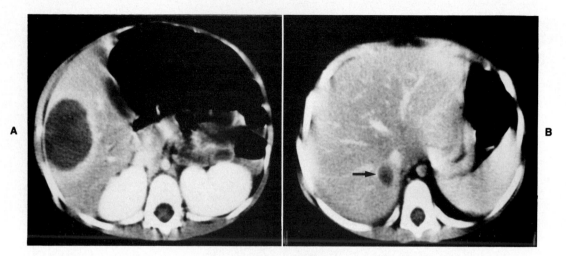

Fig. 71-3 Amebic liver abscesses in 4-year-old girl with fever of unknown origin. **A,** Large low-attenuation mass is noted in right lobe with mild rim enhancement. **B,** One of three smaller lesions *(arrow)* is noted on this scan at higher level.

flora. The abscesses are single or multiple. Percutaneous drainage is recommended for large pyogenic abscesses.

Amebic abscesses are uncommon complications of intestinal amebiasis in children. The abscesses are more often found in the right lobe of the liver; they may be single or multiple (Fig. 71-3). Most authors recommend medical treatment, although some have reported successful percutaneous drainage of amebic abscesses.[48,81,103]

Ultrasound is the screening modality of choice for both pyogenic and amebic abscesses.[18] CT (or MRI) is used to detect smaller abscesses and to assess treatment efficacy.

Tumors, cysts, and tumorlike lesions

A survey of 375 cases of primary liver tumors in children identified 252 malignant and 123 benign lesions.[37] Hepatoblastomas were the most common malignant lesions (129 cases), followed by hepatocellular carcinoma (98 cases). Other rare malignant lesions included mixed mesenchymal tumors, rhabdomyosarcomas, angiosarcomas, undifferentiated sarcomas, teratocarcinomas, cholangiosarcomas, and malignant hystiocytomas.

Hemangiomas, mesenchymal hamartomas, and infantile hemangioendotheliomas are the most common benign tumors. Hepatic adenomas and focal nodular hyperplasia can often be distinguished preoperatively using a combination of imaging modalities.[108] Other rare benign tumors include cholangiohepatomas, epithelioid epitheliomas, lymphangiomas, and eosinophilic granulomas.

Hepatoblastomas are the third most common malignant intraabdominal neoplasm in children. Most hepa-

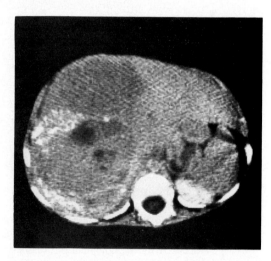

Fig. 71-4 Hepatoblastoma in 7-month-old boy first seen with failure to thrive and right upper quadrant mass. Complex mass in right lobe contains amorphous calcification and some low-attenuation areas, indicating necrotic portions of tumor. Patient is now alive and well 5 years after trisegmentectomy, chemotherapy, and several resections of pulmonary metastases. (Courtesy PE Kane, MD, Children's Hospital, Oakland, Calif.)

toblastomas initially appear as an abdominal mass in children less than 3 years of age; they are present at birth in about one third of case. The tumor is most often a single lesion and frequently contains amorphous or punctate calcification (Fig. 71-4).[26,71] Hepatocellular carcinoma, on the other hand, usually appears in children older than 3 years of age, calcifies infrequently, and is

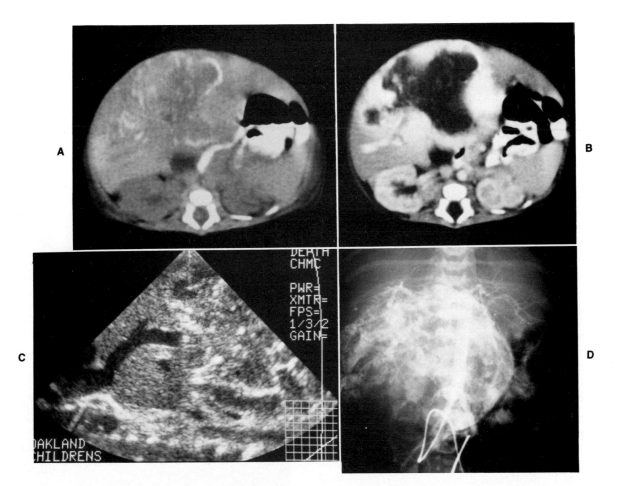

Fig. 71-5 Hemangioendothelioma in newborn boy with congestive heart failure and hyperconsumptive coagulopathy (Kasabach-Merritt syndrome). **A,** Noncontrast CT shows serpiginous calcification in large hepatic mass. **B,** On contrast-enhanced CT thick enhancing rim with central necrotic zone is noted. **C,** Longitudinal sonogram shows complex mass in inferior portion of liver with normal hepatic parenchyma and prominent hepatic veins and inferior vena cava superiorly. **D,** Aortogram through umbilical artery catheter demonstrates multiple abnormal vessels and vascular pooling. Patient died in spite of steroids, platelets, and surgical ligation of hepatic artery. Embolization was not attempted in this case.

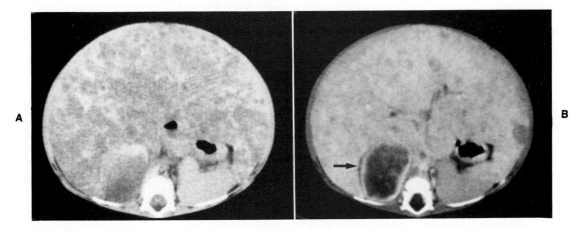

Fig. 71-6 Stage IV-S neuroblastoma in 2½-month-old girl. **A,** On noncontrast CT diffuse tumor infiltration of liver is noted. **B,** Contrast-enhanced CT demonstrates primary tumor in right adrenal with thin enhancing rim and low-attenuation center *(arrow)*. Diagnosis was confirmed by bone marrow aspiration. Patient recovered completely without any chemotherapy or surgery.

often multifocal.[105] Some conditions, such as chronic active hepatitis and a few metabolic disorders, predispose patients to hepatocellular carcinoma.

Infantile hemangioendotheliomas are highly vascular, with variable degrees of necrotic zones and calcifications (Fig. 71-5)[25,66] Mesenchymal hamartomas are usually large cystic masses with multiple septations.[44,72,85,95]

Liver metastases are seen in several childhood malignancies. Liver involvement in neuroblastoma manifests either as extensive replacement of hepatic tissue, local invasion from adjacent tumor, or focal metastases.[13] In stage IV-S type neuroblastoma (in children less than 1 year), extensive involvement frequently resolves without treatment (Fig. 71-6).[13,38] Hepatic metastases in tumors other than Wilms' are generally less common than in adults. Hemihypertrophy and precocious puberty have been reported with hepatoblastoma.[1,26,93]

Ultrasonography is generally the first imaging examination in patients with a suspected mass. Simple hepatic cysts require no further imaging unless cysts in other organs are suspected; if a solid or complex mass is detected, CT and/or MRI is recommended. Calcification, best detected on CT, is found most often in hepatoblastomas, vascular tumors, metastatic neuroblastoma, and teratomas. If segmental resection is considered, it is imperative to exclude tumor in the remaining liver. In these cases angiography is useful to demonstrate the arterial supply and venous drainage as well as the type of tumor vascularity.[102]

The angiographic features of hepatoblastomas include arteriovenous shunting and encasement of the vessels. Tumor vascular blush and extravascular pooling occur in hepatomas. An enlarged hepatic artery, the early appearance of draining veins, and a prolonged pooling of contrast medium in sinusoidal spaces are the angiographic features of angiomatous hepatic tumors.

Fatty liver

Fatty liver has been noted in patients with cystic fibrosis, Reye's syndrome, acute starvation, kwashiorkor, malabsorption syndromes, high-dose steroid therapy, glycogen storage disease, exposure to toxins, acute hepatitis, and cholesterol ester storage disease (Fig. 71-7).[19,42,114] The radiolucent fatty densities of the liver and properitoneal fat produces a distinct interface with the more radiodense abdominal musculature. Blurring of the medial margin of the right properitoneal fat stripe is probably the earliest plain film radiographic change. On noncontrast CT the vessels are denser than the hepatic parenchyma. Increased echogenicity of the liver is noted on ultrasound; occasionally, there is relative sparing of the periportal regions, which can mimic a focal mass (Fig. 71-8).[111]

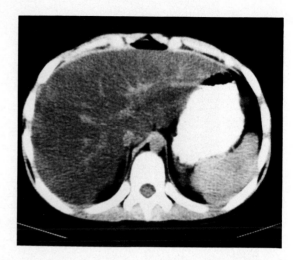

Fig. 71-7 Fatty liver in 10-year-old boy undergoing chemotherapy for leukemia. On noncontrast CT hepatic parenchyma has lower attenuation than blood vessels.

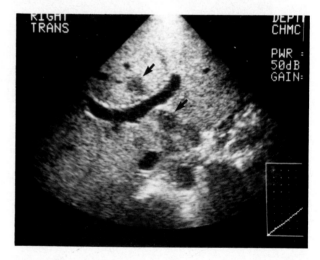

Fig. 71-8 Fatty liver with pseudomasses in 21-year-old woman with cystic fibrosis. Liver is hyperechoic with prominent beam attenuation. Hypoechoic pseudomasses are seen in periportal region and anterior to portal vein *(arrows)*.

Focal fatty infiltration may simulate a mass lesion and should be considered in the differential diagnoses of hepatic masses.

Hepatic calcifications

Hepatic calcification in neonates has been reported in cases of intrauterine infections (herpes simplex, cytomegalovirus, varicella, and toxoplasmosis), tumors (hemangioendotheliomas, hamartomas, and metastatic neuroblastomas), postumbilical catheterization (parenchymal and intravascular calcifications), and ischemic

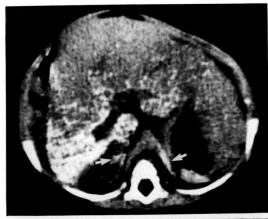

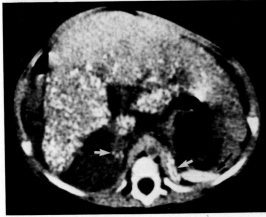

Fig. 71-9 Disseminated neonatal herpes in 8-week-old girl. **A** and **B,** Noncontrast CT scan demonstrates widespread hepatic calcification, most prominent in posterior segment of right lobe. Colon is interposed between lateral abdominal wall and small right lobe of liver. Also noted are bilateral adrenal calcifications *(white arrows)* and small spleen *(black arrows)*.

necrosis (Fig. 71-9). Subcapsular calcification in premature and stillborn infants probably represents the manifestations of portal venous thrombi.[74,90]

Hepatic calcification in children occurs in cases of chronic granulomatous disease of childhood, tuberculosis, fungal infections, parasitic diseases, cholesterol ester storage disease, intrahepatic lithiasis, amebic and pyogenic abscesses, primary neoplasms, and secondary neoplasms and after trauma.[19]

Liver transplantation

Several medical centers now perform liver transplantation in children with end-stage liver disease, most often biliary atresia. The preoperative imaging evaluation must demonstrate the vascular anatomy, particularly the portal venous system and/or the portosystemic collateral circulation.[64] Celiac and superior mesenteric arteriography are performed to evaluate the arterial supply and the portal and systemic venous systems. Splenoportography is used in selected cases. Preoperative ultrasound, scintigraphy, and percutaneous or operative cholangiography, as well as MRI or CT, often provide useful anatomic information.

Postoperative complications include transplant rejec-

tion, arterial or venous thrombosis, biliary obstruction, bile lakes, hepatic abscesses, hepatic infarction, and tumors secondary to immunosuppressant drugs. The imaging modalities chosen depend on the clinical problem that requires evaluation.[33]

Hemosiderosis and hemachromatosis

In children hemosiderosis and hemachromatosis usually result from multiple blood transfusions, most often in patients with hemoglobinopathies or other hematologic disorders, although hereditary hemachromatosis may be seen in children and adolescents.[46] The liver, heart, and pancreas are affected in these disorders. CT may show increased attenuation in the liver. MRI demonstrates decreased signal in the liver from the ferromagnetic effect of excess iron and is more sensitive than CT in detecting early stages of hemosiderosis or hemachromatosis.[96] Increased CT density has also been reported with cisplatin chemotherapy.[3]

Intrahepatic gas

Gas in the liver is in the portal veins, biliary tract, hepatic veins, or hepatic parenchyma. Portal venous gas usually results from bowel injury with collection of intramural gas and subsequent passage of gas through mesenteric veins to the portal system. In the newborn this is usually associated with necrotizing enterocolitis or related to injection of air through an umbilical venous catheter (Fig. 71-10). Gas in the biliary system is seen in postoperative biliary-enteric anastomosis, duodenal obstruction, such as duodenal atresia; or penetrating duodenal ulcer. Generally, portal venous gas extends more peripherally than biliary gas, which tends to be more central in location. Ultrasound can detect moving air bubbles in portal veins in patients with necrotizing enterocolitis, even when plain radiographs do not demonstrate portal venous gas. Air in hepatic veins is uncommon and usually associated with intravascular air elsewhere. Hepatic parenchymal gas may be posttraumatic, iatrogenic, or related to gas-forming organisms.[94]

Trauma

Patterns of liver injury in childhood have been recently described.[94] Most injuries involve the right lobe of the liver, particularly the posterior segment. Associated lung base, renal, pancreatic, and adrenal injury are seen on CT (Fig. 71-11). Most liver injuries in children are managed nonoperatively.

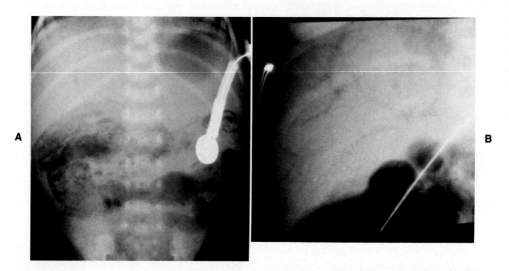

Fig. 71-10 Portal venous gas associated with neonatal necrotizing enterocolitis (NEC). **A,** Three-week-old girl with NEC. Intramural gas is noted in several bowel loops in right side of abdomen and splenic flexure. Branching intrahepatic (portal venous) gas is faintly seen. **B,** Four-week-old girl with NEC. Branching portal venous gas extends to periphery of liver (close-up view of liver, left lateral decubitus radiograph).

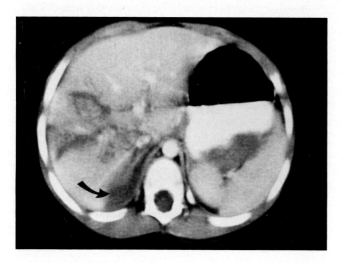

Fig. 71-11 Hepatic injury in 6-year-old boy hit by car. Complex injury is noted in right lobe of liver on this contrast-enhanced CT. Also note associated periadrenal hematoma *(arrow).*

□ TABLE 71-1

Transverse diameter of the common bile duct in normal children*

Age (years)	Range of diameter (mm)	Mean diameter (mm)
Less than 2	—	2.0
2 to 4	2 to 4	2.6
4 to 6	2 to 4	2.6
6 to 8	2 to 6	3.8
8 to 10	2 to 6	3.9
10 to 12	3 to 6	4.0
12 to 14	3 to 7	4.9

Modified from Witcombe, JB, and Cremin, BJ: Pediatr Radiol 7:147, 1978.
*The widest transverse diameter of the common bile duct is measured on an intravenous cholangiogram, ignoring the proximal 5 mm of the duct.

□ TABLE 71-2

Longitudinal axis of the gallbladder in normal children

Age (years)	Range of axis (cm)	Mean axis ± SE
2 to 4	3.1 to 5.3	4.14 ± 0.20
5 to 10	4.1 to 8.0	5.36 ± 0.34
10 to 14	4.3 to 7.5	5.91 ± 0.33
14 to 18	5.2 to 7.2	6.19 ± 0.22

Modified from Slovis, TL, et al: Pediatrics 65:789, 1980. Copyright American Academy of Pediatrics 1980.

BILIARY SYSTEM
Techniques and normal values

Oral and intravenous cholangiography are now rarely used in children. Ultrasound is usually the initial imaging modality used to evaluate the anatomy. The gallbladder is best visualized after fasting, for 3 to 4 hours in small neonates and all night in older children and adolescents.

Biliary scintigraphy, using one of the new technetium-labeled derivatives of iminodiacetic acid (IDA), is used to evaluate the function and patency of the biliary tract. Sometimes phenobarbital (5 mg/kg/day) is administered orally for at least 5 days before the scintigraphic study to stimulate bile secretion.[59]

Percutaneous transhepatic cholangiography using a 22-gauge needle and fluoroscopic control is more easily performed in the presence of dilated bile ducts.[104] The use of percutaneous cholecystography has also been reported.[40]

Intraoperative cholangiography remains an important technique, particularly in the evaluation of infants with biliary atresia or severe neonatal hepatitis. One to two cubic centimeters of contrast medium is injected into the gallbladder or bile ducts. The intrahepatic and extrahepatic ducts are outlined, and biliary patency is assessed. Retrograde linear extravasation of contrast medium along vascular channels can mimic biliary radicles and should not be confused with patent bile ducts.[116] CT and MRI are used in selected cases.

There is a close correlation between the patient's age and the diameter of the common bile duct but a poor correlation with the patient's weight (Table 71-1).[113] There is significant variation in the size of the gallbladder in children (Table 71-2).[70,92]

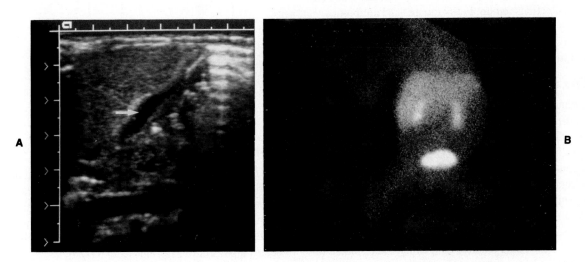

Fig. 71-12 Biliary atresia in 2-week-old girl. **A,** Ultrasonogram demonstrates small gallbladder *(arrow).* **B,** No excretion of radionuclide into GI tract is noted on biliary scan. Biliary atresia was confirmed at surgery. Patient underwent Kasai procedure and is doing well at 2 years of age.

Congenital anomalies
Biliary atresia and neonatal hepatitis

There is considerable overlap between the clinical picture and the liver biopsy findings in cases of biliary atresia and neonatal hepatitis. Prolonged obstructive jaundice and hepatomegaly are the major initial manifestations of both diseases. Some authors believe that these conditions have a common origin. Indeed, intermediate cases have been described.

Ultrasound is performed to rule out biliary obstruction and assess the size of the bile ducts and gallbladder. The gallbladder is usually small or nonvisualized in biliary atresia (Fig. 71-12).[15,106] If the hepatic duct is obliterated and the cystic and common duct are patent, the gallbladder may contract with feeding.[106] Bright periportal echoes may be present in both biliary atresia and neonatal hepatitis.

Biliary scintigraphy is very important in the differentiation of biliary atresia and neonatal hepatitis. As noted, prior administration of phenobarbital is recommended. In neonatal hepatitis hepatic uptake and excretion may be reduced, but the radionuclide should eventually pass into the intestines in all except the most severe cases. In biliary atresia the radionuclide will stay in the liver and existing bile ducts but will not be found in the intestines (Fig. 71-12, **B**). When biliary patency cannot be established, an open biopsy and operative cholangiography are recommended. The type of biliary atresia is best determined at the time of surgery (Figs. 71-13 and 71-14). Some forms are correctable, but most require a portoenterostomy (the Kasai procedure) to establish biliary drainage. The Kasai procedure is most effective when performed before the patient is 8 to 10 weeks of age. Intrahepatic bile lakes or cysts have been reported in some of these patients (Fig. 71-15). When infected, these collections require both drainage and antibiotics.[110] In many children, however, liver transplantation offers the only hope for long-term survival. Biliary atresia is sometimes associated with the polysplenia syndrome.[2]

Biliary tract stenosis or hypoplasia

Excluding the various forms of biliary atresia, there are other less common obstructive lesions of the bile ducts. These include stenosis, compression by anomalous vessels, congenital diaphragm, and stenosis of Vater's ampulla.[30,34,77,115]

Ductal dilatations can be intrahepatic or extrahepatic. Congenital stenosis occasionally results in spontaneous perforation of the bile ducts in infants.[8] Biliary hypoplasia is seen in arteriohepatic dysplasia (Alagille's syndrome), which also features congenital heart disease (in particular pulmonary artery hypoplasia or stenosis), butterfly vertebrae, and distinctive facies.[4,99]

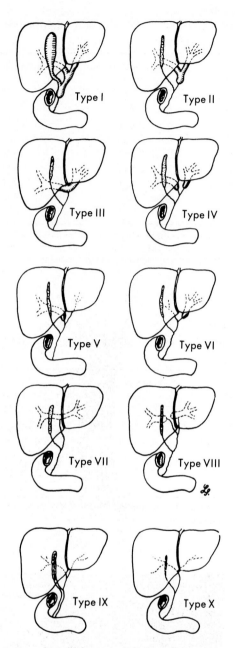

Fig. 71-13 Types of atresia of bile ducts.
(Modified from Hasse, W:Arch Dis Child 40:162, 1965.)

Cystic dilatation of bile ducts

There are many types of cystic dilatation of the biliary tract (Fig. 71-16). The most common is globular dilatation of the distal common bile duct (choledochal cyst) (Fig. 71-17). Fusiform dilatation of the common bile duct, various diverticula, and intraduodenal choledochoceles also occur (Figs. 71-18 to 71-20).[7,11,22,56,98]

The classic triad of abdominal pain, a mass, and jaundice is present in about two thirds of patients with a

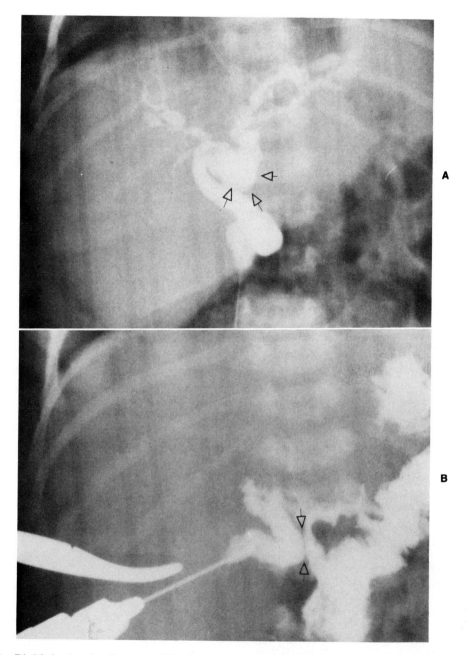

Fig. 71-14 A, Atresia of common bile duct *(arrows)* is shown by injection of contrast medium into gallbladder in 4-week-old boy. Note nonuniform dilatation of intrahepatic bile ducts. **B,** Second injection after choledochoduodenostomy shows free passage of contrast medium into duodenum.

Fig. 71-15 Bile lakes in 10-month-old with biliary atresia and Kasai procedure. CT scan (**A**) and ultrasonogram (**B**) demonstrate multiple intrahepatic bile lakes. Patient was febrile, and infection was suspected. Percutaneous aspiration and drainage of infected fluid allowed for temporary improvement of patient's condition. Patient died awaiting liver transplant.
(Courtesy KW Martin, MD, Children's Hospital, Oakland, Calif.)

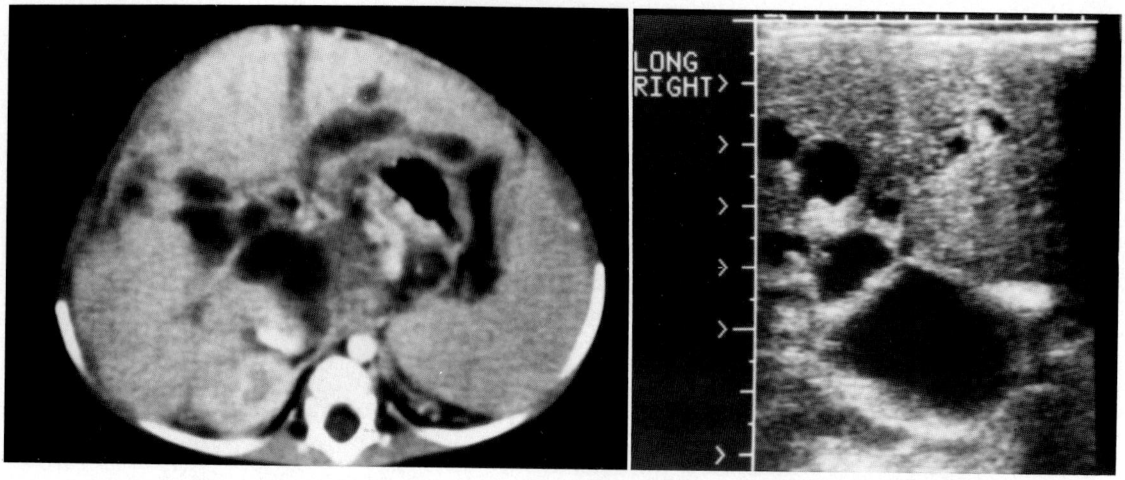

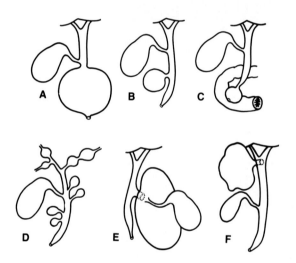

Fig. 71-16 Types of cystic dilatation of bile ducts. **A,** Cholendochal cyst. **B,** Diverticulum cyst. **C,** Choledochocele. **D,** Multiple hepatocholedochal cysts. **E,** Cystic duct cyst. **F,** Hepatic duct cyst, diverticulum type.
(Redrawn from Arthur, GW, and Stewart, JO: Br J Surg 51:671, 1964; Eisen, HB et al: Radiology 81:276, 1963; Silberman, EL and Glaessner TS: Radiology 82:470, 1964; Weinstein, C: Arch Intern Med 115:339, 1965.)

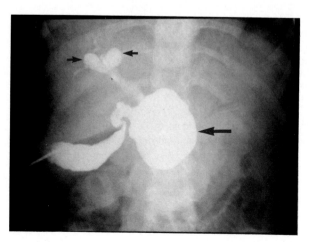

Fig. 71-17 Choledochal cyst in 3½-year-old girl. Operative cholangiogram demonstrates cystic dilatation of common bile duct (*large arrow*) and dilatation of some intrahepatic ducts (*small arrows*).

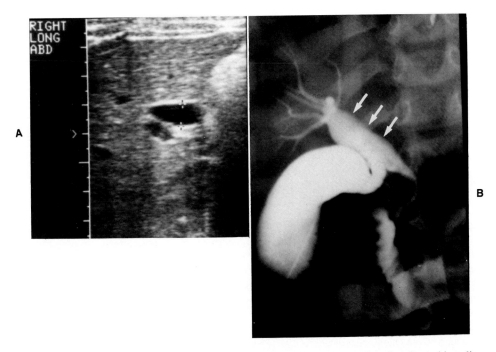

Fig. 71-18 Fusiform dilatation of common bile duct in a 2-year-old boy. He had prolonged jaundice as newborn without clear diagnosis and is now asymptomatic. **A,** Longitudinal ultrasonogram reveals dilated common bile duct *(cursors)*. Diameter is approximately 8 mm. Intrahepatic ducts were not dilated. **B,** Intraoperative cholangiogram shows fusiform dilatation of common bile duct *(arrows)* and normal intrahepatic ducts. Choledochoduodenostomy was performed, and patient is doing well.

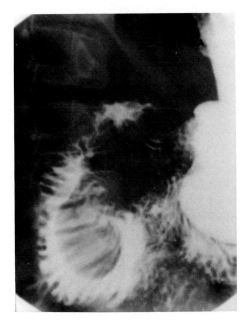

Fig. 71-19 Introduodenal choledochocele in 13-year-old boy with intermittent abdominal pain. Mobile intraluminal mass is noted in second portion of duodenum during upper gastrointestinal study.

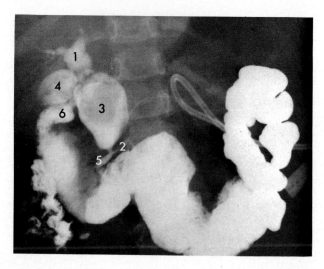

Fig. 71-20 Choledochal cyst with diverticulum of cyst in 6-year-old girl who has undergone two previous operations. In first operation choledochoduodenostomy was performed. Because of persistence of symptoms, at second operation this anastomosis was taken down, gallbladder was removed, and choledochojejunostomy was performed. Patient still remained symptomatic, and clinical manifestations of pancreatitis were present. At third operation fine catheter was introduced into pancreatic duct *(2)* and contrast medium was injected. Anomalous entrance of common bile duct into pancreatic duct *(5)* was demonstrated. In addition to cystic dilatation of common bile duct *(3)*, another cystic lesion *(4)* was opacified. On direct inspection this was found to be outpouching (diverticulum) of choledochal cyst. Previous jejunal anastomosis was to this diverticulum. *(6)*. Dilatation of hepatic duct *(1)* and branches are also shown. Some barium remains in colon from upper GI study performed on previous day. Pancreaticojejunostomy was performed, and anastomosis between cyst *(3)* and duodenum was created.

choledochal cyst. However, symptoms are frequently intermittent. Symptoms may first appear during early infancy, later in childhood, or in adulthood. Biliary cirrhosis, portal hypertension, spontaneous or traumatic rupture, stone formation, and malignant degeneration are some of the complications of choledochal cysts.[39]

An anomalous choledochopancreatic ductal junction is considered to be the most likely causative factor in the formation of cystic dilatation of the common bile duct. It is postulated that reflux of pancreatic juice into the bile ducts causes inflammation with subsequent stenosis and proximal dilatation.[7,22,56,98]

Ultrasound should be the initial imaging technique.[47] Choledochal cysts are generally anechoic masses (some low-level echoes may be present) that are contiguous with the common bile duct and separate from the gallbladder. The entire biliary ductal system should be examined for evidence of duct dilatation or diverticula. Biliary scintigraphy often provides supplementary or confirmatory information. An upper gastrointestinal barium study may demonstrate a rounded soft tissue mass that displaces the stomach downward and to the left and the duodenum downward and anterior. A choledochocele is a filling

defect in the duodenum. Percutaneous cholangiography or endoscopic retrograde cholangiopancreatography can be used in selected cases.

Caroli's disease

Caroli's disease is characterized by segmental saccular ectasia of the intrahepatic bile ducts. Association with renal cystic disease and hepatic fibrosis has been reported.[28,68] In these patients there is a marked predisposition to biliary calculi, cholangitis, and liver abscesses.

Recurrent abdominal pain, fever, intermittent jaundice related to cholangitis, and stone formation in the dilated ducts are the clinical manifestations of the disease. Percutaneous transhepatic cholangiography is an excellent method for the demonstration of the anomalous biliary tract.

Miscellaneous anomalies

A few cases of congenital bronchobiliary fistulas have been reported. In this rate entity the patient has a cough that produces foamy, bile-stained sputum and/or recurrent respiratory infections. Bronchography has been used to demonstrate the communication between the tracheo-

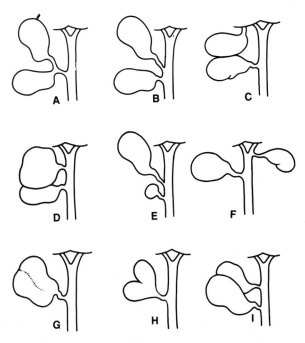

Fig. 71-21 Types of double gallbladder. **A,** Double gallbladder with single cystic duct. **B,** Double gallbladder, each with separate cystic duct. **C,** Double gallbladder, one with hepatocystic duct. **D,** Double gallbladder, one dilated. **E,** Rudimentary gallbladder in addition to normal gallbladder. **F,** Double gallbladder, one terminating into left hepatic duct. **G,** Septate gallbladder with common gallbladder neck and common cystic duct. **H,** Cleft type of double gallbladder. **I,** Two gallbladders fused externally but with two cystic ducts.
(Redrawn from Hess, W: Surgery of the biliary passages and the pancreas, Princeton, NJ, 1965, D Van Nostrand Co: Anderson, RE, and Ross, WT: Arch Surg 76:7, 1958.)

bronchial tree and the biliary tract.[21] Gas in the gallbladder has been noted in some patients with this anomaly.

Absence of the gallbladder has been reported as an isolated anomaly or in association with other anomalies of the biliary system and pancreas and polysplenia syndrome.[10] Various types of double and triple gallbladders have been demonstrated radiographically[45,86] (Fig. 71-21).

The aberrant gallbladder location may be intrahepatic, left sided, transverse, suprahepatic, or retrodisplaced. Interposition of the gallbladder is a rare anomaly characterized by the absence of the common hepatic duct and cystic duct.[97] Other rare abnormal locations are the abdominal wall and the falciform ligament.[12] Suprahepatic gallbladders can be associated with hypoplasia of the right lobe of the liver. A midline gallbladder is one finding in patients with asplenia syndrome.

A partial or complete duodenal obstruction associated with incompetence of Oddi's sphincter permits gas or contrast medium to enter the biliary system[6] (Fig. 71-22). Gas can also bypass the site of a complete duodenal obstruction through the biliary ducts. In these cases the

bifid duct has been reported to have a double termination with one orifice on each side of the obstruction. The insertion of the bile duct into a duplicate duodenum is another rare anomaly.

Acquired diseases
Cholecystitis

Cholecystitis is relatively rare in children, and it is often not considered in the initial evaluation of infants and children with acute abdominal symptoms. It is often mistaken for either appendicitis or urinary tract infection.

Unlike in adults, acalculous inflammation comprises most cases of cholecystitis in infants and children.[52] Bacterial infection is sometimes associated with sepsis. Occasionally, congenital anomalies of the gallbladder, cystic duct stenosis, or transient plugging of the bile ducts are associated with cholecystitis.[84] Ultrasonographic findings are variable. A thickened wall of the gallbladder, 3 mm or greater, is sometimes seen but is not specific. Ascites, hypoproteinemia, congestive failure, hepatitis, and other conditions also cause gallbladder wall thickening (Fig. 71-23).[75,91]

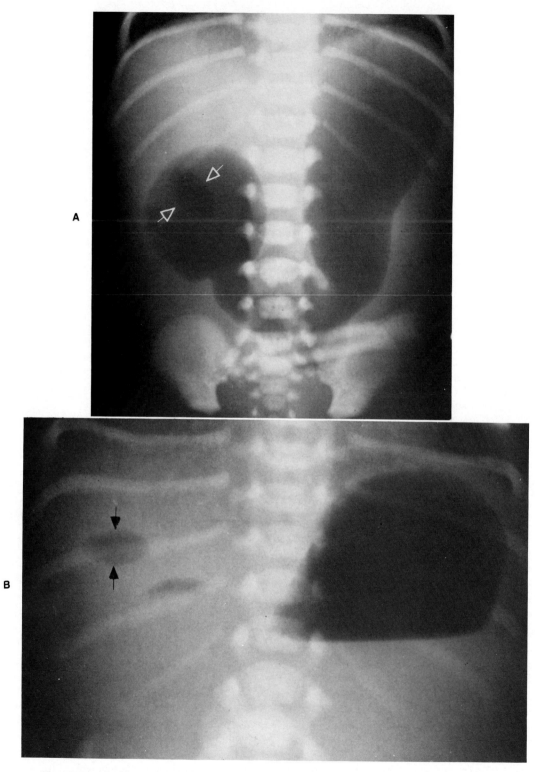

Fig. 71-22 Duodenal atresia in 2-day-old infant with marked distention of stomach and duodenum. Note presence of gas in gallbladder *(arrows)*.

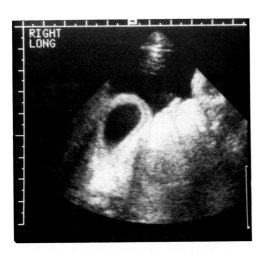

Fig. 71-23 Thick gallbladder wall in 4½-year-old girl with ascites from portal hypertension and cavernous transformation of portal veins.

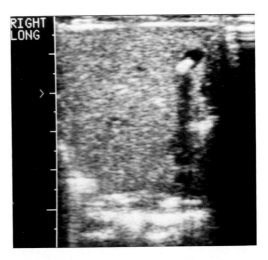

Fig. 71-24 Cholelithiasis in 3-month-old boy with bronchopulmonary dysplasia who has received parenteral alimentation and furosemide. Ultrasonogram demonstrates highly echoic structure (gallstone) in gallbladder, causing acoustic shadowing.
(Courtesy PA Nancarrow, MD, Children's Hospital, Oakland, Calif.)

Cholelithiasis

Cholelithiasis is a relatively uncommon disease in infancy and childhood. However, an increasing number of cases are being reported in premature infants and other children who receive long-term parenteral nutrition.[17,57] Chronic furosemide administration increases the incidence of both urinary tract and biliary tract calcification (Fig. 71-24).[17,82] Spontaneous resolution of gallstones has been reported in infants.[51,55] A recent report describes fetal gallstones detected prenatally by ultrasound.[61]

About 20% of the children with gallstones have hemolytic disease.[49] In patients with sickle cell disease a 27% incidence of gallstones has been reported with the use of ultrasonography.[87] In this group of 226 patients with sickle cell disease the incidence increased from 12% in children 2 to 4 years of age to 42% in patients 15 to 18 years of age (Fig. 71-25). It has been recommended that all such patients with "abdominal crisis" be investigated for cholelithiasis.[83] Hepatic and splenic infarcts or abscesses occasionally occur in sickle cell disease also and can be assessed by CT.[67]

An interruption of the enterohepatic circulation of bile salts may result in the formation of cholesterol cholelithiasis. A failure of adequate bile salt absorption from the terminal ileum, because of surgery or inflammatory bowel disease, results in a depletion of the hepatic bile salt pool. The bile becomes saturated with cholesterol, resulting in the formation of cholesterol stones.[58]

About 25% to 50% of patients with cystic fibrosis have been reported to have an abnormal gallbladder.

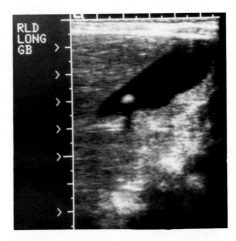

Fig. 71-25 Cholelithiasis in asymptomatic 6-year-old girl with sickle cell disease. Hyperechoic gallstone with acoustic shadowing is seen on this longitudinal ultrasonogram.

These abnormalities include microgallbladder and calculi.

Obstructive choledocholithiasis in children may be seen in the absence of cholelithiasis.[16] Other conditions associated with an increased incidence of biliary calculi in children include cardiac surgery, scoliosis surgery, short bowel syndrome, prenatal calcium supplementation, and prior surgery for congenital duodenal anomalies (Fig. 71-26).[49,78,100,101,112]

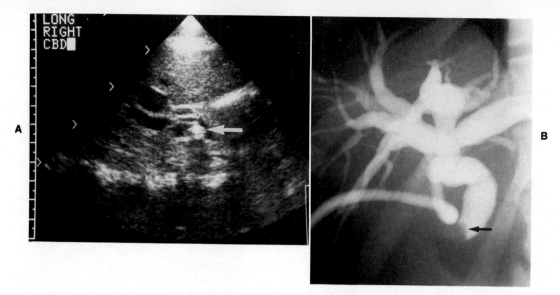

Fig. 71-26 Common bile duct stone in 14-year-old girl with right upper quadrant pain and fever. Patient had surgical repair of duodenal atresia as newborn. **A,** Longitudinal ultrasonogram demonstrates stone in dilated distal common bile duct *(arrow)*. **B,** Postoperative T-tube cholangiogram shows filling defect (stone) in distal common bile duct with complete obstruction *(arrow)*. Several weeks later stone was extracted through T-tube tract.

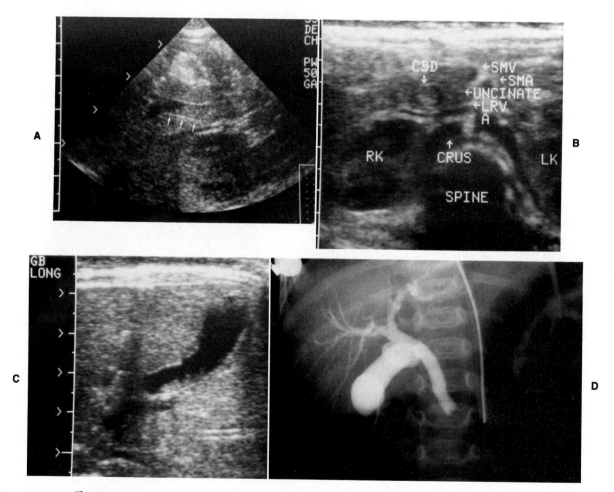

Fig. 71-27 Inspissated bile syndrome in 7-week-old girl first seen with abrupt onset of alcoholic stools. No known risk factors were identified, except for mild ABO incompatibility. There was no neonatal jaundice. **A,** Longitudinal ultrasonogram demonstrates echogenic material in dilated distal common bile duct *(arrows)*. Diameter is 4.3 mm. **B,** Transverse ultrasonogram also shows echogenic material in common bile duct. *CBD,* Common bile duct; *RK,* right kidney; *LK,* left kidney; *SMV,* superior mesenteric vein; *LRV,* left renal vein; *SMA,* superior mesenteric artery. **C,** Longitudinal ultrasonogram of gallbladder reveals some echogenic material in gallbladder. Biliary scan (not shown) demonstrated no excretion of radionuclide into GI tract. **D,** Intraoperative cholangiogram shows complete obstruction of distal common bile duct.

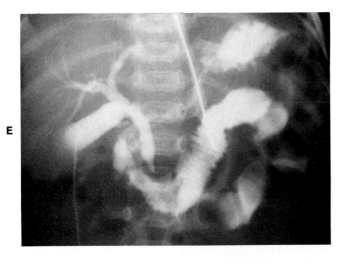

E

Fig. 71-27 cont'd E, After flushing with saline, patency is established. Material from gallbladder had appearance of gravel; analysis revealed calcium bilirubinate. Patient recovered completely and has remained asymptomatic.
(Courtesy KW Martin, MD, and E Free, MD, Children's Hospital, Oakland, Calif.)

Inspissated bile syndrome

Inspissated bile syndrome (or bile-plug syndrome) is an uncommon condition seen in young infants with signs and symptoms of biliary obstruction (Fig. 71-27). Usually there is an identifiable etiologic factor, such as hemolytic anemia, dehydration, or sepsis. Some authors believe that underlying hepatic injury must be present for the clinical syndrome to develop. Some cases spontaneously resolve. When intervention is required, irrigation of the biliary tract will usually dislodge the inspissated material and relieve the obstruction. Congenital stenosis of the bile ducts and cystic fibrosis should be considered, especially if there are no other apparent etiologic factors.[27] Dilated ducts with intraluminal echogenic material can be seen on ultrasound.[76] Biliary scintigraphy demonstrates partial or complete obstruction.

Hydrops of the gallbladder

Hydrops of the gallbladder has been associated with many conditions, including newborn sepsis, Kawasaki disease, and scarlet fever (Fig. 71-28).[20,63,73,92] The gallbladder is enlarged and usually tense and tender during the ultrasound examination. The fluid in the gallbladder is generally anechoic and not infected. The cause of the dilatation is unclear. Resolution occurs with treatment of the underlying condition. Gallbladder distention is also seen with parenteral alimentation and fasting.[9]

Rupture

In early infancy a spontaneous rupture may occur on the anterior aspect of the common bile duct or at the junction of the gallbladder and the cystic duct (Fig. 71-29). Less often, the perforation occurs in the hepatic duct.[8,34,36] The cause of the spontaneous rupture in infants and children remains unsettled in most cases. Bile plugs,

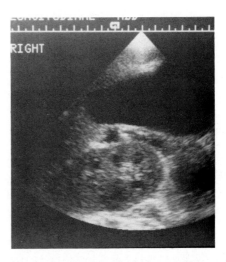

Fig. 71-28 Hydrops of gallbladder in 8-year-old boy with Kawasaki disease. Longitudinal ultrasonogram shows enlarged gallbladder that extends several centimeters inferior to lower pole of right kidney.

stones, ascarides, stenosis, and a long pancreatic-biliary channel have been reported in some infants and children.

Clinically the condition is acute or subacute. Ascites and jaundice are usually present. Signs of ascites may be present on abdominal radiographs. occasionally noted is an ill-defined mass in the right upper quadrant, which represents loculated bile near the rupture site. Ultrasonography is ideal to demonstrate ascites, bile duct dilatation, or a loculated cystic mass. Biliary scintigraphy is used to document the bile leak. Operative cholangiography usually shows the site of the rupture and, if present, the obstruction.

Traumatic rupture of the bile ducts can occur in any

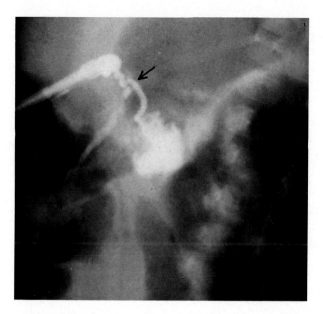

Fig. 71-29 Spontaneous rupture of common bile duct. This 2½-week-old boy was admitted with history of vomiting and abdominal distention of about 18 hours' duration. At surgery cloudy bile-stained ascites and perforation of less than 1 mm in diameter of common bile duct were found. Tube cholangiography performed 2 weeks after surgery revealed persistent leak from perforation site *(arrow)*. Repeat cholangiogram 1 week later showed that perforation had sealed.
(From Hyde, GA, Jr: Pediatrics 35:453, 1965.)

age group. Bile ascites, intrahepatic or extrahepatic bilomas, or hematobilia may result.[94]

Tumors

Primary tumors of the gallbladder and bile ducts are rare. Reported cases include rhabdomyosarcoma, hamartoma, carcinoma, cholangiosarcoma, and papilloma.[5,14,41,62,89] A rhabdomyosarcoma usually first appears with obstructive jaundice and a mass in the right upper quadrant. On ultrasound and CT a periportal mass is noted along with intrahepatic biliary duct dilatation. Operative cholangiography demonstrates the obstruction and distortion of the bile duct associated with filling defects.

Other neoplasms that cause obstructive jaundice include neuroblastoma, lymphoma, and rare pancreatic tumors (Fig. 71-30).

Sclerosing cholangitis

Sclerosing cholangitis is rare in childhood. It is characterized by the constriction of the intrahepatic and extrahepatic biliary tract from inflammation and fibrosis of the submucosa and appears with progressive obstructive jaundice. Transhepatic, operative, and endoscopic retrograde cholangiography have been used in the diagnosis of this disease. Contrast studies shown an irregular narrowing of the intrahepatic and extrahepatic bile ducts.[109] Because of the association of sclerosing cholangitis and

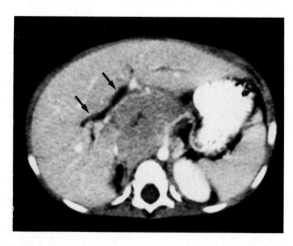

Fig. 71-30 Neuroblastoma in 9-month-old girl first seen with jaundice. CT scan demonstrates mass in portahepatis region. Note dilated hepatic duct *(arrows)*. Surgery revealed neuroblastoma arising in celiac plexus.

inflammatory bowel disease, investigation of the gastrointestinal (GI) tract is recommended.

Metachromatic leukodystrophy

Metachromatic leukodystrophy is a rare metabolic disorder caused by a deficiency of the enzyme aryl-sulfatase-A that leads to an abnormal accumulation of sulfatides

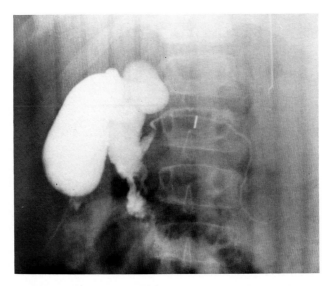

Fig. 71-31 Common bile duct stricture and portal hypertension in 14-year-old boy caused by adhesions related to right nephrectomy and radiotherapy for Wilms' tumor at 3 years of age. Hepatosplenomegaly was discovered at 14 years of age. Ultrasonography and splenoportography demonstrated biliary tract dilatation and portal vein obstruction. At laparotomy dilatation of common bile duct and venous structures related to portal hypertension were seen. Extensive adhesions were noted in periportal region. Duodenum was densely adherent to undersurface of liver and vena cava. Injection of contrast material into gallbladder shows dilated cystic duct and common duct extending down to intraduodenal portion of duct, where it is tapered and narrowed. Choledochojejunostomy and cholecystectomy were performed. Biopsy of left lobe of liver showed histologic changes consistent with large-duct biliary obstruction, portral fibrosis, and prominent bile duct proliferation.

in the central nervous system and other locations. Often the disease involves the liver parenchyma and the mucosal folds in the gallbladder. Sulfatide cholecystitis has been reported.[60] Polypoid masses containing metachromatic sulfatides have been found at autopsy.

Other causes of duct obstruction

Other acquired causes of obstructive jaundice include pancreatitis, pancreatic pseudocysts, posttraumatic or postsurgical strictures, and parasitic infestations (Fig. 71-31). Biliary ascariasis in children may be associated with abdominal pain, tenderness, vomiting, and/or jaundice. The worm has been demonstrated by cholangiography as a filling defect inside the biliary ducts. The worms can extend into the major intrahepatic ducts or the pancreatic duct.[24,80] *Ascaris* species have been implicated as a cause of intrahepatic calculi and obstruction, even after the worm has passed.[88] In Asia *Clonorchis sinesis* is a common parasite that causes biliary obstruction.

PANCREAS
Techniques and normal values

Ultrasonography is currently the imaging modality of choice in children with suspected pancreatic disease.

□ **TABLE 71-3**

Normal dimensions of the pancreas as a function of age

Patient age	No. of patients	Maximum anteroposterior dimensions of pancreas (cm ± 1 standard deviation)		
		Head	Body	Tail
<1 mo	15	1.0 ± 0.4	0.6 ± 0.2	1.0 ± 0.4
1 mo to 1 yr	23	1.5 ± 0.5	0.8 ± 0.3	1.2 ± 0.4
1 to 5 yr	49	1.7 ± 0.3	1.0 ± 0.2	1.8 ± 0.4
5 to 10 yr	69	1.6 ± 0.4	1.0 ± 0.3	1.8 ± 0.4
10 to 19 yr	117	2.0 ± 0.5	1.1 ± 0.3	2.0 ± 0.4

From Siegel, MJ, Martin, KW, and Worthington, JL: Normal and abnormal pancreas in children: US studies, Radiology 165:15, 1987.

Standards for the size of the pancreatic head, body, and tail in infants and children were recently reported (Table 71-3).[134] The echogenecity of the pancreas in normal children is generally less than in adults but is variable (Table 71-4).

CT is very useful for evaluating the pancreas, partic-

□   **TABLE 71-4**
Echogenicity of pancreas relative to liver

Patient group	Echogenicity*		
	Hypoechoic	Isoechoic	Hyperechoic
Healthy	27 (10)	145 (53)	101 (37)
With pancreatitis	1 (8)	6 (46)	6 (46)

From Siegel, MJ, Martin, KW, and Worthington, JL: Normal and abnormal pancreas in children: US studies, Radiology 165:15, 1987.
*Percentages in parentheses.

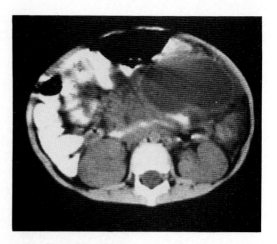

Fig. 71-32 Pancreatic pseudocyst in 3-year-old boy 2 months after motor vehicle accident. Noncontrast CT scan shows large cystic mass in region of tail of pancreas.
(Courtesy PE Kane, MD, Children's Hospital, Oakland, Calif.)

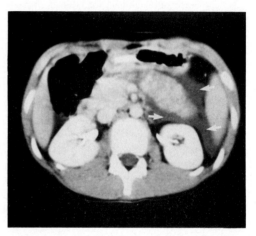

Fig. 71-33 Pancreatitis in 11-year-old girl with abdominal pain. CT scan demonstrates fluid in anterior pararenal space *(arrows)* and mild swelling of pancreatic body and tail. Scans at other levels revealed peritoneal fluid in lesser sac and pelvis.

ularly in patients with bowel gas overlying the pancreas. Careful attention to CT technique is critical. In children there is frequently little fat surrounding the pancreas, and therefore vascular opacification helps define anatomic landmarks. Also, motion artifact may seriously degrade the image.

Plain radiographs and contrast studies of the alimentary tract can demonstrate localized ileus from inflammation, a mass suggesting a pseudocyst, mucosal thickening, or pancreatic calcifications. Generally, when pancreatic disease is suspected, cross-sectional imaging techniques, such as ultrasonography and CT, are used. Endoscopic retrograde cholangiopancreatography has been used in children in selected cases to evaluate the pancreatic ducts.[119,120]

Congenital diseases

Annular pancreas is caused by abnormal rotation of the ventral pancreatic bud, which forms a ring of tissue surrounding the second portion of the duodenum. This malformation sometimes results in symptoms of upper gastrointestinal obstruction, or it may remain asymptomatic throughout life. Annular pancreas is associated with a variety of other congenital anomalies.

About 10% of patients have a persistent accessory duct (Santorini) with a more proximal orifice than the main pancreatic duct (Wirsung). Therefore, in some patients with duodenal atresia, some air passes into the distal duodenum.

Ectopic pancreatic tissue (pancreatic rests) is found in various parts of the GI tract, particularly in the duodenum, gastric antrum, jejunum, or Meckel's diverticulum.[137]

In the syndrome of exocrine pancreatic insufficiency and neutropenia (Schwachman syndrome), malabsorption and recurrent infection are frequently the initial manifestations.[138] This syndrome is associated with metaphyseal chondrodysplasis. Pancreatic lipomatosis is seen on ultrasound and CT.[133]

Pancreatitis and pancreatic injuries

In children acute pancreatitis is more common than chronic forms. The most common cause is blunt abdominal trauma (Fig. 71-32). Child abuse should be considered as a possible cause, especially in young children or those who had an unobserved accident.[135] Pseudocyst formation may occur rapidly after traumatic pancreatitis. Recurrent osteolytic lesions and subcutaneous fat necrosis have also been reported.[124]

Hereditary pancreatitis is transmitted as autosomal dominant. Recurrent episodes of acute pancreatitis often begin during childhood.[122] However, unless laboratory

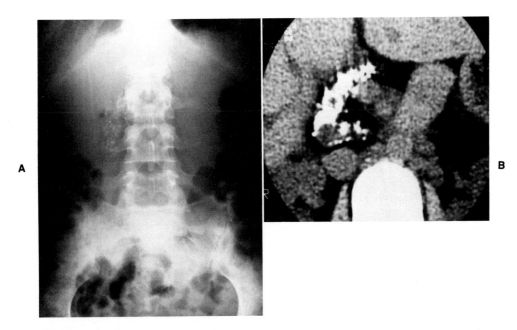

Fig. 71-34 Calcified atrophic pancreas in 23-year-old woman with cystic fibrosis. **A,** Calcifications are noted on abdominal radiograph. **B,** CT scan reveals marked atrophy and widespread calcification of pancreas.

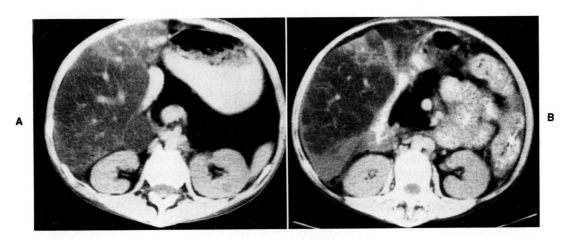

Fig. 71-35 Fatty replacement of pancreas in 29-year-old woman with cystic fibrosis shown on CT scans. Only fat density is noted in region of pancreatic body and tail **A** and pancreatic head **B.** Also noted is fatty infiltration of liver.
(Courtesy PA Nancarrow, MD, Children's Hospital, Oakland, Calif.)

and imaging tests are performed to document pancreatitis, the diagnosis can be overlooked. Calcifications in the pancreas are found frequently, and there is a high incidence of pancreatic carcinoma later in life. The cause of this disorder is unknown. Idiopathic fibrosing pancreatitis may be a cause of obstructive jaundice in childhood.[117]

Mumps infection is known to cause pancreatitis; other viruses on occasion cause pancreatitis. Drugs associated with pancreatitis include steroids and L-asparaginase.[126,132] Pancreatitis may also occur with hyperlipoproteinemia and hyperparathyroidism.

In pancreatitis the inflamed portion of the gland is swollen and is usually hypoechoic on ultrasound.[121] Edema in the anterior pararenal space is sometimes seen on CT or ultrasound (Fig. 71-33).[121]

Pseudocysts caused by pancreatitis are most often in or adjacent to the pancreas. However, pancreatic enzymes can disseminate to multiple locations in the peritoneum or to extraperitoneal sites, including the mediastinum and pleura.[131] An abscess or phlegmon can complicate the clinical course. Some pseudocysts regress, but others require drainage. Internal and external drainage procedures have been described. Increasingly, interventional radiologic techniques are being employed.

Cystic fibrosis

Acute pancreatitis is uncommon in cystic fibrosis. Rather, progressive pancreatic insufficiency is the rule. Many patients subsequently develop multiple calcifications along with fibrosis (Fig. 71-34).[125] Some will develop fatty infiltration of the pancreas (Fig. 71-35).[140] The multiple gastrointestinal and hepatobiliary manifestations are discussed elsewhere in this book.

Tumors

Cysts of the pancreas are uncommon in children but are occasionally seen in cystic diseases that affect the kidney and liver.

Insulinoma is a β islet cell tumor that causes hypoglycemia in newborns, infants, and children. The small tumors are sometimes difficult to identify on ultrasound or CT.[123,136] Arteriography may demonstrate a prominent, persistent vascular blush in the region of the tumor.[127] Nesidioblastosis, a generalized increase in insulin-producing islet cells, also appears with hypoglycemia, but there is no discrete tumor. The subcutaneous fat thickness in newborns with nesidioblastosis is increased.[130] The secreting non-β islet cell tumors are very rare in childhood.

Other primary pancreatic tumors include adenoma, carcinoma, cystadenocarcinoma, hemangioendothelioma, and sarcomas, including rhabdomyosarcoma.[118,128,129,139] All of these tumors are very rare in childhood.

REFERENCES

1. Abramson, SJ, Lack, EE, and Teele, RL: Benign vascular tumors of the liver in infants: sonographic appearance, AJR 138:629, 1982.
2. Abramson, SJ, et al: Biliary atresia and noncardiac polysplenic syndrome: US and surgical considerations, Radiology 163:377, 1987.
3. Aihara, T, Fujioka, M, and Yamamoto, K: Increased CT density of the liver due to cis-diaminedichloroplatinum (II), Pediatr Radiol 17:75, 1987.
4. Alagille, D, et al: Syndromic paucity of interlobular bile ducts: Alagille syndrome or arteriohepatic dysplasia review of 80 cases, J Pediatr 110:195, 1987.
5. Arnaud, O, et al: Embryonal rhabdomyosarcoma of the biliary tree in children: a case report, Pediatr Radiol 17:250, 1987.
6. Atkinson, GO, et al: Incompetence of the sphincter of Oddi in the newborn: report of two cases, AJR 128:861, 1977.
7. Babbitt, DP, Sharshak, RJ, and Clemett, AR: Choledochal cyst: a concept of etiology, AJR 119:57, 1973.
8. Bahia, JO, et al: Ultrasonographic detection of spontaneous perforation of the extrahepatic bile ducts in infancy, Pediatr Radiol 16:157, 1986.
9. Barth, RA, Brasch, RC, and Filly, RA: Abdominal pseudotumor in childhood: distended gallbladder with parenteral hyperalimentation, AJR 136:341, 1981.
10. Bartone, NF, and Grieco, RV: Absent gallbladder and cystic duct, AJR 110:252, 1970.
11. Bass, EM, and Cremin, BJ: Choledochal cysts: a clinical and radiologic evaluation of 21 cases, Pediatr Radiol 5:81, 1976.
12. Blanton, DE, Bream, CA, and Mandel, SR: Gallbladder ectopia: a review of anomalies of position, AJR 121:396, 1974.
13. Bousvaros, A, Kirks, DR, and Grossman, H: Imaging of neuroblastoma: an overview, Pediatr Radiol 16:89, 1986.
14. Brown, RC, and Brown, RJ: Hamartoma of the gallbladder in a child, J Pediatr 52:319, 1958.
15. Brun, P, et al: Ultrasound findings in biliary atresia in children: a study with surgical correlation in 86 cases, Ann Radiol 28:259, 1985.
16. Brunelle, F: Choledocholithiasis in children, Semin Ultrasound CT MR 8:118, 1987.
17. Callahan, J, et al: Cholelithiasis in infants: association with total parenteral nutrition and furosemide, Radiology 143:437, 1982.
18. Callen, PW, Filly, RA, and Marcus, FS: Ultrasonography and computed tomography in the evaluation of hepatic microabscesses in the immunosuppressed patient, Radiology 136:433, 1980.
19. Carter, AR, et al: Cholesterol ester storage disease: radiological features, Pediatr Radiol 2:135, 1974.
20. Chamberlain, JW, and Hight, DW: Acute hydrops of the gallbladder in childhood, Surgery 68:899, 1970.
21. Chang, CCN, and Giulian, BB: Congenital bronchobiliary fistula, Radiology 156:82, 1985.
22. Chang, et al: Congenital bile duct dilatation in children, J Pediatr Surg 21:112, 1986.
23. Chusid, MJ: Pyogenic hepatic abscess in infancy and childhood, Pediatrics 62:554, 1978.
24. Cremin, BJ, and Fisher, RM: Biliary ascariasis in children, AJR 126:352, 1976.
25. Dachman, AH, et al: Infantile hemangioendothelioma of the liver: a radiologic-pathologic-clinical correlation, AJR 140:1091, 1983.
26. Dachman, AH, et al: Hepatoblastoma: radiologic-pathologic correlation in 50 cases, Radiology 164:15, 1987.
27. Davies, C, Daneman, A, and Stringer, DA: Inspissated bile in a neonate with cystic fibrosis, J Ultrasound Med 5:335, 1986.
28. Davies, CH, et al: Congenital hepatic fibrosis with saccular dilatation of intrahepatic bile ducts and infantile polycystic kidneys, Pediatr Radiol 16:302, 1986.
29. Deligeorgis, D, et al: The normal borders of the liver in infancy and childhood: clinical and x-ray study, Arch Dis Child 45:702, 1970.
30. Devanesan, J, et al: Congenital hepatic duct obstruction with perforate diaphragms, Arch Surg 113:1452, 1978.
31. Diament, MJ, Boechat, MI, and Kangarloo, H: Interventional radiology in infants and children: clinical and technical aspects, Radiology 154:359, 1985.

32. Dittrich, M, et al: Sonographic biometry of liver and spleen size in childhood, Pediatr Radiol 13:206, 1983.

33. Dominguez, R, et al: Pediatric liver transplantation. II. Diagnostic imaging in postoperative management, Radiology 157:339, 1985.

34. Donahoe, PK, and Hendren, WH: Bile duct perforation in a newborn with stenosis of the ampulla of Vater, J Pediatr Surg 11:823, 1976.

35. Doppman, JL, et al: Computed tomography of the liver and kidneys in glycogen storage disease, J Comput Assist Tomogr 6:67, 1982.

36. Enell, H, Cavell, B, and Malmfors, G: Spontaneous perforation of the common bile duct, Acta Paediatr Scand 68:625, 1979.

37. Exelby, PR, Filler, RM, and Grosfeld, JL: Liver tumors in children in particular reference to hepatoblastoma hepatocellular carcinoma: American Academy of Pediatrics, Surgical Section Survey, 1974, J Pediatr Surg 10:329, 1975.

38. Franken, EA, Jr, et al: Hepatic imaging in Stage IV-S neuroblastoma, Pediatr Radiol 16:107, 1986.

39. Fujiwara, Y, et al: A case of congenital choledochal cyst associated with carcinoma, J Pediatr Surg 11:587, 1976.

40. Garel, LA, et al: Percutaneous cholecystography in children, Radiology 165:639, 1987.

41. Geoffray, A, et al: Ultrasonography and computed tomography for diagnosis and follow-up of biliary duct rhabdomyosarcomas in children, Pediatr Radiol 17:127, 1987.

42. Gibson, B, et al: Roentgenographically visible fatty liver in cystic fibrosis, Pediatrics 59:778, 1977.

43. Giorgio, A, et al: Ultrasound evaluation of uncomplicated and complicated acute viral hepatitis, J Clin Ultrasound 14:675, 1986.

44. Giyanani, VL, Meyers, PC, and Wolfson, JJ: Mesenchymal hamartoma of the liver: computed tomography and ultrasonography, J Comput Assist Tomogr 10:51, 1986.

45. Guyer, PB, and McLoughlin, M: Congenital double gallbladder: a review and report of two cases, BR J Radiol 40:214, 1967.

46. Haddy, TB, Castro, OL, and Rana, SR: Hereditary hemochromatosis in children, adolescents, and young adults, Am J pediatr Hematol Oncol 10:23, 1988.

47. Han, BK, Babcock, DS, and Gelfand, MH: Choledochal cyst with bile duct dilatation: sonography and ^{99m}Tc IDA cholescintigraphy, AJR 136:1075, 1981.

48. Hayden, CK, Jr: Sonographic features of hepatic amebiasis in childhood, J Can Assoc Radiol 35:279, 1984.

49. Henschke, CI, and Teele, RL: Cholelithiasis in children: recent observations, J Ultrasound Med 2:481, 1983.

50. Holder, LE, et al: Liver size determination in pediatrics using sonographic and scintigraphic techniques, Radiology 117:349, 1975.

51. Jacir, NN, et al: Cholelithiasis in infancy: resolution of gallstones in three of four infants, J Pediatr Surg 21:567, 1986.

52. Jamieson, PN, and Shaw, DG: Empyema of gallbladder in an infant, Arch Dis Child 50:482, 1975.

53. Kaplan, SL, and Feigin, RD: Pyogenic liver abscess in normal children with fever of unknown origin, Pediatrics 58:614, 1976.

54. Kaufman, RA: Liver-spleen computed tomography: a method tailored for infants and children, J Comput Assist Tomogr 7:45, 1983.

55. Keller, MS, et al: Spontaneous resolution of cholelithiasis in infants, Radiology 157:345, 1985.

56. Kimura, K, et al: Congenital cystic dilatation of the common bile duct: relationship to anomalous pancreaticobiliary ductal union, AJR 128:571, 1977.

57. King, DR, et al: Parenteral nutrition with associated cholelithiasis: another iatrogenic disease of infants and children, J Pediatr Surg 22:593, 1987.

58. Kirks, DR: Lithiasis due to interruption of the enterohepatic circulation of bile salts, AJR 133:383, 1979.

59. Kirks, DR, et al: An imaging approach to persistent neonatal jaundice, AJR 142:461, 1984.

60. Kleinman, P, Winchester, P, and Volberg, F: Sulfatide cholecystosis, Gastrointest Radiol 1:99, 1976.

61. Klingensmith, WC, III, and Cioffi-Ragan, DT: Fetal gallstones, Radiology 167:143, 1988.

62. Kulkarni, P, and Beatty, EC, Jr: Cholangiocarcinoma associated with biliary cirrhosis due to congenital biliary atresia, Am J Dis Child 131:442, 1977.

63. Kumari, S, Lee, WJ, and Barton, MG: Hydrops of the gallbladder in a child: diagnosis by ultrasonography, Pediatrics 63:295, 1979.

64. Ledesma-Medina, J, et al: Pediatric liver transplantation: I. Standardization of preoperative diagnostic imaging, Radiology 157:335, 1985.

65. Lucaya, J, et al: Congenital dilatation of the intrahepatic bile ducts (Caroli's disease), Radiology 127:746, 1978.

66. Lucaya, J, et al: Computed tomography of infantile hepatic hemangioendothelioma, AJR 144:821, 1985.

67. Magid, D, Fishman, EK, and Siegelman, SS: Computed tomography of the spleen and liver in sickle cell disease, AJR 143:245, 1984.

68. Marchal, GJ, et al: Caroli disease: high-frequency US and pathologic findings, Radiology 158:507, 1986.

69. Markisz, JA, Treves, ST, and Davis, RT: Normal hepatic and splenic size in children: scintigraphic determination, Pediatr Radiol 17:273, 1987.

70. McGahan, JP, Phillips, HE, and Cox, KL: Sonography of the normal pediatric gallbladder and biliary tract, Radiology 144:873, 1982.

71. Miller, JH, and Greenspan, BS: Integrated imaging of hepatic tumors in childhood. I. Malignant lesions (primary and metastatic), Radiology 154:83, 1985.

72. Miller, JH, and Greenspan, BS: integrated imaging of hepatic tumors in childhood. II. Benign lesions (congenital, reparative, and inflammatory), Radiology 154:91, 1985.

73. Neu, J, Arvin, A, and Ariagno, RL: Hydrops of the gallbladder, Am J. Dis Child 134:891, 1980.

74. Nguyen, DL, and Leonard, JC: Ischemic hepatic necrosis: a cause of fetal liver calcification, AJR 147:596, 1986.

75. Patriquin, HB, et al: Sonography of thickened gallbladder wall: causes in children, AJR 141:57, 1983.

76. Pfeiffer, WR, Robinson, LH, and Balsara, VJ: Sonographic features of bile plug syndrome, J Ultrasound Med 5:161, 1986.

77. Pinter, A, et al: Membranous obstruction of the common bile duct, J Pediatr Surg 10:839, 1975.

78. Powell, RW: Pure calcium carbonate gallstones in a two year old in association with prenatal calcium supplementation, J Pediatr Surg 20:143, 1985.

79. Premkumar, A, et al: The emergence of hepatic fibrosis and portal hypertension in infants and children with autosomal recessive polycystic kidney disease: initial and follow-up sonographic and radiographic findings, Pediatr Radiol 18:123, 1988.

80. Radin, DR, and Vachon, LA: CT findings in biliary and pancreatic ascariasis, J Comput Assist Tomogr 10:508, 1986.

81. Ralls, PW, et al: Medical treatment of hepatic amebic abscess: rare need for percutaneous drainage, Radiology 165:805, 1987.

82. Ramey, SL, and Williams, JL: Nephrolithiasis and cholelithiasis in a premature infant, J Clin Ultrasound 14:203, 1986.

83. Rennels, MB, et al: Cholelithiasis in patients with major sickle hemoglobinopathies, Am J Dis Child 138:66, 1984.

84. Robinson, AE, et al: Cholecystitis and hydrops of the gallbladder in the newborn, Radiology 122:749, 1977.

85. Ros, PR, et al: Mesenchymal hamartoma of the liver: radiologic-pathohlogic correlation, Radiology 158:619, 1986.

86. Ross, RJ, and Sachs, MD: Triplication of the gallbladder, AJR 104:656, 1968.

87. Sarnaik, S, et al: Incidence of cholelithiasis in sickle cell anemia using the ultrasound gray scale technique, J Pediatr 96:1005, 1980.

88. Schulman, A: Non-Western patterns of biliary stones and the role of ascariasis, Radiology 162:425, 1987.

89. Shabot, MD, et al: Benign obstructing papilloma of the ampulla of Vater in infancy, Surgery 78:560, 1975.

90. Shackelford, GD, and Kirks, DR: Neonatal hepatic calcification secondary to transplacental infection, Radiology 122:753, 1977.

91. Shlaer, WJ, Leopold, GR, and Scheible, FW: Sonography of the thickened gallbladder wall: a nonspecific finding, AJR 136:337, 1981.

92. Slovis, TL, et al: Sonography in the diagnosis and management of hydrops of the gallbladder in children with mucocutaneous lymph node syndrome, Pediatrics 65:789, 1980.

93. Smith, WL, Ballantine, RVN, and Gonzalez-Crussi, F: Hepatic mesenchymal hamartoma causing heart failure in the neonate, J Pediatr Surg 13:183, 1978.

94. Stalker, HP, Kaufman, RA, and Towbin, R: Patterns of liver injury in childhood: CT analysis, AJR 147:1199, 1986.

95. Stanley, P, et al: Mesenchymal hamartomas of the liver in childhood: sonographic and CT findings, AJR 147:1035, 1986.

96. Stark, DD, et al: Magnetic resonance imaging and spectroscopy of hepatic iron overload, Radiology 154:137, 1985.

97. Stringer, DA, et al: Interposition of the gallbladder or the absent common hepatic duct and cystic duct, Pediatr Radiol 17:151, 1987.

98. Suarez, F, et al: Bilio-pancreatic common channel in children: clinical, biological and radiological findings in 12 children, Pediatr Radiol 17:206, 1987.

99. Summerville, DA, Marks, M, and Treves, ST: Hepatobiliary scintigraphy in arteriohepatic dysplasia (Alagille's syndrome): a report of two cases, Pediatr Radiol 18:32, 1988.

100. Tchirkow, G, Highman, LM, and Shafer, AD: Cholelithiasis and cholecystitis in children after repair of congenital duodenal anomalies, Arch Surg 115:85, 1980.

101. Teele, RL, et al: Cholelithiasis after spinal fusion for scoliosis in children, J Pediatr 111:857, 1987.

102. Tonkin, ILD, Wrenn, EL, Jr, and Hollabaugh, RS: The continued value of angiography in planning surgical resection of benign and malignant hepatic tumors in children, Pediatr Radiol 18:35, 1988.

103. vanSonnenberg, E, et al: Intrahepatic amebic abscesses: indications for and results of percutaneous catheter drainage, Radiology 156:631, 1985.

104. vanSonnenberg, E, et al: Percutaneous diagnostic and therapeutic interventional radiologic procedures in children: experience in 100 patients, Radiology 162:601, 1987.

105. Weinberg, AG, Mize, CE, and Worthen, HG: The occurrence of hepatoma in the chronic form of hereditary tyrosinemia, J Pediatr 88:434, 1976.

106. Weinberger, E, Blumhagen, JD, and Odell, JM: Gallbladder contraction in biliary atresia, AJR 149:401, 1987.

107. Weinreb, JC, et al: Imaging the pediatric liver: MRI and CT, AJR 147:785, 1986.

108. Welch, TJ, et al: Focal nodular hyperplasia and hepatic adenoma: comparison of angiography, CT, US, and scintigraphy, Radiology 156:593, 1985.

109. Werlin, SL, et al: Sclerosing cholangitis in childhood, J Pediatr 96:433, 1980.

110. Werlin, SL, et al: Intrahepatic biliary tract abnormalities in children with corrected extrahepatic biliary atresia, J Pediatr Gastroenterol Nutr 4:537, 1985.

111. White, EM, et al: Focal periportal sparing in hepatic fatty infiltration: a cause of hepatic pseudomass on US, Radiology 162:57, 1987.

112. Williams, HJ, and Johnson, KW: Cholelithiasis: a complication of cardiac valve surgery in children, Pediatr Radiol 14:146, 1984.

113. Witcombe, JB, and Cremin, BJ: The width of the common bile duct in childhood, Pediatr Radiol 7:147, 1978.

114. Yousefzadeh, DK, Lupetin, AR, and Jackson, JH, Jr: The radiographic signs of fatty liver, Radiology 131:351, 1979.

115. Yousefzadeh, DK, Soper, RT, and Jackson, JH: Obstructive jaundice due to congenital stenosis of the ampulla of Vater, Gastrointest Radiol 4:379, 1979.

116. Yousefzadeh, DK, Vanhoutte, JJ, and Jackson, JH: A potential pitfall of operative cholangiography in infants, Pediatr Radiol 8:151, 1979.

117. Atkinson, GO, Jr, et al: Idiopathic fibrosing pancreatitis: a cause of obstructive jaundice in childhood, Pediatr Radiol 18:28, 1988.

118. Bienayme, J, and Gross, P: Tumeurs malignes du pancreas chez l'enfant, Ann Chir Infan 17:131, 1975.

119. Blustein, PK, et al: Endoscopic retrograde cholangiopancreatography in pancreatitis in children and adolescents, Pediatrics 68:387, 1981.

120. Filston, HC, et al: Improved management of pancreatic lesions in children aided by ERCP, J Pediatr Surg 13:143, 1978.

121. Fleischer, AC, et al: Sonographic findings of pancreatitis in children, Radiology 146:151, 1983.

122. Ghisan, FK, et al: Chronic relapsing pancreatitis in childhood, J Pediatr 120:514, 1983.

123. Günther, RW, et al: Islet-cell tumors: detection of small lesions with computed tomography and ultrasound, Radioology 148:485, 1983.

124. Hollingsworth, P, Isaac, D, and Bydder, G: Recurrent osteolytic lesions and subcutaneous fat necrosis in association with a developmental pancreatic cyst, Arch Dis Child 54:790, 1979.

125. Iannaccone, G, and Antonelli, M: Calcification of the pancreas in cystic fibrosis, Pediatr Radiol 9:85, 1980.

126. Jordan, SC, and Ament, ME: Pancreatitis in children and adolescents, J Pediatr 91:211, 1977.

127. Kirkland, J, et al: Islet cell tumor in a neonate: diagnosis by selective angiography and histologic findings, Pediatrics 61:790, 1978.

128. Mares, AJ, and Hirsch, M: Congenital cysts of the head of the pancreas, J Pediatr Surg 12:547, 1977.

129. Masterson, JB, et al: Carcinoma of the pancreas occurring in a child, J Clin Ultrasound 6:143, 1978.

130. Oestrich, AE, and Oppermann, HC: Abnormal fat thickness in newborns with nesidioblastosis, Radiology 141:679, 1981.

131. Raptopoulos, V, et al: Renal fascial pathway: posterior extension of pancreatic effusions within the anterior pararenal space, Radiology 158:367, 1986.

132. Riccardi, VM: Pancreatitis in children, J Pediatr 92:685, 1978.

133. Robberecht, E, et al: Pancreatic lipomatosis in the Shwachman-Diamond syndrome: identification by sonography and CT-scan, Pediatr Radiol 15:348, 1985.

134. Siegel, MJ, Martin, KW, and Worthington, JL: Normal and abnormal pancreas in children: US studies, Radiology 165:15, 1987.

135. Slovis, TL, Von Berg, VJ, and Mikelic, V: Sonography in the diagnosis and management of pancreatic pseudocysts and effusions in childhood, Radiology 135:153, 1980.

136. Stark, DD, et al: Ct of pancreatic islet cell tumors, Radiology 150:491, 1984.

137. Taybi, H: Pseudoneoplastic masses (pseudotumors) in children, Med Radiogr Photogr 54:24, 1978.

138. Taybi, H, Mitchell, AD, and Friedman, GD: Metaphyseal dysostosis associated syndrome of pancreatic insufficiency and blood disorders, Radiology 93:563, 1969.

139. Tunnell, WP: Hemangioendothelioma of the pancreas obstructing the common bile duct and duodenum, J Pediatr Surg 11:827, 1976.

140. Wilson-Sharp, RC, et al: Ultrasonography of the pancreas, liver and biliary system in cystic fibrosis, Arch Dis Child 59:923, 1984.

72 *Sonography*

HENRIETTA KOTLUS ROSENBERG
BARRY B. GOLDBERG

High-resolution real-time sonography has emerged as a veritable noninvasive laparoscope suitable for the evaluation of a wide gamut of abdominal and pelvic abnormalities. As a nonionizing imaging modality with no known biologic effects, it is ideal for examining infants and children. Real-time technology may be thought of as a fluoroscopic approach to imaging, whereby one can use respiratory motion, vascular pulsations, duplex or Doppler, and the presence or absence of peristaltic motion to localize and characterize disease processes. Static or linear array images can complete the sonographic study by serving as overhead films. This technology allows for a more global cross-sectional representation of the relationship of anatomic or pathologic structures too large to be shown on a single real-time scan. Although one does not ordinarily consider ultrasound as the modality of choice for imaging gas-filled structures, there are, in fact, many applications for sonography of the gastrointestinal (GI) tract in the pediatric age group.*

TECHNIQUE

To reduce the amount of gas in the GI tract, the patients fast before the sonogram. Babies less than 1 year old are studied at the time they are due for a feeding. Toddlers and older children fast for at least 8 hours before the examination. If the pelvis is to be examined as well as the abdomen, the distended bladder is used as a sonic window. Sedation is reserved for children who are unable to cooperate (usually less than 3 years of age) in whom there is suspicion of a mass or retroperitoneal adenopathy. Chloral hydrate is generally sufficient, but not infrequently sodium pentobarbital (Nembutal) is required. However, the children must be carefully monitored. We find that colorful wall posters, mobiles, interesting books, and a videocassette recorder to show cartoons and movies help to maximize the child's comfort and confidence. A promised prize from a treasure chest and a Tootsie Pop can serve as rewards for good cooperation. Having family members present during the sonogram has been enormously helpful as well.[2]

We routinely perform the ultrasound examinations

---

*References 34, 37, 45, 56, 59, 60, 87, 89, 93.

with real-time in-line multifrequency scan heads, using the highest frequency possible, including frequencies of 3, 5, 7.5, and 10 MHz. If the pelvis is to be included in the examination, we begin with this part of the anatomy, since it is not unusual for an untrained child to inadvertently empty the bladder with very little stimulation. If necessary, sterile water may be used as a contrast agent to outline the bladder (catheterization), vagina (water vaginography), rectum (water enema technique)[79] or by catheterization of other structures, such as a cloaca or utricle, and observing the filling of these structures during real-time sonography.[84] In patients with either a very small or absent urinary bladder who require visualization of the pelvis, endovaginal[82] or endorectal[77] scanning may be performed. For the evaluation of the upper GI tract, one often employs water contrast sonography, either in the form of sugar water or clear juice.[83] Retained aqueous contrast material or fluid-filled bowel loops may serve as a contrast medium for the evaluation of the small and large intestine. Plain radiographs of the neck, chest, and/or abdomen may help to narrow the differential diagnosis. Frontal and lateral plain radiographs of the abdomen help to localize a mass by demonstrating an area of soft tissue fullness and displacement of bowel loops. Upright, left lateral decubitus, or cross-table lateral views may demonstrate an obstructive pattern.[34,93] Vertebral anomalies may be identified in patients with neuroenteric cysts; permeative or sclerotic skeletal abnormalities may be present in children with lymphoma or neuroblastoma; chunky calcifications may be seen in teratomas; and more curvilinear calcification may be observed in meconium cysts or pancreatic pseudocysts.

ESOPHAGUS

The proximal and distal ends of the esophagus are the more easily imaged portions of this tubular structure because of the lack of interposed air between the transducer and the esophagus. The mid esophagus, however, is more

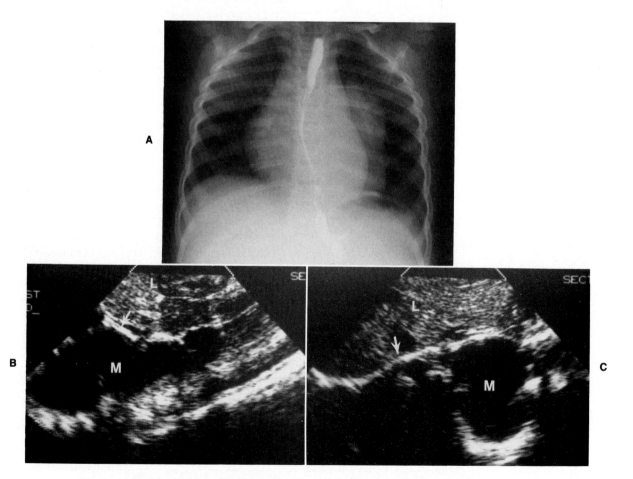

Fig. 72-1 Esophageal duplication; 2-year-old white girl with left posterior chest mass. **A,** chest radiograph shows lobulated soft tissue mass in left hemithorax, displacing esophagus to right. **B** and **C,** Sagittal and transverse sonographic views of mass show it to be lobulated and cystic and to extend to level of gastroesophageal junction. *Arrow,* Diaphragm; *L,* liver; *M,* mass.
(From Rosenberg, HK: RadioGraphics 6:427, 1986.)

difficult to visualize, but in some cases the heart or a posteriorly located mass may serve as a sonic window.

The phrenic ampulla appears as a tubular structure located slightly anteromedial to the aorta just below the diaphragm.[17,80] The thin sonolucent outer wall represents the esophageal muscle, whereas the echogenic inner rim represents the mucosa and submucosa and the contained mucus. By observing the region of the gastroesophageal junction while the patient is drinking, the esophagus can be more precisely localized. After a liquid meal, real-time ultrasound can be used to observe the opening of the gastroesophageal junction and the reflux of gastric contents, including air and liquid into the esophagus.[68] Since one cannot use ultrasound to quantitate the degree of gastroesophageal reflux, this problem is better evaluated with radionuclide and barium studies. In patients with plain film findings suggestive of an intrathoracic stomach, water-contrast sonography can help to confirm the diagnosis. Sonography is quite reliable for the evaluation of masses related to the esophagus, such as esophageal duplications and neuroenteric canal cysts[8,78] (Fig. 72-1) These lesions may be purely cystic but may contain echogenic material (mucus). A barium swallow is helpful in demonstrating the contiguity with the esophagus as well as any communication with that part of the GI tract. In the presence of vertebral anomalies, magnetic resonance imaging (MRI) should be done to demonstrate communication with the spinal canal.

STOMACH

In patients with situs solitus the stomach is identified in the left upper quadrant, anterior to the pancreas, posterolateral to the left lobe of the liver, and medial to the spleen, appearing as a brightly echogenic area because of contained mucus and gas. Appropriate positioning of the real-time transducer can demonstrate the hyperechoic mucosal lining and the hypoechoic muscle wall.[10,88] Using water-contrast material and changing the patient's position during scanning aid in the differentiation of wall lesions from mobile retained gastric contents (Fig. 72-2). The normal gastric wall should be less than 4 mm thick. A diameter greater than 5 mm may be an indication of abnormalities such as gastroenteritis, ulceration (usually 1 to 2 cm hyperechoic eccentric thickening in the antral region)[37] (Fig. 72-3) lymphoid hyperplasia, Henoch-Schönlein purpura, Crohn's disease, chronic granulomatous disease of childhood (circumferential wall thickening)[49] (Fig. 72-4) or ectopic pancreas. Gastric wall masses are unusually rare in children but may be shown with ultrasound.[61,96] Intramural hematomas, such as may occur in hemophiliacs, may appear as a focal relatively complex lesion. Cystic anechoic benign masses include duplication cysts and teratomas.[44,63,97] Gastric duplications are usually located on the greater curvature in the region of the gastric antrum and account for 4% of gastrointestinal duplications. The inner rim of a duplication cyst (mucosa) is often hyperechoic, whereas the outer rim (muscular wall) is likely to be hypoechoic. Stranding and echogenic debris may be present because of contained mucus. [99m]Tc pertechnetate radionuclide scan may be used to detect ectopic gastric mucosa when the initial symptom is bleeding from ulceration. Teratomas are likely to contain calcifications. Hamartomas, on the other hand, generally cause marked mural thick-

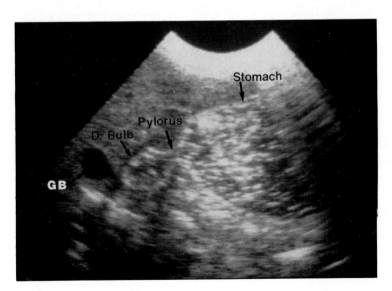

Fig. 72-2 Water contrast for gastrointestinal sonography. Small white echogenic foci within lumen of stomach, pylorus, and duodenal bulb represent microbubbles in ingested sugar water. *GB,* Gall bladder.

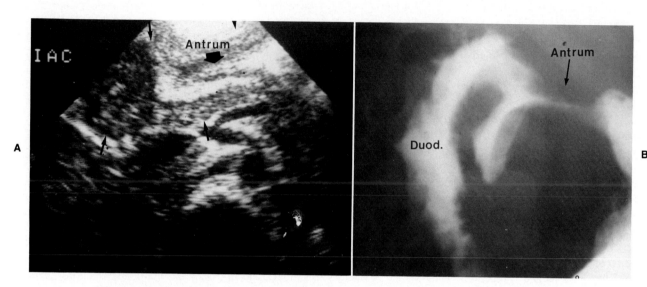

Fig. 72-3 Gastric antral ulcer; 8-year-old with epigastric pain and fullness. **A,** Transverse sonogram demonstrates antral narrowing with marked thickening of gastric wall, suggesting edema *(arrows)*. **B,** Barium examination confirms impression of severe antral narrowing and swelling of gastric antral wall.

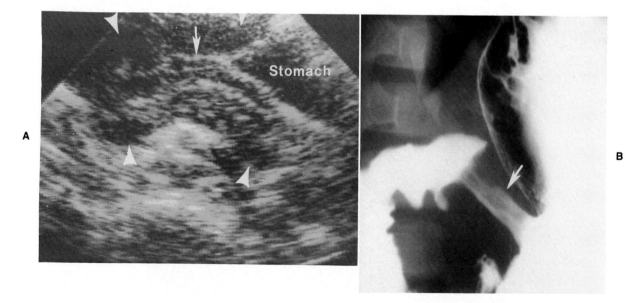

Fig. 72-4 Chronic granulomatous disease of childhood. Two-year-old boy presented with vomiting and known chronic granulomatous disease of childhood. **A,** Water contrast sonography showed narrowing of gastric antrum *(arrows)* caused by significant thickening of antral wall *(arrowheads)*. **B,** Upper GI series showing narrowed antrum and pyloric channel *(arrow)*.

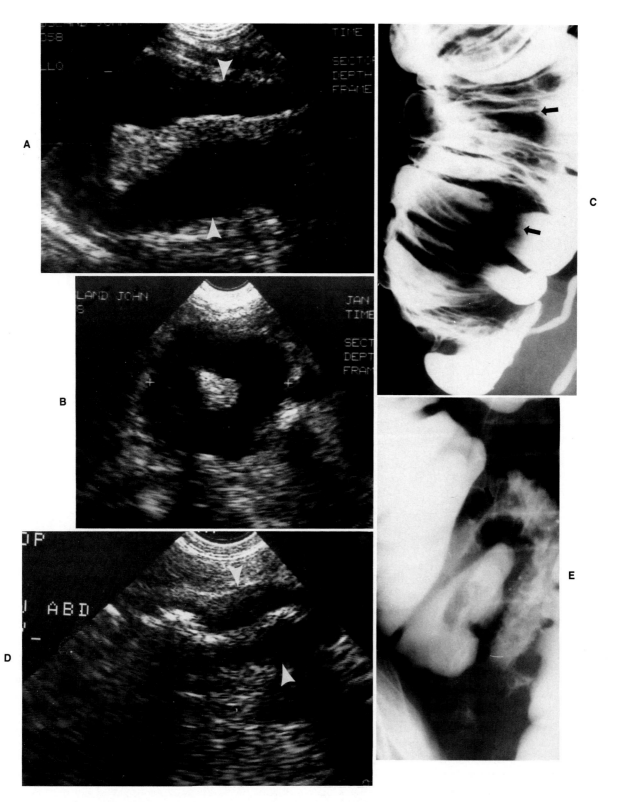

Fig. 72-15 Burkitt's lymphoma; 12-year-old boy with abdominal pain and vomiting. **A,** Sagittal sonogram demonstrating anechoic bowel wall *(arrowheads)* in region of distal ileum with poor through transmission, which was highly suggestive of lymphomatous infiltration. **B,** Cross-sectional view of bowel loop demonstrated in **A** showing asymmetric anechoic bowel wall thickening. **C,** Barium enema demonstrating large coiled spring filling defect caused by intussusception *(arrows)*. Terminal ileum could not be filled. At surgery, biopsy of thickened distal ileal loop demonstrated Burkitt's lymphoma. **D,** Follow-up sonogram several weeks after initiation of chemotherapy showed decreased thickness and improved echogenicity in infiltrated bowel loop *(arrowheads)*. **E,** Follow-up barium enema showing narrowing *(arrow)* of terminal ileum in abnormal area demonstrated sonographically.

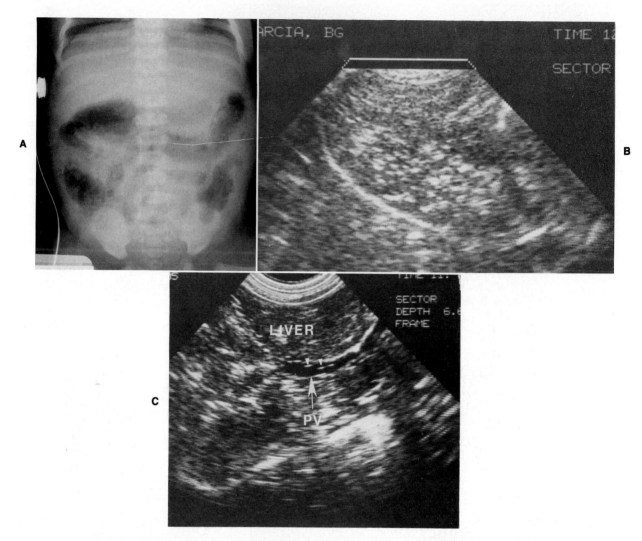

Fig. 72-16 Necrotizing enterocolitis. **A,** Plain film demonstrating generalized moderate distension of bowel with linear as well as mottled lucencies consistent with pneumatosis intestinalis. **B,** Sagittal view of liver demonstrating multiple small echogenic foci consistent with gas in portal venous system. **C,** Arrowheads point to small echogenic foci within portal vein *(PV),* which show dramatic motion during real-time observation.

conium cyst are well-known complications of both of these entities.[11,15,18] Because of distal ileal obstruction in utero, the bowel may perforate, and consequently meconium is extruded into the peritoneal cavity. Meconium peritonitis, a diffuse inflammatory process in the peritoneal cavity, results in characteristic calcific flecks on plain radiographs and a widespread, highly echogenic flocky pattern (snowstorm sign).[51] In some infants the spilled meconium may become walled off by adherent bowel loops and fibrous granulation tissue, forming a meconium cyst (Fig. 72-18). At times the cyst encases bowel loops, resulting in a persistent communication with the bowel, producing an air- and fluid-filled giant meconium cyst. Meconium cysts are predominantly cystic

complex masses with scattered areas of echogenicity in the cyst and echogenic walls. Calcifications may be seen in the wall of the cyst.

The most common gastrointestinal mass in the neonate is a bowel duplication (enteric cyst), which may appear later in the first decade with symptoms of obstruction[8,50,83,91,92] (Fig. 72-19). They may be spherical or tubular. Although they may involve any part of the GI tract, they are most frequently encountered on the mesenteric border of the terminal ileum. Their appearance is similar to the duplication cysts previously described in the more proximal parts of the GI tract.

The most common congenital anomaly of the GI tract is Meckel's diverticulum.[57] This is another type of cystic

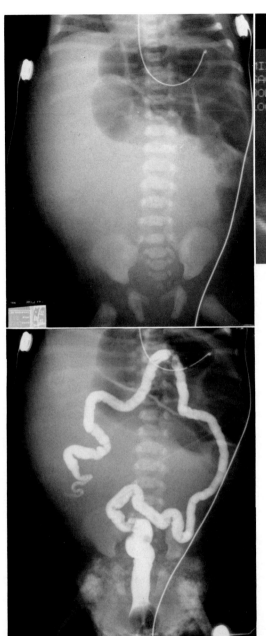

A

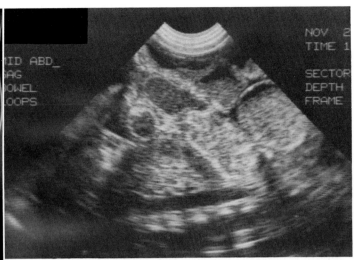

B

Fig. 72-17 Complicated meconium ileus: volvulus. **A,** Newborn with failure to pass meconium. Plain radiograph demonstrating large mass effect in right and mid-abdomen with displacement of dilated bowel loops. Calcific densities are artifactural. **B,** Sonogram of mid-abdomen shows multiple dilated bowel loops filled with thick echogenic meconium. **C,** Gastrografin enema filling unused colon and appendix.

Fig. 72-18 Meconium cyst. Newborn with passage of meconium and large abdominal mass. Sonography revealed large cystic mass occupying virtually entire abdomen and containing large amount of debris and fluid (*arrow-RK*, right kidney; *arrow-LK*, left kidney). Contrast enema following sonogram showed unused colon with no filling of distal ileum. At surgery, ileal perforation complicating ileal atresia and volvulus was found.

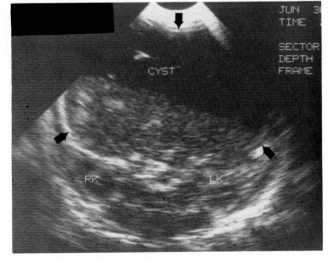

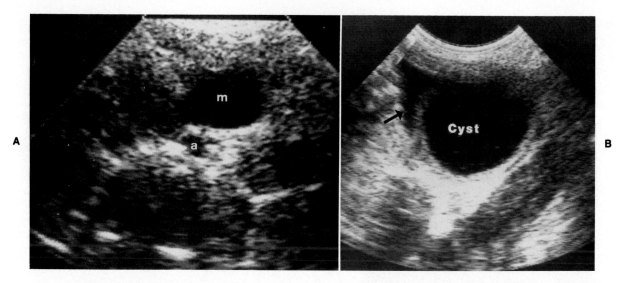

Fig. 72-19 Duplication cysts of the small bowel. **A,** Two-year-old girl with multiple duplication cysts including esophagus, duodenum, and jejunum. Cystic mass *(m)* was noted deep in mesentery anterior to aorta *(a),* proven at surgery to be jejunal duplication cyst. **B,** Newborn with suspicion of obstruction and right lower quadrant mass. Rounded cystic mass in right lower quadrant has strong back wall and good through transmission. Echogenicity noted in dependent position is consistent with debris or mucous. Mass is contiguous with dilated fluid-filled bowel loop *(arrow).*

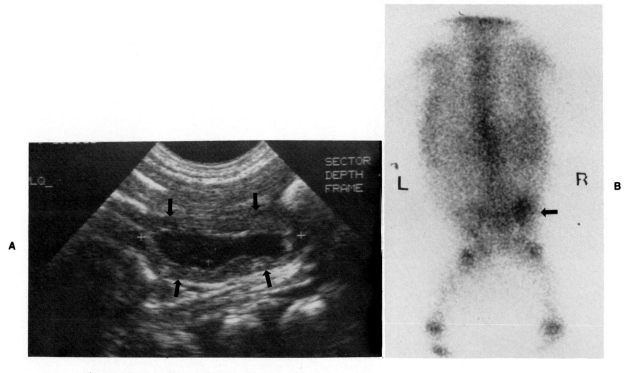

Fig. 72-20 Infected Meckel's diverticulum; young infant with fever and suspicion of intraabdominal abscess. **A,** Sonography reveals cystic structure in right lower quadrant with compressible, moderately echoic thick wall *(arrows).* Hypoechoic fluid was noted within this structure, suggesting possibility of superimposed infection. Abscess is unlikely in view of compressible walls and thickness of wall, suggesting that this was noncommunicating portion of gastrointestinal tract. Thickness and echogenicity of wall makes duplication cyst unlikely. **B,** Gallium scan showing increased uptake *(arrow)* in right lower quadrant in region of infected Meckel's diverticulum.

mass, generally in the right lower quadrant, which is a remnant of the vitelline duct persisting on the antimesenteric border of the ileum. Although the most common clinical manifestation of a Meckel's diverticulum is gastrointestinal bleeding, it has the potential for small bowel obstruction by causing volvulus, intussusception, or solely by its large size. The cystic nature of the mass and the well-defined muscular wall may be shown by ultrasound (Fig. 72-20). ^{99m}Tc pertechnetate radionuclide scan can be used to detect ectopic gastric mucosa in a Meckel's diverticulum when bleeding is the initial symptom.

The modality of choice for the examination of children with suspicion of intussusception is the contrast enema. However, there are patients who have a palpable abdominal mass without the classic signs of intussusception

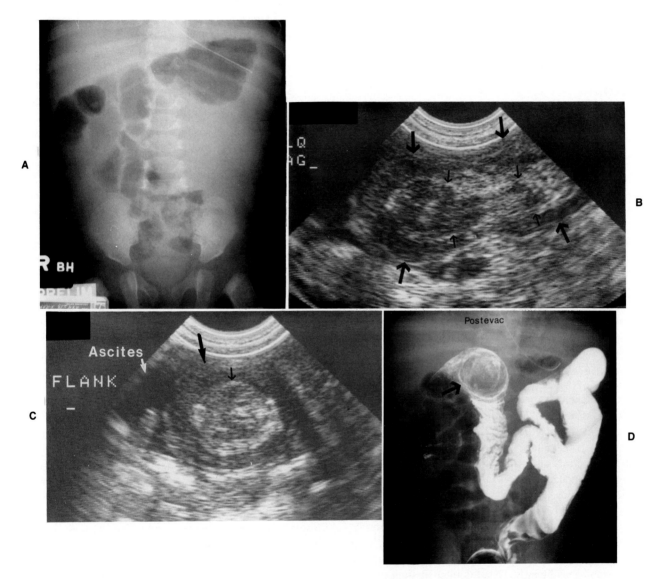

Fig. 72-21 Intussusception; 4-month-old boy with left lower quadrant mass. Plain radiograph showing paucity of gas in left mid and lower abdomen, dilated right-sided bowel loops, bulging flanks, and poor soft tissue landmarks, suggesting ascites. **A,** Kidney, ureter, and bladder film shows paucity of gas in left abdomen with several dilated bowel loops occupying right abdomen and pelvis. Bowel loops are separate, suggesting ascites. **B,** Sagittal scan of left lower quadrant demonstrating "pseudo-kidney" sign due to edematous intussuscepiens (*large arrows*) and edematous intussusceptum (*small arrows*). **C,** Sector scan of left flank showing "double doughnut" sign, indicating bowel wall edema of both the intussusceptum (*small black arrow*) and intussuscepiens (*large black arrow*). **D,** Postevacuation film demonstrating irreducible intussusception (*arrow*).

(currant jelly or bloody stools, bilious vomiting, episodes of severe abdominal pain). Sonography can establish the diagnosis of intussusception by identifying the characteristic bull's eye or target lesion.* The thickened hypoechoic rim represents the edematous wall of the intussusceptum, surrounding the hyperechoic center because of the interfaces of the compressed mucosa. When the wall of the intussuscipiens is not edematous, it is likely that the blood supply to the bowel is intact. However, double hypoechoic rings suggest edematous entering and returning walls of the intussusceptum. When the intussuscipiens is edematous and ascites is present, there is a high likelihood of compromise to the vascular supply of the bowel (Fig. 72-21).

COLON

Acute appendicitis is the most common cause of emergency surgery in children. This entity ranks second only to gastroenteritis as the most common acute abdominal inflammatory process in childhood (rare in infancy). In sexually active teenagers it may be difficult to differentiate appendicitis from pelvic inflammatory disease, and in infants and young children an imaging work-up may be necessary if the classic findings are not apparent. High-resolution real-time sonography can be very sensitive for identifying the inflamed appendix, particularly when the graded compression technique is used.[1,73,74,75] The appendix appears as a tubular structure with a blind end. The most central portion is hypoechoic, whereas the inner lining of the appendiceal wall is echogenic and the outer wall hypoechoic. When the appendix is inflamed, it appears on longitudinal imaging as a sausage-shaped, blind-ending structure with rigid hypoechoic thick walls; lacks peristalsis; and does not compress when the examiner gently compresses the abdominal wall with the transducer. On transverse imaging it appears as a target lesion (Fig. 72-22). Sonographic signs of periappendicitis include appendiceal wall thickening (often asymmetric) and irregular, hypoechoic formations around the appendix. Ultrasound plays an important role in demonstrating the complications of perforated appendix, such as abscess formation and pus accumulation in the pelvis, along the psoas muscle, in Morrison's pouch, and in the subphrenic spaces.[5,19,46] Very rarely one may find portal vein thrombosis or liver abscess caused by rupture and pylephlebitis. The ultrasound findings in periappendiceal abscess are a nonspecific complex cystic mass with generally thin walls (Figs. 72-23 and 72-24). Although they are most often confined to the right lower quadrant, they may be multiple in other distant areas

*References 13, 64, 66, 72, 85, 90.

(Fig. 72-25). Gas in the abscess may produce a highly echogenic mass with acoustic shadowing. An important pitfall to avoid is confusing a dilated fluid-filled bowel loop with an abscess. Careful observation for peristaltic motion and delayed scanning are useful for clarification. Often the bowel is paralyzed in the presence of appendiceal perforation and can be quite aperistaltic. The coffee bean sign—a cystic mass with or without internal echogenic debris—surrounding a fingerlike hyperechoic projection—the inflamed appendix—has also been reported.[54] Sonography is also helpful in the detection and follow-up evaluation of postappendectomy fluid collections. In addition, real-time ultrasound can be used for guidance during percutaneous drainage of periappendiceal abscesses or collection.[4] In older teenagers transvaginal aspiration or collections adjacent to the vaginal vault can be sonographically directed.

Hypoechoic thickening of the colonic wall may be identified in necrotizing enterocolitis, amebiasis, antibiotic-induced pseudomembranous colitis, and Behçet's syndrome.[59] The bowel wall may also be thickened in portions that are contiguous with an abscess, loops that are adjacent to inflamed bowel loops. Marked bowel wall thickening is seen with toxic megacolon. Pronounced concentric bowel wall thickening and lumenal narrowing may be seen sonographically in the presence of adenocarcinoma, whereas lymphomatous infiltration is quite anechoic with asymmetric thickening.

Metabolic or toxic states may cause a colonic ileus (Fig. 72-26). In children with dermatomyositis and mixed collagen disease states, one may observe marked dilatation of the colonic lumen, thinning of the bowel wall, and markedly reduced peristalsis during real-time observation.[59]

Ultrasound can be used to differentiate between high and low rectal pouch in infants with imperforate anus[70,81] (Fig. 72-27). The appropriate surgical procedure depends on the position of the distal rectal pouch in relation to the puborectalis muscle of the levator sling. A direct perineal exploration is used for low lesions that pass through the levator sling. The treatment for high lesions shown to be above the sling is early decompressive colostomy, followed later by a colon pull-through operation. There is a strong association of renal and spinal anomalies as well as rectogenitourinary fistulas with high inperforate anus. Although one can evaluate the rectal pouch by using the urinary bladder as a sonic window, the actual pouch-perineum distance can be measured using a perineal approach and high-resolution sonography. A pouch-perineum distance of less than 1.5 cm indicates a low imperforate anus. In high lesions the rectal pouch does not pass below the base of the bladder on sagittal images.

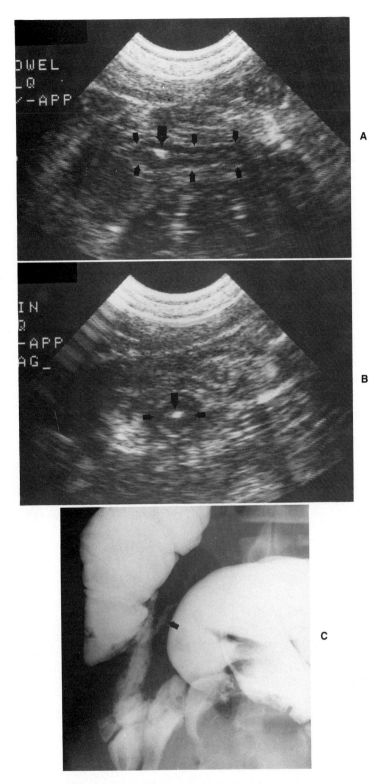

Fig. 72-22 Acute appendicitis; 17-year-old boy with right lower quadrant pain, fever, and vomiting. **A** and **B,** Sagittal and transverse views of right lower quadrant demonstrating hypoechoic thick-walled edematous appendix *(small arrows),* containing small, echogenic focus consistent with appendicolith *(large arrow).* **C,** Barium enema on this patient showed partial filling of irregular-appearing appendix *(arrow).*

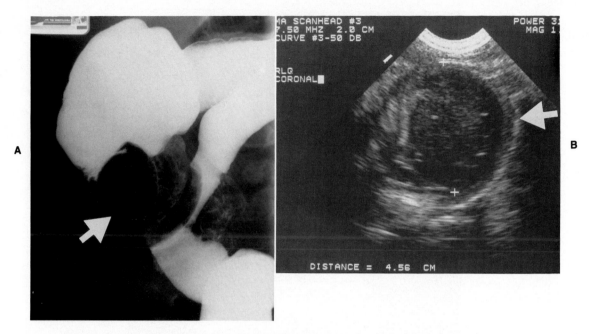

Fig. 72-23 Appendiceal abscess; 2-year-old boy with right-sided abdominal pain and fever. **A,** Barium enema shows large, rounded filling defect in region of cecum *(arrow)* with no filling of appendix. **B,** Large, rounded, thick walled, complicated cystic mass *(arrow)* noted in area of interest in right lower quadrant. Heterogenous echogenicity is superimposed suggesting infected material. Tenderness was obvious during scanning.

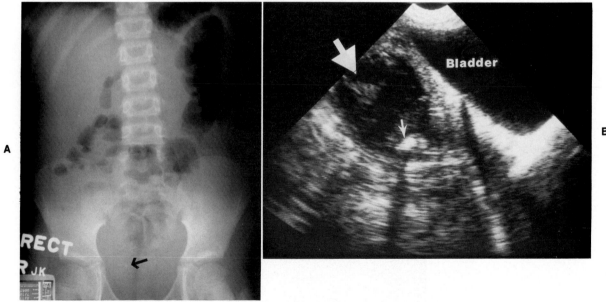

Fig. 72-24 Appendiceal abscess with appendicolith; 8-year-old girl with right lower quadrant pain, vomiting, and fever. **A,** Plain film of abdomen shows paucity of gas in right lower quadrant and pelvis, and small calcific density overlying right pelvis inferomedially *(arrow)*. **B,** Sagittal sonogram using bladder as sonic window shows complex cystic mass *(large arrow)* containing scattered areas of echogenicity, suggesting infected fluid. Echogenic focus shadowing ultrasound beam *(small arrow)* is consistent with appendicolith.

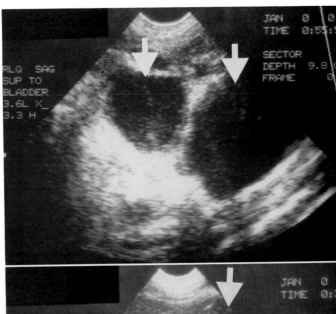

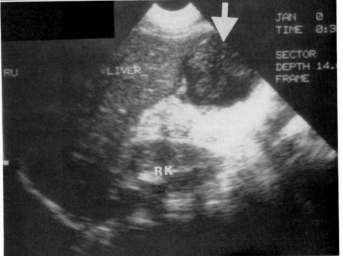

Fig. 72-25 Multiple abscesses complicating acute appendicitis. 6-year-old girl with fever, right upper quadrant pain, and right upper quadrant mass. **A,** Two rounded, tender, complex, mainly cystic masses were noted in right lower quadrant superior to bladder *(arrows)*. Irregular, slightly thickened walls were noted. **B,** In area of clinically palpable right upper quadrant mass, additional rounded, well-defined, complex, mainly cystic mass was identified with good through transmission, consistent with third abscess. *RK,* Right Kidney.

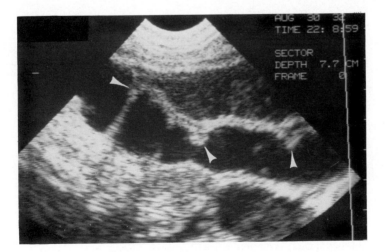

Fig. 72-26 Ileus. Coronal view of left flank in child with dynamic ileus demonstrates moderately dilated fluid-filled colon with haustral markings clearly seen *(arrowheads)*.

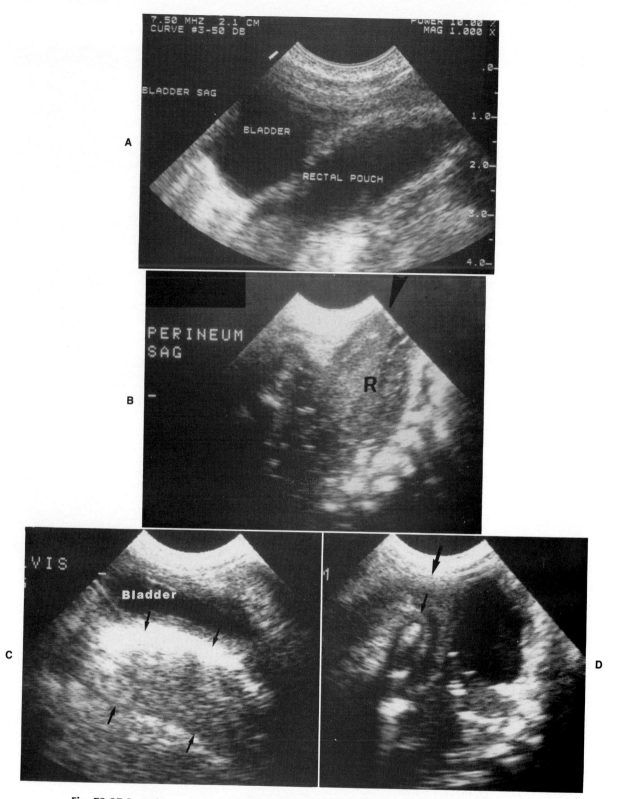

Fig. 72-27 Imperforate anus. **A,** Fluid-filled rectal pouch could be identified extending through well-distended bladder quite inferiorly, implying low imperforate anus. **B,** Perineal scan of same newborn as in **A,** showing that rectal pouch is in fact "covered anus" *(arrowhead). R,* Rectum. **C,** Consistent with clinical imperforate anus with large amount of gas in overdistended rectal pouch, extending quite inferiorly *(arrows).* **D,** Intermediate imperforate anus; perineal scan of newborn with imperforate anus. Large arrow indicates anal dimple. Small arrow shows distal end of rectal pouch, which was more than 1.5 cm from anal dimple, implying intermediate or high imperforate anus.

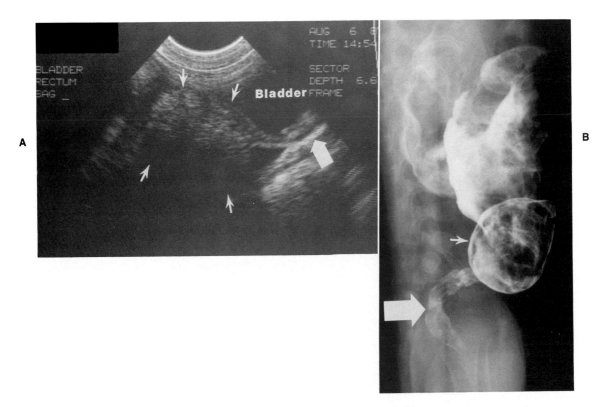

Fig. 72-28 Hirschsprung's disease; 9-month-old boy with hypotonia, weakness, and normocytic anemia, and large abdomen, had sonogram to exclude mass. **A,** Sagittal view of pelvis shows narrow, unfilled rectum *(large arrow)*. Above this area was massively distended sigmoid *(small arrows)* filled with tremendous fecal boluses, which shadowed ultrasound beam. **B,** Barium enema demonstrating collapsed aganglionic segment *(large arrow)* and distended feces-filled sigmoid colon *(small arrow)*.

Duplications of the colon and rectum may be demonstrated with sonography. At times the use of a water enema technique will help to confirm the diagnosis.

Sonography may also play a role in the diagnosis of Hirschsprung's disease in children with abdominal distention and constipation by demonstrating the aganglionic segment either with or without use of a water enema (Fig. 72-28). In newborn infants suspected of having meconium problems associated with an unused colon, ultrasound can help confirm the diagnosis by showing the distal unfilled rectum in association with the dilated meconium-filled loops of small bowel.

MISCELLANEOUS CONDITIONS

Sonography can be useful in evaluating abnormalities of the mesentery. A congenital mesenteric cyst (Fig. 72-29) or retroperitoneal lymphangioma (Fig. 72-30) represents a benign neoplasm of the lymphatic system.* It may be seen initially as gradual abdominal enlargement,

*References 31, 32, 33, 36, 62, 69, 71, 85.

a painless abdominal mass, or a small bowel obstruction. Many are nonpalpable because of their flaccid, mobile nature. Rarely acute symptoms caused by torsion, infection, hemorrhage, or rupture may be the initial sign. Because of the thin wall surrounding the cyst, they may mimic ascites. Their sonographic appearance is variable, ranging from a unilocular hypoechoic mass with back-wall enhancement to a multiloculated mass containing debris and septations. They are usually quite compressible with the ultrasound transducer.

Acquired cysts of the mesentery and omentum may be due to encystment of the distal end of ventriculoperitoneal shunt tubes[3,14,30] (Fig. 72-31). Children with a CSF-ocele (pseudocyst) may seek medical help because of headache, palpable abdominal mass, and often abdominal pain as well. The presence of septations and internal debris in the cyst, particularly in children with an elevated white blood cell count, infected cerebrospinal fluid, and/or fever, suggests an infected meningocele.

Cystic teratomas may also arise in the mesentery and omentum[12,37] (Fig. 72-33). Sonographically one may

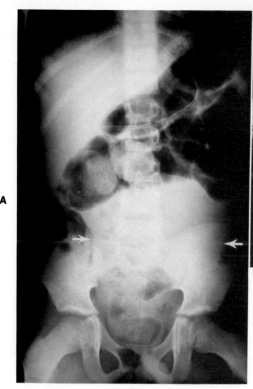

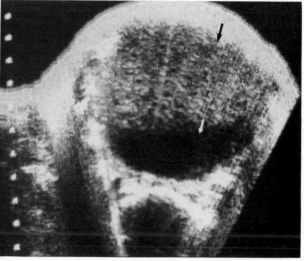

Fig. 72-29 Mesenteric cyst; 6-year-old with lower abdominal pain and constipation. **A,** Large soft tissue mass *(arrows)* in mid–lower abdomen and pelvis displacing feces-filled dilated colon. **B,** Static longitudinal scan of anterior abdomen showing well-defined rounded cystic mass, unrelated to solid organs, with strong back wall and increased through transmission. Note fat level (echogenic material, *black arrow*) and fluid level (anechoic, *white arrow*) within mass.

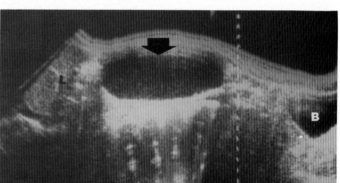

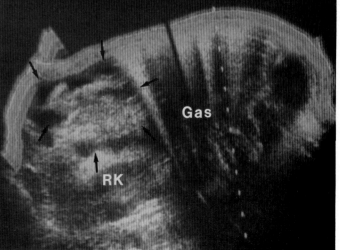

Fig. 72-30 Lymphangioma. **A,** Young girl with compressible mass in right upper and mid-abdomen. Static sagittal scan demonstrating oval cystic mass *(arrow)* with good through transmission containing hypoechoic fluid. Mass was compressible. *L,* Liver; *B,* bladder. Echogenic material is consistent with chyle. **B,** Young boy with compressible right upper quadrant mass. Transverse static sonogram demonstrates complex mass *(arrows)* in right upper quadrant, which was compressible and contained large amount of dense solid tissue. Large portion of left mid and upper abdomen was filled with gas-filled bowel loops. *RK,* Right kidney.

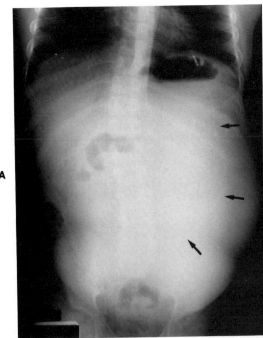

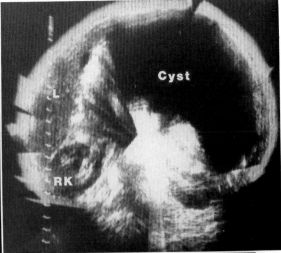

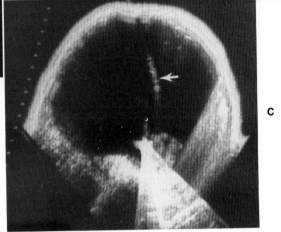

Fig. 72-31 CSF-ocele; young boy with left-sided ventricular peritoneal shunt presented to emergency room with headache, abdominal pain, and large abdominal mass. **A,** Huge abdominal mass displacing gas-filled bowel loops to right laterally and inferiorly. Arrows indicate course of left-sided ventricular peritoneal shunt tube. **B,** Transverse sonogram demonstrating liver *(L)*, right kidney *(RK)*, and large cystic mass. **C,** Transverse scan more inferiorly demonstrates shunt tube *(arrow)* coursing through large pseudocyst.

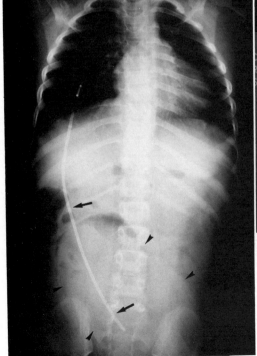

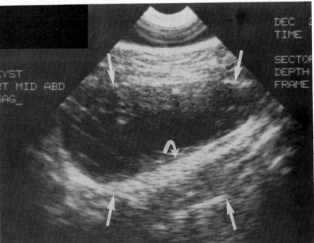

Fig. 72-32 Infected CSF-ocele. **A,** Young child with headache, abdominal pain, and right abdominal and pelvic mass *(arrowheads)*. Shunt tube *(arrows)* terminates in inferior aspect of mass. **B,** Sector sagittal scan of mass via step-off pad shows well-defined cystic mass *(straight arrows)* containing echogenic debris and shunt tube. Shunt tube indicated by curved arrow.

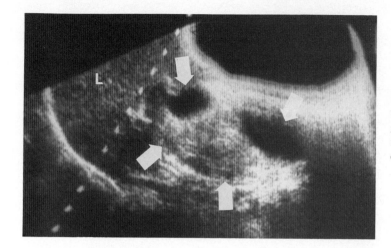

Fig. 72-33 Benign teratoma; young boy with asymptomatic right abdominal mass. Sagittal static sonogram shows complex mass *(arrows)* in right abdomen inferior to liver *(L)*, which contains two anechoic cystic areas as well as large solid component.

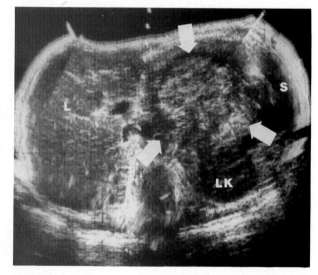

Fig. 72-34 Recurrent neuroblastoma. Asymptomatic abdominal mass noted in 6-year-old treated with surgery, chemotherapy, and bone marrow transplant for stage III left adrenal neuroblastoma. Large solid mass *(arrows)* noted deep in the mesentery on routine follow-up sonogram. *LK,* Left kidney; *S,* spleen; *L,* liver.

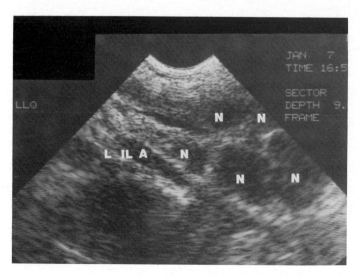

Fig. 72-35 Atypical microbacterial infection; 14-year-old boy with abdominal pain and tenderness, malaise, and splenomegaly. Sagittal sonogram in region of mass demonstrates multiple matted lymph nodes *(N)* anterior to left iliac artery *(L IL A).*

demonstrate peripheral calcification and floating echogenic debris suggesting fat. Other rare mesenteric tumors include benign fibromatosis, neurofibroma, mesenchymoma, lipoma, mesothelioma, and metastatic deposits (Figs. 72-34 and 72-35). In children with abdominal trauma ultrasound may identify a mesenteric hematoma.

REFERENCES

1. Abu-Yousef, MM, et al: High-resolution sonography of acute appendicitis, AJR 149:53, 1987.
2. Adler, DD, Samuels, BI, and Blane, CE: Sonographic diagnosis of neonatal diaphragmatic inversion, J Clin Ultrasonogr 12:166, 1984.
3. Agha, FP, et al: Unusual abdominal complications of ventriculoperitoneal shunts, Radiology 146:323, 1983.
4. Bagi, P, and Dueholm, S: Nonoperative management of the ultrasonically evaluated appendiceal mass, Surgery 101:602, 1987.
5. Baker, DE, et al: Postappendectomy fluid collections in children: incidence, nature, and evolution evaluated using US, Radiology 161:341, 1986.
6. Ball, TI, Atkinson, GO, Jr, and Gay, BB, Jr: Ultrasound diagnosis of hypertrophic pyloric stenosis: real-time application and the demonstration of a new sonographic sign, Radiology 147:499, 1983.
7. Barki, Y, and Bar-Ziv, J: Meconium ileus: ultrasonic diagnosis of intraluminal inspissated meconium, J Clin Ultrasonogr 13:509, 1985.
8. Bauer, RJ, Sieber, WK, and Kiesewetter, WB: Alimentary tract duplications in children, Am Surg 188:669, 1978.
9. Blumhagen, JD, and Coombs, JB: Ultrasound in the diagnosis of hypertrophic pyloric stenosis, J Clin Ultrasonogr 9:289, 1981.
10. Blumhagen, JD, and Weinberger, E: Pediatric gastrointestinal ultrasonography. In Sanders, RC, and Hills, M, editors: Ultrasound annual, New York, 1986, Raven Press.
11. Bowen, A, et al: Cystic meconium peritonitis: ultrasonographic features, Pediatr Radiol 14:18, 1984.
12. Bowen, B, et al: Gastrointestinal teratomas: CT and US appearance with pathologic correlation, Radiology 162:431, 1987.
13. Bowerman, RA, Silver, TM, and Jaffe, MH: Realtime ultrasound diagnosis of intussusception in children, Radiology 143:527, 1982.
14. Briggs, JR, Hendry, GM, and Minns, RA: Abdominal ultrasound in the diagnosis of cerebrospinal fluid pseudocysts complicating ventriculoperitoneal shunts, Arch Dis Child 59:661, 1984.
15. Brugman, SM, et al: Sonographic findings with radiologic correlation in meconium peritonitis, J Clin Ultrasonogr 7:305, 1979.
16. Brzuchalski, RK, Rosenberg, HK, and Deiling, K: Sonography of hypertrophic pyloric stenosos, J Diagn Med Sonogr 2:251, 1986.
17. Callen, PW, Filly, RA, and Sarti, DA: Ultrasonography of the diaphragmatic crura, Radiology 130:721, 1979.
18. Carroll, BA, and Moskowitz, PS: Sonographic diagnosis of neonatal meconium cyst, AJR 137:1262, 1981.
19. Carroll, B, et al: Ultrasonography and indium-111 white blood cell scanning for the detection of intraabdominal abscesses, Radiology 140:155, 1981.
20. Derchi, LE, et al: Sonographic staging of gastric cancer, AJR 140:273, 1983.
21. Derchi, LE, et al: The sonographic appearance of duodenal lesions, J Ultrasound Med 5:269, 1986.
22. Dinkle, E, et al: Realtime ultrasound in Crohn's disease: characteristic features and clinical implications, Pediatr Radiol 16:8, 1986.
23. Dubbins, RA: Ultrasound demonstration of bowel wall thickness in inflammatory bowel disease, Clin Radiol 35:227, 1984.
24. Fakhry, J, and Berk, R: The target pattern: characteristic sonographic features of stomach and bowel abnormalities, AJR 137:969, 1981.
25. Fleischer, AC, Muhletaler, CA, and James, AE: Sonographic patterns arising from normal and abnormal bowel, Radiol Clin North Am 18:145, 1980.
26. Fleischer, AC, Muhletaler, CA, and James, AE: Sonographic assessment of the bowel wall, AJR 136:887, 1981.
27. Fleischer, AC, et al: Sonographic patterns of distended fluid filled bowel, Radiology 133:681, 1979.
28. Fleischer, AC, et al: Realtime sonography of bowel. In Winsberg, F, editor: Clinics in diagnostic ultrasound, New York, 1982, Churchill Livingstone.
29. Fried, AM, Pulmano, CM, and Mostowyca, L: Duodenal duplication cyst: sonographic and angiographic features, AJR 128:863, 1977.
30. Fried, AM, et al: Ventriculoperitoneal shunt function: evaluation by sonography, AJR 134:967, 1980.
31. Garel, L, Pariente, D, and Sauvegrain, J: US in infancy and childhood, Clin Gastroenterol 13:161, 1984.
32. Geer, LL, et al: Mesenteric cyst: sonographic appearance with CT correlation, Pediatr Radiol 14:102, 1984.
33. Gordon, MD, and Sumner, TE: Abdominal ultrasonography in a mesenteric cyst presenting as ascites, Gastroenterology 698:761, 1975.
34. Grossman, H: The evaluation of abdominal masses in children with emphasis on noninvasive methods: a roentgenographic approach, Cancer 35:884, 1975.
35. Haller, JO, and Cohen, H: Hypertrophic pyloric stenosis: diagnosis using US, Radiology 161:335, 1986.
36. Haller, JO, et al: Sonographic evaluation of mesenteric and omental masses in children, AJR 130:269, 1978.
37. Hayden, CK, and Swischuk, LE: The gastrointestinal tract. In Hayden, CK, and Swischuk, LE, editors: Pediatric ultrasonography, Baltimore, 1987, Williams & Wilkins.
38. Hayden, CK, et al: Combined esophageal and duodenal atresia: US findings, AJR 140:225, 1983.
39. Hayden, CK, Jr, et al: Sonographic demonstration of duodenal obstruction with midgut volvulus, AJR 143:9, 1984.
40. Hayden, CK, et al: Ultrasound: the definitive imaging modality in pyloric stenosis, RadioGraphics 4:517, 1984.
41. Holt, S, and Samuel, E: Gray scale ultrasound in Crohn's disease, Gut 20:590, 1979.
42. Jackson, G, et al: Sonography of combined esophageal and duodenal atresia, J Ultrasound Med 2:473, 1983.
43. Kaftori, JK, Pery, M, and Kleinhaus, U: Ultrasonography in Crohn's disease, Gastrointest Radiol 9:137, 1984.
44. Kangarloo, H, et al: Ultrasonic evaluation of abdominal gastrointestinal tract duplication in children, Radiology 131:191, 1979.
45. Kirks, DR, et al: Diagnostic imaging of pediatric abdominal masses: an overview, Radiol Clin North Am 19:527, 1981.
46. Knochel, JQ, et al: Diagnosis of abdominal abscesses with computed tomography, ultrasound, and In-111 leukocyte scans, Radiology 137:425, 1980.
47. Kodroff, M, Hartenberg, M, and Goldschmidt, R: Ultrasonographic diagnosis of gangrenous bowel in neonatal necrotizing enterocolitis, Pediatr Radiol 14:168, 1984.
48. Komaiko, MS: Gastric neoplasm: ultrasound and CT evaluation, Gastrointest Radiol 4:131, 1979.
49. Kopen, PA, and McAlister, WH: Upper gastrointestinal and ultrasound examinations of gastric antral involvement in chronic granulomatosis disease, Pediatr Radiol 14:91, 1984.
50. Lamont, A, Starinsky, R, and Cremin, B: US diagnosis of duplication cysts in children, Br J Radiol 57:463, 1984.
51. Lawrence, PW, and Chrispin, A: Sonographic appearances in two neonates with generalized meconium peritonitis: the "snowstorm" sign, Br J Radiol 57:340, 1984.

73 *Overview*

CHARLES A. GOODING

Recent advances in imaging technology provide the opportunity to learn more than ever before about health and disease in childhood. Historically, pediatricians have been rather conservative about the application of new imaging technology to their patients because of the fear of possible unrecognized harmful effects of the new devices. Modern pediatric practice, however, now uses the unique information that is obtained noninvasively from studies such as ultrasound, computed tomography (CT), magnetic resonance imaging (MRI), and nuclear medicine. The goal of this chapter is to provide an overview of recent advances in imaging technology as applied to children.

LOW-DOSE RADIOGRAPHY AND FLUOROSCOPY

Despite the tremendous proliferation and acceptance of high-technology modalities in the diagnosis of diseases of children, 82% of all examinations at a large children's hospital are simple radiographs.[54] Several methods are available to keep the radiation dose low while maintaining a high-quality image. New film-screen combinations, new phosphor grain configurations, and new phosphors have resulted in much lower radiation dose than ever before available. For example, Wesenberg[54] found that DuPont's Kevlar fiber-front cassettes have high x-ray photon transmission characteristics that allow a 23% to 34% reduction in radiation exposure over that typically found with conventional cassettes. Carbon fiber has slightly better x-ray photon transmission than Kevlar; however, cassettes made of carbon fiber are expensive and brittle and tend to crack or even shatter if dropped. Erbium or yttrium filters can reduce the dose even further. Using yttrium filtration, the radiation exposure in the newborn ranges from 570 μR (microrad) for an anteroposterior chest film to 610 μR for the lateral projection.[54]

Radiation exposure can also be reduced during fluoroscopy.[55] Attempts to reduce fluoroscopic radiation exposure have included pulse fluoroscopy,[27] increased primary beam filtration,[25] installation of a variable aperture iris into the optical chain,[38] and addition of a digital noise reducer into the television chain.[1] Wesenberg[54] has developed a custom-modified fluoroscopy unit that will allow fluoroscopic procedures on the newborn at less than 1 μR/minute.

ULTRASONOGRAPHY

Spectacular advances in real-time and Doppler ultrasound, coupled with the reasonable cost of ultrasound hardware, make ultrasonography one of the most cost-effective imaging techniques for the investigation of abdominal disease in children.[35] Ultrasound is the primary screening modality for intraabdominal and pelvic pathology in children (Figs. 73-1 to 73-3). It can detect gastrointestinal masses, such as pyloric stenosis[4,22,24] and intussusception, and inflammatory conditions[33,34] such as appendicitis.[29,31,56] In addition, sonography is replacing the conventional gastrointestinal barium series in a variety of other gastrointestinal lesions. This does not mean that ultrasound will replace the plain film in the evalu-

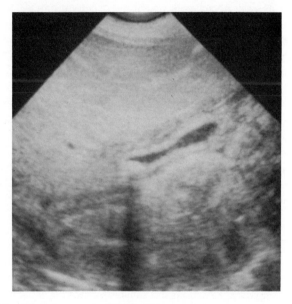

Fig. 73-1 Ultrasound of newborn with hemolysis demonstrates gallstones that cast acoustic shadow.

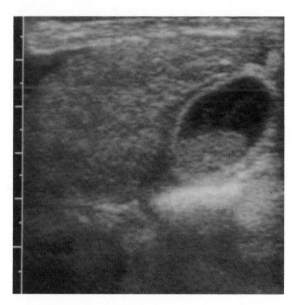

Fig. 73-2 Ultrasound of child with chronic liver disease shows sludge in gallbladder.

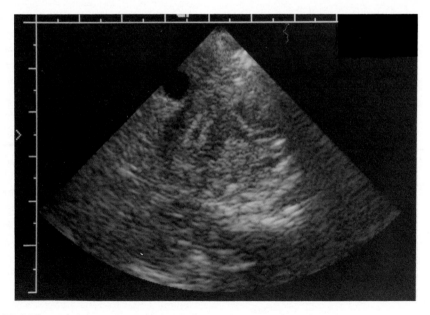

Fig. 73-3 Ultrasound demonstrates that pyloric muscle is thickened circumferentially in newborn with pyloric stenosis.

ation of acute abdominal problems in children, but it undoubtedly can provide very useful supplemental information.

In a prospective study of ultrasound in the diagnosis of idiopathic hypertrophic pyloric stenosis in 200 patients, Stunden and co-workers[48] used criteria that included measurement of the pyloric diameter, muscle thickness, and canal length and observation of the function of the pylorus and gastric peristalsis in real time. Using these ultrasonic criteria, they assessed 112 infants with pyloric stenosis and 88 as normal. The follow-up on all the infants showed that the method was 100% accurate with no false-positive or false-negative results. Ultrasound is not only accurate but also rapid and safe, and it should replace barium examination in the diagnosis of pyloric stenosis when the diagnosis is in doubt.

Haller and Cohen[23] determined that pyloric diameter measured in cross sections of 15 mm or greater is considered abnormal. This is the least reliable measurement. For pyloric muscle thickness, obtained from longitudinal and cross-sectional views, 4 mm or more is a key positive finding and a reliable sign of pyloric stenosis. A pyloric length of 1.8 cm or greater obtained from the longitudinal view is considered positive.

High-resolution real-time ultrasonography with graded compression is valuable in assessing the child thought to have appendicitis. Jeffrey and co-workers[29] report a sensitivity of 89% and a specificity of 95% in a study of 90 patients with clinically suspected appendicitis. When interpreted in light of the clinical examination, sonography should significantly reduce the rate of false-negative appendectomies.

Ultrasonography also has been shown to be valuable in the detection of intussusception. Swischuck and associates[49] reviewed the literature and findings on 14 of their patients and concluded that it should be used as a screening procedure. They believe that ultrasonography establishes the diagnosis quickly and also provides information regarding the potential reducibility of the lesion.

Positive sonographic findings consisting of circumferential bowel wall thickening have been reported in children with chronic granulomatous disease.[32] In one patient, an intramural hematoma caused a focal complex lesion involving the body of the stomach.[21]

Over the past few years, duplex Doppler ultrasonography has become established as an excellent diagnostic modality in children as well as in adults.[36] Because this method is less invasive than angiography, it is especially useful in children.

Real-time ultrasound images of the pancreas of 273 children without pancreatic disease and 13 patients with pancreatitis were analyzed by Siegel and co-workers.[44] The presence of a dilated main pancreatic duct was the most useful feature in suggesting an abnormality. Evaluation of pancreatic size, configuration, and echogenicity was not reliable in the differentiation of the normal from the abnormal pancreas.

Ultrasound also has a definite role in pediatrics as a guidance system for interventional procedures such as drainage of abscesses.[50]

NUCLEAR MEDICINE

Nuclear medicine diagnostic procedures in children are safe, sensitive, and only minimally invasive. Often they provide information not obtainable by other diagnostic methods. An advantage of radionuclide studies compared to other studies is that, in addition to providing morphologic information, they may provide accurate quantitative functional information about several organs. Advances in the fields of radiopharmaceuticals and instrumentation have contributed to the growing application of nuclear medicine techniques to detect diseases of childhood.

Radiopharmaceutical research has generated a number of radionuclide-labeled pharmaceuticals with a short physical half-life (technetium-99m, iodine-123, thallium-201, iridium-191m). These agents result in acceptably low patient radiation exposure. They do not produce toxic effects or allergic reactions and result in no hemodynamic or osmotic overload.[52]

Newer gamma cameras provide higher spatial resolution, better field uniformity, and magnification techniques that facilitate the evaluation of children. Pinhole collimators in conjunction with these cameras permit magnification with compound spatial resolution that has reasonable sensitivity.

Hepatic scintigraphy in children can complement the information provided by ultrasound and CT. Indications for hepatobiliary scintigraphy are distinguishing biliary atresia from neonatal hepatitis, evaluating the cause of right upper quadrant pain, performing postoperative evaluation, and evaluating masses such as choledochal cyst. Changes in the distribution of ^{99m}Tc sulfur colloid may give information about normal or altered liver function. A limitation of hepatic scintigraphy is that it can detect only lesions 1.5 to 2 cm or larger. Chervu and co-workers[13] have described radiopharmaceuticals used for hepatobiliary imaging.

Scintigraphy gives information about liver size, congenital abnormalities such as asplenia and polysplenia, and diffuse or focal liver disease. Enlargement of a child's liver may be seen in glycogen storage disease, biliary obstruction, congestive heart failure, infection, leukemia, Hodgkin's disease, or diffuse tumor infiltration from hepatoblastoma, metastatic Wilm's tumor, or neuroblastoma. Trauma to the child's liver also may be detected with scintigraphy.

Selective splenic imaging is possible after intravenous administration of ^{99m}Tc heat-damaged red blood cells.[17] Splenomegaly in children may be detected and is seen in a variety of conditions, including portal hypertension (cirrhosis, cystic fibrosis), Gaucher's disease, leukemia, lymphoma, anemia, congestive heart failure, bacterial endocarditis, pyelonephritis, metastatic disease, hepatitis, granulomatous disease, hemolytic disease, glycogen storage disease, and systemic infections. Relatively increased ^{99m}Tc sulfur colloid uptake in the spleen with or without splenomegaly may be seen in severe liver dysfunction, including hepatic cirrhosis, chemotoxicity, storage disease, and trauma with edema of the liver. Focal splenic defects may be found in splenic rupture, tumor, abscess, cyst, leukemia, infarction, and histiocytosis. In a review of 2000 ^{99m}Tc sulfur colloid liver spleen scans, Freeman and Tonkin[19a] found focal splenic defects in 18 (six infarcts, six metastases, five lymphomas, and one inflammation).

Gastroesophageal scintigraphy has been advocated as an alternative noninvasive study of gastroesophageal reflux (GER) requiring no sedation.[26,39] Data concerning gastric emptying are frequently recorded simultaneously with examination for GER. Arasu and co-workers[3] have described the comparative accuracy of diagnostic methods used to detect GER. GER is an important entity in pediatric patients because it occurs frequently and may lead to severe complications such as recurrent episodes of pneumonia.[6]

Meckel's diverticulum is the most common cause of lower gastrointestinal hemorrhage in previously healthy infants. A Meckel's diverticulum usually contains ileal mucosa, but it has been found to contain gastric, duodenal, jejunal, or colonic mucosa or pancreatic tissue. Because Meckel's diverticulum cannot be diagnosed reliably by other imaging techniques, scintigraphy is currently the best nonsurgical method of diagnosis.[43] Abdominal scintigraphy does not detect the Meckel's diverticulum per se, but it will reveal uptake of the radiopharmaceutical by functioning ectopic mucosa within the diverticulum. (Fig. 73-4) ^{99m}Tc sodium pertechnetate is the radiotracer used to identify a Meckel's diverticulum. Concentration of the radiotracer in ectopic mucosa can be increased with drugs such as pentagastrin, thereby enhancing the imaging. Among the surgically proved cases of Meckel's diverticulum in the literature, the accuracy of ^{99m}Tc pertechnetate scintigraphy is 90%.[43] Barium studies of the gastrointestinal tract should not be performed within a few days before abdominal scintigraphy because the contrast material can prevent detection of the Meckel's diverticulum by shielding the gamma rays of [99m]Tc. Other conditions in the abdomen that accumulate pertechnetate include intestinal obstruction, intussusception, inflammation (Fig. 73-5), vascular malformations, ulcers, some tumors, and various urinary tract abnormalities that interrupt urinary excretion of the pertechnetate.

COMPUTED TOMOGRAPHY

CT plays a valuable role in assessment of several childhood abdominal diseases (Figs. 73-6 and 73-7).[10] The development of ultrafast CT, sometimes referred to as cine-CT, makes this technique particularly attractive since it is possible to image the child without resorting to sedation.[9] Furthermore, the ultrafast CT technique has a 0.05- to 0.1-second image acquisition time, which eliminates motion artifacts associated with spontaneous respiration or bowel peristalsis.[12] Another advantage of ultrafast CT compared with conventional CT scanning is that the total time of the examination is reduced, thus diminishing the risks to the infant from hypothermia and absence from the neonatal nursery environment.

CT is valuable in assessing hepatic and splenic injury in children. Of 274 children who were examined with abdominal CT after blunt abdominal trauma by Birch and co-workers,[8] CT demonstrated parenchymal injuries in 36 patients (13%), or 20 livers and 21 spleens. Hemoperitoneum was detected in 27 of 36 patients (75%). These authors conclude that the decision for laparotomy should not be based on the extent of injury as shown on

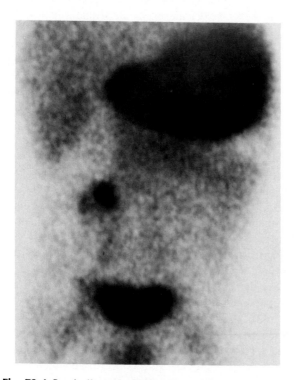

Fig. 73-4 Surgically proved Meckel's diverticulum produces increased isotopic accretion in right lower quadrant on ^{99m}Tc scan of child with abdominal pain.

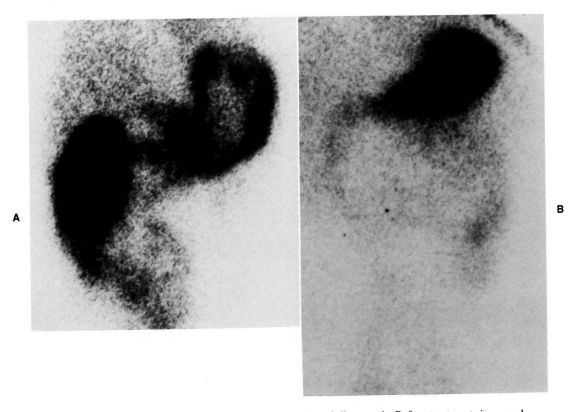

Fig. 73-5 ^{99m}TcO$_4$ scan demonstrates inflammatory bowel disease. **A,** Before treatment, increased isotopic accretion. **B,** After steroid treatment, much less isotopic accretion.

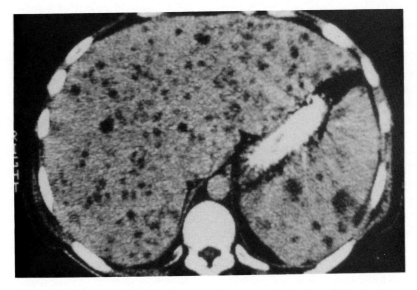

Fig. 73-6 CT demonstrates multiple microabscesses in patient with leukemia.

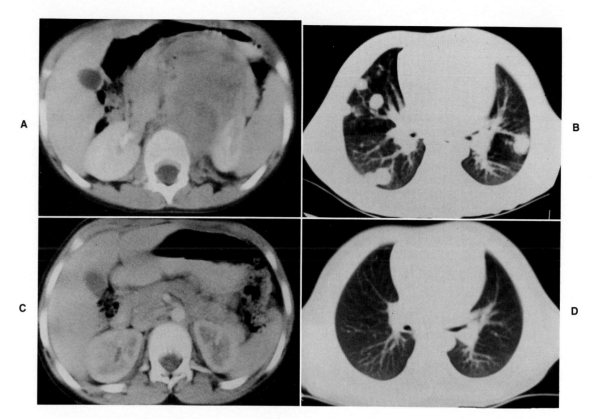

Fig. 73-7 Rhabdomyosarcoma in child appeared as large abdominal mass seen on CT **(A)** in association with multiple pulmonary mestastasis **(B)**. Four years later, no evidence of disease in the abdomen **(C)** or in the chest **(D)**.

CT, but on the child's physiologic condition. This conclusion supports the work of Berger and Kuhn.[7]

CT also has a role in patient management studies in inflammatory bowel diseases. Fishman and associates[19] found significant previously unsuspected findings that led to a change in medical or surgical management in 22 (28%) of the 80 patients studied. Although these authors do not suggest that CT can approach the diagnostic accuracy of air contrast examination for mucosal disease, CT can provide information about the extent of bowel and mesenteric disease.

Riddlesberger[37] used CT to study 10 children with inflammatory bowel disease. He correctly points out that although most children with inflammatory bowel disease do not need a CT scan, when the course becomes complicated it is often necessary to evaluate occurrences outside the bowel lumen. CT can demonstrate the presence and extent of abscesses and fistulas.

Recently the role of CT has been described in the assessment of the acquired immunodeficiency syndrome (AIDS).[28] The intraabdominal manifestations of AIDS are numerous and affect liver, spleen, bowel, mesentery, and retroperitoneum. Because of frequent nonspecificity of findings, CT-guided fine-needle aspiration biopsy is often essential for precise diagnosis. Although chemotherapy for AIDS-related neoplasms often has limited effectiveness, serial abdominal CT imaging is often useful to assess the cause of therapy.

ANGIOGRAPHY

Angiography or digital subtraction angiography has a role in the diagnosis of pediatric as well as adult disease. Angiography is helpful in planning surgical resection of benign and malignant hepatic tumors in children. Tonkin and co-workers[51] believe that sonography, CT, or MRI can be used as the initial procedure for evaluating tumor size, location, and hepatic vascularity. CT scanning demonstrates intrahepatic vascular areas with dynamic scanning; however, the exact vascular anatomy demonstrated by angiography in children is more accurate and is often needed before surgical resection of primary liver tumors. Angiography is superior in demonstrating relatively common extrahepatic arterial variations and for detecting additional small, focal hepatic lesions before surgical resection or biopsy. Angiography should differentiate benign from malignant tumors in a high percentage of

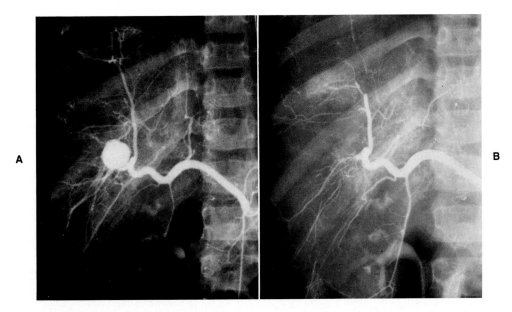

Fig. 73-8 Posttraumatic hepatic artery aneurysm in child with hemobilia after automobile accident. **A,** Before embolization, angiography demonstrates aneurysm. **B,** After embolization, aneurysm is occluded.

patients. After the diagnosis of vascular intrahepatic abnormalities such as tumor or aneurysm has been established, ablation of the abnormal vessels may be achieved by therapeutic transcatheter embolization (Fig. 73-8).[45]

PERCUTANEOUS FINE-NEEDLE BIOPSY

Percutaneous fine-needle biopsy (PFNB) has received increasing acceptance in recent years with the appreciation of its accuracy, safety, and cost effectiveness.[5,15,40] Diament and co-workers[16] found 16 true positives in 17 patients with proved malignancy. The major indication for PFNB is suspected metastatic disease or diagnosis of primary malignancy when radiation or chemotherapy is planned before surgical resection. No significant morbidity results from this procedure. Some PFNB procedures have been done on an outpatient basis, yielding considerable cost savings.

MAGNETIC RESONANCE IMAGING

Although conventional imaging modalities are used to begin the diagnostic imaging evaluation of a child's abdomen, MRI has much to offer (Fig. 73-9). MRI provides higher contrast resolution than CT and offers the opportunity to image the abdomen in coronal and sagittal as well as axial planes. No ionizing radiation is required, and use of intravenous or oral contrast media is unnecessary.

Suspected abnormalities related to the pancreas or the hepatobiliary system are best imaged first in the axial plane. Mesenteric lymphadenopathy and splenomegaly are sometimes better appreciated in the coronal plane. On T_1-weighted sequences, the liver parenchyma, the common bile duct, and the origin of the celiac axis and superior mesenteric artery, as well as the portal vein, can be evaluated.

Congenital anomalies of the hepatobiliary system such as choledochal cyst and polycystic liver disease are first

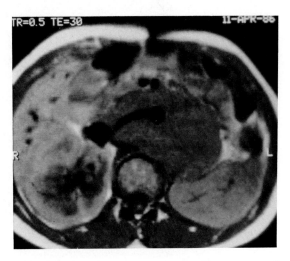

Fig. 73-9 MRI demonstrates recurrent neuroblastoma extending across midline of abdomen anterior to spine and encasing visceral vessels.

evaluated by ultrasound, but when that examination proves inconclusive, MRI can provide valuable additional information. Generalized liver disease in children such as hemochromatosis or cirrhosis are well evaluated by MRI. Hemochromatosis resulting from transfusion hemosiderosis produces an extremely lower liver intensity because the iron deposition prolongs the T_1 relaxation time (Fig. 73-10).[11] The cirrhotic liver appears small with nonhomogeneous regional intensity.[46]

MRI is especially useful in children with its ability to depict portal venous anatomy.[18] It also can depict obstructions of the inferior vena cava and/or the hepatic view (Budd-Chiari syndrome).[47] In children with severe liver disease who are candidates for liver transplantation, MRI can potentially obviate the need for angiography by demonstrating detailed vascular anatomy. Day and coworkers[14] used MRI to evaluate nine pediatric liver transplant candidates. MRI demonstrated portal vein patency in three cases, which was not seen by angiography, and confirmed portal vein patency in one patient, when it was questionably identified on sonography. Depiction of the anatomy and documentation of vascular patency are essential in evaluation of patients before liver transplantation. MRI also has a role in the diagnosis of intrahepatic lesions such as cysts, abscesses, and tumors. The most important type of liver pathology to be elucidated by MRI is hepatic neoplasia.

MRI provides information about the extent of the lesion and the potential for surgical resection. The most common hepatic neoplasms in children are hepatoma, hepatoblastoma, and lymphoma. These lesions usually have low signal intensity on T_1-weighted images. On T_2-weighted images, lymphomas usually show only a slight increase in signal intensity, whereas hepatoma and hepatoblastoma usually have a higher signal intensity.

Weinreb and associates[53] used MRI and CT to evaluate the livers of 27 children, 2 weeks to 16 years old. These authors concluded that MRI has the potential to replace CT as a technique for imaging the liver, especially in infants and young children.

The pancreas in children with cystic fibrosis has high signal intensity because of the fatty infiltration.[20] Pancreatic neoplasms are rare in children, but MRI is of value in such instances in demonstrating obstruction of the common bile duct secondary to pancreatic neoplasm.

Evaluation of the spleen is best appreciated on coronal T_1-weighted images. The normal spleen and the spleen in sickle cell anemia have been studied by MRI, with the results recently reported.[2] Lesions that infiltrate the mesentery, such as lymphoma or pancreatitis, are best imaged in the axial or sagittal plane. Thickened mesentery has a higher signal intensity than an air-filled bowel lumen and has a similar signal intensity to that of the bowel wall. Thickened mesentery is best appreciated on T_1-weighted images.

MAGNETIC RESONANCE SPECTROSCOPY

Magnetic resonance spectroscopy (MRS) has proved to be a useful technique for the assessment of phosphorus-

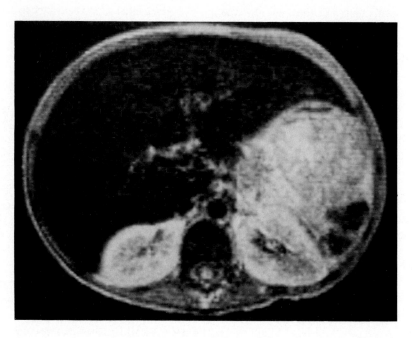

Fig. 73-10 MRI demonstrates hemochromatosis in child resulting from transfusional hemosiderosis. Liver has very low signal intensity because iron deposition (Fe^{+3}) produces long T_1 relaxation time.

containing metabolites and intracellular pH (pHi). Although most MRS research to date has been in animal models, MRS is now being applied to conditions in human beings. ^{31}P MRS can monitor intracellular ratios of adenosine triphosphate (ATP) and inorganic phosphate (Pi). Hypoxia or ischemia results in hydrolysis of ATP to adenosine diphosphate (ADP) and Pi, resulting in an increase in the Pi/ATP ratio.[30,41] The chemical shift of the ^{31}P signal can be used to monitor pHi. Since hypoxia is usually accompanied by a reduction in pH from in-

creased lactate production, then monitoring pHi provides an independent assessment of ischemia.

The intestine is a good organ to study with ^{31}P MRS because ATP levels in intestinal epithelial cells are high and the turnover of ATP in intestinal mucosal cells is also high (6 to 7 times/minute). We have shown that ^{31}P MRS can readily differentiate normal from ischemic intestine (Fig. 73-11).[30] This capability might have profound pragmatic implications in the diagnostic evaluation of entities such as neonatal enterocolitis.

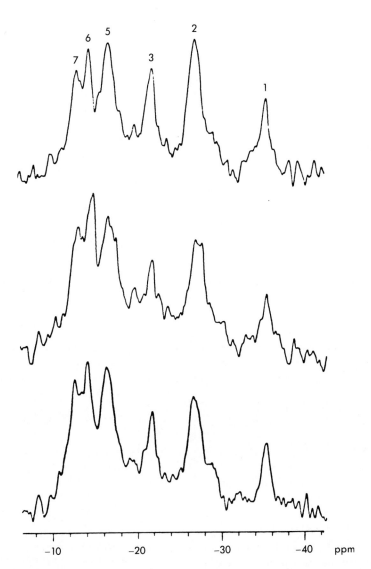

Fig. 73-11 ^{31}P MR spectra obtained from liver of infant rabbit. **A,** During normoxic conditions, with partial arterial oxygen pressure (Pao_2) approximately 100 torr, and **B,** 30 minutes after reduction of Pao_2 to about 25 torr (hypoxia). Decrease occurs in adenosine triphosphate (ATP) and increase in inorganic phosphate *(Pi)* resonance area after transition to hypoxia. **C,** Partial return of *Pi* and ATP 10 minutes after transition to hyperoxia (recovery). Peaks: *1,* β-ATP; *2,* å-ATP and NAD(H); *3,* γ-ATP; *5,* PD; *6, Pi; 7,* MP.

(From Schmidt, HC, et al: Pediatr Radiol 16:146, 1986. Reproduced with permission.)

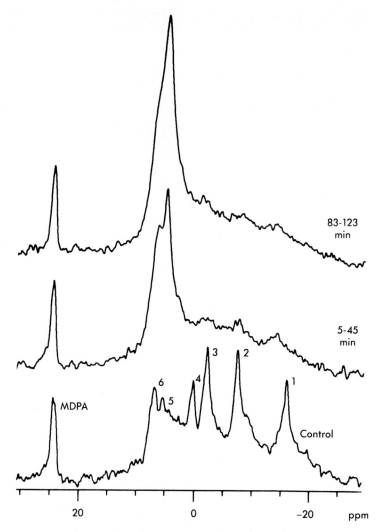

Fig. 73-12 ^{31}P spectra of rat intestine before induction of ischemia and after 5 to 45 and 83 to 123 minutes of ischemia. Chemical shifts were referenced to external parameter of methylenediphosphonic acid (MDPA), which was set to 24.3 parts per million (ppm). Peaks: *1, 2,* and *3* assigned to β-, å-, and γ-ATP; *4,* phosphocreatine; *5,* inorganic phosphate; *6,* phosphomonoesters.
(From Kass, DA, et al: Magn Reson Med 4:85, 1987. Reproduced with permission.)

In vivo studies of ^{31}P MRS spectra from the liver may eventually result in clinical application. Recently we have shown that ^{31}P MRS can disclose changes in the phosphorus metabolism in the liver after a short period of hypoxia (Fig. 73-12).[42]

New techniques will be developed to localize spectra and make them suitable and valuable in the clinical environment. At that time clinicians will be able to use a new sphere of information to answer noninvasively many metabolic and physiologic questions concerning their patients.

REFERENCES

1. Ablow, RC, et al: Fluoroscopic dose reduction using a digital television noise-reduction device, Radiology 148:313, 1983.

2. Adler, DD, Glazer, GM, and Aisen, AM: MRI of the spleen: normal appearance and findings in sickle cell anemia, Am J Roentgenol 147:843, 1986.

3. Arasu, TS, et al: Gastroesophageal reflux in infants and children: comparative accuracy of diagnostic methods, J Pediatr 96:798, 1980.

4. Ball, TI, Atkinson, GO, Jr, and Gay, BB, Jr: Ultrasound diagnosis of hypertrophic pyloric stenosis: real-time application and the demonstration of a new sonographic sign, Radiology 147:503, 1983.

5. Baran, GW, et al: CT guided percutaneous biopsies in pediatric patients, Pediatr Radiol 14:161, 1984.

6. Berquist, WE, et al: Gastroesophageal reflux associated recurrent pneumonia and chronic asthma in children, Pediatrics 68:29, 1981.

7. Berger, PE, and Kuhn, JP: CT of blunt abdominal trauma in childhood, Am J Roentgenol 136:105, 1981.

8. Birch, SH, et al: Hepatic and splenic injury in children: role of CT in the decision for laparotomy, Radiology 165:643, 1987.

9. Brasch, RC: Ultrafast computed tomography for pediatric diagnosis. In Margulis, AR, and Gooding, CA, editors: Diagnostic radiology, Berkeley, 1987, University of California.

10. Brasch, RC, Boyd, DP, and Gooding, CA: Computed tomographic scanning in children: comparison of radiation dose and resolving power of commercial CT scanners, Am J Roentgenol 131:95, 1978.

11. Brasch, RC, et al: Magnetic resonance imaging of transfusional hemosiderosis complicating thalassemia major, Radiology 150: 767, 1984.

12. Brasch, RC, et al: Upper airway obstruction in infants and children: evaluation with ultrafast CT, Radiology 165:459, 1987.

13. Chervu, LR, Nunn, AD, and Loberg, MD: Radiopharmaceuticals for hepatobiliary imaging, Semin Nucl Med 12:5, 1982.

14. Day, DI, et al: MR evaluation of the portal vein in pediatric liver transplant candidates, Am J Roentgenol 147:1027, 1986.

15. Diament, MJ, Boechat, MI, and Kangarloo, H: Interventional radiology in infants and children: clinical and technical aspects, Radiology 154:359, 1985.

16. Diament, MJ, Stanley, P, and Taylor, S: Percutaneous fine needle biopsy in pediatrics, Pediatr Radiol 15:409, 1985.

17. Eurlich, CP, et al: Splenic scintigraphy using Tc-99m labelled heat denatured red blood cells in pediatric patients, J Nucl Med 23:209, 1982.

18. Fisher, MR, et al: Hepatic vascular anatomy in magnetic resonance imaging, Am J Roentgenol 144:739, 1985.

19. Fishman, EK, et al: CT evaluation of Crohn's disease: effect on patient management, Am J Roentgenol 148:537, 1987.

19a. Freeman, MH, and Tonkin, AK: Focal splenic effects, Radiology, 121:689, 1976.

20. Gooding, CA, et al: Magnetic resonance imaging in cystic fibrosis, J Pediatr 105:384, 1984.

21. Gordon, RA, et al: Intramural gastric hematoma in a hemophiliac with an inhibitor, Pediatrics 67:417, 1981.

22. Green, LL, et al: Evolution of pyloric stenosis in the first week of life, Pediatr Radiol 15:205, 1985.

23. Haller, JO, and Cohen, HL: Hypertrophic pyloric stenosis: diagnosis using US, Radiology 161:335, 1986.

24. Hayden, CK, Jr, Swischuk, LE, and Lobe, TE: Ultrasound: the definitive imaging modality in pyloric stenosis, Radiographics 4:517, 1984.

25. Heinrich, H, and Shuster, W: Reduction of dose by filtration in pediatric fluorscopy and fluorography (abstract), Radiology 122:285, 1977.

26. Heyman, S, et al: An improved method for the diagnosis of gastroesophageal reflux and aspiration in children (milk scan), Radiology 131:479, 1979.

27. Hynes, DM, et al: Clinical experience with combined video fluorography and pulsed fluoroscopy, Radiology 145:505, 1982.

28. Jeffrey, RB, et al: Abdominal CT in acquired immunodeficiency syndrome, Am J Roentgenol 146:7, 1986.

29. Jeffrey, RB, Laing, FC, and Lewis, FR: Acute appendicitis: high resolution real-time ultrasound findings, Radiology 16:311, 1987.

30. Kass, DA, et al: ^{31}P Magnetic resonance spectroscopy of mesenteric ischemia, Magn Reson Med 4:83, 1987.

31. Kodroff, MB, Hartenberg, MA, and Goldschmidt, RA: Ultrasonographic diagnosis of gangrenous bowel in neonatal necrotizing enterocolitis, Pediatr Radiol 14:168, 1984.

32. Kopen, PA, and McAlister, WH: Upper gastrointestinal and ultrasound examinations of gastric antral involvement in chronic granulomatous disease, Pediatr Radiol 14:91, 1984.

33. Malin, SW, et al: Echogenic intravascular and hepatic microbubbles associated with necrotizing enterocolitis, J Pediatr 103:637, 1983.

34. Merritt, CRB, Goldsmith, JP, and Sharp, MJ: Sonographic detection of portal venous gas in infants with necrotizing enterocolitis, Am J Roentgenol 143:1059, 1984.

35. Miller, JJ, and Kernherling, CR: Ultrasound scanning of the gastrointestinal tract in children, Radiology 152:671, 1984.

36. Patriquin, H, et al: Surgical portosystemic shunts in children: assessment with Duplex Doppler US, Radiology 165:25, 1987.

37. Riddlesberger, MM, Jr: CT of complicated inflammatory bowel disease in children, Pediatr Radiol 15:384, 1985.

38. Rossi, RP, Wesenberg, RL, and Hendee, WR: A variable aperture fluoroscopic unit for reduced patient exposure, Radiology 129:799, 1978.

39. Rudd, TG, and Christie, DL: Demonstration of GER in children by RN gastroesophagography, Radiology 131:483, 1979.

40. Schaller, RT, Jr, et al: The usefulness of percutaneous fine needle aspiration biopsy in infants and children, J Pediatr Surg 18:398, 1983.

41. Schmidt, HC, et al: Comparison of in vivo ^{31}P MR spectroscopy of the brain, liver, and kidney of adult and infant animals, Pediatr Radiol 16:144, 1986.

42. Schmidt, HC, Gooding, CA, and James, TC: In vivo ^{31}P magnetic resonance spectroscopy of the liver in the infant rabbit to study the effect of hypoxia on the phosphorus metabolites and intracellular pH, Invest Radiol 21:156, 1986.

43. Sfakianakis, GN, and Conway, JJ: Detection of ectopic gastric mucosa in Meckel's diverticulum and in other aberrations by scintigraphy. I. Pathophysiology and 10 year clinical experience, J Nucl Med 22:642, 1981.

44. Siegel, MJ, Martin, KW, and Worthington, JL: Normal and abnormal pancreas in children: US studies, Radiology 165:15, 1987.

45. Stanley, P, et al: Therapeutic embolization of infantile hepatic hemangioma with polyvinyl alcohol, Am J Roentgenol 141:1047, 1983.

46. Stark, DD, et al: Chronic liver disease evaluation by magnetic resonance, Radiology 150:149, 1984.

47. Stark, DD, et al: MRI of the Budd-Chiari syndrome, Am J Roentgenol 146:1141, 1986.

48. Stunden, RJ, LeQuesne, GW, and Little, KET: The improved ultrasound diagnosis of hypertrophic pyloric stenosis, Pediatr Radiol 16:200, 1986.

49. Swischuk, LE, Hayden, CK, and Boulder, T: Intussusception: indications for ultrasonography and an explanation of the donut and pseudo kidney signs, Pediatr Radiol 15:388, 1985.

50. Taguchi, T, et al: Percutaneous drainage for post-traumatic hepatic abscess in children under ultrasound imaging, Pediatr Radiol 18:85, 1988.

51. Tonkin, ILD, Urenn, EL, Jr, and Hollabaugh, RS: The continued value of angiography in planning surgical resection of benign and malignant hepatic tumors in children, Pediatr Radiol 18:35, 1988.

52. Treves, ST: Pediatric nuclear medicine, New York, 1985, Springer-Verlag.

53. Weinreb, JC, et al: Imaging the pediatric liver: MRI and CT, Am J Roentgenol 147:785, 1986.

54. Wesenberg, RL: Limiting radiation exposure a boon to pediatric imaging, Diagn Imaging, May 1987, p. 138.

55. Wesenberg, RL, and Amundson, GM: Fluoroscopy in children: low-exposure technology, Radiology 153:243, 1984.

56. Wilson, DA, and Vanhoutte, JJ: The reliable diagnosis of hypertrophic pyloric stenosis, JCU 12:201, 1984.

PART XVI

SPECIAL PROCEDURES

74 *Angiography of the Alimentary Tract*

FREDERICK S. KELLER
JOSEF RÖSCH

GENERAL CONSIDERATIONS

Since the last edition of this book, indications for diagnostic angiography of the abdominal viscera have decreased as a result of the expanding role of noninvasive imaging modalities. Currently, visceral angiography is requested to localize and frequently treat bleeding, palliate tumors, delineate vascular lesions, precisely demonstrate arterial anatomy before contemplated surgery, and further define known or suspected lesions when re-

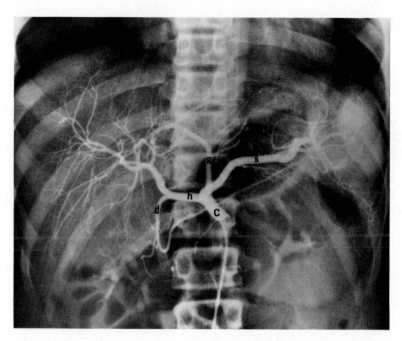

Fig. 74-1 Normal celiac arteriogram. Catheter is in celiac artery *(C)*. Splenic *(s)*, left gastric *(g)*, common hepatic *(h)*, and gastroduodenal *(d)* branches are demonstrated. In this patient, supply to left lobe of liver originates from left gastric artery.

sults of noninvasive imaging studies are conflicting or inconsistent with the patient's clinical findings. The angiographic features of many abnormalities in the alimentary tract have been well documented and may be encountered during angiographic studies performed for other reasons. Therefore it is important for the radiologist to recognize these angiographic findings and diagnose the pathologic conditions with which they are associated.

TECHNICAL NOTES

Before elective angiography the patient should be visited by the radiologist to explain the details of the examination and its potential risks and complications. Informed consent should be obtained at this time. A brief physical examination noting the quality of the femoral pulses and the presence of peripheral pulses is performed. The patient's chart is reviewed, and a note is placed in it stating that the patient understands the risks of the procedure and agrees to it. Circumstances that may increase the chance of complications, such as preexisting renal failure, hypertension, or coagulopathy, should be noted along with the reasons for proceeding with the angiogram in view of increased risk. In addition to routine preprocedure orders, a thorough bowel preparation can eliminate unwanted stool, gas, or barium and is useful when the examination is done to look for small, subtle visceral lesions. The patient is kept well hydrated before and after the angiogram.[26] All previous pertinent radio-

logic and ultrasound studies should be reviewed by the radiologist before the angiogram. Because visceral angiography is an expensive examination associated with a low but definite risk, it is essential that every effort be made to maximize diagostic information and patient benefit.

Visceral angiography is performed with the patient under local anesthesia. The retrograde femoral approach is most frequently used; however, in patients with either severe iliofemoral obstructive disease or vascular anatomy unsuitable for selective visceral catheterization from the femoral artery, the axillary approach is a suitable alternative.[3] A wide variety of preformed visceral angiographic catheter shapes are available for selective catheterization. In many angiographic facilities, steam or boiling water is used to tailor catheters to the patient's vascular anatomy when commercially available catheter shapes are unsuitable.

The basic technique in arteriography of the alimentary tract is *selective* catheterization and injection into the primary visceral branches of the aorta—the celiac, superior mesenteric, and inferior mesenteric arteries. Selective celiac arteriography demonstrates the liver, stomach, spleen, gallbladder, and portions of the duodenum and pancreas (Fig. 74-1). Superior mesenteric angiography opacifies the arteries supplying the remainder of the duodenum and pancreas as well as the small intestine and ascending and transverse colon (Fig. 74-2). Angi-

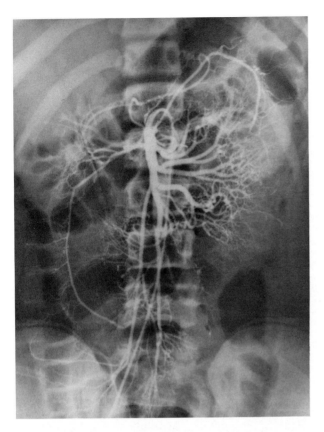

Fig. 74-2 Normal superior mesenteric arteriogram.

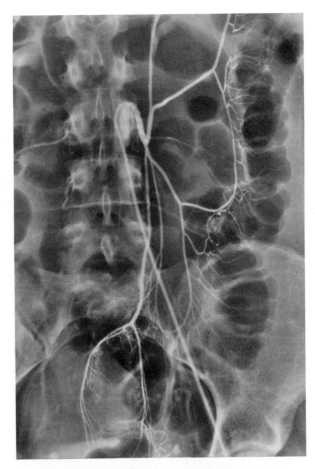

Fig. 74-3 Normal inferior mesenteric arteriogram.

ography of the inferior mesenteric artery visualizes the descending and sigmoid portions of the colon and rectum. (Fig. 74-3).

Selective arteriograms are often sufficient for diagnosis; however, when more detailed evaluation of specific vascular beds is required, *superselective* studies, with advancement of the catheter into secondary or tertiary branches of the visceral arteries, are necessary. Superselective catheterization with direct injection into the common hepatic or individual left and right hepatic branches; the left gastric, splenic, gastroduodenal arteries; or individual jejunal, ileal, or colic arteries yields better filling and visualization of arteries in these specific areas without the confusion of other superimposed arteries. This allows diagnosis of smaller lesions in their early stages[90] (Fig. 74-4). In the pancreas, which is fed by multiple arteries, superselective arteriography of some or occasionally all of the individual pancreatic arteries may be necessary.[80]

Further enhancement of diagnostic visceral angiography may be achieved using supplementary radiologic and pharmacologic methods. These include magnification arteriography for better spatial resolution and visualization of small vessels and subtraction techniques for increased contrast resolution.* Pharmacologic vasoactive drugs, both arterial dilators and constrictors, can be injected through the angiographic catheter immediately before injection of contrast material, either increasing or decreasing blood flow to the specific vascular bed under study.[32,79] Vasoconstriction frequently helps differentiate vasosensitive vessels of normal tissue from nonreactive vessels found in tumors.[38]

For visualization of the visceral veins, (portal system) *arterial portography* is most commonly used (Fig. 74-5). It consists of high-dose splenic or superior mesenteric arteriography with special attention directed to the venous phases. Either the splenic or superior mesenteric vein is opacified, depending on which artery was injected, with subsequent opacification of the main portal vein and its intrahepatic branches. Enhancement in portal vein opacification can be achieved by injection of tolazoline (25 to 50 mg) into the superior mesenteric artery 30 seconds before delivery of contrast material.[79] This drug causes

---

*References 16, 33, 41, 42, 68, 98.

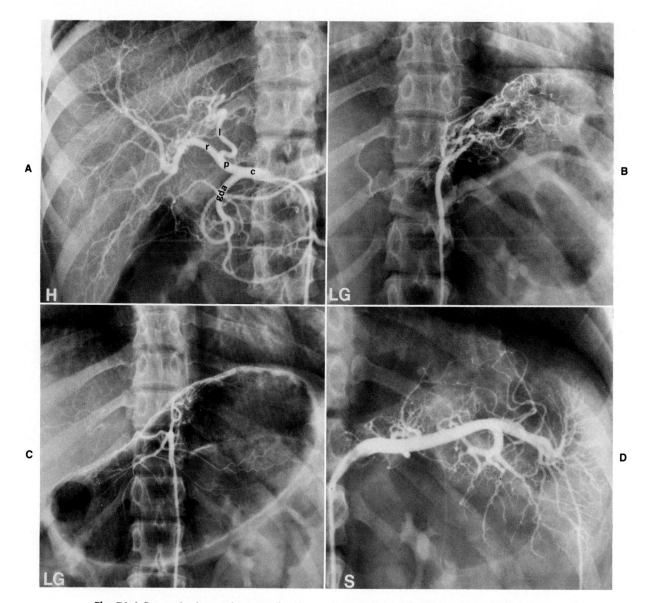

Fig. 74-4 Superselective angiograms of celiac artery branches. **A,** Normal common hepatic arteriogram. Catheter is in common hepatic artery *(c)*. Proper hepatic *(p)*, right hepatic *(r)*, left hepatic *(l)* and gastroduodenal *(gda)* arteries are demonstrated. **B,** Normal left gastric angiogram. **C,** Left gastric angiogram following gastric insufflation. **D,** Normal splenic angiogram.

dilatation of small submucosal arteriovenous connections, resulting in more rapid and denser opacification of the portal vein (Fig. 74-6).

Complications

In experienced hands, the complication rate of visceral angiography should be less than 0.5%.[43,45,106] Potential complications can be divided as to site of occurrence, that is, the vascular entry, the catheterized vessel, or systemic. Entry site complications include hematoma, vascular spasm, occlusion, pseudoaneurysm, and arteriovenous fistula. In the catheterized artery, complications of spasm, embolism, and subintimal dissection can occur. The radiologist must be prepared to treat vasovagal episodes, which are a common occurrence, as well as serious, life-threatening contrast reactions, which fortunately are unusual with intraarterial contrast administration. The systemic complication of renal failure results from administration of large amounts of contrast material. With adequate patient preparation, the risk of contrast-induced renal failure can be minimized. Such measures include mainly good hydration; judicious admin-

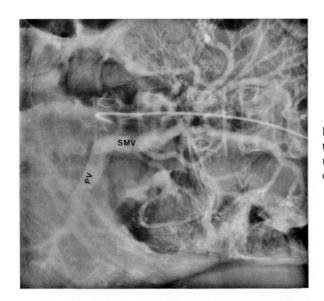

Fig. 74-5 Normal arterial portogram. Venous of superior mesenteric pharmacoangiography using tolazoline demonstrates prominent jejunal, ileal, and colic veins that empty into superior mesenteric vein *(SMV)*, which drains into portal vein *(PV)*.

Fig. 74-6 Cavernomatous transformation of portal vein. Extrahepatic portal vein occlusion is present. Multiple hepatopetal collaterals in liver hilus *(arrows)* drain into small intrahepatic portal branches. Large gastroesophageal varices are filled by hepatofugal flow in enlarged left gastric vein *(arrowheads)*.

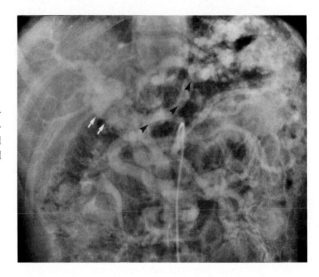

istration of contrast material; and, when indicated, dividing the angiographic study into two sessions in high-risk patients or not scheduling angiography immediately after another examination in which high doses of contrast material are given, such as computed tomography (CT).

GASTROINTESTINAL HEMORRHAGE

In 1960, arteriography was first reported to be useful in demonstrating a lesion responsible for recurrent gastrointestinal (GI) bleeding that had not been detected by conventional radiologic studies.[61] Since then it has played an important role in both the diagnosis and therapy of patients with GI hemorrhage.[5,88] Investigation of acute or chronic GI bleeding is one of the more common indications for angiography of the alimentary tract.

ACUTE GASTROINTESTINAL HEMORRHAGE

In the early 1960s, after angiography was initially introduced for localization of the site of acute GI hemorrhage, it was frequently the first procedure performed. This approach did not take into account the fact that approximately 75% to 80% of patients with acute GI hemorrhage will cease bleeding with bed rest and medical therapy consisting of blood and fluid replacement and correction of any coagulation defects. Today, the endoscope is the primary diagnostic modality for upper GI bleeding, and if varices are found, sclerotherapy can be initiated. Arteriography is only required if medical therapy is unsuccessful in controlling hemorrhage. In most patients who continue to bleed from the upper GI tract, the diagnosis has usually been established by endoscopy,

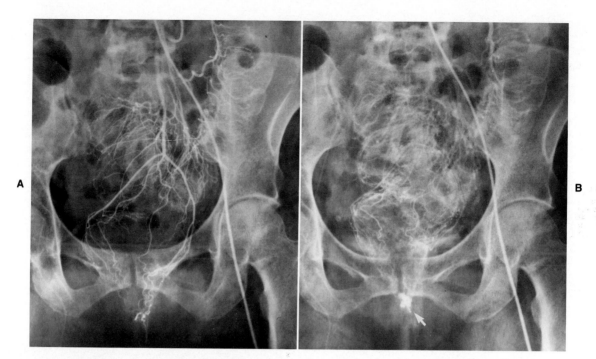

Fig. 74-7 Acute lower GI hemorrhage from distal rectum. During episodes of acute lower GI hemorrhage, blood travels both proximally and distally in alimentary tract. Flexible sigmoidoscopy performed during acute bleeding failed to localize this lesion on two separate occasions; fresh blood was reported to be visualized each time as high as splenic flexure. **A,** Early phase of selective IM arteriogram. **B,** Late phase. Extravasation *(arrow)* in distal rectum identifies bleeding site.

and the arteriogram is requested for catheter hemostasis. Endoscopy is less effective in diagnosing lesions responsible for acute lower GI hemorrhage, especially during an episode of active bleeding, and angiography is performed to localize as well as treat the bleeding lesion (Fig. 74-7).

Acute GI bleeding is frequently intermittent, and for the angiogram to be positive, the patient must be bleeding actively when contrast material is injected.[107] Therefore proper timing is crucial for successful localization of the artery responsible for hemorrhage and subsequent therapy. If the patient has ceased bleeding at a minimum rate of 0.5 ml/min when the contrast material is injected, the arteriogram will be negative.

In the upper GI tract, extent of bleeding is fairly easy to assess by means of lavage with a large-bore nasogastric tube: active bleeding is present if the lavage fluid continues to return bright red or pink after evacuation of clots. Other signs indicating active hemorrhage are tachycardia, hypotension, and a falling hematocrit after initial resuscitation.

In patients with acute lower GI bleeding it is more difficult to be certain that active bleeding is present at the time of angiography. Radionuclide scanning with technetium-labeled red blood cells or technetium-sulfur colloid can indicate the presence of active hemorrhage

at a rate of 0.1 ml/min.[1,2,62] Therefore if the radionuclide scan is negative, emergency arteriography need not be done. Isotope scanning thus has the potential to decrease the number of negative arteriograms and substantially increase the efficiency of angiography in patients with lower GI bleeding. If, however, the nuclear scan reveals a site of acute hemorrhage, emergency arteriography is indicated to determine the nature of the responsible lesion and institute some form of catheter therapy.

Because of its intermittent, minute-to-minute nature, acute lower GI bleeding often stops or decreases between a positive radionuclide scan and arteriography, or during the angiogram itself. If clinically active lower GI bleeding is present just before a negative arteriogram, recurrent active bleeding can sometimes be deliberately induced by injection of vasodilators, anticoagulants, or fibrinolytics.[96,97] These aggressive diagnostic interventions should be reserved for patients who pose severe diagnostic problems and for whom the risk of prolonging or reactivating hemorrhage is outweighed by the potential diagnostic benefits. Interventions to prolong or reactivate bleeding should be carried out only after discussion with the patient's gastroenterologist or surgeon and only on patients who are hemodynamically stable and for whom replacement blood is available.

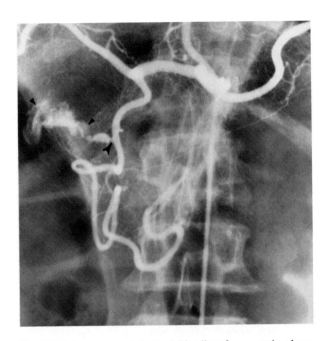

Fig. 74-8 Acute gastrointestinal bleeding from peptic ulcer. The ulcer has eroded into gastroduodenal artery *(large arrowhead)* causing extravasation of contrast material into lumen of duodenum *(small arrowheads)*.

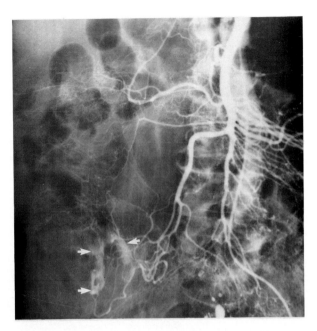

Fig. 74-9 Acute gastrointestinal bleeding from colonic diverticulum. Superior mesenteric arteriography demonstrates acute extravasation of contrast material *(arrows)* from bleeding cecal diverticulum.

Arterial bleeding—diagnosis

The angiographic diagnosis of acute arterial bleeding rests on the visualization of direct extravasation of contrast material into the GI lumen (Fig. 74-8). When bleeding is from a large artery, such as in peptic ulcers or colonic diverticuli, it is readily demonstrated by selective arteriograms (Fig. 74-9). If, however, bleeding is from a minor source or multiple capillary sites, such as in erosive gastritis or multiple stress ulcers, selective studies may not be sufficient to demonstrate the hemorrhage. Superselective studies are required in these instances.

Venous bleeding—diagnosis

Diagnosis of acute variceal hemorrhage is for the most part made by endoscopy, and the majority of these patients only undergo visceral angiography before a contemplated surgical portosystemic shunt procedure. In the unusual instance when endoscopy cannot be performed, acute upper GI bleeding from esophageal varices can be diagnosed by angiography. Because extravasation of contrast material is not demonstrable by simple arterial portography, the angiographic diagnosis of variceal hemorrhage is based on the following criteria: (1) visualization of varices during the venous phases of splenic injection or superior mesenteric or left gastric pharmacoangiograms following administration of tolazoline, and

(2) exclusion of arterial or capillary bleeding sites[82] (Fig. 74-10). The latter is important, because in some series it has been shown that approximately 40% of bleeding episodes in cirrhotic patients with known varices are caused by arterial or capillary sources such as Mallory-Weiss tears, gastritis, or peptic ulcers.

ANGIOGRAPHIC CONTROL OF ACUTE GASTROINTESTINAL HEMORRHAGE

Precise localization of the bleeding artery is the first step in catheter therapy of acute GI hemorrhage. It has been shown in patients with gastric hemorrhage that supply to the bleeding lesion was from the left gastric artery in 85% of cases.[27] The right gastric and short gastric arteries each supplied the bleeding site in 5% of cases. The remaining 5% of cases had supply from the gastroepiploeic arteries (3%), gastroduodenal artery (1%), and phrenic artery (1%).[52] Duodenal bleeding may be supplied by either the gastroduodenal or inferior pancreatiocodeuodenal artery or a combination of these. Small bowel and colonic hemorrhage originate from the various branches of the superior and inferior mesenteric arteries that supply the area of the bleeding lesion. Distal rectal or anal bleeding may have a dual supply: superior hemorrhoidal branches of the inferior mesenteric artery and/or middle hemorrhoidal branches of the internal iliac arteries.

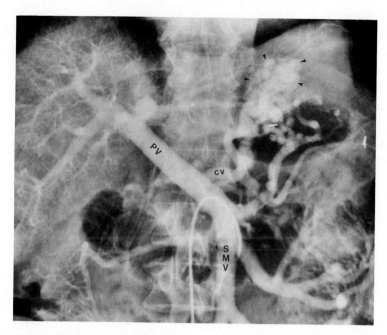

Fig. 74-10 Demonstration of portal hypertension and esophageal varices in patient with upper GI hemorrhage. Venous phase of superior mesenteric pharmacoangiography with tolazoline reveals hepatopetal flow in superior mesenteric vein *(SMV)* and portal vein *(PV)* and hepatofugal flow in coronary vein *(cv)* leading to gastroesophageal varices *(arrowheads)*.

Vasoconstrictive infusion therapy

Vasopressin, an octapeptide produced in the neurohypophysis, has a variety of pharmacologic actions. One of these, smooth muscle contraction, is most important for its use in controlling GI bleeding. Vasopressin-induced smooth muscle contraction in the walls of arterioles causes vasoconstriction, and smooth muscle contraction in the bowel wall compresses the penetrating blood vessels. Vasopressin is infused selectively into the bleeding artery at a dose ranging from 0.1 to 0.4 U/min depending on the rate of bleeding and arterial size. Infusion is continued over 12 to 36 hours while the dose is gradually tapered. If there is no recurrence of bleeding, the catheter is kept open with normal saline or 5% dextrose solution for an additional 12 hours before its removal. Vasopressin infusion is frequently successful in controlling bleeding from superficial gastric lesions such as Mallory-Weiss tears, hemorrhagic gastritis, and stress ulcers.[6,25,49,53] Diverticula and angiodysplasias, the lesions most commonly responsible for massive acute colonic hemorrhage, are both quite responsive to vasopressin infusion[6,49,53] (Fig. 74-11). Once hemorrhage from a bleeding diverticulum has been controlled, its recurrence is unlikely, and surgery can often be avoided. Angiodysplasias tend to rebleed periodically, and therefore resection is usually indicated after hemorrhage has been controlled and the patient stabilized. If the bleeding lesion is near the splenic flexure its blood supply may come from both the superior and inferior mesenteric arteries. In such instances infusions of both arteries may be required to control active bleeding.

Vasoconstrictive infusion therapy is substantially less effective in controlling hemorrhage from the duodenum than from the stomach, small bowel, or colon.[118] Three reasons have been proposed for this difference in effectiveness. One is the dual blood supply to the duodenum from the celiac and the superior mesenteric arteries; infusion of only one limb of the arcade is frequently ineffective, because the lesion continues to bleed from the opposite side. Second, vasopressin has its greatest effect on small vessels; however, duodenal hemorrhage often is caused by erosion of larger arteries that do not respond with vasoconstriction when exposed to vasopressin. Finally, chronic inflammation caused by peptic disease limits the ability of arteries in close proximity to the ulcer to constrict as well as impairing the contractility of the adjacent duodenal wall.

If endoscopic control of bleeding with either electrocoagulation or the heater probe has been attempted, vascular contractility in the area of the lesion will be impaired, rendering vasopressin infusion ineffective. The radiologist who performs visceral angiography for diagnosis and management of GI bleeding should be familiar with the potential side effects and complications of vasopression therapy. These include hyponatremia, oliguria, hypertension, fluid overload, arrhythmias, and ischemia of the myocardium, bowel, or distal extremities.

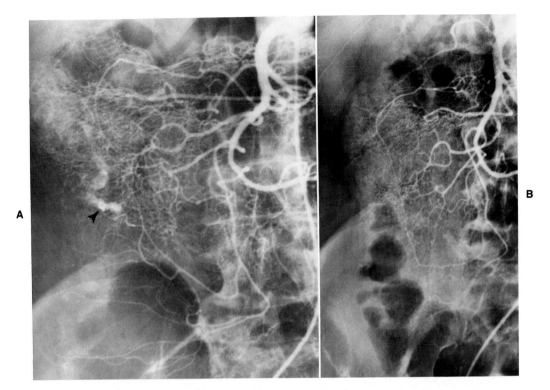

Fig. 74-11 Bleeding diverticulum of ascending colon controlled with vasopressin infusion: **A,** Active hemorrhage is present on initial arteriogram *(arrowhead)*. **B,** Following infusion of 0.3 units of vasopressin for 20 minutes, no hemorrhage is evident. Branches of superior mesenteric artery are constricted.

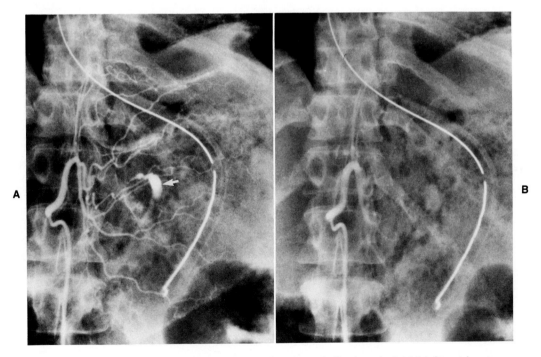

Fig. 74-12 Control of acutely bleeding gastric ulcer by embolization. **A,** Initial left gastric arteriogram demonstrates acute hemorrhage from ulcer on posterior gastric wall *(arrow)*. **B,** Follow-up arteriography after embolization with Gelfoam particles shows occlusion of major branches of left gastric artery. Bleeding has ceased.

Embolotherapy

Since its introduction as a therapeutic modality in the management of GI bleeding in the early 1970s, the indications for embolization have broadened.[40,58,59] Initially reserved as a last-ditch measure in high-risk patients, embolization without an initial trial of vasoconstrictive therapy is now preferred by many radiologists.[40] The goal of embolotherapy is to decrease the blood pressure at the site of the bleeding lesion and allow a stable clot to form without causing tissue ischemia or necrosis. Compared to vasopressin infusion, embolotherapy has the advantages of being completed rapidly and avoiding the problems of long-term arterial catheters and the multiple undesirable pharmacologic side effects of vasopressin (Fig. 74-12). However, embolization is not without risk, and unlike vasopressin, which can be decreased or discontinued at the first signs of untoward side effects, embolic particles cannot be retrieved once they are injected.

Embolic materials vary with the preference of the individual radiologist. Because GI hemorrhage is usually caused by benign, self-limiting lesions, surgical gelatin or Gelfoam, a temporary vasoocclusive agent, is widely used. Recanalization usually occurs in 1 to 3 weeks. Cut into small pieces and mixed with contrast medium, the Gelfoam is slowly injected under fluoroscopic control. Permanent embolic materials are usually reserved for hemorrhage from invasion of the GI tract by primary or secondary malignancies.

Until recently, embolotherapy for the management of acute GI hemorrhage has been limited to the upper GI tract (gastroesophageal junction, stomach, and duodenum). Because of its rich collateral supply, individual branches can be occluded with an almost negligible risk of ischemic complications. However, if collateral blood supply has been compromised by previous surgical ligations or severe atherosclerotic obstructive disease, the risk of infarction is increased.

The dual blood supply and large arteries involved in duodenal bleeding makes successful embolotherapy more difficult. Frequently, simple embolization of the gastroduodenal artery will be sufficient to control bleeding. However, when peptic erosion has caused large defects in the gastroduodenal artery, small paticles of Gelfoam are frequently ineffective, because they pass directly through the hole in the artery into the duodenal lumen. When this occurs, placement of coil springs distal and proximal to the arterial defect or sealing it with cyanoacrylate is often successful in stopping hemorrhage (Fig. 74-13).

In the mesenteric circulation, collateral pathways are less well developed than in the upper GI tract. Thus embolization has traditionally been reserved for life-threatening lower GI hemorrhage in high-risk surgical patients who fail to respond to vasopressin therapy. However, in the last decade careful embolization of lesions responsible for lower GI bleeding has been advocated by

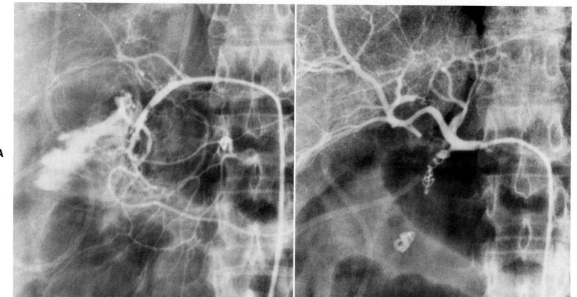

Fig. 74-13 Control of acute hemorrhage from duodenal ulcer. **A,** Marked extravasation caused by massive bleeding is present on initial gastroduodenal arteriogram. Patient is in hypovolemic shock as evidenced by intense vasoconstriction of common hepatic artery. **B,** Follow-up arteriogram after placement of coilspring occluders both distal and proximal to the peptic erosion of gastroduodenal artery reveals control of hemorrhage. Clinically, bleeding had ceased, and caliber of hepatic artery is now normal.

some radiologists.[15,36,76] Good results have been achieved in controlling lower GI hemorrhage, especially from diverticuli that have not rebled after embolization.[36] Because the incidence of ischemic complications following mesenteric embolization is significantly greater than after embolization in the upper GI tract, patients are closely monitored for several days after embolotherapy for signs of peritoneal irritation, suggesting transmural infarction and requiring operation.[70] If surgery is necessary, the patient will have already been hemodynamically stabilized and the operation will be done on an elective basis rather than as an emergency procedure on an acutely bleeding, unstable patient.

Variceal hemorrhage—therapy

Selective infusions of low doses (0.2 to 0.4 U/min) of vasopressin into the superior mesenteric artery were originally demonstrated to be effective in decreasing portal pressure and blood flow and successful in stopping hemorrhage in a significant number of patients with portal hypertension and bleeding esophageal varices.[73] Several years later it was proven both in experimental animals and in randomized clinical trials with patients bleeding from esophageal varices that low-dose peripheral intravenous infusions of vasopressin are as effective in reducing portal pressure and blood flow as selective superior mesenteric arterial infusion.[8] Therefore selective arterial vasopressin has been replaced by simpler, less invasive, intravenous administration.

Transhepatic obliteration of bleeding gastroesophageal varices was introduced in 1974 as a better alternative than emergency portosystemic shunting to stop variceal hemorrhage when medical therapy has failed.[54,59,115] This technique involves transhepatic portal vein catheterization and venographic demonstration of the portal anatomy. All branches feeding the gastroesophageal varices are then selectively catheterized and occluded. The rationale for transhepatic variceal obliteration is that occlusion of the life-threatening portosystemic collaterals, the esophageal varices, will promote formation of new or enlargement of preexisting, beneficial, less ominous portosystemic pathways.

Visceral arteriography should be performed before transhepatic variceal obliteration to exlude portal vein occlusion or a hypervascular liver lesion in the proposed catheter tract. Occlusion of the portal vein seen on the venous phase of splenic or superior mesenteric arteriography is a contraindication to transhepatic variceal obliteration, because advancement of the catheter from the intrahepatic into the extrahepatic portal venous system would not be possible.

Though transhepatic variceal obliteration has been shown to be successful in controlling variceal hemorrhage in 85% to 100% of patients, technical difficulties involved in its performance and a high incidence of re-

current variceal hemorrhage have prevented its widespread use. With the development of endoscopic sclerosis of esophageal varices, the indications for transhepatic variceal obliteration have declined. Currently, the technique is reserved for those who fail endoscopic sclerotherapy and continue to bleed. Successful transhepatic obliteration of varices in this group of patients buys valuable time for stabilization of hemodynamic and metabolic parameters in preparation for elective portosystemic shunt surgery.

CHRONIC GASTROINTESTINAL HEMORRHAGE

Unlike acute GI bleeding, with its dramatic presentations of hematemesis, hematochezia, or melena, patients with chronic GI hemorrhage present with occult fecal blood and iron deficiency anemia. Occasionally, recurrent, brief episodes of massive hemorrhage are present. Usually the diagnosis of some type of tumor is made in these patients by barium or endoscopic examinations of the upper GI tract and colon. Angiography is used only for patients who continue to bleed despite negative barium and endoscopic studies. For patients with chronic GI bleeding, a positive angiogram will usually reveal some form of hypervascular lesion rather than extravasation of contrast material into the lumen of the GI tract. A significant number of patients with chronic or recurrent lower GI bleeding will remain undiagnosed even after competently performed arteriography.[104]

Angiodysplasia

Known variously as telangiectasias, angiomas, vascular ectasias, angiodysplasias, and arteriovenous malformations, these lesions are commonly responsible for lower GI bleeding, especially in the elderly.[9,101,109] They are seen more frequently in patients with aortic and mitral valvular disease or with hereditary hemorrhagic telangiectasia (Fig. 74-14). Pathologically, angiodysplasias are clusters of ectatic submucosal vascular spaces. These lesions are not visible on barium examinations; however, they can occasionally be seen during colonoscopy. Their angiographic appearance varies with their size. Slight dilatation of the distal portion of the feeder with a minimally enlarged early draining vein may be quite subtle, and may be the only findings in smaller lesions (Fig. 74-15). Larger angiodysplasias have a tangle of vessels, the vascular tuft or nidus, which is opacified in the early arterial phase of the angiogram and empties into a prominent, early, and dense vein that fills and drains (Fig. 74-16).

Discovery of an angiodysplasia does not imply that it is the source of recurrent hemorrhage, because this type of lesion is often present in elderly patients who are not bleeding. The lesion may also be entirely coincidental in

Text continued on p. 1886.

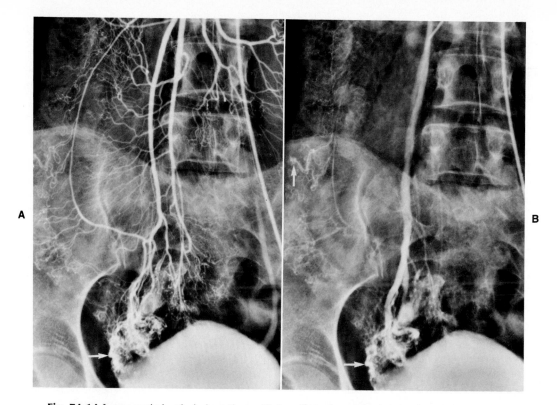

Fig. 74-14 Large angiodysplasia in patient with hereditary hemorrhagic telangiectasia. Early **(A)** and intermediate **(B)** phases of superior mesenteric arteriogram demonstrate large angiodysplasia *(large arrow)* in cecum. Venous drainage is prominent and early, while remainder of colon is still in late arterial phase. Another, much smaller angiodysplasia *(small arrow)* is present in ascending colon.

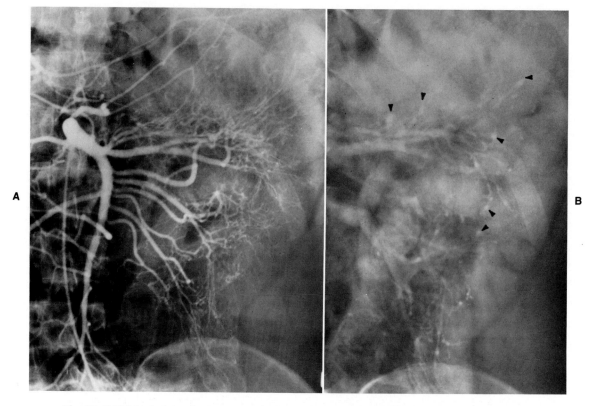

Fig. 74-15 Multiple jejunal telangiectasias. **A,** Arterial phase of superior mesenteric arteriogram is normal. **B,** Early venous drainage from jejunal branches with multiple small telangiectasias (some marked by *arrowheads*) present in distribution of proximal jejunum during late arterial phase. Following segmental jejunal resection, patient's chronic lower GI tract bleeding was cured.

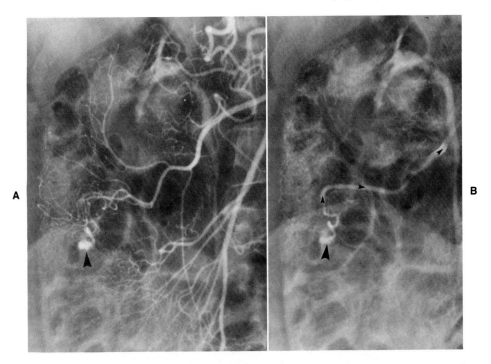

Fig. 74-16 Angiodysplasia of right colon. Early **(A)** and intermediate **(B)** phases of superior mesenteric arteriogram reveal vascular tuft *(large arrowhead)* of angiodysplasia. Prominent and intense venous drainage *(small arrowheads)* is present from angiodysplasia, while remainder of colon is still in late arterial phase of angiogram.

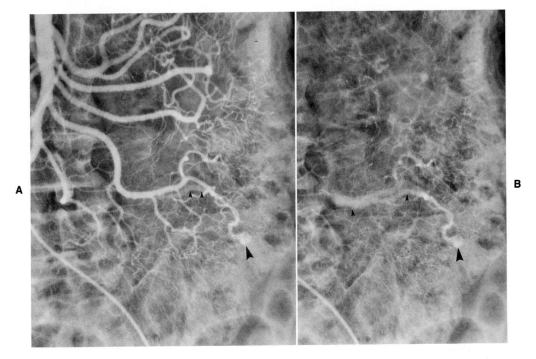

Fig. 74-17 Small bowel angiodysplasia. Early **(A)** and intermediate **(B)** arterial phases of superior mesenteric arteriography reveal vascular tuft *(large arrowhead)* of angiodysplasia. Early draining vein is present in early arterial phase *(small arrowheads)* and seen from better advantage during middle arterial phase. Incidentally, in **A,** standing waves in several jejunal branches are noted.

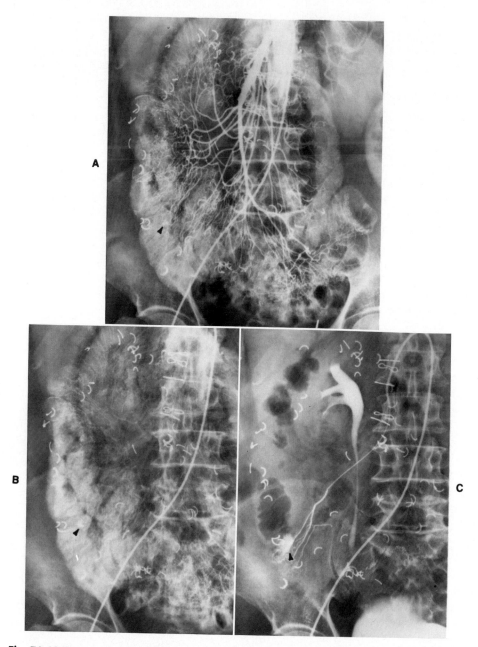

Fig. 74-18 Preoperative localization of small bowel angiodysplasia in patient with chronic lower GI bleeding following right and left hemicolectomy. Early (**A**) and late (**B**) arterial phases of superior mesenteric arteriogram reveal small angiomatous lesion *(arrowhead)* that is bleeding slowly. **C,** Immediately before surgery, No. 3 French catheter was placed into ileal branch that supplied area of bleeding lesion.

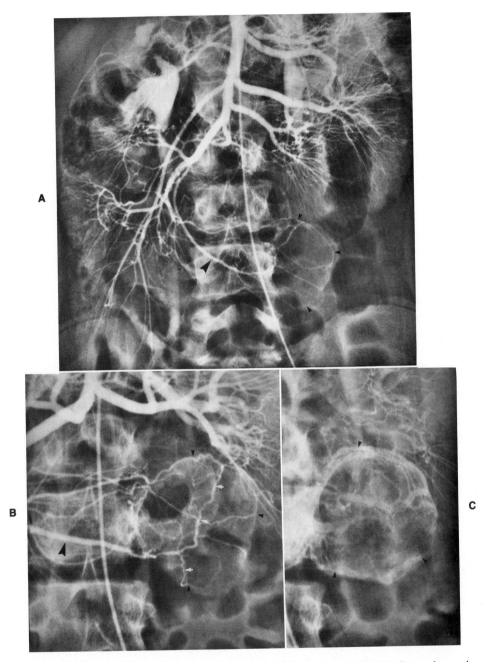

Fig. 74-19 Meckel's diverticulum in young patient with chronic lower GI tract hemorrhage. **A,** Selective superior mesenteric arteriogram demonstrates enlarged, nonbranching embryonic ileal artery (*large arrowhead,* also in **B**) leading to Meckel's diverticulum *(small arrowheads).* **B,** Early phase of superselective magnification arteriogram of ileal artery supplying diverticulum demonstrates irregular arteries in wall of Meckel's diverticulum *(small white arrows),* remnants of vitelline arteries. **C,** Late phase reveals increased parenchymal blush in wall of Meckel's diverticulum *(small arrowheads)* caused by accumulation of contrast material in its lining (gastric mucosa).

patients with chronic hemorrhage. The entire angiogram should therefore be carefully examined for any other lesion that may be the source of bleeding; if none is found, the area containing the angiodysplasia should be resected.

Precise preoperative localization of angiodysplasias is required, because these lesions can neither be seen or palpated at surgery. The diagnostic angiogram is usually sufficient for localization of colonic angiodysplasias, since the colon is a fixed structure. Jejunal and ileal angiodysplasias are often difficult to find at surgery, because once the bowel is eviscerated for inspection at surgery, the spatial relationships between individual bowel loops change (Fig. 74-17). Therefore, for these angiodysplasias, intraoperative localization is usually necessary to prevent resection of uninvolved bowel. It is performed by placing a small, No. 3 French catheter into the main feeding artery of the angiodysplasia just before surgery (Fig. 74-18). After angiographic confirmation of correct positioning of the catheter, the patient is taken to surgery. With the bowel exposed, 1 ml of methylene blue dye is injected into the catheter to stain the segment of bowel containing the angiodysplasia.[7]

Surgical resection is the primary form of therapy for angiodysplasias causing recurrent GI bleeding. Acute bleeding episodes can almost always be controlled with vasopressin infusion, but rebleeding usually occurs. Rebleeding from angiodysplasias treated by embolization has also been reported.[102]

Meckel's diverticulum

Meckel's diverticulum is a common cause of both chronic and acute lower GI bleeding in young patients.[65] Because of the ectopic gastric mucosa found in many Meckel's diverticuli, patients frequently present with melena even though the lesion is located in the distal ileum. Extravasation of contrast material is demonstrated in the distal small bowel on arteriography performed during an episode of acute hemorrhage from Meckel's diverticulum. If the angiogram is performed when the paient is not actively bleeding, an enlarged, long, nonbranching, embryonic ileal artery leading to the diverticulum is often present. Additional angiographic findings include irregular arteries in the wall of the diverticulum, remnants of vitelline arteries, and an increased parenchymal blush from the lining of gastric mucosa (Fig. 74-19).

VASCULAR DISEASES OF THE GASTROINTESTINAL TRACT
Atherosclerosis

Visceral atherosclerosis, though frequently seen during arteriography in older patients, is generally considered an incidental finding and of little clinical significance (Fig. 74-20). Narrowing of the arterial lumen from ath-

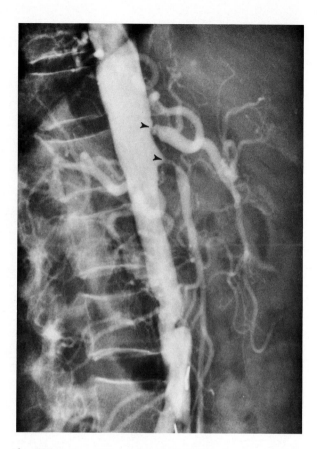

Fig. 74-20 A and B Asymptomatic visceral artery stenoses. Lateral aortography demonstrates significant stenoses of celiac and superior mesenteric arteries *(arrowheads)*. Despite these stenoses and occlusion of inferior mesenteric artery, patient was asymptomatic.

erosclerotic plaque and arterial dilatation, eventually leading to aneurysm formation, are the characteristic angiographic changes of atherosclerotic disease.

Stenoses or occlusions of individual visceral arteries can result from atherosclerotic plaque developing in the artery itself, by aortic plaque encroaching on the arterial ostia, or from involvement of the arterial origins by an abdominal aortic aneurysm. The latter mechanism is responsible for the high percentage of occluded inferior mesenteric arteries seen in patients with aneurysms of the abdominal aorta. Occlusion of any visceral vessel is not likely to cause ischemia as long as the others remain free from obstruction because of the excellent collateral circulation between them (Fig. 74-21). Collateral flow to the inferior mesenteric artery, the branch most frequently occluded, is from the superior mesenteric artery through anastomoses between the middle and left colic arteries via the marginal artery of Drummond, as well as from the internal iliac arteries through middle hemorrhoidal branches. Collateral circulation through the

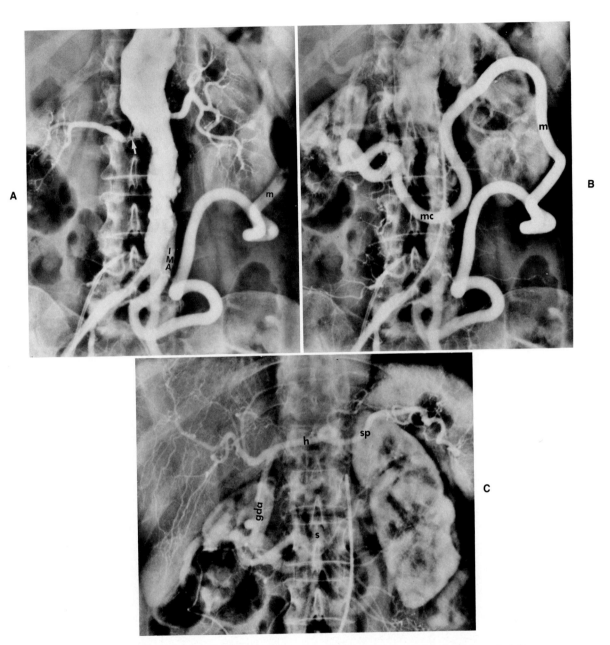

Fig. 74-21 Visceral artery occlusions. **A,** Abdominal aortography demonstrates suprarenal abdominal aortic aneurysm with occlusion of celiac and superior mesenteric arteries. High-grade stenosis *(arrow)* of right renal artery is decreased in size. Inferior mesenteric artery *(IMA)* is markedly enlarged with retrograde flow through marginal artery *(m)*. **B,** During later phase of angiographic sequence marginal artery *(m)* supplies blood in retrograde direction to middle colic (mc) artery. **C,** Later films in aortographic sequence demonstrate retrograde filling of superior mesenteric artery *(s)* via middle colic artery and gastroduodenal artery *(gda)*, which feeds hepatic *(h)* and splenic *(sp)* arteries.

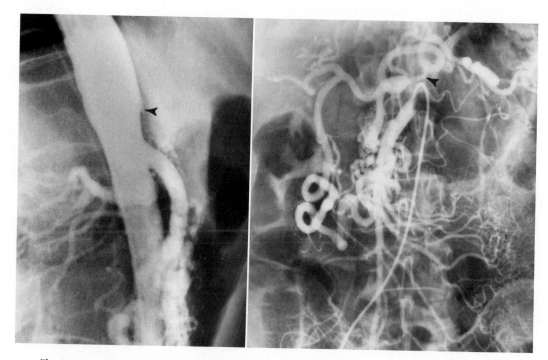

Fig. 74-22 Celiac occlusion with collaterals from superior mesenteric artery. **A,** Lateral aortography demonstrates celiac occlusion *(arrowhead).* **B,** Celiac artery and its branches are filled by selective superior mesenteric arteriography through prominent pancreaticoduodenal collaterals. Occluded celiac fills in retrograde fashion to its origin *(arrowhead).*

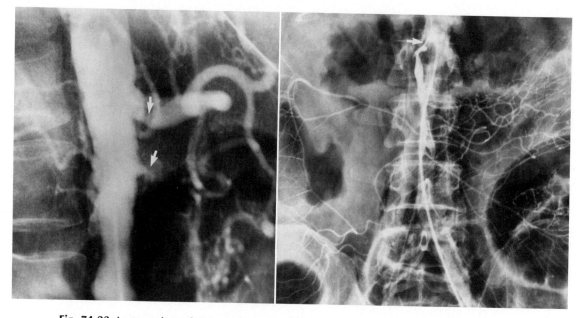

Fig. 74-23 Aortography and superior mesenteric arteriography in patient with abdominal angina. **A,** Lateral aortogram reveals tight stenosis *(arrow)* of celiac artery and occlusion *(arrow)* of superior mesenteric artery. **B,** Selective superior mesenteric arteriography with catheter tip inserted just distal to occlusion reveals marked stenosis near origin of superior mesenteric artery *(arrow)* with attenuated superior mesenteric arterial branches.

pancreaticoduodenal arcades and other pancreatic arteries supplies either the celiac or superior mesenteric arteries whenever the origin of one develops a significant stenosis or occlusion (Fig. 74-22). Nonsplanchnic collaterals to an obstructed celiac artery can originate from the phrenic and adrenal arteries.

Abdominal angina

The syndrome of abdominal angina is characterized by abdominal pain after eating that is often relieved by nitroglycerine, weight loss, anorexia, diarrhea, and occasionally nausea and vomiting. It occurs when increased postprandial visceral blood flow requirements cannot be met because of fixed obstructions (tight stenoses or occlusions) of two or more visceral arteries. Occasionally it can signal imminent bowel infarction.

In patients with suspected abdominal angina, the angiographic examination should begin with a lateral aortogram. A positive study usually reveals stenoses or occlusions of one or more splanchnic branches without evidence of well-developed collateral circulation (Fig. 74-23). Selective angiography of less involved visceral branches helps to assess collateral circulation when major obstructive disease is present on the lateral aortogram. It should be emphasized that similar aortographic findings of tight stenoses or occlusion of one or more visceral branches may be found serendipitously in asymptomatic patients. This discrepancy between the severity of vascular disease and the presence or absence of clinical symptoms makes angiographic evaluation of patients with suspected abdominal angina more difficult.

Traditionally, treatment for abdominal angina has been surgical endarterectomy of the celiac or superior mesenteric arteries or bypass to the superior mesenteric and occasionally to the hepatic arteries[120] (Fig. 74-24). Recently, transluminal angioplasty of stenotic visceral branches has been successfully used to treat patients with abdominal angina[19,37] (Fig. 74-25).

Visceral embolism

Most acute emboli to the visceral circulation originate from cardiac sources, either mural thrombi or diseased prosthetic valves. Smaller emboli travel distally until they lodge, usually at arterial branching points (Fig. 74-26). Large emboli occlude major arterial trunks.[51] Angiographic findings of emboli are an abrupt cutoff of the column of contrast material or a filling defect in the lumen of the artery with contrast streaming around it. Contrast material frequently stays in the occluded artery proximal to the embolus, and parenchymal filling downstream is decreased (Fig. 74-27). Acute mesenteric embolus is usually a surgical emergency. Fibrinolytic therapy has been used successfully to treat mesenteric emboli.[29] How-

ever, if the degree of intestinal ischemia is sufficiently severe, the time required for adquate fibrinolysis may be too great to prevent intestinal infarction.

Nonocclusive mesenteric ischemia

Intense vasoconstriction of the mesenteric arteries without evidence of obstruction is the primary angiographic finding in nonocclusive mesenteric ischemia.[105] It is found in elderly patients with low cardiac flow states and often leads to intestinal infarction. Nonocclusive mesenteric ischemia is associated with myocardial infarctions, congestive heart failure, or recent major abdominal or thoracic surgery. Frequently, a history of digitalis ingestion is present. Because of the high mortality associated with this condition, early diagnosis is essential.

Angiography in patients with nonocclusive mesenteric ischemia demonstrates severe vasoconstriction of the superior mesenteric artery and its branches. Peripheral mesenteric branches fill very slowly or not at all, and segments of bowel appear to lack perfusion. A beaded appearance of individual superior mesenteric arterial branches with areas of constriction and dilatation can be seen as the syndrome progresses. Treatment consists of aggressive medical therapy to increase cardiac output and correction of decreased intravascular fluid volume. Tolazoline, 50 mg, may be injected into the superior mesenteric artery and the angiogram repeated to look for a vasodilatory response. Relief of vasospasm seen on the angiogram after tolazoline is given is a good indication that the process is still reversible. Vasodilator therapy with papaverine infused at 1 mg/min is then continued for 24 to 36 hours, while the patient is closely monitored for clinical signs of bowel infarction[105] (Fig. 74-28). On the other hand, lack of response to the initial injection of tolazoline suggests that irreversible ischemic changes have already occurred.

Median arcuate ligament syndrome

Occasionally the median arcuate ligament of the diaphragm compresses the proximal portion of the celiac artery. The compression is maximal in full expiration, and there is a decrease in or even a disappearance of the narrowing during inspiration.[81] Median arcuate ligament syndrome is most often seen in slender young females and is frequently associated with an epigastric bruit that may change in character during the respiratory cycle. Findings of this syndrome are either celiac occlusion or a concave stenosis along the superior aspect of the celiac artery close to its origin seen on lateral aortography performed during maximum expiration (Fig. 74-29). If the aortogram is repeated during deep inspiration, the ob-

Text continued on p. 1894.

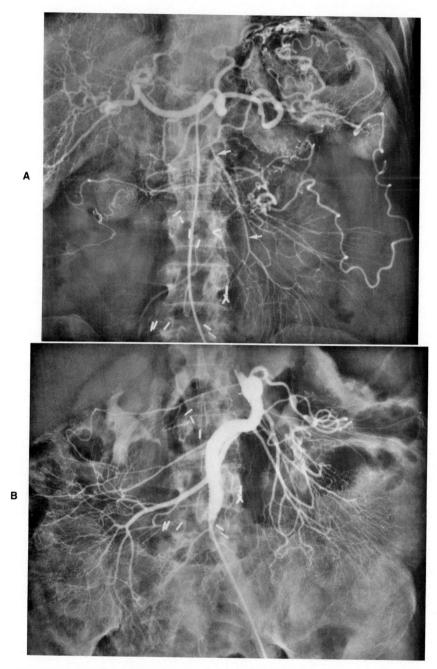

Fig. 74-24 Abdominal angina treated by superior mesenteric arterial bypass grafting. **A,** Selective celiac arteriography demonstrates collateral filling of attenuated superior mesenteric artery *(arrows)*. All branches of superior mesenteric artery are small and underperfused. **B,** Following distal aortic-to-superior mesenteric bypass, main superior mesenteric arterial trunk is normal in caliber, and its branches are well filled.

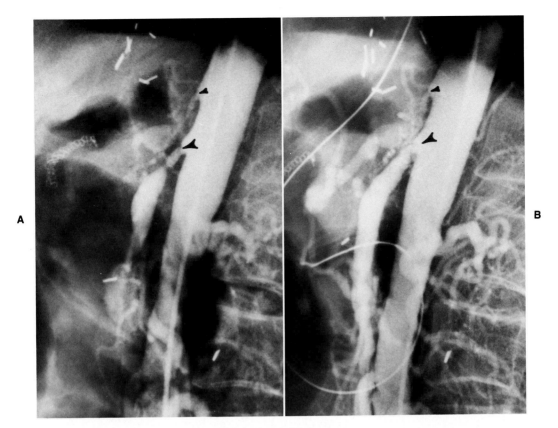

Fig. 74-25 Abdominal angina treated by transluminal angioplasty. **A,** Control lateral aortography demonstrated occlusion of celiac artery *(small arrowhead,* also in **B)** with very tight stenosis of superior mesenteric artery *(large arrowhead).* **B,** Following percutaneous transluminal angioplasty, stenosis of superior mesenteric artery is considerably reduced *(large arrowhead).*

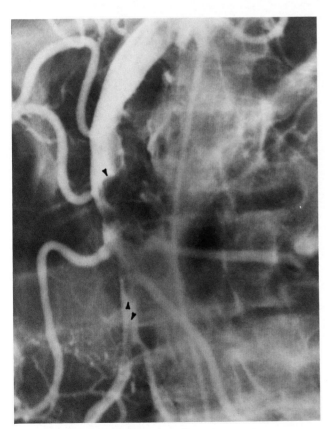

Fig. 74-26 Partially occluding mesenteric embolus. Superior mesenteric arteriography demonstrates multiple filling defects *(arrowheads)* within main trunk of superior mesenteric artery and extending into its branches.

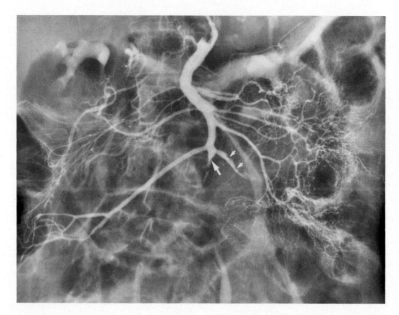

Fig. 74-27 Mesenteric embolus. There is abrupt occlusion of ileocolic branch of superior mesenteric artery *(large arrow)*. Occlusion of large ileal branch is also present *(small arrows)*.

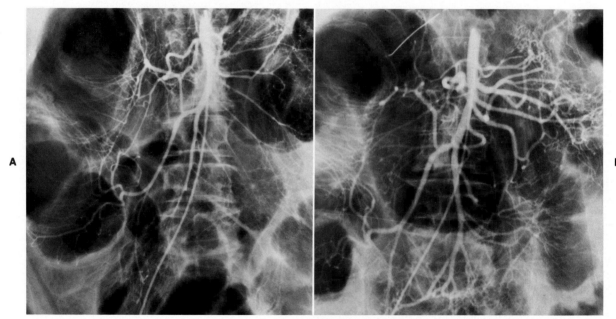

Fig. 74-28 Nonocclusive mesenteric ischemia. **A,** Superior mesenteric arteriogram in patient following coronary artery bypass reveals intense peripheral vasoconstriction of jejunal and ileal branches. **B,** Follow-up arteriogram 24 hours after infusion of papaverine reveals relief of vasospasm with normal caliber of jejunal and ileal branches and excellent perfusion of small bowel.

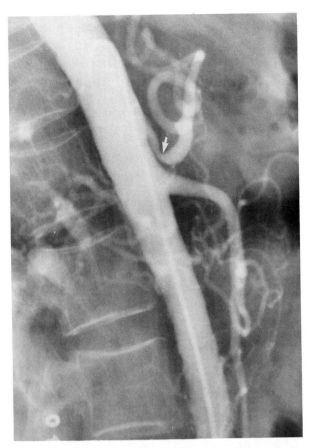

Fig. 74-29 Median arcuate ligament syndrome. Lateral aortography reveals smooth, concave stenosis along superior aspect of proximal portion of celiac artery *(arrow)*.

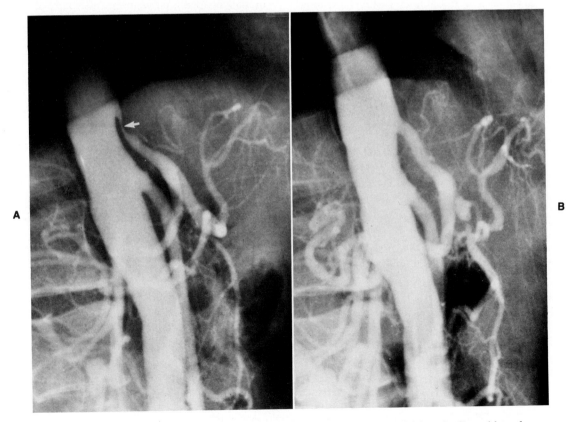

Fig. 74-30 Median arcuate ligament syndrome before and after surgery division. **A,** Control lateral aortogram demonstrates concave stenosis *(arrow)*, which is characteristic for median arcuate ligament syndrome, along proximal portion of superior mesenteric artery. **B,** Following surgical division of median arcuate ligament, aortography demonstrates relief of stenosis.

struction is less prominent.[81] Despite well-documented angiographic findings, the clinical significance of the median arcuate ligament syndrome remains controversial (Fig. 74-30).

Aneurysms

Because most abdominal aortic aneurysms originate distal to the renal arteries, the celiac and superior mesenteric arteries are not commonly affected by the aneurysm. In contrast, occlusion of the inferior mesenteric artery is a common finding; however, adequate collaterals are ordinarily present, and the patient is asymptomatic. Dissections of the aorta that originate in the aortic arch and extend distally to involve the distal aorta may occlude visceral artery origins. In patients with dissection, abdominal aortography can reveal lack of filling of visceral branches. However, if the catheter is advanced proximally to the aortic arch and a thoracic aortogram is performed, visceral branches frequently fill from the false lumen. Infarction of GI organs or rupture of the false lumen into the GI tract are rare complications of aortic dissections.

Individual aneurysms of the celiac or superior mesenteric arteries are rarely encountered (Fig. 74-31). They are usually asymptomatic unless they compress adjacent structures, rupture, or attain sufficient size to become clinically apparent as a pulsatile epigastric mass (Fig. 74-32). Splenic artery aneurysms can be caused by atherosclerosis or pancreatitis with autodigestion of the ar-

terial wall. Seen more frequently in females, atherosclerotic splenic artery aneurysms have a greater propensity for spontaneous rupture, especially during pregnancy (Fig. 74-33). Most hepatic artery aneurysms are located in the extrahepatic portion of the hepatic artery. If large enough they can compress the adjacent bile duct, resulting in obstructive jaundice. Rupture of hepatic artery aneurysms is rare and usually accompanied with massive hemorrhage. Occasionally, a hepatic artery aneurysm will spontaneously rupture into the portal vein or a splenic artery aneurysm into the splenic vein, thus creating an unusual cause of portal hypertension. Aneurysms of visceral arterial branches are for the most part atherosclerotic in nature. Occasionally they rupture; if this occurs in the mesentery, a mesenteric hematoma results (Fig. 74-34). Rupture of the aneurysm into the intestinal lumen causes acute or chronic GI bleeding.

Arteritis

Involvement of the GI tract arteries by autoimmune vasculitis is usually part of a generalized systemic process. In polyarteritis nodosa, aneurysms are seen in medium-sized and small arterial branches (Fig. 74-35). Usually these aneurysms are small (2 to 3 mm in diameter), and the arteriogram must be carefully scrutinized to find them. However, occasionally they become quite large. In patients with polyarteritis nodosa, the aneurysms sometimes spontaneously rupture with ensuing peritoneal or retroperitoneal hemorrhage (Fig. 74-36). The liver is

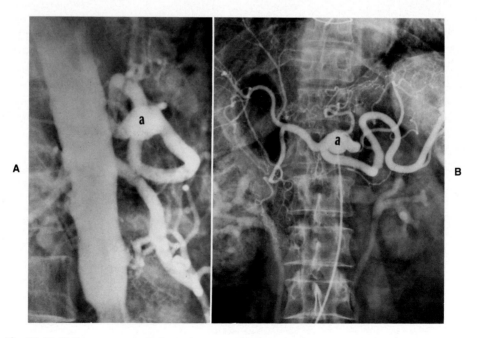

Fig. 74-31 Celiac aneurysm. **A,** Lateral aortography demonstrates 3 cm aneurysm *(a)* originating from proximal portion of celiac artery. **B,** Same aneurysm is seen on celiac arteriogram.

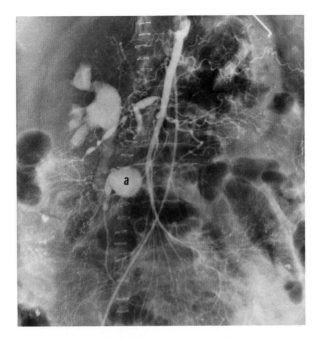

Fig. 74-32 Ruptured superior mesenteric artery aneurysm. Superior mesenteric arteriography in 67-year-old woman who presented with shock and intraabdominal hemorrhage demonstrates large aneurysm *(a)* of ileal branch. At surgery it was discovered that rupture of this aneurysm was responsible for intraperitoneal bleeding. Bizarre dilatation of right colic branch is also caused by atherosclerotic disease.

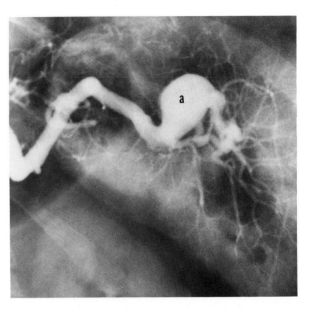

Fig. 74-33 Splenic artery aneurysm. Aneurysm *(a)* is located in distal portion of splenic artery.

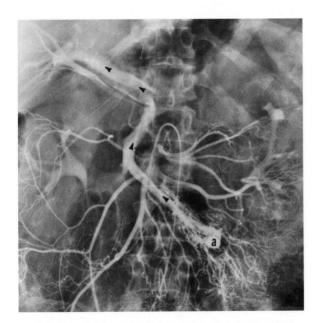

Fig. 74-34 Mesenteric arterial-venous fistula from rupture of jejunal artery aneurysm into adjacent vein. Superior mesenteric arteriography in this 53-year-old man demonstrates small aneurysm *(a)* of distal jejunal artery that has spontaneously ruptured into adjacent jejunal vein. Early, rapid, and dense filling of jejunal vein, superior mesenteric vein, and portal vein is present *(arrowheads)*.

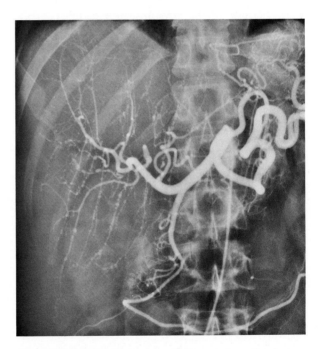

Fig. 74-35 Polyarteritis nodosa. Celiac arteriography demonstrates multiple small aneurysms of intrahepatic arteries.

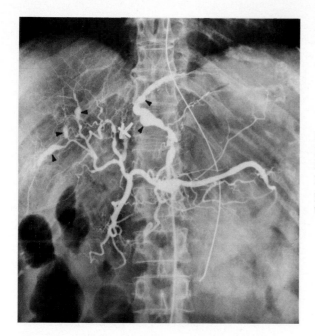

Fig. 74-36 Polyarteritis nodosa with intraperitoneal rupture of hepatic artery aneurysm. Celiac arteriography demonstrates bizarre arterial dilatations of multiple branches of intrahepatic arteries and left gastric artery *(arrowheads)*. This patient presented with hypovolemic shock caused by intraperitoneal hemorrhage from ruptured left hepatic artery aneurysm that has been surgically clipped.

involved in approximately two thirds and the intestines in one half of these patients. Arterial occlusions may result from the inflammatory component of the arteritis, causing ischemia or even infarction of the involved organs. Because of the high incidence of renal (80%), hepatic, and intestinal involvement in patients with polyarteritis nodosa, arteriography plays an important role in its diagnosis and in the determination of its extent[28] (Fig. 74-37).

Angiographic and pathologic changes similar to those seen with polyarteritis nodosa are present in necrotizing angiitis. Intravenous drug abuse, especially of amphetamines, is a common cause of this type of arteritis (Fig. 74-38).

Unlike the small and medium-sized arterial changes seen in polyarteritis nodosa, Takaysau's arteritis affects major aortic branches, usually at or close to their origin. Known as "pulseless disease," it was originally thought to be limited to aortic arch branches, but it is now evident that the abdominal aorta and its major branches may also be affected.[101] Takayasu's arteritis is most often seen in young women and is usually progressive for several years before eventually becoming quiescent. Stenosis or occlusion of the abdominal aorta or any of its major visceral branches may occur.

Malrotation, herniation, and intussusception

Normally, visceral branches originate from the celiac and superior mesenteric artery in an orderly fashion and extend toward the organs they supply in a smooth, direct, yet relaxed course. However, when these branches follow an abnormal route, supplying an organ that is not in its usual anatomic position, congenital malrotation or acquired herniation should be suspected (Fig. 74-39). Often acute angulation close to the origin of a visceral branch or an abrupt change in direction along its course indicates an internal hernia or entrapment by adhesions (Fig. 74-40). If strangulation occurs, stasis in the artery supplying the strangulated bowel loop with poor distal perfusion is seen (Fig. 74-41).

Though it is commonly seen in children, intussusception is an infrequent finding in adult patients. In adults, intussusceptions are almost always caused by a tumor of sessile or pedunculated nature. Though visceral angiography is not indicated for the diagnosis of intussusception, arteriographic findings are characteristic. The mesenteric branches supplying the intussusceptum are stretched distally and encircled by the arteries supplying the intussuscipiens. Frequently, a hypervascular tumor, the lead point, can be visualized (Fig. 74-42).

Standing waves

The regular beaded appearance of standing waves is quite characteristic (Fig. 74-43). This phenomenon is a normal finding caused by the pressure of the injection and the resistance of the vascular system. Standing waves should not be confused with pathologic conditions such as tumor encasement or medial fibromuscular dysplasia.

INFLAMMATORY DISEASE OF THE ALIMENTARY TRACT

Arteriography is rarely used in the primary evaluation of inflammatory disease of the alimentary tract; however,

Text continued on p. 1900.

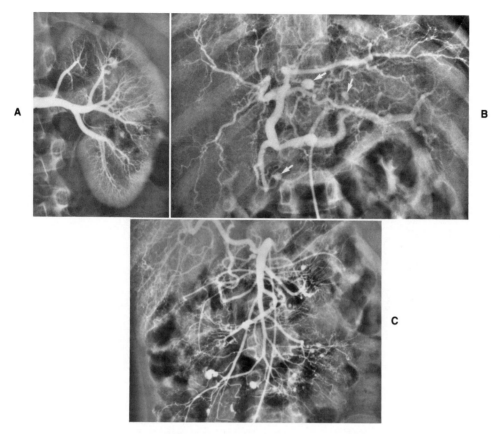

Fig. 74-37 Renal **(A),** hepatic **(B),** and mesenteric **(C)** involvement with polyarteritis nodosa. Typical microaneurysms are well seen in **B** (arrows).

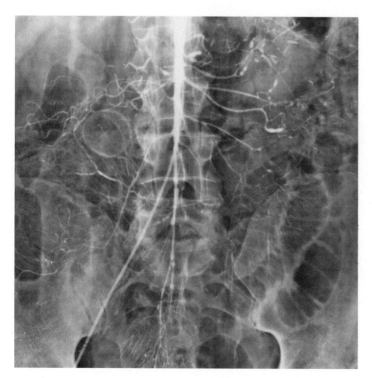

Fig. 74-38 Necrotizing angiitis in a 27-year-old man with a history of intravenous methedrine abuse.

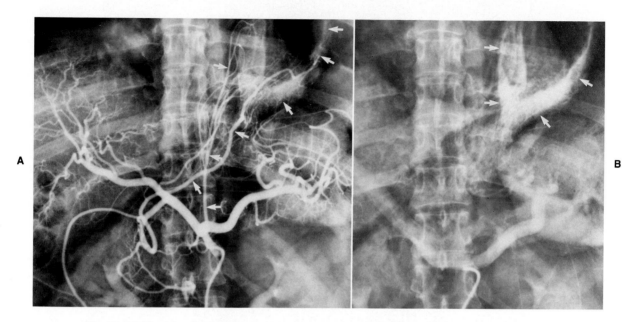

Fig. 74-39 Hiatal hernia. **A,** Branches of left gastric and right gastroepiploic arteries *(arrows)* are stretched superiorly and extend well above diaphragm. **B,** Late phase of celiac arteriogram demonstrates blush in gastric fundus wall *(arrows),* which is intrathoracic.

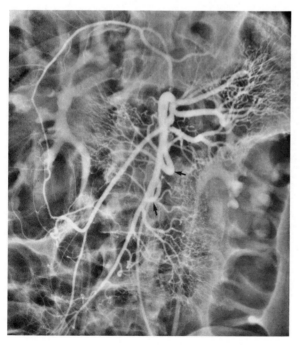

Fig. 74-40 Internal hernia. Acute angulation of two jejunal branches *(arrows).* These branches pass through internal paraduodenal hernia with their corresponding loops of jejunum located in right upper quadrant.

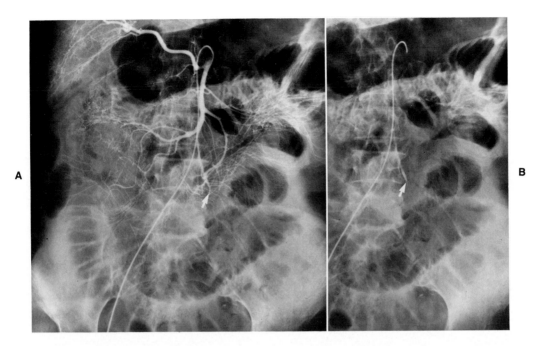

Fig. 74-41 Strangulated loop of bowel secondary to adhesions. **A,** Branches of superior mesenteric artery are vasoconstricted. There is an acute kink of a distal ileal branch *(arrow)*. **B,** Stasis in artery that is supplying strangulated loop *(arrow)*.

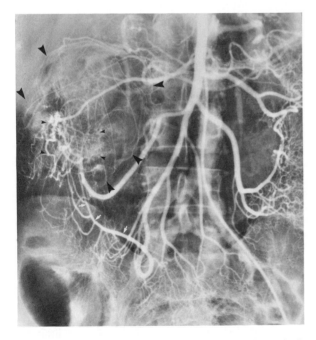

Fig. 74-42 Cecal carcinoma causing cecal-ascending colonic intussusception. Ileocolic artery *(white arrows)* is stretched superiorly, supplying a hypervascular lesion with multiple crowded arteries: the intussusceptum *(small arrowheads)*. Right colic artery branches *(large arrowheads)* are stretched around intussusceptum.

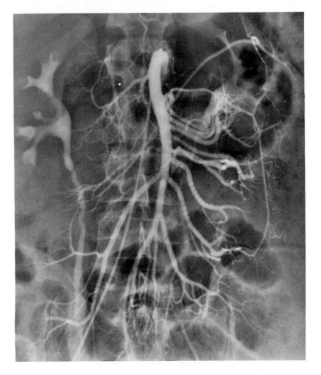

Fig. 74-43 Standing waves. Several jejunal branches of superior mesenteric artery demonstrate an irregular, beaded appearance that is characteristic of standing waves.

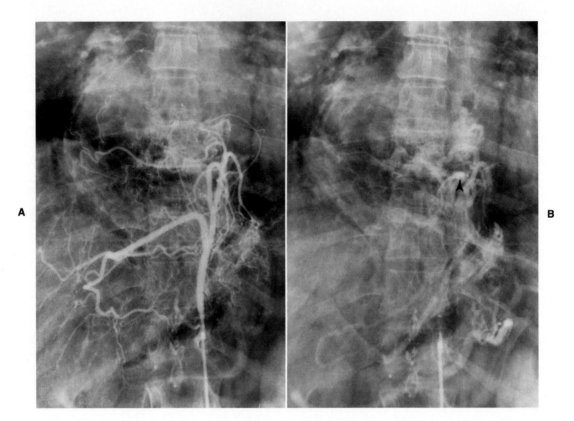

Fig. 74-44 Gastritis in hiatal hernia. **A,** During early phase branches of left gastric artery extend well above diaphragm. Hypervascularity exists in region of hiatal hernia. **B,** Extravasation *(arrowhead)* is seen on late phase with marked hypervascularity in hiatal hernia and prominent venous drainage.

because abnormal findings caused by inflammatory disease may be encountered during angiography performed for other indications, their recognition is important.

Gastritis and duodenitis

Mucosal hypervascularity with an intense parenchymal blush and prominent venous drainage are the angiographic findings in gastritis and duodenitis. When severe enough to cause active hemorrhage, diffuse extravasation of contrast material from multiple patchy areas can be seen (Fig. 74-44).

Inflammatory bowel disease

Typical angiographic findings in inflammatory bowel disease are enlarged arteries supplying a hypervascular thickened bowel wall. The venous drainage is usually early and intense (Fig. 74-45). These changes can be limited to a small area of the bowel or may involve major segments[13] (Fig. 74-46). These angiographic changes are of little aid in distinguishing one type of inflammatory bowel disease from another. Control of acute hemorrhage is usually the only indication for visceral angiography in patients with inflammatory bowel disease. Ischemic colitis is a type of inflammatory bowel disease seen fol-

lowing low perfusion states. Decreased blood flow to the colon leads to necrosis of the mucosa with sloughing. The angiographic appearance of ischemic colitis is nonspecific and consists of hypervascularity with prominent accumulation of contrast in the bowel wall and dense venous drainage[83] (Fig. 74-47). Diagnosis of ischemic colitis is almost always made by endoscopy, and angiography has a limited role in this disease.

Diverticulitis

Localized hyperemia with dense accumulation of contrast in the wall of the involved segments of colon and early draining veins are the findings of diverticulitis. In essence, they are the same angiographic findings present in all inflammatory bowel diseases. Displacement of individual arterial branches usually indicates the presence of a pericolonic abscess (Fig. 74-48). In diverticular disease, the indications for angiography are limited to localization and treatment of acute bleeding.

ALIMENTARY TRACT TUMORS
Angiographic characteristics of GI neoplasia

Both benign and malignant GI neoplasms demonstrate characteristic changes in the angiographic appearance of

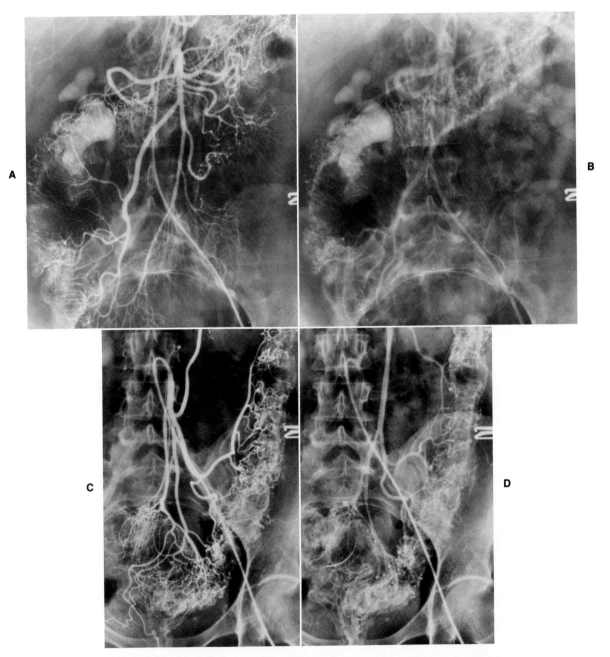

Fig. 74-45 Granulomatous colitis. Early phases (**A** and **C**) and late phases (**B** and **D**) of superior and inferior mesenteric arteriograms demonstrate hypervascularity of bowel wall with prominent intense venous drainage.

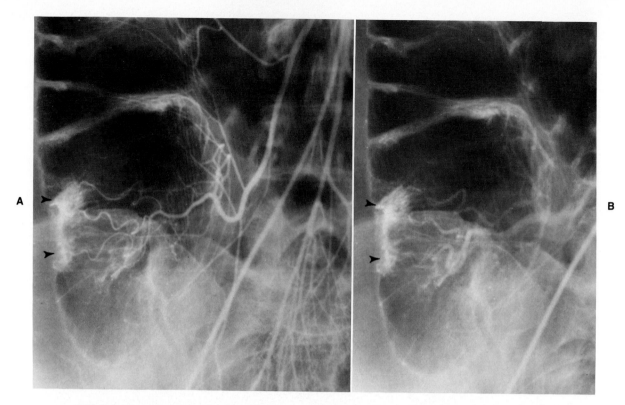

Fig. 74-46 Localized granulomatous colitis. **A,** Superior mesenteric arteriogram reveals focal area of granulomatous colitis involving lateral wall of cecum. **B,** Venous drainage is prominent. This lesion was responsible for chronic GI tract bleeding.

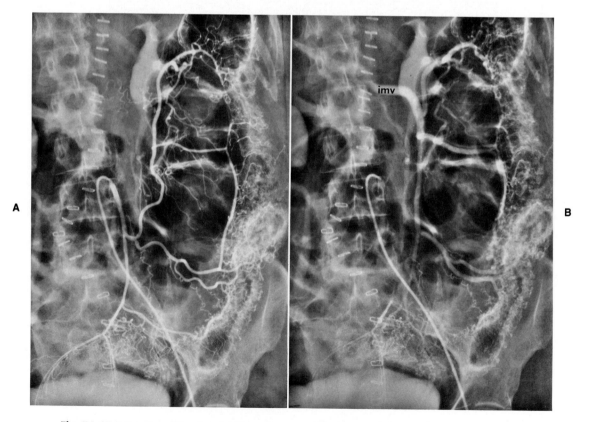

Fig. 74-47 Ischemic colitis. Arterial (**A**) and venous (**B**) phases of inferior mesenteric angiogram demonstrate hypervascularity of bowel wall with dense parenchymal blush and early, dense opacification of inferior mesenteric vein *(imv)* and its branches.

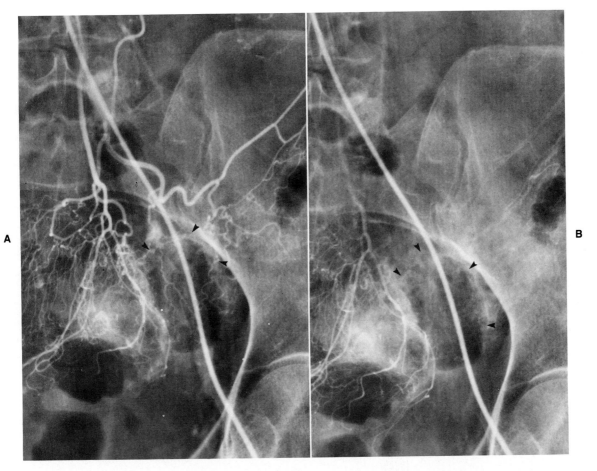

Fig. 74-48 Diverticulitis with parasigmoidal abscess. **A,** Inferior mesenteric angiography demonstrates irregularity and displacement of sigmoid branches *(arrowheads)*. **B,** During late phase, increased blush *(arrowheads)* is present where sigmoid colon is displaced by parasigmoidal abscess.

the involved arteries and veins. These angiographic changes include vascular invasion or encasement, vascular displacement, neovascularity or formation of new tumor vessels, and increased accumulation of contrast material within the tumor (tumor blush). The specific angiographic findings associated with various types of GI tumors are usually influenced by their histologic nature.

Though vascular displacement clearly outlines masses, it is rather nonspecific and may appear similar when caused by cysts, abscesses, or benign or malignant neoplasms (Fig. 74-49). Sometimes vascular displacement is the most striking abnormality on the arteriogram and serves to direct attention to other less apparent but more specific findings.

Vascular encasement is a reliable sign of malignant neoplasia. Encasement of vessels results from the scirrhous nature of many GI tumors and their ability to evoke a desmoplastic reaction in the tissues they invade. Encased arteries have either a serpiginous or serrated ap-

pearance, and with extensive encasement arterial or venous occlusion occurs (Fig. 74-50). Though encasement cannot differentiate between histologically different types of tumors, it is a very reliable sign of infiltrating, scirrhous, malignant neoplasms.

Angiogenesis, or new vessel formation, is characteristic of many nonscirrhous malignant and sometimes benign tumors. Neovasculature, often called tumor vessels, lack a normal vascular endothelium and muscular wall and therefore do not exhibit the typical vasoconstrictive response to epinephrine. They appear as short, irregular vascular channels with changing luminal dimensions and abrupt angulations. Their origins and terminations are obscure and often seen to be without connection to any native vessel (Fig. 74-51).

Increased accumulation of contrast material within the substance of the tumor during the parenchymal phase of the arteriogram is called tumor blush (Fig. 74-52). This finding is usually seen with vascular neoplasms and occasionally with infiltrating, scirrhous tumors. Tumor

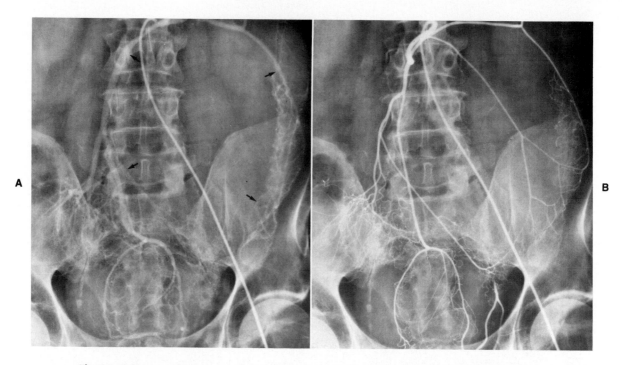

Fig. 74-49 Vascular displacement. **A,** Inferior mesenteric artery demonstrates displacement *(arrows)* of multiple inferior mesenteric arterial branches by large mesenteric cyst. **B,** Venous phase reveals marked venous displacement also.

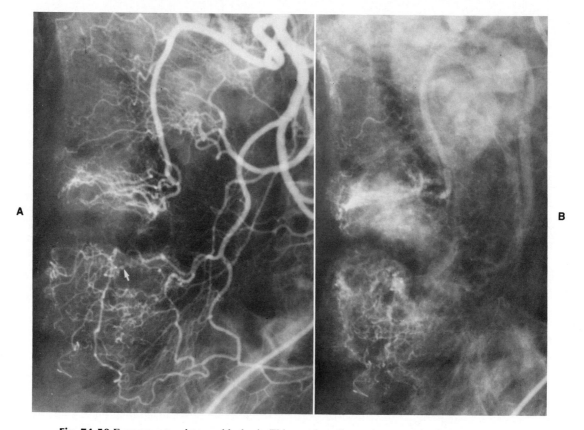

Fig. 74-50 Encasement and tumor blush. **A,** This cecal carcinoma has caused encasement *(arrow)* of individual branches of ileocolic artery. **B,** Late phase shows increased accumulation of contrast material within tumor *(tumor blush)* and prominent draining vein.

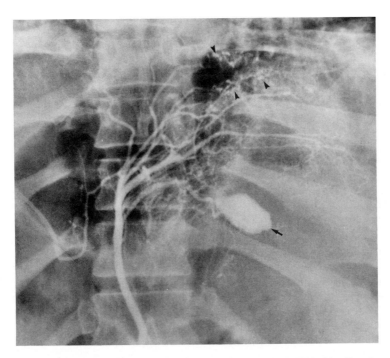

Fig. 74-51 Neovascularity. Left gastric angiography demonstrates acutely bleeding *(arrow)* leio-myosarcoma with neovascularity *(arrowheads)*.

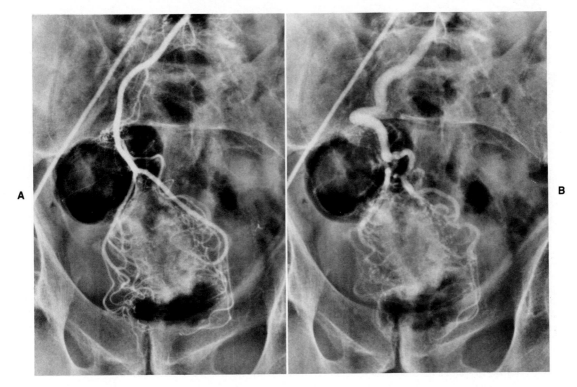

Fig. 74-52 Tumor blush. Dense accumulation of contrast material, tumor blush, is present in this rectal carcinoma in arterial **(A)** and venous **(B)** phases of inferior mesenteric arteriogram.

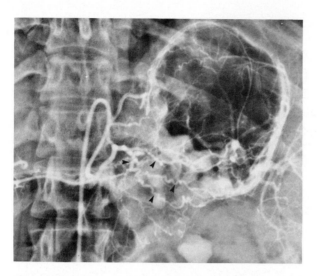

Fig. 74-53 Gastric carcinoma. Stomach has been insufflated with air, however, area involved with tumor does not distend. Marked vascular encasement *(arrowheads)* of left gastric arterial branches in region of carcinoma is present.

blush is not a specific finding for neoplasm, becuase it is frequently present in inflammatory processes.

Adenocarcinoma

Adenocarcinoma is the most frequently occurring tumor of the alimentary tract. Gastric adenocarcinomas are primarily scirrhous; thus the angiographic findings are predominantly vascular encasement and few if any tumor vessels[13,14] (Fig. 74-53). On the other hand, colon carcinomas usually exhibit marked tumor vascularity, a prominent tumor blush, and vascular encasement. Invasion of the mesenteric arteries by carcinoma of the colon or small bowel or of the gastroepiploic artery by gastric carcinoma indicates tumor extension beyond the primary site (Fig. 74-54).

Myomatous tumors

Leiomyoma and leiomyosarcoma are tumors of smooth muscle and can arise anywhere in the alimentary tract. In the small intestine they account for 23% of

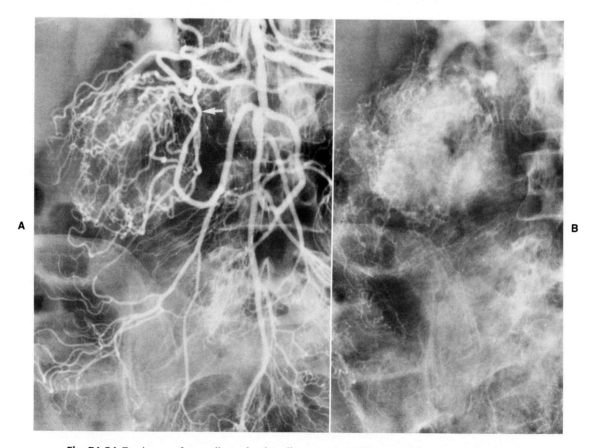

Fig. 74-54 Carcinoma of ascending colon invading mesentery. Hypervascular tumor with vascular encasement and tumor blush is present in ascending colon. Encasement of mesenteric arterial branch *(arrow)* indicates tumor invasion of mesentery. **A,** Early phase and **B,** late phase of *SM* arteriogram.

neoplasms (Fig. 74-55). Clinically, patients with myomatous tumors often present with chronic recurrent bleeding and episodes of massive acute hemorrhage (Fig. 74-56). Angiographically these tumors are usually hypervascular with abundant tumor vessels, a vascular blush, and dense venous drainage; however, occasionally they may be hypovascular[112,121] (Fig. 74-57). Myomatous tumors of the stomach may become very large before they are discovered, and their large size often makes it impossible to determine their site of origin by noninvasive imaging studies. Gastric origin is easy to recognize on

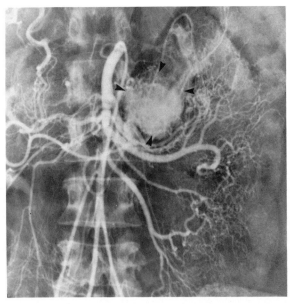

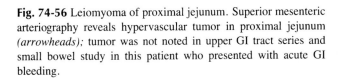

Fig. 74-56 Leiomyoma of proximal jejunum. Superior mesenteric arteriography reveals hypervascular tumor in proximal jejunum *(arrowheads);* tumor was not noted in upper GI tract series and small bowel study in this patient who presented with acute GI bleeding.

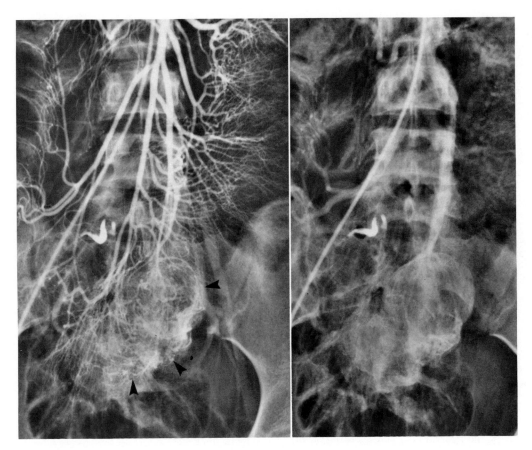

Fig. 74-55 Leiomyoma of ileum. **A,** Hypervascular tumor *(arrowheads)* is present in distal ileum. **B,** Tumor blush with dense venous drainage is present.

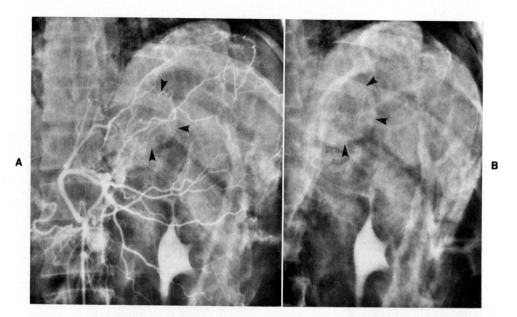

Fig. 74-57 Hypovascular leiomyoma of stomach. Left gastric arteriogram demonstrates displacement of arterial branches *(arrowheads)* in early phase **(A)** and subtle tumor blush *(arrowheads)* during parenchymal phase **(B).**

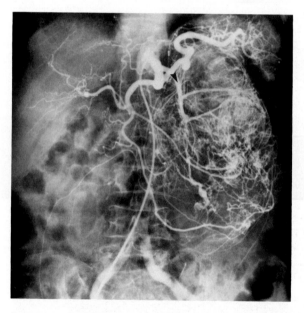

Fig. 74-58 Large leiomyosarcoma. On CT scan, left-sided abdominal mass was present; however, its origin was unclear. Celiac arteriography demonstrates enlarged left gastric artery *(arrowhead)* supplying very large hypervascular tumor with marked neovascularity and tumor puddling inside it.

the angiogram by the marked enlargement of either the gastroepiploic artery with greater curvature lesions or the left gastric artery with those arising from the lesser curvature (Fig. 74-58). With leiomyomas, the tumor blush is often homogeneous and well circumscribed, whereas

leiomyosarcomas tend to be larger, more irregular, and disorganized. Exact angiographic and at times even pathologic differentiation between benign and malignant myomatous tumors can be difficult. The presence of arterial encasement in a myomatous tumor indicates malignancy; however, its absence is not a sign of benignity.

Carcinoid tumors

Carcinoid tumors of the alimentary tract arise in the distal ileum and become detectable angiographically once the mesentery has been invaded. Frequently these lesions will ulcerate into the ileum, and the patient presents with acute lower GI hemorrhage. Because of their extremely desmoplastic nature, carcinoid tumors cause mesenteric thickening and retraction with prominent kinking of individual arterial branches adjacent to involved portions of the mesentery (Fig. 74-59). Frequently the distorted arteries are retracted toward a central point, producing the so-called "sunburst" appearance[12] (Fig. 74-60). Carcinoid metastasis to the liver appear as multiple, hypervascular, well-circumscribed nodules.

Metastases to the alimentary tract

Most metastases to the alimentary tract are usually by direct extension from adjacent cancers. Of the malignancies that metastasize to the stomach or intestines by the hematogenous route, melanoma and choriocarcinoma are the most common (Fig. 74-61). GI hemorrhage is the most common presenting symptom in patients with alimentary tract metastases.

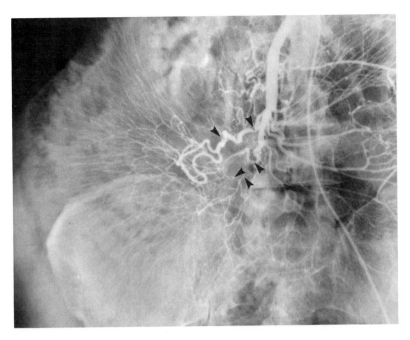

Fig. 74-59 Carcinoid tumor of distal ileum. Occlusion of several distal ileal branches and marked kinking of other *(arrowheads)* indicate desmoplastic nature of this tumor.

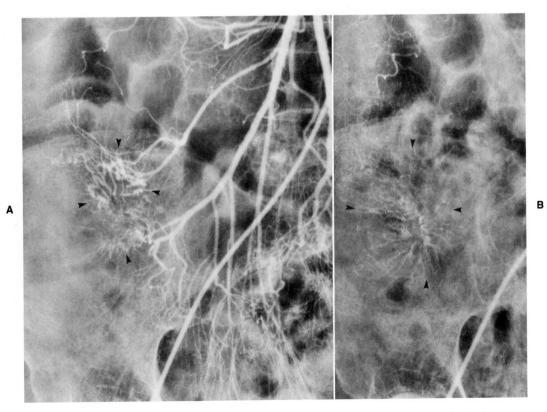

Fig. 74-60 Small carcinoid tumor of distal ileum. **A,** Early lesion *(arrowheads)* just beginning to invade mesentery causes marked vascular retraction, giving "sunburst" appearance *(arrowheads)* in late phase **(B).**

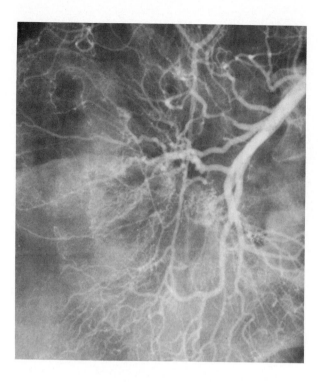

Fig. 74-61 Melanoma metastatic to distal ileum. Multiple encased vessels and areas of neovascularity are present in this segment of distal ileum.

PANCREATIC ANGIOGRAPHY

With the introduction of and rapid improvement in noninvasive imaging, predominantly ultrasound and CT, the role of pancreatic angiography has changed considerably. Once used as a primary method of screening patients with suspected pancreatic disease, pancreatic arteriography is now reserved for cases in which the results of noninvasive imaging studies and percutaneous needle biopsy are inconclusive or negative despite clinical evidence of pancreatic disease, especially pancreatic carcinoma.[44]

Technique and accuracy

It has been established that the degree of visualization and filling of small intrapancreatic arteries is an index to the adequacy of the pancreatic arteriogram and closely correlates with its diagnostic accuracy.[27] If the arteriogram is limited to selective study of the celiac and superior mesenteric arteries it will demonstrate larger, more advanced processes; however, small lesions may not be detected because of lack of filling and visualization of small intrapancreatic arteries. With pancreatic carcinoma, it has been demonstrated that only 60% of tumors are likely to be shown when only selective studies are performed. The diagnostic accuracy of pancreatic angiography increases to over 90% with the use of superselective arteriography, which includes catheterization and injection of second- and third-order aortic branches such as the splenic, hepatic, gastroduodenal, dorsal pancreatic, and inferior or superior pancreaticoduodenal ar-

teries.[92] Superselective studies afford excellent visualization of small intrapancreatic arterial branches without the confusion of other superimposed arteries (Fig. 74-62). Furthermore, superselective injections, by distending small intrapancreatic arteries, make more apparent the fixed, nondistensible luminal irregularities often caused by pancreatic carcinomas. Besides proper performance of the pancreatic angiogram, proper interpretation is essential. When these are combined, superselective pancreatic arteriography is a highly sensitive radiologic means of detecting pancreatic tumors in their early stages, while they are still small and confined within the pancreas and thus potentially resectable.[4,27,91,92]

When there are atherosclerotic obstructions of the celiac or superior mesenteric arteries or of vascular anatomy unsuitable for superselective catheterization, pancreatic pharmacoangiography with the use of vasodilators (tolazoline and papaverine), vasoconstrictors (epinephrine and angiotensin), and agents that stimulate pancreatic function (secretin) can be used to improve diagnostic accuracy.[91]

Pancreatic adenocarcinoma

Adenocarcinomas of the pancreas demonstrate angiographic changes reflecting their hypovascular, infiltrating, and scirrhous character. Vascular encasement and occlusion are the predominant findings seen with carcinoma of the pancreas (Fig. 74-63). In small or early lesions, only the small intrapancreatic arteries are affected with focal serrated or serpiginous encasement

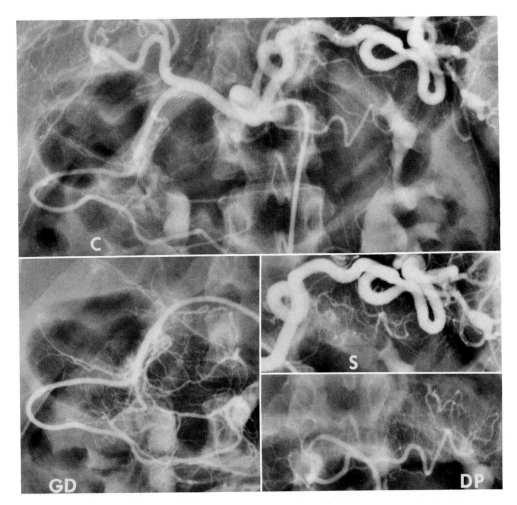

Fig. 74-62 Selective arteriography versus superselective arteriography in pancreas evaluation. Selective celiac *(C)* arteriogram results in only minimal opacification of intrapancreatic arteries. Superselective gastroduodenal *(GD)*, splenic *(S)* and dorsal pancreatic *(DP)* arteriograms result in excellent distention and opacification of small intrapancreatic arteries in head, tail, and body of pancreas, respectively.

(Fig. 74-64). As the tumor progresses, vascular encasement eventually develops into occlusion. Extension of the carcinoma beyond the confines of the pancreas results in invasion (encasement) of larger peripancreatic arteries, that is, the gastroduodenal, hepatic, and splenic arteries (Fig. 74-65). These encased arteries are fixed and have irregular, serrated contours (Fig. 74-66).

In addition to arterial encasement, pancreatic carcinoma frequently causes changes in major venous structures in or nearby it.[17] These consist of displacement, encasement, or occlusion and are best demonstrated on the venous phases of splenic angiography and superior mesenteric pharmacoangiography. Carcinomas of the body and tail of the pancreas commonly occlude the splenic vein and cause extensive venous collateral circulation, usually gastric varices along the lesser curvature

or an enlarged gastroepiploic vein along the greater gastric curvature (Fig. 74-67). Cancers in the pancreatic head often encase and occasionally occlude the superior mesenteric or portal veins (Fig. 74-68). Besides vascular encasement, neovascularity, another arteriographic sign of neoplasia, can be demonstrated by superselective angiography in approximately 50% of patients with pancreatic carcinoma.

In addition to making a diagnosis of carcinoma, arteriography helps differentiate cancer from nonneoplastic pancreatic masses, especially pancreatitis.[91] In the presence of pancreatic carcinoma, arteriography is useful in determining tumor resectability. Small tumors confined to the pancreas with encasement of only intrapancreatic arteries are usually resectable (Fig. 74-69). However, invasion of larger peripancreatic arteries or major trib-

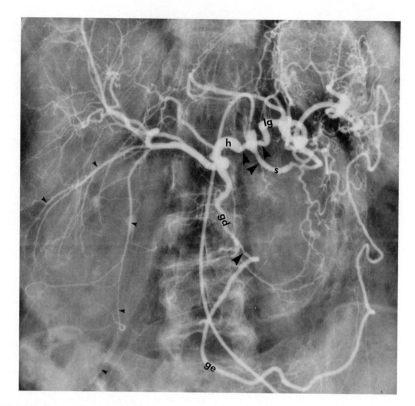

Fig. 74-63 Large pancreatic carcinoma. There is extensive vascular encasement *(large arrowheads)*. Encasement is particularly well seen in proximal splenic *(s)*, left gastric *(lg)*, hepatic *(h)*, and gastroduodenal *(gd)* arteries. Encasement of splenic artery is so severe that collateral flow to spleen is present through left gastric and gastroepiploic *(ge)* arteries. Markedly enlarged gallbladder *(small arrowheads)* indicates that pancreatic carcinoma has occluded common bile duct.

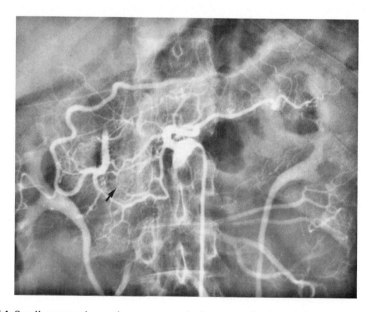

Fig. 74-64 Small pancreatic carcinoma seen only by superselective angiography. Focal area of encasement *(arrow)* is present on dorsal pancreatic arteriogram, indicating that small pancreatic cancer has invaded only intrapancreatic arteries and not extended beyond confines of pancreas. This lesion was resectable.

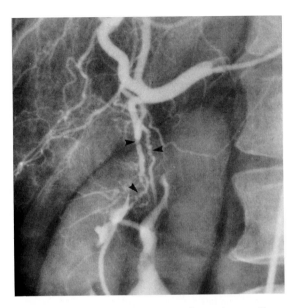

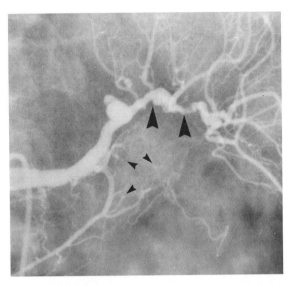

Fig. 74-65 Small unresectable pancreatic carcinoma. Encasement of gastroduodenal artery and superior pancreatico-duodenal artery *(arrowheads)* is present. Encasement of gastroduodenal artery indicates tumor extension beyond confines of pancreas. This lesion was unresectable.

Fig. 74-66 Small pancreatic cancer invading splenic hilum. Vascular occlusion of intrapancreatic branches *(small arrowheads)* and encasement of splenic artery *(large arrowheads)* are diagnostic of pancreatic carcinoma. Involvement of major peripancreatic artery such as the splenic artery indicates nonresectability.

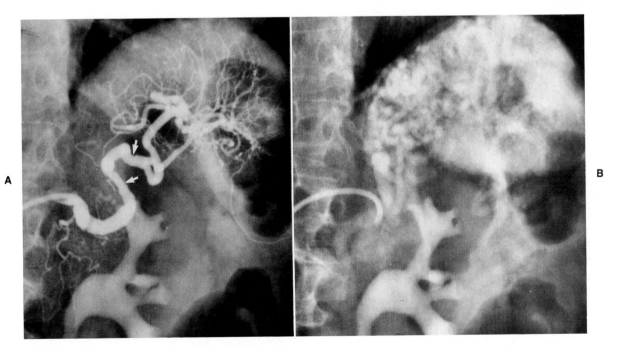

Fig. 74-67 Pancreatic carcinoma with splenic vein occlusion. **A,** Splenic arteriography demonstrates encasement of splenic artery *(arrows).* **B,** During venous phase splenic vein is not opacified, and gastric varices are noted along lesser curvature of stomach.

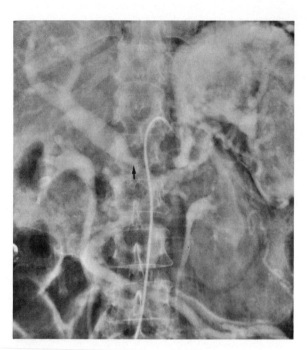

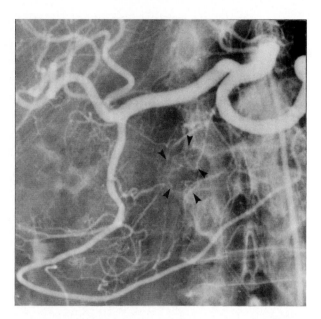

Fig. 74-68 Portal vein occlusion by pancreatic carcinoma. Venous phase of superior mesenteric pharmacoangiography with tolazoline reveals occlusion of portal vein *(arrow)*.

Fig. 74-69 Small resectable pancreatic carcinoma. Celiac arteriography demonstrates good filling of intrapancreatic arteries of pancreatic head. Several arteries are occluded, and encasement of small intrapancreatic arterial branch is present *(arrowheads)*. Compare size of pancreatic carcinoma with adjacent intervertebral disc space. This lesion was not visible on CT scan or ultrasonograph.

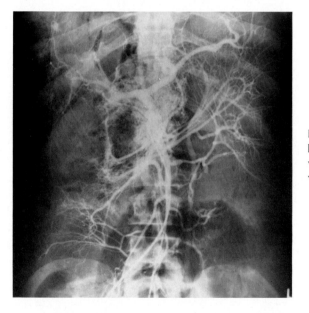

Fig. 74-70 Acute necrotizing hemorrhagic pancreatitis. Marked hypervascularity in pancreatic head and body region is present with early filling of portal vein. Air is seen in intrahepatic portal vein branches.

utaries of the portal vein indicates nonresectability. If major surgery is contemplated, arteriography can help by demonstrating vascular anomalies of the visceral circulation which, undetected, could cause difficulties during resection.

Pancreatitis

Pancreatitis and its sequelae are readily identified by ultrasound and CT, and therefore the role of angiography in its diagnosis is limited. However, because it may sometimes be difficult to distinguish between inflammatory and neoplastic pancreatic masses by noninvasive imaging alone and because the angiographic findings in these diseases are different, pancreatic arteriography can be useful in making this crucial differentiation.

The angiographic changes in pancreatitis parallel the disease process. In acute necrotizing hemorrhagic pancreatitis, marked hypervascularity with arteriovenous

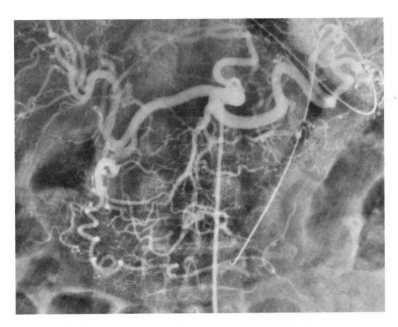

Fig. 74-71 Subacute pancreatitis. Celiac arteriogram demonstrates enlargement and hypervascularity involving entire pancreas. Changes are far less extensive than those seen with acute necrotizing, hemorrhagic pancreatitis.

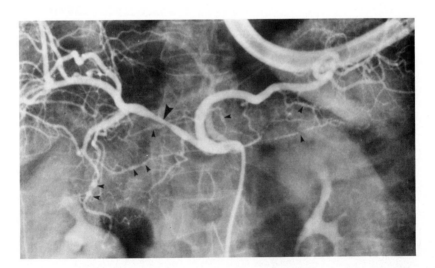

Fig. 74-72 Chronic pancreatitis. Celiac arteriogram reveals multiple findings typical of chronic pancreatitis. Entire pancreas is involved, and there is beading *(small arrowheads)* and aneurysms *(small arrowheads)* of multiple intrapancreatic arteries. Smooth, long segment cuffing of larger peripancreatic arteries and hepatic artery *(large arrowhead)* is also typical of chronic pancreatitis.

shunting is present[86] (Fig. 74-70). Edema and swelling with moderate hypervascularity are seen in less severe instances of acute pancreatitis and subacute pancreatitis (Fig. 74-71). The angiographic findings vary in chronic pancreatitis, but generally there is involvement of all or most of the pancreas in contrast to the more focal abnormalities seen in pancreatic carcinoma. Beaded intrapancreatic arteries with short dilated segments alternating with a normal lumen or narrowed segments are the typical angiographic findings in chronic pancreatitis. Small aneurysms are often present in the intrapancreatic arteries. Occasionally, larger peripancreatic branches are involved in the inflammatory process with smooth narrowing over long segments (Fig. 74-72). This appearance differs from that of neoplastic encasement, which is serrated and usually more focal. Occlusion of the splenic vein is also

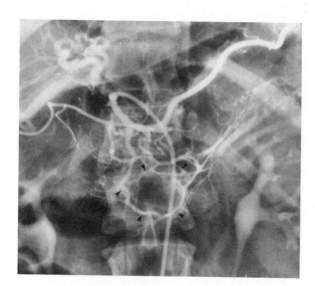

Fig. 74-73 Small pancreatic pseudocyst. Avascular area causes displacement of pancreatic arteries in uncinate process *(arrowheads)*.

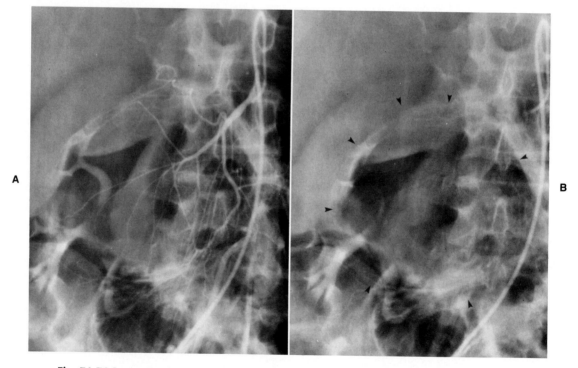

A

B

Fig. 74-74 Large pseudocyst extending outside of pancreas. **A,** Inferior pancreaticoduodenal arteriography demonstrates avascular mass with stretching of arterial branches in pancreatic head in early phase. **B,** Pseudocyst wall is hypervascular *(arrowheads)*, and is best appreciated during parenchymal phase.

A   B   C

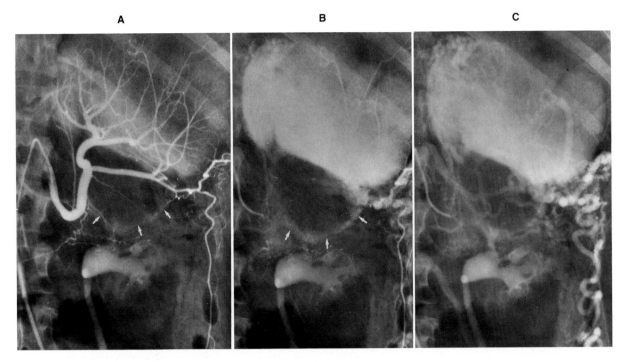

Fig. 74-75 Large pancreatic pseudocyst occluding splenic vein. **A,** Splenic arteriography demonstrates displacement and stretching of intrapancreatic arteries *(arrows).* **B,** In intermediate arterial phase, pseudocyst wall blushes *(arrows).* **C,** Late phase shows collateral veins in gastric fundus and retroperitoneum indicating splenic vein occlusion.

occasionally seen in association with chronic pancreatitis or adjacent pseudocysts. Long-standing chronic pancreatitis leads to pancreatic atrophy with widespread attenuation and beading of arterial branches. Pancreatic enzymes released during repeated exacerbations of chronic pancreatitis damage adjacent vascular walls, leading to the development of pseudoaneurysms.[47] These may rupture, causing acute GI or retroperitoneal hemorrhage.

Pancreatic pseudocyst

Pseudocysts are a common complication of pancreatitis and abdominal trauma. They are well imaged by ultrasound and CT. The arteriographic findings of small pseudocysts are avascular masses with stretching and displacement of intrapancreatic arteries (Fig. 74-73). Large pseudocysts cause displacement and stretching of peripancreatic visceral baranches (Fig. 74-74). The splenic vein is frequently occluded by pseudocysts in the pancreatic tail (Fig. 74-75). Occasionally a pseudocyst erodes into a pancreatic artery and fills with contrast material during angiography.[116] Attempted surgical or percutaneous drainage of a pseudocyst that has unexpectedly eroded into a large artery can be complicated by fulminant hemorrhage.

Islet cell tumors

Pancreatic islet cell tumors may be either secretory or nonfunctioning. Secretory tumors cause clinical syndromes determined by the hormones produced. Insulin-producing beta cell tumors (insulinomas) are the most commonly occurring islet cell tumor, accounting for 60% of these neoplasms. Alpha-1 islet cell tumors that secrete gastrin are responsible for Zollinger-Ellison syndrome and are fairly common. Islet cell tumors that produce glucagon (alpha-2 cell), vasoactive intestinal peptide (nonbeta cell), and somatostatin (D cell) are rare. The diagnosis of functioning islet cell tumors is usually made clinically on the basis of characteristic syndromes and confirmed by biochemical assay. Because most benign islet cell adenomas are small and similar in tissue consistency to the normal pancreas, they are frequently difficult to detect by noninvasive imaging studies or to find at surgery. Blind subtotal pancreatectomy done without prior localization of the adenoma often results in excision of normal pancreas but not of that part containing the adenoma.

Most islet cell tumors have a typical arteriographic appearance regardless of their cell type or hormonal activity. They are usually hypervascular, well-circumscribed lesions that opacify early in the arterial phase,

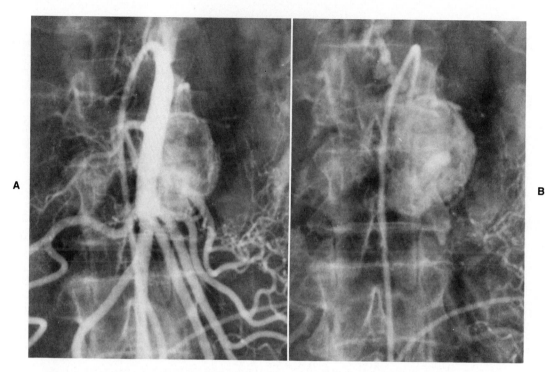

Fig. 74-76 Large islet cell adenoma. Superior mesenteric arteriography shows islet cell adenoma, 3 cm in diameter, in uncinate process of pancreas. It is hypervascular, with blush that starts in early arterial phase **(A)** and persists into late venous phase **(B).**

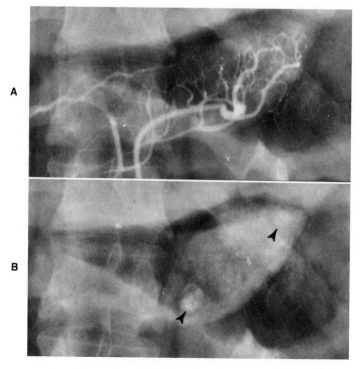

Fig. 74-77 Demonstration of two small islet cell tumors causing Zollinger-Ellison syndrome by superselective pancreatica magna arteriography. **A,** Injection into pancreatica magna artery causes excellent distention and opacification of arteries in pancreatic tail. **B,** During parenchymal phase two small islet cell adenomas *(arrowheads)* are demonstrated.

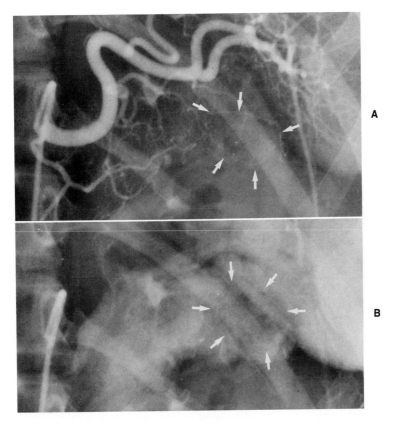

Fig. 74-78 Avascular glucagon-secreting islet cell tumor. **A,** Avascular islet cell adenomas are demonstrated by displacement of intrapancreatic arteries during arterial phase *(arrows).* **B,** During parenchymal phase lucent area compared to adjacent normal pancreatic tissue is present in tumor region *(arrows).*

blush densely, and stay opacified into the venous phase[21,24,35] (Fig. 74-76). Because adenomas may be quite small, superselective angiography is often required for their demonstration (Fig. 74-77). Islet cell tumors are occasionally avascular and detected on the angiogram by spreading and displacement of intrapancreatic arteries during the arterial phase and by a hypovascular lucent area compared to normal adjacent pancreatic tissue in the parenchymal phase (Fig. 74-78). Differentiation between benign and malignant islet cell tumors can be difficult; however, size is one criterion. If the lesion exceeds 5 cm in diameter, it is more likely to be malignant. If a malignant lesion is suspected, hepatic arteriography should be performed, because liver metastases from islet cell carcinoma are very hypervascular and thus can be detected when quite small. Occasionally the tail of the pancreas visualized *en face* can be mistaken for an islet cell adenoma because of the apparent increased blush. An accessory spleen is another potential source of false-positive diagnosis of islet cell tumors. However, differentiation between islet cell adenoma and accessory spleen can be made by close attention to the parenchymal phase,

which in the case of accessory spleen appears at the same time in the angiographic sequence and is of the same intensity as that of the normal spleen (Fig. 74-117).

Insulinomas occur as discrete hypervascular lesions in approximately three fourths of cases, and therefore angiography is frequently successful in their localization (Fig. 74-79). Gastrinomas, on the other hand, are less often hypervascular and may be multiple or exist in the form of generalized alpha-1 hyperplasia. In the latter instance, pancreatic arteriography will not demonstrate a discrete, well-circumscribed lesion. Approximately 10% to 15% of gastrinomas will have an extrapancreatic location, most often in the duodenum (Fig. 74-80).

If a good pancreatic arteriogram with adequate visualization of the pancreas fails to demonstrate an islet cell adenoma in a patient with strong clinical and biochemical evidence for one, transhepatic catheterization with selective sampling of individual pancreatic veins, splenic vein, superior mesenteric vein, and portal vein is indicated.[60] If a focal adenoma is present, a step-up in the concentration of the appropriate hormone will indicate the site of the lesion.

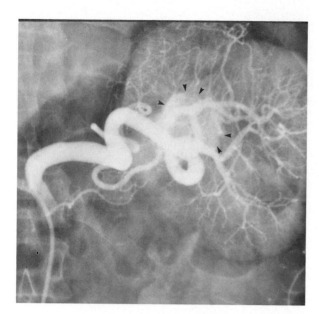

Fig. 74-79 Islet cell adenoma in splenic hilum. Splenic arteriography demonstrates 2 cm islet cell adenoma *(arrowheads)* located in hilum of spleen.

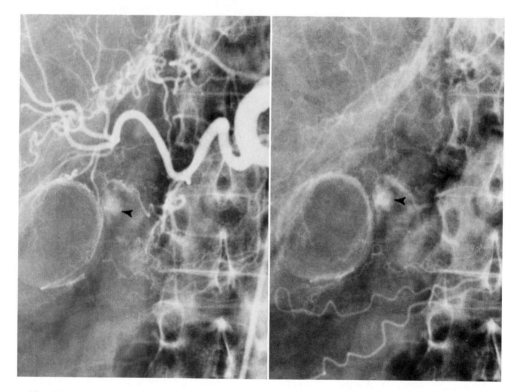

Fig. 74-80 Islet cell adenoma located in wall of first portion of duodenum. Celiac arteriography demonstrates islet cell adenoma *(arrowheads)* in duodenum wall adjacent to gallbladder in patient with Zollinger-Ellison syndrome.

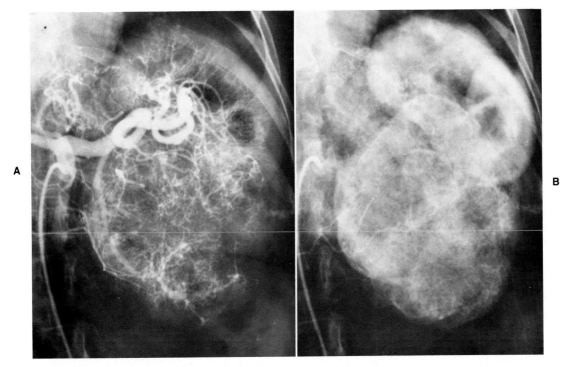

Fig. 74-81 Cystadenoma of pancreas. **A,** Expansile hypervascular mass with tumor vessels is noted on splenic arteriogram. **B,** During parenchymal phase lucent areas indicate cystic nature of this lesion.

Cystic pancreatic tumors

Cystadenomas and cystadenocarcinomas of the pancreas are rare tumors that lack early clinical signs and therefore are not usually diagnosed until quite large in size. It is difficult to differentiate cystadenoma from cystadenocarcinoma unless metastases are present. Both of these tumors appear as hypervascular neoplasms containing many lucencies, the cystic component best appreciated on the parenchymal phase of the arteriogram[31] (Fig. 74-81).

HEPATIC ANGIOGRAPHY

Angiographic demonstration of the entire liver can be achieved by common hepatic arteriography in approximately 60% of patients. In the remainder, variations in hepatic arterial anatomy require injections of the left gastric artery, which supplies all or part of the left hepatic lobe in about 20% of cases, and/or the right hepatic artery, whose origin is partially or completely replaced to the superior mesenteric artery in approximately 25% of cases. Occasionally, the entire blood supply to the liver originates from the superior mesenteric artery or directly from the aorta.[66,67] These anatomic variations must be recognized, particularly when it is necessary for complete angiographic visualization of the liver.

Diffuse hepatic parenchymal disease

Most diffuse hepatocellular diseases are diagnosed clinically, confirmed by liver biopsy, and then treated medically. Therefore arteriography is used infrequently in the management of these diseases.

Cirrhosis

The angiographic findings in cirrhotic patients vary with the stage of disease and the degree of hepatic atrophy. Usually the liver is hypervascular, with enlargement and occasionally tortuousity of the hepatic artery. Early in the disease process enlargement of the liver causes elongation and straightening of intrahepatic arteries. However, when atrophy develops, the arteries have a typical tortuous, corkscrew appearance that begins in the periphery and, with continued shrinkage of the liver, eventually involves the larger arteries (Fig. 74-82). In advanced cirrhosis reversal of portal flow (visualization of the portal vein on the late phase of hepatic arteriography) may occur.[11,34] When macroregenerative nodules develop in the cirrhotic liver they can be confused with hepatocellular carcinoma.[78] The nodules themselves displace surrounding branches and can be hypervascular or hypovascular in appearance, with irregular vessels inside them (Fig. 74-83). Displacement of the liver from the

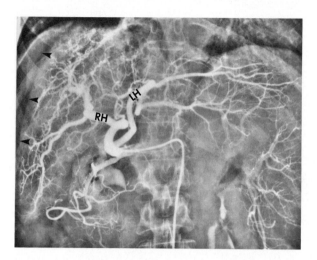

Fig. 74-82 Selective hepatic arteriogram in patient with cirrhosis. There is atrophy of right liver lobe as evidenced by tortuousity and "corkscrewing" of branches of right hepatic artery *(RH)*. There has been hypertrophy of left lobe with stretching of branches of left hepatic artery *(LH)*. Right edge of liver is separated from right lateral abdominal wall *(arrowheads)* by ascitic fluid.

lateral abdominal wall in cirrhotic patients with portal hypertension indicates the presence of ascitic fluid (Fig. 74-84).

Hepatitis

Similar to cirrhosis, the angiographic findings of hepatitis parallel the disease process. In the acute, active stage the liver is enlarged and hypervascular (Fig. 74-85). There is stretching of major intrahepatic branches and a suffusion of indistinctly outlined small arteries throughout the hepatic parenchyma. These small arteries may be duplicated and have a "railroad track" appearance.[99] Chronic hepatitis has various angiographic appearances. The liver can look normal or, depending on the degree of necrosis, may resemble advanced cirrhosis (Fig. 74-86).

Budd-Chiari syndrome

Occlusion of the hepatic veins, Budd-Chiari syndrome, is often seen as a complication of inferior vena caval thrombosis by neoplasms, typically renal or hepatocellular carcinoma. Other causes are oral contraceptives, hypercoagulable states, and, most frequently, idiopathic appearance. Angiographic findings are nonspecific and consist of stretching, narrowing, and minimal

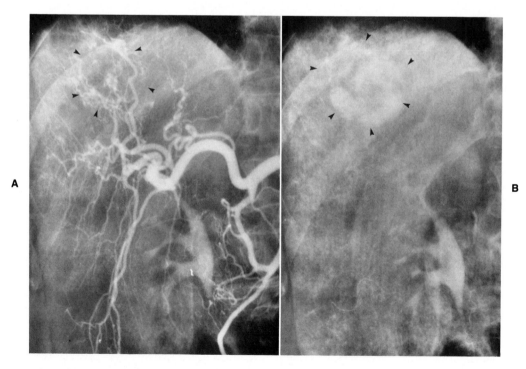

Fig. 74-83 Macro-regenerative nodule. **A,** Area of increased vascularity with slightly irregular vessels *(arrowheads)* indicates presence of regenerative nodule in superior lateral aspect of right liver lobe. **B,** There is an increased accumulation of contrast material *(arrowheads)* in regenerative nodule.

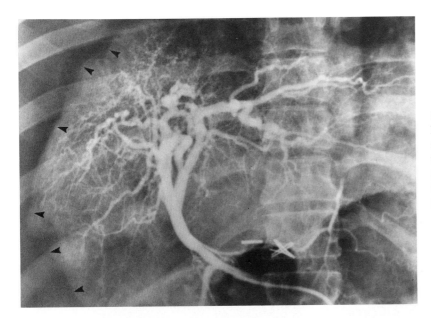

Fig. 74-84 Severe, end-stage cirrhosis. Hepatic arteriography demonstrates small, shrunken, atrophic liver with marked tortuousity and "corkscrewing" of intrahepatic arteries. Liver edge is nodular *(arrowheads)* and separated from lateral abdominal wall by large amount of ascitic fluid.

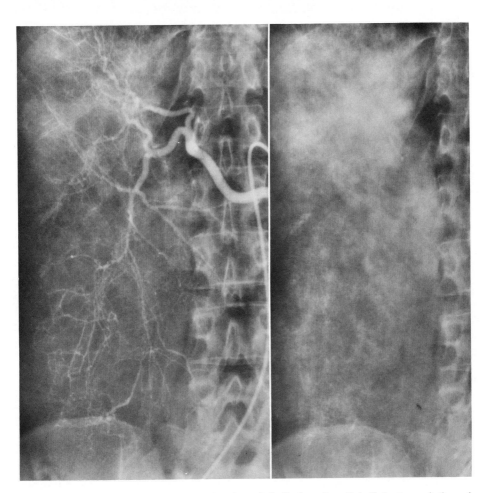

Fig. 74-85 Acute alcoholic hepatic. Liver is enlarged. Suffusion of small, indistinct vessels throughout hepatic parenchyma causes moderately hypervascular appearance. Parenchymal phase is inhomogeneously mottled.

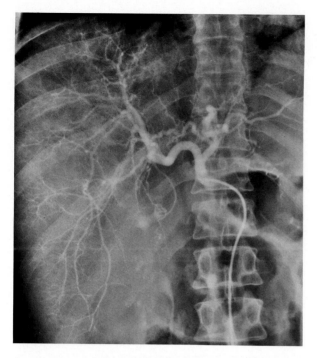

Fig. 74-86 Chronic active hepatitis. Selective hepatic arteriography demonstrates atrophy of left lobe with tortuousity and "corkscrewing" of vessels. Right lobe is enlarged with multiple, small, indistinctly outlined vessels.

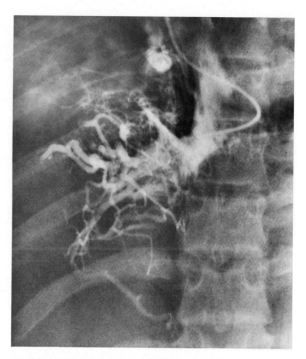

Fig. 74-87 Wedged hepatic venogram in patient with Budd-Chiari syndrome. Inferior vena cava was thrombosed, therefore wedged hepatic venogram was done via transjugular approach. Hepatic veins are occluded. Typical "spider-web" appearance is present as result of multiple tortuous collateral veins that drain toward hepatic capsule and inferior vena cava.

displacement of intrahepatic arteries caused by marked hepatic congestion. Definitive diagnosis is achieved by wedged hepatic venography, which demonstrates myriad tortuous collateral hepatic veins that drain toward hepatic capsular veins and the inferior vena cava.[56] These findings are pathognomonic of Budd-Chiari syndrome and have been called the "spiderweb" appearance (Fig. 74-87). Dilatation of hepatic venous webs and stenoses or re-canalization of focally occluded hepatic veins or of the intrahepatic portion of the inferior vena cava with trans-luminal angioplasty balloons has been successful in treating patients with Budd-Chiari syndrome[13] (Fig. 74-88).

Peliosis hepatis

Peliosis hepatis is an unusual disease that has been associated with ingestion of anabolic steroids. The characteristic angiographic finding is multiple, small accumulations of contrast ranging from barely perceptible to one cm in size. These appear in the late arterial phase of the angiogram and become more prominent in the parenchymal and venous phases. There is neither enlargement nor displacement of the feeding arteries[77] (Fig. 74-89). Histologically, peliosis hepatis is characterized

by multiple blood-filled, endothelium-lined vascular spaces that communicate with the hepatic sinusoids.

Cholangitis

In cholangitis, hypervascularity of multiple small vessels surrounding the bile ducts, the peribiliary plexus, is present.[20] Occasionally, when involved by severe inflammation, the walls of the major biliary ducts will be demonstrated during the parenchymal phase of the angiogram (Fig. 74-90).

HEPATIC NEOPLASMS
Benign hepatic neoplasms
Cavernous hemangioma

Cavernous hemangioma, the most common benign hepatic tumor, is seen frequently in middle-aged women. Its angiographic characteristics are very distinctive.[30,48] Regardless of size, the feeding arteries are normal in caliber. Groups of irregular dilated spaces inside the hemangioma begin to fill with contrast material during the mid arterial phase of the angiogram. Contrast material is retained undiluted in these spaces and persists there, appearing like "cotton wool," late into the venous phase

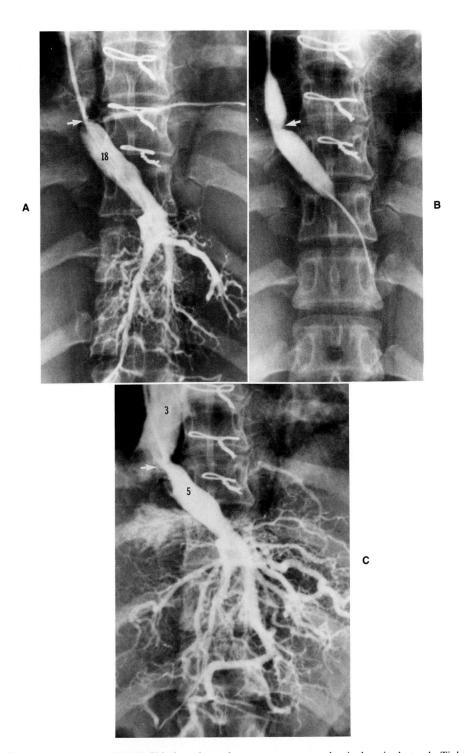

Fig. 74-88 Treatment of Budd-Chiari syndrome by percutaneous transluminal angioplasty. **A,** Tight focal stenosis is present at origin of left hepatic vein *(arrow)*. Pressure in hepatic vein was 18 mm/Hg. **B,** There is a definite waist in angioplasty balloon *(arrow)* at site of stenosis. **C,** Left hepatic venogram following angioplasty reveals significantly increased flow from left hepatic vein to inferior vena cava. Although stenosis has not been completely eliminated *(arrow)*, follow-up pressure in left hepatic vein was 5 mm/Hg and 3 mm/Hg in inferior vena cava, indicating that no significant pressure gradient remained following transluminal angioplasty.

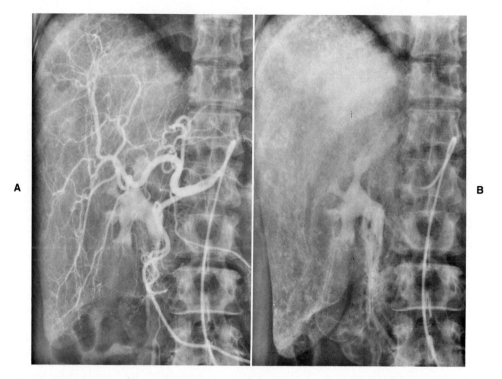

Fig. 74-89 Peliosis hepatis. **A,** Arterial phase of hepatic arteriogram is normal. **B,** Multiple small, distinct, accumulations of contrast material corresponding to endothelial lined vascular spaces found in peliosis hepatis are evident during parenchymal phase.

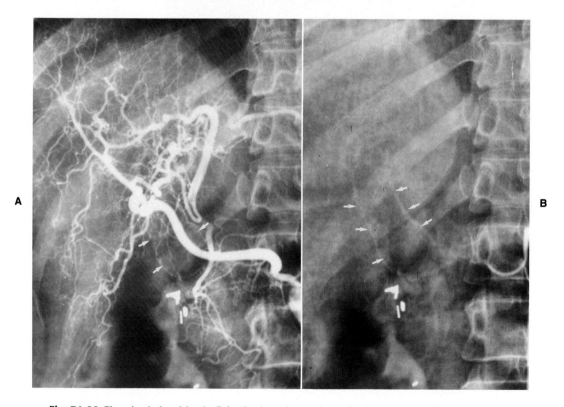

Fig. 74-90 Chronic cholangitis. **A,** Selective hepatic arteriography demonstrates dilated arteries of peribiliary plexus *(arrows)* in distribution of common bile duct. **B,** During parenchymal phase there is increased accumulation of contrast in common bile duct walls *(arrows)*.

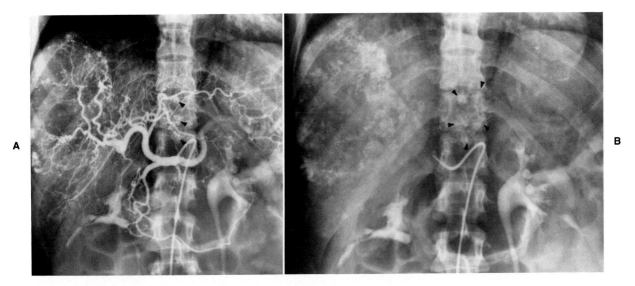

Fig. 74-91 Cavernous hemangiomas. **A,** Groups of dilated vascular spaces in right liver lobe and in medial segment of left liver lobe *(arrowheads)* begin to fill with contrast material during early arterial phase. **B,** These vascular spaces (arrowheads) retain contrast material late into parenchymal phase.

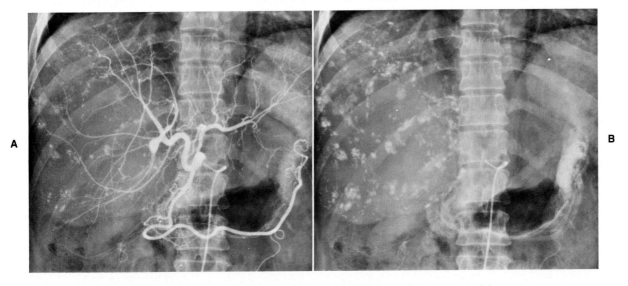

Fig. 74-92 Giant cavernous hemangioma. Multiple accumulations of contrast material are present in early arterial phase **(A)** and remain late into parenchymal phase **(B).** Stretching of right hepatic arterial branches indicates large size of this lesion. Despite its large size and vascular nature, feeding arteries are not enlarged, and AV shunting is not present.

(Fig. 74-91). With large hemangiomas, adjacent arteries and branches of the portal vein may be displaced. Vascular encasement or occlusion does not occur, and arteriovenous shunting is rare. Unless they become sufficiently large to compress adjacent structures or cause discomfort by expansion of the liver capsule, most cavernous hemangiomas are asymptomatic and discovered serendipitously (Fig. 74-92). Rupture of large cavernous hemangiomas with massive intraabdominal hemorrhage can occur but is unusual. Surgical resection, or more recently transcatheter embolization, has been reserved for very large or symptomatic hemangiomas.

Hemangioendothelioma

Hemangioendothelioma is a benign hepatic tumor that occurs predominantly in infants. These are extremely

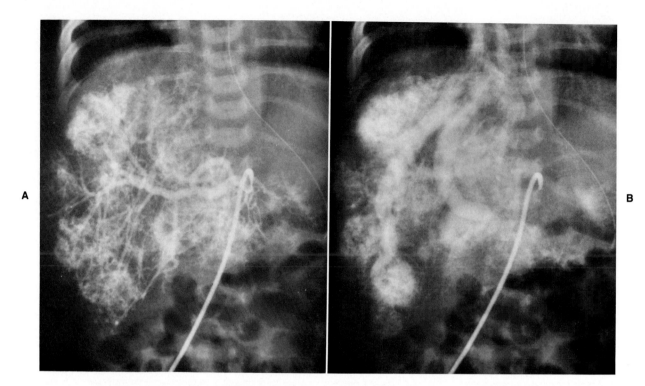

Fig. 74-93 Hemangioendothelioma. This infant presented with high-output heart failure. Selective hepatic arteriography demonstrates intensely hypervascular lesion involving entire liver with enlarged feeding arteries and prominent arterial-venous shunting.

vascular lesions with large amorphous spaces that fill with contrast, similar to those seen in cavernous hemangiomas. However, unlike in cavernous hemangiomas, the feeding arteries are markedly enlarged, blood flow is very rapid without persistence of contrast material in the vascular spaces, and arteriovenous shunting is a prominent feature[72] (Fig. 74-93). Hemangioendothelioma usually presents after birth as an abdominal mass or with high output or congestive heart failure. If heart failure can be managed, the lesions usually involute within a year; however, resection and hepatic artery ligation or hepatic embolization have been used to control severe cardiac failure.

Focal nodular hyperplasia

Focal nodular hyperplasia is a benign, harmless hepatic lesion that occurs in children and adults of both sexes. This tumor has a stellate configuration with multiple fine septae that radiate peripherally from a central core of fibrotic tissue. Histologically, the lesion is composed of normal hepatocytes, proliferating bile ducts, and fibrous septae arranged in a disorganized fashion. Kupffer cells are present in sufficient quantity to take up technetium-99m–sulfer colloid in about half the lesions. In such cases, isotope scanning permits a specific diagnosis.[18,39,64]

Focal nodular hyperplasia has characteristic angiographic findings. It is usually hypervascular, with arteries penetrating directly into the central portion of the tumor and then dividing into a group of radiating branches. There is a dense homogeneous blush during the parenchymal phase, which is often granular in nature (Fig. 74-94). Frequently, a linear lucency, the central scar, is noted in the parenchymal phase (Fig. 74-95). Focal nodular hyperplasia may be single or multiple and also can be pedunculated.[18,39,64] Once the diagnosis of focal nodular hyperplasia has been established, no treatment is required; however, differentiation of focal nodular hyperplasia from hepatic adenoma, which has a much less benign natural history, is important.[119]

Hepatic adenoma

Unlike focal nodular hyperplasia, hepatic adenomas do not have a benign clinical course but frequently present with massive abdominal hemorrhage from spontaneous rupture. These tumors usually occur in young women and have been associated with the use of oral contraceptives.[55] Though it has not been established that degeneration of hepatic adenomas into hepatocellular carcinoma occurs, the high incidence of bleeding associated with hepatic adenomas is an indication for their resection.

Hepatic adenomas are hypervascular lesions supplied

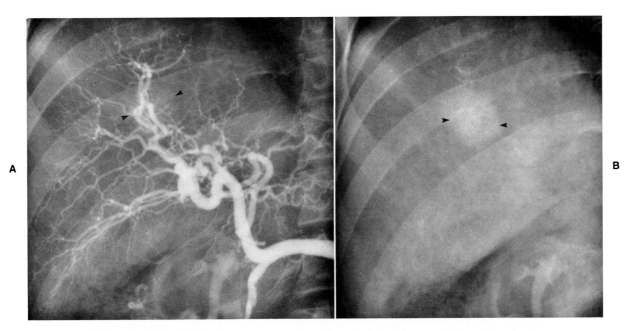

Fig. 74-94 Focal nodular hyperplasia. **A,** Arterial phase demonstrates minimal tumor blush *(arrowheads)* in mid portion of right liver lobe. **B,** During parenchymal phase, stellate configuration of this homogeneously blushing lesion *(arrowheads)* is evident.

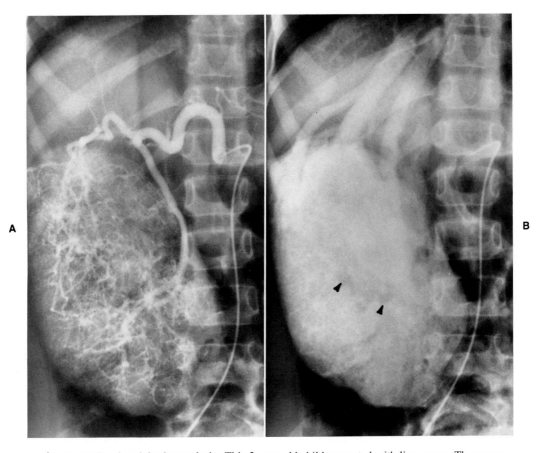

Fig. 74-95 Focal nodular hyperplasia. This 3-year-old child presented with liver mass. There was some uptake of sulfur colloid within lesion on radionuclide scan. **A,** Selective hepatic arteriography demonstrates enlarged hepatic artery feeding large hypervascular lesion with multiple disorganized arteries within it. **B,** During parenchymal phase lesion has dense, fairly homogeneous tumor blush. Linear lucency *(arrowheads)* indicates region of central scar. There is dense, but not early, filling of hepatic veins.

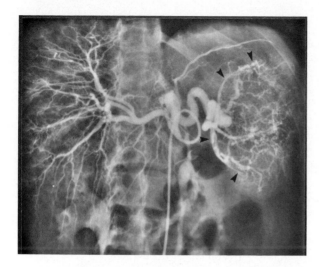

Fig. 74-96 Hepatic adenoma. Hypervascular lesion is present in lateral segment of left liver lobe *(arrowheads)*. Feeding arteries penetrate lesion from circumferential branches. Coarse neovascularity without AV shunting is present.

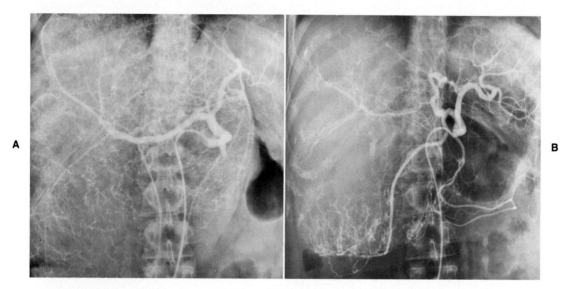

Fig. 74-97 Giant, unresectable hepatic adenoma treated by transcatheter embolization with Ivalon. **A,** Selective hepatic angiography demonstrates massive hypervascular lesion of liver involving entire right lobe and medial segment of left lobe. Feeding arteries arise from circumferential branches and marked neovascularity is present. Open surgical biopsy on two occasions revealed hepatic adenoma. **B,** Six months following embolization with Ivalon particles lesion has shrunken tremendously. There is some recanalization of vessels in right lobe, and interval hypertrophy of lateral segment of left lobe has occurred.

primarily by enlarged branches of the hepatic artery that extend around the periphery of the lesion. From these circumferential arteries, multiple penetrating branches penetrate toward the center, where coarse neovascularity is often present (Fig. 74-96). Portal branches are displaced by larger adenomas but are not invaded. Arteriovenous shunting is not a feature of this lesion. Once hemorrhage has occurred, the hematoma appears as an avascular area within the adenoma[18,39,119] Transcatheter embolization has been used successfully to treat acute

hemorrhage from ruptured hepatic adenomas and as primary therapy for lesions that cannot be approached surgically (E. Finck, M.D., personal communication, 1987) (Fig. 74-97).

Mesenchymal hamartoma

Hepatic mesenchymal hamartoma is a rare lesion that presents as an abdominal mass in young children. It usually undergoes cystic degeneration. The angiogram reveals marked displacement and stretching of individual

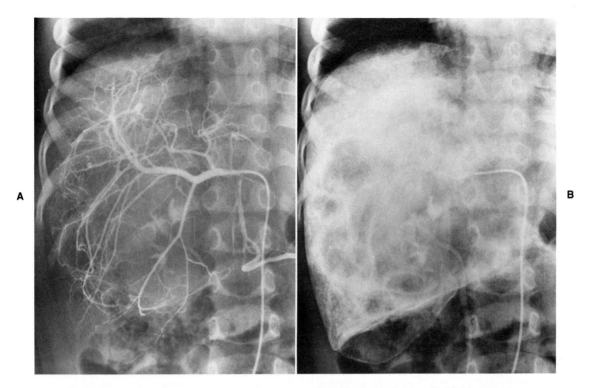

Fig. 74-98 Mesenchymal hamartoma. **A,** Hepatic arteriography in this 4-year-old child demonstrates stretching of multiple intrahepatic arterial branches in right liver lobe. **B,** Large lucent spaces during parenchymal phase that correspond to cystic component of this tumor.

hepatic arterial branches around the lesion. There is minimal hypervascularity in the arterial phase; however, large avascular areas corresponding to the cystic components of the tumor are present in the parenchymal phase (Fig. 74-98). Vascular encasement and arteriovenous shunting are not seen with this lesion.[63] Treatment for mesenchymal hamartoma is surgical resection.

Simple cyst, echinococcus cyst, biliary cystadenoma, and abscess

Unless associated with polycystic disease of the kidneys, simple cysts of the liver are uncommon (Fig. 74-99). Parasitic infection with *Echinococcus* organisms is responsible for most of the liver cysts seen in North America (Fig. 74-100). All types of hepatic cysts are readily diagnosed by ultrasound. Displacement of adjacent arteries is the most striking angiographic finding in liver cysts. Other findings include compression of adjacent parenchyma and an avascular area in the capillary phase of the angiogram.[95]

Biliary cystadenomas are benign, septated, cystic tumors that originate from intrahepatic biliary ducts and occur predominantly in females. Rarely they degenerate into biliary cystadenocarcinoma. Except for a few fine tumor vessels in the cyst wall, the angiographic findings

in biliary cystadenoma are similar to those of simple hepatic cysts (Fig. 74-101).

Because hepatic abscesses are easily demonstrated by CT and ultrasound, angiography is rarely used for their diagnosis. Angiographic findings in liver abscess vary with the duration and degree of inflammation. With indolent infection, the abscess may have the same angiographic appearance as a simple cyst with displacement of adjacent arteries and portal vein branches and an avascular zone during the parenchymal phase. More virulent pathogens evoke a greater inflammatory response, with multiple small, fine vessels around the periphery of the abscess. During the capillary phase, there is a marked blush in the wall of the lesion, and the abscess itself may increase in density. Because the angiographic findings of abscesses are nonspecific, the patient's clinical history is very important in interpreting the arteriogram and arriving at an accurate diagnosis.

Malignant hepatic neoplasms
Hepatocellular carcinoma

Hepatocellular carcinoma can appear as a single, discrete hepatic mass (unifocal hepatoma), multiple well-circumscribed tumor nodules of various sizes (multifocal hepatoma), or generalized, infiltrating involvement of the

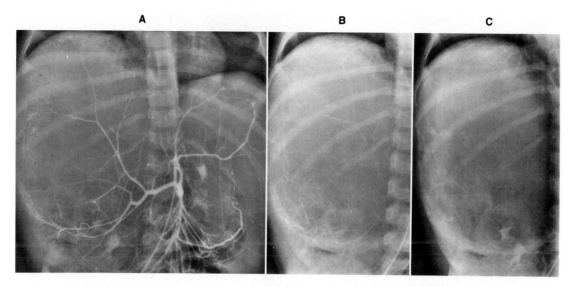

Fig. 74-99 Simple liver cyst. **A,** Hepatic artery is replaced to superior mesenteric artery. There is marked stretching of intrahepatic arterial branches with no evidence of neovascularity or tumor blush. **B,** During late arterial phase, zone of compressed parenchyma adjacent to cyst wall is present. **C,** In parenchymal phase cyst area is lucent compared with normal liver parenchyma.

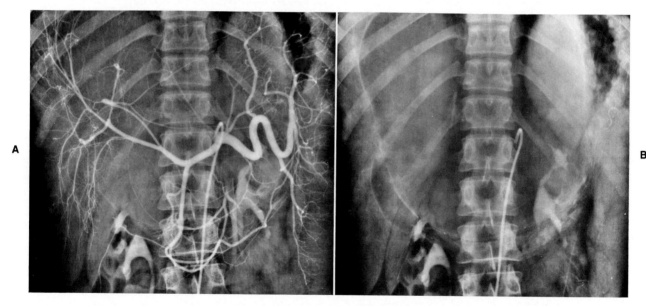

Fig. 74-100 Echinococcus cyst. **A,** Celiac arteriogram demonstrates stretching of intrahepatic arteries in arterial phase. **B,** Large avascular area with compressed adjacent hepatic parenchyma during capillary phase.

majority of liver parenchyma (diffuse hepatoma). Most hepatocellular carcinomas are hypervascular, with enlarged feeders supplying multiple abnormal, dilated arteries within the neoplasm. Bizarre appearing tumor vessels and vascular puddling are frequently seen (Fig. 74-102). Hepatic artery to portal vein shunting is present in approximately one third of hepatomas and is a good angiographic indicator of the diagnosis, because it is rarely

seen in other types of primary or metastatic hepatic tumors (Fig. 74-103).

Because hepatomas frequently invade and occlude branches of the portal vein, arterial portography readily demonstrates portal venous encasement or amputation[85] (Fig. 74-104). Tumor extension into the portal or hepatic venous systems can also be manifested by a discrete tumor nodule or a linear, striated appearance of multiple

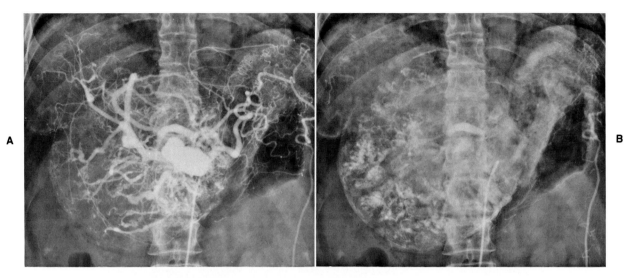

Fig. 74-101 Biliary cystadenoma. **A,** Hepatic arteriography demonstrates stretching of right hepatic artery branches and displacement during arterial phase. **B,** There is minimal blush in cystadenoma wall during parenchymal phase.

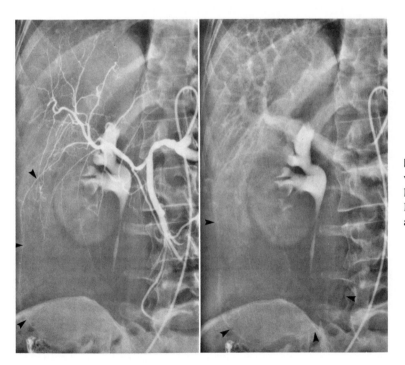

Fig. 74-102 Unifocal hepatoma. Large hypervascular mass with irregular, bizarre neovascularity and puddling of contrast material is present. Both lobes of liver are involved. **A,** early phase and **B,** late phase of celiac arteriogram.

small arteries extending along the expected course of the vein. The latter finding is called the "thread and streak" sign and represents arterial blood supply to that portion of tumor growing inside the vein.[74] Hepatic venous involvement by hepatoma may extend into and eventually occlude the inferior vena cava. When this occurs, inferior cavography may be necessary for complete angiographic evaluation.

Arteriography is very useful in determining the resectability of hepatocellular carcinoma and should be performed on all patients before the contemplated resection. Because the tumor is usually hypervascular, small satellite lesions are frequently detected by angiography in the lobe or segment that was previously found to be tumor free by CT and ultrasound.[110] Furthermore, in patients who are candidates for resection of hepatocellular

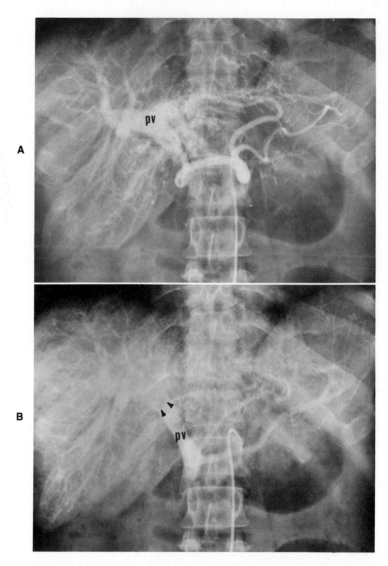

Fig. 74-103 Hepatoma with arterial-portal shunting and invasion of portal vein. **A,** Early phase of celiac arteriography demonstrates hypervascular lesion in hilum of liver with early dense opacification of portal vein *(pv)*. Left gastric artery is markedly enlarged because left hepatic artery, which also supplies this hypervascular tumor, originates from it. **B,** Later phase of celiac arteriography demonstrates retrograde flow in portal vein *(pv),* coronary vein, and splenic vein resulting from portal hypertension from arterial-venous shunt through tumor. Filling defect *(arrowheads)* represents tumor within portal vein.

carcinoma, preoperative angiography precisely demonstrates the arterial supply to the liver and delineates any vascular anomalies that, undetected, could cause difficulty during surgery.

Hepatoblastoma

Hepatoblastoma is the most commonly encountered liver tumor in children under the age of 3. Angiographically, it has an appearance similar to but usually less aggressive than that of hepatocellular carcinoma. Tumor vessels inside the lesion are generally less bizarre in appearance than those found in hepatomas, and arteriovenous shunting or venous invasion is not so common (Fig. 74-105).

Cholangiocarcinoma

Cholangiocarcinoma or primary bile duct carcinoma is scirrhous and infiltrating in nature. Generally less vascular than hepatoma, primary bile duct carcinomas usually encase rather than displace hepatic artery branches (Fig. 74-106). The feeding arteries are not enlarged, and there is no arterioportal shunting present with this tu-

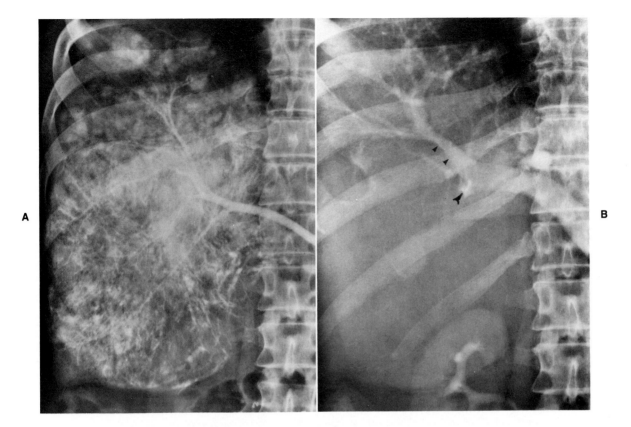

Fig. 74-104 Multifocal hepatocellular carcinoma amputating branches of portal vein. **A,** Hepatic arteriography demonstrates large hypervascular mass in right liver lobe with multiple hypervascular "satellite" lesions around it. **B,** During venous phase there is amputation of major portal venous branch *(large arrowhead)* in region of hepatoma. Compression of right portal vein is also present *(small arrowheads).*

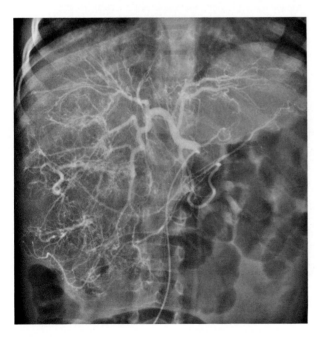

Fig. 74-105 Hepatoblastoma. Hypervascular tumor is present in right liver lobe. Multiple areas of neovascularity are noted; however, AV shunting is absent. Tumor vessels and hepatoblastoma appear less wild and bizarre than those of most hepatocellular carcinomas.

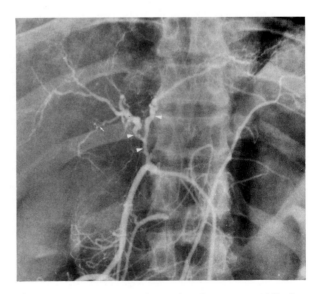

Fig. 74-106 Cholangiocarcinoma invading common bile duct and gallbladder. Hepatic arteriography demonstrates serrated encasement of proper hepatic, right hepatic, and left hepatic arteries *(arrowheads).* There is also encasement of cystic artery *(arrow),* indicating involvement of gallbladder.

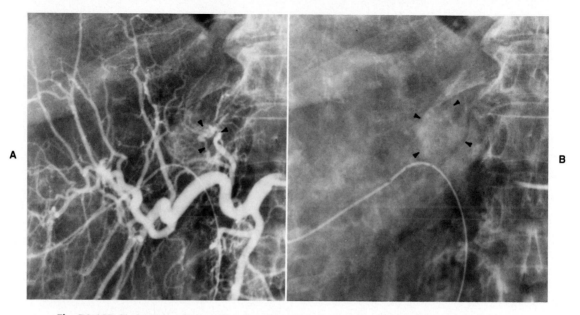

Fig. 74-107 Cholangiocarcinoma. Transhepatic biliary drainage has been established. Arteriogram was requested to determine whether cholangiocarcinoma extended outside biliary ductal system into hepatic parenchyma. **A,** Multiple encased vessels are present in region of tumor, indicating extension into hepatic parenchyma. **B,** Moderate tumor blush *(arrowheads)*.

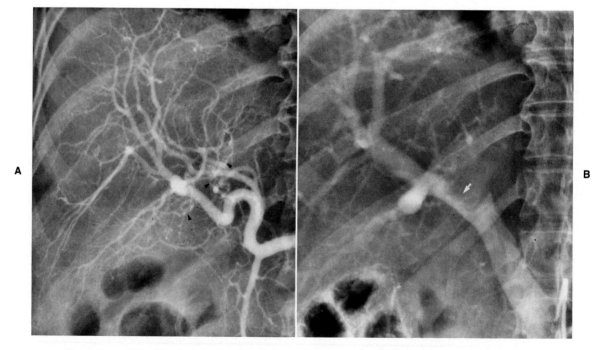

Fig. 74-108 Cholangiocarcinoma invading portal vein. **A,** Hepatic arteriography demonstrates multiple small encased arteries *(arrowheads)*. **B,** Invasion of portal vein *(arrow)* is evident on venous phase and indicates nonresectability.

mor.[50,84,117] Because cholangiocarcinoma grows by infiltration rather than by creating a mass effect, CT and ultrasound are usually not very sensitive in determining its extent (Fig. 74-107). When central in location, bile duct carcinomas cause obstructive jaundice early and are discovered while still small. On the other hand, peripheral lesions can become quite large before diagnosis. Serrated encasement of intrahepatic arteries indicates tumor progression from the ductal system into hepatic parenchyma. Besides determining the lesion's extent, angiography is useful in assessing resectability. Encasement of the main portal vein, proper hepatic artery, or major arteries of both lobes are signs the lesion cannot be resected (Fig. 74-108).

Hepatic metastases

In view of the many different types of primary malignancies that metastasize to the liver, it is not surprising that metastases are the most common malignant hepatic tumors. The vascularity of hepatic metastases often reflects that of their primary. Relative to normal hepatic parenchyma, they can appear as hypervascular, hypovascular, or isodense. Hypervascular metastases are very noticeable against the relatively homogeneous background of liver parenchyma during the capillary phase of the angiogram and thus can be detected when quite

small. In contrast, hypovascular metastases are more difficult to diagnose by conventional angiography. Therefore an infusion hepatic angiogram should be done to study the liver in patients with primary tumors known to have hypovascular metastases. Performed by a long, slow injection of contrast over 12 to 15 seconds with filming every other second carried out over 24 to 30 seconds, infusion hepatic arteriography makes hypovascular metastases stand out relative to normal hepatic parenchyma, which appears less dense because of dilution of contrast material in the hepatic sinusoids from portal vein inflow[94] (Fig. 74-109). Selective hepatic angiography with separate infusion angiograms of both right and left lobe arteries should be considered before hepatic lobectomy is done for presumed unilobar metastatic disease, because additional metastases are frequently revealed in the lobe that was initially found to be free of tumor by noninvasive imaging studies.

Angiography can be useful in the therapy of patients with liver metastases. Redistribution of hepatic arterial blood flow by placement of coil spring occluders in replaced hepatic arterial branches permits infusion of the entire liver with chemotherapeutic agents through a single arterial catheter.[22] For patients with severe clinical syndromes caused by liver metastases from endocrine tumors, hepatic embolization has been successful in pro-

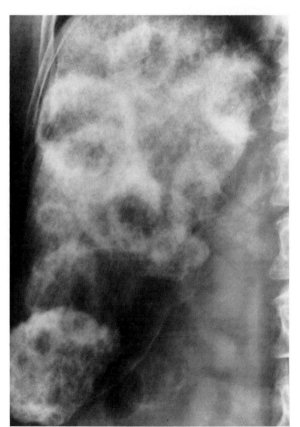

Fig. 74-109 Infusion hepatic arteriogram in patient with hepatic metastasis from colon carcinoma. Multiple metastases with hypervascular rims and necrotic centers are very evident.

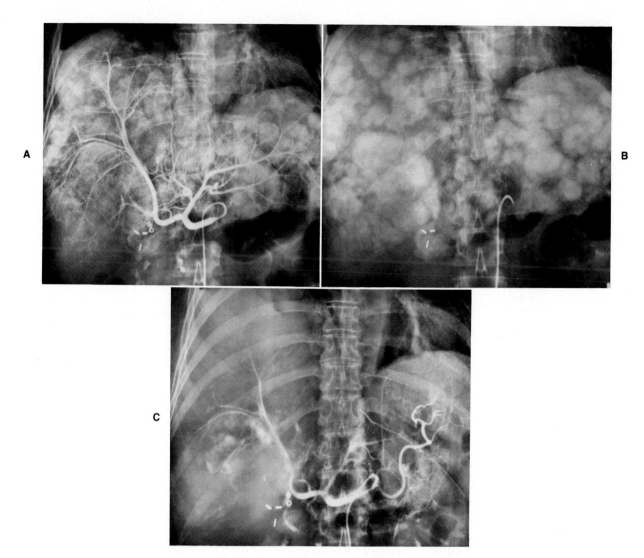

Fig. 74-110 Carcinoid metastasis to liver causing carcinoid syndrome and treated by transcatheter embolotherapy. Early (**A**) and late (**B**) phases of infusion hepatic arteriography demonstrate multiple hypervascular liver metastases from primary carcinoid tumor of distal ileum. **C**, Hepatic arteriography after embolization reveals essentially no arterial flow to liver. Patient's symptoms from carcinoid syndrome were well palliated.

viding long-term palliation[71] (Fig. 74-110). Embolotherapy is effective without infarction of normal liver tissue, because primary and secondary hepatic tumors receive their entire blood supply from the hepatic artery, whereas 80% of the blood supply to normal liver parenchyma comes from the portal vein. Hepatic embolization has also provided palliation for patients with nonendocrine metastases that have not responded to chemotherapy.[23] Before hepatic embolization for metastatic disease is performed, portal vein patency must be demonstrated.

HEPATIC TRAUMA

Though rarely indicated for initial evaluation of patients with liver trauma, angiography is useful whenever vascular complications are suspected or hemorrhage persists following hepatic injury. With liver contusion the arteriogram reveals stretching and straightening of intrahepatic arterial branches with slow flow through them (Fig. 74-111). If active bleeding is present in the contused area, extravasation of contrast material is visualized. Hepatic or subcapsular hematoma appears as an avascular zone either within the liver itself (intrahepatic hematomas) or adjacent to the liver, causing displacement of hepatic parenchyma (subcapsular hematoma) (Fig. 74-112). Contrast material will extravasate into the hematoma if active hemorrhage is present during the arteriogram (Fig. 74-113).

Hepatic lacerations may cause pseudoaneurysm for-

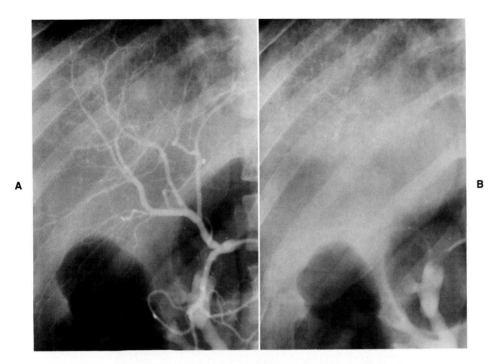

Fig. 74-111 Hepatic contusion. **A,** Branches of hepatic artery are slightly stretched. **B,** Flow through hepatic artery branches is slow, evidenced by contrast material lingering in them during parenchymal phase.

mation, arterioportal venous fistula, or arterial occlusion (Fig. 74-114). In recent years, lacerating injuries of intrahepatic arteries are being seen more frequently because of the increasing number of invasive diagnostic and therapeutic procedures involving the liver.[93] Fistulas between the hepatic artery and portal vein will usually close spontaneously. However, they occasionally persist and enlarge, eventually causing a hyperdynamic circulatory state in the portal system that results in portal hypertension[10] (Fig. 74-115). Arterial pseudoaneurysms may thrombose spontaneously or erode into adjacent biliary ducts to cause hemobilia.[114] Pseudoaneurysms of the hepatic artery can also erode into a portal venous branch, resulting in a hepatic arterioportal venous fistula. In addition to being the primary method for diagnosing the vascular complications of liver trauma, hepatic angiography with therapeutic catheter embolization of pseudoaneurysms that cause hemobilia or persistent hepatic arterioportal venous fistulae is the method of choice for their treatment[69,114] (Fig. 74-116).

SPLENIC ANGIOGRAPHY
Splenomegaly

Enlargement of the spleen is often seen in patients with portal hypertension and hematologic diseases. In such cases the spleen is diffusely enlarged with slight stretching but no displacement of intrasplenic arteries.

The capillary phase is homogeneous in density. With massive splenomegaly, demonstration of the splenic vein may be difficult because of the marked dilution of contrast material that occurs in the enlarge spleen. Partial splenic embolization has been effective in returning platelet and white blood cell counts to normal levels in patients with hypersplensim.[57,75,108] It can also help control recurrent variceal hemorrhage when splenic or portal vein thrombosis is present in patients who are not surgical candidates.[75]

Accessory spleen

Accessory spleens have the angiographic appearance of small, sharply marginated, round densities that are found in close proximity to the spleen. Their blood supply is from the splenic artery. In the parenchymal phase the density and timing of contrast accumulation is similar to that of the spleen itself (Fig. 74-117). Accessory spleens are unusual findings with no clinical importance; however, they should not be mistaken for islet cell adenomas or areas of splenic contusion.

Splenic cysts and abscesses

The majority of splenic cysts are caused by trauma and develop from an intrasplenic hematoma that has not ruptured. Congenital splenic cysts do occur but are rare.

Text continued on p. 1945.

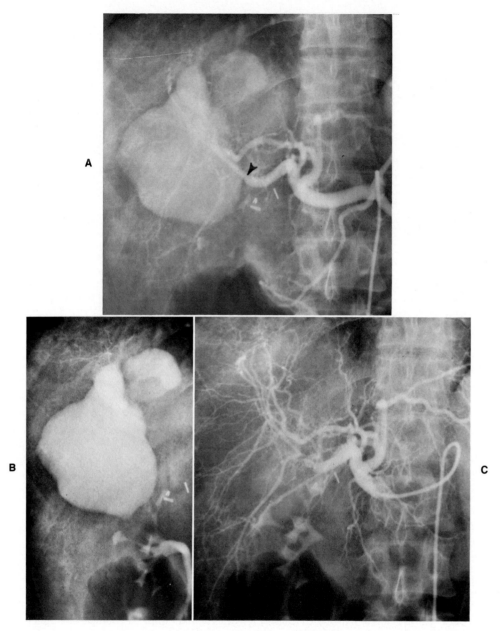

Fig. 74-112 Large intrahepatic pseudoaneurysm causing hemobilia and treated by transcatheter embolization. **A** and **B,** Early and late phase of hepatic arteriogram demonstrate large pseudo-aneurysm in right liver lobe. It originates from right hepatic artery *(arrowhead)* and resulted from machete wound to right upper quadrant. **C,** Following transcatheter embolization with coil spring, pseudoaneurysm no longer fills. After embolization, patient had no further recurrence of hemobilia.

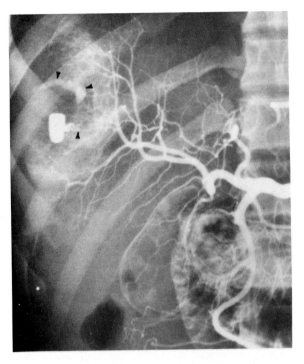

Fig. 74-113 Hepatic hematoma with active hemorrhage. There is displacement and stretching of intrahepatic arteries in region of liver injury. Active bleeding is indicated by extravasation of contrast material *(arrowheads).*

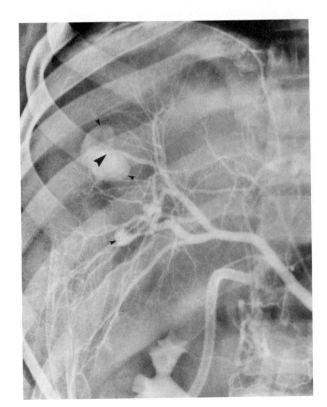

Fig. 74-114 Hepatic lacerations with pseudoaneurysm formation. Hepatic arteriography demonstrates disruption of large intrahepatic arterial branch *(large arrowhead)* with resultant pseudoaneurysm *(small arrowheads).* Another smaller pseudoaneurysm *(small arrowhead)* is present.

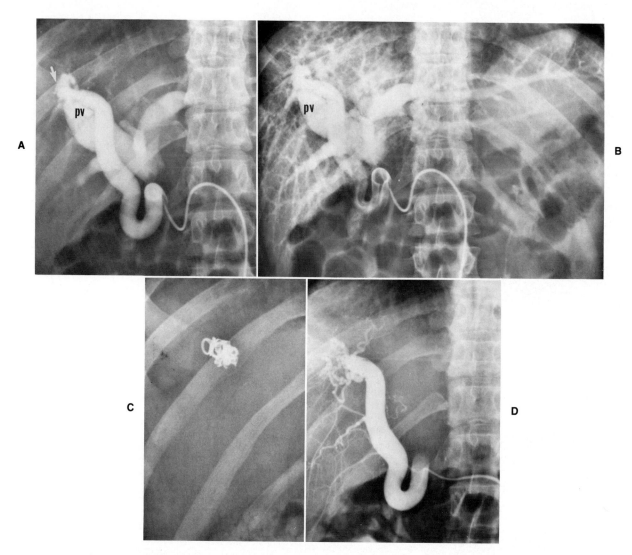

Fig. 74-115 Hepatic artery-to–portal vein fistula following liver injury. This 26-year-old man was involved in automobile accident 10 years previously and received liver trauma. **A,** Early phase of replaced right hepatic arteriography demonstrates marked enlargement of replaced right hepatic artery with early and dense filling of portal vein *(pv)* from an AV fistula *(arrow)*. **B,** Slightly later phase in replaced right hepatic arteriogram demonstrates extensive opacification of portal venous system. **C,** Multiple coil springs placed at site of hepatic artery-to–portal vein fistula. **D,** Arteriography following embolization of hepatic artery-to–portal vein fistula demonstrates that there is no longer filling of portal vein. Multiple small intrahepatic branches that previously did not fill because of steal phenomenon associated with fistula are now opacified.

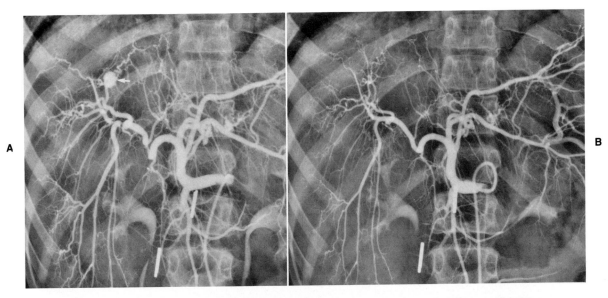

Fig. 74-116 Hepatic injury resulting in hemobilia treated by transcatheter embolotherapy. This 10-year-old girl suffered liver laceration when horse she was riding rolled on top of her. During the ensuing 6 months she had four episodes of upper GI tract hemorrhage. **A,** Hepatic angiography demonstrates pseudoaneurysm *(arrow)* in superior portion of right liver lobe, which was responsible for hemobilia. **B,** Follow-up arteriogram 6 weeks after occlusion of pseudoaneurysm demonstrates that it has been successfully obliterated. Patient has had no recurrent hemobilia for 10 years.

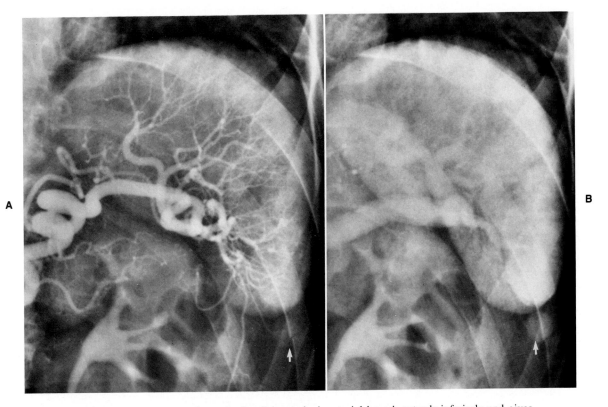

Fig. 74-117 Accessory spleen. **A,** Small intrasplenic arterial branch extends inferiorly and gives supply to accessory spleen *(arrow)*, which is starting to blush. Incidentally noted is rib fracture. **B,** During parenchymal phase, accessory spleen *(arrow)* blushes with same intensity as normal spleen.

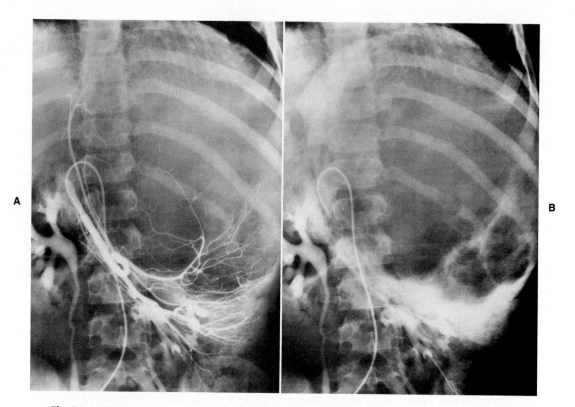

Fig. 74-118 Splenic cyst. Branches of splenic artery are markedly displaced **(A)**. In capillary phase **(B)**, large avascular mass is present that displaces and compresses normal adjacent splenic tissue.

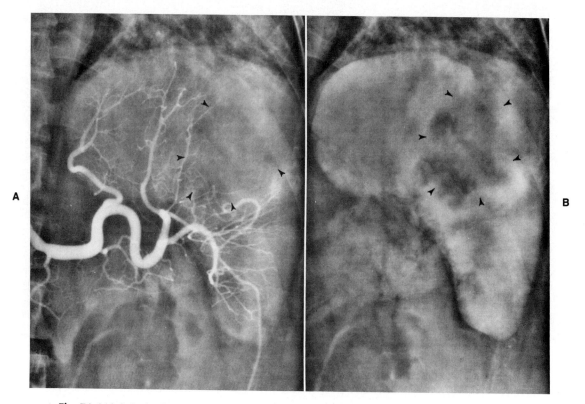

Fig. 74-119 Splenic abscess. Avascular mass is present in central portion of spleen *(arrowheads)*. Minimal hypervascularity is present on arterial phase **(A)**. During capillary phase **(B)**, avascular area has hypervascular rim *(arrowheads)* and lobulated margins.

The angiographic appearance of splenic cysts is similar to that of cysts of other organs. The splenic artery branches are stretched and displaced around the periphery of a round, avascular area that is sharply bordered in the capillary phase by normal spleen (Fig. 74-118). Splenic vein branches are also displaced.[103] Neovascularity, vascular invasion, and arteriovenous shunting are not present. Splenic cysts are easily detected by noninvasive imaging studies, and angiography is rarely indicated for their diagnosis.

There is little to differentiate the angiographic findings of splenic abscess from those of splenic cysts. Abscesses also appear as sharply marginated avascular masses that displace intrasplenic arteries. Occasionally, hypervascularity of arteries adjacent to the abscess or stretching of the epiploic artery toward the spleen, indicating migration of the omentum, gives some clue to the inflammatory nature of the lesion[46] (Fig. 74-119). Also, like splenic cysts, splenic abscesses are readily diagnosed by noninvasive imaging.

Splenic tumors

Benign splenic neoplasms are rare and usually discovered incidentally. Cavernous hemangioma is the most common benign splenic tumor. Its angiographic features are similar to those of cavernous hemangiomas of the liver. Unless they are large and produce portal hypertension, splenic cavernous hemangiomas need not be treated. Other benign splenic tumors include hamartoma or splenadenoma and lymphangiomas.[87]

Malignant splenic neoplasms can be divided into reticuloendothelial tumors and metastatic lesions (Fig. 74-120). Metastases to the spleen may result from direct extension of malignancies from adjacent organs, such as the stomach or pancreas, or they can originate from distant primary sites and metastasize to the spleen via the hematogenous route.[87]

Splenic trauma

Of all intrabdominal organs, the spleen is the most commonly injured in blunt abdominal trauma. CT is usu-

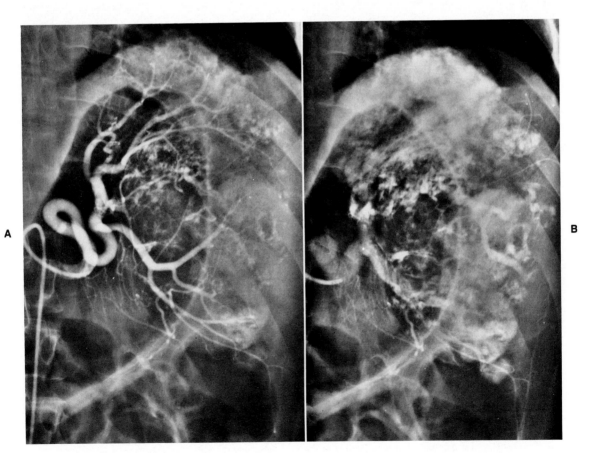

Fig. 74-120 Histiocytic lymphoma involving spleen. Early (**A**) and late (**B**) arterial phases of splenic arteriogram demonstrate hypervascular tumor with displacement of intrasplenic branches, neovascularity, and puddling of contrast material.

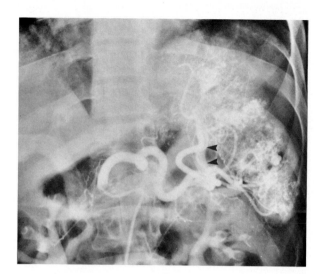

Fig. 74-121 Splenic trauma. Selective splenic arteriography performed in left posterior oblique position separates intrasplenic branches from short gastric branches. There is diffuse extravasation of contrast material into splenic parenchyma. Early filling of splenic vein *(arrowheads)* indicates AV shunting.

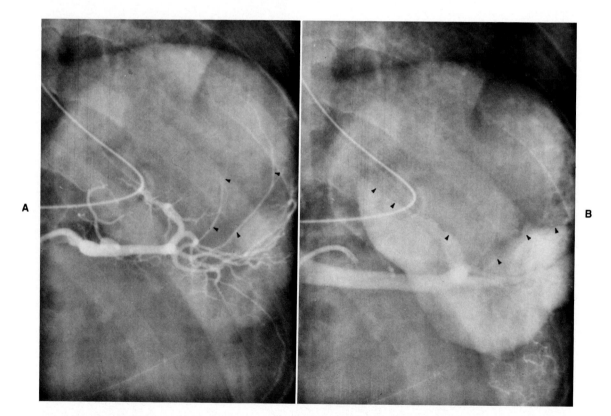

Fig. 74-122 Splenic subcapsular hematoma. **A,** Displacement of intrasplenic branches around avascular mass *(arrowheads)* is present on arterial phase of splenic angiogram. **B,** During venous phase there is displacement of intrasplenic veins by hematoma, which does not blush—in comparison with remainder of spleen *(arrowheads)*.

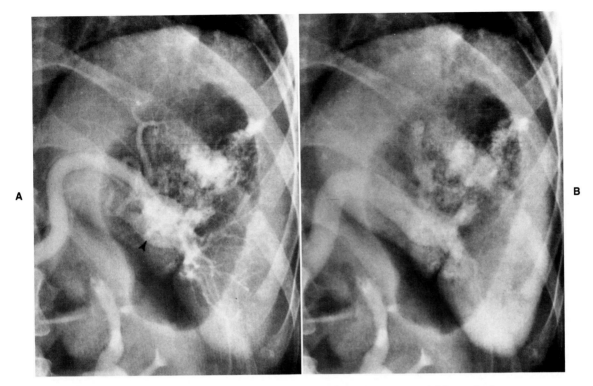

Fig. 74-123 Splenic contusion. **A,** Marked extravasation of contrast material into splenic parenchyma is present, and splenic vein is beginning to fill *(arrowhead)* during arterial phase. **B,** Extravasated contrast remains within splenic parenchyma during capillary phase.

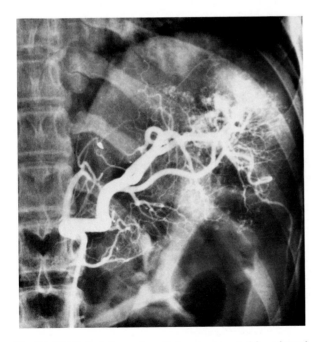

Fig. 74-124 Splenic laceration. Spleen is separated from lateral abdominal wall by hemoperitoneum. There is extensive extravasation of contrast material into splenic parenchyma.

ally the initial radiologic examination performed in evaluation of the patient with blunt abdominal trauma, and angiography is generally reserved for patients in whom serious vascular injury is suspected. Aside from the routine anteroposterior view, splenic angiography often needs to be performed in the left posterior oblique position to project the overlying stomach away from the spleen and permit complete evaluation (Fig. 74-121).

Depending on the extent of injury to the spleen, angiographic findings will vary. Irregular patchy areas of increased density in a portion of the spleen indicate splenic contusion. In subcapsular hematoma, the spleen is enlarged and the splenic artery and vein are displaced medially. Intrasplenic arterial branches are stretched and displaced around the hematoma, which appears as an avascular mass (Fig. 74-122). The angiographic findings of splenic rupture include extravasation of contrast into the splenic parenchyma; early, dense visualization of the splenic vein; occlusion of intrasplenic arterial branches; and avascular areas within the spleen (Fig. 74-123). One of these findings or a combination of several is sufficient to diagnose splenic rupture (Fig. 74-124).

Traditional therapy for splenic subcapsular hematoma or rupture has been immediate splenectomy. In recent years, however, because of the spleen's important immunologic and hematologic functions, trauma surgeons have attempted to preserve splenic function by performing splenorrhaphy or partial splenectomy.[111] Angiographic occlusion of the splenic artery with coil spring occluders achieves similar results. Splenic arterial occlusion decreases arterial inflow and blood pressure at the bleeding site, allowing a stable clot to form at the site of injury.[100] Rich collateral supply through the gastroepiploic and left gastric arteries maintains arterial blood flow to the spleen and thus preserves its viability and function.

REFERENCES

1. Alavi, A: Scintigraphic demonstration of acute gastrointestinal bleeding, Gastrointest Radiol 5:205, 1980.
2. Alavi, A, and Ring EJ: Localization of gastrointestinal bleeding: superiority of ^{99m}Tc sulfur colloid compared with angiography, AJR 137:741, 1981.
3. Antonovic, R, Rösch, J, and Dotter, CT: Complications of percutaneous transaxillary catheterization for arteriography and selective chemotherapy, AJR 126:386, 1976.
4. Ariyama, J, et al: The diagnosis of the small resectable pancreatic carcinoma, Clin Radiol 28:437, 1977.
5. Athanasoulis, CA: Therapeutic application of angiography, N Engl J Med 302:1117, 1980.
6. Athanasoulis, CA, et al: Angiography: its contribution to the emergency management of gastrointestinal hemorrhage, Radiol Clin North Am 14:265, 1976.
7. Athanasoulis, CA, et al: Intraoperative localization of small bowel bleeding sites with combined use of angiographic methods and methylene blue injection, Surgery, 87:77, 1980.
8. Barr, WE, Lakin, PC, and Rösch, J: Similarity of arterial and intravenous vasopressin on portal and systemic hemodynamics, Gastroenterology, 69:13, 1975.
9. Baum, S, et al: Angiodysplasia of the right colon: a cause of gastrointestinal bleeding, AJR 129:789, 1977.
10. Bedell, JE, Keller, FS, and Rösch, J: Iatrogenic intrahepatic arterial-portal fistula, Radiology 151:79, 1984.
11. Boijsen, E: Selective angiography of the celiac axis and superior mesenteric artery in portal hypertension, Rev Intern Hepatol 15:323, 1965.
12. Boijsen, E, Kaude, J, and Tyler, V: Radiologic diagnosis of ilial carcinoid tumors, Acta Radiol (Diagn) (Stockh) 15:165, 1974.
13. Boijsen, E, and Reuter, SR: Mesenteric angiography in the evaluation of inflammatory and neoplastic disease of the intestine, Radiology 87:1082, 1966.
14. Boijsen, E, Wallace, S, and Kanter, IE: Angiography in tumors of the stomach, Acta Radiol (Diagn) (Stockh) 4:306, 1966.
15. Bookstein, JJ, Naderi, JJ, and Walter JR: Transcatheter embolization for lower gastrointestinal bleeding, Radiology 127:345, 1978.
16. Bookstein, JJ, and Voegeli, E: Critical analysis of magnification angiography, Radiology 98:23, 1971.
17. Buranasiri, S, and Baum, S: The significance of the venous phase in celiac and superior mesenteric arteriography in evaluating pancreatic carcinoma, Radiology 102:11, 1972.
18. Casarella, WJ, et al: Focal nodular hyperplasia and liver cell adenoma: radiologic and pathologic differentiation, AJR 131:393, 1978.
19. Castaneda-Zuniga, WR, et al: Transluminal angioplasty in the management of mesenteric angina, Förtschr Röntgenstr 137:330, 1982.
20. Cho, KJ, and Lunderquist, A: The peribiliary vascular plexus: the microvascular architecture of the bile duct in the rabbit and in clinical cases, Radiology 147:357, 1983.
21. Cho, KJ, Wilcox, CW, and Reuter, SR: Glucagon producing islet cell tumor of the pancreas, AJR 129:159, 1977.
22. Chuang, VP, and Wallace, S: Hepatic arterial redistribution for intraarterial infusion of hepatic neoplasms, Radiology 135:295, 1980.
23. Chuang, VP, and Wallace, S: Hepatic artery embolization in the treatment of hepatic neoplasms, Radiology 140:51, 1981.
24. Clouse, ME, et al: Subselective angiography in localizing insulinomas of the pancreas, AJR 128:741, 1977.
25. Eckstein, MR, et al: Gastric bleeding: therapy with intraarterial vasopressin and embolization, Radiology 152:563, 1984.
26. Eisenberg, RL, Bank, WO, and Hedgcock, MW: Renal failure after major angiography can be avoided with hydration, AJR 136:859, 1981.
27. Finlay, DBL, and Herlinger, H: The intrapancreatic anatomy as an index of adequacy of pancreatic arteriography, Clin Radiol 28:595, 1977.
28. Fisher, RG, et al: Polyarteritis nodosa and hepatitis-B surface antigen: role of angiography in diagnosis, AJR 129:77, 1977.
29. Flickinger, EG, et al: Local streptokinase for superior mesenteric artery thromboembolism, AJR 140:771, 1983.
30. Freeny, PC, Vimont, TR, and Barnett, DC: Cavernous hemangioma of the liver: ultrasonography, arteriography, and computed tomography, Radiology 132:143, 1979.
31. Freeny, PC, et al: Cystic neoplasms of the pancreas: new angiographic and ultrasonographic findings, AJR 131:795, 1978.
32. Friedman, J, et al: Optimal use of tolazoline in arteriography, AJR 142:817, 1984.
33. Friegman, PJ, and Greespan, RH: Observations on magnification radiology, Radiology 92:549, 1969.
34. Fuchs, WA, et al: Hepatic arteriography in cirrhosis of the liver and portal hypertension, Invest Radiol 7:369, 1972.
35. Gold, RP, et al: Radiologic and pathologic characteristics of the WDHA syndrome, AJR 127:397, 1976.
36. Goldberger, LE, and Bookstein, JJ: Transcatheter embolization in the treatment of diverticula hemorrhage, Radiology 122:613, 1977.
37. Golden, DA, et al: Percutaneous angioplasty in the treatment of abdominal angina, AJR 139:247, 1982.
38. Goldstein, HM, and Miller, M: Angiographic evaluation of carcinoid tumors of the small intestine: the value of epinephrine, Radiology 114:23, 1975.
39. Goldstein, HM, et al: Angiographic findings in benign liver cell tumors, Radiology 110:339, 1974.
40. Gomes, AS, Lois, JF, and McCoy, RD: Angiographic treatment of gastrointestinal hemorrhage: comparison of vasopressin infusion and embolization, AJR 146:1031, 1986.
41. Hale, J, and Miskin, MM: Serial direct magnification cerebral angiography, AJR 107:616, 1969.
42. Hanafee, W, and Shinno, JM: Second-order subtraction and simultaneous bilateral carotid, internal carotid injections, Radiology 86:334, 1966.
43. Haut, G, and Amplatz, K: Complication rates of transfemoral and transaortic catheterization, Surgery 63:594, 1968.
44. Herlinger, H, and Finlay, DBL: Evaluation and follow-up of pancreatic arteriograms: a new role for angiography in the diagnosis of carcinoma of the pancreas, Clin Radiol 29:277, 1978.

45. Hessel, SJ, Adams, DF, and Abrams, HL: Complications of angiography, Radiology 138:273, 1981.

46. Jacobs, RP, et al: Angiography of splenic abscesses, AJR 122:419, 1974.

47. Jhaveri, HS, et al: Value of arteriography in the evaluation of sonolucent pancreatic mass, Cardiovasc Radiol 2:55, 1979.

48. Johnson, CM, et al: Computed tomography and angiography of cavernous hemangioma of the liver, Radiology 138:115, 1981.

49. Kadir, S, and Athanasoulis, CA: Angiographic management of gastrointestinal bleeding with vasopressin, Fortschr Röntgenstr 127:111, 1977.

50. Kaude, J, and Rian, R: Cholangiocarcinoma, Radiology 100:573, 1971.

51. Kaufman, SL, Harrington, DB, and Siegelman, SS: Superior mesenteric artery embolization: an angiographic emergency, Radiology 124:625, 1970.

52. Kelemouridis, V, Athanasoulis, CA, and Waltman, AC: Gastric bleeding sites: an angiographic study, Radiology 149:643, 1983.

53. Keller, FS, and Rösch, J: Angiography in the diagnosis and therapy of acute upper gastrointestinal bleeding, Schweiz med Wschr 109:586, 1979.

54. Keller, FS, et al: Embolization in the treatment of bleeding gastroesophageal varices, Semin Roentgenol 16:103, 1981.

55. Klatskin, G: Hepatic tumors: possible relationship to use of oral contraceptives, Gastroenterology 73:386, 1977.

56. Kreel, L, Feston, JW, and Clain, D: Vascular radiology in the Budd-Chiari syndrome, Br J Radiol 40:755, 1967.

57. Kumpe, DA, Rumack, CM, and Pretorius, DH: Partial splenic embolization in children with hypersplenism, Radiology 155:357, 1985.

58. Lieberman, DA, et al: Arterial embolization for massive upper gastrointestinal tract bleeding in poor surgical candidates, Gastroenterology 86:876, 1984.

59. Lunderquist, A, and Vang, J: Transhepatic catheterization and obliteration of the coronary vein in patients with portal hypertension and esophageal varices, N Engl J Med 291:646, 1974.

60. Lunderquist, A, et al: Selective pancreatic vein catheterization for homone assay in endocrine tumors of the pancreas, Cardiovasc Radiol 1:117, 1978.

61. Margulis, AR, Heinbecker, P, and Bernard, HR: Operative mesenteric arteriography in the search for the site of bleeding in unexplained gastrointestinal hemorrhage, Surgery 48:534, 1960.

62. McKuscik, KA, et al: ^{99m}Tc Red blood cells for detection of gastrointestinal bleeding: experience with 80 patients, AJR 137:1113, 1981.

63. McLoughlin, MJ, and Phillips, MJ: Angiographic findings in multiple bile duct hamartomas of the liver, Radiology 116:41, 1975.

64. McLoughlin, MJ, et al: Focal nodular hyperplasia of the liver: angiography and radioisotope scanning, Radiology 107:257, 1973.

65. Meyerovitz, MF, and Fellows, KE: Angiography in gastrointestinal bleeding in children, 143:837, 1984.

66. Michels, NA: Blood supply and anatomy of the upper abdominal organs, Philadelphia, 1955, JB Lippincott.

67. Michels, NA: Newer anatomy of the liver and its collateral circulation, Am J Surg 112:337, 1981.

68. Mistretta, CA, Crumny, AB, and Strother, CM: Digital angiography: a perspective, Radiology 139:273, 1981.

69. Mitchell, SE, et al: Biliary catheter drainage complicated by hemobilia: treatment by balloon embolotherapy, Radiology 157:645, 1985.

70. Mitty, HA, Efremidis, S, and Keller, RJ: Colonic stricture after transcatheter embolization for diverticular bleeding, AJR 133:519, 1979.

71. Mitty, HA, et al: Control of carcinoid syndrome with hepatic artery embolization, Radiology 155:623, 1985.

72. Mortenson, W, and Pettersson, H: Infantile hepatic hemangioendothelioma, Acta Radiol (Diagn) (Stockh) 20:161, 1979.

73. Nusbaum, M, et al: Pharmacologic control of portal hypertension, Surgery 62:299, 1967.

74. Okuda, K, et al: Demonstration of growing casts of hepatocellular carcinoma in the portal vein by celiac angiography: the thread and streak sign, Radiology 117:303, 1975.

75. Owman, JT, et al: Embolization of the spleen for treatment of splenomegaly and hypersplenism in patients with portal hypertension, Invest Radiol 14:457, 1979.

76. Palmaz, JC, Walter, JF, and Cho, KJ: Therapeutic embolization of small bowel arteries, Radiology 152:377, 1984.

77. Pliskin, M: Peliosis hepatis, Radiology 114:23, 1975.

78. Rabinowitz JG, Kinkabwala, M, and Ulreich, S: Macroregenerating nodule in the cirrhotic liver, AJR 121:140, 1974.

79. Redman, HC, Reuter, SR, and Miller, SJ: Improvement of superior mesenteric and portal vein visualization with tolazoline, Invest Radiol 4:24, 1969.

80. Reuter, SR: Superselective pancreatic angiography, Radiology 92:74, 1967.

81. Reuter, SR: Accentuation of celiac compression by the median arcuate ligament of the diaphragm during deep expiration, Radiology 98:561, 1971.

82. Reuter, SR, and Atkin, TW: High dose left gastric angiography for demonstration of esophageal varices, Radiology 105:573, 1972.

83. Reuter, SR, Kanter, IE, and Redman, HC: Angiography in reversible colonic ischemia, Radiology 97:371, 1970.

84. Reuter, SR, Redman, HC, and Bookstein, JJ: Angiography in carcinoma of the biliary tract, Br J Radiol 44:636, 1971.

85. Reuter, SR, Redman, HC, and Siders, DB: The spectrum of angiographic findings in hepatoma, Radiology 94:89, 1970.

86. Roe, M, and Greenough, WG: Marked hypervascularity and arteriovenous shunting in acute pancreatitis, Radiology 113:47, 1974.

87. Rösch, J: Tumors of the spleen: the value of selective angiography, Clin Radiol 17:183, 1966.

88. Rösch, J, Antonovic, R, and Dotter, CT: Current angiographic approach to diagnosis and therapy of acute gastrointestinal bleeding, Fortschr Röntgenstr 125:301, 1976.

89. Rösch, J, Dotter, CT, and Brown, MS: Selective arterial embolization, Radiology 102:303, 1972.

90. Rösch, J, and Grollman, JH, Jr: Superselective arteriography in the diagnosis of abdominal pathology: technical considerations, Radiology 92:1008, 1969.

91. Rösch, J, and Keller, FS: Pancreatic angiography in early diagnosis of pancreatic cancer, K Kawai (ed.) Tokyo, 1980, Igaku-Shoin.

92. Rösch, J, Keller, FS, and Bilbao, MK: Radiologic diagnosis of pancreatic cancer, Semin Oncol 6:318, 1979.

93. Rösch, J, Putnam, JS, and Keller, FS: Diagnosis and management of hemobilia, Semin Intervent Radiol 5:49, 1988.

94. Rösch, J, et al: Infusion hepatic angiography in the diagnosis of liver metastases, Cancer 38:2278, 1976.

95. Rösch, J, et al: Vascular benign liver cyst in children: report of two cases, Radiology 126:747, 1978.

96. Rösch, J, et al: Pharmacoangiography in the diagnosis of recurrent massive lower gastrointestinal bleeding, Radiology 145:615, 1982.

97. Rösch, J, et al: Interventional angiography in the diagnosis of lower gastrointestinal hemorrhage, Eur J Radiol 6:136, 1986.

98. Rossi, P, et al: Digital celic angiography, Radiology 154:229, 1985.

99. Rourke, JA, Bosniak, MA, and Ferris, EJ: Hepatic angiography in alcoholic hepatitis, Radiology 91:290, 1968.

100. Scalfani, SJA: Angiographic hemostasis: its role in salvage of the injured spleen, Radiology 141:645, 1981.

101. Scully, RE, Mark, EJ, and McNeely, BU: Case records of the Massachussetts General Hospital, N Engl J Med 305:391, 1981.

102. Sebrechts, C, and Bookstein, JJ: Embolization in the management of lower gastrointestinal hemorrhage, Semin Intervent Radiol 5:39, 1988.

103. Shanser, JD, et al: Angiographic evaluation of cystic lesions of the spleen, AJR 119:166, 1973.

104. Sheedy, PF, Fulton, RE, and Atwell, DT: Angiographic evaluation in patients with chronic gastrointestinal bleeding, AJR 123:338, 1975.

105. Siegelman, SS, Sprayregen, S, and Boleys, J: Angiographic diagnosis of mesenteric arterial vasoconstriction, Radiology 112:533, 1974.

106. Sigstedt, B, and Lunderquist, A: Complications of angiographic examinations, AJR 130:455, 1978.

107. Sos, TA, et al: Intermittent bleeding from minute to minute in acute massive gastrointestinal hemorrhage: arteriographic demonstration, AJR 131:1015, 1978.

108. Spigos, DG, et al: Splenic embolization, Cardiovasc Intervent Radiol 3:282, 1980.

109. Sprayregen, S, and Boley, SJ: Vascular ectasias of the right colon, JAMA 239:962, 1977.

110. Takashima, T, and Matsui, O: Infusion hepatic angiography in the detection of small hepatocellular carcinomas, Radiology 136:321, 1980.

111. Traub, Ac, and Perry, JF, Jr: Splenic preservation following splenic trauma, J Trauma 22:496, 1982.

112. Uflacker, R, et al: Angiography in primary myomas of the alimentary tract, Radiology 139:361, 1981.

113. Uflacker, R, et al: Percutaneous transluminal angioplasty of the hepatic veins for treatment of Budd-Chiari syndrome, Radiology 143:53, 1984.

114. Vaughan, R, et al: Treatment of hemobilia by transcatheter vascular occlusion, Eur J Radiol 4:183, 1984.

115. Viamonte, M, Jr, et al: Transhepatic obliteration of gastroesophageal varices: results in acute and nonacute bleeders, AJR 129:237, 1977.

116. Vujic, I, Seymour, EQ, and Meredith, HC: Vascular complications associated with sonographically demonstrated cystic epigastric lesions: an important indication for angiography, Cardiovasc Intervent Radiol 3:75, 1980.

117. Walker, JF, Bookstein, JJ, and Bouffard, EV: Newer angiographic observations in cholangiocarcinoma, Radiology 118:19, 1976.

118. Waltman, AC, et al: Pyloroduodenal bleeding and intraarterial vasopressin: clinical results, AJR 133:643, 1979.

119. Welch, TJ, et al: Focal nodular hyperplasia and hepatic adenoma: comparison of angiography, CT, US, and scintigraphy, Radiology 156:593, 1985.

120. Zelenock, GB, et al: Splanchnic arteriosclerotic disease and intestinal angina, Arch Surg 115:497, 1980.

121. Zollikofer, CL, et al: Angiographic appearance of leiomyomas of the small intestine: report of two cases, Cardiovasc Radiol 2:131, 1979.

75 *Venography*

PATRICK C. FREENY

The venous system of the upper abdominal visceral organs and gastrointestinal tract is important in both diagnostic and interventional radiology. It may be studied by a variety of techniques, including direct percutaneous venography, indirect arterial portography, computed tomography (CT), ultrasonography, and magnetic resonance (MR).

NORMAL VENOUS ANATOMY
Inferior vena cava

The inferior vena cava is formed by the junction of the left and right iliac veins (Fig. 75-1). It ascends within the retroperitoneum to the right of the aorta, receiving branches from multiple lumbar veins, the kidneys and adrenal glands, the right gonadal vein, and the hepatic veins. It is located ventral to the caudate lobe of the liver and for a short distance is intrahepatic. The hepatic veins enter the inferior vena cava ventrally and laterally in its subdiaphragmatic suprahepatic or intrahepatic segment.

A variety of congenital or developmental anomalies of the inferior vena cava has been described and may be found in the excellent monograph by Ferris and co-workers.[53]

Hepatic veins

There are three major hepatic veins—left, right, and middle (Figs. 75-2, 75-3, and 75-4). The anatomy of the hepatic veins has been described in several monographs.[46,122,128] The *right hepatic vein* is located within the right hepatic intersegmental fissure, which separates the anterior and posterior setments of the right lobe of the liver. It enters the right ventrolateral surface of the inferior vena cava. The *middle hepatic vein* is within the main hepatic lobar fissure, which divides the left and right hepatic lobes or, more specifically, the anterior segment of the right lobe and the medial segment of the left lobe. It enters the ventral surface of the inferior vena cava. The *left hepatic vein* is within the left hepatic intersegmental fissure, which separates the medial and lateral segments of the left lobe of the liver, and enters the inferior vena cava along its left ventromedial surface. The *caudate lobe* of the liver is drained separately by one or more small veins that enter the ventral surface of the vena cava.

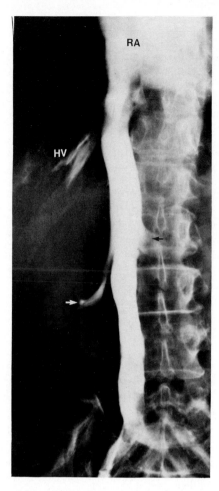

Fig. 75-1 Normal inferior vena cavagram. Inferior vena cavagram shows reflux of contrast into hepatic veins *(HV)* and renal veins *(arrows)*. *RA,* Right atrium.

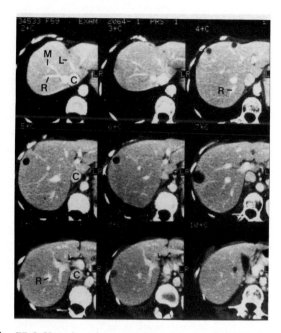

Fig. 75-2 Hepatic veins: computed tomography (CT). Incremental bolus–dynamic computed tomograms of liver show normal contrast enhancement of hepatic veins (*L,* left; *M,* middle; *R,* right) and inferior vena cava *(C).* Incidental hepatic cyst in right lobe.

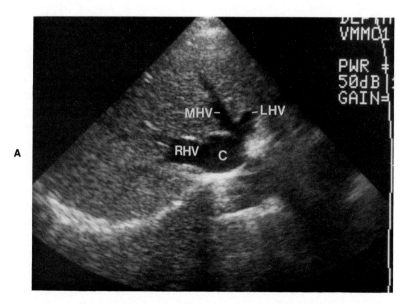

Fig. 75-3 Inferior vena cava and hepatic veins: sonography. Axial (**A** and **B**) and sagittal (**C** and **D**) real-time sonograms of liver show normal hepatic venous anatomy. *C,* Inferior vena cava; *RHV,* right hepatic vein; *MHV,* middle hepatic vein; *LHV,* left hepatic vein; *A,* anterior segmental right hepatic vein; *P,* posterior segmental right hepatic vein; *MPV,* main portal vein; *L,* left portal vein.

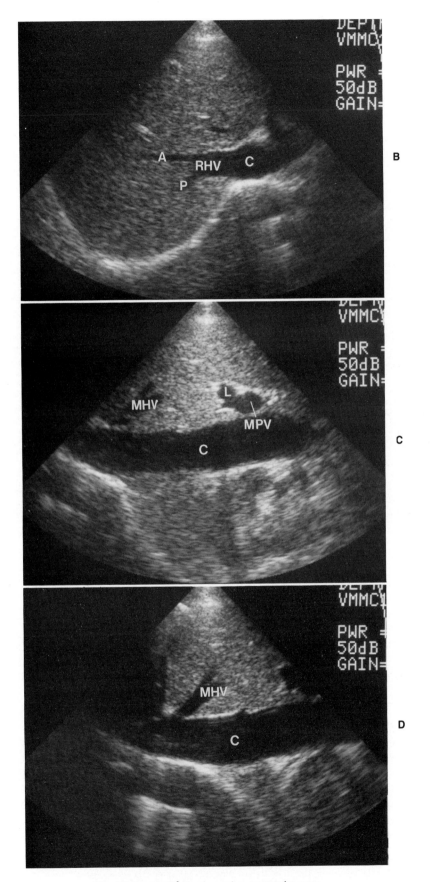

Fig. 75-3, cont'd For legend see opposite page.

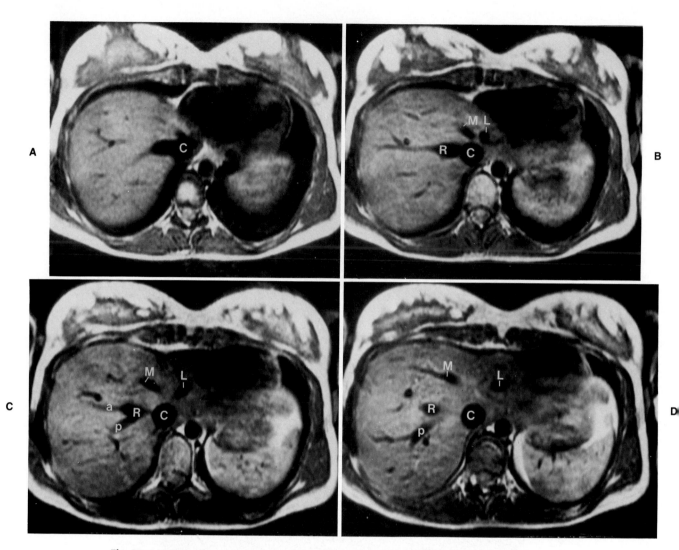

Fig. 75-4 Hepatic veins: magnetic resonance (MR). Sequential MR images show inferior vena cava *(C)* and main hepatic veins *(L,* left; *R,* right; *M,* middle; *a,* anterior segmental branch of right hepatic vein; *P,* posterior segmental branch of right hepatic vein). Veins are seen as areas of signal void because of flowing blood.

Specific evaluation of the hepatic venous system can be accomplished by a variety of techniques, including ultrasound, CT, MR, selective hepatic venography, and percutaneous parenchymal hepatography[29,114,173,182] (Figs. 75-2, 75-3, and 75-4). The hepatic veins may be visualized during the venous phase of selective hepatic arteriography, although in the experience of Glickman and Handel[69] this occurred in only 3 to 50 normal hepatic arteriograms.

Selective hepatic venography may be performed by several techniques. *Free hepatic venography* is accomplished by catheterizing the hepatic veins from the inferior vena cava. The catheter is placed in the orifice of the vein, and 10 to 30 ml of contrast medium is injected at a rate of 5 to 10 cm/second (Fig. 75-5). *Wedged hepatic venography* may be accomplished by advancing the catheter peripherally until the tip is wedged in a small vein or by using an occlusion balloon catheter.[31] In either case the catheter may be used to measure corrected sinusoidal pressure (wedged hepatic vein pressure minus inferior vena cava pressure), which accurately reflects portal venous pressure, and to obtain a segmental venogram (Fig. 75-5). *Parenchymal hepatography* is performed by percutaneously placing a small needle into the hepatic parenchyma and injecting 8 to 12 ml of contrast medium.[173] This technique now is rarely used.

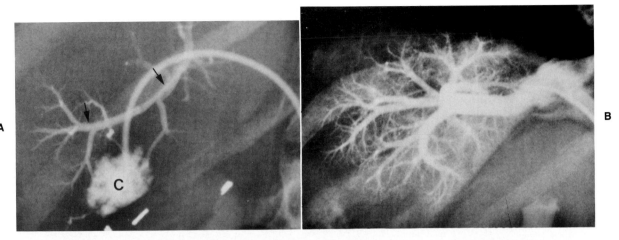

Fig. 75-5 Hepatic venography. **A,** Normal wedged hepatic venogram shows hepatic parenchymal stain *(C)* and reflux of contrast into small portal vein branches *(arrows)*. **B,** Normal free hepatic venogram shows major segmental vein and peripheral branches.

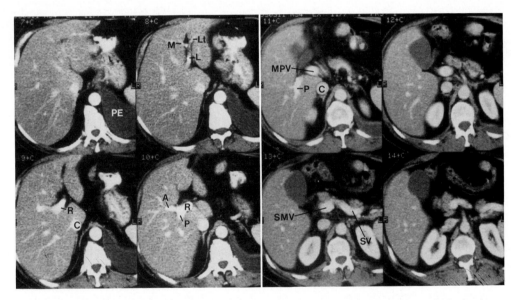

Fig. 75-6 Portal venous system: CT. Sequential bolus–dynamic computed tomograms show superior mesenteric vein *(SMV)* and splenic vein *(SV)* confluence forming main portal vein *(MPV)* and the intrahepatic branches of the main portal vein (*L,* left portal vein; *M,* medial segmental branch of left portal vein; *Lt,* lateral segmental branch of left portal vein; *R,* right portal vein; *A,* anterior segmental branch of right portal vein; *P,* posterior segmental branch of right portal vein). *C,* Inferior vena cava; *PE,* left pleural effusion.

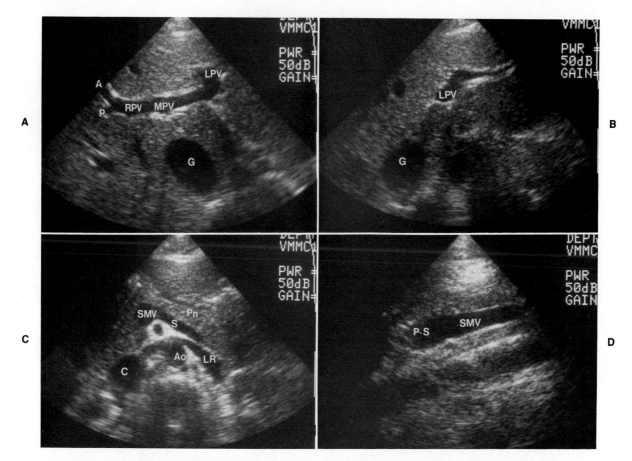

Fig. 75-7 Portal venous system: sonography. **A,** Axial scan at level of main portal vein. **B,** Axial scan at level of left portal vein. **C,** Axial scan at level of pancreas. **D,** Sagittal scan through superior mesenteric vein. *MPV,* Main portal vein; *LPV,* left portal vein; *RPV,* right portal vein; *A,* anterior segmental right portal vein; *P,* posterior segmental right portal vein; *G,* gallbladder; *Pn,* pancreas; *SMV,* superior mesenteric vein; *S,* splenic vein; *C,* inferior vena cava; *Ao,* aorta; *LR,* left renal vein; *P-S,* confluence of portal and splenic veins.

Portal venous system

The portal venous system is formed by the confluent drainage of the superior and inferior mesenteric veins and the splenic vein.[47,122] The *splenic vein* leaves the splenic hilum and courses to the right in a smooth arc to join the superior mesenteric vein. The confluence of these two veins forms an easily identifiable landmark during ultrasound, MR, and CT (Figs. 75-6, 75-7, and 75-8). The splenic vein usually lies within a groove along the posterocranial aspect of the pancreas. It receives the left gastric (coronary) vein in about 20% of cases. In the remaining instances the left gastric vein drains into the main portal vein or into the splenic–superior mesenteric venous confluence.

The *superior mesenteric vein* is formed by the confluence of jejunal, ileal, and right colic veins. It passes anterior to the duodenum and posterior to the pancreas to join the splenic vein. The *inferior mesenteric vein* is formed by the superior hemorrhoidal, sigmoid, and left colic veins. It drains into the splenic vein in about 40% of cases and into the superior mesenteric vein or splenic–superior mesenteric venous confluence in the remaining cases.[46,122] It is usually a single vessel, but rarely it may be composed of two or three major trunks.

The small tributaries of the portal venous system include the left and right gastroepiploic veins, short gastric veins, and pancreaticoduodenal veins. The anatomy of the *pancreatic veins* is important for performing selective pancreatic venous sampling for localization of endocrine tumors[26,106] (Fig. 75-9). The head of the pancreas is drained by two major venous arcades, the anterior and posterior pancreaticoduodenal arcades. The posterior superior arcade drains into the main portal vein, and the anterior superior arcade drains into the gastrocolic trunk.

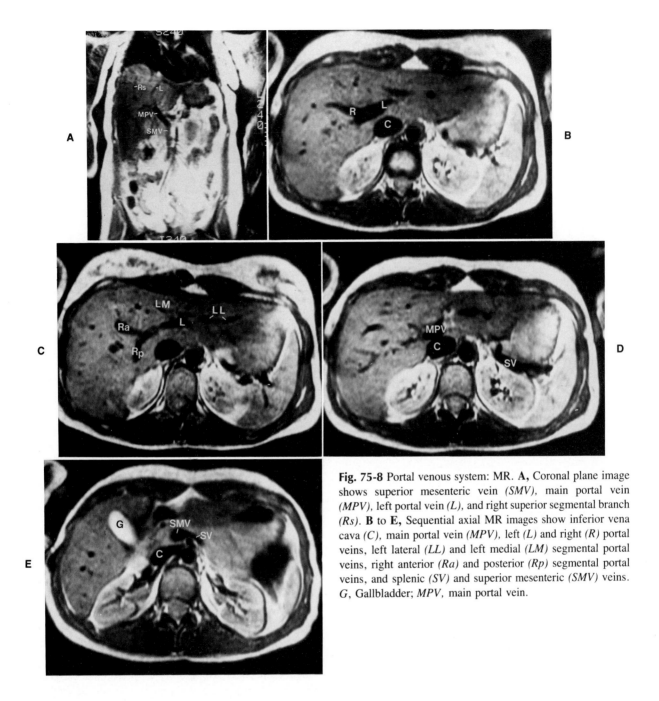

Fig. 75-8 Portal venous system: MR. **A,** Coronal plane image shows superior mesenteric vein *(SMV)*, main portal vein *(MPV)*, left portal vein *(L)*, and right superior segmental branch *(Rs)*. **B** to **E,** Sequential axial MR images show inferior vena cava *(C)*, main portal vein *(MPV)*, left *(L)* and right *(R)* portal veins, left lateral *(LL)* and left medial *(LM)* segmental portal veins, right anterior *(Ra)* and posterior *(Rp)* segmental portal veins, and splenic *(SV)* and superior mesenteric *(SMV)* veins. G, Gallbladder; *MPV,* main portal vein.

The inferior arcades usually anastomose with the first jejunal vein. The body and tail of the gland are drained by the transverse pancreatic vein and by multiple small tributaries that enter the splenic vein.

The *main portal vein* is formed by the splenic–superior mesenteric venous confluence, which is usually located just dorsal to the head of the pancreas (Figs. 75-6, 75-7, and 75-8). It runs obliquely toward the liver hilum, passes posterior to the duodenum, and divides into the main left and right portal veins within the liver or porta hepatis.

Several anomalous communications may exist between the intrahepatic and extrahepatic portal venous systems. These include a segmental left hepatic portal vein draining directly into the left gastric (coronary) vein and anastomotic transhepatic veins connecting the left portal vein and esophageal veins[48,49,149] (see Fig. 75-15, C). Recognition of these anomalous connections is im-

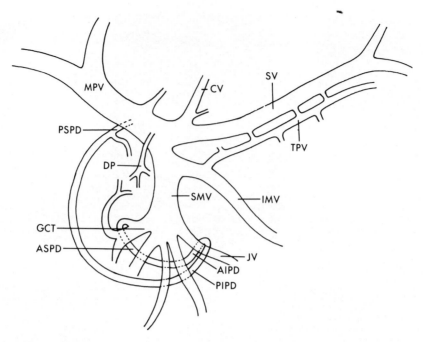

Fig. 75-9 Pancreatic venous system. Line drawing shows normal pancreatic venous system. *MPV*, Main portal vein; *SV*, splenic vein; *SMV*, superior mesenteric vein; *IMV*, inferior mesenteric vein; *CV*, coronary vein; *JV*, jejunal vein; *PSPD, ASPD*, posterior and anterior superior pancreatico- duodenal veins; *PIPD, AIPD*, posterior and anterior pancreaticoduodenal veins; *GCT*, gastrocolic trunk; *DP*, dorsal pancreatic vein; *TPV*, transverse pancreatic vein.

portant during the time when venous studies in pa- tients with portal hypertension and varices are interpreted and when transhepatic embolization of varices is per- formed.[95]

Congenital absence of the portal vein is a rare anomaly that has been reported in only several patients.[112] In one case the superior mesenteric and splenic veins drained directly into the left renal vein.[112] Other anomalies of the portal vein include duplication and a preduodenal loca- tion.[82,113,183]

PORTAL VENOGRAPHY

Portal venography may be performed by the tech- niques of splenoportography, transhepatic or transjugular portography, indirect arterial portography, umbilical por- tography, and wedged hepatic venography, with retro- grade filling of the portal vein. Indirect arterial portog- raphy and transhepatic portography currently are the most widely used methods.

Splenoportography

Splenoportography is performed by direct percuta- neous puncture of the spleen with a large-bore 18-gauge needle or catheter-sheathed needle. A total of 40 to 50

ml of contrast medium is then injected into the splenic parenchyma, resulting in antegrade filling of the splenic vein, collateral vessels, and portal venous system[160] (Fig. 75-10).

Transhepatic portography

The techniques of percutaneous transhepatic portog- raphy were described initially by Bierman in 1952. Sev- eral investigators subsequently expanded these tech- niques, and the transhepatic route is now widely used for direct portography and selective catheterization of the tributaries of the portal venous system.[105,106,142,206]

Transhepatic portography is performed by percuta- neous catheterization of a right portal vein branch through a right lateral intercostal approach[22,198] (Fig. 75-11). A 23-gauge needle and 0.015-inch guidewire are used for the initial puncture of the portal vein and selective cath- eterization. Once a portal vein branch has been entered, the small guidewire is inserted through the needle and carefully maneuvered into the main portal vein. Curved catheters and troque-controlled guidewires are then used to catheterize the primary and secondary tributaries of the portal venous system. Pressure measurements, con- trast portal venograms, venous sampling, and selective

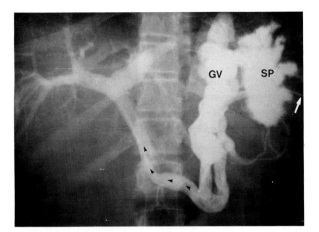

Fig. 75-10 Splenoportogram in patient with portal hypertension shows hepatopetal flow in portal vein *(arrowheads)* and retrograde filling of large gastric varices *(GV)*. Needle *(arrow)*; splenic parenchymal stain *(SP)*.

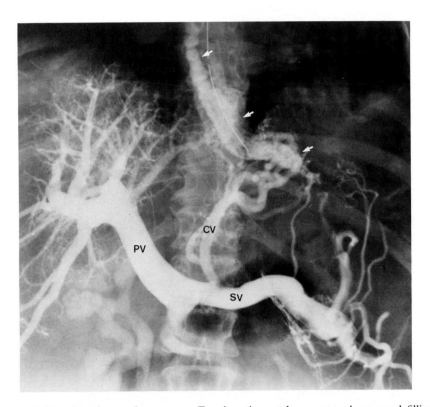

Fig. 75-11 Transhepatic portal venogram. Transhepatic portal venogram shows good filling of splenic *(SV)* and portal *(PV)* veins and retrograde flow into network of gastroesophageal varices *(arrows)* by way of coronary vein *(CV)*.

venous embolization can be performed by way of the transhepatic route.

Transjugular portography

Access to the portal venous system may be accomplished by using a percutaneous transjugular route. This technique originally was described by Hanafee and Weiner[79] for cholangiography but was expanded by Rösch and co-workers[161,163,164] for numerous other uses, including portal venography. Descriptions of the technique can be found in several excellent monographs.[70,161] Although now infrequently used, the transjugular approach may serve as an alternative to the transhepatic route if the latter is not adequate because of abnormal bleeding parameters or massive ascites.

Arterial portography

Selective splenic and superior and inferior mesenteric angiography provides excellent opacification of the main tributaries and intrahepatic branches of the portal vein.[130,145] The degree of opacification can be improved substantially by using a large volume of contrast (50 to 70 ml in the superior mesenteric artery and 40 to 60 ml in the splenic artery) and a vasodilator, such as tolazoline (Priscoline)[148] (Fig. 75-12). A dose of 25 to 50 mg of tolazoline, diluted to a total volume of 10 ml with saline, is injected into the superior mesenteric artery over a 30- to 45-second period. Following a 30-second delay, an intraarterial bolus of contrast (50 to 70 ml at 10 to 12 ml/second) is injected, and the filming sequence is extended to cover 31 seconds, usually 1 film/second for 7 seconds and then 1 film every third second for 24 seconds. The volume and rate of injection must be determined for each individual patient, depending on the size of the artery, the presence of splenomegaly, and the estimated rate of flow in the vessel. In my colleagues' and my experience, tolazoline has not been of value for enhance-

ment of the venous phase of the selective splenic arteriogram. However, it has been useful in the left gastric and mesenteric arteries.

Selective high-dose left gastric arterial injections also have been found to be valuable for opacifying the left gastric (coronary) vein and for identifying gastroesophageal varices[152] (see Fig. 75-22).

Umbilical portography

The umbilical vein drains into a branch of the left portal vein, which communicates with one of the central hepatic veins by way of the ductus venosus. Following birth, the ductus venosus closes and the umbilical vein collapses but remains patent. In the adult the vein usually can be catheterized through a transcutaneous cutdown in the midline of the abdomen just above the umbilicus. A catheter can then be threaded up the umbilical vein and into the left portal vein for pressure measurements and contrast portal venography.[35,137] This technique now is rarely used.

LIVER
Portal hypertension

The normal portal venous system has a pressure of about 5 to 10 mm Hg and an average flow of 1000 to

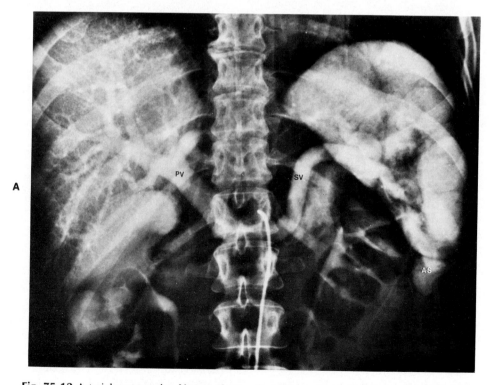

Fig. 75-12 Arterial portography. Venous phases of selective splenic, superior mesenteric, inferior mesenteric, and left gastric arteriograms show normal portal venous system. **A,** Selective splenic artery injection shows normal splenic *(SV)* and portal veins *(PV)*. Note small accessory spleen *(AS)*.

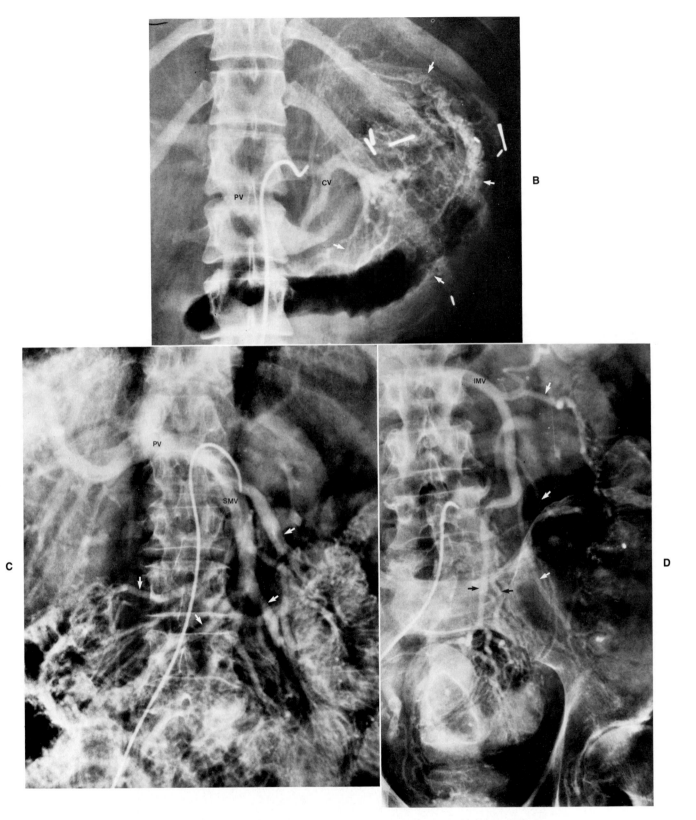

Fig. 75-12, cont'd B, Selective left gastric artery injection shows plexus of gastric veins *(arrows)* emptying into coronary vein *(CV)*. Main portal vein *(PV)* also is seen. **C,** Selective tolazoline-augmented superior mesenteric artery injection shows main portal vein *(PV)*, superior mesenteric vein *(SMV)*, and its main tributaries *(arrows)*. **D,** Selective inferior mesenteric arteriogram shows inferior mesenteric vein *(IMV)* and its major tributaries, left colic veins *(white arrows)*, and sigmoid and hemorrhoidal veins *(black arrows)*.

1200 ml/minute.[154] Since pressure is the product of flow and resistance, portal hypertension may develop as a result of increased portal flow (hyperkinetic portal hypertension) or increased resistance within the portal venous system.

Hyperkinetic portal hypertension

Hyperkinetic portal hypertension usually is caused by an intrahepatic or extrahepatic arterioportal fistula. The cause of the fistula may be traumatic, congenital, atherosclerotic, or idiopathic. A review of 61 arterioportal fistulas by Van Way and co-workers[193] found that 32 were traumatic, usually the result of surgery or a penetrating abdominal wound, 25 were caused by splenic or hepatic artery aneurysms, usually atherosclerotic in origin, and only 4 were congenital. Congenital fistulas may be associated with hepatic or splenic artery aneurysms, Osler-Weber-Rendu disease (hereditary hemorrhagic telangiectasia), or arteriovenous malformations in the pancreas or duodenum.[37,75] In the case of Osler-Weber-Rendu disease, the most common type of fistula is a hepatic artery–hepatic vein communication.[78] Only a few cases of arterioportal fistulas have been reported.[37]

The most common symptoms caused by arterioportal fistulas of less than 1 year duration are postprandial abdominal pain, diarrhea, gastrointestinal bleeding caused by congestive vascular enteritis, and ascites.[184] Fistulas that have been present for greater than 1 year usually are asymptomatic but occasionally may cause gastrointestinal hemorrhage resulting from varices.

Arterioportal fistulas are best evaluated by selective arteriography.[37,75,184,193] The most common vessels involved are the hepatic, splenic, and superior mesenteric arteries or one of their branches.[184] The inferior mesenteric artery is only infrequently involved. Angiography may show a direct communication between the artery and vein (Fig. 75-13), or it may demonstrate a racemose collection of vessels representing an arteriovenous malformation (see Fig. 75-41). The feeding artery is invariably dilated and tortuous, and the draining veins show early, dense opacification. Fistulas and malformations may be treated by surgical resection or by selective transcatheter embolization.[96]

Increased portal venous resistance

The most common cause of portal hypertension is increased resistance to flow within the portal venous circulation. The abnormality causing the increased resis-

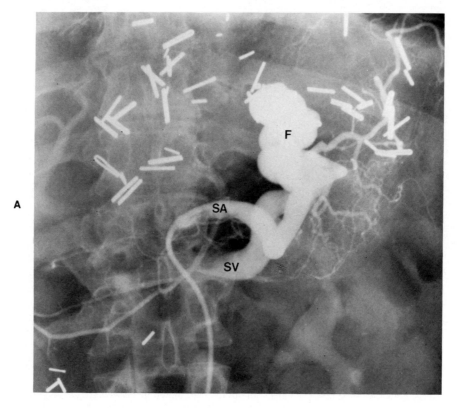

Fig. 75-13 Hyperkinetic portal hypertension. Selective splenic artery *(SA)* injection in patient with intractable variceal bleeding following gastric devascularization procedure and splenectomy. Early phase, **A,** shows filling of large pseudoaneurysm and fistula *(F)* with early opacification of splenic vein *(SV)*. (Courtesy Dr. Josef Rösch.)

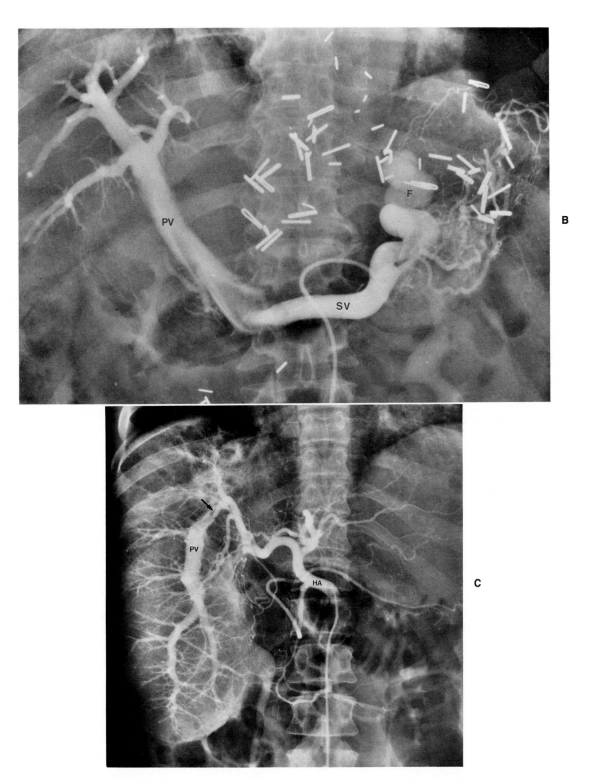

Fig. 75-13, cont'd Late phase, **B,** shows dense opacification of splenic and portal veins *(PV).* **C,** Selective hepatic artery *(HA)* injection in different patient shows diffuse hepatomegaly and hepatoportal fistula *(arrow)* caused by previous liver biopsy. Note intense opacification of large portal vein *(PV).*

tance may be intrahepatic or extrahepatic (see following outline).

Intrahepatic portal hypertension

Intrahepatic portal hypertension may be subdivided into presinusoidal and postsinusoidal causes.

Presinusoidal causes

Increased resistance within the intrahepatic portal venous system may be caused by presinusoidal lesions such as schistosomiasis or congenital hepatic fibrosis. These abnormalities are rare and usually are diagnosed by liver biopsy.[134,180]

Postsinusoidal causes

The most common cause of portal hypertension is hepatic cirrhosis. Cirrhosis causes increased portal vein pressure by obstructing hepatic venous outflow. This may result from extrinsic compression of the hepatic veins by nodules of regenerating liver tissue or from obliteration of the central veins by extensive fibrosis.

The spectrum of hemodynamic changes caused by cirrhosis is complex. During the early stage of the cirrhotic process, normal hepatic portal venous inflow is maintained by an increase in portal vein perfusion pressure. Eventually, however, outflow hepatic vein resistance becomes too great, and portal venous flow decreases. Hepatic artery flow usually increases in proportion to the decrease in portal vein flow. In the normal liver, about 75% of total blood flow comes from the portal vein and only 25% is supplied by the hepatic artery.[154] In advanced cirrhosis, hepatic venous outflow resistance may be so great that all or part of the portal venous flow may be diverted away from the liver—so-called hepa-

tofugal flow. In this case the hepatic artery dilates and may supply up to 100% of total liver blood flow. However, hepatic artery flow cannot compensate completely for the lack of portal venous flow, and thus total hepatic blood flow decreases.

Hepatofugal portal venous flow results in retrograde flow through numerous collateral routes, the most common of which surround the stomach and esophagus or develop within the retroperitoneum. These collateral channels represent portosystemic shunts, which divert blood around the liver and directly into the systemic veins. The most common metabolic consequence of these shunts is portosystemic encephalopathy.

Radiologic evaluation of intrahepatic portal hypertension

Radiologic evaluation of patients with known or suspected cirrhosis and portal hypertension may be used to (1) establish the diagnosis, (2) define the portal vascular anatomy for surgical portosystemic shunts or other therapeutic maneuvers, and (3) evaluate the patency of surgical portosystemic shunts. In addition, interventional angiographic techniques, such as transhepatic embolization of gastroesophageal varices, may be efficacious for nonsurgical management of patients with portal hypertension.

BARIUM STUDIES

Portal hypertension results in increased flow through a variety of portosystemic collateral vessels. Some of these vessels are located within the walls of the gastrointestinal tract and can be identified by barium studies (Fig. 75-14). Knowledge of their presence and extent is important in the evaluation of patients with portal hypertension and gastrointestinal bleeding (Fig. 75-15).

COMPUTED TOMOGRAPHY, SONOGRAPHY, AND MAGNETIC RESONANCE IMAGING

Both CT and ultrasound are useful imaging modalities for evaluating patients with cirrhosis and portal hypertension. Although the CT and ultrasound appearance of the cirrhotic liver may be normal, a variety of abnormal findings usually can be seen. These include ascites, splenomegaly, alterations in the hepatic parenchymal texture or attenuation pattern, discrete enlargement of the caudate lobe relative to the right lobe, and surface irregularities caused by regenerating nodules or focal scarring[55,81,144] (Fig. 75-16). The presence of primary (hepatocellular carcinoma) or metastatic hepatic tumor can be detected by CT or ultrasound, and the patency of the portal venous system and the presence of portosystemic collateral varices also can be demonstrated by CT

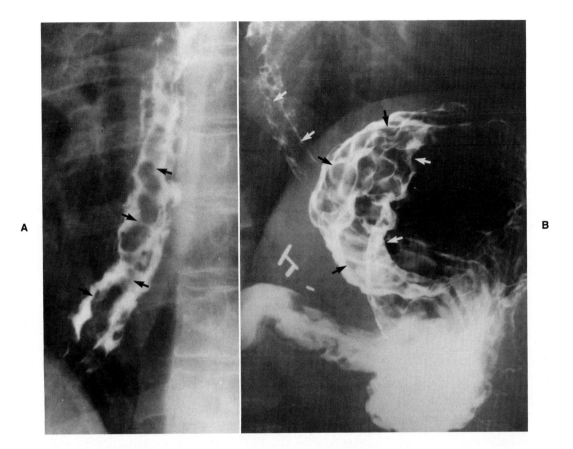

Fig. 75-14 Gastroesophageal varices. Barium studies of esophagus, **A,** and stomach, **B,** show numerous serpentine filling defects representing varices *(arrows).*

and by real-time and Doppler ultrasound* (Figs. 75-16 and 75-17).

MR imaging (MRI) is now being shown to be an important modality for both preoperative and postoperative evaluation of patients with portal hypertension. Its main advantages are its ability to image the liver and portal venous system in multiple planes, to determine patency of the portal vein and its main tributaries, to detect portosystemic collateral vessels, and to assess the patency of surgical shunts[12,41,136,190,209] (Fig. 75-18).

ANGIOGRAPHY

Selective visceral angiography continues to be an important modality for the diagnostic evaluation of patients with portal hypertension. Reuter and co-workers[154] have defined four roles for angiography: (1) identification of nonvariceal causes for gastrointestinal bleeding in patients with portal hypertension, (2) evaluation of hemo-

dynamic changes of the hepatic artery and portal vein, (3) exclusion of coexisting hepatoma, and (4) definition of portal venous anatomy and portosystemic collateral vessels.

The increasing use of the noninvasive modalities (CT, ultrasound, MR) have replaced angiography for exclusion of hepatocellular carcinoma and for definition of portal venous anatomy and patency and portosystemic collateral vessels. However, angiography continues to be useful for grading of portal hypertension and for assessment of portal venous hemodynamics before and after shunt surgery[12,190] (see Figs. 75-26 and 75-27).

From 20% to 30% of patients with portal hypertension and gastrointestinal hemorrhage bleed from nonvariceal lesions, particularly hemorrhagic gastritis, esophageal Mallory-Weiss tears, and gastric or duodenal ulcers. Angiography is useful for both diagnosis and transcatheter therapy of these lesions.

Hepatic portal venous flow and hepatic arterial flow are inversely related in patients with hepatic cirrhosis and portal hypertension. As the cirrhotic process progresses,

---

*References 39, 42, 51, 67, 91, 175, 185.

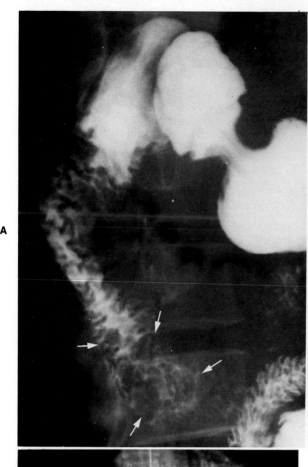

A

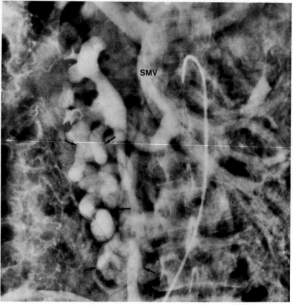

B

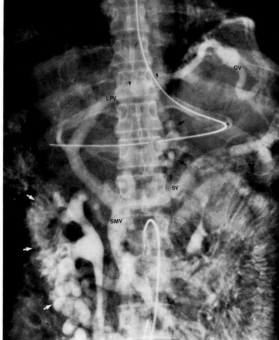

C

Fig. 75-15 Bleeding duodenal varices. **A,** Barium study shows irregular, tortuous filling defects in wall of duodenum *(arrows).* **B,** Venous phase of selective superior mesenteric artery injection shows large duodenal varix *(arrows). SMV,* Superior mesenteric vein. **C,** Later film shows contrast extravasation into lumen of duodenum due to massive variceal hemorrhage *(white arrows).* Note transhepatic collateral vein *(arrowheads)* from left portal vein *(LPV)* to gastric veins *(GV).* Gastric varices also are filled *(black arrows). SV,* Splenic vein.

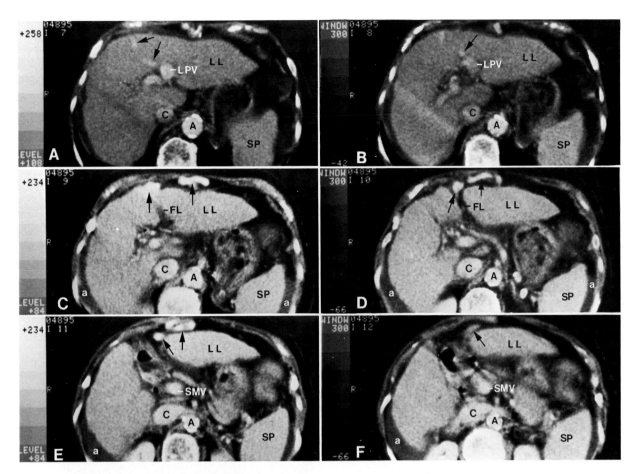

Fig. 75-16 Recanalized umbilical vein: CT. Consecutive contrast-enhanced computed tomograms of liver show patent umbilical vein. **A,** and **B,** Scans show umbilical vein *(arrows)* arising from left portal vein *(LPV)*. **C** and **D,** Lower scans show umbilical vein within falciform ligament *(FL)* and anterior to liver *(arrows)*. **E** and **F,** Lower scans show tortuous umbilical vein anterior to liver *(arrows)*. *A,* Aorta; *C,* cava; *LL,* left lobe of liver; *a,* ascites; *SP,* spleen; *SMV,* superior mesenteric vein.

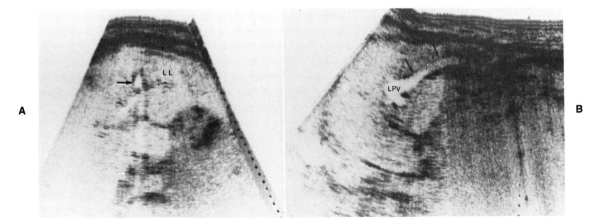

Fig. 75-17 Recanalized umbilical vein; ultrasonography. **A,** Axial ultrasonogram of left lobe of liver *(LL)* shows patent umbilical vein *(arrow)* within falciform ligament. **B,** Sagittal ultrasonogram of left lobe of liver shows patent umbilical vein *(arrows)* arising from left portal vein *(LPV)*.

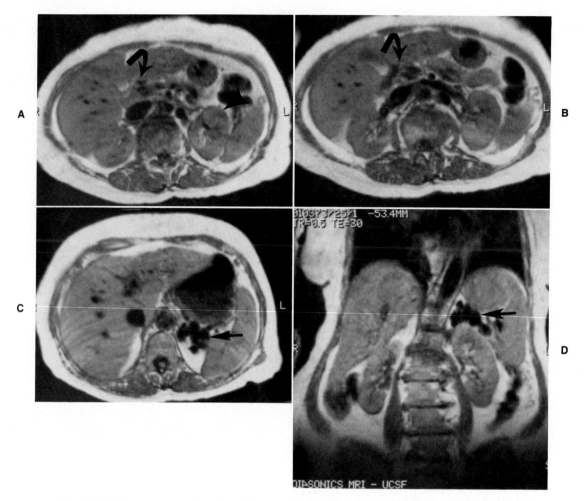

Fig. 75-18 Cavernous transformation of the portal vein: MRI. **A** and **B,** MR images (PS 500/30) show cavernous transformation of portal vein *(curved arrow).* Normal anterior upper pole of kidney is prominent *(arrowhead).* **C** and **D,** Confluence of splenic varicosities in left suprarenal area *(arrow).*
(Courtesy Thomas J. Gilbert, MD, San Francisco.)

portal venous flow to the liver decreases and hepatic arterial flow increases. These hemodynamic changes may be demonstrated by selective angiography.[172,195]

The wide variety of portosystemic shunts that may develop in patients with portal hypertension have been described in detail by several investigators.[48,49,170] These shunts are of two types—tributary collaterals and developed collaterals[170] (Figs. 75-19 and 75-20). *Tributary collaterals* are the normally occurring tributaries of the portal venous system. These include the coronary or left gastric vein, short gastric veins, and the superior and inferior mesenteric veins. They reach the systemic veins by way of the azygos and hemiazygos systems and the retroperitoneal and mesenteric venous plexi. *Developed*

collaterals are those that form from preexisting vessels that normally do not function as collaterals and are not considered to be tributaries of the portal venous system. These include the paraumbilical vein and splenorenal and splenoretroperitoneal collateral vessels.

Selective splenic, left gastric, and superior mesenteric arteriography can be used to define portal venous anatomy, identify varices, and evaluate the status of portosystemic shunts and collateral vessels. Vasodilators, such as tolazoline, and high-volume injections may be used to enhance the venous phase of the injections.[177] Varices most often are located in the distal esophagus and gastric fundus. They usually may be demonstrated by selective splenic or superior mesenteric arteriography (Fig. 75-21)

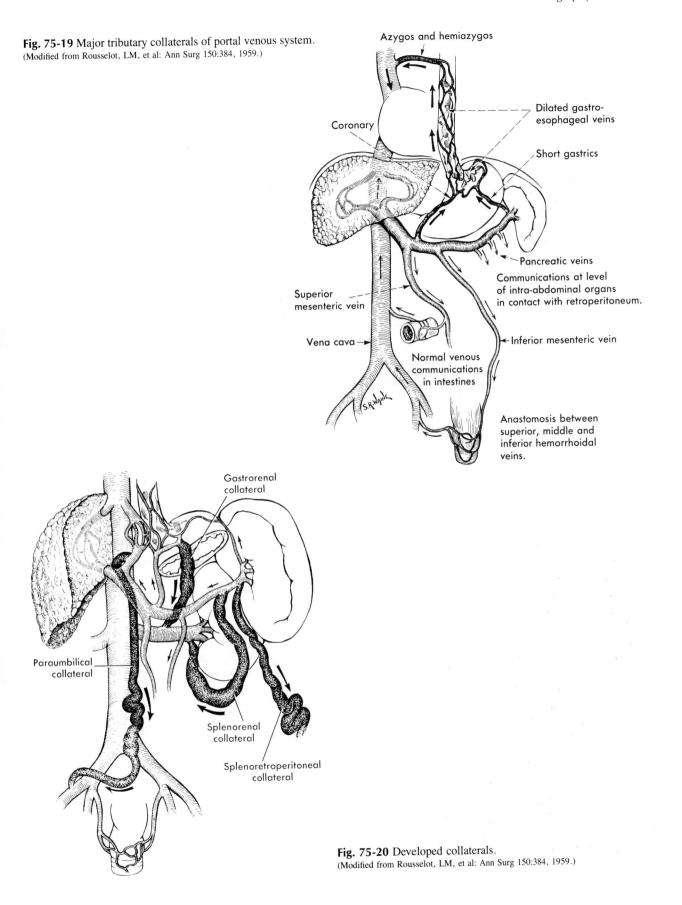

Fig. 75-19 Major tributary collaterals of portal venous system.
(Modified from Rousselot, LM, et al: Ann Surg 150:384, 1959.)

Azygos and hemiazygos

Coronary

Dilated gastro-esophageal veins

Short gastrics

Pancreatic veins

Communications at level
of intra-abdominal organs
in contact with retroperitoneum.

Superior
mesenteric vein

Inferior mesenteric vein

Vena cava

Normal venous
communications
in intestines

Anastomosis between
superior, middle and
inferior hemorrhoidal
veins.

Gastrorenal
collateral

Paraumbilical
collateral

Splenorenal
collateral

Splenoretroperitoneal
collateral

Fig. 75-20 Developed collaterals.
(Modified from Rousselot, LM, et al: Ann Surg 150:384, 1959.)

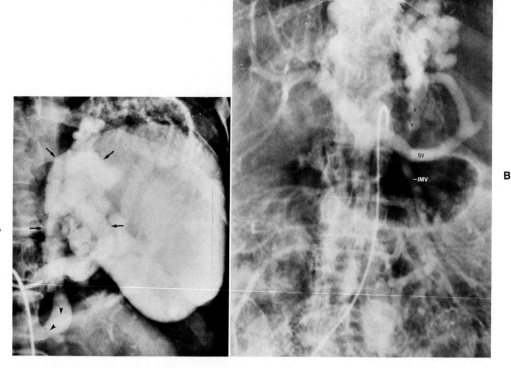

Fig. 75-21 Arterial portography: varices. Venous phases of selective splenic, **A,** and superior mesenteric, **B,** arteriograms in two different patients show gastroesophageal varices *(arrows)*. Note retrograde flow into spontaneous splenorenal shunts *(arrowheads)* in both cases and into splenic *(SV)* and inferior mesenteric *(IMV)* veins in **B.**

but rarely may be seen only during the venous phase of a selective left gastric injection[152] (Fig. 75-22). Duodenal, umbilical, and colonic varices are less common but also may be seen during the venous phases of selective mesenteric angiography (Fig. 75-15).

Patients with cirrhosis have an increased incidence of hepatocellular carcinoma (hepatoma). Sudden changes in the clinical status of patients with known cirrhosis may result from acute alcoholism or other hepatic insults, but a developing hepatoma must also be considered. In addition, the presence of hepatoma must be excluded in patients who are candidates for surgical or angiographic treatment of portal hypertension.

SPLENOPORTOGRAPHY

Splenoportography has been used successfully and with a low incidence of complications for definition of portal venous anatomy[171] (Fig. 75-10). However, it has largely been replaced by the techniques of arterial portography and direct transhepatic catheterization of the portal vein.

HEPATIC VENOGRAPHY AND MANOMETRY

Hepatic cirrhosis causes morphologic changes in the hepatic veins that can be demonstrated by free or wedged selective hepatic venography. The wedged hepatic venous catheter also can be used to measure the sinusoidal pressure within the liver.

The effect of hepatic cirrhosis on the appearance of the hepatic veins as demonstrated by free hepatic venography has been described by several investigators.[132,177,178] In general, as the severity of cirrhosis increases, the hepatic veins show progressive loss or pruning of the peripheral branches and marginal irregularities of the larger ventral veins (Fig. 75-23). The veins may be virtually obliterated in advanced, end-stage cirrhosis. The appearance of the hepatic veins, parenchymal stain, and flow into peripheral hepatic and portal veins during wedged hepatic venography has received considerable attention, and attempts have been made to correlate both the degree or severity of cirrhosis and the type of cirrhosis with the morphologic changes of the wedged hepatic venogram.[15,62,154,196,197] Although some correlation exists

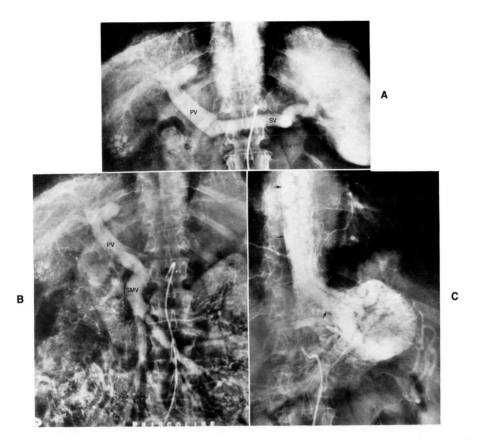

Fig. 75-22 Arterial portography: value of selective left gastric arteriography. Venous phases of selective splenic, **A,** and tolazoline-augmented superior mesenteric, **B,** arteriograms show hepatopedal portal venous flow and no evidence of varices. Venous phase of selective left gastric arteriogram, **C,** shows filling of gastroesophageal varices *(arrows)* by way of numerous short gastric veins. *PV,* Portal vein; *SMV,* superior mesenteric vein; *SV,* splenic vein.

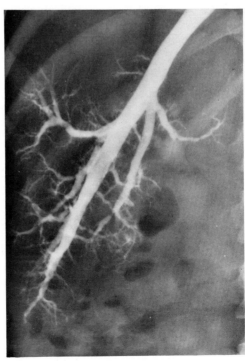

Fig. 75-23 Hepatic cirrhosis. Free hepatic venogram in patient with moderately advanced cirrhosis shows loss of normal tapering, pruning of primary and secondary branches, and marked irregularity of small peripheral branches.
(Courtesy Josef Rösch, MD.)

between the severity of cirrhosis and the wedged venographic changes, prediction of the type of cirrhosis is somewhat tenuous.[137] This is partly because of the subjective nature of the interpretation of borderline changes in the parenchymal stain morphology and the different changes that can be produced if the contrast injection rate and volume are varied.

The measurement of wedged hepatic venous pressure is a reliable indication of portal venous pressure.[155,156] The most clinically useful determination is corrected sinusoidal pressure (CSP), which is the wedged hepatic venous pressure minus the inferior vena caval pressure. The normal wedged venous pressure is 40 to 150 mm of water, and the normal CSP is less than 100 mm of water.[154] Patients with mild, moderate, and severe portal hypertension usually have CSP measurements in the range of 100 to 200, 200 to 300, and greater than 300 mm water, respectively. In general, variceal hemorrhage is rare if CSP is less than 200 mm water.[154,194]

TRANSJUGULAR AND TRANSHEPATIC PORTAL VENOGRAPHY

Direct access to the portal venous system can be accomplished by percutaneous transjugular or transhepatic portal vein catheterization.[161,198] These techniques can be used for diagnostic evaluation and for transcatheter occlusive therapy of gastroesophageal varices.

Selective catheterization of the portal vein may be used to demonstrate the location and extent of both intrahepatic and extrahepatic portosystemic shunts.[23,24,25,133,140] (Fig. 75-11). Current studies indicate that the size of the collateral venous shunts is unrelated to the frequency or severity of variceal hemorrhage. The most important predictive findings are the presence of hepatofungal flow and contrast opacification of the inferior vena cava. The latter finding indicates the existence of large, spontaneous portosystemic shunts and is believed to be associated with fewer bleeding episodes.[93,204]

Preoperative and postoperative portosystemic shunt evaluation

Surgical portosystemic shunts are effective methods for decompression of the hypertensive portal venous system and for control of bleeding from gastroesophageal varices. Although a variety of shunts exist, only two are functional types: total shunts and selective shunts. Total shunts, such as the portocaval or mesocaval shunt, decompress both the portal system and the variceal system, whereas selective shunts, such as the splenorenal or coronocaval shunt, decompress the varices and are believed not to affect either portal venous pressure or flow.[110,111]

The selection of patients for total or selective shunts remains controversial.[126] However, data are accumulating

to suggest that selective shunts are equally as effective as total shunts in protecting against variceal hemorrhage and have a decreased incidence of postshunt encephalopathy.[63,64,150,157]

PREOPERATIVE EVALUATION

Several hemodynamic criteria may be helpful for preoperative selection of patients who are surgical candidates for portosystemic shunts.

Total shunts. It has been demonstrated that hepatic portal venous perfusion ceases following interposition mesocaval or side-to-side portocaval shunts.[61] If preoperative portal venous flow is hepatopedal, sudden cessation of flow following a total shunt may produce portosystemic encephalopathy. Thus patients who already have established hepatofugal flow would appear to be the best hemodynamic candidates for a total shunt.[131]

Preoperative evaluation of patients before shunt surgery can be accomplished with a variety of modalities, including sonography (real-time and Doppler), dynamic CT, MR, and angiography.

Sonography can be employed to determine the patency of the portal vein and its main tributaries, the inferior vena cava, and the renal veins and to determine the direction of portal vein blood flow, that is, hepatofugal or hepatopedal.[3,55,123,214] The presence and direction of flow are determined by assessing the positive or negative shift of the Doppler signal from baseline.[123]

Dynamic CT and MR can give similar information and can be used to determine the patency of the portal vein and to assess the presence of collaterals.[55,136,151,190,209]

Angiography continues to be an important method for precise evaluation of portal venous anatomy and patency and for grading of flow before shunt surgery.[131,190] Portal venous anatomy and hemodynamics are best displayed using selective splenic or superior mesenteric arterial injections.[131] However, it is important to prevent reflux of contrast into the hepatic artery to avoid misinterpretation of retrograde hepatic artery–portal vein opacification as prograde or hepatopedal flow.[61] In addition, angiographic demonstration of patency of the superior mesenteric and portal veins and the inferior vena cava and exclusion of a coexisting malignant hepatic neoplasm (hepatoma) also may be accomplished.

Other hemodynamic criteria, such as corrected sinusoidal pressure or the appearance of the wedged hepatic venogram, may provide useful information regarding the portal venous pressure and severity of the cirrhotic process. If the pressure difference between the portal vein and inferior vena cava does not exceed 10 mm Hg, shunt surgery is believed to be contraindicated because of the low probability of long-term shunt patency.[207]

Selective shunts. Selective shunts include the splenorenal shunt with splenectomy, distal splenorenal shunt with preservation of the spleen, and the coronocaval shunt. In each type preoperative identification of venous anomalies, such as aberrant or duplicate left gastric veins or an unusually small splenic vein, and demonstration of the patency of the splenic or coronary (left gastric) veins and left renal vein are imperative.[127,207] This may be accomplished by selective splenic, superior mesenteric, or left gastric arteriography and selective renal venography. In some cases transhepatic portal venography also has been used.[127,207] Evaluation of the inferior vena cava may be accomplished at the time of renal venography to determine patency, absence of anatomic anomalies, and infrahepatic caval pressure. Stenosis or occlusion of the suprarenal cava or elevation of caval or renal vein pressure resulting from causes such as constrictive pericarditis or chronic congestive heart failure would signifi-

cantly influence the selection of the type of shunt. A gradient of greater than 5 mm Hg between the renal vein and inferior vena cava indicates that a splenocaval anastomosis rather than a splenorenal shunt should be performed. Patients with hepatopetal portal venous flow are believed to be the best candidates for a selective shunt.[131]

POSTOPERATIVE EVALUATION

The primary indication for postoperative angiographic evaluation of patients with portosystemic shunts is determination of shunt patency if recurrent variceal hemorrhage occurs. This can be accomplished with arteriography, selective catheterization of the shunt, dynamic CT, sonography, or MR.[36,55,68]

Several hemodynamic changes occur following portosystemic shunts. Total shunts (portocaval) result in

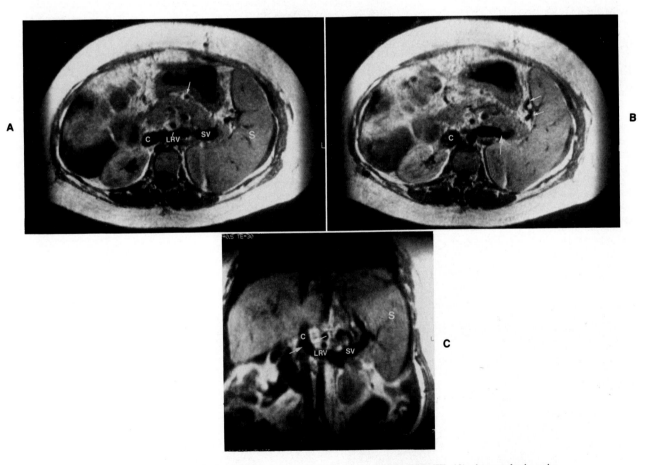

Fig. 75-24 Splenorenal shunt: MR. **A** and **B,** Axial scans (TR 1000/TE 40) show splenic vein *(SV)*–left renal vein *(LRV)* shunt *(arrow* in **A**). Signal void in veins indicates shunt patency (flowing blood). Spleen *(S)* is enlarged, and perigastric varices *(small arrows)* are noted. *C,* Inferior vena cava. **C,** Scan in coronal projection shows patency of splenic–left renal vein anastomosis. Junction of left renal vein *(LRV)* and inferior vena cava *(C)* is well seen *(arrows)*. *S,* Spleen; *C,* inferior vena cava; *SV,* splenic vein.
(Courtesy Paul Weatherall, MD, and Helen Redman, MD, Dallas.)

complete loss of hepatic portal venous flow.[61] An unusual appearance of the hepatic veins also has been described following side-to-side portocaval shunts, consisting of narrowing of the hepatic veins, attenuation of the peripheral branches, and multiple small round collections of contrast arranged along the main venous channels.[153]

Selective shunts generally do not alter portal venous pressure so that hepatopedal portal venous flow is maintained postoperatively. However, postoperative angio-

graphic studies have shown reversal of portal venous flow in some patients following distal splenorenal shunts as early as 1 week following surgery.[126,127,192,201,207] Similar findings have been reported by Rikkers and co-workers,[157] who studied patients 3 to 6 years following splenorenal shunt surgery.

Patency of portosystemic shunts may be evaluated by sonography, CT, MR, selective mesenteric arterial portography, direct catheterization of the shunt through the

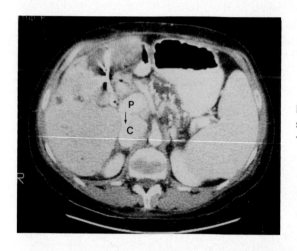

Fig. 75-25 Portocaval shunt: CT. Bolus-dynamic computed tomogram shows patent portocaval shunt *(arrow)*. *C,* Inferior vena cava; *P,* portal vein. Patient also has splenomegaly and chronic calcific pancreatitis.

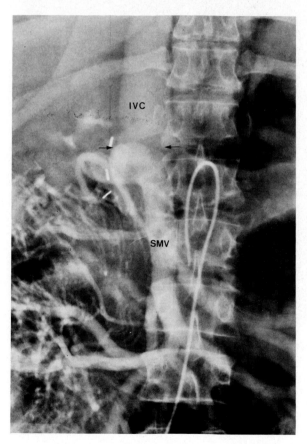

Fig. 75-26 Patent portosystemic shunt. Venous phase of tolazoline-augmented superior mesenteric arteriogram in patient with portocaval shunt demonstrates shunt patency *(arrows)* and contrast opacification of inferior vena cava *(IVC)*. *SMV,* Superior mesenteric vein.

inferior vena cava, or transhepatic catheterization of the portal vein.[12,41,68]

MR or duplex Doppler sonography are the most efficacious methods for initial evaluation of shunt patency.[12,41] MR can be used to assess patients with either portocaval or splenorenal shunts (Fig. 75-24). A potential problem is that slow flow in the portal vein or shunt can cause increased MR signal intensity, incorrectly indicating vessel thrombosis. However, slow flow usually can be differentiated from thrombosis by evaluation of the signal intensity on second echoes (spin-echo pulse sequence).[190] Slow flow produces an increase in signal intensity on the second echo (even-echo rephasing), whereas signal decreases in cases of thrombosis.[17] Patients with inconclusive or confusing MR studies also can be evaluated by Doppler sonography, dynamic CT, or angiography[68,116,214] (Fig. 75-25).

Mesenteric portography usually can demonstrate flow of contrast into the vena cava from the superior mesenteric or portal veins (Fig. 75-26). If the shunt is occluded, flow is absent (Fig. 75-27). In some cases, direct catheterization of the shunt may be necessary for diagnosis (Fig. 75-28).

Extrahepatic portal hypertension

Extrahepatic portal hypertension may result from abnormalities of the portal venous system proximal to the liver (prehepatic) or from abnormalities of the hepatic venous outflow tract (posthepatic).

Posthepatic hypertension

Posthepatic causes of portal hypertension include hepatic vein or inferior vena cava obstruction or elevated canal and hepatic vein pressure caused by congestive heart failure or constrictive pericarditis.

Hepatic venous obstruction (Budd-Chiari syndrome)

Hepatic venous obstruction (Budd-Chiari syndrome) is characterized by a constellation of clinical findings that

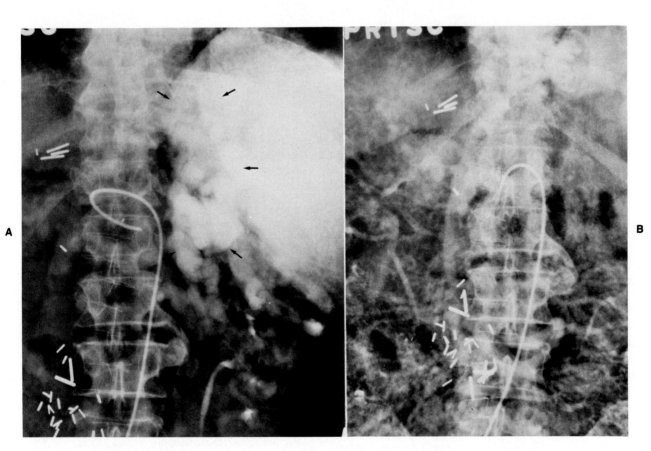

Fig. 75-27 Occluded portosystemic shunt. Venous phases of selective splenic, **A,** and tolazoline-augmented superior mesenteric, **B,** arteriograms in patient with previous portocaval and mesocaval portosystemic shunts show no evidence of shunt patency. There are large gastric (*arrows* in **A**) and mesenteric, **B,** varices.

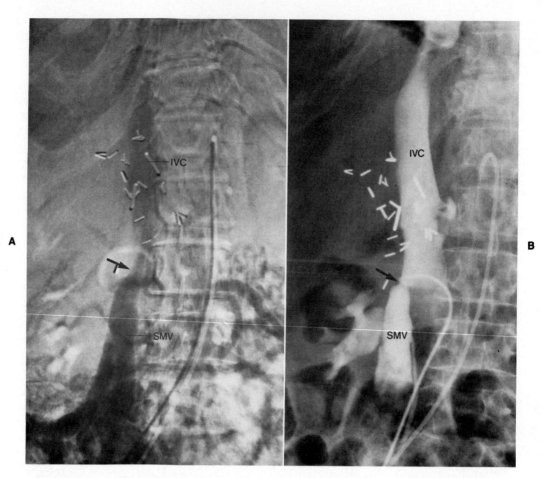

Fig. 75-28 Stenotic mesocaval portosystemic shunt. **A,** Venous phase of selective superior mesenteric arteriogram shows patent shunt *(arrow)* and opacification of inferior vena cava. However, superior mesenteric vein is dilated. **B,** Selective study of mesocaval shunt through inferior vena cava shows stenosis *(arrow)* at anastomosis. *IVC,* Inferior vena cava; *SMV,* superior mesenteric vein.

include abdominal pain, hepatomegaly, ascites, jaundice, and gastrointestinal bleeding.* The onset usually is chronic but may be acute, in which case the disease is often rapidly fatal.[98]

Hepatic vein occlusion may be caused by a variety of factors, such as membranous obstruction of the inferior vena cava or ostia of the hepatic veins, venous thrombosis associated with polycythemia rubra vera, pregnancy, or the use of various drugs (oral contraceptives, azathioprine), tumor invasion of the inferior vena cava or hepatic veins, and trauma.* An interesting variety of plants that contain pyrrolizidine alkaloids also have been incriminated as etiologic agents in hepatic venoocclusive dis-

ease. These are largely found in the West Indies, Africa, India, South America, and the Middle East.[85,107]

Radiologic diagnosis may be made by ultrasound CT, MR, selective venography of the inferior vena cava or hepatic veins, selective hepatic angiography, and hepatic scintigraphy.

COMPUTED TOMOGRAPHY, ULTRASONOGRAPHY, AND MAGNETIC RESONANCE

CT, ultrasound, and MR have been found to be quite accurate in determining the patency of the inferior vena cava and in detecting an intraluminal soft tissue mass caused by primary caval neoplasm or extension from a contiguous site (renal, adrenal, hepatic) (Fig. 75-29).

The CT and sonographic findings of Budd-Chiari syndrome include hepatomegaly, enlargement of the caudate lobe with increased contrast enhancement (dynamic CT), absent or thrombosed hepatic veins, and ascites.[6,9,117]

---

*References 32, 38, 50, 84, 98, 108.
*References 32, 38, 50, 84, 98, 108, 115, 176.

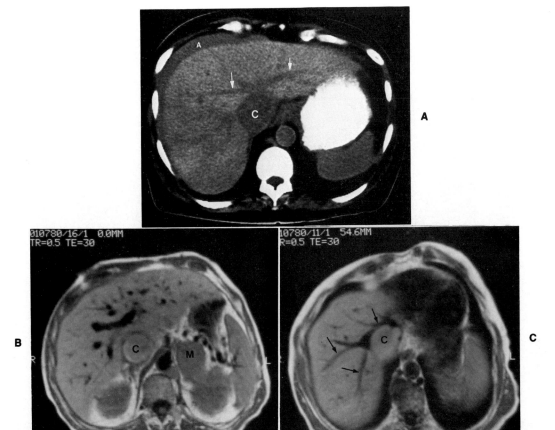

Fig. 75-29 Vena caval obstruction. **A,** Leiomyosarcoma of inferior vena cava. Computed tomogram shows that tumor-filled inferior vena cava *(C)* and hepatic veins *(arrows)* have similar attenuation. Lack of contrast enhancement of hepatic veins is caused by tumor obstruction. *A,* Ascites. **B** and **C,** Papillary renal adenocarcinoma invading inferior vena cava. MR image **(B)** (PS 500/30) shows tumor thrombus in expanded vena cava *(C)*. *M,* Left adrenal metastasis. Higher image in **C** shows tumor thrombus in cava *(C)* extending to level of hepatic veins *(arrows)*.
(Courtesy Thomas J. Gilbert, MD, San Francisco.)

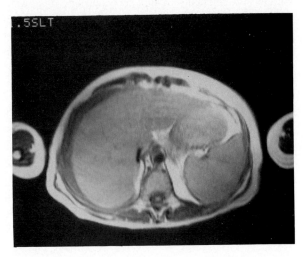

Fig. 75-30 Budd-Chiari syndrome: MR. MR image of liver (SE: TR 2000/TE 30) shows marked narrowing of inferior vena cava *(arrowhead)* and absence of hepatic veins. Spleen is enlarged and ascites present around liver.
(Courtesy David D. Stark, MD, Boston.)

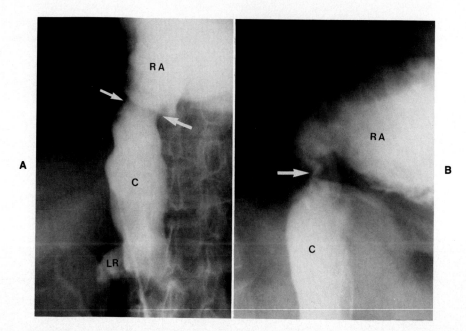

Fig. 75-31 Budd-Chiari syndrome. Anterior **(A)** and lateral **(B)** views of inferior vena cavagram show partial membranous obstruction *(arrows)* of inferior vena cava *(C)*–right atrium *(RA)* junction. Caval pressure was elevated, and patient had typical clinical Budd-Chiari syndrome. *LR,* Left renal vein.

MR has been shown to be quite accurate in diagnosis of patients with suspected Budd-Chiari syndrome. The findings include absent or severe reduction in caliber of hepatic veins, "comma-shaped" intrahepatic collateral vessels, and luminal narrowing of the intrahepatic segment of the inferior vena cava[125,182] (Fig. 75-30). Other findings include hepatomegaly, caudate lobe enlargement, and ascites.

INFERIOR VENA CAVOGRAPHY

Selective venography of the inferior vena cava may show severe narrowing or stenosis of the retrohepatic and intrahepatic segments, complete occlusion, or a well-defined membrane located at or just cephalad to the hepatic vein ostia[43,50,186] (Fig. 75-31). Intraluminal caval obstruction also may be caused by tumor extension from the kidneys, adrenal glands, or liver. In these latter cases tumor neovascularity often may be demonstrated within the cava.

HEPATIC VENOGRAPHY

Selective hepatic venography may show thrombus within major veins or complete venous occlusion. If the catheter can be advanced peripherally to a wedged position, a characteristic venographic pattern consisting of a "spider-web" plexus of veins may be demonstrated[15,19,101,109] (Fig. 75-32). This pattern is thought to be virtually pathognomonic of the Budd-Chiari syn-

drome.[101] Occasionally the veins may be seen to drain into azygos collateral vessels.[186] Similar findings may be seen by direct percutaneous needle puncture of the hepatic parenchyma (intraparenchymal venography).[147]

ANGIOGRAPHY

Selective hepatic angiography of patients with hepatic vein occlusion shows hepatomegaly, stretching, and attenuation of the intrahepatic arteries and retrograde filling of the portal venous system[45,109,146,186] (Fig. 75-33). Selective splenic injections usually show splenomegaly and either delayed hepatopetal portal venous flow or reversed flow (hepatofugal) into the mesenteric or retroperitoneal vessels.

SCINTIGRAPHY

Sulfur colloid scintigraphy often shows a characteristic central localization of the radionuclide within the caudate lobe.[30,80,118,143,186] This is believed to result from sparing of the veins of the caudate lobe, which has a separate venous drainage into the vena cava through multiple small veins.

A partial form of the Budd-Chiari syndrome, referred to as *unilobar vasoocclusive disease,* has been described by Galloway and co-workers[65] and by Maguire and Doppman.[109] In this disease the veins of only one or two lobes are occluded. Portal venous flow to the occluded lobe decreases, the lobe atrophies, and the portal flow is then

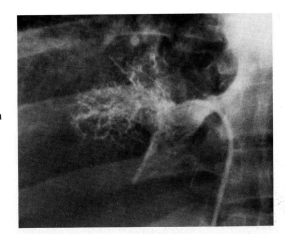

Fig. 75-32 Budd-Chiari Syndrome. Wedged hepatic venogram shows typical spider-web pattern of Budd-Chiari syndrome. (Courtesy Dr. Josef Rösch.)

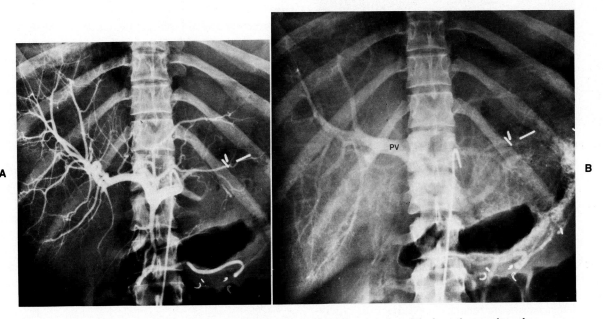

Fig. 75-33 Budd-Chiari syndrome. Selective hepatic arteriogram. Arterial, **A,** and parenchymal, **B,** phases of selective hepatic arteriogram show hepatomegaly, stretching, and attenuation of intrahepatic arteries and intense retrograde opacification of portal vein *(PV)* (arterioportal shunting) caused by hepatic venous outflow obstruction.

diverted to the normal lobes, which undergo hypertrophic enlargement. These pathophysiologic changes produce a series of interesting venographic and arteriographic findings that may be confused with intrahepatic neoplasm. The atrophic lobe shows crowding and tortuosity of the intrahepatic arteries, whereas the arteries in the normal, hypertrophied lobe show stretching and attenuation. However, selective wedged hepatic venography of the atrophied lobe shows the typical spider-web venous network of hepatic venous occlusion.

The prognosis of patients with Budd-Chiari syndrome is generally poor, with death usually occurring within several days or a few years of the initial diagnosis.[98,186] Occasionally patients may be treated effectively by resection of membranous obstructions of the inferior vena cava or by portocaval shunts.[34,87,141] Percutaneous balloon angioplasty can be used to treat Budd-Chiari syndrome caused by membranous obstruction of the intrahepatic inferior vena cava or hepatic vein ostia.[88,212]

Prehepatic hypertension

Prehepatic (extrahepatic) portal hypertension may be caused by portal vein occlusion or thrombosis. The cause of the occlusion frequently is related to infection, usually

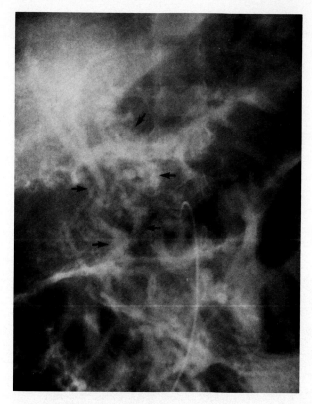

Fig. 75-34 Cavernous transformation of portal vein. Venous phase of selective superior mesenteric arteriogram in a 4-year-old child shows occlusion of extrahepatic portal vein and filling of intrahepatic portal venous branches through numerous tortuous collateral vessels *(arrows).*

omphalitis or a complication of umbilical vein catheterization in the neonatal period or inflammatory visceral disease in adults, such as ulcerative colitis or appendicitis. Other causes are trauma, blood dyscrasias (polycythemia rubra vera, myelofibrosis), use of oral contraceptives, postoperative complication of portocaval shunt, tumor invasion of the portal vein, and advanced hepatic cirrhosis.[28,33,74,199,203] Many cases also are idiopathic.

Occlusion of the extrahepatic portal vein produces hypertension in the region of proximal venous drainage, sometimes referred to as *regional portal hypertension.* Collateral venous channels develop that are similar to those that occur in response to intrahepatic causes of portal hypertension. These include gastric, esophageal, mesenteric, and retroperitoneal veins. Extensive hepatopedal collaterals also form within the porta hepatis in the hepatoduodenal and hepatocolic ligaments, around the gallbladder, and over the surface of the liver.[162] This extensive network of collateral vessels, which replaces the portal vein, is referred to as *cavernous transformation* of the portal vein (Fig. 75-34).

Diagnostic evaluation of patients with regional or prehepatic portal hypertension may be accomplished with CT, ultrasound, MR, and selective angiography and venography (Fig. 75-34).

ULTRASONOGRAPHY, COMPUTED TOMOGRAPHY, AND MAGNETIC RESONANCE

The superior mesenteric and portal veins are routinely seen during ultrasound, CT, and MR (see Figs. 75-2 to 75-6 and 75-8). Recent reports have shown that thrombosis or tumor invasion of these veins may be demonstrated by these techniques* (see Fig. 75-18).

ANGIOGRAPHY AND VENOGRAPHY

Selective splenic or superior mesenteric angiography, splenoportography, and transhepatic portal venography may be used for diagnosis of extrahepatic portal vein obstruction and for precise definition of collateral venous channels.[23,162,189,200] Although splenoportography has been used efficaciously, the current use of arterial portography and direct transhepatic portal venography has largely replaced splenoportography.[23] Arterial portography requires the use of selective injections and pharmacoangiographic techniques for achieving adequate opacification of the portal venous system.[154] Widrich and co-workers[205] have reported a 93% success rate in visualization of the portal and superior mesenteric veins using papaverine for augmentation of the venous phase. Similar results may be obtained with tolazoline.[148]

Hepatic venography is of little use in the evaluation of prehepatic portal hypertension. Wedged hepatic venous pressure is usually normal, and the absence of liver disease in most patients precludes the diagnostic value of wedged venography.

TREATMENT

Portal vein thrombosis may be treated by conventional portosystemic shunt (portocaval or mesocaval) of by a selective distal splenorenal shunt.[76,202] However, 30% to 50% of children with portal vein occlusion may be successfully managed nonsurgically and appear to have significantly fewer bleeding episodes as they become older.[56] Persistent hemorrhage, however, is believed to be an indication for a shunt.

Direct tumor invasion of the portal vein

Primary and metastatic hepatic neoplasms may obstruct the portal vein by direct invasion or extrinsic compression.[83] Direct invasion may be demonstrated by sonography, CT, MR, and angiography.[57,135,154] Portal

---

*References 5, 39, 57, 121, 159, 182, 190.

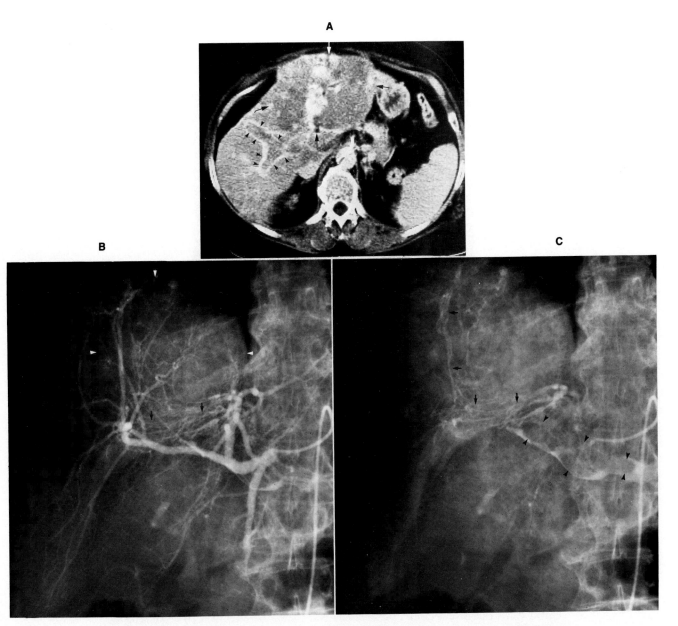

Fig. 75-35 Hepatocellular carcinoma: tumor invasion of portal vein. **A,** Axial computed tomogram during selective hepatic artery contrast medium infusion shows filling defect in portal vein *(arrowheads)* caused by direct invasion by hepatocellular carcinoma *(arrows)*. Arterial, **B,** and parenchymal, **C,** phases of selective hepatic arteriogram show hepatoma in superior aspect of liver *(white arrowheads)*, arterioportal shunting, and tumor thrombus within portal vein *(black arrowheads)*. Note thread and streaks sign of portal vein tumor invasion *(arrows)*.

vein tumor is seen angiographically as the "thread and streaks" sign (Fig. 75-35).

It is thought that tumor thrombus within the portal vein has its own blood supply originating from the vasa vasorum of the wall of the vein.[129] The thread and streaks sign is believed to represent contrast opacification of the vasa vasorum.[15,138,139]

Other angiographic manifestations of portal vein tumor involvement include extrinsic obstructive and arterioportal shunting. Extrinsic obstruction typically results from metastatic neoplasm but can also be caused by primary hepatocellular carcinoma or cholangiocarcinoma.[83] Arterioportal shunting is common in hepatocellular carcinoma, as seen in about 60% of cases reported by Kido

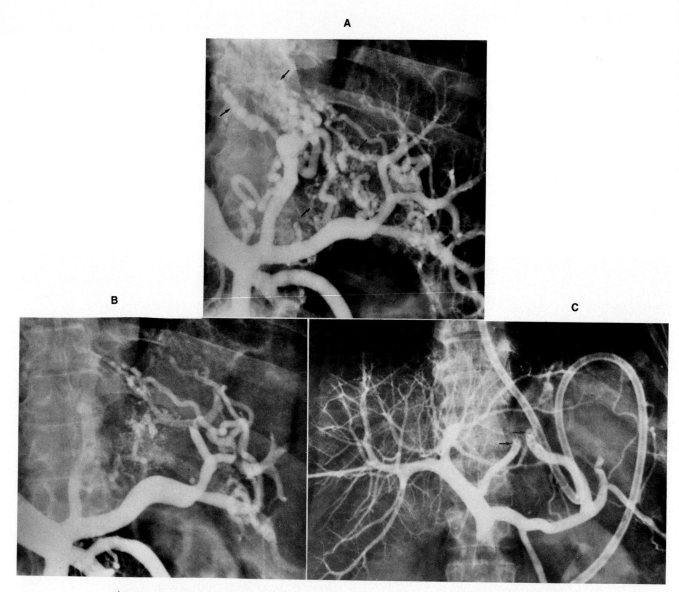

Fig. 75-36 Selective transhepatic variceal obliteration. **A,** Initial transhepatic portal venogram (THPV) shows extensive network of gastroesophageal varices *(arrows).* **B,** THPV following selective obliteration of varices with isobutyl 2-cyanoacrylate (Bucrylate) shows occlusion of majority of varices. **C,** THPV in different patient with varices shows obliteration of varices by selective obstruction of coronary and short gastric veins with steel coils *(arrows).*

and co-workers[99] and by Okuda and associates,[139] but is distinctly less common with metastatic tumors.[2,83,92]

Interventional radiologic techniques for treatment of variceal hemorrhage and portal hypertension

Vasopressin infusion

Intraarterial vasopressin controls variceal hemorrhage by lowering portal venous pressure. However, Barr and

co-workers[7] demonstrated that systemic venous infusions of vasopressin in dogs at rates similar to those used for arterial infusions (0.2 to 0.4 units/minute) result in an equal fall of portal venous pressure during the infusion. Subsequent clinical trials in humans comparing systemic and intraarterial infusions showed both techniques to be similarly efficacious in controlling variceal hemorrhage.[94] It is now well accepted that variceal hemorrhage can be controlled effectively by systemic venous infusion and that the severity of the underlying liver disease is the primary factor that influences overall success.

Transhepatic variceal obliteration

Transhepatic catheterization of the portal vein and selective obliteration of gastroesophageal varices have been used, including sclerosing agents reported by several investigators. Several embolic agents (sotradecol, absolute alcohol), Gelfoam, Ivalon sponge, steel coils, and isobutyl 2-cyanoacrylate[58,95,105,142,208] (Fig. 75-36).

Selective variceal embolization is an appropriate technique for acute control of hemorrhage if conservative therapeutic modalities fail and the patient is not considered an acceptable risk for immediate portosystemic shunt surgery. However, the results even for acute control are similar to those for vasopressin control; that is, they are best in patients with Child's class A or B cirrhosis (approximately 80% to 90% success) and those who have hepatopedal portal venous flow. Similarly, results are poor in patients with Child's class C cirrhosis and those who have hepatofugal flow (about 0% to 30% success). Second, long-term control of bleeding is poor, and overall mortality rate from recurrent hemorrhage or underlying liver disease may be as high as 50% during the first 4 weeks following embolization.[206] In the report by Mendez and Russell,[119] 21 of 29 patients who were not considered to be surgical candidates for shunts died during their hospitalization for variceal hemorrhage following transhepatic embolization. Failure to achieve long-term control of bleeding results from several factors, including persistent portal hypertension, inexorable progression of underlying liver disease, formation of new variceal collateral vessels, and recanalization of previously obliterated varices.[97,105]

Complications of transhepatic variceal obliteration include portal or splenic vein thrombosis, hemoperitoneum or subcapsular hepatic hematoma resulting from the hepatic puncture site, hemothorax or pneumothorax, fever and sepsis, and ascitic fluid leak from the percutaneous entry site. Portal vein thrombosis and intraperitoneal hemorrhage are the most significant complications and may occur in as many as 14% and 7% of cases, respectively.[10,206] However, considering the overall mortality rate of these patients when treated by balloon tamponade or emergency portosystemic shunt, the complication rate is acceptable.

Splenic and left gastric artery embolization

Some patients with recurrent variceal hemorrhage from extrahepatic portal hypertension caused by cavernous transformation of the portal vein are poor candidates for portosystemic shunt surgery and do not have a per-cutaneous access route for transhepatic variceal obliteration. In these cases selective splenic and left gastric artery embolization may be of value by decreasing portal venous flow.[20,97]

Percutaneous portosystemic shunt

Several investigators have actively pursued percutaneous transcatheter creation of intrahepatic portosystemic shunts.[27,167,168] The techniques of transjugular portography, which consist of passing a catheter from an hepatic vein through the intervening liver parenchyma and into a branch of the portal vein, essentially establish a portosystemic communication. Attempts to maintain this communication by placing a stent or conduit within the hepatic parenchyma in laboratory animals show promise.[168]

Endoscopic sclerotherapy

Endoscopic sclerotherapy consists of the direct injection of a sclerosing agent (sodium morrhuate) into distal esophageal varices using a fiberoptic endoscope.[188] The values of this technique are its relative simplicity and the ability to repeat the injections on multiple occasions. The success rate for control of acute hemorrhage is approximately 90%. A dual approach using transhepatic variceal embolization and sclerotherapy also may prove efficacious.[169]

PANCREAS AND SPLEEN
Pancreatic islet cell tumors

The primary role of the radiologic evaluation of patients with functioning islet cell tumors is preoperative localization of the neoplasms. This may be accomplished by ultrasound or CT and by selective pancreatic angiography. However, many clinically symptomatic islet cell tumors are too small to be imaged by ultrasound or CT and are hypovascular and thus undetectable by angiography. In the past these patients often underwent exploratory laparotomy and blind resection of the head or tail of the pancreas in an attempt to remove the tumor. Unfortunately blind resection may miss as many as 80% of tumors.[120] More recently the technique of transhepatic pancreatic vein catheterization has permitted endocrine tumor localization by selective venous sampling and radioimmunoassay techniques.[106,158]

The technique of pancreatic venous catheterization has been described by Göthlin and co-workers.[73] Venous samples are obtained from individual veins in the head, body, and tail of the gland, and radioimmunoassay is then performed for the hormone in question (insulin, gastrin, and so on). A focal area of increased hormone concentration has been shown to correlate with the location of islet cell tumors, facilitating surgical resection.[26,89,90,100]

Pancreatitis and pancreatic carcinoma

The splenic, portal, and superior mesenteric veins may be occluded or narrowed by retropancreatic extension of tumor or inflammatory disease of the pancreas. The importance of the evaluation of the venous phase of diagnostic pancreatic angiography has been emphasized by numerous investigators.[59,60,71,165,166]

Pancreatic carcinoma usually causes focal arterial changes (encasement, obstruction) with contiguous changes in the corresponding veins. Occasionally, however, the arterial changes may be relatively subtle, whereas the venous changes are more obvious, the latter finding facilitating diagnosis (Fig. 75-37). In addition, tumor involvement of major extrapancreatic veins (splenic, superior mesenteric, or portal) is a reliable angiographic criterion of tumor unresectability.[59,60,191]

Pancreatitis usually causes more diffuse arterial changes than carcinoma but also may result in occlusion or narrowing of the major extrapancreatic veins.[86] Occlusion of the splenic vein resulting in splenomegaly and gastric varices is the most common venous abnormality.[21,102] However, collateral venous circulation may also produce varices in the duodenum and colon.[21] Gastric varices caused by isolated splenic vein obstruction are an important angiographic diagnosis, since variceal hemorrhage may be cured by splenectomy.[4,174]

The most precise methods for evaluating the peripancreatic veins are arterial and direct transhepatic portography. In most cases arterial portography is favored because of the added diagnostic information gained from evaluation of the arteries. More recently, ultrasound and CT have been used to evaluate the portal venous system. These studies may demonstrate venous involvement and varices and may add valuable information about the spleen, pancreas, and liver.*

---

*References 39, 51, 67, 86, 91, 175.

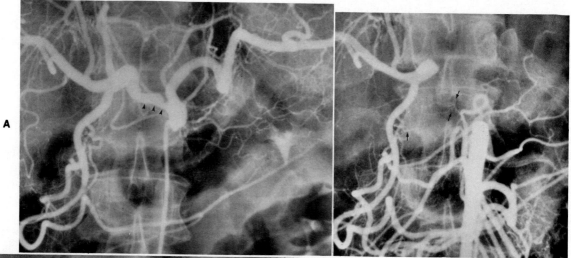

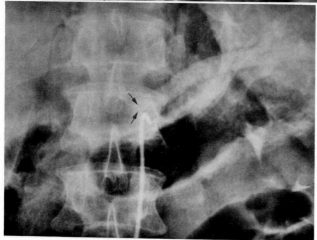

Fig. 75-37 Pancreatic carcinoma: value of venous phase. Arterial phases of selective celiac, **A,** and superior mesenteric, **B,** arteriograms show only subtle eccentric effacement of hepatic artery *(arrowheads),* minimal small vessel irregularity *(arrows),* and hypovascularity in head of pancreas. Although arterial phases are abnormal, venous phase of celiac injection, **C,** is most important. It shows complete occlusion of splenic vein *(arrows),* indicating extrapancreatic tumor extension and thus unresectability.

Splenic vein obstruction

The most common causes of splenic vein obstruction are pancreatitis and pancreatic carcinoma. Less frequent causes include idiopathic thrombosis, portal hypertension, trauma, retroperitoneal hematoma or tumor, and hematologic disorders such as myeloproliferative disease.[11,40]

An unusual cause of splenic vein obstruction is wandering spleen, a congenital abnormality resulting from failure of formation of the normal splenic ligaments. In this abnormality excessive splenic mobility may result in torsion of the vascular pedicle and subsequent venous obstruction or splenic infarction.[72,179,181]

STOMACH, SMALL BOWEL, AND COLON
Stomach

The veins of the stomach serve as important collateral vessels in cases of portal hypertension and splenic vein obstruction. The radiologic evaluation of gastric varices is discussed in detail in the preceding sections of this chapter (see Figs. 75-14, 75-18, 75-21, and 75-22).

The venous phases of selective left gastric and gastroduodenal injections also may be valuable in the eval-

uation of patients with arteriovenous malformations or hereditary hemorrhagic telangiectasia.

Small bowel and duodenum

The venous phases of selective gastroduodenal and superior mesenteric arterial injections are important in the evaluation of patients with inflammatory bowel disease (regional enteritis, radiation enteritis), arteriovenous malformations of the duodenum or small bowel, primary or metastatic small bowel tumors, and mesenteric venous thrombosis.

Although the diagnosis of inflammatory disease of the small bowel primarily is made by barium studies, some patients may undergo selective angiography for diagnosis and control of gastrointestinal bleeding. The angiographic findings during the acute inflammatory stage of regional enteritis and radiation enteritis may be similar and include severe hypervascularity of the wall of the small bowel and dense, early opacification of the veins[18,44,104] (Fig. 75-38). Hemorrhage may be detected by demonstration of active contrast extravasation and may be treated by selective intraarterial vasopressin infusion.

Arteriovenous malformations may occur within the

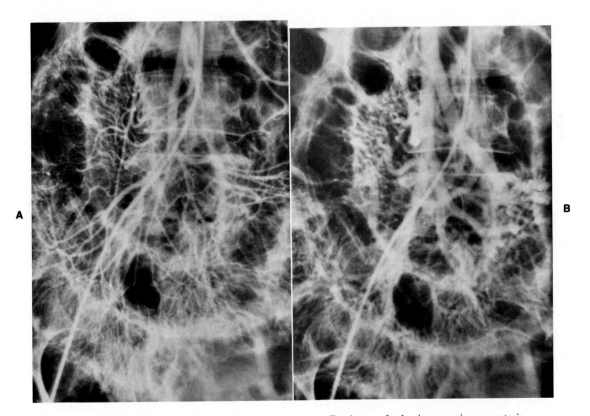

Fig. 75-38 Radiation enteritis. Arterial, **A,** and venous, **B,** phases of selective superior mesenteric arteriogram show severe hypervascularity of wall of small bowel and intense opacification of veins. Note dilated vasa recta in small bowel.

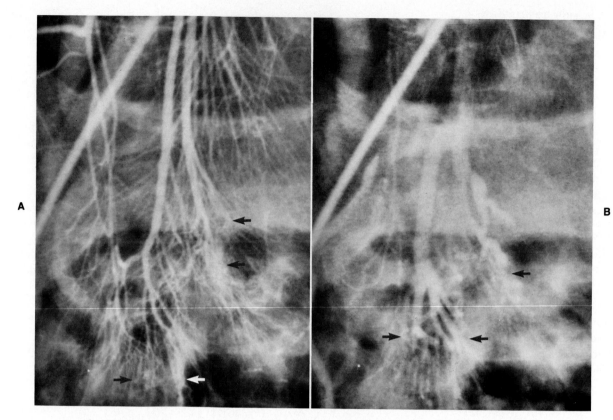

Fig. 75-39 Arteriovenous malformation of small bowel. Selective (×2) magnification, superior mesenteric arteriogram. **A,** Arterial phase shows only subtle changes in vasa recta of small bowel *(arrows).* **B,** Venous phase shows early contrast opacification of ectatic veins arising from localized segment of small bowel *(arrows).* Pathologic examination of resected bowel showed arteriovenous malformation.

duodenum and small bowel. Angiographic findings include a dilated feeding artery, a racemose tangle of vessels in the bowel wall, and densely opacified, early draining veins. In some cases the venous findings may be the most important for diagnosis (Fig. 75-39).

Primary and metastatic small bowel tumors also may cause changes in the venous phase during selective superior mesenteric angiography. Some tumors are hypervascular, such as leiomyomas and leiomyosarcomas, and may show early and dense opacification of the veins draining the neoplasms. Other tumors, such as carcinoids and primary or metastatic adenocarcinomas that involve the mesentery, may obstruct the venous drainage of the involved segment of the small bowel.

Primary mesenteric venous occlusion disease is a rare and often fatal disorder. It may occur spontaneously in the absence of any underlying disease but usually is the result of cirrhosis and portal hypertension, hypercoaguable hematologic disorders such as polycythemia rubra vera, sickle cell disease, or migratory thrombophlebitis

caused by a tumor such as pancreatic carcinoma. Other causes include intraabdominal sepsis resulting from abscess, appendicitis, diverticulitis, or inflammatory bowel disease, hypoperfusion syndrome, and drug abuse.

Most patients with mesenteric venous occlusion undergo emergency laparotomy because of physical signs and symptoms of an acute abdomen. Radiologic evaluation usually consists only of a conventional radiograph of the abdomen. It may be normal or may show signs of bowel ischemia, including dilatation, mucosal edema, or gas in the bowel wall or portal vein. The latter finding invariably indicates an infarcted, gangrenous bowel, and more than 90% of these patients die. Rarely, however, gas has been reported in the portal vein in the absence of infarction.[187] In these cases the pathogenesis of the gas is uncertain, although some reports suggest that it results from gas-forming bacteria that enter the portal venous system through a small tear in the mucosa.[211]

The angiographic findings of mesenteric venous thrombosis include delayed arterial filling and lack of

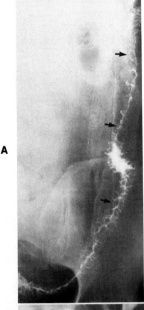

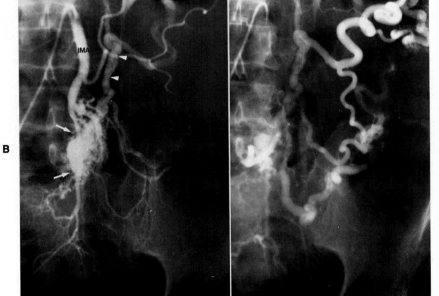

Fig. 75-40 Arteriovenous malformation of distal left (descending sigmoid) colon. **A,** Barium examination of colon shows numerous intramural filling defects in wall of descending colon *(arrows).* **B** and **C,** Selective inferior mesenteric *(IMA)* arteriogram. Arterial phase, **B,** shows dilated IMA feeding racemose collection of vessels *(arrows).* Note early draining vein *(arrowheads).* Venous phase, **C,** shows early, intense opacification of numerous, ectatic draining veins.
(Courtesy Dr. L. John Davis.)

venous opacification within the segment of infarcted small bowel.[189] CT, MR, and sonography also can be used to diagnose thrombosis of the superior mesenteric and portal veins.[117,123,213]

Colon

The venous drainage of the colon is important in the evaluation of arteriovenous malformations or angiodysplasias, inflammatory bowel disease (ulcerative colitis and Crohn disease), portal hypertension with colonic varices, and varices caused by adhesions.

Colonic arteriovenous malformations and angiodys-

plasias (vascular ectasias) are common causes of occult lower gastrointestinal bleeding. These two lesions appear to be different. Whereas malformations are congenital lesions and may be seen in young patients, angiodysplasias are believed to be developmental and most often are found in older patients.[13,14] Thus the term *dysplasia* is a misnomer, and the lesions are more correctly referred to as vascular *ectasias*. Arteriovenous malformations are characterized by dilated feeding arteries, a large tangle of vessels representing the malformation, and densely opacified, early draining ectatic veins (Fig. 75-40). Vascular ectasias usually are smaller lesions. The feeding

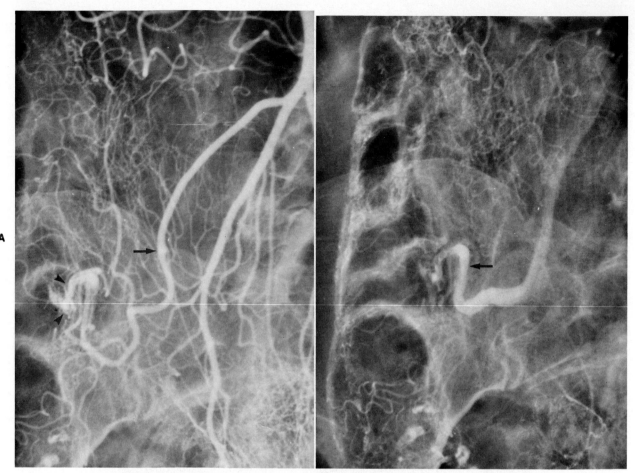

A   B

Fig. 75-41 Cecal vascular ectasia (angiodysplasia). **A** and **B,** Selective superior mesenteric arteriogram. Arterial phase, **A,** shows normal-sized ileocolic artery *(arrow)* and small vascular tuft in wall of cecum *(arrowheads)*. Venous phase, **B,** shows early, intense opacification of vein *(arrow)* draining from tuft.

artery may be of normal size or slightly dilated, the vascular ectasia is seen as a small capillary tuft, and the draining vein appears early but often is of normal size[8,14] (Fig. 75-41). Vascular ectasias are most often found in the cecum or right colon and have been noted to have an increased prevalence in patients with aortic stenosis.[66,210]

The active or acute stages of both granulomatous colitis (Crohn's colitis) and ulcerative colitis are characterized by intense hypervascularity of the wall of the colon, lack of normal tapering of the vasa recta, and densely opacified early draining veins.[18,44,104] These angiographic findings are similar to those seen in inflammatory bowel disease involving the small intestine (Fig. 75-38).

Colonic varices may result from generalized portal hypertension resulting from intrahepatic or posthepatic causes or from regional portal hypertension (prehepatic) caused by splenic vein occlusion.[21,52,54,77,103] The formation of varices within the colon is capricious and depends on the particular route of collateral venous drainage that occurs in each patient. The ectatic veins may be demonstrated by barium studies, CT, and transhepatic or arterial portography (Fig. 75-40).

Mesenteric varices occasionally may form within postoperative adhesions. This entity is most likely to occur in patients with coexisting portal hypertension and can be the source of massive colonic or enteric hemorrhage.[16,124] The diagnosis may be established by selective mesenteric angiography, and treatment consists of lysis of the adhesion and resection of the involved segment of bowel[124] (Fig. 75-42).

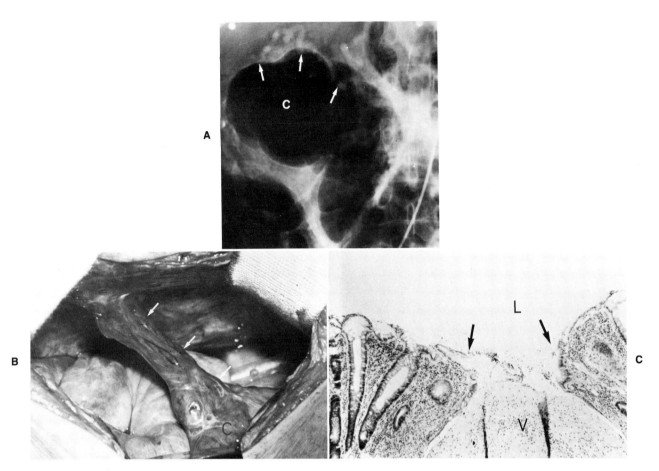

Fig. 75-42 Colonic varices caused by postoperative adhesion. **A,** Venous phase of selective superior mesenteric arteriogram in patient with recurrent episodes of lower gastrointestinal bleeding shows collection of ectatic veins *(arrows)* in area of hepatic flexure of colon *(C)*. Arterial phase was normal. **B,** Photograph taken during surgery shows thick adhesion *(arrows)* extending from abdominal wall to colon *(C)*. **C,** Photomicrograph of resected colon shows venous varix *(V)*, which has eroded through colonic mucosa *(arrows)*. *L,* Lumen of colon.

REFERENCES

1. Abernethy, J: An account of two instances of uncommon formation in the viscera of the human body, Philos Trans R Soc Lond (Biol) 17:292, 1980.

2. ~~Allen~~ ...
ology 129:315, 1978.

3. Alpern, MB, et al: Porta hepatis: doppler ultrasound with angiographic correlation, Radiology 162:53, 1987.

4. Babb, RR: Splenic vein obstruction: a curable cause of variceal bleeding, Am J Dig Dis 21:512, 1976.

5. Babcock, DS: Ultrasound diagnosis of portal vein thrombosis as a complication of appendicitis, AJR 133:317, 1979.

6. Baert, AL, et al: Early diagnosis of Budd-Chiari syndrome by computed tomography and ultrasonography: report of 5 cases, Gastroenterology 84:587, 1983.

7. Barr, JW, Lakin, RC, and Rösch, J: Similarity of arterial and intravenous vasopressin on portal and systemic hemodynamics, Gastroenterology 69:13, 1975.

8. Baum, S, et al: Angiodysplasia of the right colon: a cause of gastrointestinal bleeding, AJR 129:789, 1977.

9. Becker, CD, Scheidegger, J, and Marineck, B: Hepatic vein occlusion: morphologic features on computed tomography and ultrasonography, Gastrointest Radiol 11:305, 1986.

10. Bengmark, S, et al: Obliteration of esophageal varices by PTP:

11. Bergentz, SE, et al: Thrombosis in the superior mesenteric and portal veins: report of a case treated with thrombectomy, Surgery 76:286, 1974.

12. Bernardino, ME, et al: Shunts for portal hypertension: MR and angiography for determination of patency, Radiology 158:57, 1986.

13. Boley, SJ, et al: On the nature and etiology of vascular ectasias of the colon: degenerative lesions of aging, Gastroenterology 72:650, 1977.

14. Boley, SJ, et al: The pathophysiologic basis for the angiographic signs of vascular ectasias of the colon, Radiology 125:615, 1977.

15. Bookstein, JJ, et al: Histological-venographic correlates in portal hypertension, Radiology 116:565, 1975.

16. Börjesson, B, Olsson, AM, and Varig, JO: Hemorrhage from portal-systemic venous shunt with unusual localization in a case of portal hypertension, Scand J Gastroenterol 9:571, 1974.

17. Bradley, WG, Jr, and Walach, V: Blood flow: magnetic resonance imaging, Radiology 154:443, 1985.

18. Brahme, F, and Hildell, J: Angiography in Crohn's disease revisited, Am J Roentgenol 126:941, 1976.

19. Brink, AJ, and Botha, D: Budd-Chiari syndrome: diagnosis by hepatic venography, Br J Radiol 28:330, 1955.

20. Bücheler, E, et al: Catheter embolization of the splenic artery as treatment for acute bleeding from varices, Fortschr Roentgenstr 122:224, 1975.

21. Burbige, EJ, et al: Colonic varices: a complication of pancreatitis with splenic vein thrombosis, Am J Dig Dis 23:752, 1978.

22. Burcharth, F: Percutaneous transhepatic portography. I. Technique and application, AJR 132:177, 1979.

23. Burcharth, F, Nielbo, N, and Andersen, B: Percutaneous transhepatic portography. II. Comparison with splenoportography in portal hypertension, AJR 132:183, 1979.

24. Burcharth, F, Sørensen, TIA, and Andersen, B: Percutaneous transhepatic portography. III. Relationship between portosystemic collaterals and portal pressure in cirrhosis, AJR 133:1119, 1979.

25. Burcharth, F, Sørensen, TIA, and Andersen, B: Findings in percutaneous transhepatic portography and variceal bleeding in cirrhosis, Surg Gynecol Obstet 150:887, 1980.

26. Burcharth, F, et al: Localization of gastrinomas by transhepatic portal venous catheterization and gastrin assay, Gastroenterology 77:444, 1979.

27. Burgener, FA, and Gutierrez, OH: Nonsurgical production of intrahepatic portosystemic venous shunts in portal hypertension with the double lumen balloon catheter, Fortschr Roentgenstr 130:686, 1979.

28. Capron, JP, et al: Gastrointestinal bleeding due to chronic portal vein thrombosis in ulcerative colitis, Am J Dig Dis Sci 24:232, 1979.

29. Carlsen, EN, and Filly, RA: Newer ultrasonographic anatomy in the upper abdomen. I. The portal and hepatic venous anatomy, J Clin Ultrasound 4:85, 1976.

30. Carulli, N, et al: Liver scans in the Budd-Chiari syndrome, JAMA 223:1161, 1972.

31. Cavaluzzi, J, et al: Hepatic venography and wedge hepatic vein pressure measurements in diffuse liver disease, AJR 129:441, 1977.

32. Chamberlain, DW, and Walter, JB: The relationship of Budd-Chiari syndrome to oral contraceptives and trauma, Can Med Assoc J 101:618, 1969.

33. Chambers, JSW, and Goodbody, RA: Portal phlebothrombosis in the puerperium, Br Med J 2:1104, 1963.

34. Chapman, JE, and Ochsner, JL: Iliac-mesenteric-atrial shunt procedure for Budd-Chiari syndrome complicated by inferior vena caval thrombosis, Ann Surg 188:642, 1978.

35. Chiandussi, L, et al: Hepatic portography by direct catheterization of the portal vein through the round ligament of the liver (ligamentum teres), Am J Roentgenol 99:625, 1967.

36. Chuang, VP, Lunderquist, A, and Herlinger, H: Portal hypertension. In Herlinger, H, Lunderquist, A, and Wallace, S, editors: Clinical radiology of the liver, New York, 1983, Marcel Decker.

37. Chuang, VP, et al: Angiography in pancreatic arteriovenous malformation, AJR 129:1015, 1977.

38. Clain, D, et al: Clinical diagnosis of Budd-Chiari syndrome: report of six cases, Am J Med 43:544, 1967.

39. Clark, KE, et al: CT evaluation of esophageal and upper abdominal varices, J Comput Assist Tomogr 4:510, 1980.

40. Clatworthy, HW: Extrahepatic portal hypertension, Major Probl Clin Surg 14:243, 1973.

41. Cohen, JM, Weinreb, JC, and Redman, HC: Postoperative assessment of splenorenal shunts with MRI: preliminary investigation, AJR 146:597, 1986.

42. Dach, JL, et al: Sonography of hypertensive portal venous system: correlation with arterial portography, AJR 137:511, 1981.

43. Datta, DV, et al: Diagnostic value of combined transhepatic venography and inferior vena cavography in chronic Budd-Chiari syndrome, Am J Dig Dis 23:1031, 1978.

44. Dencker, H, et al: Mesenteric angiography in patients with radiation injury of the bowel after pelvic irradiation, Am J Roentgenol 114:476, 1972.

45. Deutch, V, et al: Budd-Chiari syndrome: study of angiographic findings and remarks on etiology, Am J Roentgenol 116:430, 1962.

46. Doehner, GA: The hepatic venous system: its normal roentgen anatomy, Radiology 90:1119, 1968.

47. Doehner, GA, et al: The portal venous system: its roentgen anatomy, Radiology 64:675, 1955.

48. Doehner, GA, et al: The portal venous system: on its pathological roentgen anatomy, Radiology 66:206, 1956.

49. Edwards, EA: Functional anatomy of the porta-systemic communications, Arch Intern Med 88:137, 1951.

50. Espana, P, et al: Membranous obstruction of the inferior vena cava and hepatic veins: Budd-Chiari syndrome? A treatable disease, Am J Gastroenterology 73:28, 1980.

51. Fakhry, J, Gosink, BB, and Leopold, GR: Recanalized umbilical vein due to portal vein occlusion documented by sonography, AJR 137:410, 1981.

52. Federle, M, and Clark, RA: Mesenteric varices: a source of mesosystemic shunts and gastrointestinal hemorrhage, Gastrointest Radiol 4:331, 1979.

53. Ferris, EJ, et al: Venography of the inferior vena cava and its branches, Baltimore, 1969, Williams & Wilkins.

54. Fleming, RJ, and Seaman, WB: Roentgenographic demonstration of unusual extra-esophageal varices, Am J Roentgenol 103:281, 1968.

55. Foley, WD, et al: Dynamic computed tomography and duplex ultrasonography: adjuncts to arterial portography, J Comput Assist Tomogr 7:77, 1983.

56. Fonkalsrud, EW: Discussion. In Warren, WD, et al, editors: Noncirrhotic portal vein thrombosis: physiology before and after shunts, Ann Surg 192:341, 1980.

57. Freeny, PC: Portal vein tumor thrombus: demonstration by computed tomographic arteriography, J Comput Assist Tomogr 4:263, 1980.

58. Freeny, PC, and Kidd, R: Transhepatic portal venography and selective obliteration of gastroesophageal varices using isobutyl 2-cyanoacrylate (Bucrylate), Am J Dig Dis 24:321, 1979.

59. Freeny, PC, and Lawson, TL: Radiology of the pancreas, New York, 1983, Springer-Verlag, New York.

60. Freeny, PC, et al: Pancreatic ductal adenocarcinoma: diagnosis and staging with dynamic CT, Radiology 166:125, 1988.

61. Fulenwider, JT, et al: Portal pseudoperfusion: an angiographic illusion, Ann Surg 189:257, 1979.

62. Futagawa, S, et al: Hepatic venography in noncirrhotic idiopathic portal hypertension: comparison with cirrhosis of the liver, Radiology 141:303, 1981.

63. Galambos, JT, Rudman, D, and Warren, WD: Portal hypertension: a new beginning for an old problem, Am J Dig Dis 21:827, 1976.

64. Galambos, J, et al: Selective and total shunts in the treatment of bleeding varices: a randomized controlled trial, N Engl J Med 295:1089, 1976.

65. Galloway, S, Casarella, WJ, and Prince, JB: Unilobar veno-occlusive disease of the liver: angiographic demonstration of intrahepatic competition simulating hepatoma, Am J Roentgenol 119:89, 1973.

66. Gelfand, ML, et al: Gastrointestinal bleeding in aortic stenosis, Am J Gastroenterol 71:30, 1979.

67. Glazer, GM, et al: Sonographic demonstration of portal hypertension: the patient umbilical vein, Radiology 136:161, 1980.

68. Gleysteen, JJ, et al: Patency evaluation of distal splenorenal shunt with dynamic computed tomography, Surg Gynecol Obstet 154:689, 1982.

69. Glickman, MG, and Handel, SF: Opacification of hepatic veins during celiac and hepatic angiography, Radiology 103:565, 1972.

70. Goldman, ML, Fajman, W, and Galambos, J: Transjugular obliteration of the gastric coronary vein, Radiology 118:453, 1976.

71. Goldstein, HM, Neiman, HL, and Bookstein, JJ: Angiographic evaluation of pancreatic disease: a further appraisal, Radiology 112:275, 1974.

72. Gordon, D, et al: Wandering spleen—the radiological and clinical spectrum, Radiology 125:39, 1977.

73. Göthlin, J, Lunderquist, A, and Tylén, U: Selective phlebography of the pancreas, Acta Radiol (Diagn) (Stockh) 15:474, 1974.

74. Graef, V, et al: Venous thrombosis occurring in nonspecific ulcerative colitis: a necropsy study, Arch Intern Med 117:377, 1966.

75. Grannis, FW, et al: Diagnosis and management of an arteriovenous fistula of pancreas and duodenum, Mayo Clin Proc 48:780, 1973.

76. Graver, SE, and Schwartz, SI: Extrahepatic portal hypertension: a retrospective analysis, Ann Surg 189:566, 1979.

77. Gray, RK, and Groelman, JH: Acute lower gastrointestinal bleeding secondary to varices of the superior mesenteric venous system, Radiology 111:559, 1974.

78. Halpern, M, Turner, AF, and Citron, BP: Hereditary hemorrhagic telangiectasia: an angiographic study of abdominal visceral angiodysplasias associated with gastrointestinal hemorrhage, Radiology 90:1143, 1968.

79. Hanafee, WM, and Weiner, M: Transjugular percutaneous cholangiography, Radiology 88:35, 1967.

80. Hanelin, LG, Uszler, JM, and Sommer, DG: Liver scan "hot-spot" in hepatic venoocclusive disease, Radiology 117:637, 1975.

81. Harbin, WP, Robert, NJ, and Ferrucci, JT, Jr: Diagnosis of cirrhosis based on regional changes in hepatic morphology: a radiological and pathological analysis, Radiology 135:273, 1980.

82. Harell, G: Ventral portal vein, Am J Roentgenol 121:369, 1974.

83. Heaston, DK, et al: Metastatic hepatic neoplasms: angiographic features of portal vein involvement, AJR 136:897, 1981.

84. Hepner, GW, Steiner, RE, and Benthall, HH: Hepatic venous occlusion associated with intrahepatic narrowing of the inferior vena cava, Br J Surg 56:245, 1969.

85. Hill, KR: The world-wide distribution of seneciosis in man and animals, Proc R Soc Med 53:281, 1960.

86. Hofer, BO, Ryan, JA, Jr, and Freeny, PC: Surgical significance of vascular changes in chronic pancreatitis, Surg Gynecol Obstet 164:499, 1987.

87. Huguet, C, et al: Interposition mesocaval shunt for chronic primary occlusion of the hepatic veins, Surg Gynecol Obstet 148:691, 1979.

88. Ida, M, et al: Therapeutic hepatic vein angioplasty for Budd-Chiari syndrome, Cardiovasc Intervent Radiol 9:187, 1986.

89. Ingemansson, S, Lunderquist, A, and Holst, J: Selective catheterization of the pancreatic vein for radioimmunoassay in glucagon-secreting carcinoma of the pancreas, Radiology 119:555, 1976.

90. Ingemansson, S, et al: Pancreatic vein catheterization with gastrin assay in normal patients and patients with the Zollinger-Ellison syndrome, Am J Surg 134:558, 1977.

91. Ishikawa, T, et al: Venous abnormalities in portal hypertension demonstrated by CT, AJR 134:271, 1980.

92. Itzchak, Y, et al: Intrahepatic arterial portal communications: angiographic study, Am J Roentgenol 121:384, 1974.

93. Jackson, FC: "Directional" flow patterns in portal hypertension, Arch Surg 87:307, 1963.

94. Johnson, WC, et al: Control of bleeding varices by vasopressin: a prospective randomized study, Ann Surg 186:369, 1977.

95. Keller, FS, Dotter, CT, and Rösch, J: Percutaneous transhepatic obliteration of gastroesophageal varices: some technical aspects, Radiology 129:327, 1978.

96. Keller, FS, Rösch, J, and Dotter, CT: Bleeding from esophageal varices exacerbated by splenic arterial-venous fistula: complete transcatheter obliterative therapy, Cardiovasc Intervent Radiol 3:97, 1980.

97. Keller, FS, et al: Embolization in the treatment of bleeding gastroesophageal varices, Semin Roentgenol 16:103, 1981.

98. Khuroo, MS, and Datta, CV: Budd-Chiari syndrome following pregnancy: report of 16 cases, with roentgenologic, hemodynamic and histologic studies of the hepatic outflow tract, Am J Med 68:113, 1980.

99. Kido, C, Sasaki, T, and Kameko, M: Angiography of primary liver cancer, Am J Roentgenol 113:70, 1971.

100. Kingham, JGC, et al: Vipoma: localization by percutaneous portal venous sampling, Br Med J 2:1682, 1978.

101. Kreel, L, Freston, JW, and Clain, D: Vascular radiology in the Budd-Chiari syndrome, Br J Radiol 40:755, 1967.

102. Longstreth, G, Newcomer, AD, and Green, P: Extrahepatic portal hypertension caused by chronic pancreatitis, Ann Intern Med 75:903, 1971.

103. Lopata, HL, and Berling, L: Colon varices: a rare cause of lower gastrointestinal bleeding, Radiology 87:1048, 1966.

104. Lunderquist, A, and Knutsson, H: Angiography in Crohn's disease of the small bowel and colon, Am J Roentgenol 101:338, 1967.

105. Lunderquist, A, et al: Istobutyl 2-cyanoacrylate (Bucrylate) in obliteration of gastric coronary vein and esophageal varices, AJR 130:1, 1978.

106. Lunderquist, A, et al: Selective pancreatic vein catheterization for hormone assay in endocrine tumors of the pancreas, Cardiovasc Radiol 1:117, 1978.

107. Lyford, CL, Vergara, GG, and Moeller, DD: Hepatic venoocclusive disease originating in Ecuador, Gastroenterology 70:105, 1976.

108. MacMahon, HE, and Ball, HG: Leiomyosarcoma of the hepatic vein and the Budd-Chiari syndrome, Gastroenterology 61:219, 1971.

109. Maguire, R, and Doppman, JL: Angiographic abnormalities in partial Budd-Chiari syndrome, Radiology 122:629, 1977.

110. Malt, RA: Portasystemic venous shunts. I, N Engl J Med 295:24, 1976.

111. Malt, RA: Portasystemic venous shunts. II, N Engl J Med 295:80, 1976.

112. Mardis, D, et al: Congenital absence of the portal vein, Mayo Clin Proc 54:55: 1979.

113. Marks, C: Developmental basis of the portal venous system, Am J Surg 117:671, 1969.

114. Marks, WM, Filly, RA, and Callen, PW: Ultrasonic anatomy of the liver: a review with new applications, J Clin Ultrasound 7:137, 1979.

115. Marubbio, AT, and Danielson, B: Hepatic veno-occlusive disease in a renal transplant patient receiving azathioprine, Gastroenterology 69:739, 1975.

116. Mathieu, D, Vasile, N, and Greiner, P: Portal thrombosis: dynamic CT features and course, Radiology 154:737, 1985.

117. Mathieu, D, et al: Budd-Chiari syndrome: dynamic CT, Radiology 165:409, 1987.

118. Meindok, H, and Langer, B: Liver scan in Budd-Chiari syndrome, J Nucl Med 17:365, 1976.

119. Mendez, G, Jr, and Russell, E: Gastrointestinal varices: percutaneous transhepatic therapeutic embolization in 54 patients, AJR 135:1045, 1980.

120. Mengoli, L, and LeQuesne, LP, Blind pancreatic resection for suspected insulinoma: review of problem, Br J Surg 54:749, 1967.

121. Merritt, CB: Ultrasonographic demonstration of portal vein thrombosis, Radiology 133:425, 1979.

122. Michels, NA: Blood supply and anatomy of the upper abdominal organs, Philadelphia, 1955, JB Lippincott.

123. Miller, VE, and Berland, LL: Pulsed doppler duplex sonography and CT of portal vein thrombosis, AJR 145:73, 1985.

124. Moncure, AC, et al: Gastrointestinal hemorrhage from adhesion-related mesenteric varices, Ann Surg 183:24, 1976.

125. Murphy, FB, et al: The Budd-Chiari syndrome: a review, AJR 147:9, 1986.

126. Nasbeth, DC: The distal splenorenal shunt: an enigma, Am J Surg 141:579, 1981.

127. Nasbeth, DC, et al: Flow and pressure characteristics of the portal system before and after splenorenal shunts, Surgery 78:739, 1975.

128. Nakamura, S, and Tsuzuki, T: Surgical anatomy of the hepatic veins and the inferior vena cava, Surg Gynecol Obstet 152:43, 1981.

129. Nakashima, T: Vascular changes and hemodynamics in hepatocellular carcinoma. In Okuda, K, and Peters, RL, editors: Hepatocellular carcinoma, New York, 1976, John Wiley & Sons.

130. Nebesar, RA, and Pollard, JJ: Portal venography by selective arterial characterization, Radiology 97:477, 1966.

131. Nordlinger, BM, et al: Angiography in portal hypertension: clinical significance in surgery, Am J Surg 139:132, 1980.

132. Novak, D, Butzow, GH, and Becker, K: Hepatic occlusion venography with a balloon catheter in portal hypertension, Radiology 122:623, 1977.

133. Nunez, D, et al: Portosystemic communications studied by transhepatic portography, Radiology 127:75, 1978.

134. Obeid, FN, et al: Bilharzial portal hypertension, Arch Surg 118:702, 1983.

135. Ohtomo, K, et al: Magnetic resonance imaging of portal vein thrombosis in hepatocellular carcinoma, J Comput Assist Tomogr 9:328, 1985.

136. Ohtomo, K, et al: Portosystemic collaterals on MR imaging, J Comput Assist Tomogr 10:751, 1986.

137. Okuda, K, and Iio, M: Radiological aspects of the liver and biliary tract: x-ray and radioisotope diagnosis, Chicago, 1976, Year Book Medical Publishers.

138. Okuda, K, et al: Angiographic assessment of gross anatomy of hepatocellular carcinoma: comparison of celiac angiograms and liver pathology in 100 cases, Radiology 123:21, 1977.

139. Okuda, K, et al: Angiographic demonstration of intrahepatic arterioportal anastomoses in hepatocellular carcinoma, Radiology 122:53, 1977.

140. Okuda, K, et al: Percutaneous transhepatic catheterization of the portal vein for the study of portal hemodynamics and shunts: a preliminary report, Gastroenterology 73:279, 1977.

141. Orloff, MJ, and Johansen, KH: Treatment of Budd-Chiari syndrome by side-to-side portacaval shunt: experimental and clinical results, Ann Surg 188:494, 1978.

142. Pereiras, R, et al: New techniques for interruption of gastroesophageal venous blood flow, Radiology 124:313, 1977.

143. Picard, M, et al: Budd-Chiari syndrome: typical and atypical scintigraphic aspects, J Nucl Med 28:803, 1987.

144. Piekarski, J, et al: Difference between liver and spleen CT numbers in the normal adult: its usefulness in predicting the presence of diffuse liver disease, Radiology 137:727, 1980.

145. Pollard, JJ, and Nebesar, RA: Catheterization of splenic artery for portal venography, N Engl J Med 271:234, 1964.

146. Pollard, JJ, and Nebesar, RA: Altered hemodynamics in the Budd-Chiari syndrome demonstrated by selective hepatic and selective splenic angiography, Radiology 89:236, 1967.

147. Ramsay, GC, and Britton, RC: Intraparenchymal angiography in the diagnosis of hepatic veno-occlusive diseases, Radiology 90:716, 1968.

148. Redman, HC, Reuter, SR, and Miller, WJ: Improvement of superior mesenteric and portal vein visualization with tolazoline, Invest Radiol 4:24, 1969.

149. Reichardt, W, Butzow, GH, and Erbe, W: Anomalous venous connections involving the portal system, Cardiovasc Radiol 2:41, 1979.

150. Reichle, FA, and Owen, OE: Hemodynamic patterns in human hepatic cirrhosis: a prospective randomized study of the hemodynamic sequelae of distal splenorenal (Warren) and mesocaval shunts, Ann Surg 190:523, 1979.

151. Renig, JW, Sanchez, FW, and Vujic, I: Hemodynamics of portal blood flow shown by CT portography, Radiology 154:473, 1985.

152. Reuter, SR, and Atkin, TW: High-dose left gastric angiography for demonstration of esophageal varices, Radiology 105:573, 1972.

153. Reuter, SR, Berk, RN, and Orloff, MJ: An angiographic study of the pre- and postoperative hemodynamics in patients with side-to-side portacaval shunts, Radiology 116:33, 1975.

154. Reuter, SR, Redman, HC, and Cho, KJ: Gastrointestinal angiography, ed 2, Philadelphia, 1986, WB Saunders.

155. Reynolds, TB: Portal venography and pressure measurement. In Bockus, HL, editor: Gastroenterology, Philadelphia, 1976, WB Saunders.

156. Reynolds, TB, Redecker, AG, and Geller, HM: Wedged hepatic venous pressure: a clinical evaluation, Am J Med 22:341, 1957.

157. Rikkers, L, et al: A randomized controlled trial of the distal splenorenal shunt, Ann Surg 188:271, 1978.

158. Roche, A, Raisonnier, A, and Gillion-Savouret, MC: Pancreatic venous sampling and arteriography in localizing insulinomas and gastrinomas: procedure and results in 55 cases, Radiology 145:621, 1982.

159. Ros, PR, et al: Demonstration of cavernomatous transformation of the portal vein by magnetic resonance imaging, Gastrointest Radiol 11:90, 1986.

160. Rösch, J: Roentgenology of the spleen and pancreas, Springfield, Ill, 1967, Charles C Thomas.

161. Rösch, J, Antonovic, R, and Dotter, CT: Transjugular approach to the liver, biliary system, and portal circulation, Am J Roentgenol 125:602, 1975.

162. Rösch, J, and Dotter, CT: Extrahepatic portal obstruction in childhood and its angiographic diagnosis, Am J Roentgenol 112:143, 1971.

163. Rösch, J, Goldman, ML, and Dotter, CT: Experimental catheter obstruction of gastric coronary vein: possible technique for percutaneous intravascular tamponade of gastroesophageal varices, Invest Radiol 10:206, 1975.

164. Rösch, J, Hanafee, WN, and Snow, H: Transjugular portal venography and radiologic portacaval shunt: experimental study, Radiology 92:1112, 1969.

165. Rösch, J, and Judkins, MP: Angiography in the diagnosis of pancreatic disease, Semin Roentgenol 3:296, 1968.

166. Rösch, J, and Keller, FS: Pancreatic arteriography, transhepatic pancreatic venography, and pancreatic venous sampling in diagnosis of pancreatic cancer, Cancer 47:1679, 1981.

167. Rösch, J, et al: Transjugular intrahepatic portocaval shunt, Am J Surg 121:588, 1971.

168. Rösch, J, et al: Experimental intrahepatic portocaval Gianturco stents, Radiology 162:481, 1987.

169. Rösch, W: Control of bleeding esophageal varices by endoscopic sclerotherapy, Cardiovasc Intervent Radiol 3:307, 1980.

170. Rousselot, LM, Moreno, AR, and Panke, WF: Studies of portal hypertension. IV. The clinical and physiopathologic significance of self-established (nonsurgical) portal systemic venous shunts, Ann Surg 150:384, 1959.

171. Rousselot, LM, Ruzicka, FF, and Doehner, GA: Portal venography via the portal and percutaneous splenic routes: anatomic and clinical studies, Surgery 34:557, 1953.

172. Russell, E, et al: An angiographic approach to hepatobiliary diseases, Surg Gynecol Obstet 143:414, 1976.

173. Ruzicka, FF, et al: The hepatic wedge pressure and venogram vs the intraparenchymal liver pressure and venogram, Radiology 102:253, 1972.

174. Salam, AA, Warren, D, and Tyras, DH: Splenic vein thrombosis: a diagnosable and treatable form of portal hypertension, Surgery 74:961, 1973.

175. Schabel, SI, et al: The "bulls-eye" falciform ligament: a sonographic finding of portal hypertension, Radiology 136:157, 1980.

176. Sequeira, FW, et al: Budd-Chiari syndrome caused by hepatic torsion, AJR 137:393, 1981.

177. Smith, GW: An assessment of the validity of preoperative hemodynamic studies in portal hypertension, Surgery 47:130, 1973.

178. Smith, GW, Westgaard, T, and Björn-Hansen, R: Hepatic venous angiography in the evaluation of cirrhosis of the liver, Ann Surg 173:469, 1971.

179. Smulewicz, JJ, and Clement, AR: Torsion of the wandering spleen, Am J Dig Dis 20:274, 1975.

180. Sniderman, KW, and Sos, TA: Hepatic schistosomiasis: a case with intrahepatic shunting and extrahepatic portal vein occlusion, AJR 130:565, 1978.

181. Sorgen, RA, and Robbins, DI: Bleeding gastric varices secondary to wandering spleen, Gastrointest Radiol 5:25, 1980.

182. Stark, DD, et al: MRI of the Budd-Chiari syndrome, AJR 146:1141, 1986.

183. Stevens, JC, et al: Preduodenal portal vein: two cases with differing presentation, Arch Surg 113:311, 1978.

184. Stone, HH, et al: Portal arteriovenous fistulas: review and case report, Am J Surg 109:191, 1965.

185. Takashima, T, et al: Diagnosis and screening of small hepatocellular carcinomas: comparison of radionuclide imaging, US, CT, hepatic angiography, and alpha-1-fetoprotein assay, Radiology 145:635, 1982.

186. Tavill, AS, et al: The Budd-Chiari syndrome: correlation between hepatic scintigraphy and the clinical, radiological, and pathological findings in nineteen cases of hepatic venous outflow obstruction, Gastroenterology 68:509, 1975.

187. Tedesco, FJ, and Stanley, RJ: Hepatic portal vein gas without bowel infarction or necrosis, Gastroenterology 69:240, 1975.

188. Terblanche, J, et al: A prospective evaluation of injection sclerotherapy in the treatment of acute bleeding from esophageal varices, Surgery 85:239, 1979.

189. Tey, PH, et al: Mesenteric vein thrombosis: angiography in two cases, AJR 136:809, 1981.

190. Torres, WE, et al: Correlation between MR and angiography in portal hypertension, AJR 148:1109, 1987.

191. Tylén, U, and Arnesjo, B: Resectability and prognosis of carcinoma of the pancreas evaluated by angiography, Scand J Gastroenterol 8:691, 1973.

192. Tylén, U, Simert, G, and Vang, J: Hemodynamic changes after distal splenorenal shunt studied by sequential angiography, Radiology 121:585, 1976.

193. Van Way, CW, III, et al: Arteriovenous fistula in the portal circulation, Surgery 70:876, 1971.

194. Viallet, A, et al: Hemodynamic evaluation of patients with intrahepatic portal hypertension, Gastroenterology 69:1297, 1975.

195. Viamonte, M, Jr, Warren, WD, and Fomon, JJ: Liver panangiography in the assessment of portal hypertension in liver cirrhosis, Radiol Clin North Am 8:147, 1970.

196. Viamonte, M, Jr, et al: Angiographic investigations in portal hypertension, Surg Gynecol Obstet 130:37, 1970.

197. Viamonte, M, Jr, et al: The hemodynamics of diffuse liver disease, Semin Roentgenol 10:187, 1975.

198. Viamonte, M, Jr, et al: Selective catheterization of the portal vein and its tributaries: preliminary report, Radiology 114:457, 1975.

199. Vorhees, AB, Jr, and Price, JB, Jr: Extrahepatic portal hypertension: a retrospective analysis of 127 cases and associated clinical implications, Arch Surg 108:338, 1974.

200. Wales, LR, Morishima, MS, and Allan, TNK: Portal vein thrombosis: diagnosis via percutaneous transhepatic needle, AJR 134:842, 1980.

201. Warren, WD, et al: Spontaneous reversal of portal blood flow in cirrhosis, Surg Gynecol Obstet 126:315, 1968.

202. Warren, WD, et al: Non-cirrhotic portal vein thrombosis: physiology before and after shunts, Ann Surg 192:341, 1980.

203. Webb, LJ, and Sherlock, S: The aetiology, presentation and natural history of extrahepatic portal venous obstruction, Q J Med 48:627, 1979.

204. Wexler, MJ, and MacLean, LD: Massive spontaneous portal systemic shunting without varices, Arch Surg 110:995, 1975.

205. Widrich, WC, Nordahl, DL, and Robbins, AH: Contrast enhancement of the mesenteric and portal veins using intra-arterial papaverine, Am J Roentgenol 121:374, 1974.

206. Widrich, WC, Robbins, AH, and Nabseth, DC: Transhepatic embolization of varices, Cardiovasc Intervent Radiol 3:298, 1980.

207. Widrich, WC, et al: Portal hypertension changes following selective splenorenal shunt surgery: evaluation by percutaneous transhepatic portal catheterization, venography and cinefluorography, Radiology 121:295, 1976.

208. Widrich, WC, et al: Pitfalls of transhepatic portal venography and therapeutic coronary vein occlusion, AJR 131:637, 1978.

209. Williams, DM, et al: Portal hypertension evaluated by MR imaging, Radiology 157:703, 1985.

210. Williams, RC, Jr: Aortic stenosis and unexplained gastrointestinal bleeding, Arch Intern Med 108:859, 1961.

211. Wiot, JF, and Felson, B: Gas in the portal venous system, Am J Roentgenol 86:920, 1961.

212. Yamada, R, et al: Segmental obstruction of the hepatic IVC treated by transluminal angioplasty, Radiology 149:91, 1983.

213. Zirinsky, K, et al: MR imaging of portal venous thrombosis: correlation with CT and sonography, AJR 150:283, 1988.

214. Zoli, M, et al: Echo-Doppler measurement of splanchnic blood flow in control and cirrhotic subjects, JCU 14:429, 1986.

76 *Percutaneous Transhepatic Cholangiography*

JOE ARIYAMA

Percutaneous transhepatic cholangiography (PTC) with a thin needle has proved to be a safe and preferable approach to evaluating patients with jaundice and biliary tract disorders. PTC is simple to perform and less costly than other invasive modalities. It also provides the opportunity to visualize the entire biliary tract to assess the cause of obstructive jaundice.

Since the introduction of the fine needle, PTC has been accomplished with an extremely low incidence of serious complications. The need for scheduling the patient for possible surgical intervention after the procedure is no longer mandatory before the study period. PTC has become an important part of an integrated approach to the diagnosis and treatment of biliary tract disorders and is used in conjunction with ultrasonography, computed tomography (CT), surgery, and interventional procedures.[6,17,52]

HISTORICAL REVIEW

The method of percutaneous bile duct injection was originally described by Burchhardt and Müller[7] in 1921. They injected contrast medium directly into the gallbladder in three patients. A lateral approach was used as the needle was introduced through the liver parenchyma, and the gallbladder was punctured. With the advent of oral cholecystography, however, interest in this method of visualizing the gallbladder and bile ducts was lost. The second report of direct cholangiography was made by Kalk[32] in 1934. He directly punctured the gallbladder under laparoscopic observation and opacified the biliary tract.

The first report of percutaneous transhepatic puncture of the intrahepatic bile ducts was made by Huard and Do-Xuan-Hop[27] in 1937. In 1952 Carter and Saypol[10] stressed the importance of this method in the diagnosis of obstructive jaundice. This was followed by a number of other reports.* Arner and co-workers[4] and Glen and co-workers[22] were successful in puncturing the nondilated intrahepatic ducts under fluoroscopy with image intensification.

---

*References 16, 23, 33, 36, 49, 51.

Since 1969 Kubota and co-workers,[38] Ohto and co-workers,[46] and Ariyama[2] have modified the technique of PTC. Instead of the large sheathed needle, a thin flexible needle (with an outside diameter of 0.7 mm and an inside diameter of 0.5 mm) was used to puncture the intrahepatic bile ducts. The incidence of complications has been remarkably reduced. Okuda and co-workers[47] described this method as a "fine (Chiba) needle transhepatic cholangiography," and since 1974 PTC has been repopularized. A large number of reports on fine-needle transhepatic cholangiography have been published.* This method has become rapidly accepted as a safe and successful procedure in the diagnosis of biliary tract disease and in the differentiation of jaundice.

TECHNIQUE
Patient preparation

A bleeding diathesis must be excluded. If abnormal coagulation is detected, it is treated with an infusion of fresh-frozen plasma and platelets, and the procedure is postponed until the coagulation is restored to normal. On the day of examination, the patient is required to fast. Selection of premedication and explanation of the procedure to the patient are important, because anxiety and

---

*References 3, 18, 20, 26, 30, 31, 43, 45, 48, 53.

an easily reactive patient may interfere with the success of the procedure. In my department 10 mg of diazepam is given intramuscularly 30 minutes before the examination. The skin at the puncture site is prepared and infiltrated with 1% hydrochloride. Routine antibiotic premedication is recommended.

Puncture site

Studies done on the anatomy of the intrahepatic bile ducts with intravenous cholangiography and PTC have shown that in the lateral projection the left hepatic duct lies more anteriorly than the right.[8] There is a relationship between the hepatic duct junction and the distance between the xiphoid process of the patient and the tabletop (Fig. 76-1). When PTC is performed under fluoroscopic control, the puncture site is selected on the basis of the data in Table 76-1. With fluoroscopic evaluation of hepatic size and configuration, a puncture site is usually selected at the level of the seventh or eighth intercostal space.

Puncture technique

The fine needle with stylet is introduced horizontally and parallel to the tabletop. The patient is required to suspend breathing in expiration, and under fluoroscopic control the needle is advanced during apnea in a relatively cephalic direction, 2 cm to the right of the vertebral column. If the visualization of the bile duct is not successful at the first puncture, serial needle passes in small incremental angles in a more caudal direction are performed (Fig. 76-2). The needle should not be directed too caudally, because this may result in puncture of the gallbladder or extrahepatic bile ducts. The stylet is then removed, and the patient is instructed to breathe gently. A syringe filled with contrast medium (iodamide meglumine, 65%) is connected to the needle, the needle is withdrawn slowly, and a small amount of contrast medium is continuously injected. Various structures in the liver other than the bile duct may be punctured. If the liver parenchyma is punctured, an intrahepatic deposit of contrast medium will result. Puncture of a radicle of

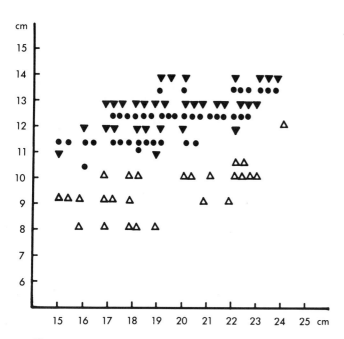

Fig. 76-1 Distribution of bilateral intrahepatic bile ducts in lateral projection. *Vertical axis,* Distribution of bilateral intrahepatic bile ducts from fluoroscopy tabletop. *Horizontal axis,* Distance between xiphoid process of patient and fluoroscopy tabletop. *Inverted black triangle,* left intrahepatic duct; *white triangle,* right intrahepatic duct; *black dot,* junction.

☐ **TABLE 76-1**
Site of puncture in PTC

Distance between xiphoid process and tabletop	Puncture site (distance from fluoroscopy tabletop)
Less than 18 cm	10.5 cm
18 to 20 cm	11 cm
20 to 23 cm	12 cm
More than 23 cm	13 cm

the portal vein results in filling of a structure resembling the biliary tree, but the contrast medium flows away rapidly. Puncture of the hepatic vein can be recognized by the rapid flow of contrast medium in a left cranial direction. A lymphatic channel appears as a thin thread-like opacity in the liver hilum. When the biliary tree is punctured, contrast medium remains and outlines the in-

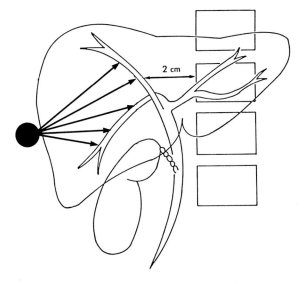

Fig. 76-2 Site of puncture in PTC and sequence of needle passes into liver parenchyma.

trahepatic ducts, the common hepatic duct, and then the common bile duct. After the needle is withdrawn, radiographs are obtained with the patient in the supine, prone, and oblique position. It is particularly important to obtain a radiograph with the patient in the prone position to assist demonstration of the left intrahepatic ducts and the gallbladder.

PTC may be performed using a real-time scanner to localize the tip of a fine needle in the bile duct. This has several advantages. The puncture can be performed without using fluoroscopy. There is no radiation to the operator's hands, which is becoming a problem for many radiologists specializing in interventional work. The portal vein lies posterior to the bile duct. Since the tip of the needle can be followed during insertion, inadvertent puncture of the portal bacteremia and endotoxin shock. With a real-time scanner the left intrahepatic bile duct is usually punctured (Fig. 76-3).

SUCCESS RATE

The success rates of PTC using a fine needle in 2604 cases collected from the literature is listed in Table 76-2. The overall success rate was 99% for dilated bile ducts and 85% for nondilated ducts. The high success rate of entry into dilated bile ducts signifies that PTC is the most reliable method in the differentiation of jaundice.

With a real-time scanner all patients who had a duct

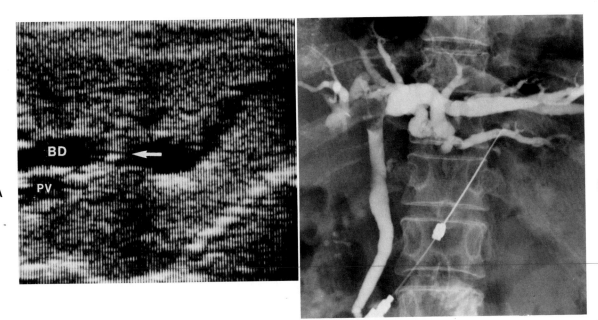

Fig. 76-3 A, Fine needle has been inserted using ultrasonography to check its position. Tip of needle *(arrow)* is seen in left intrahepatic bile duct *(BD)*. *PV,* portal vein. **B,** Contrast medium has been injected. PTC shows growth of tumor thrombus of hepatocellular carcinoma as negative filling defect in bile duct at liver hilum.

☐ **TABLE 76-2**

Success rate of PTC using fine needle

Study	Total procedures	Success rate in dilated bile ducts		Success rate in nondilated bile ducts	
Kubota, Wagai, and Hasegawa[38]	109	104/109	(95%)	—	
Ohto et al[46]	660	335/357	(97%)	257/303	(84%)
Pereiras et al[48]	131	86/86	(100%)	43/45	(95%)
Jaques, Mauro, and Scatliff[31]	94	43/45	(95%)	34/49	(69%)
Mueller et al[43]	450	353/355	(99%)	70/95	(74%)
Juntendo University[3]	1160	534/535	(99%)	626/722	(87%)
Total	2604	1475/1487	(99%)	1030/1214	(85%)

☐ **TABLE 76-3**

Complications of PTC using fine needle

Study	Total procedures	Bile leakage	Hemorrhage	Sepsis	Miscellaneous	Death
Ohto et al[46]	660	4	1	5	2	0
Okuda et al[47]	314	5	2	11	0	2
Jain et al[30]	80	0	0	0	5	0
Pereiras et al[48]	131	0	0	3	0	0
Fraser et al[18]	102	2	2	3	0	0
Jaques, Mauro, and Scatliff[31]	94	0	0	0	2	0
Juntendo University[3]	1160	2	0	18	2	0
Total	2541	13 (0.5%)	5 (0.2%)	40 (1.5%)	11 (0.4%)	2 (0.07%)

diameter of more than 5 mm were successfully punctured after one or two puncture attempts.

COMPLICATIONS

The complications of PTC using a fine needle are listed in the Table 76-3. Serious complications of PTC include bile leakage, hemorrhage, and endotoxin shock.[34,35] Bile leakage is most often associated with puncture of the extrahepatic bile ducts.[49] Intraperitoneal hemorrhage is usually associated with laceration of the liver capsule. Hemorrhage into the biliary tract may cause hemobilia. In patients with extrahepatic obstructive jaundice, direct communications exist between bile canaliculi and the liver sinusoid.[28] Biliary venous reflux may occur during PTC with bacteremia and endotoxin shock. Complications are reduced by routine antibiotic administration and percutaneous drainage following PTC.

Other complications of PTC are puncture of the lung, colon, duodenum, or stomach. Puncture of the lung may cause pneumothorax and can be avoided by careful determination of the puncture site under fluoroscopic control. Arteriovenous fistulas of the liver and subcapsular hematomas are occasionally found after PTC but are usually clinically silent and of no serious consequence.

INDICATIONS AND ILLUSTRATED EXAMPLES

The relative indications for PTC and ERCP are becoming better defined. PTC is less costly and relatively simple, whereas ERCP is less invasive and enables opacification of both the biliary tract and pancreatic ducts.

In patients with suspected malignant bile duct obstruction, PTC should be the examination of first choice. Transhepatic biliary drainage can be performed immediately after the visualization of the bile ducts with higher success rate than endoscopic retrograde biliary drainage.[11] If bile duct obstruction is caused by stone, ERCP is indicated. Endoscopic sphincterotomy can be performed after demonstration of choledocholithiasis.

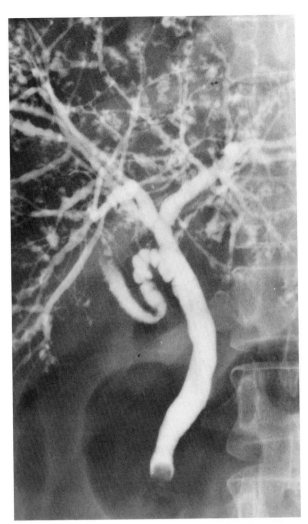

Fig. 76-4 Patient with high fever and jaundice. Small stone impacted at distal common bile duct with multiple communicating abscess cavities. External catheter drainage was instituted.

Duct stones

Stones in the bile ducts vary in number and size, and the bile ducts may or may not be dilated. It is usually possible to differentiate an impacted calculus from tumor (Fig. 76-4). The cystic duct may be completely occluded with a stone. Intrahepatic gallstones are rare in Europe and the United States but common in Japan and China.[5] The cause of this disease is not clear. Obstruction or stenosis of the intrahepatic ducts resulting from congenital anomaly, postoperative stricture, or neoplasm has been described.[21]

PTC is useful for the preoperative assessment of intrahepatic gallstones. In some cases left intrahepatic ducts are not demonstrated because of stone impaction,[19] and selective puncture of intrahepatic duct by PTC using a real-time scanner is mandatory (Fig. 76-5). Surgical treatment of this disease is difficult.[40] Stones may be removed by cholangioscope via the transhepatic biliary drainage tract. Nonfilling of the left hepatic duct may also be caused by the rare condition of aplasia of the left lobe of the liver.[42]

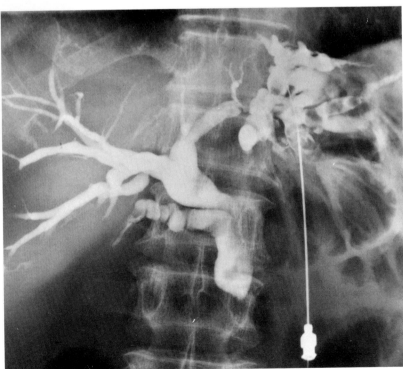

Fig. 76-5 Selective puncture of left intrahepatic bile duct using real-time scanner demonstrates intrahepatic gallstones.

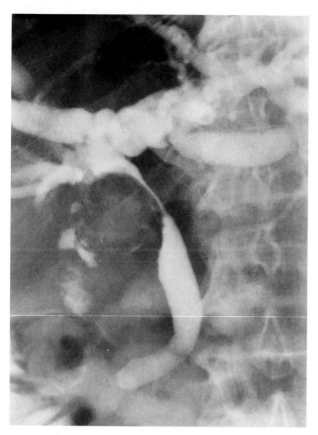

Fig. 76-6

Fig. 76-6 Mirizzi syndrome caused by impacted stone in cystic duct. PTC shows narrowing and displacement of common hepatic duct.

Fig. 76-7 Bile duct carcinoma at liver hilum. Transhepatic bile duct catheterization was performed both in right and left intrahepatic bile ducts. Complete obstruction of bile ducts at liver hilum.

Fig. 76-8 Early cancer of bile duct. PTC shows polypoid carcinoma of common hepatic duct. Histology of resected specimen disclosed mucosal cancer. Five-year survival rate after resection of mucosal bile duct cancers is 100%.

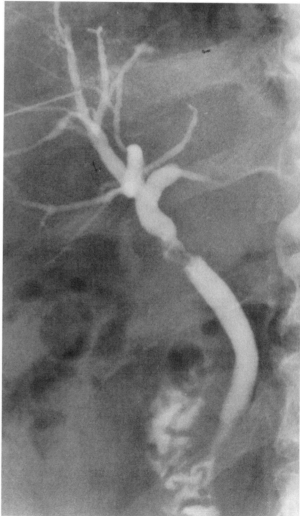

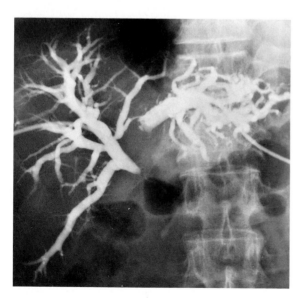

Fig. 76-7

Fig. 76-8

Mirizzi syndrome

Impaction of a gallstone in the cystic duct or neck of the gallbladder may cause common hepatic duct stenosis or obstruction. This is known as the Mirizzi syndrome.[12,13] PTC shows stenosis and displacement of the common hepatic duct (Fig. 76-6). Compression usually occurs from the right side of the duct. Gallbladder carcinoma may produce similar defects in the common hepatic duct.

Biliary duct carcinoma

PTC is useful in the preoperative diagnosis of bile duct carcinoma.[44] The characteristic bile duct deformities produced by primary bile duct carcinoma are a rattail stricture, concave obstruction, or polypoid luminal tumor margin (Figs. 76-7 and 76-8).

Pancreatic carcinoma

Carcinoma of the head of the pancreas causes obstruction of the intrapancreatic segment of the common bile duct and produces obstructive jaundice.[50] Several cholangiographic patterns may be associated with this tumor. Configuration of the duct at the point of obstruction may show a rattail, concave, tapered, or rounded obstruction (Fig. 76-9).

Papillary carcinoma

Carcinoma of Vater's papilla causes obstruction of the distal end of the common bile duct. The PTC shows an uneven, serrated margin at the site of obstruction (Fig. 76-10). Sometimes tumors produce a meniscus margin. Endoscopic diagnosis and biopsy establish the diagnosis and differentiation from benign papillary stenosis.

Chronic pancreatitis

The typical cholangiographic findings in patients with chronic pancreatitis are a long, smooth stricture of the common bile duct and moderate dilatation of the bile duct above the stricture (Fig. 76-11).

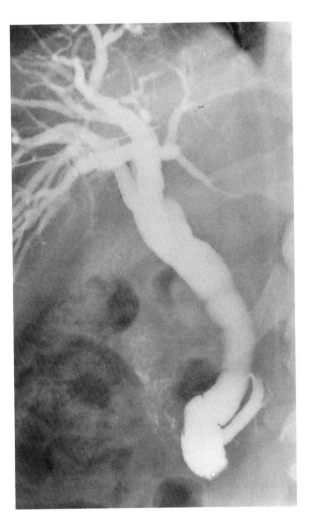

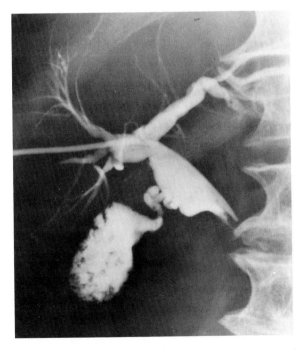

Fig. 76-9 Carcinoma of head of pancreas producing tapered obstruction of common bile duct.

Fig. 76-10 Carcinoma of Vater's papilla. PTC demonstrates uneven margin at distal end of common bile duct. Main pancreatic duct is partially opacified and dilated.

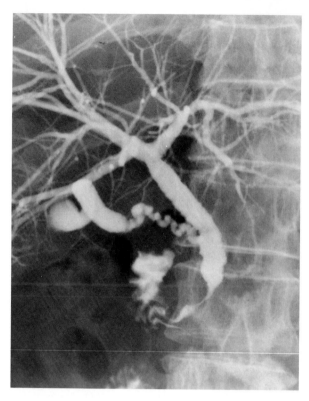

Fig. 76-11 Long smooth stricture of common bile duct and moderate dilatation of bile duct above stricture caused by chronic pancreatitis.

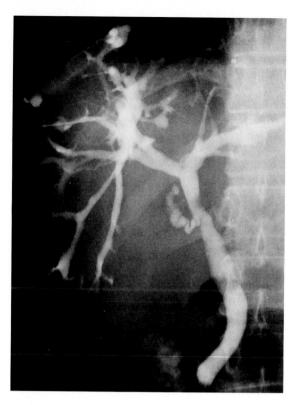

Fig. 76-12 Caroli's disease. PTC demonstrates segmental saccular dilatation of intrahepatic bile ducts. (Courtesy Dr. Saburo Nakazawa.)

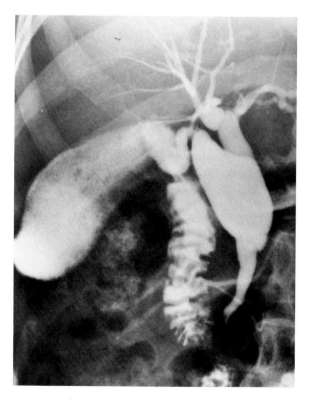

Fig. 76-13 Choledochal cyst with anomalous pancreaticobiliary union.

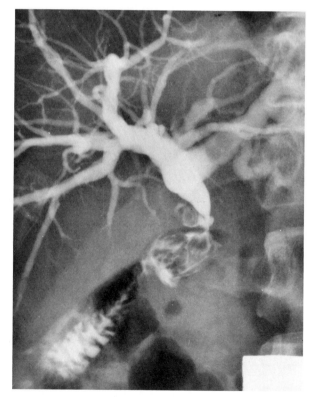

Fig. 76-14 Postoperative bile duct stricture at hepatojejunostomy. Stricture was negotiated by transhepatic balloon catheter dilatation.

Congenital abnormalities

Caroli's disease

Caroli's disease is defined as congenital dilatation of the intrahepatic bile ducts.[9] There are two forms of this disease: (1) a simple type, which is not associated with hepatic fibrosis,[41] and (2) segmental dilatation of the intrahepatic ducts with medullary spongelike kidney disease, congenital periportal fibrosis with splenomegaly, and portal hypertension.[25]

PTC demonstrates segmental saccular dilatation of the intrahepatic bile ducts. Cystic spaces varying in size communicating with the intrahepatic bile ducts are demonstrated (Fig. 76-12). The differential diagnosis includes multiple abscesses communicating with the bile ducts.

Choledochal cyst

A choledochal cyst is a congenital anomaly of cystic dilatation of the common bile duct. The portion of cystic dilatation may involve entire bile ducts, the intrahepatic ducts, or part of the common bile duct.[1,15,24,39] Anomalous insertion of the common bile duct into the pancreatic duct is present in almost all cases.[37]

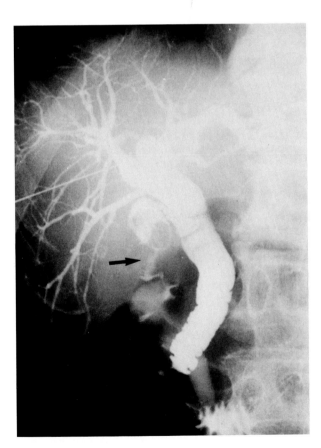

Fig. 76-15 Cholecystoduodenal fistula. PTC demonstrates stones in gallbladder and common bile duct. Contrast medium injected into bile duct is seen to enter duodenum via gallbladder.

PTC is useful for demonstrating the site, size, and extent of the cystic dilatation and the presence of calculi or carcinoma (Fig. 76-13). However, a choledochal cyst may be more easily demonstrated by ERCP in patients with anomalous junction of the common bile duct and pancreatic duct.

POSTOPERATIVE PROBLEMS

Postoperative strictures of the bile ducts are usually at the level of a prior enteric anastomosis (Fig. 76-14). Residual or recurrent gallstones are usually quite easily demonstrated by PTC.

Fistulas formed between the biliary tract and various segments of gastrointestinal tract are the cholecystoduodenal, cholecystocolic, or choledochoduodenal types.[14,29]

PTC is useful for the demonstration of fistulas, with contrast medium seen to enter the gastrointestinal tract (Fig. 76-15).

REFERENCES

 1. Alonso-Lej, F, Rever, WB, and Pessagno, DJ: Congenital choledochal cyst, with a report of 2 and analysis of 94 cases, Surg Gynecol Obstet 108:1, 1959.
 2. Ariyama, J: Percutaneous transhepatic cholangiography. In Saitoh, et al, editors: Clinical x-ray diagnosis, Tokyo, 1971, Igaku-Shoin.
 3. Ariyama, J, et al: Experience with percutaneous transhepatic cholangiography using Japanese needle, Gastrointest Radiol 2:359, 1978.
 4. Arner, O, Hagberg, S, and Seldinger, SI: Percutaneous transhepatic cholangiography: puncture of dilated and nondilated bile ducts under roentgen television control, Surgery 52:561, 1962.
 5. Balasegram, M: Hepatic calculi, Ann Surg 175:149, 1972.
 6. Berk, RN, et al: Radiology of the bile ducts, Radiology 145:1, 1982.
 7. Burchhardt, H, and Müller, W: Versuche uber die Punktion der Gallenblase und ihre Roentgendarstellung, Dtsch Z Chir 161:168, 1921.
 8. Burhenne, HJ, and Li, DK: Needle orientation for transhepatic cholangiography, Gastrointest Radiol 5:143, 1980.
 9. Caroli, J: Diseases of the intrahepatic biliary tree, Clin Gastroenterol 2:147, 1973.
10. Carter, RH, and Saypol, GM: Transabdominal cholangiography, JAMA 148:253, 1952.
11. Classen, M, and Hagenmüller, F: Biliary drainage, Endoscopy 15:221, 1983.
12. Clemett, AR, and Lowman, RM: The roentgen features of the Mirizzi syndrome, AJR 94:480, 1965.
13. Dietrich, KF: Die Hepatikusstenose bei Gallenbalsenhals und Zystikussteinen (Mirizzi syndrome), Bruns Beitr Klin Chir 206:9, 1963.
14. Dowse, JL: Cholecysto-duodenocolic fistulae due to gallstones, Br J Surg 50:776, 1963.
15. Esguerra-Gomez, G, and Riveros-Gomboa, E: A case of multidiverticular cystic dilatation of the common and hepatic ducts, AJR 94:477, 1965.
16. Evans, JA, et al: Percutaneous transhepatic cholangiography, Radiology 78:362, 1962.
17. Ferruci, JT, Jr, et al: Advance in the radiology of jaundice: a symposium and review, AJR 141:1, 1983.
18. Fraser, GM, et al: Percutaneous transhepatic cholangiography with the Chiba needle, Clin Radiol 29:101, 1978.

19. Gibney, RG, et al: Segmental biliary obstruction: false negative diagnosis with direct cholangiography without US guidance, Radiology 164:27, 1987.

20. Gibson, RN, et al: Bile duct obstruction: radiologic evaluation of level, cause, and tumor resectability, Radiology 160:43, 1986.

21. Glenn, F, and Moody, FG: Intrahepatic calculi, Ann Surg 153:711, 1961.

22. Glenn, F, et al: Percutaneous transhepatic cholangiography, Ann Surg 156:451, 1962.

23. Göthlin, J, Mansoor, M, and Tranberg, KG: Combined percutaneous transhepatic cholangiography (PTC) and selective visceral angiography (SVA) in obstructive jaundice, AJR 117:419, 1973.

24. Grewe, H: Idiopathische Papillenzyste in Duodenum, Chirurg 35:463, 1964.

25. Grumbach, R, Bourillon, J, and Auvert, JP: La maladie fibrokynetique du foie avec hypertension portale chez l'enfant, Arch Anat Pathol 74:30, 1954.

26. Harbin, WP, Mueller, PR, and Ferrucci, JT, Jr: Transhepatic cholangiography: complications and use patterns of the fine-needle technique: a multi-institutional survey, Radiology 135:15, 1980.

27. Huard, P, and Do-Xuan-Hop: La ponction transhepatique des canaux biliares, Bull Soc Med Chir Indoch 15:1090, 1937.

28. Hultborn, A, Jacobsson, B, and Rosengren, B: Cholangiovenous reflux during cholangiography: an experimental and clinical study, Acta Chir Scand 123:111, 1962.

29. Hutchings, VZ, Wheeler, JR, and Puestow, CB: Cholecystoduodenal fistula complicating duodenal ulcer, Arch Surg 73:830, 1943.

30. Jain, S, et al: Percutaneous transhepatic cholangiography using the "Chiba" needle: 80 cases, Br J Radiol 50:175, 1977.

31. Jaques, PF, Mauro, MA, and Scatliff, JH: The failed transhepatic cholangiogram, Radiology 134:33, 1980.

32. Kalk, H: Laparoskopische Cholezysto- und Cholangiographie, Dtsch Med Wochenschr 77:590, 1952.

33. Kaplan, AA, Brodsky, L, and Rumball, JM: Percutaneous transhepatic cholangiography, Am J Dig Dis 5:450, 1960.

34. Keighly, MRB, Drysdale, RB, and Quoraishi, AH: Antibiotics in biliary disease: the relative importance of antibiotics concentrations in the bile and serum, Gut 17:495, 1976.

35. Keighly, MRB, Lister, DM, and Jacobs, SI: Hazards of surgical treatment due to microorganisms in the bile, Surgery 75:578, 1974.

36. Kidd, HA: Percutaneous transhepatic cholangiography, Arch Surg 72:262, 1956.

37. Kimura, K, et al: Congenital cystic dilatation of the common bile duct: relationship to anomalous pancreaticobiliary ductal union, AJR 128:571, 1977.

38. Kubota, H, Wagai, K, and Hasegawa, M: The gallbladder and bile ducts. In Shirakabe, H, and Ichikawa, H, editors: Gastrointestinal radiology, Tokyo, 1969, Kanehara & Co.

39. Lorenzo, GA, Seed, RW, and Beal, JM: Congenital dilatation of the biliary tract, Am J Surg 121:510, 1971.

40. Maki, T, Sato, T, and Matsushiro, T: A reappraisal of surgical treatment for intrahepatic gallstones, Ann Surg 175:155, 1972.

41. Martin, E, Corcos, V, and Albano, O: La dilatation congenitale des voies biliares intrahepatiques segmentaries (Maladie de J Caroli), Press Med 73:2565, 1965.

42. Merrill, GG: Complete absence of the left lobe of the liver, Arch Pathol 42:232, 1946.

43. Mueller, PR, et al: Fine-needle transhepatic cholangiography: reflections after 450 cases, AJR 136:85, 1981.

44. Nichols, AN, MacCarty, RL, and Gaffey, TA: Cholangiographic evaluation of bile duct carcinoma, AJR 141:1291, 1983.

45. Nilsson, U, et al: Percutaneous transhepatic cholangiography and drainage: risk and complications, Acta Radiol 24:433, 1983.

46. Ohto, M, et al: Percutaneous transhepatic cholangiography, Tokyo, 1973, Igaku-Shoin.

47. Okuda, K, et al: Nonsurgical, percutaneous transhepatic cholangiography: diagnostic significance in medical problems of the liver, Am J Dig Dis 19:21, 1974.

48. Pereiras, R, Jr, et al: Percutaneous transhepatic cholangiography with the "skinny" needle, Ann Intern Med 86:562, 1977.

49. Seldinger, SI: Percutaneous transhepatic cholangiography, Acta Radiol 253:1, 1966.

50. Shapiro, TM: Adenocarcinoma of the pancreas: a statistical analysis of biliary bypass vs. Whipple resection in good risk patients, Ann Surg 182:751, 1975.

51. Wiechel, KL: Percutaneous transhepatic cholangiography: technique and application, Acta Chir Scand 330:1, 1964.

52. Wild, SR, et al: Grey-scale ultrasonography and percutaneous transhepatic cholangiography in biliary tract disease, Br Med J 281:1524, 1980.

53. Zajko, AB, et al: Percutaneous transhepatic cholangiography and biliary drainage after liver transplantation: a five-year experience, Gastrointest Radiol 12:137, 1987.

77 Radiographic-Endoscopic Correlations in the Gastrointestinal Tract

HENRY I. GOLDBERG
HOWARD A. SHAPIRO

ESOPHAGEAL DISEASE

GASTRIC DISEASE

PYLORODUODENAL DISEASE

COLON DISEASE

The importance of radiographic-endoscopic correlation cannot be stressed strongly enough. Much of our understanding of the radiographic findings of gastrointestinal disease has come from correlating those findings with autopsy and pathologic specimens and with the surface features of the disease in the living patient, as noted by the endoscopist. In this chapter, endoscopic and radiographic correlations to the morphologic changes in the gastrointestinal tract will be reviewed. To adopt proper approaches to the use of both radiography and endoscopy, it is necessary to examine the factors that influence the choice of the given test, such as the expertise of examiner, the equipment available, the cost of the studies, the risks, the complications, and the benefits. Endoscopic-radiographic correlation in esophageal, gastric, pyloroduodenal, and colonic disease are clearly influenced by the technique of the radiographic and endoscopic examinations. In many instances the single contrast barium study does not provide the same degree of correlation as the double contrast study. Likewise, the endoscopic data based on flexible fiberoptic endoscopy will provide more information than the straight sigmoidoscopic or esophagoscopic examination. Much of the data in this chapter is based on the state of the art of both studies—mainly double contrast radiography and flexible fiber optic endoscopy. Differences in correlation between these studies and more conventional modalities will be noted wherever possible.

ESOPHAGEAL DISEASE

Because the esophagram is ordinarily obtained before endoscopy when a question of esophageal disease arises, this section and subsequent ones are organized so that the morphologic features detected on single and double contrast radiographs are presented first, followed by endoscopic correlations in relationship to morphologic features.

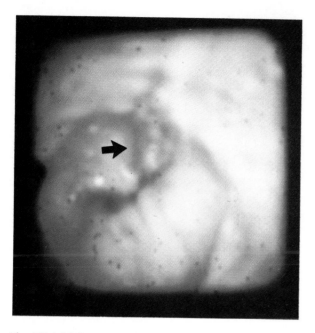

Fig. 77-1 Mallory-Weiss tear of esophageal mucosa at cardioesophageal junction *(arrow)*. Esophagram was normal in this patient, as it is in almost all such cases.

A normal esophagram using a full-column single contrast technique appears as a smooth tube of barium with no distinguishable mucosal surface features. If the pleural reflection can be noted in the left posterior oblique position, it is possible to determine the thickness of the wall of the esophagus, which should be less than 4 mm when distended.[25] Wall thickness can also be detected by computed tomography (CT).[52] Endoscopy cannot evaluate wall thickness. With a double contrast study, a smooth appearance to the mucosa is seen *en face*. Occasionally, thin longitudinal folds may be detected, numbering less than five and measuring less than 5 mm in width when the esophagus is partially collapsed. Several abnormalities in the esophagus may be detected endoscopically in the presence of a normal esophageal radiograph. Erythema, abnormalities of vascular pattern, mild edema, and superficial erosions may be present and not detected by either single or double contrast studies. These are seen in mild or grade I to II esophagitis.[36] In addition, early superficial cancer, subtle stricture, and small varices may also elude detection even with the best air contrast technique. Tears of the esophageal mucosa at the cardioesophageal junction are almost never detected by

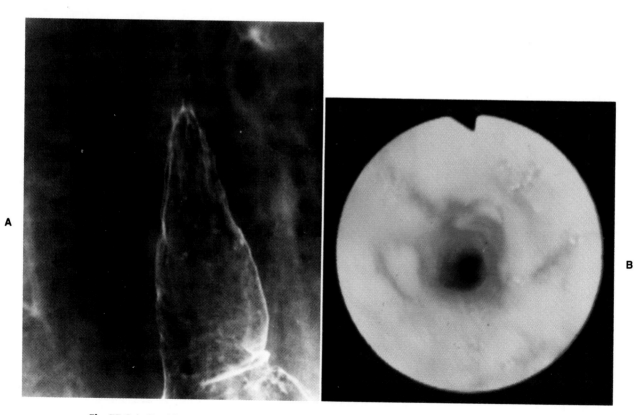

Fig. 77-2 A, Double contrast radiograph of cardioesophageal region shows many punctate collections of barium superimposed on slightly roughened mucosal surface. These are radiographic features of mild esophagitis. **B,** Endoscopic examination shows linear erythematous streaks and isolated punctate ulcers on lateral wall—endoscopic features of early esophagitis.

esophagram but are invariably found by endoscopy (Fig. 77-1).

Small punctate collections of barium seen on double contrast studies correspond to small superficial erosions measuring only 1 or 2 mm when viewed endoscopically. These, along with a granular surface pattern, represent the earliest features of esophagitis that can be recognized on a double contrast radiographic study[39] (Fig. 77-2). Early signs of esophagitis also include replacement of the normally smooth mucosal surface by a granular, somewhat lumpy appearance that is most prominent near the cardioesophageal junction. This radiographic finding correlates endoscopically with the presence of mucosal edema exudate, superficial ulcerations, and sometimes mucosal sloughing with pseudomembrane. The process of ulceration may become more severe, resulting in a radiographic appearance of interlacing linear ulcers and nodular defects seen en face. On double contrast studies this produces an appearance similar to that of tree bark (Fig. 77-3). This more advanced form of esophagitis

correlates with the endoscopic appearance of thickened folds, exudate, nodular granularity, linear ulcerations, sloughing of mucosa, and pseudomembrane formation. Single or multiple large ulcers of the esophagus may be characterized radiographically as round, oval, or in many instances linear.[39] These often project beyond the lumen in profile, and when seen *en face* appear similar to ulcers and other portions of the gastrointestinal tract, with mounds of edema and radiating folds. There is excellent correlation between the radiographic and endoscopic appearance.

Single or multiple plaquelike, shallow elevations of the mucosal surface seen on double contrast radiography may be caused by monilial esophagitis[21,39] and leukoplakia, a benign condition often seen in chronic smokers. In addition, nodular plaquelike lesions may be seen with herpes simplex infection, cytomegalovirus infection, glycogenic acanthosis, bullous pemphigoid, ectopic sebaceous glands, squamous papillomas, esophagitis cystica, and superficial spreading esophageal cancer.[29] Many of

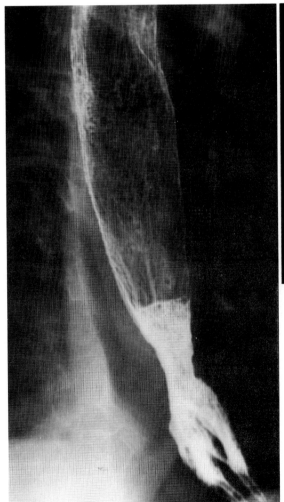

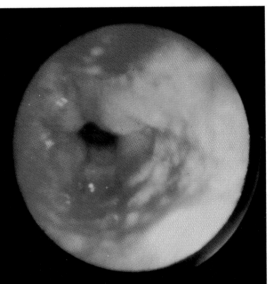

Fig. 77-3 A, In addition to stricture of cardioesophageal junction region, double contrast esophagram demonstrates extensive roughening of surface mucosal pattern above stricture, indicative of severe esophagitis. **B,** Endoscopic view demonstrates marked thickening of esophageal mucosa, confluent patches of exudate that, when stripped, show underlying superficial ulceration.

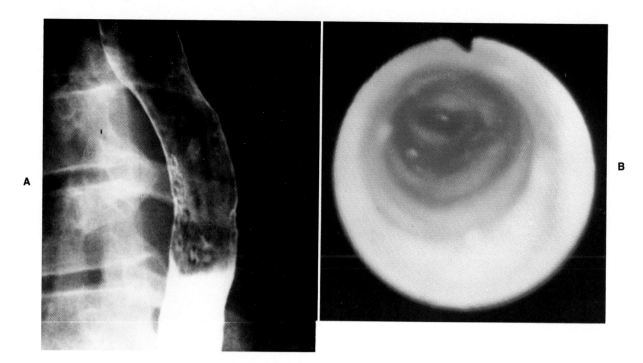

Fig. 77-4 A, Double contrast esophagram demonstrates several plaquelike lesions and at least one ulceration, occurring on background of smooth surface mucosal pattern. **B,** Plaquelike lesions seen at endoscopy are white. Brush cytology and biopsy showed mycelia typical of candidiasis.

these cannot be differentiated radiographically in the absence of clinical information. However, when plaquelike lesions are seen on more than one film, and do not represent artifacts such as undissolved gas tablets or bubbles, the correlation between endoscopic and radiographic detection is high. The actual nature of the plaquelike lesions can be determined on endoscopy, sometimes by the appearance of the lesions and certainly by biopsy (Fig. 77-4).

Focal narrowing of the esophagus can be evaluated both with single and double contrast studies, and the narrowing can be characterized as to length, smoothness of the edges, contour in the narrowed area, and symmetry or eccentricity of the narrowing. The radiographic appearance of strictures correlates well with the endoscopic appearance. However, though no specific data are available on frequency, it has been reported that strictures may be present in the esophagus but not detected by radiography[2,31,75] or endoscopy.[26] In some instances, the esophageal wall may be abnormally thickened or damaged in such a way that, though the caliber is not abnormal when liquids are swallowed, the area acts as a stricture and fails to distend when a bolus of solid material is ingested. These strictures may be detected by air insufflation during endoscopic examination so that such nondistensible areas become apparent. Radiographic detection of these lesions requires the use of barium and

solid material. On the other hand, occasionally a stricture clearly demonstrated by radiographic examination is not detected by endoscopy.[26]

Shallow polypoid or plaquelike flat lesions on one side of the esophageal wall may either have a smooth surface or an irregular contour as detected by double contrast radiography. If the surface is entirely smooth, both in profile and *en face,* then radiographic differential diagnosis includes submucosal lesions such as a leiomyoma or fatty tumor, an extramural lesion indenting the esophagus, or a varix. These shallow, smooth lesions with normal overlying mucosa may be difficult to characterize by visual inspection, unless discoloration is seen or a submucosal vessel identified. However, if the mound or plaque is irregular and ulcerated, a monilial plaque or early cancer is more likely. In the case of cancer, retraction of the esophageal wall beneath a tumor may be detected on single and double contrast radiography but often is not appreciated at endoscopic examination.

The radiographic features of advanced esophageal carcinoma are well known. On single and double contrast studies esophageal carcinomas are seen as lesions that produce an irregular malignant stricture, a bulky endophytic growth, large ulcerating lesions, or combinations of these.[44] There is a high correlation between the radiographic and endoscopic findings in advanced cancer. In obstructing lesions the radiographic study shows the extent of the lesion better than endoscopy, because the endoscope cannot be passed beyond the proximal margin of the lesion. CT has provided further sensitivity in staging the extent of esophageal tumor as determined by wall thickness, invasion of adjacent structures, and lymph node enlargement.[52,54,68,83] CT is often used to complement endoscopy for complete staging of esophageal cancer, because the CT scan provides information about the extent and spread of tumor that endoscopy does not.

The correlation of radiography and endoscopy in detection of early esophageal cancer is difficult to document. The earliest radiographic findings are small, plaquelike, ulcerated lesions along one side of the wall; small depressions; or areas of localized stiffness.[30,35,51] Most patients with early or superficial esophageal cancer have dysphagia.[30] Double contrast radiography is the most sensitive method to detect these subtle lesions.[30,35] The endoscopic correlation has not been fully elucidated. The major problem is finding small lesions endoscopically in the absence of discoloration or ulceration of the mucosa. Another is that the biopsy specimen of suspected lesions may yield evidence of tumor in a variable number of cases, between 50% and 100% on the initial biopsy.[13,70] In evaluation of adult-onset achalasia, the major goal of the radiographic examination is to detect carcinoma at the cardioesophageal junction. In some instances the area may be eccentric and ulcerated, suggesting tumor. Areas of the lower esophagus may be symmetrically narrowed as the result of submucosal infiltration by adenocarcinoma. If a flexible fiberoptic endoscope can pass through the narrowed cardioesophageal junction, the gastric cardia can be visualized by retroflexion of the endoscope and the adenocarcinoma detected. If the endoscope cannot be passed, then tumor or stricture is a certainty. In this case brush cytology and biopsy are generally diagnostic.[84] Single and double contrast radiography also provide information about the peristaltic activity of the esophagus. Motility disorders may be detected by radiographic monitoring yet not detected by endoscopy, because the esophagus is artificially dilated with air and pharmacologically altered from its normal motility pattern.

The correlation between radiography and endoscopy is particularly high in the evaluation of moderate to severe esophagitis, large varices, advanced cancer, and severe monilial infection. A history of dysphagia, or heartburn that is refractory to standard therapy, warrants endoscopic evaluation. Endoscopy is more likely to detect small punctate ulcers, grade I or II esophagitis, and early stricture formation, small varices, and early esophageal cancer.

In the radiographic evaluation of reflux esophagitis, moderate or severe forms of esophagitis (grade III or IV) are seen, characterized by thickened folds, irregular contour and ulceration, limited distensibility, and stricture. These are detected in one half to three fourths of patients[36,47,61] by single contrast radiography. However, if all grades of esophagitis are included in the evaluation, radiographic sensitivity and accuracy decrease. In one study, in which single and double contrast esophagrams were compared for detection of esophagitis, the double contrast study alone detected the changes of Grade II and III esophagitis in three fourths of cases. When single and double contrast studies were used in combination, the detection rate was 90%.[36] The rate of false positive diagnosis also rises with the double-contrast study.[36] We estimate, however, that a properly performed diagnostic double contrast esophagram can only be done in approximately 75% of patients. Thus the success of the double contrast technique may influence overall detection. The best radiographic approach to detect esophageal lesions would seem to be a combination of double and single contrast radiographs.

In Barrett's esophagus (columnar-lined esophagus) radiographic findings of thickened esophageal folds, hiatus hernia, strictures, ulcers, and granular mucosal pattern have all been described. Radiography is sensitive in detecting the most indicative features (midesophageal stricture, ulcer, distal widening).[8] However, because many of the radiographic features are nonspecific, endoscopy may be necessary to confirm the presence of columnar lining in the esophagus and to distinguish between Barrett's esophagus and simple reflux esophagitis.

GASTRIC DISEASE

In the past, most patients with suspected upper gastrointestinal disease underwent a radiographic study of the stomach and duodenum before endoscopy. However, esophagogastroscopy is currently used as the first diagnostic test in many instances. Even the most carefully performed radiographic study of the stomach, either single or double contrast or a combination of the two, may fail to detect certain disease processes that can be diagnosed only by endoscopy. All of the following may evade detection by radiographic studies: the erythema associated with mild forms of gastritis; minute punctate erosions in gastritis; some forms of early gastric cancer, particularly the Japanese type 2; some scars from healed ulcers; and shallow duodenal erosions associated with a mild form of duodenitis. Accordingly, patients with radiographically negative dyspepsia that is refractory to symptomatic therapy should be examined endoscopically.

For the most part, the fine reticular network of interlacing lines seen in the antrum, body, and sometimes the fundus of the stomach on double contrast examination is not seen during endoscopy. This network, called the areae gastricae (see Chapter 22) is the organizational

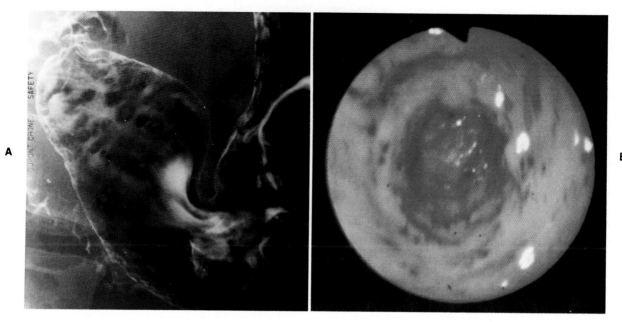

Fig. 77-5 A, Many small superficial erosions are seen on double contrast radiograph of antrum. These are surrounded by lucent halos representing tissue reaction to gastric erosions. **B,** Endoscopic view of distal antrum shows multiple punctate hemorrhagic erosions as well as edema and erythema of intervening mucosa. Patient had developed erosive gastritis as result of chronic salicylate ingestion.

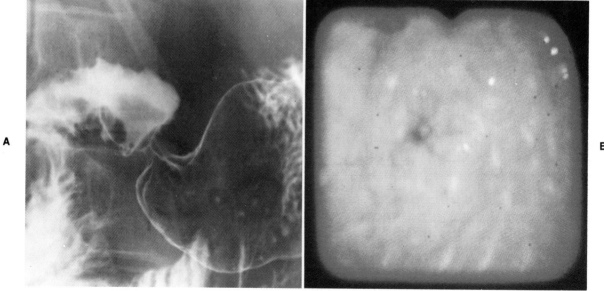

Fig. 77-6 A, Several small ulcerations with surrounding lucent halo indicate presence of antral erosions in otherwise normal-appearing antral mucosa. These erosions are identical to aphthous lesions seen in colon in early Crohn's disease (see Fig. 77-15). This patient had ileocolic Crohn's disease. **B,** Mucosa in prepyloric area has granular appearance with multiple superficial ulcers with yellow bases that appear confluent in some areas. This appearance is characteristically seen with Crohn's disease. Biopsy specimens of these aphthous lesions demonstrated features of Crohn's disease.

pattern of the surface mucosa of the stomach and is seen in approximately 50% of patients. This fine lacy pattern may appear coarse, with the units that make up the area measuring 3 to 4 mm or more. In some of these patients endoscopy and biopsy may show that the mucosa has undergone intestinal metaplasia, a process associated with gastric atrophy or severe inflammation.[3] However, because of the frequency with which the areae gastricae is seen, and the fact that it has been associated with metaplasia in some patients and gastritis in others, the significance of this finding is not understood and remains to be elucidated.

In well-performed double contrast studies, small (1 to 4 mm), superficial erosions may be detected. Some of these erosions represent punctate collections of barium with very little tissue reaction around them. In others, there is a mound of tissue with an ulcer in the center (Fig. 77-5). This is particularly true in some of the erosions produced by chronic salicylate use, alcohol abuse, herpetic gastritis, and Crohn's disease (the so-called aphthoid lesion)[43] (Fig. 77-6). Viewed endoscopically, some superficial erosions seen in gastritis have almost no swelling around them, though others have a significant mound. This mound correlates very well with the lucent halo seen around punctate lesions, particularly those produced by Crohn's disease.

The radiographic detection of gastritis may be difficult. In one series,[50] most of the errors on double as well as single contrast examinations of the stomach ocurred in the detection of gastritis. The overall error rate when gastritis was excluded fell from 27% to 17%. In another series, 11% of patients referred for gastric endoscopy showed superficial erosions with gastritis, but only 2% showed erosions on double contrast study.[39] In another study erosions were detected in as many as 10% of patients examined by double contrast study.[58] The combination of enlarged gastric rugae and superficial erosions permits the radiographic designation of gastritis.[16] In the absence of erosions, the term *gastritis* should probably not be used, even if thickened folds, spasm, and irregular contour suggest it.

Thickened and tortuous gastric rugae are nonspecific findings on double or single contrast study (Fig. 77-7). Folds may be identified, polypoid lesions on top of folds recognized, and superficial ulcerations detected, in addition to the fold enlargement. In peptic ulcer disease, large gastric folds are often seen in the presence of high acid output.[72] Large folds may accompany erosions in gastritis, and almost always appear in Zollinger-Ellison syndrome. However, these findings do not permit a specific radiographic diagnosis. The same difficulties may be present with endoscopic inspection. Endoscopy adds

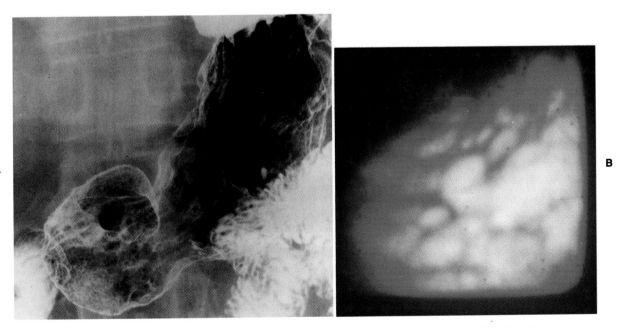

A   **B**

Fig. 77-7 A, Double contrast spot film shows prominent areae gastricae associated with enlarged gastric folds. These folds are seen in fundus and body of stomach. No erosions could be detected. **B,** In tangential view of body of stomach, folds are enlarged, edematous, and do not efface completely with air insufflation. Diagnostic considerations include hypertrophic gastritis, Menetrier's disease, and infiltration in submucosa by lymphoma or carcinoma. Diagnosis of chronic severe nonspecific gastritis was made on endoscopic biopsy material. Full-thickness gastric wall biopsy confirmed this diagnosis.

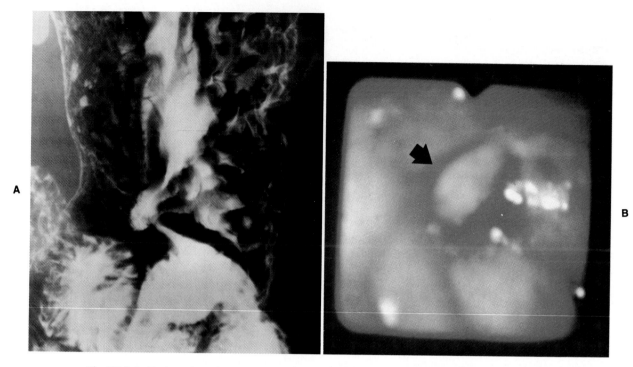

Fig. 77-8 A, *En face* view of ulcer crater containing barium demonstrates nature of folds converging on ulcer. These folds are smooth and have round, tapered end—findings typical of benign ulcer. **B,** Clean, yellow base is seen in benign ulcer, with smooth folds radiating into sharply circumscribed ulcer crater *(arrow).* Some clot is adherent to rim of ulcer—indicative of recent bleeding.

the ability to detect erythema and to appreciate the presence of excessive proteinaceous and mucous excretions. However, many of the processes that produce thickened folds also produce nonspecific or uninformative mucosal biopsies. Deep-snare biopsies that include the submucosal and brush cytologic specimens improve the diagnostic yield. This is true for all causes of large gastric folds, including hypertrophic gastritis, lymphoma, or even underlying gastric carcinoma.[5] The use of CT to evaluate the thickness of the gastric wall may add a new dimension to the radiographic evaluation of these patients. It has been found[53] that distended normal gastric wall does not exceed 1 cm in thickness when examined by CT. Patients with lymphoma often have a greatly thickened gastric wall, up to 4 cm, whereas those with gastric cancer may have thickened walls greater than 1 cm but not as thick or extensive as in lymphoma. However, CT does not appear to be able to differentiate between gastric cancer and lymphoma on the basis of gastric wall thickening alone.

The radiographic features of benign and malignant gastric ulcers are well described in Chapter 24. The *en face* radiographic features of ulcers, particularly on double contrast study, will completely reflect what is seen at endoscopy, as will the profile view. The *en face* view permits the evaluation of the radiating folds, the mound

of tissue around the ulcer, and the presence of nodularity or irregularity at the margin of the ulcer or at the tips of these folds (Figs. 77-8 and 77-9). However, the profile view may demonstrate undercutting and irregularity of the base of the ulcer, which may not be visible through the endoscope. The ring shadows and crescent-shaped lines seen in double contrast views often represent gastric ulcers on the nondependent wall of the stomach when viewed endoscopically. These ulcers are unfilled or incompletely filled with barium on the double contrast study. Double contrast radiography can be used to follow the healing process once a benign ulcer is discovered. Complete healing or residual scar formation are readily shown, and endoscopy need not be performed unless the lesions fail to heal.[46]

The appearance of a smooth, featureless stomach with loss of rugal folds is often associated with the endoscopic appearance of gastric atrophy, in which the mucosa is thin and submucosal vessels are visible. The radiographic detection of a polypoid lesion on a stalk correlates well with endoscopic confirmation of a benign polyp. The specificity of radiography in evaluating a sessile smooth-surfaced lesion is lower, particularly when lesions contain a central collection of barium, suggesting either metastatic melanoma, pancreatic rest, or leiomyoma (Fig. 77-10). However, it is not always possible to distinguish

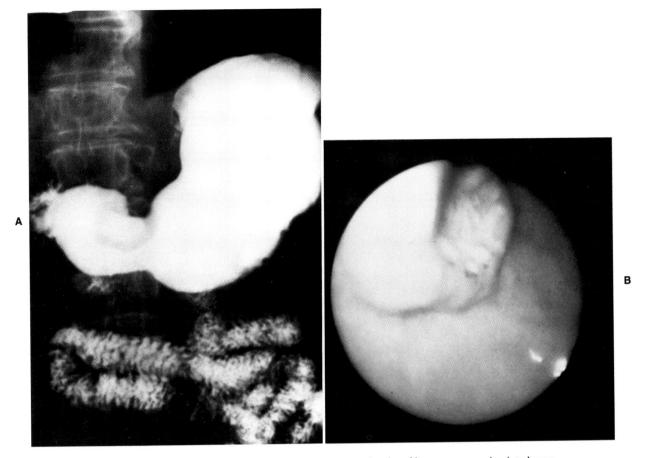

Fig. 77-9 A, Thickened ring of tissue in antrum represents border of large mass growing into lumen with ulcer crater in center, typical of ulcerating neoplasm. **B,** Endoscopic appearance of this gastric ulceration is that of ulcer within and endophytic mass protruding into gastric lumen. Margins are irregular and nodular, as is base. These findings are characteristic of malignant ulcer.

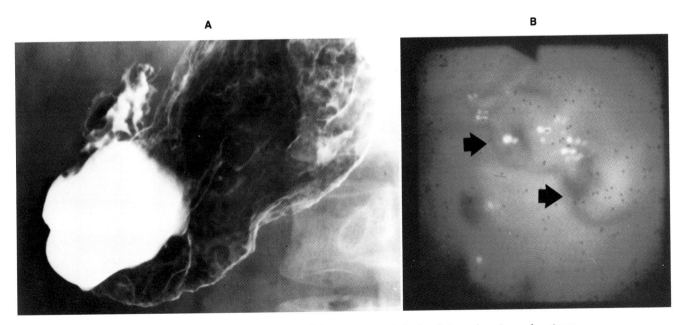

Fig. 77-10 A, Multiple large smooth nodules are present in body of stomach, seen *en face* (open arrow) and in profile (closed arrow). **B,** Several submucosal nodules are present *(arrows),* with dark centers. Biopsy tissue revealed metastatic melanoma.

between adenocarcinoma or hyperplastic sessile polyps. The double contrast technique has added sensitivity to the radiographic evaluation; multiple polyps are more commonly encountered with double contrast studies of the stomach than single contrast.[39] Furthermore, some authors feel that the fine surface detail of the polypoid lesion aids in identifying its nature. The smooth surface of a polyp indicates a higher likelihood of hyperplastic polyp, and lobulated surface indicates an adenomatous polyp.[48] Endoscopic gastric polypectomy is both diagnostic and curative.

Stiffening of the gastric wall caused by either benign or malignant infiltrative disease is often detected radiographically, because infiltration produces both a morphologic change in the contour of the gastric wall and a motility change, manifested by the failure of peristaltic waves to progress through the stiffened area. Depending on whether or not the infiltrative process involves the mucosa, endoscopy may not be able to detect changes in the mucosal pattern. However, distention of the stomach by air during endoscopy and observation of antral peristalsis may bring out such areas of stiffness. When the antrum is irregularly narrowed and contains large folds, radiographic detection of ulcers and nodules may be particularly difficult. In such instances, endoscopic evaluation is of particular value.

In the evaluation of the postoperative stomach, particularly after resection and anastomosis, single contrast radiography has been limited in detection of pathologic changes. This is especially true of anastomotic or marginal ulcers,[71,71] for which detection rates are near 50%. In addition, false positive diagnoses occur, because barium trapped between surgical plication defects may stimulate ulcers.[10] The double contrast technique has improved detection of marginal ulcers and erosions associated with severe bile reflux gastritis[56,57] (Fig. 77-11). In one study,[56] double contrast radiographic evaluation of the anastomosis agreed with endoscopic evaluation in 32 of 37 cases (86%). In another study the correlation was 33 of 40 (82%).[20] Small (less than 4 mm) marginal ulcers and erosions may elude radiographic detection. However, large irregular gastric folds, often indicating gastritis, are frequently detected by double contrast radiography.[56] Nevertheless, endoscopy should be performed if there is any question about the radiographic study in a symptomatic patient. Radiography provides additional information about the appearance of the afferent and efferent loop and the dynamics of emptying of liquid in the erect and horizontal position that endoscopy does not.

Radiography has a distinct advantage over endoscopy in evaluating motility disorders that result in poor gastric

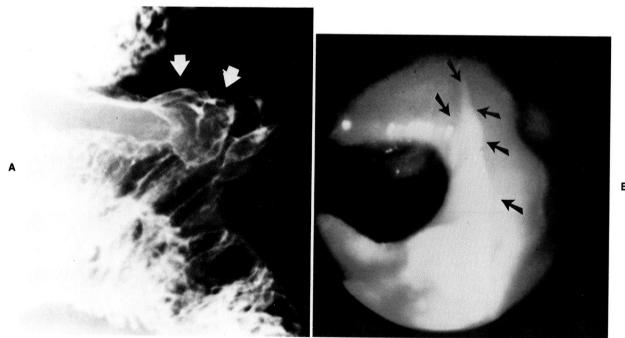

Fig. 77-11 A, Double contrast spot film of gastrojejunal anastomosis demonstrates mass straddling stoma, containing irregular-shaped, jagged ulceration *(arrows).* **B,** This view of gastric side of Billroth II anastomosis shows large marginal ulceration of edematous stoma. Spurlike extension of ulcer can also be seen *(arrows).*

emptying, such as those in diabetics, in partial gastric obstruction caused by benign or malignant disease, and following gastric surgery. In radiography a real-time study is done in which the motion of the stomach is observed fluoroscopically and may be recorded on videotape. Physiologic meals labeled either with barium or isotopes may be used to monitor the emptying process. Motility disorder can only be inferred during the endoscopic examination by the finding of debris and food in the stomach, that is, a bezoar. However, endoscopy may reveal subtle ulcers or tumors at the gastric outlet that are not apparent radiographically. Endoscopy should therefore be considered in patients with symptoms of persistent gastric outlet obstruction.

Several studies have shown the advantage of double contrast over single contrast technique to detect benign or malignant ulcers. When only single contrast technique was used, false negative determinations of gastric ulcer have been reported in varying percentages—18% (20 of 112),[55] 38% (12 of 31),[40] 50% (7 of 14),[24] 54% (7 of 13),[79] and 77% (7 of 9)[47]—when compared to endoscopy. The double contrast technique has improved ulcer detection. One examiner experienced a 20% error rate with single contrast radiography, which decreased to 9% when the examiner adopted the double contrast radiography.[75] When double contrast technique was employed, false negative determinations have been noted in 11% (1 of 9),[34] 10% (17 of 19),[81] and 17% (2 of 12).[40] However, others have found the two techniques to be similar in ulcer detection if ulcers less than 5 mm are excluded.[62,65] The causes of failure to detect gastric ulcers include the type of technique, poor mucosal coating, technical failure to distend the stomach with air, inability to use compression in barium-filled areas, presence of large folds obscuring ulcers, ulcer size (usually less than 1 cm),[7,62,65,73] and observer error.

False positive errors also occur both with single and double contrast techniques. As detection of gastric ulceration improves, an appreciable number of false positive determinations occur because of the peculiarities of the double contrast technique itself. Small clumps of precipitated barium, strands of viscous barium between the anterior and posterior gastric walls (stalactitie phenomenon), small barium collections between gastric folds may be misinterpreted as evidence of erosion or ulceration. Reports of false positive results have included 8%[22,35] and 11%[34] with double contrast technique and 13%,[27] 17%,[67] and 35%[40] with single contrast technique. In a large prospective study of benign and malignant ulcers of the stomach and duodenum using double and single contrast radiographic examination and fiberoptic endoscopy, findings for the detection of gastric carcinomas were in almost perfect agreement. For gastric ulcers, radiography and endoscopy agreed substantially.

Agreement became perfect if small ulcers (under 5 mm) were excluded.[73]

The level of accuracy to which double contrast radiographic study of the stomach has risen is best illustrated by the fact that this technique was chosen as the primary method for screening for early gastric cancer in Japan. In that screening, routine double contrast studies detected 86% of all lesions.[74] To achieve a high level of diagnostic accuracy for gastric cancer, gastric ulcers should be confirmed endoscopically and biopsied. When inspection, brush cytology, and biopsy are combined, the accuracy in detecting cancer approaches 96%.[11]

PYLORODUODENAL DISEASE

Very shallow punctate erosions, erythema, and mild edema may be evident endoscopically in peptic ulcer disease but not radiographically, even with double contrast or biphasic techniques.[73] However, depending on their size and extent, duodenal erosions can readily be detected radiographically, either as punctate collections of barium without swelling or small collections of barium with lucent halos, similar to those seen in the stomach. The endoscopic findings of a nondistensible duodenal bulb with irregular indentations correspond to the radiographic detection of deformed duodenal bulb, either the typical cloverleaf deformity of chronic ulcer disease or flattening of the fornices of the bulb. Deformity of the pyloric channel and base of the bulb may result in a fixed collection of barium (pseudodiverticulum), which simulates an ulcer. Endoscopy is very useful in evaluating this type of abnormal duodenum. The overall extent of the deformity is better seen with radiography than with endoscopy. False negative determination of duodenal ulcer occurs in the presence of bulb deformity—35% in one series[7]—because large folds and scarring may obscure an ulcer. This problem is occasionally encountered by endoscopists (Fig. 77-12). Barium trapped between deformed irregular folds may simulate an ulcer radiographically, producing false positive determinations.

Though radiographic study demonstrates thickened folds in the duodenal bulb, endoscopy provides further information about the folds. They may be thickened and erythematous with punctate ulcerations and erosions, indicating a duodenitis, Crohn's disease, or pancreatitis, or the fold thickening may be intrinsic to the duodenum without inflammation, as in lymphoma. It is only when thick folds, small punctate ulcers, and granular nodular mucosal pattern are seen together that a radiographic diagnosis of duodenitis can be made. This was the case in less than 25% of patients with endoscopically detected peptic duodenitis in one study.[37] However, in another study the overall sensitivity and specificity of the radiographic diagnosis was approximately 75% when both single and double contrast techniques were used.[18]

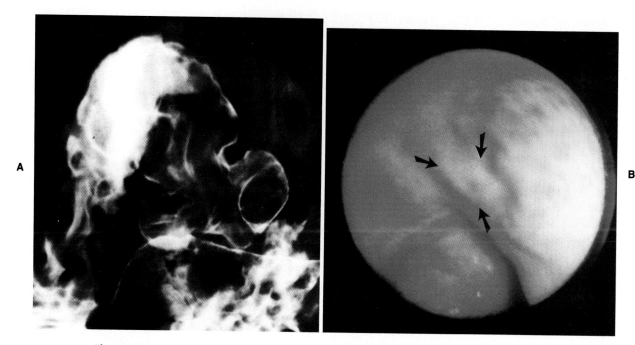

Fig. 77-12 A, Although bulbar deformity is shown and thickened folds detected, no ulcer is seen. **B,** Endoscopic examination of this deformed bulb shows sharply circumscribed 4 mm ulcer at junction of superior duodenal angle and anterior wall *(arrows)*. Extensive erythema is present with some superficial erosions indicative of severe duodenitis.

Overall, endoscopy is superior to radiography in detecting duodenal bulb ulcers.[73] In a recent study, the positive predictive value of a diagnosis of duodenal ulcer, taking into account the true positive and the false positive determinations, was 57% amongst several radiologists, with a variation in sensitivity between 44% and 80%.[63] The ability to detect erosions or small ulcers on double contrast radiography exceeds that of the single contrast technique, which can detect only ulcers 3 to 4 mm or larger. This may be why single contrast technique has been reported to fail in detecting ulcers in up to 50% of cases,[47,79] while in one series double contrast radiography failed to detect only 10%.[34] However, double contrast radiography has an inherent disadvantage in detecting anterior wall ulcers of duodenal bulb, the most common form of ulceration,[76] as well as some pyloric channel ulcers (Fig. 77-13). In these situations, barium empties out of the crater when the patient is in the supine position, leaving a ring shadow or a crescentic line as the only indication of an ulcer. On the other hand, these ulcers are usually detected by single contrast radiography if compression spots are used to trap barium in the crater. In one series of 22 patients with duodenal disease, double contrast study failed to detect six ulcers; single contrast missed none and endoscopy missed three.[27] It is therefore imperative that the radiologist recognize this limitation when examining the duodenal bulb by adding compres-

sion views with barium in the duodenum to the study to detect such anterior wall ulcerations. Occasionally, false negative interpretations are made in the endoscopic evaluation of duodenal ulcers,[9,27] usually in the setting of large edematous duodenal folds or extensive scarring with deformity.

When the diagnosis of duodenal ulcer is questionable, endoscopy should be performed before specific medical or surgical therapy is initiated.

COLON DISEASE

Colonoscopy and double contrast radiography were introduced in North America at approximately the same time, and both techniques have been extensively used and compared. This body of data* has enhanced our understanding of the gross morphologic changes in the colon that produce radiographic features—such as diffuse and local narrowing, loss of haustra, isolated and multiple ulcers, erosions and shallow ulcerations, fine granular and coarse irregular mucosal patterns, cobblestone appearance, and plaquelike sessile and pedunculated polypoid masses.

Radiographic and endoscopic evaluation of colonic disease both depend on proper colon cleansing for suc-

*References 1, 4, 6, 12, 15, 19, 28, 38, 41, 42, 45, 49, 59, 60, 78, 80, 82, 85, 88.

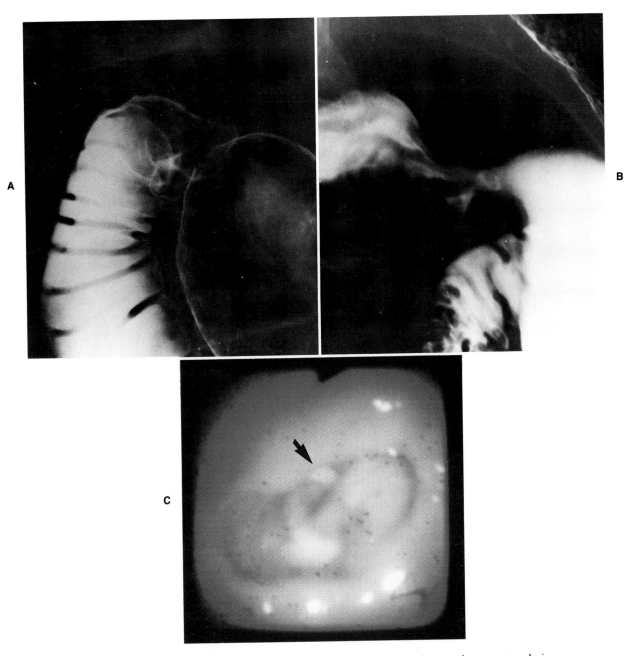

Fig. 77-13 A, Double contrast radiograph of duodenal bulb and antrum does not demonstrate pyloric ulcer. Pylorus is not seen in profile. **B,** Compression spot film of pyloroduodenal area, with barium in antrum and bulb, demonstrates pyloric channel ulcer. **C,** Pyloric channel is deformed with white base of ulcer seen within channel *(arrow)*.

cessful visualization. Patient compliance with colonic preparation can greatly effect the overall accuracy of both techniques.

The most important application of endoscopic-radiographic correlation is currently polyp and cancer detection. The complementary role of these techniques is also seen in the evaluation of all forms of colitis, particularly those in which small, shallow ulcerations are present. Conflicts in interpretation of confusing radiographs in diverticular disease and strictures may be resolved.

Fibrosis and extensive changes in the caliber of the colon, particularly caused by inflammation with spasm and edema, are best determined by initial radiographic evaluation. Thickening of haustra, loss of haustral pat-

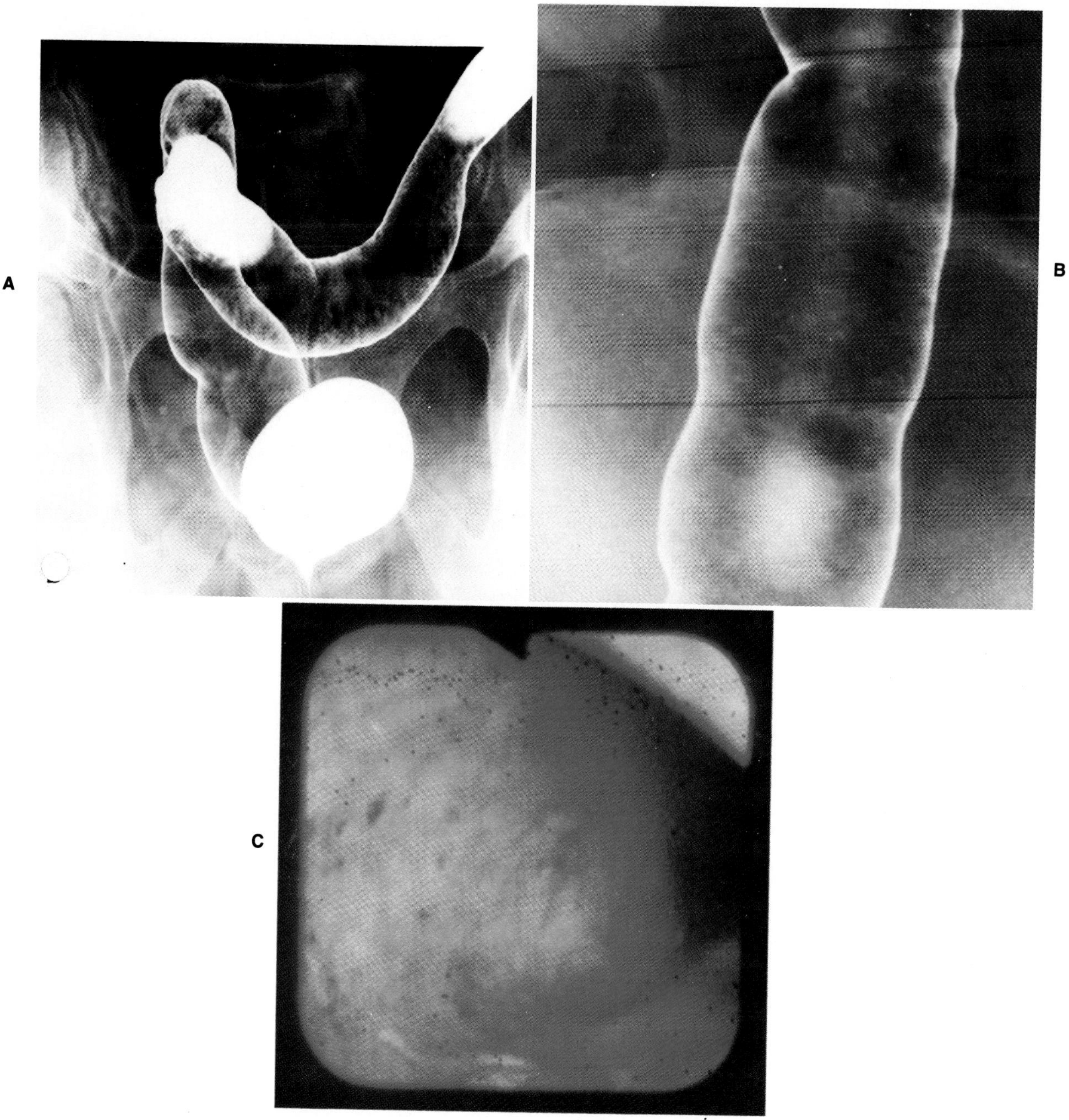

Fig. 77-14 A, Caliber of rectosigmoid colon is diminished. Small collections of barium can be seen on mucosal surface. This pattern is seen in mild colonic inflammation. **B,** Enlargement of sigmoid–left colon junction in **A** demonstrates punctate collections of barium representing superficial erosions. These cannot be seen to project beyond surface. **C,** Endoscopic view of sigmoid colon shows lack of haustra. Mucosa is hyperemic with areas of punctate hemorrhage. Normal vascular pattern is absent because of mucosal edema. These features are typical of mild ulcerative colitis.

tern, overall decrease in the diameter of the colon over a long segment, and foreshortening are all more clearly seen on radiographic studies, because all parts of the colon can be compared at the same time. However, colonoscopy is a complementary study in this setting. It adds information about the presence of subtle superficial mucosal changes, which help explain the underlying radiographic findings. These findings may include the presence of melanosis associated with an ahaustral pattern in cathartic colon or edema and erythema from superficial inflammatory processes.

With the use of double contrast barium enemas, small (1 to 3 mm) punctate barium collections can be seen *en face* as well as in profile. These represent shallow ulcerations seen in idiopathic ulcerative colitis, Crohn's disease, tuberculosis, amebiasis, *Yersinia enterocolitica* infection, and Beçhet's disease.[39] The ability to demonstrate these lesions radiographically depends on the technical quality of the examination. If quality is high, then a high degree of correlation exists between the radiographic features and the endoscopic detection of inflammatory bowel disease[28] (Figs. 77-14 and 77-15). However, endoscopy is more sensitive in detecting the degree and extent of the superficial inflammatory process; the mucosa between ulcerations is more completely evaluated. Also appreciated is the associated erythematous, granular quality to the appearance of the mucosa, caused by edema, loss of normal vascular pattern, and shallow pseudomembranes.[41]

In radiographic studies of idiopathic ulcerative colitis, it is sometimes difficult to distinguish between shallow ulcerations in the ulcerative phase and the contour irregularity caused by so-called granularity pattern of edema and erythema without ulcers. This is particularly true when single contrast barium enema is used, where only the profile of the bowel is used to make the determination.[6] In this setting, direct endoscopic examination of the colon surface will permit differentiation. In the early phases of idiopathic ulcerative colitis the double contrast study generally underestimates the severity of the disease when compared to colonoscopic evaluation and specimens examined after surgical resection.[38,39,41] It has been shown, however, that the single contrast study is even less sensitive than double contrast barium enema in both ulcerative colitis and Crohn's disease.[15]

The more advanced forms of inflammatory disease produce deep ulcerations, either single or confluent, associated with the granular pattern of mucosal irregularity. These are easily detected by radiography and reflect multiple ulcers, pseudomembranes, edema, and erythema seen on endoscopic examination. In the cobblestone pattern of Crohn's disease, the radiographic features are linear ulcers and transverse lines seen *en face*, with oval, round, and rectangular lucent areas between the crossing

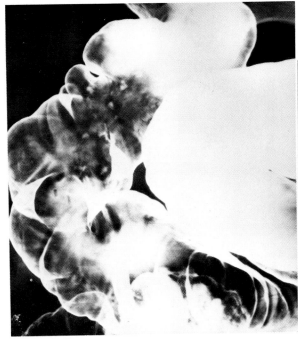
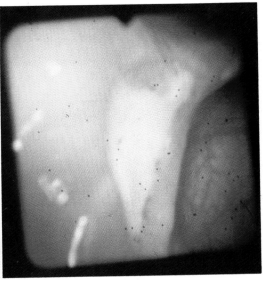

Fig. 77-15 A, Small, well-circumscribed collections of barium are seen in sigmoid colon representing ulcers. Surface pattern of surrounding mucosa seems normal. Each ulcer is typical of aphthous lesions in Crohn's disease. **B,** Shallow ulceration is present on top of plaquelike mucosal elevation. This is typical endoscopic appearance of early Crohn's disease.

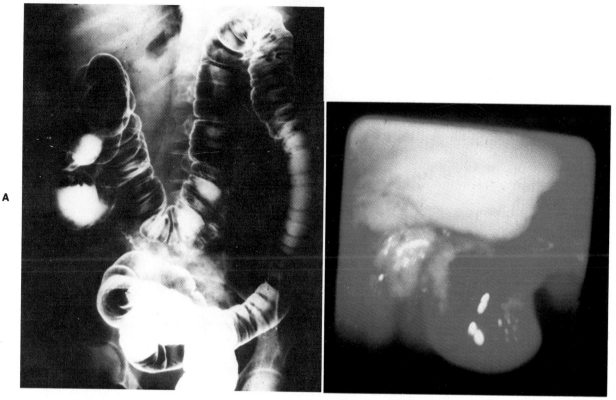

Fig. 77-16 A, Pneumocolon study in patient with persistent guaiac-positive stools failed to demonstrate sigmoid polyp. Redundancy in sigmoid, which could not be alleviated even with radiographs obtained in various positions, was thought to be responsible for this error. **B,** Colonoscopic examination revealed bleeding polyp 50 cm from anal verge. It was removed by electrocautery technique and had histologic characteristic of adenomatous polyp.

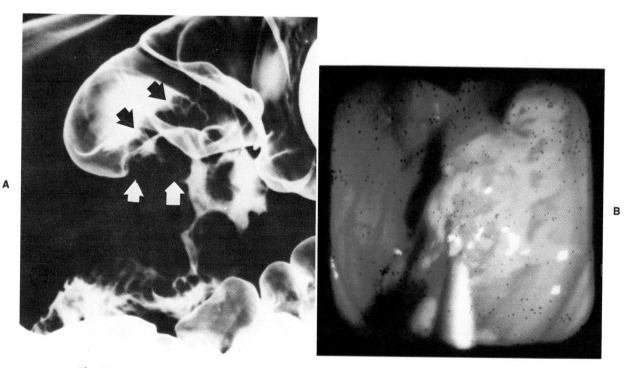

Fig. 77-17 A, Pneumocolon examination disclosed presence of lobulated polypoid mass *(arrows)* projecting into medial wall of cecum and measuring 2 to 3 cm. Size and appearance were those of malignant neoplasm. **B,** Colonoscopic view of medial wall of cecum shows 2 × 3 cm exophytic lobulated mass. Biopsy forceps (2 mm in diameter) are in field of view in preparation for target biopsy. Some surface features of polypoid lesion are obscured by liquid stool.

lines. In profile, both flat and deep ulcerations are seen. The endoscopic correlations to these features are serpiginous linear ulcers, transverse fissures in the mucosa with mounds of tissue between. Fingerlike polypoid lesions develop in the colon during the healing phase of inflammatory processes such as chronic ulcerative colitis, Crohn's disease, amebiasis, and tuberculosis. These lesions, best seen on double contrast radiographic study, are postinflammatory filiform polyps a few millimeters in width and varying in length up to 1 cm. They are often found radiographically in what appears to be a nonulcerative mucosa. Endoscopy may reveal that polyps actually occur in an area of subtle inflammation, manifested by erythema, edema, and punctate erosions.

The complementary nature of endoscopy and radiography is well illustrated in the evaluation of focal narrowing of the colon. For example, though radiography detects strictures and even characterizes the proximal and distal margins, the actual mucosal pattern within the stricture itself is often difficult to evaluate. The colonoscope or sigmoidoscope, however, may be able to enter the stricture and allow visual evaluation of the surface pattern. Endoscopy can determine the presence of ulcerations or endopytic growth and biopsy can confirm the disease process. When the colonoscope cannot enter the stricture, however, radiography becomes the more sensitive method of determining the extent of the stricture. Eccentricity of the strictures, as may be seen in endometriosis or metastasis, is better evaluated radiographically. However, the presence of ulceration in a stricture segment and the nature of the nodular appearance at the abrupt margin may be better determined colonoscopically with a visually directed biopsy.

Comparison of radiographic and colonoscopic examination for the detection of polyps and polypoid cancers has occupied considerable effort and energy by many investigators in the 1980s.[33] Colon cancer is one of the major malignancies of the North American adults, and malignant transformation of adenomatous polyps is recognized.[19,85] Evidence suggests that early detection of colon neoplasms may significantly affect cure and survival. If lesions are detected and removed before they penetrate the colon wall and involve lymph nodes, survival is improved.[86]

Most studies that compare radiographic and endoscopic methods for polyp and cancer detection compare the initial radiographic examination (either single or double contrast) with a subsequent endoscopic examination. It is therefore important to recognize that these two examinations are used in conjunction with one another as complementary studies—a situation that recognizes the proper role of the two techniques in polyp-cancer detection.[1,12]

To judge the expected rate of detection of polypoid lesions in the colon by radiographic studies, it is important to know the true incidence of polyps. Depending on whether lesions of 5 mm in size or less are included, the incidence in the general population varies widely. In a large autopsy series, the incidence of polyps larger than 5 mm was approximately 8%.[4] In a review of several autopsy series, the average incidence of polyps was 12.4%.[59] Because the incidence of polyps in the general population is known to increase with age, with an overall incidence in the range of 12%, it is possible to estimate the expected detection rate in single and double contrast radiographic studies. The frequency of polyps seen with single contrast enemas has been reported to be 1% to 7.8%; use of double-contrast technique improves detection by 9.8% to 13%.[59] Double contrast enemas are more sensitive in polyp detection, approaching detection rates expected from the known incidence of polyps in autopsy series.[69] In groups of patients examined by the same examiners, single contrast barium enema missed 45% but double contrast only 11.7% of all polyps detected colonoscopically.[82]

The significance of polyp detection must also be considered when evaluating the endoscopic and radiographic correlations. Though polyps 5 mm in size are more likely hyperplastic with an incidence of malignancy under 1%,[59] there is increasing evidence that a significant number of polyps 5 mm in size or less are adenomatous and therefore have malignant potential.[14,23,64] If polypoid lesions of 5 mm in size or less are excluded, the detection rate of radiographic studies is closer to that of colonoscopic detection.[45,80] Lesions greater than 1 cm in size are the most important ones to detect because of their higher incidence of malignancy—over 5%. In lesions of this size, double contrast barium enema and colonoscopy are quite comparable. The overall accuracy in detection of polypoid lesions of the colon using double-contrast radiography compared to colonoscopic findings is in the range of 90%.* When polyps under 1 cm in size are excluded, the well-performed single contrast barium enema with extensive compression of the barium-filled colon yields a rate detection approaching that of double contrast studies.[66] Errors are most often related to the distribution of the polypoid lesions and to technical difficulties in both examinations. Perception errors also play a role in the overall error rate.[32] Perhaps the main reason why colonoscopy does not detect all polypoid lesions is that polyps may be distributed in redundant areas of the colon or flexures, precluding adequate visual inspection. However, these areas also present difficulties in radiographic evaluation (Fig. 77-16).

---

*References 42, 45, 59, 60, 80, 82.

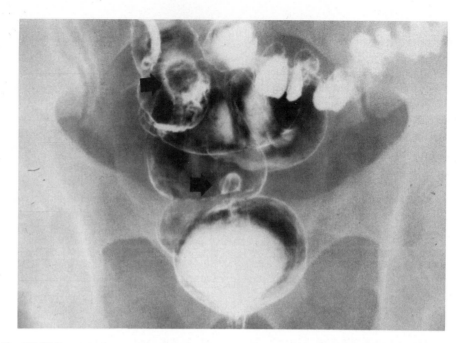

Fig. 77-18 Pneumocolon examination showed two polyps *(arrows)*, one sessile lesion adjacent to rectal valve, and one lesion on stalk in sigmoid colon. Colonoscopic examination failed to detect lesion on proximal side of rectal valve. This area is difficult to visualize with either straight or flexible sigmoidoscopy.

Polyps may be missed by direct vision in the rectum and the cecum—in the rectum because of the rectal valves and in the cecum because of technical failure of the colonoscope to reach the area[42,49,82] (Figs. 77-17 and 77-18). Thoeni found that the colon could not be reached by colonoscopy in 10% of cases.[80] His error rates in polyp detection are comparable in both double contrast radiography and colonoscopy in sigmoid colon, splenic flexure, and hepatic flexure. Evidence suggests that the error rate is higher with a rigid sigmoidoscope than with a flexible sigmoidoscope or colonoscope.[78,87] Other factors that affect detection of polyps include the presence of extensive diverticular disease or strictures, patient intolerance to the procedure, and poor colon cleansing. The highest incidence of undetected polyps both by double contrast barium enema and colonoscopy, is in the rectosigmoid area.* The presence of a polypoid lesion in association with diverticular disease produces difficulties in interpretation on the double contrast enema and difficulties of perception for the endoscopist. When an area

of narrowing and irregularity is located in a zone of extensive diverticular disease, it may be difficult to distinguish between diverticulitis and cancer. In these instances, endoscopy may be of great value by permitting direct visualization.

The complementary nature of the radiographic-endoscopic techniques has been well established. In the setting of evaluation of a high risk group for colon cancer (age, family history, guaiac-positive stools, known polyps, inflammatory bowel disease of long duration) a double contrast barium enema should be performed. If this is normal, or if areas of suspicion are detected, endoscopy should follow. If the double contrast enema is positive for polyps less than 5 mm in size, then no further study may be needed. However, if larger polyps are detected, then endoscopy is an important next study.

Flexible sigmoidoscopy accompanied by air contrast barium enema would seem to provide complementary information for the detection of polyps and cancers in patients being screened because of positive occult fecal blood test or because of high-risk factors.

*References 42, 45, 49, 60, 77, 78, 82.

REFERENCES

1. Amberg, JR, et al: Colonic polyp detection: role of roentgenography and colonoscopy, Radiology 125:255, 1977.

2. Anselm, K: Comparison of endoscopy and barium swallow in the diagnosis of esophageal stricture, Gastrointest Endosc 25:95, 1979.

3. Aoyama, D: Radiological diagnosis of chronic gastritis. In Recent advances in gastroenterology, Proceedings of the Third World Congress of Gastroenterology, Tokyo, 1967, Nankodo.

4. Arminski, TC, and McLean, DW: Incidence and distribution of adenomatous polyps of the colon and rectum based on 1,000 autopsy examinations, Dis Colon Rectum 7:249, 1964.

5. Balthazar, EJ, and Davidian, MM: Hyperrugosity in gastric carcinoma: radiographic, endoscopic and pathologic feature, AJR 136:531, 1981.

6. Bartrum, CI, and Walmesley, K: A pathologic and radiological correlation of the mucosal changes in ulcerative colitis, Clin Radiol 29:323, 1978.

7. Cameron, AJ, and Ott, B: The value of gastroscopy in clinical diagnosis, Mayo Clin Proc 52:806, 1977.

8. Chen, YM, et al: Barrett esophagus as an extension of severe esophagitis, AJR 145:275, 1985.

9. Classen, M: Endoscopy in benign peptic ulcer, Clin Gastroenterol 2:315, 1973.

10. Cotton, PB, et al: Diagnostic yield of fiberoptic endoscopy in the operated stomach, Br J Surg 60:629, 1973.

11. Dekker, W, and Tytgut, G: Diagnostic accuracy of fiberendoscopy in detection of upper intestinal malignancy, Gastroenterology 73:710, 1977.

12. Dodds, WJ, Stewart, ET, and Hogan, WJ: Role of colonoscopy and roentgenology in the detection of polypoid colonic lesions, Dig Dis 22:646, 1977.

13. Edwards, DAW: Carcinoma of the esophagus and fundus, Postgrad Med J 50:223, 1974.

14. Feczko, PJ, et al: Small colonic polyps: a reappraisal of their significance, Radiology 152:301, 1984.

15. Fraser, GM, and Findlay, JM: The double contrast enema in ulcerative colitis and Crohn's disease, Clin Radiol 27:103, 1976.

16. Frik, W: Roentgenbefunde am Faltenund feurelief des Magens bei chronescher Gastritis, Radiologe 4:69, 1964.

17. Gabrielsson, N: Gastric ulceration revealed only by gastrophotography, Acta Radiol 12:59, 1972.

18. Gelfand, DW, Dale, WJ, and Ott, DJ: Duodenitis: endoscopic-radiographic correlation in 272 patients, Radiology 157:577, 1985.

19. Gilbertsen, VA: Proctosigmoidoscopy and polypectomy in reducing the incidence of rectal cancer, Cancer 34:936, 1974.

20. Gohel, VK, and Laufer, I: Double contrast examination of the postoperative stomach, Radiology 129:601, 1978.

21. Goldberg, HI, and Dodds, WJ: Cobblestone esophagus due to monilial infection, AJR 104:608, 1968.

22. Goldberg, HI, et al: UGI endoscopy versus radiography: is radiography obsolete? Gastroenterology 80:626, 1981.

23. Grangrist, S, Gabrielson, N. and Sundelin, B: Diminutive colonic polyps: clinical significance and management, Endoscopy 11:36, 1979.

24. Greenlaw, R, et al: Gastroduodenitis: a broader concept of peptic ulcer disease, Dig Dis Sci 25:660, 1980.

25. Halber, MD, Daffner, RH, and Thompson, WM: CT of the esophagus. I. Normal appearance, AJR 133:1047, 1979.

26. Halpert, RD, et al: Radiological assessment of dysphagia with endoscopic correlation, Radiology 157:599, 1985.

27. Hedemand, N, et al: X-ray examination or endoscopy? A blind prospective study including barium meal, double contrast examination, and endoscopy of the esophagus, stomach and duodenum, Gastrointest Radiol 1:331, 1977.

28. Hilldell, J., Lindstrom, C., and Wenckert, A: Radiographic appearance in Crohn's disease. I. Accuracy of radiograph methods, Acta Radiol 20:609, 1979.

29. Itai, Y, et al: Diffuse finely nodular lesions of the esophagus, AJR 128:563, 1977.

30. Itai, Y., et al: Superficial esophageal carcinoma, Radiology 126:597, 1978.

31. Kelley, J: The marshmallow as an aid to radiological examination of the esophagus, N Eng J Med 265:1306,1961.

32. Kelvin, FM, Gardiner, R, and Vas, N: Colorectal carcinoma missed on double contrast barium enema study: a problem in perception, AJR 137:307, 1981.

33. Kelvin, FM, and Maglinte, DDT: Colorectal carcinoma: a radiologic and clinical review, Radiology 164:1, 1987.

34. Keto, P, et al: Double contrast examination of the stomach compared with endoscopy, Acta Radiol 20:762, 1979.

35. Koehler, RE, Moss, AA, and Margulis, AR: Early radiographic manifestations of carcinoma of the esophagus, Radiology 119:1, 1976.

36. Koehler, RE, Weymann, PJ, and Oakley HF: Single and double contrast techniques in esophagitis, AJR 135:15, 1980.

37. Kunstlinger, FC, et al: The radiographic appearance of erosive duodenitis: a radiographic endoscopic correlative study, J Clin Gastroenterol 2:205, 1980.

38. Laufer, I: Air contrast studies of the colon in inflammatory bowel disease, CRC Crit Rev Diagn Imaging 9:421, 1977.

39. Laufer, I, editor: Double contrast gastrointestinal radiology with endoscopic correlation, Philadelphia, 1979, WB Saunders.

40. Laufer, I, Mullens, JE, and Hamilton, J: The diagnostic accuracy of barium studies of the stomach and duodenum correlation with endoscopy, Radiology 115:569, 1975.

41. Laufer, I, Mullen, JE, and Hamilton, J: Correlation of endoscopy and double contrast radiography in the early stages of ulcerative and granulomatous colitis, Radiology 118:1, 1976.

42. Laufer, I, Smith, NCW, and Mullens, JE: The radiological demonstration of colorectal polyps undetected by endoscopy, Gastroenterol 70:1670, 1976.

43. Laufer, I, Truemen, T, and de Sa, D: Multiple superficial gastric erosions due to Crohn's disease of the stomach, radiologic and endoscopic diagnosis, Br J Radiol 49:726, 1976.

44. Laufer, I, and Yamada, A: Tumors of the esophagus. In Laufer, I, editor: Double contrast gastrointestinal radiology with endoscopic correlation, Philadelphia, 1979, WB Saunders.

45. Leinicke, JL, et al: A comparison of colonoscopy and roentgenography for detecting polypoid lesions of the colon, Gastrointest Radiol 2:125, 1977.

46. Levine, MS, et al: Benign gastric ulcers: diagnosis and followup with double-contrast radiography, Radiology 164:9, 1987.

47. Martin, TR, et al: A comparison of upper gastrointestinal endoscopy and radiography, J Clin Gastroenterol 2:21, 1980.

48. Maruyama, M: Early gastric cancer. In Laufer, I, editor: Double contrast gastrointestinal radiography, Philadelphia, 1979, WB Saunders.

49. Miller, RE, and Lehman, G: Polypoid colonic lesions undetected by endoscopy, Radiology 129:295, 1978.

50. Montagne, JP, Moss, AA, and Margulis, AR: Doubleblind study of single and double contrast upper gastrointestinal examinations using endoscopy as a control, AJR 130:1041, 1978.

51. Moss, AA, Koehler, RE, and Margulis, AR: Initial accuracy of esophagograms in detection of small esophageal carcinoma, AJR 127:909, 1976.

52. Moss, AA, et al: Esophageal carcinoma: pretherapy staging by computed tomography, AJR 136:1051, 1981.

53. Moss, AA, et al: Gastric adenocarcinoma: a comparison of the accuracy and economics of staging by computed tomography and surgery, Gastroenterology 80:45, 1981.

54. Munyer, TP, et al: Post-inflammatory polyposis (PIP) of the colon: the radiologic-pathologic spectrum, Radiology 145:607, 1982.

55. Nelson, RS, Urrea, LH, and Lanza, FL: Evaluation of gastric ulceration, Am J Dig Dis 21:389, 1976.

56. Ominsky, SH, and Moss, AA: The postoperative stomach: a comparative study of double contrast barium examinations and endoscopy, Gastrointest Radiol 4:17, 1979.

57. Op den Orth, JO: The postoperative stomach. In Laufer, I, editor: Double contrast gastrointestinal radiography, Philadelphia, 1979, WB Saunders.

58. Op den Orth, JO, and Dekker, W: Gastric polyps or erosions, AJR 128:357, 1977.

59. Ott, DJ, and Gelfand, DW: Colorectal tumors: pathology and detection, AJR 131:691, 1978

60. Ott, DJ, Gelfand, DW, and Ramquest, NA: Causes of error in gastrointestinal radiology. II. Barium enema examination, Gastrointest Radiol 5:99, 1980.

61. Ott, DJ, Gelfand, DW, and Wu, WE: Reflex esophagitis: radiographic and endoscopic correlation, Radiology 130:583, 1979.

62. Ott, DJ, Gelfand, DW, and Wu, WC: Detection of gastric ulcer: comparison of single and double-contrast examination, AJR 139:93, 1982.

63. Ott, DJ, et al: Positive predictive value and examiner variability in diagnosing duodenal ulcer, AJR 145:1207, 1985.

64. Ott, DJ, et al: How important is radiographic detection of diminutive polyps of the colon? AJR 146:875, 1986.

65. Ott, DJ, et al: Radiographic efficacy in gastric ulcer: comparison of single-contrast and multiphasic examinations, AJR 147:697, 1986.

66. Ott, DJ, et al: Single-contrast vs. double-contrast barium enema in detection of colonic polyps, AJR 146:993, 1986.

67. Papp, JP: Endoscopic experience in 100 consecutive cases with the Olympus GIF endoscope, Am J Gastroenterol 60:466, 1973.

68. Quint, LE, et al: Esophageal carcinoma: CT findings, Radiology 155:171, 1985.

69. deRoos, A, et al: Colon polyps and carcinomas: prospective comparison of the single- and double-contrast examination in the same patient, Radiology 154:11, 1985.

70. Rosech, W: Carcinoma of the esophagus and cardia-endoscopy, Postgrad Med J 50:227, 1974.

71. Schulman, A: Anastomotic gastrojejunal ulcer: accuracy of radiological diagnosis in surgically proven cases, Br J Radiol 33:422, 1971.

72. Shaw, D, et al: Gastric secretion and coarse mucosal folds, Clin Radiol 23:508, 1972.

73. Shaw, PC, et al: Peptic ulcer and gastric carcinoma: diagnosis with biphasic radiography compared with fiberoptic endoscopy, Radiology 163:39, 1987.

74. Shirakabe, H, et al: Comparison of x-ray endoscopy and biopsy examinations for the diagnosis of early gastric cancer, Jpn J Clin Oncol 12:93, 1972.

75. Stevenson, GW: Who needs radiology? Gastrointest Endosc 26:119, 1980.

76. Stevenson, GW, and Laufer, I: Duodenum. In Laufer, I, editor: Double contrast gastrointestinal radiography, Philadelphia, 1979, WB Saunders.

77. Stroehlein, JR, Goulston, K, and Hunt, RH: Diagnostic approach to evaluating the cause of a positive fecal occult blood test, Cancer 34:148, 1984.

78. Tedesco, FJ, et al: Diagnostic implications of the spatial distribution of colonic mass lesions (polyps and cancers): a prospective colonoscopic study, Gastrointest Endosc 26:95, 1980.

79. Tedesco, F, et al: Skinny upper gastrointestinal endoscopy, the initial diagnostic tool: a prospective comparison of upper gastrointestinal and radiology, J Clin Gastroenterol 2:27, 1980.

80. Thoeni, RF: Double-contrast bariums enema and colonoscopy: where do we stand? In Margulis, AR, and Gooding, CA, editors: Diagnostic radiology, San Francisco, 1981, University of California.

81. Thoeni, RF, and Cello, JP: A critical look at the accuracy of endoscopy and double contrast radiography of the upper gastrointestinal (UGI) tract in patients with substantial UGI hemorrhage, Radiology 135:305, 1980.

82. Thoeni, RF, and Menuck, L: Comparison of barium enema and colonoscopy in the detection of small colonic polyps, Radiology 124:631, 1977.

83. Thompson, WM, et al: Computed tomography for staging esophageal and gastroesophageal cancer: re-evaluation, AJR 141:951, 1983.

84. Tucker, HJ, Snape, WJ, and Cohen, S: Achalasia secondary to carcinoma: manometry and clinical features, Ann Intern Med 89:315, 1978.

85. Welch, CE, and Hedberg, SE: Polypoid lesions of the gastrointestinal tract, ed 2, Philadelphia, 1975, WB Saunders.

86. Winawer, SJ, and Sherlock, P: Malignant neoplasms of the small and large intestine. In Sleisenger, MG, and Fordtran, JS, editors: Gastrointestinal disease, ed 3, Philadelphia, 1983, WB Saunders.

87. Winawer, SJ, et al: Comparison of flexible sigmoidoscope with other diagnostic techniques in the diagnosis of rectocolon neoplasia, Dig Dis Sci 24:277, 1979.

PART XVII

INTERVENTIONAL RADIOLOGY

78 *Interventional Radiology of the Alimentary Canal*

E.J. RING

GENERAL CONSIDERATIONS

Interventional radiology primarily utilizes catheterization methods used for angiographic procedures. Percutaneous routes of access and methods of manipulation were developed for interventions in tubular structures such as the bile ducts and renal collecting system. With the development of cross-sectional imaging, controlled percutaneous entry became feasible for drainage of fluid collections in both the abdomen and the chest.

Despite the widespread application of these interventional radiologic techniques, alimentary tract pathology has not generally been considered very amenable to radiologically guided intervention. Percutaneous bowel puncture was largely avoided because of concern about the risks of leakage and contamination of the peritoneal cavity and the inherent problems associated with puncturing the highly mobile alimentary organs. Transluminal manipulation within the gastrointestinal (GI) tract can also be more difficult than in other tubular structures because the channel is much larger, longer, and more tortuous. Peristalsis and the irregularity of the mucosal surface of the bowel inhibit free passage of standard catheters and guidewires. Ever since radiologists first began reducing intussusceptions, however, great interest has developed in treating GI diseases by radiologic methods, and several interventional procedures applicable to GI tract pathology are now available.

STRICTURE DILATATION

Esophageal strictures were treated for many years by the blind passage of a series of graded dilators. More recently, dilatation has been accomplished by the Eder-Pustow olive-tipped or mercury-filled bougies. During the dilatation with these devices, a longitudinal force is applied, increasing the risk of rupture. In addition, when endoscopic guidance is used for dilatation, only the proximal end of the strictured lumen is visualized, and a false tract can easily develop when an irregular channel must be negotiated.

The low-compliance balloon catheters developed for angioplasty offer a much safer alternative for esophageal dilatation. A relatively small-diameter balloon catheter (10 French) can be used to achieve dilatation to a diameter as large as 30 mm. Balloon catheters are positioned and inflated under fluoroscopic guidance to ensure an intraluminal location. The force of dilatation is perpendicular to the stricture, and the fixed inflation diameter of the balloon avoids overdistention of the thin-walled, dilated segment above the stricture.

Since the first report of the use of fluoroscopically guided balloon catheters to treat symptomatic strictures in 1980,[9] several series have confirmed the safety and efficacy of this technique.[5,19] Initial success rates for balloon dilatation of benign strictures have consistently been greater than 90%. McLean et al.,[16] reporting on the long-term efficacy of stricture dilatation, found that 83% of patients remained symptom free for 1 year and 69% for 2 years. The results of balloon dilatation of malignant strictures have been much less encouraging. Only 20% of patients have any lasting positive results, and the only significant complications reported from balloon dilatation have been ruptures of esophageal malignancies.[17]

TECHNIQUE OF BALLOON DILATATION

The technique of dilatation of the esophagus is an adaptation of the dilatation methods used for stenoses in the arterial system, bile ducts, and ureter. After spraying the throat with a topical anesthetic, a nasogastric tube is advanced through the mouth, into the esophagus, and up to the area of the stricture. A guidewire is manipulated through the nasogastric tube. In most cases the guidewire advances with little difficulty through the stricture into the distal esophagus.

For unusually complex strictures, the nasogastric tube is exchanged over the guidewire for an angiographic catheter that has a gentle curve at its tip. This catheter is then used to direct the guidewire through the stricture. Once the angiographic catheter has been advanced into the stomach, it is exchanged for the dilatation balloon catheter. Generally a 15 or 20 mm balloon is used for the dilatation. The balloon is inflated in the strictured area using dilute contrast material with increasing pressure until the deformity in the balloon is effaced (Fig. 78-1). The balloon is then deflated and removed. Generally only 2 or 3 atm pressure are required.

Because of its simplicity and safety, balloon dilatation therapy has also been employed for strictures elsewhere in the GI tract. For example, strictures at anastomotic sites in the colon and at gastroenterostomy anastomoses can be effectively dilated in approximately 50% of cases (Fig. 78-2). The limiting factor appears to be the ability to access and manipulate into the area of the stricture. Long-term results for nonesophageal GI stricture dilatation recorded by McLean et al.[16] indicate that more than 70% of patients in whom successful dilatation can be accomplished will remain symptom free for longer than 1 to 2 years.

GASTROINTESTINAL INTUBATION

GI intubation has become a routine procedure in the management of several GI disorders. Although traditionally placed for the relief of small bowel obstruction, tubes are now also being widely used for enteric alimentation

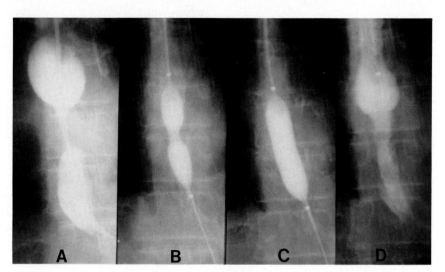

Fig. 78-1 Balloon dilatation of benign esophageal stricture. **A,** Angiographic catheter is positioned in dilated esophagus just above stricture. **B,** Guidewire is manipulated across strictured segment, and angiographic catheter is exchanged for 15 mm dilatation balloon catheter. As balloon is inflated, it is initially constricted by stricture. **C,** With increasing pressure, balloon expands to its full diameter. **D,** Contrast study confirms that satisfactory dilatation has been achieved.

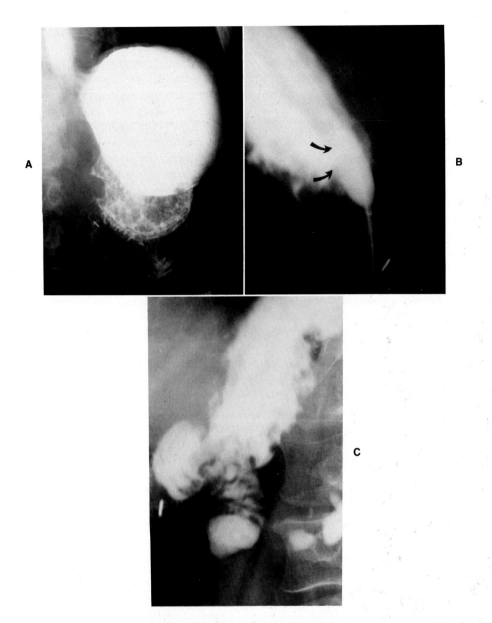

Fig. 78-2 Dilatation of gastroenterostomy anastomosis. **A,** Upper GI series demonstrates dilatation of gastric remnant and poor gastric emptying. **B,** A 20 mm balloon *(arrows)* is inflated in anastomosis. **C,** Follow-up upper GI series 2 days later shows widely patent anastomosis and free gastric emptying.

and occasionally for cytologic and microbiologic examinations. Placement of conventional tubes has relied on both gravity and intestinal peristalsis to carry a weighted tip from the stomach through the pylorus and duodenum into the small bowel. When tubes fail to advance passively into the desired location, radiologists may use catheter and guidewire technique to place the tube into appropriate position.[12]

TECHNIQUE OF GASTROJEJUNAL INTUBATION

Many methods of gastrojejunal intubation have been described. We employ an approach that employs modifications of angiographic catheter and guidewire technique.[4] Usually a nasogastric tube is already in place and is exchanged over a guidewire for an angiographic catheter. If no tube is present, a 10 French feeding tube is placed into the esophagus and a guidewire then passed through the lumen of the feeding tube and out a distal side hole or a precut end hole. The nasogastric tube is then removed, and an angiographic catheter with a gentle curve at its tip is introduced over the guidewire. The tip of the catheter is advanced under fluoroscopic guidance toward the pylorus.

Two guidewires are extremely helpful in manipulating

through the GI tract. A 15 mm J guidewire with a long, tapered mandril is very useful because it tends to buckle and form a long loop when it encounters an irregular mucosal wall. The rounded edge of the loop advances easily, spreading open the bowel lumen. After this guidewire has been manipulated for a distance of several centimeters, it is held in position and the catheter advanced over it. When a narrow lumen is encountered, or when crossing through the pylorus, a biliary torque guidewire* can be extremely helpful. A right-angle curve is placed at the tip of the torque-control guidewire, and the wire is rotated to probe the areas adjacent to the catheter tip. When the guidewire jumps forward into the pyloric channel or through an obstruction, the catheter is advanced over it. Excessive force should be avoided when using this guidewire because its relatively stiff end tends to catch on mucosal surfaces.

Once the catheter has been advanced to the desired position at the Treitz' ligament, a long exchange guidewire (260 cm) is placed through the angiographic catheter, which is removed. Standard feeding tubes do not have an open end hole and have been difficult to place over a guidewire. A feeding tube was developed for use with catheter-guided techniques.† This feeding tube has a weighted tip and an open end hole so that it can be advanced directly over the guidewire to the appropriate location (Fig. 78-2). Before introducing any tube through the nose, both the guidewire and the feeding tube should be coated with a lubricating jelly.

MANAGEMENT OF ENTEROCUTANEOUS FISTULAS

Enterocutaneous fistulas usually occur as a complication of complex alimentary tract surgery. Most fistulas originating in the duodenum, jejunum, and ileum are classified as high-output fistulas and may drain as much as 4000 ml or more of intestinal contents daily. The problems posed by such losses of fluids are formidable, and management is frequently complicated by one or more intraabdominal abscesses.

Surgical management of enterocutaneous fistulas has traditionally included (1) nutritional support, (2) diversion of enteric contents to control the fistula, and (3) drainage of all associated abscesses. The evolution of various interventional radiologic catheterization techniques has made safe and detailed exploration of fistulous tracts possible and has allowed a new nonsurgical option to accomplish these goals.[13]

Technique of catheterization

The procedure begins by passing a blunt, steerable catheter into the fistula opening. Contrast is then injected

---

*L-R Torque Guide, Cook, Inc., Bloomington, Ind.
†McLean-Ring Feeding Tube, Cook, Inc., Bloomington, Ind.

to fill the fistula (Fig. 78-3). As the tract is demonstrated in more detail, the steerable catheter is advanced farther into the fistula. Additional injections of contrast medium in the fistula will demonstrate the exact site of the fistula as well tracts into any associated abscesses. Guidewires can then be manipulated up to the site of leakage as well as to the abscess cavities. Large-bore sump drainage tubes are then placed over the guidewires and positioned immediately adjacent to the site of leakage and into dependent areas in the abscesses. Continuous suction is applied to all drainage tubes for several days.

When the abscesses have been completely collapsed, a single large tube is left in the tract immediately adjacent to the bowel opening. In a relatively short time, usually 1 to 2 weeks, a mature fibrous tract forms around the drainage tube. Removing the tube from the mature fistulous tract is comparable to removing a tube from a mature jejunostomy or T-tube tract, and the tract closes rapidly. In our experience with 14 consecutive, high-output enterocutaneous fistulas, closure was accomplished in every case.[14] Based on previous surgical experience, however, this approach is probably not effective when distal bowel obstruction exists and may be less effective when intrinsic bowel disease such as radiation enteritis or Crohn's disease (regional enteritis) is present.

For patients with postoperative esophageal leaks and major mediastinal and pleural abscesses, drainage can also be accomplished transnasally.[11] In these cases an angiographic catheter is manipulated through the leak and into the cavity. A large-bore Salem sump tube is then placed over the guidewire into a dependent location in the abscess. A second sump tube is then passed through the other nostril and positioned within the esophageal lumen at the site of the leak. The second tube is used to control swallowed saliva and any refluxed gastric contents. Once the abscesses have resolved, the esophageal tube is kept in place until the dehiscence has healed (Fig. 78-4).

Enteric leaks may appear with only abdominal abscesses and no cutaneous fistula. In these cases percutaneous puncture of the abscess and insertion of a drainage tube under computed tomography (CT) or ultrasound guidance is a well-established procedure. Close follow-up with injections of contrast through the tube will demonstrate the communication to the GI tract in a high percentage of cases. In our experience fistulous communications were found on sinography in 38 of 81 postsurgical abscesses.[8] Treatment of the leakage in these cases is similar to that of enterocutaneous fistulas; once a connection to the bowel is identified, a second guidewire is introduced and manipulated to a point immediately adjacent to the opening in the bowel. A second drainage tube is placed over the guidewire to control the leakage of enteric contents (Fig. 78-5).

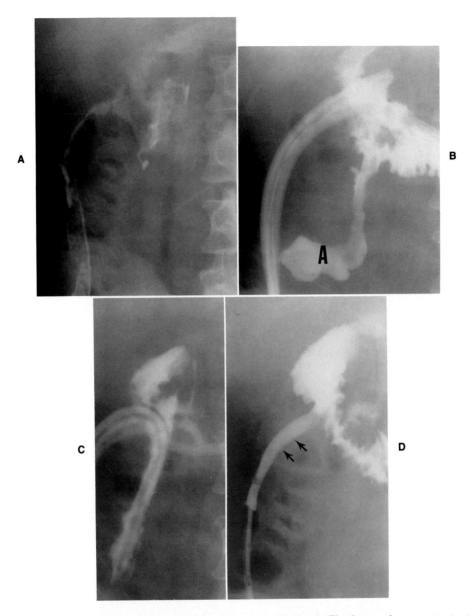

Fig. 78-3 Management of high-output duodenocutaneous fistula. **A,** Fistulagram demonstrates tract with minimal contrast entering duodenum. **B,** Steerable catheter is manipulated through tract. Injection of contrast close to fistula shows open communication to duodenum and dependent abscess *(A).* **C,** Large-bore sump tube is positioned in abscess, and drain is placed into duodenum to control flow of duodenal contents. **D,** Drains are removed after abscess has cleared and mature fibrous tract has formed *(arrows).*

PERCUTANEOUS PUNCTURE OF ALIMENTARY TRACT
Percutaneous gastrostomy

Nutritional support by gastrostomy feeding is an important therapeutic adjunct for patients with swallowing difficulty secondary to neurologic problems or obstructive neck or esophageal tumors. Although nutrition can often be provided for these patients by nasoenteric tubes,

transnasal tubes are uncomfortable and not usually well tolerated for long periods. Transnasal tubes also create a cosmetic problem and add to the psychologic difficulty of patients already burdened with a malignancy and poor prognosis. Patients with neurologic disorders are often uncooperative, and it is generally difficult to keep a nasal tube in place for long periods.

Gastrostomy feeding is therefore usually preferred

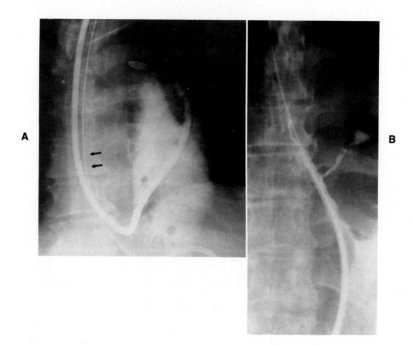

Fig. 78-4 Transluminal management of major postoperative esophageal leak. **A,** Large-bore drainage tube has been manipulated through one nostril, down esophagus, and across dehiscence into large pleural collection. Salem sump tube *(arrows)* is placed through other nostril and positioned so that its side holes are located immediately above and below leakage site. **B,** After 2 weeks of continuous drainage, abscess sump is removed; only thin tract remains. Several days later nasoesophageal drainage is discontinued and tract closed completely.

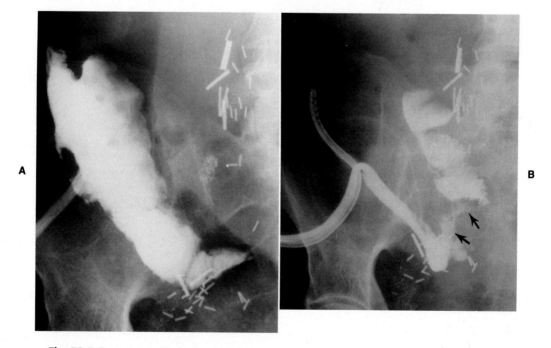

Fig. 78-5 Percutaneous drainage of abscess associated with low-output, small bowel fistula. **A,** Abscess in right lower quadrant is drained under ultrasound guidance. Contrast injection after emptying abscess cavity demonstrates its full extent. **B,** Repeat sinogram performed 3 days later demonstrates fistula to small bowel *(arrows)*. Second tube is placed immediately adjacent to fistula.

when long-term nutritional support is required. Although a relatively minor procedure, surgical gastrostomy still usually requires general anesthesia and has a mortality of 1% to 6%.[22] Percutaneous gastrostomy has evolved as a safe and relatively simple alternative.[6] Not only can a feeding tube be directly placed into the stomach by percutaneous methods, but it can also be readily advanced through the pylorus and into the proximal jejunum, where feeding can begin immediately in the most optimal location.[15]

Technique

Several methods of percutaneous gastrostomy have been described. In some centers the procedure is performed in combination with endoscopy. A gastroscope is passed into the stomach and flexed, tenting the stomach against the anterior abdominal wall. The stomach is then punctured by aiming the needle at the endoscopic light seen through the abdominal wall, and a guidewire is passed into the stomach. In one technique the guidewire is ensnared and brought out through the endoscope, and the gastrostomy tube is fed through the endoscope, over the guidewire, and out the percutaneous hole.[20] In another technique the guidewire is coiled in the stomach, and the tract is dilated to 14 French. A Foley catheter is then placed through a "peel-away" sheath. The sheath is removed, and the tube is affixed to the patient's abdominal wall.[18]

Considerable experience now indicates that gastroscopy is not needed to perform the procedure and that it can be done safely using fluoroscopic guidance alone.[21] Several modifications of a percutaneous technique have been described. We employ the method described by Alzate et al.[1]

First, the left lobe of the liver is identified using ultrasound, and the stomach and transverse colon are localized fluoroscopically. In most cases the stomach is then distended with air or dilute contrast medium introduced through a nasogastric tube. After anesthetizing the skin and subcutaneous tissue, the stomach is punctured along the greater curvature. Although some authors recommend use of a direct trocar approach, most prefer a modified Seldinger technique (Fig. 78-6). We generally puncture the stomach with a 5 F needle sheath. A guidewire is then advanced through the sheath and into the stomach, usually up into the fundus. The tract is dilated sequentially with angiographic dilators until a peel-away sheath can be passed over the guidewire into the stomach. Once the peel-away sheath is in place, an angiographic catheter and torque-control guidewire are manipulated through the pylorus, across the duodenum, and into the proximal jejunum. The feeding tube is then placed over the guidewire. Once positioned, the external portion of the feeding tube is sutured to the patient's abdominal

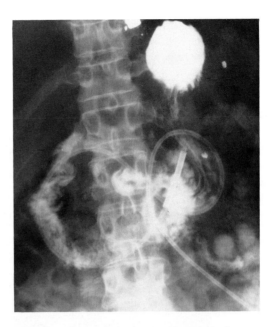

Fig. 78-6 Percutaneous gastrostomy. After puncturing stomach, feeding tube is advanced through pylorus into distal duodenum so that enteric nutrition can begin immediately after procedure.

wall. The contents of the stomach are then evacuated through the nasogastric tube, which is removed. Feeding can begin immediately.

The main technical problem encountered during this procedure occurs when the guidewire buckles into the peritoneal cavity as the dilators are being introduced. The buckle develops because the thick muscular stomach wall offers considerable resistance to the dilators, and the mobile stomach moves away from the dilators. Buckling of the guidewire can usually be avoided by using a very rigid wire and advancing the dilators with a short, thrusting motion. A device has recently been developed to provide tension on the stomach wall, thereby facilitating passage of dilators and catheters.[3] This device is basically a T-bar, which is introduced first through the puncture needle. It is attached to a suture that is grasped externally to hold the stomach wall and prevent movement during insertion of catheters and dilators.

Complications from percutaneous gastrostomy result mainly from inadvertent puncture of other organs, such as the spleen, left lobe of the liver, or colon. This problem can be minimized using proper guidance with ultrasound and fluoroscopy.

Percutaneous puncture of small bowel

Although occasional reports have described the use of percutaneous intubation for temporary decompression in patients with bowel obstruction, not enough experience yet exists to confirm the safety and utility of this method.[7] We have used percutaneous decompression, however, for three patients with acute obstruction of an afferent loop after gastric surgery. In each case percutaneous catheter drainage avoided rupture of the stump of the afferent limb and allowed the patient's condition to improve before surgical revision (Fig. 78-7).

Percutaneous transjejunal puncture of Roux-en-Y choledochojejunostomies

Patients with complex biliary tract pathology are often treated surgically by construction of a Roux-en-Y biliary jejunal anastomosis. Recent reports have documented the usefulness of constructing the Roux-en-Y loop with an extraperitoneal segment that is marked with metal clips.[2]

The extraperitoneal segment can then be punctured percutaneously and catheterization into the biliary tree readily accomplished. This approach offers considerable advantage for patients with chronic biliary tract pathologies such as sclerosing cholangitis and Oriental cholangiohepatitis who require frequent intervention. We have also had experience puncturing Roux-en-Y loops that were not specifically constructed with an extraperitoneal segment.[10] In 14 patients we were able to identify the loop at CT or fluoroscopy and determine a safe pathway through which a needle could be inserted. The Roux-en-Y was then punctured and a catheter advanced up to the biliary tree for biliary intervention (Fig. 78-8).

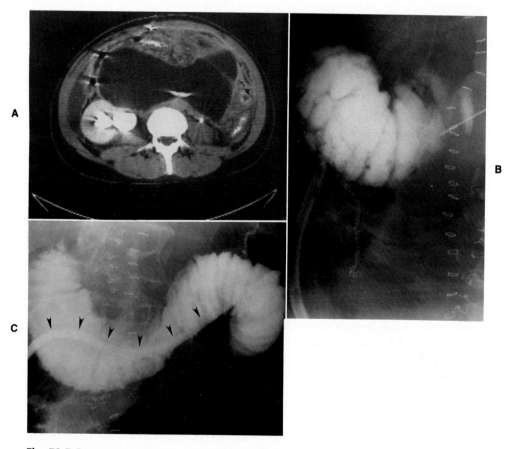

Fig. 78-7 Percutaneous drainage of obstructed afferent loop following partial gastrectomy with Billroth II anastomosis. **A,** CT scan demonstrates large fluid collection. **B,** Collection is punctured with thin needle. Injection of contrast demonstrates bowel mucosa in obstructed loop. **C,** Large-bore sump catheter *(arrows)* is placed percutaneously to decompress loop and avoid rupture of duodenal stump until surgery can be performed.

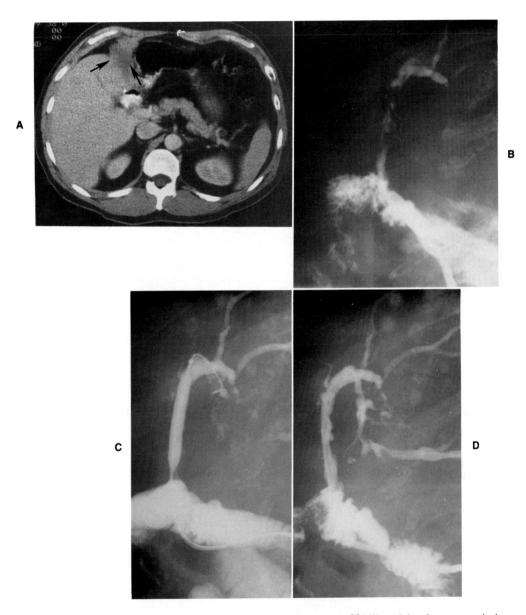

Fig. 78-8 Percutaneous transjejunal catheterization of Roux-en-Y biliary jejunal anastomosis in patient with sclerosing cholangitis. **A,** CT scan demonstrates Roux loop to be located anteriorly *(arrows)*. **B,** Bowel loop is punctured and catheter manipulated to anastomosis. Cholangiogram through catheter shows high-grade stricture. **C,** Catheter is advanced through stricture and exchanged for balloon catheter, which is inflated in diseased segment. **D,** Cholangiogram following dilatation shows considerable improvement in ductal lumen at site of stricture. Transjejunal catheter was removed 48 hours later.

REFERENCES

1. Alzate, GD, et al: Percutaneous gastrostomy for jejunal feeding: new technique, AJR 147:822, 1986.

2. Barker, EM, and Winkler, M: Permanent-access hepatico-jejunostomy, Br J Surg 71:188, 1984.

3. Brown, AS, and Mueller, PR: Controlled percutaneous gastrostomy: nylon T-fastener for fixation of the anterior gastric wall (letter reply), Radiology 160:278, 1986.

4. Cardoza, JD, and Jeffrey, RB, Jr: Nasojejunal feeding tube placement in immobile patients, Radiology 166:893, 1988.

5. Dawson, SL, et al: Severe esophageal strictures: indications for balloon catheter dilatation, Radiology 153:637, 1984.

6. Gauderer, MWL, Ponsky, JL, and Izant, RJ, Jr: Gastrostomy without laparotomy: a percutaneous endoscopic technique, J Pediatr Surg 15:872, 1980.

7. Hoddick, WK, Demas, BE, and Moss, AA: CT-guided percutaneous bowel loopogram, AJR 143(5):1098, 1984.

8. Kerlan, RK, et al: Abdominal abscess with low-output fistula: successful percutaneous drainage, Radiology 155(1):73, 1985.

9. London, RL, et al: Dilatation of severe esophageal strictures by inflatable balloon catheters, Gastroenterology 80:173, 1980.

10. Maroney, TP, and Ring, EJ: Percutaneous transjejunal catheterization of Roux-en-Y biliary-jejunal anastomoses, Radiology 164:151, 1987.

11. Maroney, TP, et al: The role of interventional radiology in the management of major esophageal leaks, Am J Surg. (In press.)

12. McLean, GK, Ring, EJ, and Freiman, DB: Applications and techniques of gastrointestinal intubation, J Cardiovasc Interv Radiol 5:108, 1982.

13. McLean, GK, Rosen, RJ, and Ring, EJ: Miscellaneous interventional procedures. In Ring, EJ, and McLean, GK, editors: Interventional radiology: principles and techniques, Boston, 1981, Little, Brown & Co.

14. McLean, GK, et al: Enterocutaneous fistulae: interventional radiologic management, AJR 138:615, 1982.

15. McLean, GK, et al: Transgastrostomy jejunal intubation for enteric alimentation, AJR 139(6):1129, 1982.

16. McLean, GK, et al: Radiologically guided balloon dilation of gastrointestinal strictures. Part I. Technique and factors influencing procedural success, Radiology 165:35, 1987.

17. McLean, GK, et al: Radiologically guided balloon dilation of gastrointestinal strictures. Part II. Results of long-term follow-up, Radiology 165:41, 1987.

18. Ponsky, JL, Gauderer, MWL, and Stellato, TA: Percutaneous endoscopic gastrostomy: review of 150 cases, Arch Surg 118(8):913, 1983.

19. Starck, E, et al: Esophageal stenosis: treatment with balloon catheters, Radiology 153:637, 1984.

20. Strodel, WE, et al: Early experience with endoscopic percutaneous gastrostomy, Arch Surg 118:449, 1983.

21. vanSonnenberg, E, et al: Percutaneous gastrostomy and gastroenterostomy. 1. Techniques derived from laboratory evaluation, AJR 146:577, 1986.

22. Wasiljew, BK, Ujiki, GT, and Beal, JM: Feeding gastrostomy: complications and mortality, Am J Surg 143:194, 1982.

79 *Vascular System*

ANDERS LUNDERQUIST

New diagnostic imaging modalities have decreased the diagnostic importance of angiography. I rarely perform gastrointestinal angiography at present for diagnostic purposes. The exception might be cases in which vessels are suspected to be occluded or narrowed, or when I am looking for sources of occult hemorrhage. Thus there is a reduced need for superselective catheterization and magnification angiography to demonstrate the tiny vascular changes that were once important for the diagnosis.

After the report of Dotter and Judkins[13] in 1964 on the interventional dilatation of vessels and the report of Nusbaum and co-workers[30] in 1969 on the treatment of gastrointestinal hemorrhages by intraarterial vasopressin infusion, angiographers became more and more occupied with the treatment of patients, leading to a wide spectrum of interventional vascular procedures. The decrease in diagnostic vascular procedures has reduced the opportunities for the angiographer to maintain the high technical skill that is so important when small vascular branches are to be catheterized.

This chapter will discuss how interventional radiology can be applied in the vascular system of the gastrointestinal tract and replace previous conventional ways of treatment.

THE LIVER AND PORTAL SYSTEM
Trauma

Trauma to the liver can be blunt or penetrating and can cause severe intraperitoneal hemorrhage. Computed tomography (CT) has been widely used to diagnose the extent of damage to intraabdominal organs; ultrasonography has been less accurate in emergency cases. Many surgeons still claim that peritoneal lavage is the most accurate technique to demonstrate hemorrhage in the peritoneal cavity that requires laparotomy, whereas others prefer a more conservative approach. Too frequently laparotomy demonstrates blood in the peritoneum, a fractured liver, but no actual hemorrhage. When blood clots in the fractured liver are removed to obtain better visualization of the damage, the hemorrhage often starts again, and a lobe resection or ligation of the hepatic artery might be necessary. Since the blood clots are excellent substrate for bacteria, postsurgical abscesses are not infrequent.

Surgeons who favor a more conservative treatment are satisfied with contrast-enhanced CT of the abdomen to map the damage. If there are clinical signs of continuous hemorrhage and the patient's condition does not necessitate immediate laparotomy, angiography should be performed. The bleeding can be localized and selective embolization done (Fig. 79-1). Frequently laparotomy can be prevented and the patient treated conservatively and followed with CT or ultrasonography.

Superselective catheterization and embolization of bleeding intrahepatic vessels is often technically difficult if only the bleeding artery is to be obliterated. Too extensive obliteration of the hepatic artery may cause damage to the bile ducts and produce cystic changes in the liver.[12]

The most elegant way to obliterate the bleeding vessel is to introduce a detachable balloon,[50] which does not need to be detached until its position is correct. The high cost of these balloon catheters has prevented their more extensive use; therefore other embolization materials have been used, such as Gelfoam, Ivalon, and Gianturco coils.* To facilitate superselective catheterization, F5 catheters with soft and long tapered tips can be used or a coaxial system with the Teflon F3 catheter advanced through the guiding catheter. In combination with a 0.018-inch Teflon guidewire or Cope's platinum-tipped

*References 14, 18, 20, 22, 34, 40, 49.

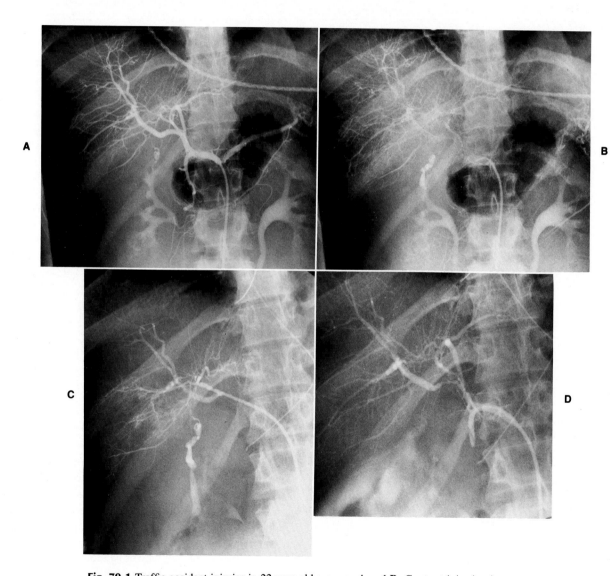

Fig. 79-1 Traffic accident injuries in 22-year-old woman. **A** and **B,** Contrast injection in common hepatic artery shows extravasation of contrast from branch of middle hepatic artery. **C,** Catheter is advanced into artery that is occluded with pieces of Gelfoam. **D,** Angiogram after embolization shows no further extravasation. Other arterial branches are patent. Spasm of first part of right hepatic artery.

ultrathin guidewire with quite good torque control, the F3 catheter can in most cases be placed in correct position for embolization. Embolization through the F3 catheter can be performed either with Gianturco mini coils or bucrylate mixed with Ethiodol. Finally, an open-ended guidewire has become available that can be used in embolization of small, tortuous arterial branches.[6]

The ability to control hemorrhage in the traumatized liver by hepatic artery embolization has been well documented. In the collected material presented by Wagner and co-workers[47] five of 41 patients died. Two patients died from uncontrolled hemorrhage. Three patients had congestive jaundice and died from liver failure.

A few words of caution are needed. First, one has to make sure that the portal vein is patent before embolization is performed. Second, iatrogenic hemorrhage caused by percutaneous transhepatic cholangiography (PTC) in patients with obstructive jaundice should be treated with embolization of only the bleeding vessel (Fig. 79-2). Dilated bile ducts can cause compression of the adjacent portal venous branches in the portal triad. Since the excretion pressure in the obstructed bile ducts can rise to more than 30 cm of water, the obstruction to the portal blood flow can become quite significant. Embolization of too many hepatic arterial branches in that combination may result in liver failure.[12]

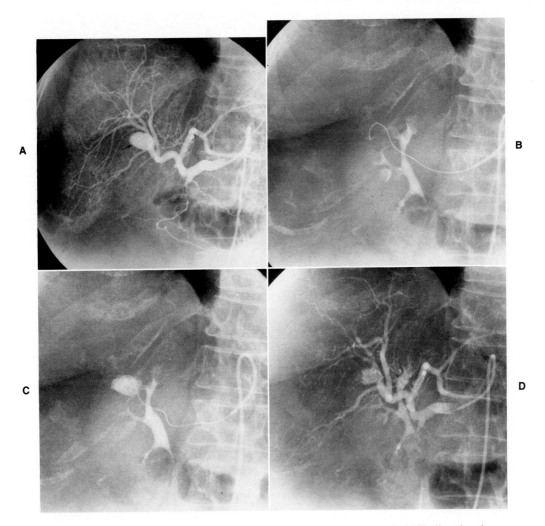

Fig. 79-2 Nonresectable pancreatic carcinoma in 75-year-old woman. Surgical biliodigestive shunt anostomosis after PTC with drainage for 2 weeks. Postsurgical intestinal hemorrhage. **A,** Common hepatic angiography demonstrates large aneurysm of branch of right hepatic artery caused by previous PTC. **B,** Coaxial catheterization of aneurysm. **C,** Aneurysm is obliterated with bucrylate mixed with Lipiodol. **D,** Postembolization angiogram shows obliterated aneurysm and patent other vessels.

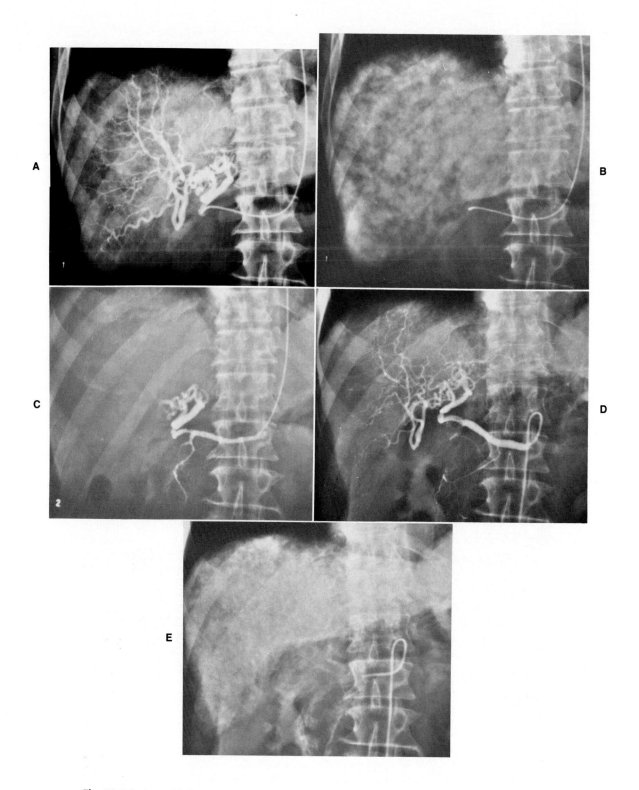

Fig. 79-3 Patient with liver metastases from carcinoid tumor and carcinoid syndrome. **A,** Selective catheterization of proper hepatic artery, arterial phase. **B,** In parenchymal phase whole liver is filled with hypervascular metastases. **C,** After embolization with Gelfoam powder, blood flow to liver is obliterated. **D,** One month later vessels are recanalized and, **E,** metastases are less vascular. Patient became free from carcinoid syndrome 2 days after embolization and remained symptom free for 9 months.

Liver tumors

Treatment of primary liver tumors and metastatic tumors from colorectal carcinoma by hepatic arterial infusion of cytotoxic drugs through either percutaneously placed catheters or surgically placed catheters connected with subcutaneous infusion chambers[2] have not given the expected dramatic improvement. Intermittent arterial occlusion combined with drug infusion also seems to have failed.[4]

Patients with carcinoid syndrome associated with liver metastases have, on the other hand, been successfully treated with hepatic artery embolization[1,27,36] (Fig. 79-3). Symptoms of the carcinoid syndrome almost immediately disappear and may be absent for several months to more than a year. The quality of life of these patients is markedly improved, but survival time is only slightly prolonged.

When hepatic artery embolization is to be performed, it is first important to ascertain that extensive tumor growth has not occluded the portal vein. Fatal liver necrosis can otherwise occur. If cholecystectomy has not been previously performed, the patient must be carefully watched for gallbladder necrosis.[10] Fortunately this complication is rare.

Recent reports from Japan on hepatic artery embolization with Ethiodol mixed with cytotoxic drugs have given some positive results. Patients with hepatocellular carcinoma have been embolized with 10 to 20 ml of Ethiodol mixed with doxorubicin (Adriamycin), cisplatin, or neocarzinostatin (SMANCS).[22,23]

I have performed vital microscopic examinations of the rat liver during Lipiodol injection into the hepatic artery, which has shown that Lipiodol passes from the artery over arterioportal connections into the portal vein. Lipiodol also passes through the sinusoids into the hepatic veins for further embolization to other organs. This has made me more reluctant to use the technique for treatment of liver tumors.

Portal hypertension

Bleeding from esophagogastric varices in patients with portal hypertension has for many years been treated with the Sengstaken-Blakemore tube and intravenous vasopressin infusion. Infusion of vasopressin into the superior mesenteric artery reduces the portal venous pressure only slightly more than intravenous administration.[3] The effect of vasopressin infusion cannot be totally explained by lowering the portal venous pressure. Increased muscular tonus in the distal esophagus has been suggested in the mechanism, but recordings of the lower esophageal sphincter pressure demonstrate a reduced tonus during vasopressin infusion.[28]

Transhepatic embolization of the left and short gastric veins was introduced in the treatment of patients whose bleeding could not be controlled otherwise.[25] This obliteration of varices has been performed with Gelfoam and sodium tetradecyl sulphate,[33,46,51] bucrylate,[4,15,26] Gelfoam and stainless steel coils,[16,52] and absolute alcohol.[44] Acute variceal bleeding has thus been controlled in 43% to 95% of patients for varying periods. This method has sufficed for changing the patient's status from that of emergency to elective surgery.

The most serious complications reported with this procedure have been portal vein thrombosis and severe intraperitoneal bleeding.[5,51]

Transhepatic obliteration of esophageal varices has been replaced by endoscopic sclerosing injections into the varices. Repeated, such treatments will in most cases control the bleeding and make emergency portal caval shunt operation unnecessary.

When a portal systemic shunt operation becomes the only way to save the patient from life-threatening hemorrhages, it is made either as a portal caval, splenorenal, or mesocaval shunt. Not infrequently a stenosis may develop and reduce the function of this shunt, and the patient can again suffer from bleeding varices. In these cases balloon dilatation has proved very useful to reopen the shunt and restore the blood flow[9] (Fig. 79-4).

THE PANCREAS
Hemorrhage in pancreatitis

Pancreatitis with pseudocyst or abscess formation sometimes produces erosion of the splenic or pancreatic arteries with hemorrhage into the pseudocyst or into the pancreatic duct.[42] Angiography can demonstrate the extravasation into the pseudocyst or pancreatic duct, but sometimes an aneurysm or only an irregularity of an artery may suggest the origin of the intermittent bleeding. Depending on the location of the damaged vessels, the approach is different.

If the main stem of the splenic artery is eroded, a catheter is advanced to the place of erosion, and that part of the vessel is obliterated with a large Gianturco coil or bucrylate (Fig. 79-5). Small coils or pieces of Gelfoam should not be used, as they will move into the spleen, and the eroded part of the splenic artery will not be obliterated until the whole spleen is infarcted. Large coils or bucrylate delivered to the splenic artery can produce only a segmental occlusion of the artery. Splenic infarction is prevented by collateral arterial supply. An intrapancreatic arterial erosion bleeding into the pancreatic duct is usually supplied by a widened pancreatic branch. This has to be selectively catheterized and can be obliterated with either a small coil or bucrylate.

THE SPLEEN

It has become clear that the spleen has to be saved to protect the body from life-threatening infection. Septi-

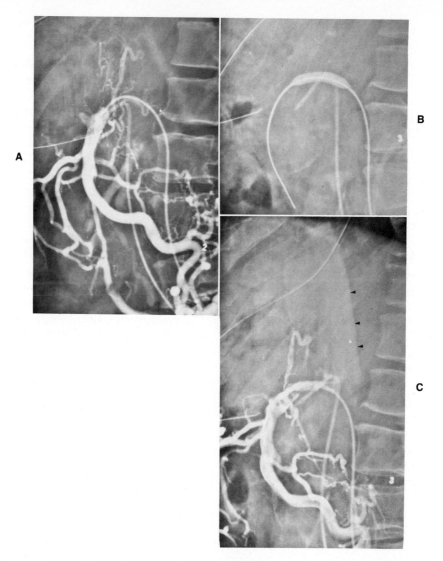

Fig. 79-4 Patient with portal hypertension and occluded mesocaval shunt. **A,** Contrast injection through catheter passed from inferior vena cava through occlusion and into superior mesenteric vein. There was no contrast flow into inferior vena cava. **B,** Balloon dilatation of occlusion. **C,** Postdilatation superior mesenteric vein injection shows flow into inferior vena cava *(arrowheads)*.

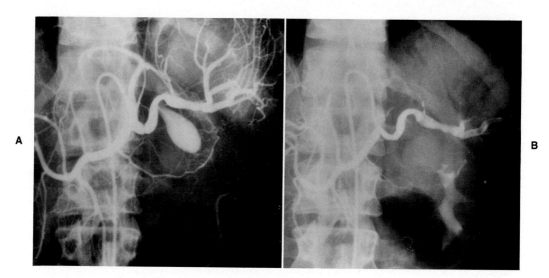

Fig. 79-5 Pancreatitis and intestinal hemorrhage in 38-year-old woman. **A,** Celiac angiography demonstrates large pseudoaneurysm extending into pancreas. **B,** Splenic artery obliterated with bucrylate mixed with Ethiodol. Hemorrhage was stopped.

cemia is 50% to 70% more frequent in patients who have had the spleen removed for one reason or another.[11,24] Moreover, surgical complications combined with splenectomy are common. In patients with hypersplenism combined with portal hypertension, the enormous col-

lateral venous network around the spleen explains the frequent appearance of postsplenectomy hematomas. The vicinity of the tail of the pancreas to the hilum of the spleen is another explanation for complications from splenectomy. In more than 80% of the cases the distance

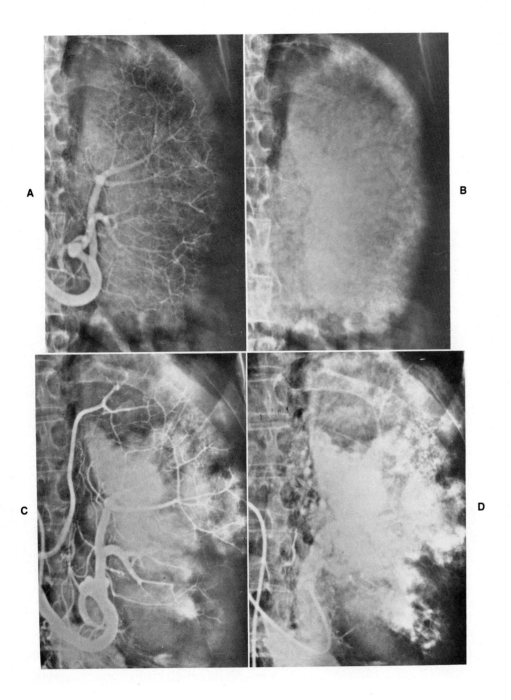

Fig. 79-6 Hypersplenism in patient with portal hypertension and markedly enlarged spleen. **A,** Arterial phase. **B,** Parenchymal phase. After embolization with pieces of Gelfoam, only parts of splenic parenchyma are perfused. **C,** Arterial phase. **D,** Parenchymal phase.

between the tail of the pancreas and the spleen is less than 5 mm, and frequently the tip of the pancreatic tail is removed with the spleen, causing leak of pancreatic juice into the surrounding tissue and a pancreatic pseudocyst (see 79-7, *D*).

During the last few years treatment with transcatheter splenic artery embolization for partial splenic infarction has been used in patients with hypersplenism to improve the tolerance to immunosuppressive drugs in renal transplant candidates and in patients with hematologic disorders.[17,19,31,35] Infarction of only 20% to 30% of the splenic parenchyma produces an immediate rise in thrombocyte and white cell counts (Fig. 79-6). If too much of the spleen is infarcted, there is a risk for formation of an abscess in the spleen, but 20% to 30% infarction of the spleen is found to be safe. Still, up to 65% infarction of the spleen carries no more complications than does

surgical splenectomy.[29] The infarction of the spleen is performed by injection of pieces of Gelfoam through a catheter placed in the splenic artery. The catheter should not be placed far out in the splenic artery. The pieces of Gelfoam only go to the spleen because other branches are too small to allow them to enter. Small steel coils have also been used, but they are unnecessarily expensive. In some cases Gelfoam powder has resulted in severe complications with pancreatitis. These small particles do not only go to the spleen but also to pancreatic arterial branches, which become obliterated, and ischemic necrosis of the pancreatic tail can occur.

Partial splenic embolization causes a marked increase in the platelet and white blood cell counts within a few days. If symptoms recur, embolization can be repeated as early as 1 month later. Side effects from the procedure are left upper quadrant pain, transient left pleural effu-

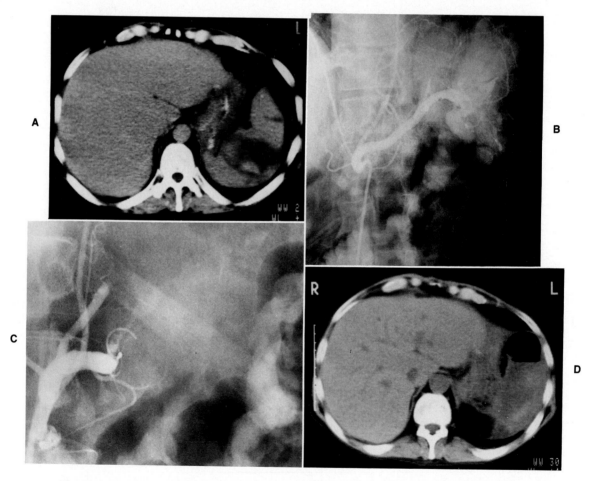

Fig. 79-7 A, CT scan demonstrates ruptured spleen. **B,** Selective splenic angiogram demonstrates extravasation in spleen. **C,** After splenic artery embolization with Gianturco coil, hemorrhage stops. However, surgery with splenectomy was performed 2 weeks later. Specimen included spleen with tip of pancreatic tail. Postsurgical abscess developed. **D,** Postsurgical CT demonstrates left-sided subphrenic abscess. This was subsequently drained percutaneously.

sion, and small atelectases in the left lower lobe. Development of a splenic abscess rarely occurs if the degree of embolization is limited to less than 65%.

Patients whose spleen is to be embolized must be given broad-spectrum antibiotics before, during, and after the procedure.

Splenic embolization in patients with portal hypertension has shown that the reduced splenic blood flow produced by the embolization sometimes has little influence on the portal venous pressure.[53] Portal hypertension without hypersplenism is thus no indication for splenic embolization.

Blunt trauma to the abdomen causing fracture of the spleen is not a clear indication for surgery and splenectomy. During the last few years surgeons have used a conservative treatment much more often and followed their patients with ultrasonography or CT, depending on the patient's condition, to document the healing. When surgery is performed, the surgeon often tries not to remove the spleen but to suture the ruptured capsule.

It is surprising that transcatheter embolization of the splenic artery is not more frequently used in cases of splenic trauma. Recently Chuang and Reuter[8] experimentally demonstrated the effectiveness of embolization to stop hemorrhage from a damaged spleen. This treatment has been tried at other institutions and found useful.[54] However, it is important to know how this embolization is performed to avoid complications. Embolization with pieces of Gelfoam will cause full infarction of the spleen before the bleeding has stopped, and an abscess will ensue. The embolization must be done with steel coils large enough to obliterate the main stem of the splenic artery (Fig. 79-7). As the fracture of the spleen usually goes through rather avascular parenchyma, the reduction of the flow caused by obliteration of the main stem of the splenic artery will in most cases stop the hemorrhage. Splenic infarction is prevented by numerous collaterals over pancreatic and gastric arteries.

GASTROINTESTINAL HEMORRHAGE
Stomach

Hemorrhage into the stomach from peptic ulcers, Mallory-Weiss tears, gastric erosions, or surgical anastomoses are best treated with intraarterial infusion of vasopressin.[21] The dose most commonly used is 0.2 IU/min, and a control angiography is performed after 20 minutes to see if the bleeding has stopped. If not, the infusion rate of vasopressin can be increased to 0.4 IU/min.

If vasopressin cannot control the hemorrhage, the bleeding artery can be embolized. The embolization is usually performed with pieces of Gelfoam in the left gastric artery. If the bleeding originates from branches of the gastroduodenal artery, vasopressin is rarely effec-

tive. The gastroduodenal artery is then obliterated with one or several Gianturco coils. If Gelfoam is used in the gastroduodenal artery, the embolization material goes far into the peripheral branches, and the desired effect is not achieved until the whole gastroepiploic artery is filled. Many radiologists prefer not to use vasopressin in the left gastric artery; they embolize the artery with particles of Gelfoam to avoid the indwelling catheter for vasopressin infusion.

Small bowel and colon

Hemorrhage is the most common indication for interventional radiology in the small bowel and colon. After the site of hemorrhage has been localized, the bleeding can frequently be stopped by selective intraarterial vasopressin infusion. Again the same concentration and injection rate of vasopressin is used as for hemorrhage in the stomach. When intraarterial vasopressin infusion is done, the patient should be carefully watched in the intensive care unit. Potential complications are fluid retention caused by the antidiuretic effect of vasopressin, bowel infarction, and superior mesenteric vein thrombosis[37,41] as a consequence of the severe vasoconstriction.

Some patients do not respond to vasopressin infusion and have clinical conditions too poor for surgical intervention. In these selected cases embolization of the bleeding artery has to be performed and then on vital indication knowing that bowel necrosis may ensue. In one series Rosenkrantz and co-workers[38] reported 13% postembolic infarction of the bowel wall. Among 13 patients, Uflacker[45] found two with bowel necrosis, both in the colon.

This embolization is done with the catheter as close to the bleeding vessel as possible for two reasons. First, if embolization is started with particles of Gelfoam too far from the source of bleeding, too many vessels will be obliterated, and the risk for bowel infarction will increase. Second, if embolization is done with coils, a localized obliteration of the vessel may be too far from the bleeding point, and the hemorrhage may continue, fed by collaterals.

The level at which to occlude the mesenteric arterial branches is, however, controversial. Some authors advocate a more central occlusion to reduce the risk of bowel wall ischemia and necrosis.[7,48]

ARTERIOVENOUS FISTULA

Trauma to the abdomen—blunt, penetrating, or iatrogenic—may cause arteriovenous fistulae. In the liver a fistula between the hepatic artery and the portal vein usually closes spontaneously. In the mesentery, on the other hand, these fistulae often increase in size, and a "steal syndrome" may develop (Fig. 79-8). These pa-

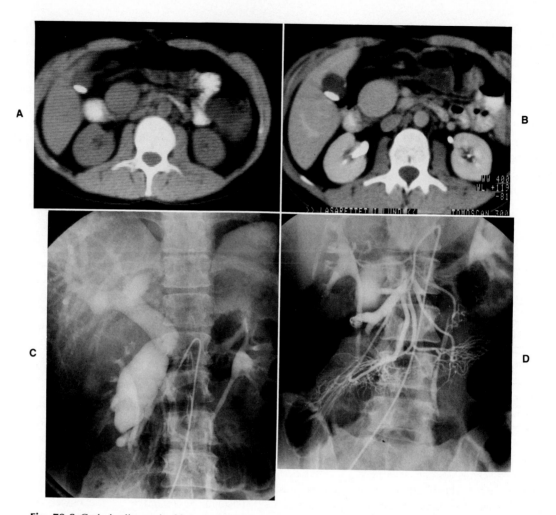

Fig. 79-8 Crohn's disease in 32-year-old man. Multiple previous bowel resections complicated with abscesses. Short bowel syndrome, possibly, and malabsorption. **A** and **B,** Unenhanced and intravenously enhanced CT scans show 6 cm wide aneurysmatic lesion ventral to vena cava. **C,** Superior mesenteric angiography demonstrates arteriovenous fistula between iliocolic artery and iliocolic vein with stealing of contrast from superior mesenteric artery branches to fistula. **D,** Fistula is obliterated with coil, and injection of contrast into superior mesenteric artery demonstrates obliterated iliocolic artery and increased flow to small bowel.

tients can initially have malabsorption, sometimes misinterpreted as celiac sprue. After an arteriovenous fistula has been angiographically localized, it can be obliterated either with a detachable balloon or with coils. In the case of a mesenteric arteriovenous fistula it is important to close the vessel at the location of the fistula to prevent damage to other mesenteric vessels.

MESENTERIC ISCHEMIA

It has been suggested that mesenteric ischemia does not develop unless two of the three large intestinal arterial branches—the celiac artery, the superior mesenteric artery, and the inferior mesenteric artery—are occluded and the one left is stenosed.

Stenosis or occlusion of only the celiac artery is sometimes suggested to be responsible for upper abdominal pain. This is hardly true unless the collateral blood flow from the superior mesenteric artery is insufficient, as is sometimes the case after surgery in that region.

Arteriosclerotic stenosis or occlusion of the first part of the superior mesenteric artery can be handled by percutaneous transluminal angioplasty (PTA) and the blood flow restored.[43] Collateral blood flow over the middle colic artery is almost always enough to supply the branches of the inferior mesenteric artery. Consequently PTA of the inferior mesenteric artery is rarely necessary. To prevent recurrent vascular narrowing after PTA, vascular stents have become available; however, these have still only been used in a few clinical trials.[32,39]

REFERENCES

1. Allison, D, Modlin, JM, and Jenkins, WJ: Treatment of carcinoid liver metastases by hepatic artery embolization, Lancet 2:1323, 1977.

2. Balch, CM, et al: A prospective phase II clinical trial of continuous FUDR regional chemotherapy for colorectal metastases to the liver using a totally implantable drug infusion pump, Ann Surg 198:567, 1983.

3. Barr, JW, Lakin, RC, and Rösch, J: Similarity of arterial and intravenous vasopressin on portal and systemic hemodynamics, Gastroenterology 69:13, 1975.

4. Bengmark, S, Jeppson, B, and Nobin, A: Arterial ligation and temporary dearterialization. In Blumgart, LH, editor: Surgery of the liver and biliary tract, vol 2, Edinburgh, 1988, Churchill Livingstone.

5. Bengmark, S, et al: Obliteration of esophageal varices by PTP: a follow-up of 43 patients, Ann Surg 190:549, 1979.

6. Caldwell, D: Hepatic embolization with an open-ended guide wire, Radiology 165:285, 1987.

7. Cho, KJ, Schmidt, RW, and Lenz, J: Effect of experimental embolization of superior mesenteric artery branch on the intestine, Invest Radiol 14:207, 1979.

8. Chuang, VP, and Reuter, SR: Selective arterial embolization for the control of traumatic splenic bleeding, Invest Radiol 10:18, 1975.

9. Cope, C: Balloon dilatation of closed mesocaval shunts, AJR 135:989, 1980.

10. DeJode, LR, Nicholls, RJ, and Wright, PL: Ischemic necrosis of the gallbladder following hepatic artery embolization, Br J Surg 63:621, 1976.

11. Dickerman, JD: Splenectomy and sepsis: a warning, Pediatrics 63:938, 1979.

12. Doppman, JL, Girton, ME, and Vermess, M: Risk of hepatic artery embolization in the presence of obstructive jaundice, Radiology 143:37, 1982.

13. Dotter, CT, and Judkins, MP: Transluminal treatment of arteriosclerotic obstruction: description of a technique and a preliminary report of its application, Circulation 30:654, 1964.

14. Fagan, EA, et al: Treatment of haemobilia by selective arterial embolization, Gut 21:541, 1980.

15. Freeny, PC, et al: Long-term radiographic-pathologic follow-up of patients treated with visceral transcatheter occlusion using isobutyl 2-cyanocrylate (Bucrylate), Radiology 132:51, 1979.

16. Funaro, A, et al: Transhepatic obliteration of esophageal varices using the stainless steel coil, AJR 133:1123, 1979.

17. Gerlock, AF, Jr, et al: Partial splenic embolization for hypersplenism in renal transplantation, AJR 138:451, 1982.

18. Jander, HP, et al: Emergency embolization in blunt hepatic trauma, AJR 129:249, 1977.

19. Jonasson, O, Spigos, DG, and Mozes, MF: Partial splenic embolization: experience in 136 patients, World J Surg 9:461, 1985.

20. Jonsson, K, Bjernstad, A, and Eriksson, B: Treatment of a hepatic artery aneurysm by coil occlusion of the hepatic artery, AJR 134:1245, 1980.

21. Kadir, S, and Athanasoulis, CA: Angiographic management of gastrointestinal bleeding with vasopressin, Fortschr Geb Rontgenstr Nuklearmed Erganzungsbad 127:11, 1977.

22. Kanno, T, et al: Effects of arterial administration of high molecular weight anticancer agent SMANCS with lipid lymphographic agent on hepatoma: a preliminary report, Eur J Cancer Clin Oncol 19:1058, 1983.

23. Kobayashi, H, et al: Intra-arterial injection of Adriamycin/Mitomycin C Lipiodol suspension in liver metastases, Acta Radiol 28:275, 1987.

24. Kumpe, DA, et al: Partial splenic embolization in children for hypersplenism, Radiology 155:357, 1985.

25. Lunderquist, A, and Vang, J: Transhepatic catheterization and obliteration of the coronary vein in patients with portal hypertension and esophageal varices, N Engl J Med 291:646, 1974.

26. Lunderquist, A, et al: Isobutyl 2-cyanoacrylate (Bucrylate) in obliteration of gastric coronary vein and esophageal varices, AJR 130:1, 1978.

27. Lunderquist, A, et al: Gelfoam powder embolization of the hepatic artery in liver metastases of carcinoid tumors, Radiologe 22:65, 1982.

28. Lunderquist, A, et al: Pharmacologic influence on esophageal varices: a preliminary report, Cardiovasc Intervent Radiol 6:65, 1983.

29. Mozes, MF, et al: Partial splenic embolization: an alternative to splenectomy—results of a prospective, randomized study, Surgery 96:694, 1984.

30. Nusbaum, M, Baum, S, and Blakemore, WS: Clinical experience with the diagnosis and management of gastrointestinal hemorrhage by selective mesenteric catheterization, Ann Surg 170:506, 1969.

31. Owman, T, et al: Embolization of the spleen for the treatment of splenomegaly and hypersplenism in patients with portal hypertension, Invest Radiol 14:457, 1979.

32. Palmaz, JC, et al: Normal and stenotic renal arteries: experimental balloon-expandable intraluminal stenting, Radiology 164:705, 1987.

33. Pereiras, R, et al: The role of interventional radiology in diseases of the hepatobiliary system and the pancreas, Radiol Clin North Am 17:555, 1979.

34. Perlberger, RR: Control of hemobilia by angiographic embolization, AJR 128:672, 1977.

35. Politis, C, et al: Partial splenic embolisation for hypersplenism of thalassaemia major: five year follow up, Br Med J 294:665, 1987.

36. Peuyo, I, et al: Carcinoid syndrome treated by hepatic embolization, AJR 131:511, 1978.

37. Renert, WA, et al: Mesenteric venous thrombosis and small bowel infarction following infusion of vasopressin into the superior mesenteric artery, Radiology 102:299, 1972.

38. Rosenkrantz, H, et al: Postembolic colonic infarction, Radiology 142:47, 1982.

39. Rousseau, H, et al: Self-expanding endovascular prosthesis: an experimental study, Radiology 164:709, 1987.

40. Rubin, BE, and Katzen, BT: Selective hepatic artery embolization to control massive hepatic hemorrhage after trauma, AJR 129:253, 1977.

41. Sherman, LM, Shenoy, SS, and Cerra, FB: Selective intra-arterial vasopressin: clinical efficacy and complications, Ann Surg 189:298, 1979.

42. Steckman, ML, et al: Major gastrointestinal hemorrhage from peripancreatic blood vessels in pancreatitis: treatment by embolotherapy, Dig Dis Sci 29:486, 1984.

43. Turrer, J, et al: Treatment of abdominal angina with percutaneous dilatation of an arteria mesenterica superior stenosis, Cardiovasc Intervent Radiol 3:43, 1980.

44. Uflacker, R: Percutaneous transhepatic obliteration of gastroesophageal varices using absolute alcohol, Radiology 146:621, 1983.

45. Uflacker, R: Transcatheter embolization for treatment of lower gastrointestinal bleeding, Acta Radiol 28:425, 1987.

46. Viamonte, M, Jr, et al: Transhepatic obliteration of gastroesophageal varices: results in acute and nonacute bleeders, AJR 129:237, 1977.

47. Wagner, WH, Lundell, CJ, and Donovan, AJ: Percutaneous angiographic embolization for hepatic arterial hemorrhage, Arch Surg 120:1241, 1985.

48. Walker, WJ, et al: Per catheter control of haemorrhage from the superior and inferior mesenteric arteries, Clin Radiol 31:71, 1980.

49. Walter, JF, Paaso, BT, and Cannon, WB: Successful transcatheter embolic control of massive hematobilia secondary to liver biopsy, AJR 127:847, 1976.

50. White, RJ, et al: Therapeutic embolization with detachable balloon, Cardiovasc Intervent Radiol 3:299, 1980.

51. Widrich, WC, Robbin, AH, and Nabseth, DC: Transhepatic embolization of varices, cardiovasc Intervent Radiol 3:298, 1980.

52. Witt, WS, et al: Interruption of gastroesophageal varices: steel coil technique, AJR 135:829, 1980.

53. Zannini, G, et al: Percutaneous splenic artery occlusion for portal hypertension, Arch Surg, 118:897, 1983.

54. Zucker, K, et al: Nonoperative management of splenic trauma: conservative or radical treatment? Arch Surg 119:400, 1984.

80 *Biliary Tract*

H. JOACHIM BURHENNE

GENERAL CONSIDERATIONS

Biliary interventional radiology began in 1972 with nonoperative extraction of retained common duct stones.[6] This new radiologic subspecialty expanded rapidly, with internal catheter drainage for the relief of obstructive jaundice described in 1974 and dilatation of biliary tract strictures in 1975.[10] The growing body of manipulative radiologic interventions (see the box on p. 2048) entails clinical judgment, manual skill, and responsibility to the patient before, during, and after the procedure.[62]

Access to the biliary tract for interventional procedures can be gained through three different routes: retrograde with gastrointestinal endoscopy, antegrade through the liver, or through the T-tube tract (Fig. 80-1). Retrograde procedures were developed by gastroenterologists, and the majority of endoscopic procedures are still performed by these specialists. The transhepatic approach was pioneered by radiologists as a further development of percutaneous needle cholangiography. It is primarily designed for bile drainage to prepare the patient for surgery or to avoid operative procedures in patients with a poor prognosis from a carcinoma of the bile ducts or pancreas. The subhepatic radiologic approach uses the postoperative drainage tracts. Procedures are performed primarily in ambulatory patients. Percutaneous extraction of retained stones is now practiced in preference to repeated surgery. This subhepatic approach also permits internal drainage of bile and a variety of other interventional radiologic techniques for diagnosis, therapy, or palliation.

Radiation exposure

Attention has been drawn to the possibility of an excessive radiation dose to the radiologist's finger during procedures such as percutaneous transhepatic cholangiography.[27] By means of thermoluminescent monitors taped to the index finger of the hand holding the needle butt, it was found that radiologists might approach or exceed the maximum permissible dose for extremities. The number of examinations that one radiologist can safely perform in a year is limited, even if the screening diaphragm is coned to a field of about 10 × 10 cm throughout the course of each examination.

Interventional radiologic procedures of the biliary

☐ **INTERVENTIONAL BILIARY RADIOLOGY** ☐

1. Nonoperative removal of retained stones	Subhepatic—1962[76] Retrograde—1974[22] Transcholecystic—1974[69] Transhepatic—1979[31]	
2. Restoration of tube patency	Subhepatic—1975[63]	
3. Biliary shockwave lithotripsy	Intracorporeal—1975[11] Extracorporeal—1986[96]	Prosthesis—1964[114]
4. Internal bile	Subhepatic—1974[8] Transhepatic	Catheter—1974[74]
5. Stricture dilatation	Subhepatic—1974[8,10] Transhepatic—1978[75]	
6. Biopsy	Subhepatic—1975[9,84] Transhepatic—1979[71]	

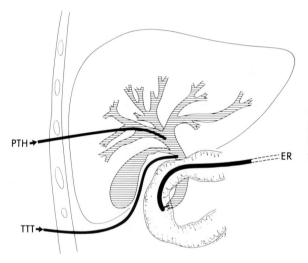

Fig. 80-1 Nonoperative routes of access to biliary tract. *PTH*, Percutaneous transhepatic; *TTT*, trans T-tube tract (other subhepatic access routes are via cholecystostomy or enterostomy tract); *ER*, endoscopic retrograde.

tract may involve more fluoroscopy time than percutaneous cholangiography. Strict attention to radiation protection is therefore mandatory, with the following precautions:

1. Fingers should never be in the primary beam.
2. Collimation should be to the smallest possible field, preferably 3 × 5 cm.
3. The Roentgen ray tube should be under the table.
4. Under-table collimation is ideal.
5. A lead apron with a window should be draped over the patient.
6. Instruments should be moved between fluoroscopy procedures.
7. Radiation-resistant sterile gloves* can be used.

*Available from Arco Medical Products Co., Leechburg, PA

8. Radiation exposure to fingertips should be periodically monitored with a thermoluminescent monitor.
9. The number of procedures performed annually, total screening time, and extrapolations of total radiation dose to the radiologist's finger should be recorded.

Endoscopy

Retrograde endoscopic intervention in the treatment of common duct stones using endoscopic papillotomy was described in 1974.[22] This technique is detailed in Chapter 81. It is the procedure of choice in high-risk patients with common duct stones.[54] The overall mortality is 1.2%.[94] If the T-tube remains in place, the antegrade interventional technique through the T-tube tract

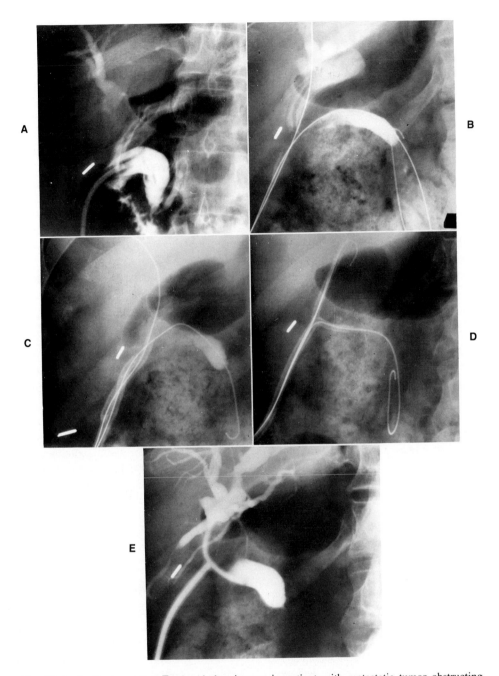

Fig. 80-2. A, Postoperative T-tube cholangiogram in patient with metastatic tumor obstructing common hepatic duct. Common duct is dilated because of previous stone disease. Patient requires catheter placement for internal drainage and relief of jaundice. **B,** Proximal and distal guide wires have been placed with steerable catheter. **C,** T-tube is being advanced through sinus tract. **D,** T-tube has been placed beyond obstruction. **E,** In final cholangiogram, ampullary portion is spastic from catheter instrumentation. Patient was maintained on internal drainage for 16 months until death.

is therefore the procedure of choice for the removal of postoperatively retained biliary tract stones.[23,111]

Biliary tract prostheses can be inserted endoscopically via the papilla of Vater.[102] A combined radiologic and endoscopic intervention is useful for patients with difficult endoscopic access to the biliary tract.[38] The same approach can also be used for patients with stenosis of the papilla of Vater.[66] Endoscopic sphincterotomy and common duct stone removal provides relief of obstruction in patients without T-tube access. Cholecystectomy, however, should be advocated whenever possible after endoscopic shincterotomy because of the high incidence of acute cholecystitis in patients with gallstones.[104]

Percutaneous antegrade electropapillotomy was first described as another feasible radiologic interventional technique in animals.[42] Transcholecystis sphincterotomy was then applied in humans[18] and modified for percutaneous transhepatic approach for successful relief of mechanical obstructive jaundice.[25] The transhepatic approach can be extended to biliary endoscopic procedures.[100]

Nonsurgical removal of retained biliary calculi is also accomplished by endoscopic methods through the T-tube tract.[116] It requires hospitalization of the patient and is technically more difficult than stone removal with the steerable catheter, particularly if stones are lodged in the distal common duct or in intrahepatic radicles. In my experience, calculi in the intrahepatic and extrahepatic bile ducts are more easily visualized during fluoroscopic cholangiography than by endoscopy. Endoscopic techniques are more suitable, however, for biopsy procedures accomplished through the T-tube tract.[78]

Tube replacement

Indwelling tubes may require replacement because of dislodgement, inadvertent extraction, or obstruction by an encrustation of bile sediment. Restoration of the tube's patency was originally accomplished by passing guidewires through the obstructed T-tube.[63] Insertion of a torque guidewire under fluoroscopic control can successfully disimpact the occlusion.[50] The obstruction of draining tubes by sediment and bile encrustation, however, is a recurring problem, and I prefer to replace the obstructed tube by placing a new and clean catheter into the bile ducts. This can readily be accomplished even with a T-tube. Nonoperative replacement of a T-tube in the common duct after inadvertent removal was first described in 1971, accomplished by use of the Seldinger technique.[30] Replacement has also been described with the steerable catheter.[49] T-tubes have been modified for this purpose.[91] Reinsertion over a guidewire[28] or over a stiffer Teflon dilator[101] has been described.

I have found that the insertion of a T-tube is easier with the use to two guidewires (Fig. 80-2). Separate guidewires are placed through the T-tube tract into the proximal and distal bile ducts, and the two short arms of the T-tube are then inserted over the guidewires separately. Both guidewires are then fed through the long arm of the T-tube. The critical catheter width is at the junction of the short and long arms, where the two short arms are folded alongside of each other. T-tubes with short arms smaller than the long arms[7] are available for this purpose.* It is important to insert the largest possible T-tube to maintain a satisfactory T-tube tract. Dilatation of the sinus tract with Grüntzig balloons may be required before insertion of the T-tube.

The skin fixation of an indwelling tube is accomplished by using the conventional method with a stitch at the skin level. This technique, however, may lead to infection at the skin level and painful subsequent instrumentation. I prefer stitching the tube to a Stomahesive wafer.†

T-tubes may be converted into transhepatic U-tubes by a percutaneous approach.[17] This is useful in patients with multiple intrahepatic stones that require multiple sessions for removal and in patients with bile duct strictures for long-term stenting. The steerable catheter is used for the replacement of U-tubes following their inadvertent removal.[49]

Anesthesia

Intravenous analgesia is rarely required during nonoperative basket retrieval of retained common duct stones. Other interventional radiologic biliary procedures such as catheter drainage, however, usually cause pain, discomfort, and anxiety, making sedation, analgesia, or even anesthesia necessary.[59] Intravenous application of fentanyl and diazepam usually suffices in otherwise painful interventional procedures.[73] Pain control after biliary drainage is well treated with local infiltration anesthesia.[58]

BILIARY DRAINAGE

Biliary drainage can be accomplished via the transhepatic or subhepatic route, and in the vast majority of cases is performed in patients with malignant obstruction of the extrahepatic bile ducts.[47] Interventional relief of biliary tract obstruction allows bile to pass normally from the liver through the ducts into the gut. The technique was first described in the surgical literature in 1964[114] with the use of a prosthesis and was modified by radiologists in 1974[74] (Figs. 80-3 to 80-5).

---

*Whelan-Moss T-tube, available from Davol Inc., Cranston, RI.
†Stomahesive wafer No. 4288, available from Squibb, Princeton, NJ.

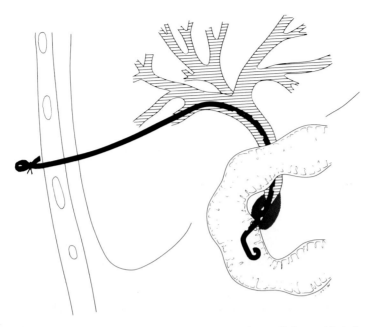

Fig. 80-3 Transhepatic internal bile drainage with pigtail catheter. Catheter side holes are placed in common hepatic duct above obstructing carcinoma of pancreas.

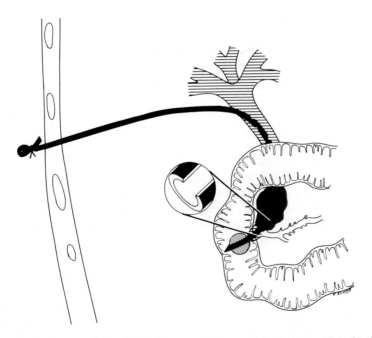

Fig. 80-4 Catheter placement through T-tube tract for internal bile drainage. Note fixation at skin level and in duodenum. Enlarged cutout section shows lateral groove in drainage catheter for internal pancreatic drainage.

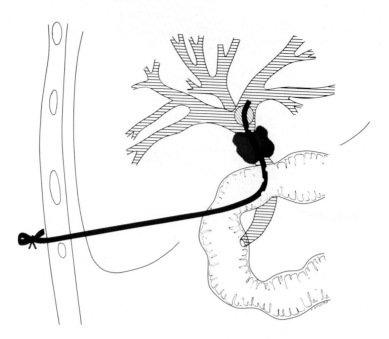

Fig. 80-5 Internal catheter drainage of malignant common hepatic duct stricture using postoperative subhepatic T-tube tract. Retention is maintained by balloon above lesion and closure at skin level.

External bile drainage

The extension of transhepatic cholangiography from a diagnostic role to therapeutic external bile drainage was initiated in Argentina. The transhepatic needle was left in place 7 days for drainage, and small catheters were used in subsequent patients to provide an external bile fistula.[89] Pruritus and jaundice usually improved within a few days.[45]

Percutaneous transhepatic cholangiography and percutaneous transhepatic external biliary drainage may necessitate two separate punctures of the intrahepatic biliary tract. Performing fine-needle cholangiography as the first step facilitates fluoroscopically directed catheterization of the bile duct most suitable for subsequent introduction of the drainage catheter.[107] The catheter remains in place for external drainage into a bile bag. As with transhepatic cholangiography, the routine use of antibiotics is recommended.

Preoperative bile drainage

Previous publications have indicated that preoperative biliary decompression reduces the incidence of postoperative complications and death in patients undergoing surgery for obstructive jaundice.[28,41] However, more recent randomized studies to determine the effect of preoperative drainage on operative mortality, morbidity, hospital stay, and hospital cost have shown no reduced operative risk but an increase in hospital cost.[86] Preoperative drainage diminishes serum bilirubin levels but

does not reduce perioperative morbidity, and the justification for routine use of preoperative biliary drainage has been questioned.[46] I do not perform routine preoperative biliary decompression but employ percutaneous transhepatic biliary drainage as the initial treatment of choice in selected patients with acute cholangitis.[85] Though preoperative drainage does not affect mortality or postoperative complications, it is the alternative nonsurgical procedure for patients in whom surgical decompression is not indicated.[61]

Internal bile drainage

Percutaneous decompression of obstructive jaundice for internal drainage was a logical extension of percutaneous transhepatic cholangiography and external drainage. It was first described in 1974.[74] A catheter is advanced through the obstructing lesion in the bile duct over a guidewire to act as a conduit. Internal drainage catheters may be placed transhepatically or subhepatically through a benign or malignant stricture. Side holes are placed above and an end hole below the lesion. Successful internal drainage was achieved in 75% of 200 patients.[81] Drainage catheters can also be placed for intrahepatic biliary obstruction caused by cholangiocarcinoma or sclerosing cholangitis.

The right upper lateral abdomen is prepared and draped. Fine-needle cholangiography is performed as the first stage. After the obstruction is identified and the indications for internal drainage are considered, a larger

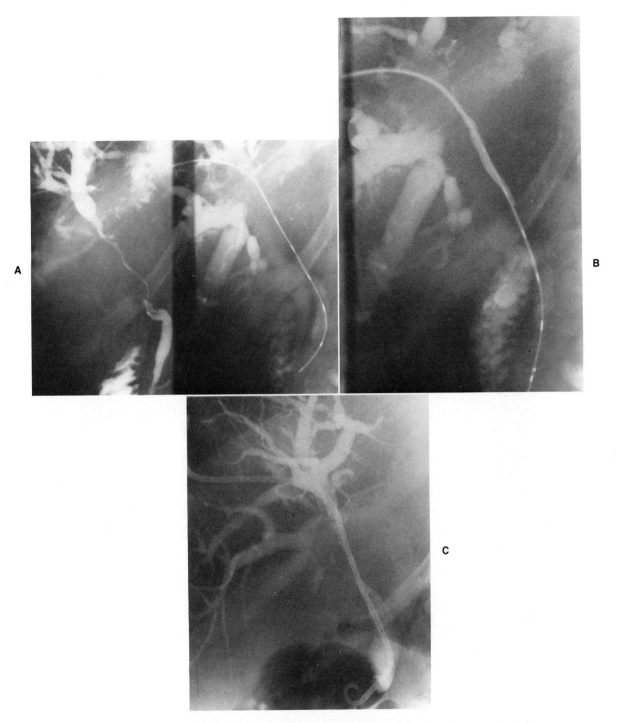

Fig. 80-6 A, Transhepatic cholangiogram shows long malignant stricture caused by cholangiocar-cinoma involving porta hepatis and common hepatic duct. Torque wire has been placed through stricture. **B,** Stricture was dilated with 4-mm Grümtzig balloon catheter with several inflations. **C,** Pigtail catheter in place for internal bile drainage. Note that other right hepatic radicles show involvement by tumor at porta hepatis. Pigtail catheter is being withdrawn from duodenum on this cholangiogram obtained 3 days after instrumentation. Left hepatic duct required additional internal drainage 2 weeks later.

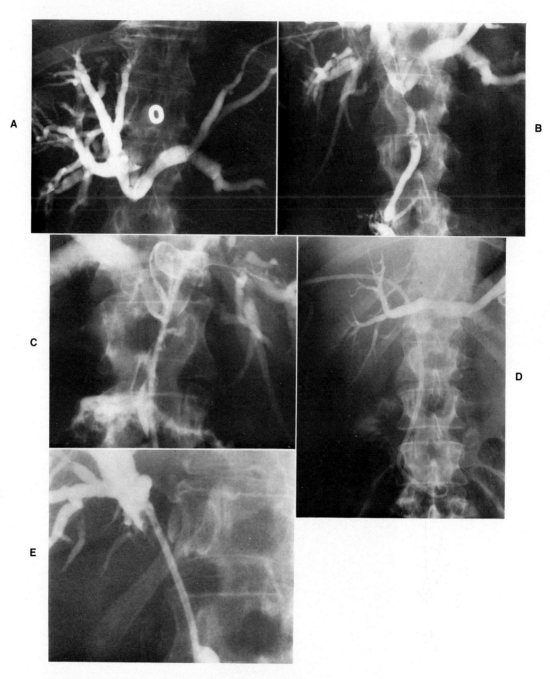

Fig. 80-7 A, Transhepatic cholangiogram showing complete obstruction at proximal common hepatic duct. **B,** Small catheter has been wedged into rattail of Klatzkin tumor. Forceful injection of undiluted contrast medium now results in demonstration of malignant stricture extent. **C,** Filling defect in hepatic ducts on day of instrumentation demonstrates hemobilia. Follow-up study 3 days later showed blood clots resolved. **D,** Pigtail catheter in place for internal bile drainage. **E,** Follow-up cholangiogram 3 months after internal drainage procedure shows tumor extension into right hepatic duct.

18-gauge needle with a thin-wall polyethylene sheath is directed under fluoroscopic guidance toward a hepatic duct with straight access to the common hepatic duct. Once the hepatic duct has been punctured, a variable-size J-torque wire is used for placement of the sheathed catheter further into the region of the obstruction. A common practice is to puncture the desired hepatic duct, withdraw the needle, and then slowly withdraw the sheath until the free flow of bile has been obtained. This indicates the intraductal position. If a guidewire cannot be advanced through the obstruction, the drainage catheter is left in place. After 48 hours of external drainage, it is often possible to advance the guidewire through the point of obstruction to accomplish internal stenting and bile drainage (Fig. 80-6).

It is my practice to wedge a catheter into the rattail of the obstruction, give a small forceful injection of undiluted contrast medium for visualization of the stricture channel, and pass a torque guide* through it at the first interventional session (Fig. 80-7).

Once the guidewire is seen to enter the duodenum, it is replaced by a drainage catheter. A modified pigtail catheter is now commonly used.[90] Side holes above and below the obstruction provide for the internal drainage of bile. The catheter is secured at the skin with sutures or by sutering it to a Stomahesive wafer (Fig. 80-7).

Daily flushing of the catheter with bacteriostatic saline has been recommended.

The use of a modified 45-cm long Chiba needle† often permits placement in a single-stage procedure. The initial transhepatic cholangiogram is directed more posteriorly toward the right hepatic ducts. The sheath over the Chiba needle is then inserted into the ducts; the needle is removed, and catheters of increasing sizes are placed over guidewires. A No. 6 French dilator may have to be moved over the guidewire, and further dilators are required if a drainage catheter larger than a No. 8 French polyethylene catheter is to be placed. Most radiologists now use the COOK*-COPE biliary drainage set.

As described for transhepatic cholangiography, antibiotics are administered before the procedure is started. The platelet count and prothrombin time are determined and should be within normal limits. Care must be taken that the side holes of the catheter do not lie within hepatic parenchyma. As with other percutaneous transhepatic procedures, the complications are sepsis, bile leakage, hemorrhage, and possible bile peritonitis.

For additional drainage through the left hepatic duct

---

*THG 100678, available from Cook Inc., Bloomington, IN.
†Available from Cook Inc., Bloomington, IN.

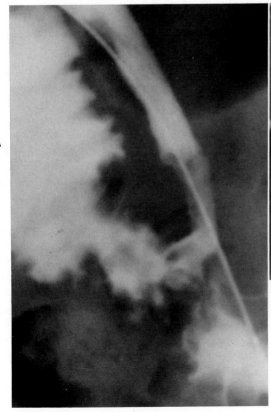

A

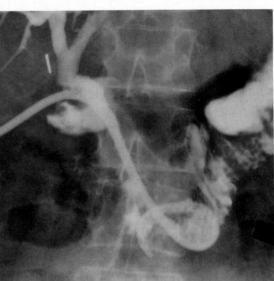

B

Fig. 80-8 A and B, Internal drainage procedure performed for distal common duct lesion with short malignant stricture at choledochoduodenal junction. Note tumor mass invading duodenum. Biopsy through drainage tract revealed adenocarcinoma at papilla of Vater. Patient underwent surgical resection with Whipple procedure.

system in cases with an obstruction at the porta hepatis, the procedure involves a 45-degree angle approach under the left costal margin toward the area of the porta hepatis. As with external biliary fistulas, incomplete drainage may result in cholangitis, sepsis, and abscess formation.

Insertion of the catheter for internal drainage may be difficult and time consuming. Placing the patient in a cradle or using a C-arm is most useful for fluoroscopic direction of the sheathed needle into the desired intrahepatic duct. Anteroposterior and lateral films may be required if this equipment is not available.

Percutaneous transhepatic internal biliary drainage is the treatment of choice for patients with a malignant bile duct obstruction caused by unresectable lesions originating in the pancreas or common duct or with an obstruction caused by metastatic disease surrounding the porta hepatis. This indication applies particularly to the large number of technically difficult patients in whom surgical bypass is not possible.[40]

Computed tomography (CT) may demonstrate iatrogenic hepatic lesions following percutaneous transhepatic instrumentation.[106] Hepatic CT is indicated with patients scheduled for surgical bypass of obstructing malignant bile duct lesions. If metastases are present, transhepatic internal drainage is certainly preferable to surgery. Upper gastrointestinal studies and endoscopy are required to identify tumors of the papilla of Vater because these lesions are better treated by resection, and a possible cure may be overlooked if internal catheter drainage is performed (Fig. 80-8).

Internal bile drainage is technically easier with the subhepatic approach than with the percutaneous transhepatic procedure. It requires previous surgical access to the bile ducts but has the following advantages: (1) a large-diameter catheter can be placed, providing better long-term drainage; (2) less technical skill and time are required and radiation exposure is decreased; (3) structures are more easily dilated with Grüntzig balloons: (4) inadvertent tube removal is less likely because of easier tube retention; (5) complications of the transhepatic approach, such as a fluid leak at the capsule, hemorrhage, or parenchymal damage are avoided; (6) added internal pancreatic drainage is more readily provided; and (7) softer rubber catheters may be used for patient comfort in long-term indwelling tubes (Fig. 80-4).

Subhepatic internal drainage can be performed in a retrograde fashion as described in a 1974 case involving a stricture at the site of hepatojejunostomy[8] (Fig. 80-9). The obstructing benign stricture at the anastomosis was entered with a guidewire through a jejunostomy tract, the stricture was distended with a balloon catheter, and a Silastic-coated balloon catheter was placed to splint the previous stricture. An end hole above and side holes

below the lesion provided for internal drainage. The catheter was clamped at the skin.

The same technique may be applied through the T-tube tract in cases of malignant lesions close to the porta hepatis from a duct carcinoma or metastasis, and in cases of obstructing carcinomas in the distal common duct (Figs. 80-10 and 80-11). The retention balloon is then placed into the duodenum. No skin fixation of the closed catheter is necessary. Internal biliary drainage catheters have also been placed via the transcystic duct approach.[97]

I place bilateral or multiple drainage catheters only if required because of hepatic abscess formation or cholangitis and only if a single catheter is insufficient to provide palliation. Cross-connection for bilateral percutaneous biliary drainage in patients with multisegmental obstruction of the bile ducts avoids the disadvantage of external biliary drainage.[3] Biliary drainage catheters can be converted from external to internal drainage with the use of an additional catheter advanced through a gastrostomy opening.[77]

The reports on complications from percutaneous biliary drainage vary greatly. Major complications can be as low as 5%[44,117] and as high as 35%.[83] It appears to depend greatly on the experience of the interventional radiologist and whether mortality figures are assessed during the conventional 3-week period or less. Endoscopically performed biliary drainage has been reported to carry a lower mortality than percutaneous transhepatic catheter placement.[103]

Biliary endoprosthesis

Placement of an internal biliary drainage prosthesis avoids some the problems of bile leakage, infection, catheter displacement, and patient intolerance often associated with catheter drainage. Following routine transhepatic cholangiography, a sheathed needle is passed with a lateral approach in the seventh or eighth intercostal space in midaxillary line to enter a distended bile duct. A flexible guidewire is then passed under fluoroscopic control into the hepatic or common bile duct and advanced through the obstruction. Bending the guidewire at the tip and rotating it is usually successful for passage of the stricture. If initial instrumentation into the duodenum is not successful, the procedure is repeated after external drainage for several days. Insertion of the endoprosthesis is performed with the help of an introducer of the same diameter. The endoprosthesis is centered in the obstruction with sufficient extension for drainage both above and below. An anterior subcostal approach from the left may also be employed to place an endoprosthesis through the left main hepatic radicle. The soft endoprosthesis by Carey-Coons is my preferred drainage device.[26]

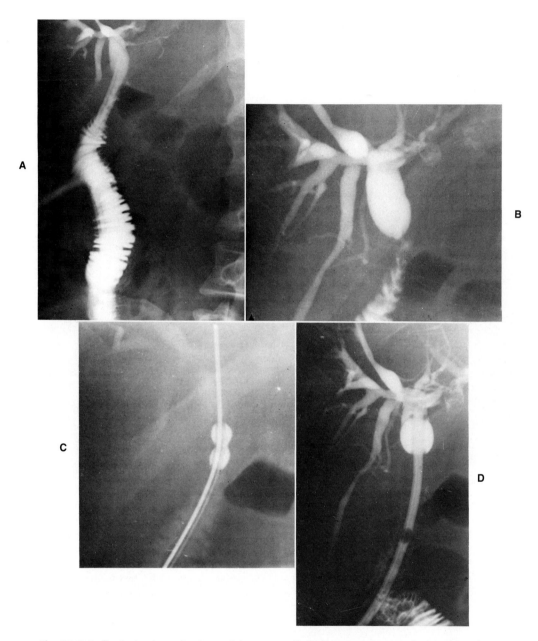

Fig. 80-9 A, T-tube in place after hepatojejunostomy. **B,** Stricture at anastomosis site with patients jaundiced 3 weeks after short arm of T-tube slipped back into jejunum. **C,** Balloon catheter placed over guide wire through jejunostomy is seen distended with contrast medium during stricture dilatation. **D,** Retention catheter in place after stricture dilatation with retention balloon inflated in common hepatic duct above hepatojejunostomy. Side hole in Silastic catheter provides for internal drainage with catheter closed at skin. Note narrowing of intrahepatic ducts from previous cholangitis. Stones ratained in left hepatic duct were removed in subsequent session. Catheter remained in place for 2½ years to maintain and splint previous stricture. This 1974 case was first instance of interventional radiology for nonoperative stricture dilatation and internal drainage.

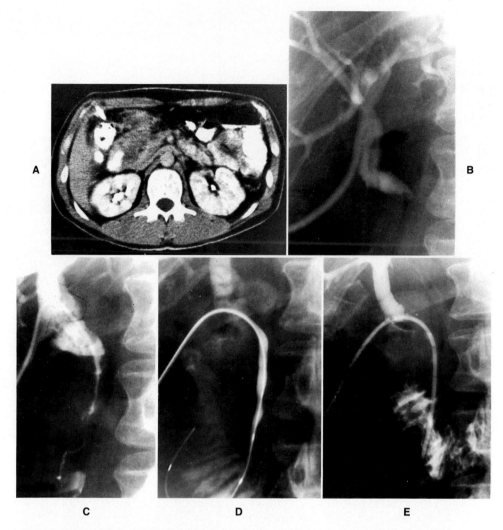

Fig. 80-10 A, Carcinoma of head of pancreas as seen on CT scan with involvement of uncinate process and obliteration of vena cava plane. Surgical exploration for resection was attempted. **B,** Postoperative T-tube cholangiogram shows complete obstruction by unresectable tumor in head of pancreas. Lesion was considerably larger than seen on CT. T-tube was placed. **C,** Interventional procedure 3 weeks after exploration demonstrated malignant stricture with catheter wedged in rattail and with forced contrast injection. **D,** Dilatation of malignant stricture with Grüntzig balloon. **E,** Internal bile drainage catheter in place via subhepatic approach with side holes above malignant stricture. Retention balloon catheter in duodenum was then inflated with saline.

Obstruction and migration of the endoprosthesis and also duodenal perforation may occur.[39,79] Clinical overall satisfaction, however, is better with endoprosthesis than with catheter drainage.[112]

Placement of an internal stent via the percutaneous transhepatic route is now less commonly used because of the advances that have occurred in endoscopic approaches. The advent of the larger duodenoscope allows for the placement of large-bore prosthesis, minimizing the problem of early cholangitis and clogging of the endoprosthesis. The choice of endoprosthesis placement depends on the availability of local expertise (Fig.

80-12). Expandable stents constructed of stainless steel wire are more recent innovation and hold promise for use in the biliary tract.[21]

Local radiotherapy

With widespread acceptance of percutaneous transhepatic drainage as an established technique, localized internal radiotherapy using iridium-192 wire by means of transhepatic catheter has been described. Patients may receive either internal radiation alone or in combination with external irradiation. An increase in mean survival time with this technique has been reported,[52] though more

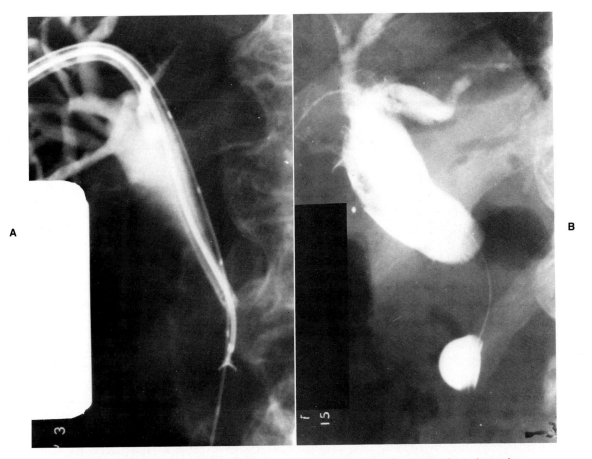

Fig. 80-11 A, Endoscopic wire forceps are placed through steerable catheter into obstructing malignant stricture. Torque wire indicates position of narrowed common duct. Biopsy tissue shows carcinoma of pancreas. Previous surgical open needle biopsy and repeated percutaneous needle biopsy under ultrasonography had negative results. **B,** Subhepatic internal drainage catheter in place with retention balloon inflated in duodenum. Balloon inflation with saline is preferred because contrast withdrawal and balloon deflation may become difficult with long-term indwelling catheter drainage.

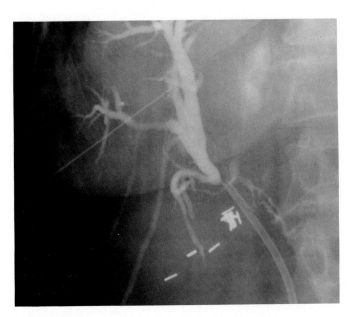

Fig. 80-12 Transhepatic cholangiogram demonstrating distal migration of endoprosthesis 3 weeks after initial placement. Note filling of lymphatics. Prosthesis was extracted by endoscopy and replaced.

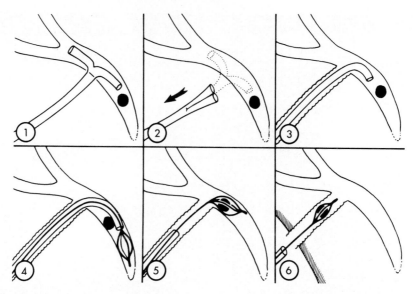

Fig. 80-13 Technical steps of subhepatic stone extraction. *1*, T-tube cholangiogram shows retained common duct stone. *2*, Catheter is extracted. *3*, Steerable catheter is manipulated through sinus tract into common duct. *4*, Tip of steerable catheter is advanced beyond stone, and wire stone basket is opened distally to stone. *5*, After partial withdrawal of steerable catheter, retained stone is snared in open basket. *6*, Stone is withdrawn through sinus tract.

clinical experience with this adjuvant irradiation therapy is required to obtain evidence of efficacy.[72]

INTERVENTION FOR CHOLELITHIASIS
Stone extraction

The retention of biliary tract stones, as seen with postoperative T-tube cholangiography, after what the experienced surgeon considered to be a thorough removal continues to be an exasperating problem. Routine operative cholangiography[51] has reduced the number of retained stones, but the incidence of false-negative completion cholangiograms is still at least 5% of patients after common duct exploration.[60] This amounts to 3000 patients in the United States annually. The additional use of biliary endoscopy may reduce this figure.[98]

This problem is not new. More than 70 years ago William Halsted,[43] who performed one of the earliest operations on the gallbladder, stated that a simple, reliable method was needed to determine accurately the presence of stones in the common bile duct. Twenty years later, Dr. Halsted was himself to die of complications after the removal of a retained common duct stone.[60]

Retained stones can be treated by nonoperative extraction, by irrigation techniques, by chemical dissolution, or by surgical removal. The radiologic intervention technique of percutaneous removal through the T-tube tract is the method of choice at present.[23] Percutaneous extraction of retained stones via the common duct is

widely practiced; its success rate is 95%.[13,36] The success of this interventional procedure is the result of three developments: the use of the postoperative sinus tract described in 1962,[76] the method of extraction with the Dormia ureteral stone basket added in 1969,[55] and the addition of the steerable catheter in 1972[6] (Fig. 80-13).

The necessary equipment for nonoperative stone extraction includes steerable catheters in three sizes, stone baskets in different sizes from different manufacturers, a steering handle or a wobble plate for catheter manipulation, J-tipped guidewires with a removable core, and a variety of straight catheters for placement in multiple sessions (Fig. 80-14).

The majority of patients are ambulatory at the time of the procedure and receive no premedication. If the patient has a history of postoperative infection or pancreatitis, the patient is admitted and receives preinstrumentation medication of antibiotics (250 mg of cephalexin [Keflex] by mouth every 6 hours). Of 661 patients undergoing stone extraction at my institution, 38 received antibiotic therapy.[13]

The T-tube is extracted as the initial step of the procedure. Cholangiograms are then obtained with use of the steerable catheter. Selective cholangiograms may be required for adequate visualization of anatomic variations and identification of the location of retained stones. The cholangiograms include those made with selective contrast injections of the intrahepatic ducts.

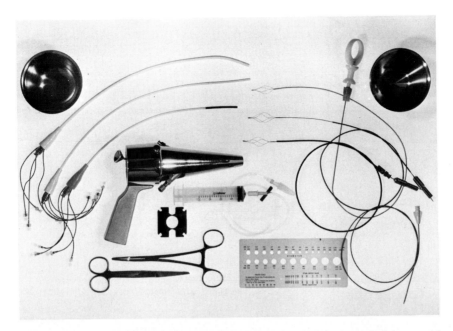

Fig. 80-14 Equipment for percutaneous stone procedure. *Left, top to bottom,* Stainless steel bowl for contrast: 13, 10, and 8 French steerable catheters; control handle; syringe and tubing for hand injection; wobble plate for steerable catheter; hemostat; surgical scissors. *Right, top to bottom,* Stainless steel bowl for saline; Meditech, Dormia, and Cook stone extraction baskets; Fogarty balloon catheter; measuring templet.

The stone basket is maneuvered through the steerable catheter beyond the location of the biliary stones. The steerable catheter is partially withdrawn, and the stone basket is opened. I no longer close the stone basket after the stone has been engaged, because closure often results in the fragmentation or disengagement of the stone. Even small stones remain in the basket tip during a continuous extraction through the duct system and sinus tract. Hesitant withdrawal, however, may permit small stones to fall out the side of the basket. The details of my stone extraction technique were described in 1980.[13]

Small stones and fragments about 3 mm in diameter frequently pass spontaneously through the ampullary part of the common duct into the duodenum. If the short arms of the T-tube prevent retained small stones in the common hepatic duct from moving distally, the T-tube is exchanged for a straight tube early in the postoperative period. This facilitates the spontaneous passage of small stones. The expulsion of biliary stones into the duodenum may be accomplished with the use of catheters; this technique was described in 1970.[34]

The use of a so-called pliable forceps for retraction of retained stones with good success has also been described.[68] This technique is still used today in Argentina.

It may be difficult to advance a steerable catheter beyond a retained stone if it is partially impacted. The small No. 8 steerable catheter or a Fogarty balloon is then used. Wire guides with controllable tip catheters are also in use.[2] Large stones over 6 to 8 mm in diameter cannot be extracted through the sinus tract with a No. 14 French T-tube, and fragmentation is then indicated (Fig. 80-15). In my series of 661 patients, 98 stones required fragmentation.[13] This was possible in all cases, because large retained stones are almost always relatively soft. The stone is brought with the basket to the junction of the bile duct and the sinus tract, where strong resistance is felt. Increasing and steady traction on the end of the basket wire is then applied over 1 to 2 minutes. A hemostat is clamped to the end of the wire basket for manual traction. The other hand presses against the abdominal wall over the sinus tract opening with the wire running between the fingers. No more than a pull of about 10 kg is necessary, and sudden jerks are not advisable. The steady pull results in the stone being cut by the basket wires. No common duct injury has been experienced. In 4-week follow-up studies with intravenous cholangiography in 28 of these patients, no deformity or narrowing at the common duct was seen. However, extravasation from the sinus tract occurred in six patients after stone fragmentation.

After a fragmentation procedure, only the major fragments are extracted in the same session. The patient then returns for a second session for extraction of fragments that have not passed spontaneously. Fragments lost in the sinus tract are pushed with a steerable catheter back into the duct system and then extracted. The success rate

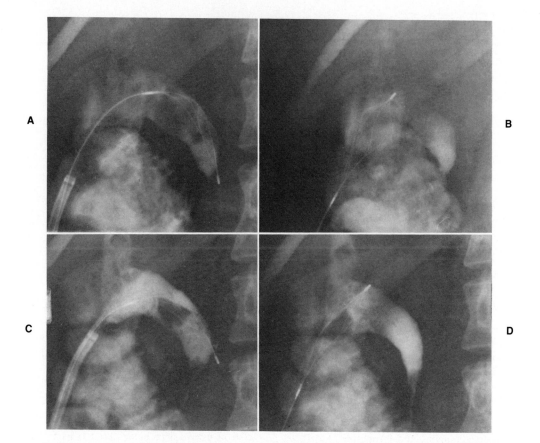

Fig. 80-15 Fragmentation of large retained stone. **A,** Large Cook stone basket has been draped over stone on greater curvature aspect of common duct. Steerable catheter has been withdrawn to sinus tract. **B,** Stone has been ensnared and brought to junction of common duct and sinus tract. Continuous strong traction has been applied to wire of basket. Note deformity of basket during traction, but there is no deviation of bile duct. **C,** Basket has been repositioned after strong fragmentation. Note clean-cut margin of stone produced by basket wire. There is another fragment in common hepatic duct and another in distal end of common duct. **D,** Large fragment has been engaged in basket for further fragmentation. After extraction of some fragments, straight catheter was placed through sinus tract into duct, and all remaining fragments were removed in second session.

of over 90% described in large series[13,36,68] is not obtained by radiologists early in their experience. A 1980 survey of 26 hospitals in England with the treatment of 131 patients revealed an overall success rate of 70% and a marked improvement in success rates with increasing experience.[65]

Impacted stones in hepatic radicles or in the distal common duct may be difficult to engage in the wire basket because their position does not permit complete opening of the basket distally to them. Impacted stones must therefore be moved; this may be accomplished with a variety of maneuvers. Sometimes waiting is beneficial; at a second session the stone may have moved. Suction through the catheter or a strong contrast injection distal to the stone is occasionally of help. If the stone cannot be moved, I proceed to use a vascular Fogarty balloon

catheter (Fig. 80-16). It is distended with contrast material for exact visualization under the fluoroscope. The balloon is inflated and eased centrally with a gentle pull. If the balloon is seen to wedge the stone sideways, no undue traction should be applied. I have not had the complication of bile duct perforation, and the total experience at my institution is now over 2000 patients undergoing radiologic basket extraction.

My survey of 612 patients in 39 institutions showed a morbidity of 5% and no mortality in patients undergoing nonoperative extraction of retained common duct stones.[12] The review of procedures performed in 26 British hospitals showed a complication rate of 9.2%, including pancreatitis, fever, and tract perforation.[65] One death has been reported from acute pancreatitis after radiologic manipulation of a common bile duct stone.[87]

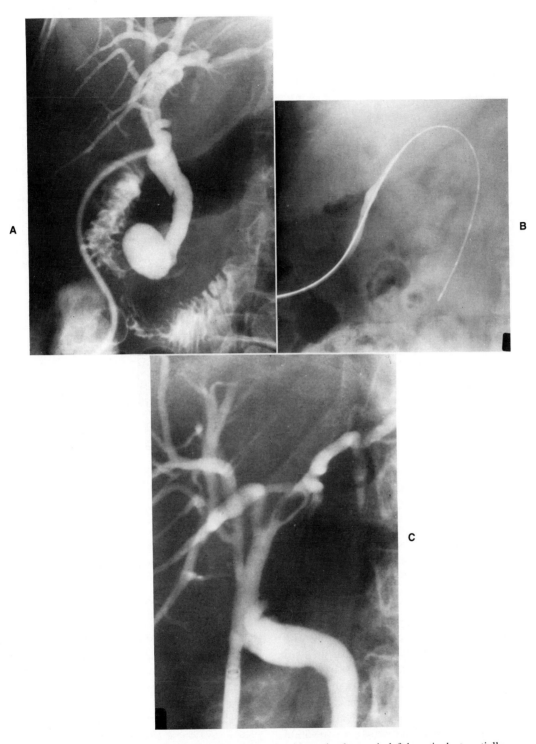

Fig. 80-16 A, Postoperative T-tube cholangiogram with retained stone in left hepatic duct partially hidden on straight projection. Note T-tube insertion in common hepatic duct with long cystic duct remnant. There is juxtapapillary duodenal diverticulum. **B,** Dilatation of T-tube tract using 4-mm Grüntzig balloon over torque wire. **C,** Steerable catheter is in place. Retained stone is now well seen on oblique film.

Continued.

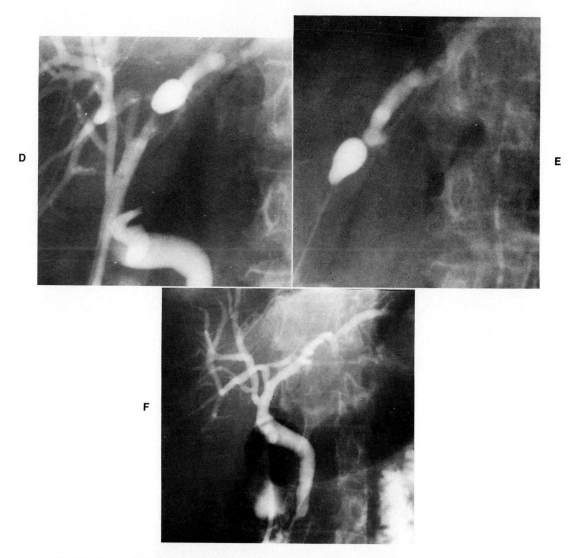

Fig. 80-16, cont'd. D, Fogarty balloon is in place above retained stone. **E,** Fogarty balloon deformity is seen during traction. This indicates wedging by retained stone and requires repositioning of balloon. **F,** Bile ducts are clear after stone removal.

The case involved a small distal common duct stone with difficult instrumentation. The radiologist had previous experience with four stone extractions. It is of interest that this patient had previous history of acute pancreatitis. As well, this patient was transferred with the instruments in place from one fluoroscopic room to another with spot film facilities. I believe that fluoroscopic visualization alone is insufficient, particularly with small stones, because the identification of small stones on the fluoroscopic screen alone can be impossible. A spot film device is mandatory.

It must be remembered that reexploration for retained stones, the previous method of choice for stone removal, carries a mortality of about 3%.[99] At this time nonsurgical removal by the radiologic interventional tech-

nique through the sinus tract remains the procedure of choice.[23,111] Other techniques such as stone dissolution or endoscopic removal have a significantly lower success rate. Endoscopic sphincterotomy for retained common bile duct stones in patients with T-tube in situ can be effective in the early postoperative period but carries at least a 7.7% complication rate, sometimes requiring reoperation.[82] However, noninvasive treatment for retained common bile duct stones in patients with the T-tube in situ, using a saline washout after intravenous medication to relax the sphincter of Oddi, is a procedure with good indication.[105]

Endoscopic sphincterotomy and basket removal of common duct stones is the method of choice if no T-tube access is available. Percutaneous transhepatic interven-

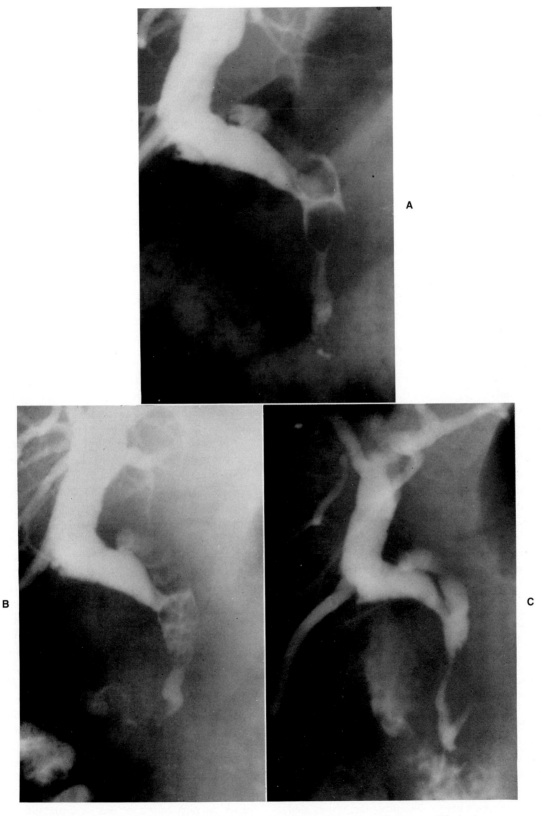

Fig. 80-17 A, Two retained stones impacted in cystic duct remnant are not accessible by interventional technique via T-tube tract. **B,** Extracorporeal shock-wave lithotripsy resulted in stone fragmentation, which permittted subsequent basket extraction. **C,** Duct system is clear of retained material.

tion for removal of bile duct stones can be performed when sphincterotomy with stone removal is technically impossible, for instance, in patients who have previously undergone choledochojejunostomy.[24] Percutaneous stone dissolution with the experimental cholesterol solvent methyl tertiary butyl ether (MTBE) is also a promising technique if basket extraction is not available or is impractical. The use of MTBE is quite time consuming, and the odor is difficult to control.[4] MTBE has been reported to induce rapid dissolution of cholesterol gallstones in the gallbladder.[1]

Shockwave lithotripsy

It was shown in 1975 that electrohydrolytic shockwaves can fragment gallstones in vitro and in vivo.[11] This intracorporeal lithotripsy approach showed 80% calculi fragmentation[64] and was also used by radiologists successfully via a percutaneous transhepatic approach.[57] The first work on extracorporeal fragmentation of gallbladder stones with shockwaves was reported in 1986.[96] Oral chemolitholysis was used as an adjuvant litholytic therapy. Gallbladder stones disintegrated with extracorporeal lithotripsy in all patients but 1 of 175.[93] Ninety percent clearance of stone fragments, however, requires 12 to 18 months.

The experience with lithotripsy of bile duct stones is more encouraging, particularly when interventional access to the biliary tract is available transhepatically, endoscopically, or via a T-tube tract or cholecystostomy.[20] As opposed to fragment passage after cholecystolithotripsy, stone fragments will readily pass through a sphincterotomy or may be amenable for fragment clearing by basket extraction. Lithotripsy of gallbladder stones, however, requires more clinical trial to investigate fragment clearance through the cystic duct and ampulla of Vater. A drawback to this form of treatment is the relatively stringent criteria currently used for selection of patients[119] (Fig. 80-17).

CHOLECYSTOSTOMY PROCEDURES

Similar to interventional access through the postoperative T-tube tract, instrumentation through cholecystostomy tracts is possible to gain access to the gallbladder or the common duct (Fig. 80-18).

Gallbladder stones

Instrumentation through the cholecystostomy tract as a radiologic interventional procedure was first described in 1974.[8] A gallstone impacted in the neck of the gallbladder was successfully removed by applying suction through the steerable catheter. This procedure is indicated for patients following drainage or acute cholecystitis if the patient's general condition does not indicate subsequent gallbladder removal. Gallbladder stones of any size may be crushed and removed through the cholecystos-

tomy tract. Initial dilatation of the sinus with Grüntzig balloon catheters permits easier instrumentation.

Bile duct stones

The same subhepatic interventional approach through the cholecystostomy tract may be used to gain access to the bile ducts. The removal of common bile duct stones through the cholecystostomy opening and cystic duct was first described in 1974.[69] This technique was successful in 9 of 13 patients in the original report. After cholecystocholangiography, curved-tip sounds with stylets were introduced through the cystic duct. The tip of the probe was rotated to negotiate the turns in the cystic duct. After the catheter entered the bile duct, cystic duct dilatation was performed. Every 2 or 3 days a larger sound was introduced. The duration of treatment ranged from 7 days to 2 months.[69]

I have used a modified technique with a steerable catheter and J-shaped guidewires. The No. 8 French steerable catheter is brought to the neck of the gallbladder with the patient in a left anterior oblique position. The tip of the guidewire is then used to negotiate each turn, followed by the steerable catheter. Once the catheter has entered the common duct, a torque guidewire is introduced, and the steerable catheter removed. Grüntzig balloon catheters are used to dilate the cystic duct in the same sitting. The extraction of stones in the common duct is then accomplished in the same manner as with percutaneous instrumentation through the postoperative T-tube tract.

Burckhardt and Muller[5] demonstrated the gallbladder cavity by direct transhepatic puncture in 1921 and transperitoneal cholecystostomy was first performed for drainage of obstructive jaundice in 1979.[33] It is now used for successful catheter drainage of gallbladder empyema under ultrasonic guidance,[88] and is performed in critically ill patients with acute acalculous cholecystitis.[32] Vagal hypotension has been reported in some patients undergoing diagnostic and therapeutic percutaneous gallbladder punctures,[109] but percutaneous gallbladder drainage is otherwise a fast and low-risk procedure well suited for the treatment of acute cholecystitis and poor surgical risk patients.[56] A specially designed catheter is available for percutaneous cholecystostomy.[70]

Percutaneous cholecystostomy for removal of gallstones started with animal work in 1982,[14,15] and percutaneous removal of gallstones as a definitive form of therapy was reported in three patients with acute cholecystitis in 1985.[53]

Patients with acute gallbladder disease who are considered at high operative risk or unsuitable for cholecystectomy can be treated with cholecystostomy catheter insertion under local anesthesia. The gallbladder is sutured into the abdominal wall, and stones from the gallbladder and biliary tract are removed subsequently by

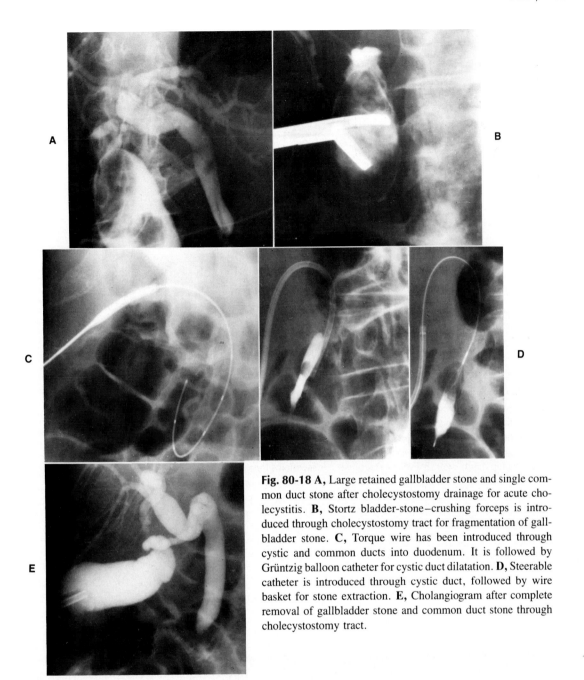

Fig. 80-18 A, Large retained gallbladder stone and single common duct stone after cholecystostomy drainage for acute cholecystitis. **B,** Stortz bladder-stone–crushing forceps is introduced through cholecystostomy tract for fragmentation of gallbladder stone. **C,** Torque wire has been introduced through cystic and common ducts into duodenum. It is followed by Grüntzig balloon catheter for cystic duct dilatation. **D,** Steerable catheter is introduced through cystic duct, followed by wire basket for stone extraction. **E,** Cholangiogram after complete removal of gallbladder stone and common duct stone through cholecystostomy tract.

interventional radiologic techniques.[19] This combined surgical and radiologic intervention for complicated cholelithiasis in high-risk patients has been reported with an overall success rate of 86%, with better results for gallbladder stones than for cystic duct stones or common bile duct stones.[37] (Figs. 80-19 and 80-20).

STRICTURE DILATATION

Interventional dilatation of benign bile duct strictures is indicated if biliary stones are retained proximally to such strictures resulting from cholangitis or previous sur-gery. I have used coaxial arterial catheters, ureteral dilators, and specially designed balloon catheters for this purpose but now believe that the Grüntzig arterial balloon catheter is best suited for this purpose.[16] The first case was reported in 1974,[5] and experience with seven patients was reported in 1975.[9] Even malignant strictures are readily dilated in one sitting to accommodate a No. 14 French catheter for internal bile drainage.[16] As well, dilatation of a narrow sinus tract is readily accomplished with the use of the Grüntzig balloon catheter.

It has been suggested that indwelling splint catheters

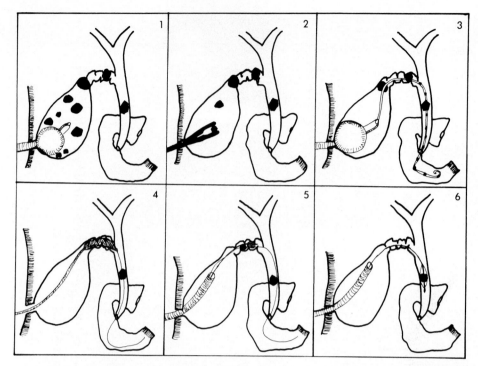

Fig. 80-19 Cholecystostomy intervention for cholelithiasis. *Top left,* Balloon catheter is in place after minicholecystostomy, with gallbladder fundus sutured to abdominal wall. Cholelithiasis affects gallbladder, cystic duct, and common duct. *Top middle,* Stones are removed from gallbladder with Mazzariello forceps under fluoroscopic control 10 days after minicholecystostomy. *Top right,* Drainage catheter with side holes has been placed through cystic and common ducts into duodenum after manipulation with 8 French steerable catheter and guide wire. Drainage catheter is placed through 24 French cholecystostomy balloon catheter between procedures. *Bottom left,* Guide wire is again manipulated into duodenum, and angiographic balloon catheter is placed into cystic duct for dilatation. *Bottom middle,* Stones in cystic duct are retrieved into gallbladder after inflation of Fogarty balloon distal to stone. Guide wire remains in place along side of Fogarty balloon for access. *Bottom right,* Final session involves catheter placement into common duct followed by stone extraction, basket positioning, and extraction of common duct stone through cystic duct and gallbladder. Cholelithiasis treatment is completed.

must remain within previous strictures for a period of 8 to 24 months for the scar to mature and stabilize.[110] I have applied indwelling splinting catheters for periods of up to 2½ years. Patients tolerate indwelling catheters well. Should the catheter become obstructed, it can be readily replaced over a guidewire.

The maturing of a previous stricture or a possible recurrence can be checked by withdrawing the catheter just outside the previous narrowing. The catheter remains in place to keep the sinus tract open. Should the stricture recur, the splint is again placed through it.

Selected benign biliary strictures have now been treated safely and successfully by percutaneous balloon dilatation in a large number of patients. Lasting patency followed removal of biliary stents in 73% of patients with biliary-enteric anastomosis and in 88% of patients

with primary ductal strictures, for an overall success rate of 78%. However, no definite conclusions can be drawn about the utility of long-term internal-external stenting after stricture dilatation.[35,80,95,113,115] Stricture dilatation as a radiologic intervention presents an alternative to surgical revision, particularly after repeat surgical stricture at the anastomosis. Balloon dilatation can be performed through a choledochojejuno-cutaneous fistula[48] or through a stomatized jejunal limb.[92] It has also been employed in strictures in symptomatic patients with primary sclerosing cholangitis[37] (Fig. 80-21).

BIOPSY

Biopsy samples of lesions in the biliary tract can be obtained with the transhepatic and subhepatic approach using the postoperative T-tube tract. This technique was

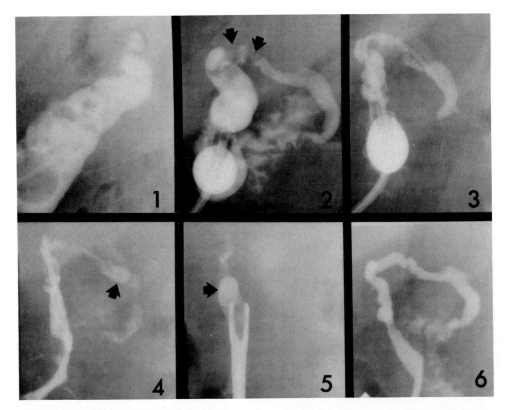

Fig. 80-20 *1,* Patient with acute cholecystitis and cholelithiasis underwent cholecystostomy tube insertion. Cystic duct is obstructed. *2,* After cholecystostomy drainage and treatment of acute cholecystitis, gallbladder stones were removed. Two cystic duct stones are visualized on chole-cystocholangiography *(arrows). 3,* Catheter has been manipulated through cystic duct into common duct. *4,* Fogarty balloon is inflated in cystic duct for cystic duct stone extraction *(arrow). 5,* Fogarty balloon has been withdrawn into gallbladder neck, previous cystic duct stone has been engaged in stone forceps. *6,* Gallbladder, cystic duct, and common ducts are clear of stone material.

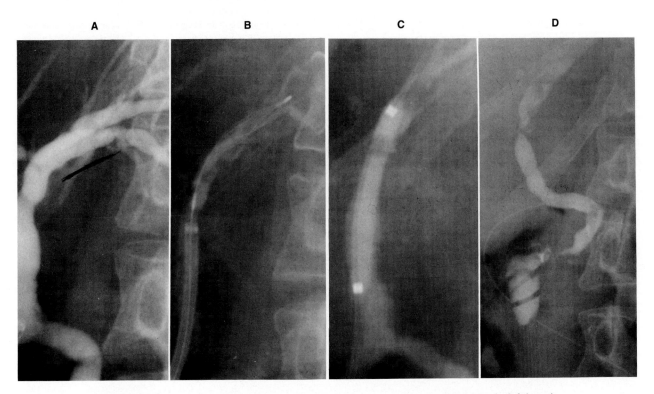

Fig. 80-21 A, Operative cholangiogram shows stricture at porta hepatis with stones in left hepatic radicle. **B,** Postoperative radiologic intervention with balloon catheter dilatation of structure. **C,** Basket extraction of retained stones. **D,** Stricture remains dilated on 8-week follow-up after radiologic intervention. Note also stricture at right hepatic takeoff.

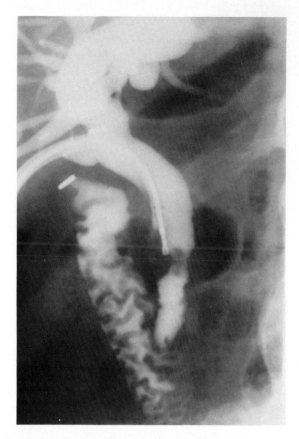

Fig. 80-22 Postoperative cholangiogram demonstrated defect in common duct. Subhepatic biopsy access through T-tube tract with flexible biopsy forceps revealed carcinoma.

first reported in 1975.[10] The biopsy forceps employed with the bronchial or duodenal fiberscope has been successfully used for this purpose[84] (Fig. 80-11).

After cholangiographic identification of the filling defect in the bile ducts, the steerable catheter is moved with its tip directly on the lesion. The endoscopic biopsy forceps is then moved through the steerable catheter and the biopsy sample obtained under fluoroscopic control. The technique is applicable for biliary masses in hepatic and extrahepatic ducts, including carcinomas of the pancreas involving the distal common duct. My biopsy experience through the subhepatic approach now involves 13 patients. No bleeding or perforation has resulted. The T-tube tract is kept open with a catheter for several days after the biopsy for drainage and to regain access if indicated (Fig. 80-22).

REFERENCES

1. Allen, MJ, et al: Rapid dissolution of gallstones by methyl tert-butyl ether, N Engl M Med 312:217, 1985.
2. Bean, WJ, and Mahorner, HR: Removal of residual biliary stones through the T-tube tract, South Med J 65:377, 1972.
3. Becker, CD, et al: External-internal cross-connection for bilateral percutaneous biliary drainage, AJR 149:91, 1987.
4. Brandon, JC, et al: Common bile duct calculi: updated experience with dissolution with methyl tertiary butyl ether, Radiology 166:665, 1988.
5. Burckhardt, H, and Muller, W: Versuche über die Punktion der Gallenblase und ihre Roentgendarstellung, Dtsch Z Chir 162:163, 1921.
6. Burhenne, HJ: Extraktion von Residualsteinen der Gallenwege ohne Reoperation, Fortschr Röntgenstr 117:425, 1972.
7. Burhenne, HJ: Nonoperative retained biliary tract stone extraction: a new roentgenologic technique, AJR 117:388, 1973.
8. Burhenne, HJ: Nonoperative roentgenologic instrumentation technics of the postoperative biliary tract, Am J Surg 128:111, 1974.
9. Burhenne, HJ: Bile duct biopsy with the stone extraction basket, Radiol Clin 44:178, 1975.
10. Burhenne, HJ: Dilatation of biliary tract strictures, Radiol Clin 44:153, 1975.
11. Burhenne, HJ: Electrohydrolytic fragmentation of retained common duct stones, Radiology 117:721, 1975.
12. Burhenne, HJ: Complications of nonoperative extraction of retained common duct stones, Am J Surg 131:260, 1976.
13. Burhenne, HJ: Percutaneous extraction of retained biliary tract stones: 661 patients, AJR 134:888, 1980.
14. Burhenne, HJ, and Hamilton, S: Nonoperative trans-cholecystic removal of common duct stones (abstract), Gastrointest Radiol 7:92, 1982.
15. Burhenne, HJ, and Hamilton, S: Percutaneous cholecystostomy for entry into the canine gallbladder and common bile duct, Radiology 149:844, 1983.
16. Burhenne, HJ, and Morris, DC: Biliary stricture dilatation: use of the Grüntzig balloon catheter, J Can Assoc Radiol 31:196, 1980.
17. Burhenne, HJ, and Peters, HE: Retained intrahepatic stones: use of the U tube during repeated nonoperative stone extractions, Arch Surg 113:837, 1978.
18. Burhenne, HJ, and Scudamore, CH: Antegrade transcholecystic sphincterotomy: canine study of a new interventional technique, Gastrointest Radiol 11:73, 1986.
19. Burgenne, HJ, and Stoller, JL: Minicholecystostomy and radiologic stone extraction in high-risk cholelithiasis patients, Am J Surg 149:632, 1985.
20. Burhenne, HJ, et al: Biliary lithotripsy by extracorporeal shockwaves: an integral part of nonoperative intervention, AJR 150:1279, 1988.
21. Carrasco, CH, et al: Expandable biliary endoprosthesis: an experimental study, AJR 145:1279, 1985.
22. Classen, M, and Demling, L: Endoskopische sphincterotomoie der papilla vateri und steinextraktion aus dem ductus choledochus, Dtsch Med Wochenschr 99:496, 1974.
23. Classen, M, and Ossenberg, FW: Nonsurgical removal of common bile duct stones, Gut 18:760, 1977.
24. Clouse, ME, et al: Bile duct stones: percutaneous transhepatic removal, Radiology 160:525, 1986.
25. Cobourn, C, et al: Percutaneous transhepatic sphincterotomy in the management of biliary tract disease, Gastrointest Radiol 11:273, 1986.
26. Coons, HG, and Carey, PH: Biliary endoprosthesis: yes or no? AJR 145:429, 1985.
27. Cruikshank, JG, Fraser, GM, and Law, J: Finger doses received by radiologists during Chiba needle percutaneous cholangiography, Br J Radiol 53:584, 1980.

28. Crummy, AB, and Turnipseed, WD: Percutaneous replacement of a biliary T tube, AJR 128:869, 1977.

29. Denning, DA, Ellison, EC, and Carey, LC: Preoperative percutaneous transhepatic biliary decompression lowers operative morbidity in patients with obstructive jaundice, Am J Surg 141:61, 1981.

30. Dorsey, TJ, Rowen, M, and Hepps, SA: Nonoperative replacement of T tube in common duct after inadvertent removal, Surgery 71:97, 1972.

31. Dotter, CT, Bilbao, MK, and Katon, RM: Percutaneous transhepatic gallstone removal by needle tract, Radiology 133:242, 1979.

32. Eggermont, AM, Laméris, JS, and Jeekel, J: Ultrasound-guided percutaneous transhepatic cholecystostomy for acute acalculous cholecystitis, Arch Surg 120:1354, 1985.

33. Elyaderani, M, and Gabriele, OF: Percutaneous cholecystostomy and cholangiography in patients with obstructive jaundice, Radiology 130:601, 1979.

34. Fennessy, JJ, and You, KD: A method for the expulsion of stones retained in the common duct, AJR 110:256, 1970.

35. Gallacher, DJ, et al: Nonoperative management of benign postoperative biliary strictures, Radiology 156:625, 1985.

36. Garrow, DG: The removal of biliary tract stones: report of 105 cases, Br J Radiol 50:777, 1977.

37. Gibney, RG, et al: Combined surgical and radiologic intervention for complicated cholelithiasis in high-risk patients, Radiology 165:715, 1987.

38. Gibney, RG, et al: Managing difficult common bile duct problems with the help of the interventional radiologist, Australas Radiol 32:77, 1988.

39. Gould, J, et al: Duodenal perforation as a delayed complication of placement of a biliary endoprosthesis, Radiology 167:467, 1988.

40. Gudjonsson, B, Livstone, EM, and Spiro, HM: Cancer of the pancreas: diagnostic accuracy and survival statistics, Cancer 42:2494, 1978.

41. Gundry, SE, et al: Efficacy of preoperative biliary tract decompression in patients with obstructive jaundice, Arch Surg 119:703, 1984.

42. Günther, RW, Klose, KJ, and Störkel, S: Percutaneous antegrade electropapillotomy: study in dogs, Cardiovasc Intervent Radiol 7:270, 1984.

43. Halsted, WS, and Finney, JMT: Excision of the gallbladder, Johns Hopkins Hosp Bull 13:54, 1902.

44. Hamlin, JA, et al: Percutaneous biliary drainage: complications of 118 consecutive catheterizations, Radiology 158:199, 1986.

45. Hansson, JA, et al: Clinical aspects of nonsurgical percutaneous transhepatic bile drainage in obstructive lesions of the extrahepatic bile ducts, Ann Surg 189:58, 1979.

46. Hatfield, AR, et al: Pre-operative external biliary drainage in obstructive jaundice: a prospective controlled clinical trial, Lancet 2:896, 1982.

47. Hoevels, J, Lunderquist, A, and Ihse, I: Percutaneous transhepatic intubation of bile ducts for combined internal-external drainage in preoperative and palliative treatment of obstructive jaundice, Gastrointest Radiol 3:23, 1978.

48. Hutson, DG, et al: Balloon dilatation of biliary strictures through a choledochojeuno-cutaneous fistula, Ann Surg 199:637, 1984.

49. Janes, JO, and McClelland, R: Fluoroscopic replacement of a choledochal U-tube using a steerable catheter, Radiology 128:828, 1978.

50. Jelaso, DV, and Hirschfield, JS: Jaundice from impacted sediment in a T tube: recognition and treatment, AJR 127:413, 1976.

51. Jolly, PC, et al: Operative cholangiography, Ann Surg 168:551, 1968.

52. Karani, J, et al: Internal biliary drainage and local radiotherapy with iridium-192 wire in treatment of hilar cholangiocarcinoma, Clin Radiol 36:603, 1985.

53. Kerlan, RK, Jr, LaBerge, JM, and Ring, EJ: Percutaneous cholecystolithotomy: preliminary experience, Radiology 157:653, 1985.

54. Koch, H, et al: Endoscopic papillotomy, Gastroenterology 73:1393, 1977.

55. Lagrave, G, et al: Lithiase biliaire résiduelle: extraction à la sonde de Dormia par de drain de Kehr, Mem Acad Chir (Paris) 95:431, 1969.

56. Larssen, TB, et al: Ultrasonically and fluoroscopically guided therapeutic percutaneous catheter drainage of the gallbladder, Gastrointest Radiol 13:37, 1988.

57. Lear JL, et al: Percutaneous transhepatic electrohydraulic lithotripsy, Radiology 150:589, 1984.

58. Lieberman, RP, and Sleder, PR: Pain control after percutaneous biliary drainage: local infiltration with bupivacaine and epinephrine, AJR 146:595, 1986.

59. Lind, LJ, and Mushlin, PS: Sedation, analgesia, and anesthesia for radiologic procedures, Cardiovasc Intervent Radiol 10:247, 1987.

60. Longmire, WP, Jr, et al: The treatment of retained gallstones, West J Med 130:422, 1979.

61. Lukes, P, et al: Evaluation of percutaneous cholangiography and percutaneous biliary drainage in obstructive jaundice, Eur J Radiol 5:267, 1985.

62. Margulis, AR: Interventional diagnostic radiology: a new subspecialty (editorial), AJR 99:761, 1967.

63. Margulis, AR, Newton, TH, and Najarian, JS: Removal of plug from T tube by fluoroscopically controlled catheter, AJR 93:975, 1965.

64. Martin, EC, et al: Use of the electrohydraulic lithotriptor in the biliary tree in dogs, Radiology 139:215, 1981.

65. Mason, R: Percutaneous extraction of retained gallstones via the T-tube tract: British experience of 131 cases, Clin Radiol 31:497, 1980.

66. Mason, RR, and Cotton, PB: Combined duodenoscopic and transhepatic approach to stenosis of the papilla of Vater, Br J Radiol 54:678, 1981.

67. May, GR, et al: Nonoperative dilatation of dominant strictures in primary sclerosing cholangitis, AJR 145:1061, 1985.

68. Mazzariello, R: Review of 220 cases of residual biliary tract calculi treated without reoperation: an eight-year study, Surgery 73:299, 1973.

69. Mazzariello, RM: Transcholecystic extraction of residual calculi in common bile duct, Surgery 75:338, 1974.

70. McGahan, JP: A new catheter design for percutaneous cholecystostomy, Radiology 166:49, 1988.

71. Mendez, G, Jr, et al: Percutaneous brush biopsy and internal drainage of biliary tree through endoprosthesis, AJR 134:653, 1980.

72. Meyers, WC, and Jones, RS: Internal radiation for bile duct cancer, World J Surg 12:99, 1988.

73. Miller, DL, and Wall, RT: Fentanyl and diazepam for analgesia and sedation during radiologic special procedures, Radiology 162:195, 1987.

74. Molnar, W, and Stockum, AE: Relief of obstructive jaundice through percutaneous transhepatic catheter: a new therapeutic method, AJR 122:356, 1974.

75. Molnar, W, and Stockum, AE: Transhepatic dilatation of choledochoenterostomy strictures, Radiology 129:59, 1978.

76. Modet, A: Técnica de la extracción incruenta de los calculos en la litiasis residual del colédoco, Bol Soc Cir Bs Aires 46:278, 1962.

77. Morita, S, et al: Biliary drainage: conversion of external to internal drainage, Radiology 167:267, 1988.

78. Moss, JP, et al: Postoperative choledochoscopy via the T-tube tract, JAMA 236:2781, 1976.

79. Mueller, PR, et al: Biliary stent endoprosthesis: analysis of complications in 113 patients, Radiology 156:637, 1985.

80. Mueller, PR, et al: Biliary stricture dilatation: multicenter review of clinical management in 73 patients, Radiology 160:17, 1986.

81. Mueller, PR, vanSonnenberg, E, and Ferrucci, JT, Jr: Percutaneous biliary drainage: technical and catheter-related problems in 200 procedures, AJR 138:17, 1982.

82. O'Doherty, DP, Neoptolemos, JP, and Carr-Lock, DL: Endoscopic sphincterotomy for retained common bile duct stones in patients with T-tube in situ in early postoperative period, Br J Surg 73:454, 1986.

83. Olak, J, Stein, LA, and Meakins, JL: Palliative percutaneous transhepatic biliary drainage: assessment of morbidity and mortality, Can J Surg 29:243, 1986.

84. Palayew, MJ, and Stein, L: Postoperative biopsy of the common bile duct via the T-tube tract, AJR 130:287, 1978.

85. Pessa, ME, Hawkins, IF, and Vogel, SB: The treatment of acute cholangitis: percutaneous transhepatic biliary drainage before definitive therapy, Ann Surg 205:389, 1987.

86. Pitt, HA, et al: Does preoperative percutaneous biliary drainage reduce operative risk or increase hospital cost? Ann Surg 201:545, 1985.

87. Polack, EP, Fainsinger, MH, and Bonnano, SV: A death following complications of roentgenologic nonoperative manipulation of common bile duct calculi, Radiology 123:585, 1977.

88. Radder, RW: Ultrasonically guided percutaneous catheter drainage for gallbladder empyema, Diagn Imaging 49:330, 1980.

89. Remolar, J, et al: Percutaneous transhepatic cholangiography, Gastroenterology 31:39, 1956.

90. Ring, EJ, et al: Therapeutic applications of catheter cholangiography, Radiology 128:333, 1978.

91. Russell, E, and Koolpe, HA: A modified T-tube for use after nonoperative biliary stone removal, Radiology 129:237, 1978.

92. Russell, E, et al: Dilatation of biliary strictures through a stomatized jejunal limb, Acta Radiol Diagn 26:283, 1985.

93. Sackmann, M, et al: Shock-wave lithotripsy of gallbladder stones: the first 175 patients, N Engl J Med 318:393, 1988.

94. Safrany, L: Duodenoscopic sphincterotomy and gallstone removal, Gastroenterology 72:338, 1977.

95. Salomonowitz, E, et al: Balloon dilatation of benign biliary strictures, Radiology 151:613, 1984.

96. Sauerbruch, T, et al: Fragmentation of gallstones by extracorporeal shockwaves, N Engl J Med 314:818, 1986.

97. Shaver, RW, and Soong, J: Percutaneous placement of a transcystic duct internal biliary drainage catheter, Gastrointest Radiol 8:149, 1983.

98. Shore, JM: Prevention of residual biliary calculi, Calif Med 114:1, 1971.

99. Smith, HW, et al: Problems of retained and recurrent common bile duct stones, Surgery 66:291, 1969.

100. Smith, TP, et al: Percutaneous transhepatic biliary endoscopic procedures, Gastrointest Radiol 12:144, 1987.

101. Sniderman, KW, et al: A modified technique for percutaneous insertion of a biliary T-tube, Radiology 131:539, 1979.

102. Speer, AG, et al: Randomised trial of endoscopic versus percutaneous stent insertion in malignant obstructive jaundice, Lancet 2:57, 1987.

103. Stanley, J, et al: Biliary decompression: an institutional comparison of percutaneous and endoscopic methods, Radiology 158:195, 1986.

104. Tanaka, M, et al: The long-term fate of the gallbladder after endoscopic sphincterotomy: complete follow-up study of 122 patients, Am J Surg 154:505, 1987.

105. Tritapepe, R, de Padova, C, and de Padova, F: Non-invasive treatment for retained common bile duct stones in patients with T tube in situ: saline washout after intravenous ceruletide, Br J Surg 75:144, 1988.

106. Tylén, U, Hoevels, J, and Nilsson, U: Computed tomography of iatrogenic hepatic lesions following percutaneous transhepatic cholangiography and portography, J Comput Assist Tomogr 5:15, 1981.

107. Tylén, U, Hoevels, J, and Vang, J: Percutaneous transhepatic cholangiography with external drainage of obstructive biliary lesions, Surg Gynecol Obstet 144:13, 1977.

108. vanSonnenberg, E, and Hofmann, AF: Horizons in gallstone therapy: 1988, AJR 150:43, 1988.

109. vanSonnenberg, E, et al: Diagnostic and therapeutic percutaneous gallbladder procedures, Radiology 160:23, 1986.

110. Warren, KW, and Whitcomb, FF, Jr: Diagnosis and treatment of benign biliary tract stricture, Hosp Pract, p 62, February 1971.

111. Way, LW: Retained common duct stones, Surg Clin North Am 53:1139, 1973.

112. Weber, J, and Höver, S: Technische Probleme der perkutanen transhepatischen Gallengangsdrainage, Fortschr Röntgenstr 143:534, 1985.

113. Weyman, PJ, and Balfe, DM: Percutaneous dilatation of biliary strictures, Semin Intervent Radiol 2:50, 1985.

114. Wiechel, KL: Percutaneous transhepatic cholangiography: technique and application, Acta Chir Scand (suppl) 330:1, 1964.

115. Williams, HJ, Jr, Bender, CE, and May, GR: Benign postoperative biliary strictures: dilation with fluoroscopic guidance, Radiology 163:629, 1987.

116. Yamakawa, T, et al: An improved choledochofiberscope and nonsurgical removal of retained biliary calculi under direct visual control, Gastrointest Endosc 22:160, 1976.

117. Yee, ACN, and Ho, C-S: Complications of percutaneous biliary drainage: benign vs malignant diseases, AJR 148:1207, 1987.

81 *Endoscopic Therapies: Biliary Tract and Pancreas*

PETER B. COTTON

The techniques and indications for endoscopic retrograde cholangiography and pancreatography (ERCP) are described in Chapter 54. This section reviews the current status of endoscopic therapy in the biliary tract and pancreas, about 15 years after the first endoscopic sphincterotomy.

SPHINCTEROTOMY

The technique of sphincterotomy[5] employs a side-viewing duodenoscope and a diathermy sphincterotome, which consists of a catheter with wire exposed near the distal tip; traction produces a cutting bow (Fig. 81-1).

The duodenoscope is maneuvered to provide an *en face* view of the papilla of Vater, and retrograde cholangiography is performed to confirm the need for incision. The standard catheter is then replaced by the sphincterotome, and its position in the bile duct checked radiologically. With the wire pointing between the 11 and 1 o'clock positions, diathermy current is applied with upward pressure to produce a sphincterotomy approximately 15 mm in length. The desirable length varies with the indication, and the safe length depends on the diameter of the bile duct and the direction of its termination at the papilla. A balloon-tipped catheter can be used to document the size of the orifice.

When standard sphincterotomy techniques fail, entrance to the bile duct can be obtained using the technique of "precutting." This involves placing a diathermy wire into the common channel and cutting upwards until the bile duct is found. This procedure is more hazardous than sphincterotomy, and should be used only when the indications are very strong.

Sphincterotomy can be more difficult in patients with peripapillary diverticula, patients with duodenal distortion or compression, and those who have undergone diversionary surgery such as Billroth II partial gastrectomy. Irreversible coagulopathy is a relative contraindication. Most patients selected for sphincterotomy are elderly and frail, and some are acutely ill. Careful medical management before and after the procedure is essential, and surgery may be required urgently if sphincterotomy fails or complications occur. The technique should therefore be applied only in institutions with appropriate specialist medical and surgical facilities. Prophylactic antibiotics

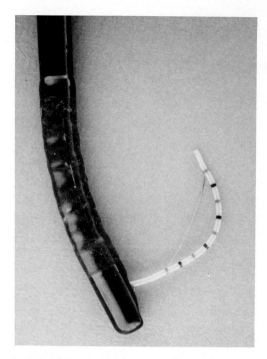

Fig. 81-1 Typical side-viewing duodenoscope and diathermy sphincterotome.

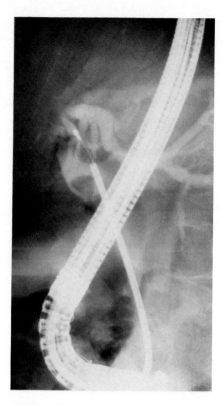

Fig. 81-2 Crushing basket in place in common hepatic duct. Large stone has been fragmented into two pieces.

are usually given, because most patients with biliary obstruction have infected bile, and instrumentation can aggravate or provoke clinical infection.

REMOVAL OF STONES

Most small stones will pass spontaneously within a few days or weeks after a standard-size sphincterotomy, but the risks of leaving stones to pass are greater than those of removing them immediately, especially in patients with cholangitis. Balloon-tipped catheters can be used to remove small stones and to confirm that the duct is clear. Baskets provide better traction (Fig. 81-2). The previous fear of stone and basket impaction is no longer a factor, because disimpaction can always be achieved by using the sleeve of a "crushing" basket (discussed later).

Stones in difficult positions (cystic duct or intrahepatic duct or behind strictures) can usually be removed with appropriate guidewire and balloon techniques.

NASOBILIARY DRAINS

When stones prove difficult to remove after sphincterotomy, it is prudent to leave a drainage catheter in the bile duct and bring it out through the patient's nose (Fig. 81-3). This virtually eliminates the risk of cholangitis and allows flushing and check cholangiography. Stents can also be placed to prevent stone impaction on a temporary or permanent basis.

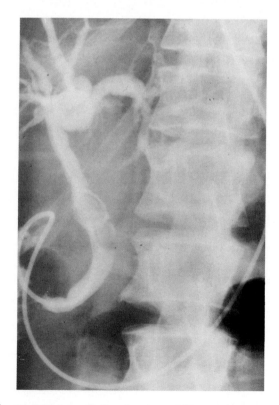

Fig. 81-3 Endoscopically placed nasobiliary drain in patient with two retained stones in large cystic duct remnant.

SUCCESS RATES FOR SPHINCTEROTOMY

Endoscopic sphincterotomy should be completed within a hour, and patients are usually discharged on the following day. The results are consistent from many countries.[1] Sphincterotomy is technically possible in 90% to 95% of attempts, and the duct is cleared in a similar percentage. The overall success rate for removing stones is therefore 85% to 90%. Extraction failures virtually always result from the size of stones, a problem that is discussed later. A second procedure—or referral to a more experienced center—may sometimes be necessary.

COMPLICATIONS

Endoscopic sphincterotomy carries the usual rare risks of ERCP. Specific complications of sphincterotomy occur in about 10% of patients; 2% to 3% require surgery urgently for these complications, and 1% die.[1,6] Bleeding is the most common problem. It is more likely with longer incisions but is largely unpredictable, presumably because of anatomic variations. Minor bleeding can be arrested by endoscopic techniques, but severe bleeding usually requires surgery—oversewing the lesion, with or without tying off the gastroduodenal artery. Angiographic embolization has been effective in a few cases,[13] but further data are required. Cholangitis occurs only when sphincterotomy and stone extraction fail and can be minimized by providing drainage with endoscopic insertion of a nasobiliary tube or by percutaneous transhepatic drainage when endoscopy fails. Pancreatitis can be caused by inadvertant damage to the pancreatic duct orifice, but also occurs rarely after apparently routine procedures. Retroperitoneal perforation is a dramatic event. Most cases can be treated conservatively, at least initially, especially if bile duct drainage is achieved by the sphincterotomy or nasobiliary drainage. Percutaneous or surgical drainage of local abscesses may be required later.

THE PROBLEM OF LARGE STONES

Stones less than 10 to 15 mm in diameter are usually easy to remove with balloons or baskets. Many different methods are now being evaluated for breaking up larger stones within the duct to facilitate their extraction.[11] "Crushing" baskets have become more effective as the size of the instrument channel of the duodenoscopes has increased, but the success rate is still disappointing. The presence of a nasobiliary tube allows infusion of chemicals to attempt dissolution. Mono-octanoin and methyl tert butyl ether (MTBE) are effective cholesterol solvents. Unfortunately, most large stones are composed mainly of pigment material, for which effective chemicals are not yet available. This method will, however, become dominant when appropriate solvents are developed, especially since it is not necessary to perform a sphincterotomy to place a nasobiliary drain. Two endo-

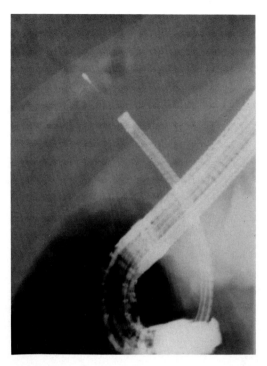

Fig. 81-4 Peroral choledochoscopy with "mother and baby" combination.

scopic probes are available for direct fragmentation of duct stones. The electrohydraulic probe is effective, but has been little used because of the potential for damage to the bile duct. Laser lithotripsy appears safer, using the tunable dye or nd-YAG lasers. Laser energy is applied under direct vision using a small choledochoscope passed through a large-channel duodenoscope (Fig. 81-4).

A further method for stone fragmentation is external shockwave lithotripsy, which has been applied effectively in many cases, using injection of contrast through a nasobiliary tube (or other drainage tube) for focusing.

INDICATIONS FOR ENDOSCOPIC TREATMENT[1,9]
Bile duct stones

Endoscopic sphincterotomy is now established as a quick, inexpensive, and relatively safe technique that is well tolerated by most patients.[4] Its application depends on the alternative treatments available to the individual patient and their relative risks.

Postcholecystectomy

The most common indication for sphincterotomy is removal of stones from the duct of a patient who has previously undergone cholecystectomy (and who does not have a T-tube drain). Surgical exploration of the duct is relatively safe in young and fit patients, but the mortality rises to 5% or 10% with increasing age and frailty.[9]

The endoscopic approach must therefore be considered as the treatment of choice in high-risk patients. In young and fit patients the short-term risks of sphincterotomy and surgery are comparable. The convenience of sphincterotomy has to be weighed against any potential long-term risks, which may not be evident for many years.[8]

Patients with T-tube drains are best treated by percutaneous extraction methods, because the risks are less than those of sphincterotomy, and the sphincter is not damaged. Endoscopic methods are used when the T-tube drain is too small or incorrectly placed or when clinical conditions demand early intervention.

Patients with gallbladders

Endoscopic treatment is increasingly used as an emergency procedure in patients with acute symptoms caused by duct stones—such as acute cholangitis and gallstone-related pancreatitis—even when the gallbladder is in place. The clinical results are usually dramatic. Simple cholecystectomy can be performed (with greatly reduced risk) after the acute illness has subsided or postponed indefinitely in patients who are in poor general condition. Follow-up studies in elderly patients indicate that less than 20% require cholecystectomy over a 5- to 10-year period.[1]

Benign noncalculus obstruction

Filling defects other than stones are sometimes seen in the bile duct. Endoscopic sphincterotomy has been used for removal of suture material, worms, shrapnel, blood clot, and retained tubes and stents.

Benign papillary stenosis

ERCP is an important diagnostic technique in patients who have symptoms after cholecystectomy. It allows detailed examination of the stomach, duodenum, papilla, and duct systems. The concept of benign stenosis at the sphincter caused by fibrosis or spasm remains controversial. By ruling out other conditions, ERCP has brought this problem into closer focus, but diagnostic difficulties remain. The size of the duct is helpful only if previous radiographs are available for comparison. Rates of bile duct emptying after ERCP are affected by instrumentation and medication. Noninvasive methods for determining duct emptying potential (ultrasound and isotope scanning) are still being evaluated. Endoscopic sphincter manometry appears helpful in some centers,[7] but its precise role is controversial.

Many experts now perform endoscopic sphincterotomy for "papillary stenosis," despite these diagnostic and conceptual difficulties. The short-term results are good in patients with classic pains associated with biochemical evidence of cholestasis, particularly if there is delayed bile duct emptying and a dilated duct. Sphincterotomy is speculative in the absence of these and other objective criteria.

Bile duct strictures

ERCP is an accurate method for detecting and delineating traumatic strictures of the bile duct. Angioplasty-type balloons are used for dilatation (Fig. 81-5). The recurrence rate is high after single dilatation, and most experts now leave a splinting stent in place for 3 to 12 months. More long-term data are required. Expert surgery probably remains the treatment of choice in most suitable cases.

Low bile duct strictures are common in patients with chronic pancreatitis. Though they can be managed by endoscopic insertion of a stent, this can only be of temporary benefit, because stents must be exchanged every few months.

Sclerosing cholangitis is recognized increasingly with the more frequent use of ERCP in patients with biochemical cholestasis, especially in the context of inflammatory bowel disease. There are now impressive anecdotal reports of endoscopic management (by sphincterotomy, with or without balloon dilatation and temporary stenting) in some of these patients. Saline lavage through

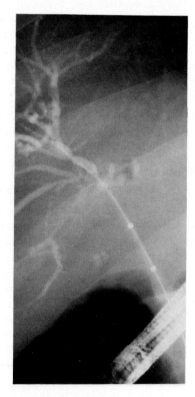

Fig. 81-5 Balloon catheter (between metal rings) being placed within high bile duct stricture.

a nasobiliary tube may be appropriate in patients with much biliary debris, and there are claims that steroid infusions into the bile duct can produce worthwhile remission.

Biliodigestive anastomoses and fistulae

Some patients with pains and cholangitis after biliary surgery are found to have a fistula above the orifice of the papilla of Vater. These fistulae result from stone migration or ill-directed surgical dilatation. Good results have been claimed for improving drainage by connecting the bile duct orifice to the fistula with endoscopic sphincterotomy.

Stenosed choledochoduodenostomies can be enlarged by balloon dilatation and stenting, but the proximity of large blood vessels renders diathermy treatment hazardous. The sump syndrome can be simply treated by standard sphincterotomy of the main papilla.

Malignant obstructive jaundice

ERCP is an excellent method for diagnosing tumors of the papilla of Vater. Sphincterotomy and laser disobliteration can provide good drainage in patients who are unsuitable or unfit for resection. Jaundice caused by malignant obstruction above the papilla can be managed by

endoscopic stenting, using a three-layer system of guidewire, catheter, and stent[2] (Fig. 81-6). Initial attempts with small (No. 7 or 8 French) stents were complicated by early blockage. Larger instruments now allow placement of No. 12 and 15 French stents (Fig. 81-7), which stay patent for 6 to 12 months—longer than the expected survival of most patients in whom they are applied. The lower tip of the stent is always left in the duodenum so that the stent can be removed (and replaced) easily when blockage occurs.

Endoscopic biliary stents provide excellent palliation in patients with tumors of the distal bile duct and pancreas, but hiler lesions are more difficult to manage. Single stents can provide drainage sufficient to normalize the bilirubin level, but there is a risk of sepsis in undrained segments. Despite the use of torque stable and deflectable tip guidewires, it is often impossible to place sufficient stents to drain all areas. In these cases, a combined percutaneous-endoscopic approach may be appropriate (discussed later).

Endoscopic biliary stents can also be used to improve a patient's condition before resection of obstructing tumors. Randomized studies are in progress to clarify whether this approach is valuable.

The relative roles of endoscopic, percutaneous, and

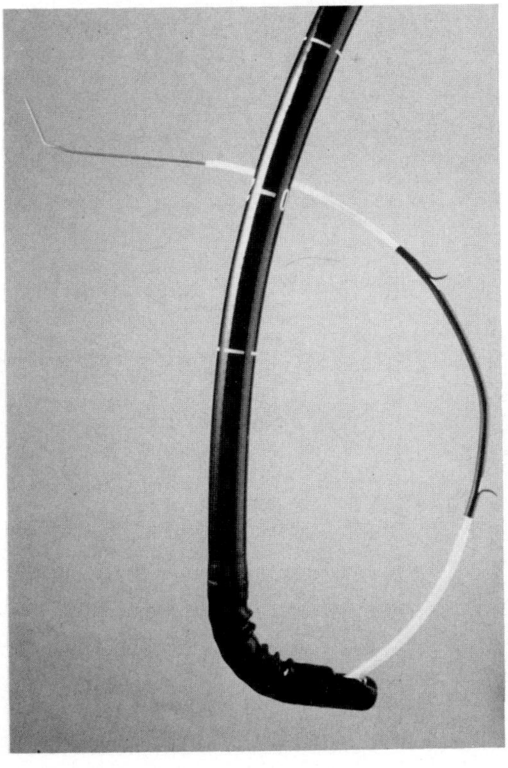

Fig. 81-6 Three-layer system for endoscopic insertion of No. 11.5 French stents—guidewire, inner catheter, and stent with terminal barbs.

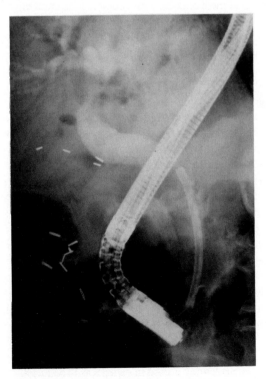

Fig. 81-7 Endoscopic placement of No. 15 French stent with experimental duodenoscope.

surgical biliary drainage are being explored. Clearly, surgery is indicated in younger and fitter patients believed to have a resectable lesion. At the other end of the spectrum there are some patients referred in the terminal phases of the disease for whom further intervention is inappropriate.

At my institution, Speer and co-workers[14] have reported the results of a randomized trial comparing the endoscopic and percutaneous insertion of indwelling biliary stents. The endoscopic approach was shown to be more successful and safer. As a result, it is now used as the primary method, and the percutaneous approach is used only when endoscopic methods fail or are not available. Surgical bypass provides good palliation in fitter patients and is necessary in those with duodenal obstruction. Further randomized studies are in progress.

Malignant biliary strictures can be treated by temporary endoscopic insertion of radioactive sources, such as iridium wires.

RADIOLOGIC-ENDOSCOPIC COLLABORATION

It is self-evident that the therapeutically ambitious endoscopist must rely heavily on colleagues in radiology to provide detailed imaging and interventional expertise. Maximum benefit can be obtained only by a team approach.

Many centers now use a "two-handed" combined approach to the bile duct, with simultaneous duodenoscopy and percutaneous transhepatic procedures.[10,12] These are particularly appropriate in patients with hilar lesions, in whom it is not possible endoscopically to drain all segments of the liver. The radiologist passes a guidewire percutaneously through the appropriate segment of the liver and into the duodenum. The large-channel duodenoscope is passed and the guidewire grasped and withdrawn through the endoscope. A standard stent can then be passed through the endoscope over this guidewire, with control at both the mouth and skin. The guidewire should be covered with a catheter to prevent damage to the liver. This "combined" approach is preferred to a simple percutaneous approach, because it is assumed (but not proven) that the brief transhepatic passage with a No. 6 French catheter is safer than more prolonged placement of a larger tube.

The same percutaneous assistance can be given to an endoscopist who has difficulties in cannulating the papilla for sphincterotomy, for example, in a patient with a large peripapillary diverticulum.

PANCREATIC DISEASE

Sphincterotomy is used in patients with acute gallstone pancreatitis, and endoscopic stenting is now established in the management of jaundice caused by tumors of the

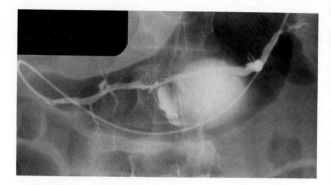

Fig. 81-8 Endoscopically placed pernasal drain in dorsal pancreatic duct in patient with pancreas divisum and pseudocyst of midbody.

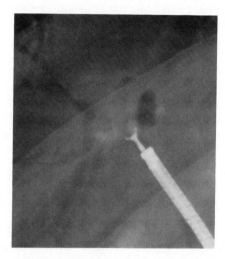

Fig. 81-9 Direct vision biopsy of hilar lesion through peroral choledochoscope.

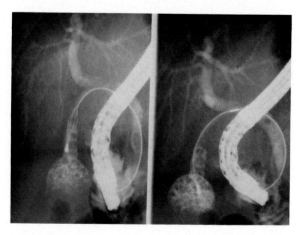

Fig. 81-10 Basket extraction of gallbladder stones via endoscopic cannulation of cystic duct.

pancreatic head. Few endoscopists have performed other therapeutic procedures on the pancreas itself. Localized stenosis at the pancreatic duct orifice is rare, and should be documented by drainage studies and endoscopic manometry before any attempted manipulation. Stones can be removed from within the duct in the pancreatic head with standard balloon catheters or baskets after sphincterotomy, but recurrence is frequent.

Pancreatic pseudocysts have been drained by endoscopic puncture through the stomach or duodenal wall with use of diathermy or laser probes. Pseudocyst resolution has also been facilitated by temporary placement of an endoscopic stent or drain (Fig. 81-8). Attempts to induce acinar atrophy of the pancreas in patients with painful chronic pancreatitis—using endoscopic injection of tissue glues—have largely proved unsuccessful.

The widespread use of ERCP has highlighted the congenital anomaly of pancreas divisum, in which the main pancreatic drainage from the dorsal pancreas is through Santorini's duct and the accessory papilla.[1] This anomaly occurs in about 7% of the population and is usually clinically irrelevent. However, there is now clear evidence that the accessory papilla orifice may be inadequate in some patients, resulting in recurrent pain and pancreatitis. Endoscopic sphincterotomy at the accessory papilla has been largely abandoned because of rapid restenosis, but the results of temporary insertion of a stent appear encouraging.

PERORAL CHOLEDOCHOSCOPY

Very small-diameter fiberscopes have been available for many years, but only recently has peroral choledochoscopy become a practical procedure. The latest instruments provide excellent views and a working channel for direct vision biopsy (Fig. 81-9) and therapeutic procedures such as insertion of guidewires, extraction of stones, and laser lithotripsy.

FUTURE PROSPECTS

Endoscopic therapy will continue to expand its popularity and frontiers, but sphincterotomy itself (with its inherent hazards) may be used less often in the future. The developing methods for lithotripsy and stone dissolution may allow duct clearance (and removal of small fragments) through the intact papilla, minimizing the complications. Sphincterotomy can be reserved for patients who have definite stenosis.

Endoscopists are beginning to explore the cystic duct and gallbladder with use of appropriate guidewires and dilating balloons. A catheter can be placed and left in the gallbladder for infusion of chemicals, and stones can be extracted directly with standard baskets (Fig. 81-10).

The field of biliary therapy continues to develop dramatically, and it will be years before the relative roles of surgical, radiologic, and endoscopic techniques can be clarified.

REFERENCES

1. Cotton, PB: Endoscopic management of bile duct stones (apples and oranges), Gut 25:587, 1984.
2. Cotton, PB: Endoscopic methods for relief of malignant obstructive jaundice. World J Surg 8:854, 1984.
3. Cotton, PB: Pancreas divisum: curiosity or culprit? Gastroenterology, 89:1431, 1985.
4. Cotton, PB, and Dineen, L: Endoscopic treatment for bile duct stones without cholecystectomy: Followup at 3-10 years. In press.
5. Cotton, PB, and Williams, CB: Practical gastrointestinal endoscopy, ed 2, Oxford, England, 1982, Blackwell Scientific Publications.
6. Cotton, PB, et al: Complications of endoscopic sphincterotomy and their management, Am J Surg, 1988. In press.
7. Geenen, JE, et al: The efficiency of endoscopic sphincterotomy in post cholecystectomy patients with sphincter of Oddi dysfunction: results of a 4 year prospective study, N Engl J Medicine, 1988. In press.
8. Hawes, RH, Vallon, AG, and Cotton, PB: Long-term followup after duodenoscopic sphincterotomy for choledocholithiasis in patients with previous cholecystectomy, Gastrointest Endosc, 1988. In press.
9. Johnson, AG, and Hosking, SW: Appraisal of the management of bile duct stones, Br J Surg 74:555, 1987.
10. Mason, RR, and Cotton, PB: Combined duodenoscopic and transpapillary approach to stenosis of the papilla of Vater, Br J Radiol 54:678, 1981.
11. Raskin, JB: The continuing direct assault on the gallstone, Gastrointest Endosc 33:262, 1987.
12. Robertson, AF, et al: Experience with a combined percutaneous and endoscopic approach to stent insertion in malignant obstructive jaundice, Lancet 2:1449, 1987.
13. Saeed, M, et al: Bleeding following endoscopic sphincterotomy; management by transcatheter embolization. In press.
14. Speer, AG, et al: Randomized trial of endoscopic versus percutaneous stent insertion in malignant obstructive jaundice, Lancet 2:57, 1987.

82 *Percutaneous Abdominal Biopsy and Drainage*

GARY M. ONIK
ROBERT KERLAN

GENERAL CONSIDERATIONS

Imaging techniques such as ultrasound, computed tomography (CT), and magnetic resonance imaging (MRI) have revolutionized the diagnosis of pathologic conditions of the abdomen and allowed the application of various therapeutic options. Percutaneous biopsy and drainage of abdominal fluid collections are now routine procedures in most hospitals and accepted as standard care. They have been shown to be both safe and effective and are preferred to open laparotomy for diagnosis and treatment. This chapter will review the indications, techniques, and complications of percutaneous biopsy and drainage procedures. Since both biopsy and drainage begin with needle placement in a lesion, some emphasis will be placed on pathologic localization and needle placement.

PERCUTANEOUS BIOPSY

Using ultrasound, CT, and now even MRI, percutaneous fine-needle biopsy has become a common practice, obviating the need for exploratory surgery in the majority of cases. A plethora of literature attests to both its safety and accuracy.* It is therefore the procedure of choice when a tissue diagnosis is needed before treatment. The main indication for a percutaneous biopsy is to make the diagnosis of any persistent radiologic abnormality that cannot be diagnosed by other noninvasive techniques. More specifically, it is indicated in patients who are marginal surgical candidates in whom a positive biopsy may lend weight to the indications for surgery and in inoperable patients in whom tissue diagnosis will support the need for radiotherapy or chemotherapy.

Percutaneous biopsy is contraindicated in uncooperative patients or patients who are refusing therapy regardless of results. Relative contraindications may include suspected vascular lesions, such as hemangiomas. In the past a suspected hemangioma used to be an absolute contraindication; however, the recent literature suggests that by using fine needles, hemangiomas can be biopsied safely without undue risk of clinically significant hemorrhage and yield a specific histologic diagnosis.[12]

---

*References 3, 5, 27, 28, 29, 31, 37, 73, 78.

Despite these reports, it seems reasonable that if a hemangioma is suspected, all efforts should be made to diagnose it before a percutaneous biopsy by looking for its characteristic findings on MRI or ^{99}Tc red blood cell studies. A bleeding diathesis is also a relative contraindication; therefore all patients should have coagulation studies before biopsy.

Percutaneous biopsy is also contraindicated when a hydatid cyst is suspected because of the possibility of leakage of the contents of the cyst, causing either anaphylaxis or spread of daughter cysts to other areas.[51] This can usually be ruled out in the abdomen by serologic tests. Also, pelvic lesions that may possibly be ovarian carcinoma should not be biopsied, again because of the possibility of peritoneal seeding of tumor. In addition, lesions that might possibly be a pheochromocytoma should not be biopsied because of the possibility of a hypertensive crisis precipitated by the procedure.[10] Lastly, when biopsy of a lesion might cause a pneumothorax, such as those in the dome of the liver, attention must be paid to whether the patient can tolerate a pneumothorax. Severe empyema or a pneumonectomy on the side contralateral to the biopsy is a relative contraindication.

Methods of lesion localization and needle placement

The specific technique of needle localization and needle placement depends on the imaging modality used. The common denominator of all the imaging modalities is that confirmation of the needle tip within the lesion has to be obtained. For abdominal biopsies fluoroscopy is of limited value and is usually reserved for chest and bone biopsies.

Ultrasound

Real-time ultrasound is fast, inexpensive, and therefore the most cost-effective means of guiding a biopsy. It is ideal for liver and pancreatic biopsies; however, it may not be possible to use in the lower abdomen if gas obscures the pathologic condition. The most common approach to ultrasound-guided biopsy is the free hand method. However, this usually necessitates multiple passes to localize a needle in the lesion, increasing procedure time and patient trauma. Some biopsy aid associated with the ultrasound transducer guiding the needle along its intended path is therefore preferred. Transducers specifically designed for biopsies are available.[68] Available now with almost all ultrasound transducers are attachable biopsy guides that hold the needle at a fixed angle in relationship to the head of the transducer (Fig. 82-1). The biopsy guide is arranged so that the placement of the needle is in the plane of the scan, and the needle can therefore be followed on its path to the lesion. All

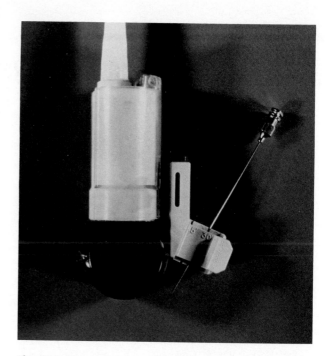

Fig. 82-1 Ultrasound transducer with attached biopsy guide. Guide holds needle in fixed relationship to head of transducer.

scanners now have software that shows the intended path the needle will take, which enables one to avoid vascular or other vital structures (Fig. 82-2). The major disadvantage of this arrangement is that for the first 2 cm of the biopsy, the area that the needle is traversing is not visualized. Although the lesion is usually deeper than 2 cm, obstructions such as ribs, which may be out of the field of visualization, can totally obstruct or deviate the needles.

The choice of needles for ultrasound-guided biopsy is a matter of preference but is influenced by what type of pathologic sample is preferred. These aspects of needle selection will be discussed in detail in a later section. However, needles with some type of echogenic coating at their tip are preferred because of the difficulty of sometimes visualizing the needle on its course (Fig. 82-3).

The results expected from percutaneous ultrasound-guided biopsies of abdominal masses using fine-needle techniques have been excellent. For solid masses the sensitivity for malignant disease has been reported to be from 79% to 95%.* The specificity is virtually 100%, with no false-positive diagnoses for malignant disease reported. The sensitivity for cystic masses, reported at 98%, is extremely high.[65]

When pathologic conditions cannot be visualized adequately by ultrasound because of intervening gas or when an added degree of safety is required (as is needed

---

*References 6, 8, 46, 52, 65, 71, 80.

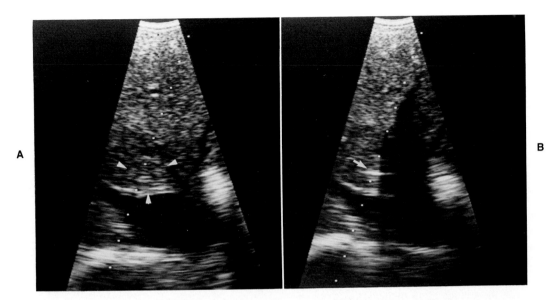

Fig. 82-2 Intraoperative ultrasound-guided biopsy showing principle of biopsy guide. **A,** Hyperechoic lesion 1 cm in diameter *(arrowheads)* just anterior to inferior vena cava adjacent to takeoff of right hepatic vein. Dotted oblique line indicates path biopsy needle will take. **B,** Bright dot *(arrow)* represents tip of biopsy needle in lesion. Note that needle has followed intended path exactly. Shadowing is seen from this 14-gauge Trucut needle.

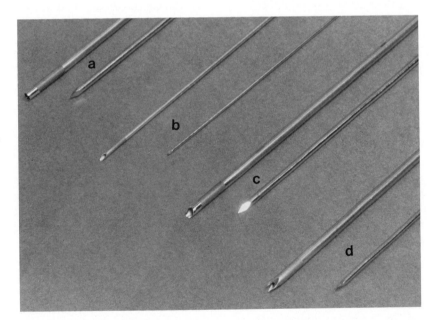

Fig. 82-3 Array of different trocar tipped and beveled tipped needles is shown. Note roughened metal portion at their tips, which makes them more echogenic than rest of needle, enabling tip to be more easily confirmed in lesion. Shown are Greene 18 G *(a)*, Chiba 22G *(b)*, Turner 18 G *(c)*, and Franseen 18 gauge *(d)*.

in abscess drainages), CT should be used for the localization and guidance of the needle placement.

Computed tomography

The traditional method of CT-guided biopsy consists of a number of steps. The first step is to visualize the lesion and plan a route to it. Four or five scans are usually needed to find a CT slice on which the lesion is visualized in its greatest diameter and to show an acceptable path to it. The entry point to the lesion is chosen on the appropriate scan slice, and its distance from a reference point that can be easily identified on the patient, usually the patient's midline, is calculated.[54] The distance from the entry point to the target point and the angle from the horizontal or the vertical are calculated using the standard CT software.

To miss the sulcus of the lung, necessary for lesions in the dome of the liver, or to miss other intervening structures, such as a rib, an entry point on a scan slice different from that of the abnormality is occasionally needed. In such the triangulation method will need to be used to calculate the angle and depth to the lesion. This method simply uses the Pythagorean theorem[75] (Fig. 82-4).

Once the path to the lesion is calculated, the level of the scan slice of interest is marked on the patient using the laser localization lights of the CT scanner. The reference point on the patient is found, and the distance to the entry point is measured. Once the entry point is found and marked, the skin is sterilized and draped. Using local anesthesia, a skin nick is made with a small No. 11 blade. A localization needle is then placed at what is felt to be the correct angle and depth to the lesion. The patient is scanned to confirm the placement of this needle. In general, when using this method, it is necessary to obtain three CT scan slices to localize the needle. It is imperative to localize the tip of the needle, which may fall outside one scan slice. If the lesion is small or in a difficult position, it may be necessary to place a short, localizing needle to confirm the correct position of the entry point and correct angulation of the needle before using the longer localization needle. Once the needle is confirmed to be in the lesion, a number of different methods, which will be discussed later, can be used to obtain the biopsy.

Although the accuracy of pathologic diagnosis and the safety of CT-guided percutaneous biopsy have been well proved in the literature, the actual placement accuracy and the difficulty of biopsy in small or difficultly placed lesions have only been alluded to in the literature.[20] A number of skin localizers, including paper clips and ball bearings, have been used to more accurately define the entry point (Fig. 82-5). A more sophisticated skin lo-

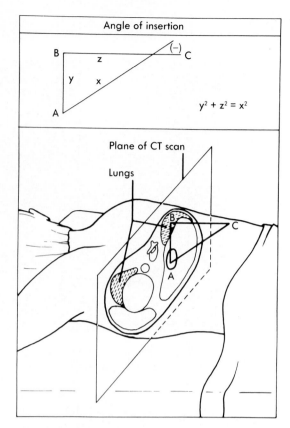

Fig. 82-4 Calculations needed to miss sulcus of lung. Needle path length, x, can be calculated using Pythagorean theorum as shown. Distance, y, can be calculated from CT scan slice on which lesion is identified. Distance, z, can be simply calculated from difference between positions of target slice and entry slice. If wanted, angle of insertion can be calculated using any trigonometric function.

calizer consists of various lengths of cut catheters in a ladder-like fashion.[20] One can localize the level of the scan slice by counting how many catheters are visualized and choosing an exact entry point. A new localizer is now available that localizes the plane of the scan slice down to an accuracy of 1 mm and allows 15 separate entry points within the plane of each scan* (Fig. 82-6).

Even if the entry point for the biopsy or drainage is correctly found, major problems with accuracy can occur because of inaccurate angulation of the needle. To solve these problems, much work has recently been done on body stereotaxis.† These methods, although they have some limitations, have shown an accuracy of placement clearly superior to the accuracy shown by the hand guid-

---

*Radionics, Inc., Burlington, Mass.
†References 16, 21, 33, 61, 62, 63, 79.

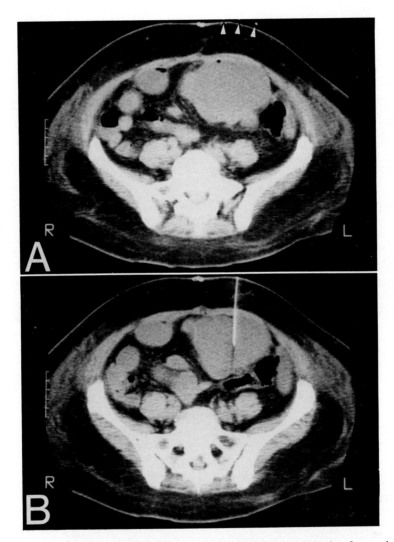

Fig. 82-5 Sixty-four-year-old woman with fever and abdominal pain 3 weeks after total pancreatectomy. **A,** Three white dots *(arrowheads)* represent straightened paper clip placed on skin as entry marker on anterior abdominal wall over large abscess. **B,** No. 5 French ring needle sheath is advanced into center of abscess after using paper clips for localization.

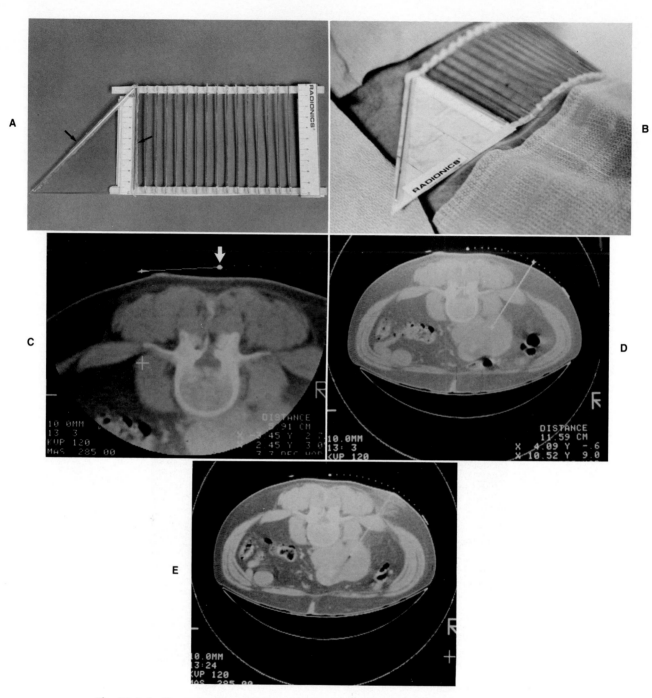

Fig. 82-6 A, Biopsy localizer. Localizer consists of plexiglass triangle with two aluminum rods attached to it, which define one of legs and hypotenuse of triangle *(arrows)*. Scale in centimeters lies next to verticle aluminum rod. Connected to triangle are 15 rods at 1 cm intervals. Triangle and aluminum rectangle at end of ladder both have double back tape to fasten them to patient. Since triangle defined by aluminum rods is equilateral right triangle, scale not only indicates distance from top of triangle but also distance between two rods in any scan plane. **B,** Localizer is placed on skin in general area of biopsy and aligned to plane of scan using laser localizer lights. **C,** Magnified image of cross-section of triangular localizer seen on CT scan. Distance measurement is taken between well-defined dot *(arrow)*, which represents verticle leg of triangle and center of line, which represents cross-section through aluminum rod making hypotenuse of triangle. **D,** Path is calculated from one bright dot, which is cross-section through one of aluminum rods of ladder, to tumor in retroperitoneum of this patient. **E,** Needle placement follows path calculated.

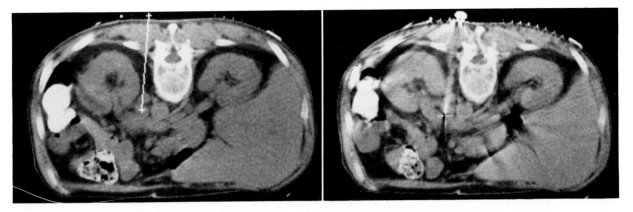

Fig. 82-7 A, Calculated path to small 1.5 cm retroperitoneal lymph node. Note that path goes just underneath transverse process and just medial to rib and kidney. **B,** Needle is noted to have followed path exactly, and biopsy was positive for lymphoma.
(From Onik, G, et al: Radiology 166:389, 1988.)

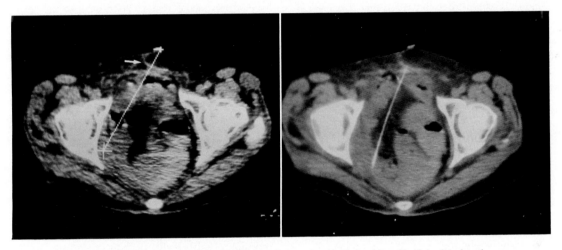

Fig. 82-8 A, Calculation of path to abnormal tissue along pelvic sidewall. Calculated path goes through scar caused by previous laparotomy *(arrow)*. **B,** Twenty-two-gauge needle has been deviated from its course by passing through scar.

Fig. 82-9 Tip of needle is deviated away from acute angle made by needle with skin. Needle entry points therefore should be as perpendicular to skin as possible. This type of deflection should be taken into account when small lesions are biopsied.

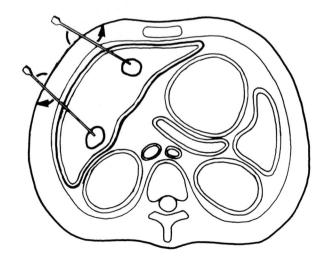

ance method.[63] Biopsies not possible by the hand method can be completed with stereotaxis (Fig. 82-7). Stereotaxis is also associated with fewer complications.[63]

Tissue inhomogeneities—either abnormal tissue, such as scars, or normal tissue planes, such as fascia—can deflect needles from their course and should be avoided when possible (Fig. 82-8). The angle of needle entry into the skin also appears to be an important factor in the placement accuracy of the needle (Fig. 82-9). The literature indicates that beveled needles track away from the bevel, greatly affecting their placement accuracy, and should be avoided if possible.[13,18,23] If one is committed to beveled needles for whatever reason, their accuracy can be enhanced by twirling the needle as it is placed. Lastly, patient respiration degrades accuracy of needle placement in a cephalocaudad direction because of the movement of internal organs. Quiet breathing is generally more reproducible than end inspiration or expiration. We tell patients to breathe easily but stress that it is critical to stop respiration at the same point in the cycle for each scan and needle placement. With careful instruction patient respiration can be greatly reduced as a factor in needle placement inaccuracy. Respiratory gating devices are difficult to use.[40]

Magnetic resonance imaging

Application of MRI-guided biopsies to the body has already begun with the development of appropriate nonferromagnetic needles.[57] At this juncture, however, MRI biopsies are more of academic interest than practical importance, since the overwhelming majority of biopsy procedures can be guided by ultrasound. CT can be used if the lesion is not well visualized by ultrasound or if additional accuracy is required.

Choice of biopsy needle

Various kinds of biopsy needles have been advocated. A controlled study by Andriole[1] examining 30 different needles on cadaver liver allows certain generalizations. First, the larger the needle, the larger the specimen. Second, the more acute the angle of a beveled needle, the better the specimen will be. Lastly, the Franseen,* Lee, and Rotex needles yield a significantly larger specimen than the beveled needles. Needle choice is dictated by other factors relating to the biopsy. For instance, for small lesions in difficult locations a trocar tip needle that tracks straighter, such as the Franseen or the E-Z-EM biopsy needle, is preferred over the beveled needles, such as the Chiba,* which will deviate. In addition, the needle chosen depends somewhat on the method of placement and

gaining a specimen—that is, whether multiple biopsies are going to be obtained coaxially through a single needle and whether the sample is going to be examined cytologically or histologically. Certain needles are designed to yield better core specimens for histologic examination.

Because of the many variables and the small samples obtained, multiple samples are usually necessary for diagnosis.[24,53] Since the time-consuming part of the biopsy is placement of the needle and confirmation in the mass, a number of methods have evolved for obtaining multiple samples without removing the localization needle. The most common is the tandem needle technique. After localizing a 22-gauge needle in the lesion, multiple punctures are made and pathologic specimens taken with another 22-gauge needle beside this localization needle, using the localization needle as a guide to the necessary entry point and angulation. An alternative to this method is obtaining multiple biopsies coaxially through the localization needle that is confirmed in the lesion. This method reduces the number of new needle punctures; however, it usually requires that localization be done with a larger needle. We have found that we can use a 19.5-gauge thin-walled needle (E-Z-EM) with a 22-gauge Chiba needle in it to obtain multiple samples. With stereotaxis this is probably the preferred method.

Recently, a combination of these two methods has been described, in which a 23-gauge needle is used to localize the lesion, minimizing trauma because of the needle's small size. The hub of the 23-gauge needle is then removed, and over this needle the 19-gauge needle is placed. Multiple biopsies can then be obtained through the 19-gauge needle.

The choice of histologic or cytologic processing of a specimen will greatly depend on the preference of the pathologist. One advantage of histologic processing is that less experienced pathologists can more easily make a diagnosis. In addition, if a good core sample is obtained, a specific diagnosis of a benign condition is often possible. This can be extremely important, since unless a specific diagnosis is made, a benign or negative biopsy has to be considered inadequate and another biopsy or a more invasive procedure must be performed. Lastly, a more specific diagnosis of malignancy can often be made from a histologic sample, which may have therapeutic implications. The major disadvantage of histologic sampling is that there is a lower yield of adequate tissue when used alone. The difference can be as great as 56% for histologic sampling and 85% for cytologic sampling, using a 22-gauge needle.[34] To raise this yield, larger needles are often needed to gain a sample, which theoretically raises the incidence of complications.

The advantages of cytologic processing are essentially

---

*Cook, Inc., Bloomington, Ind.

the opposite of the disadvantages of histologic processing. A higher yield of adequate specimens can be obtained when the specimen is looked at cytologically than histologically. A smaller needle can be used, thereby decreasing patient trauma, and adequate specimens can still be obtained.

The best approach may be a combination of these two methods, in which 1 to 2 cc of saline is kept in the biopsy syringe. The biopsy is conducted using the cutting needle designed to get a tissue core. The specimen, when obtained, is injected into a test tube and sent to the laboratory, at which time the tissue fragments are removed and histologically processed, while the supernatant is passed through a milipore filter from which the cells are recovered and examined cytologically.[26,34]

Results

The accuracy of the results of the biopsy depends on a number of factors. One of the most important is the lesion biopsied. Pancreatic carcinoma and lymphoma have demonstrated a lower sensitivity than other types of abnormalities.[4,48,66,81,82] In general, the accuracy of the results (combined sensitivity and specificity) will be increased when the size of the needle is increased, since more adequate samples will be obtained, and when a pathologist is present during the biopsy to assess the adequacy of the sample.[39] This procedure obviates the need for repeat biopsies at a second sitting, since samples can continue to be taken until the pathologist feels an adequate one has been obtained.

The expected sensitivity for malignancy is 85% to 95%. Of great importance is that false-positive diagnoses for malignancy are extremely rare.

Complications

The most important advantage of percutaneous fine-needle biopsy is that its morbidity is *extremely* low. This makes it the procedure of choice for obtaining pathologic confirmation of intraabdominal lesions. The specific complications associated with this procedure include:

1. *Death*. This is an extremely rare complication, with a published mortality rate of 0.008%. The cause of death is usually bleeding.[32]
2. *Bleeding*. Significant bleeding is extremely rare, with 27 cases of 63 of 108 cases requiring blood transfusion.[32]
3. *Infection*. Whenever a needle is placed into an organ, there is a chance for infection. This is an extremely rare complication.[32]
4. *Bile leakage*. This is a risk when a liver lesion is being biopsied in a patient who has an obstructed bile system. Although unusual, if this does occur,

it will manifest as an acute abdomen with bile peritonitis and can be treated with biliary decompression.[47]
5. *Pancreatitis*. Clinical pancreatitis associated with a pancreatic biopsy is quite unusual. One death from pancreatitis has been reported in the literature. The patient who died had a questionable pancreatic head mass and a normal pancreas biopsied.[19]
6. *Pneumothorax*. Biopsy of a lesion in the dome of the liver may be followed by pneumothorax.
7. *Tumor seeding*. Although rare cases of tumor seeding have been reported, this carries little weight in the decision-making process.[11,64]

DRAINAGE OF ABDOMINAL FLUID COLLECTIONS

CT-guided percutaneous drainage of abdominal fluid collections has become a commonly performed, safe, and effective procedure, replacing analogous open surgical drainage in most patients.[22,43,60,72,74] Although percutaneous drainage was described almost 50 years ago,[49] possible interposition of abdominal viscera and organs limited the utility of this approach in the abdomen. As CT clearly depicts parenchymal organs, bowel, and major vascular structures, a safe percutaneous approach can be identified today.

Patient selection

One of the main reasons why percutaneous drainage has gained widespread acceptance is that the procedure is applicable to most patients, regardless of the location of the fluid. Intraperitoneal, retroperitoneal, and intraparenchymal (liver, spleen, and pancreas) fluid collections can be evacuated whenever a percutaneous access route that avoids the pleural space, intervening bowel, and major vascular structures can be achieved.

Moreover, the procedure can be performed on critically ill individuals and avoids the morbidity of a major operation. In selected cases percutaneous abscess drainage may be used as a temporizing measure, followed by a more extensive surgical procedure when the clinical condition of the patient improves.[76]

The success of percutaneous abscess drainage depends on whether the majority of the infected material can be removed. Factors that influence this success include the viscosity of the fluid, the size and location of the drainage tube, and the extent of loculations in the abscess cavity.

Because particulate debris and pieces of tissue obstruct drainage tubes, serous fluid can be more efficiently removed than viscous fluid. This is why pancreatic phlegmons, some pancreatic abscesses, and infected hematomas cannot be effectively evacuated by the percutaneous route. Some investigators have recommended injection of proteolytic agents, including N-acetylcysteine (Mucomyst); hyaluronidase; or fibrolytic agents to liquify semisolid debris.[9,70,77] However, these techniques are not consistently effective,[17] and surgical debridement is often the more appropriate alternative.

The presence of multiple loculations can make percutaneous drainage more difficult. These loculations often communicate, despite the appearance on CT images, and should not deter an attempt at percutaneous therapy.[25] Even when true locules are present, they can be disrupted with catheter and guidewire manipulations.[45] The effectiveness of locule disruption can be assessed with CT sinography.

Most abdominal and pelvic fluid collections can be managed with percutaneous techniques. Operative management should be reserved for patients without safe percutaneous access route, when an adjunctive surgical procedure must be performed, or when the debris is so viscous that percutaneous aspiration is ineffective.

Patient preparation

Patients are maintained on a clear liquid diet before the procedure. If abscess is suspected, appropriate antibiotic therapy is initiated before drainage. Although this may alter the results of bacterial cultures obtained at the time of drainage, it is more important to protect the patient against massive septicemia. Bacteremia undoubtedly occurs during most percutaneous abscess drainage procedures.

Adequate analgesia is important. In most patients a narcotic analgesic combined with a hypnotic sedative intramuscularly 30 minutes before the procedure, augmented by intravenous midazolam (1 to 10 mg) at the time of the drainage, is adequate. Caution, however, must be exercised when using this agent because of reports of severe respiratory depression associated with its use.

Guidance

CT provides the best depiction of abdominal fluid collections and clearly demonstrates adjacent organs, bowel, and major vascular structures. For these reasons CT is the best available modality for planning percutaneous drainage. Subsequent catheter manipulations are better controlled with fluoroscopic imaging. For difficult cases it may be optimal to perform the initial puncture under CT and place a guidewire coil in the abscess. The patient can then be moved to the fluoroscopic suite for tract dilatation and placement of a drainage tube. In most cases, however, moving the patient is unnecessary, and the procedure can be completed under CT.

Some investigators have advocated real-time ultrasound imaging for abdominal abscess drainage.[58] Ultrasound may be a useful adjunct but is clearly more operator dependent than CT or fluoroscopy.

Selection of puncture site

The technique of CT localization has already been described; however, certain aspects of puncture site selection for drainage procedures should be discussed. If an intercostal approach is needed, care should be taken to avoid the space immediately below the rib, where the intercostal artery and nerve reside. Laceration of the artery can lead to excessive bleeding, and catheters placed adjacent to the nerve are extremely uncomfortable.

The pleural space should also be avoided. The pleural space extends well below aerated lung and is often inadvertently transgressed during biliary drainage procedures without complication. However, problems occasionally do develop, and these problems are exponentially magnified if grossly infected debris accumulates in the thoracic cavity. Therefore an entry site below the diaphragmatic insertion is optimal. To avoid the pleural space, spleen, and kidneys, it may be necessary to use the triangulation method.

Fluid collections in the lesser sac may be drained through a transhepatic approach (Fig. 82-10).[56] The only contraindication to this route is the presence of undrained biliary obstruction.

The other region where indirect percutaneous paths are not infrequently used is the pelvis. Loops of small bowel and sigmoid colon are often interposed between the abdominal wall and these dependent pelvic fluid collections (Fig. 82-11). Alternative approaches include the transvaginal, transrectal,[50,59] and transgluteal routes.[7] The

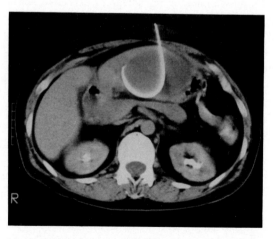

Fig. 82-10 Forty-three-year-old woman with abdominal pain. No. 10 French catheter is placed into lesser sac fluid collection through lateral segment of left hepatic lobe. Diagnosis was infected pancreatic pseudocyst.

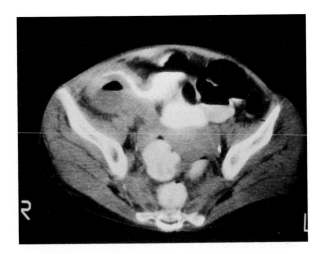

Fig. 82-11 In this patient with Crohn's disease, thickened loop of small bowel can be seen to drape over abscess. On this scan there is no safe route to this fluid collection.

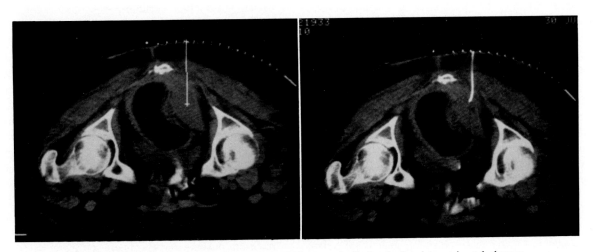

Fig. 82-12 Transgluteal approach to perirectal abscess. **A,** Path calculated to perirectal abscess. **B,** Catheter following calculated path.

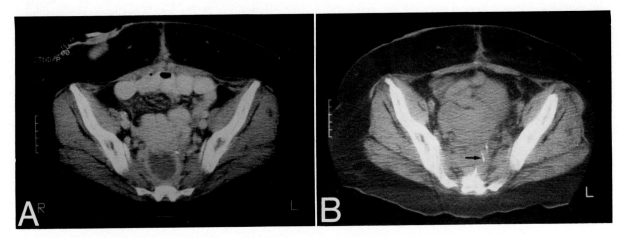

Fig. 82-13 Fifty-five-year-old woman 1 year after proctocolectomy and 1 month after laparotomy for lysis of adhesions returned with pelvic pain and fever. **A,** Pelvic CT shows presacral fluid collection, presumably representing abscess. **B,** Drainage catheter *(arrow)* is placed through transperineal approach, successfully evacuating 150 ml of purulent fluid.

transgluteal route employs the greater sciatic foramen as the access window into the pelvic peritoneal cavity (Fig. 82-12). When placing a transgluteal catheter, an attempt should be made to transgress the greater sciatic foramen as close to the sacrum and as caudally within the foramen as possible. This minimizes the chance of irritating or damaging the sciatic nerve. Other neural and vascular structures are present in this region,[35] but the incidence of significant complications appears to be quite low.

A transperineal approach is feasible in patients who have undergone proctocolectomy (Fig. 82-13). However, external stabilization of drainage tubes inserted through the perineum is difficult, and a Cope-loop type of catheter should be used.

Catheter selection and insertion

The selection of the specific type of drainage catheter is again largely a matter of personal preference. For superficial collections direct insertion of a No. 5 French needle sheath* has advantages compared with a conventional 18-gauge needle. The major advantage is that the outer No. 5 French sheath is extremely flexible and virtually atraumatic after the stylet has been removed. This flexibility becomes important when one considers the time required to move the patient back into the gantry and perform and reconstruct the CT image to confirm the position of the needle when fluid cannot be freely aspirated.

For deeper fluid collections located adjacent to vital structures many radiologists prefer using a smaller 22- or 21-gauge needle with a conversion system that allows placement of a 0.018-inch guidewire, such as the system designed by Cope.[36] Although this system can be used safely with CT guidance, buckling of the initial 0.018 guidewire occasionally presents problems.

After successful puncture of the fluid collection, 20 to 30 ml are removed and a specimen sent for aerobic and anaerobic culture. It is usually not difficult to ascertain by simple inspection whether the fluid is infected. If a question does exist on the nature of the fluid, a Gram stain is performed immediately. If the fluid is not infected, as much fluid as possible is aspirated through the needle sheath or Cope dilator, and the catheter is removed.

If a drainage tube will be placed, no additional fluid is removed. It is much more difficult to manipulate catheters in a collapsed cavity compared with a space in which some fluid remains. On the other hand, some fluid should be removed through the needle sheath or Cope dilator, as manipulations in a tense cavity increase the incidence of septicemia.

Whatever puncture system is used, a sturdy 0.035- or 0.038-inch guidewire must be coiled securely in the cavity for placement of the drainage catheter. Placement of the drainage catheter is facilitated by dilatation of the percutaneous tract to the size of the drainage tube. Angiographic or larger fascial dilators are suitable for this purpose, and dilatation may be performed in four or six French increments in most patients. Stiffening cannulas that accompany commercially available percutaneous drainage catheters should be used to insert the tube.

Single lumen tubes work best when the fluid is thin and easily aspirated. Nephrostomy tubes with a locking Cope-loop tip ranging in size from a No. 8 to No. 14 French tube are easily inserted and effective for simple gravity drainage. Continuous suction cannot be used with this type of tube, as the tissue of the abscess wall is drawn into the tube occluding it.

For the majority of abscesses with more viscous fluid and debris sump tubes ranging in size from a No. 12 to No. 24 French tube are more appropriate. The major advantage of a sump tube is that low continuous suction may be applied to more completely evacuate the cavity. When the cavity has completely collapsed, air is drawn in through the sump port. This prevents excessive suction of the tube against the cavity wall and promotes tube patency. The Ring-McLean sump* is internally vented in the true sump design. The van Sonnenberg sump† is externally vented, creating a parallel catheter system rather than a true sump. Both drainage tubes are effective in evacuating most abscess cavities, but the small sump lumens of both catheters frequently occlude, requiring recurrent flushing and eventually replacement. To avoid this problem, the Kerlan-Ring drainage tube† was developed with a replaceable sump lumen. However, the softness of this catheter makes initial insertion difficult, and the tube is prone to kinking when bent.

When exceptionally viscous fluid or fecal debris is being drained, larger No. 24 to No. 30 French tubes may be required. Tubes of this size must either be inserted through existing surgical drainage tracts, or the percutaneous tract must be widened with fascial dilators.[15] Although the Ring-McLean sump is available in a No. 24 French size, similar tubes may be created with commonly available materials. For example, a No. 24 French sump tube is easily made by suturing a No. 6 French angiographic catheter into the distal lumen of a No. 24 French Mallecot or similar drainage tube.

Regardless of the specific type of drainage tube selected, as much fluid as possible is aspirated after insertion. Fluoroscopic manipulation may be necessary to position the drainage tube in the dependent portion of com-

---

*Ring biliary drainage needle, Cook, Inc., Bloomington, Ind.

*Cook, Inc., Bloomington, Ind.
†Meditech.

plex cavities. However, in most cases confirmation of dependent positioning on the basis of the CT image alone is sufficient.

Irrigation of the cavity at the time of initial drainage has been advocated by some authors.[69] In our experience this practice leads to a higher incidence of postprocedural sepsis, even if overdistention of the cavity is carefully avoided, and is potentially dangerous.

After the fluid is aspirated, the patient is rescanned to check for undrained loculations and to confirm appropriate tube position. The tube is then externally secured and the patient returned to the ward.

Special considerations
Pancreas

Three types of fluid collections occur in the pancreas: pseudocysts, encapsulated abscesses, and phlegmons. Although there is clearly some overlap in these categories, it is useful to consider the predominant type of collection when selecting the appropriate form of therapy.

The most common type of collection is the pseudocyst. A simple pseudocyst requires no emergent intervention. In fact, spontaneous resolution of pseudocysts is well documented. If the cyst is causing intractable pain or obstructive jaundice, percutaneous drainage is warranted. Although aspiration with a 22-gauge needle will occasionally be curative, drainage tube insertion is usually required. In most patients the thin pancreatic fluid can be effectively evacuated with a No. 10 or No. 12 French nephrostomy tube.

Pseudocysts may be approached anteriorly if no intervening loops of bowel are present. When bowel is interposed, transhepatic drainage should be considered as well as an anterolateral approach between the stomach and spleen. Transgastric drainage has also been advocated to create a percutaneous cyst gastrostomy.[2,55]

Sinograms performed 3 to 5 days after pseudocyst drainage will often opacify the pancreatic duct. If the duct is obstructed, the pseudocyst will not resolve without adjunctive therapy to relieve the obstruction. When the sinogram opacifies an unobstructed pancreatic duct, rapid resolution can be anticipated.

Whenever a pseudocyst is present in a patient with fever or sepsis, an infected pseudocyst should be suspected and diagnostic aspiration performed. If infection is confirmed, the pseudocyst is drained percutaneously or surgically.

Thick-walled pancreatic abscesses can also be managed percutaneously (Fig. 82-14). In most cases these cavities are filled with frank pus rather than infected pancreatic fluid and require insertion of a moderate size (No. 12 to No. 16 French) drainage tube for complete evacuation.

Pancreatic phlegmons cannot be managed with exist-

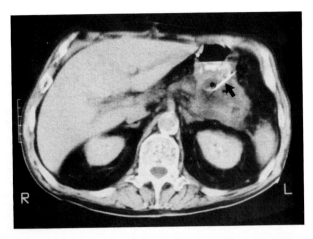

Fig. 82-14 Sixty-year-old man with abdominal distention and sepsis. Thick-walled pancreatic abscess is punctured from anterolateral approach between stomach and spleen. Subsequently No. 16 French drainage tube was placed, yielding 50 ml of thick, purulent fluid. Patient's condition improved, and surgical debridement was electively performed.

ing percutaneous techniques. Despite insertion of even large No. 24 to No. 30 French drainage catheters (Fig. 82-15), the semisolid infected debris cannot be removed. Surgical debridement has been the only effective form of therapy.

Although CT-guided percutaneous procedures involving the pancreas are being performed more commonly, the risks of percutaneous drainage of pancreatic fluid collections must always be considered. Not only is there potential for creating a pancreaticocutaneous fistula, but an inadequate percutaneous drainage can aggravate the existing infection and convert a serious surgical problem into a disastrous complication.

Spleen

Fluid collections in the spleen can be safely drained percutaneously.[30,67] However, there is an increased risk of intraperitoneal hemorrhage, and only collections that can be evacuated without traversing splenic parenchyma should be attempted (Fig. 82-16). It may be useful to use a Cope-loop type of drainage tube, as respiratory motion will tend to dislodge straight tubes. Moreover, a tube with a pigtail configuration is less likely to perforate the splenic parenchyma, reducing the chance of hemorrhage.

Liver

Heaptic abscesses are well suited for percutaneous drainage and generally preclude the necessity of a difficult open surgical procedure. Both pyogenic and amebic

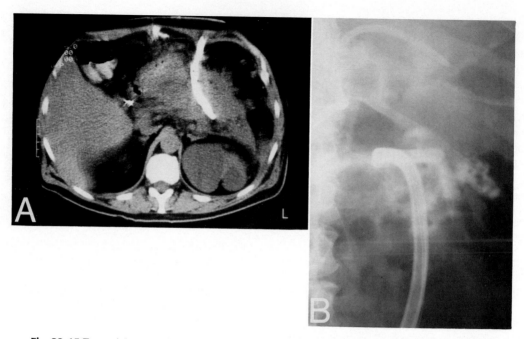

Fig. 82-15 Forty-eight-year-old man with pancreatitis and sepsis. **A,** CT scan demonstrates drainage tube in pancreatic phlegmon. **B,** Sinogram performed through No. 30 French drainage tube fails to reveal defined cavity. No. 16 French drainage tube is present in adjacent pancreatic pseudocyst. Surgical debridement was eventually required.

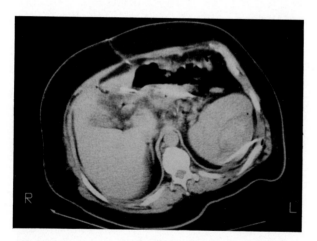

Fig. 82-16 Fifty-one-year-old man with left upper quadrant pain and fever 2 weeks after gastric stapling procedure. No. 12 French drainage catheter is inserted into peripheral low-density collection in spleen. Diagnosis was infected splenic hematoma.

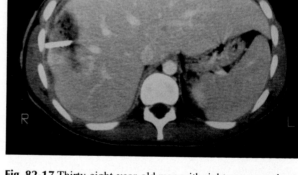

Fig. 82-17 Thirty-eight-year-old man with right upper quadrant pain and fever. No. 12 French sump tube has been inserted to drain pyogenic abscess in right lobe. Abscess resolved after 3 weeks of drainage.

abscesses (Fig. 82-17) can be successfully treated, although the latter group can be medically managed in most patients. The proximity of the pleural space often requires using the triangulation technique. In addition, the sensitivity of the hepatic capsule usually prevents initial placement of a drainage catheter larger than a No. 12 French catheter without regional or general anesthesia.

Patient management and follow-up

Hospitalized patients with indwelling catheters are seen daily or more often if necessary. Most drainage tubes require flushing to maintain patency. Routine flushing with 3 to 6 ml of sterile saline three times a day is usually sufficient.

Parenteral narcotic analgesia may be required during

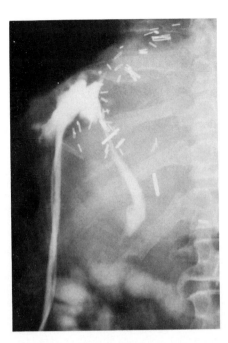

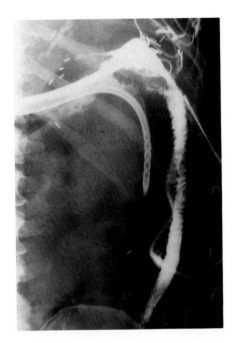

Fig. 82-18 Sixty-two-year-old man 2 weeks after percutaneous drainage of perihepatic abscess that formed after right hepatic lobectomy. Sinogram demonstrates fistula to extrahepatic bile duct through stump of right hepatic duct. Drainage catheter has been placed through fistulous opening to control bile leak.

Fig. 82-19 Fifty-one-year-old man 10 days after percutaneous drainage of interloop abscess through anterior abdominal midline incision. Sinogram demonstrates fistulous connection to descending colon. Drainage catheters have been placed adjacent to site of perforation and dependently within adjacent abscess cavity.

the initial 24 hours. After the first day, oral analgesia is adequate for most patients.

The amount of drainage should be recorded. Although variable in the first 24 hours, the amount is generally less than 50 ml in the second 24 hours. When the drainage exceeds 50 ml in 24 hours, fistulous communication should be strongly suspected.

All patients return to the fluoroscopic suite 3 to 5 days after abscess drainage for sinography.[44] Tubes are routinely replaced and repositioned in the dependent portion of the cavity at that time. If significant retained debris is present in the cavity, the tract is dilated and a larger drainage tube inserted.

Not infrequently, sinography will reveal communications to the alimentary canal, biliary tract, or pancreatic ductal system. When a fistulous communication is suspected on the basis of the quantity or quality of the drainage tube effluent, gentle exploration of the abscess cavity with a guidewire and catheter under fluoroscopic observation is warranted. The use of a steerable catheter is usually less traumatic and less time consuming. The identification of these low-output fistulous communications is important, as the cause of the abscess is often revealed. Moreover, a drainage tube may be positioned adjacent to the fistulous tract, evacuating the cavity more effectively (Figs. 82-18 and 82-19). Low-output com-

munications can be identified in 30% to 50% of patients with abdominal abscesses.[41,42]

When the discomfort of drainage tube insertion is controlled with oral analgesics, the patient is discharged home on gravity drainage to a leg bag. As an outpatient, the patient returns weekly for sinography and tube replacements. Patients without fistulous communications generally require 2 to 3 weeks of drainage. Patients with fistulous communications require 4 to 6 weeks for both the fistula and abscess cavity to heal. The drainage tube is removed when there is no output for 48 hours and the sinogram demonstrates that the cavity has healed.

REFERENCES

1. Andriole, J, et al: Biopsy needle characteristics assessed in the laboratory, Radiology 148:659, 1983.
2. Bernardino, ME, and Amerson, JR: Percutaneous gastrocystostomy: a new approach to pancreatic drainage, AJR 143:621, 1984.
3. Bree, R, et al: Abdominal fine needle aspiration biopsies with CT and ultrasound guidance: techniques, results and clinical implications, Comput Radiol 8:99, 1984.
4. Bret, P, Nicolet, V, and Labadie, M: Percutaneous fine needle aspiration biopsy of the pancreas, Diagn Cytopathol 2:5, 1986.
5. Bret, P, et al: Abdominal lesions: a prospective study of clinical efficacy of percutaneous fine needle biopsy, Radiology 159:345, 1986.
6. Bret, PM, et al: Ultrasonically guided fine needle biopsy in focal intrahepatic lesions: six years' experience, J Can Assoc Radiol 37:5, 1986.

7. Butch, RJ, et al: Drainage of pelvic abscesses through the greater sciatic foramen, Radiology 158:487, 1986.

8. Casamassima, F, et al: Percutaneous needle biopsy guided by ultrasound in the diagnosis of intraabdominal masses, Rays 12:53, 1987.

9. Casola, G, and van Sonnenberg, E: Skin damage from acetylcysteine leak during percutaneous abscess drainage, Radiology 152:232, 1984.

10. Casola, G, et al: Unsuspected pheochromocytoma: risk of blood pressure alterations during percutaneous adrenal biopsy, Radiology 159:733, 1986.

11. Caturelli, E, et al: Malignant seeding after fine needle aspiration biopsy of the pancreas, Diagn Imag Clin Med 54:88, 1985.

12. Caturelli, E, et al: Ultrasound guided fine needle aspiration biopsy in the diagnosis of hepatic hemangioma, Liver 6:326, 1986.

13. Cooley, R, and Robinson, S: Comparative evaluation of 30-gauge dental needle, Oral Surg 48:400, 1979.

14. Cope, C: Conversion from small (0.018 inch) to large (0.038 inch) guidewires in percutaneous drainage procedures, AJR 138:170, 1982.

15. Cope, C: Improved anchoring of nephrostomy catheters: loop technique, AJR 138:170, 1982.

16. Costello, P, Onik, G, and Cosman, E: Computed tomographic guided stereotaxic biopsy of thoracic lesions, J Thorac Imag 2:27, 1987.

17. Dawson, SL, Mueller, PR, and Ferrucci, JT, Jr: Mucomyst for abscesses: a clinical comment, Radiology 151:342, 1984.

18. Drummond, G, and Scott, D: Deflection of spinal needles by the bevel, Anesthesia 35:854, 1980.

19. Evans, W, et al: Fatal necrotizing pancreatitis following fine needle aspiration biopsy of the pancreas, Radiology 141:161, 1981.

20. Ferrucci, J, and Wittenberg, J: CT guided biopsy of abdominal tumors: aids for localization, Radiology 129:739, 1979.

21. Frederick, R, et al: Light guidance system to be used for CT guided biopsy, Radiology 154:535, 1985.

22. Gerzof, SG, et al: Expanded criteria for percutaneous abscess drainage, Radiology 156:270, 1985.

23. Glazener, E: The bevel and deflection of spinal needles (letter), Anesth Anal 62:371, 1983.

24. Gothlin, J, and Gadeholt, G: Percutaneous fine needle biopsy of abdominal pelvic lesions: passes necessary for secure diagnosis with fluoroscopy and CT guidance, Eur J Radiol 6:288, 1986.

25. Gray, R, et al: Percutaneous abscess drainage, Gastrointest Radiol 10:79, 1985.

26. Greene, R, et al: Supplementary tissue core histology for fine needle transthoracic aspiration biopsy, AJR 144:787, 1985.

27. Haaga, J, and Alfidi, R: Precise biopsy localization by computed tomography, Radiology 118:603, 1976.

28. Hammers, L, et al: Computed tomographic guided percutaneous fine needle aspiration biopsy: the Yale experience, Yale J Biol Med 59:425, 1986.

29. Harter, L, et al: CT guided fine needle aspirations for the diagnosis of benign and malignant disease, AJR 140:363, 1983.

30. Ho, CS, and Taylor, B: Percutaneous transgastric drainage for pancreatic pseudocyst, AJR 143:623, 1984.

31. Ho, C, et al: Guided percutaneous fine needle aspiration biopsy of the liver, Cancer 47:1781, 1981.

32. Holm, H, et al: Percutaneous fine needle biopsy, Clin Gastroenterol 14:423, 1985.

33. Hruby, W, and Muschik, H: A new belt-type device for CT guided biopsy and puncture, Ann Radiol 30:145, 1987.

34. Isler, R, et al: Tissue core biopsy of abdominal tumors with a 22-gauge cutting needle, AJR 136:725, 1981.

35. Jaques, PF, and Mauro, MA: Drainage of pelvic abscesses through the greater sciatic foramen (letter), Radiology 160:278, 1986.

36. Jeffrey, RB, Jr, Wing, VW, and Laing, FC: Real-time sonographic monitoring of percutaneous drainage, AJR 144:469, 1985.

37. Jewel, K: Computerized tomography guided percutaneous needle biopsy, J Med Soc NJ 81:297, 1984.

38. Jewel, K, and Kimler, S: Percutaneous fine needle biopsy using direct imaging techniques, J Med Soc NJ 79:731, 1982.

39. Johnsrude, I, et al: Rapid cytology to decrease pneumothorax incidence after percutaneous biopsy, AJR 144:793, 1985.

40. Jones, K: A respiratory monitor for use with CT body scanning and other imaging techniques, Br J Radiol 55:530, 1982.

41. Kerlan, RK, Jr, et al: Abdominal abscess with low-output fistula: successful percutaneous drainage, Radiology 155:73, 1985.

42. Kerlan, RK, Jr, et al: Radiologic management of abdominal abscesses, AJR 144:145, 1985.

43. Lawler, GA, Doyle, TCA, and Lavan, J: Use of computed tomography in the percutaneous drainage of abdominal abscesses, Radiology 155:275, 1985.

44. Lerner, RM, and Spataro, RF: Splenic abscess: percutaneous drainage, Radiology 153:643, 1984.

45. Lieberman, RP, et al: Loculated abscesses: management by percutaneous fracture of septations, Radiology 161:827, 1986.

46. Limber, B, Hopker, W, and Commerell, B: Histologic differential diagnosis of focal liver lesions by ultrasonically guided fine needle biopsy, Gut 28:237, 1987.

47. Livraghi, T, et al: Risk in fine needle abdominal biopsy, J Clin Ultrasound 11:77, 1983.

48. Luning, M, et al: CT guided percutaneous fine needle biopsy of the pancreas, Eur Radiol 5:104, 1985.

49. Martin, HE, and Ellis, EB: Biopsy by needle puncture and aspiration, Ann Surg 92:169, 1930.

50. Mauro, MA, et al: Pelvic abscess drainage by transrectal catheter approach in men, AJR 144:477, 1985.

51. McCorkell, S: Unintended percutaneous aspiration of pulmonary echinococcal cysts, AJR 143:123, 1984.

52. Mok, P, and Yeong, M: Ultrasound guided fine needle biopsy of abdominal mass lesions, NZ Med J 99:111, 1986.

53. Morettin, L, et al: Multiple simultaneous percutaneous needle biopsy technique for masses of the abdomen in peritoneum, Eur J Radiol 7:98, 1987.

54. Moss, A: Interventional computed tomography. In Moss, A, et al, editors: Computed tomography of the body, Philadelphia, 1983, WB Saunders.

55. Mueller, PR, van Sonnenberg, E, and Ferrucci, JT, Jr: Percutaneous drainage of 250 abdominal abscesses and fluid collections. II. Current procedural concepts, Radiology 151:343, 1984.

56. Mueller, PR, et al: Lesser sac abscesses and fluid collections: drainage by transhepatic approach, Radiology 155:615, 1985.

57. Mueller, P, et al: MR-guided aspiration biopsy: needle design and clinical trials, Radiology 161:605, 1986.

58. Nichols, DM, et al: Safe intercostal approach? Pleural complications in abdominal interventional radiology, AJR 142:1013, 1984.

59. Nosher, JL, et al: Transrectal pelvic abscess drainage with sonographic guidance, AJR 146:1047, 1986.

60. Olak, J, et al: Operative versus percutaneous drainage of intraabdominal abscesses: comparison of morbidity and mortality, Arch Surg 121:141, 1986.

61. Onik, G, et al: CT body stereotaxic instrument for percutaneous biopsy and other interventional procedures: phantom studies, Invest Radiol 20:525, 1985.

62. Onik, G, et al: CT body stereotaxis: an aid for CT guided biopsies, AJR 146:163, 1986.

63. Onik, G, et al: CT guided aspirations for the body: comparison of hand guidance with stereotaxis, Radiology 166:389, 1988.

64. Onodera, H, et al: Cutaneous seeding of hepatocellular carcinoma after fine needle aspiration biopsy, J Ultrasound Med 6:273, 1987.

65. Pelaez, J, et al: Abdominal aspiration biopsies sonographic versus computed tomographic guidance, JAMA 250:2663, 1983.

66. Phillips, V, Knopf, D, and Bernardino, M: Percutaneous hepatic biopsy in suspected pancreatic carcinoma, J Comput Tomogr 8:307, 1984.

67. Quinn, SF, et al: Interventional radiology in the spleen, Radiology 161:289, 1986.

68. Rizzatto, G, et al: Aspiration biopsy of superficial lesions: ultrasonic guidance with a linear ray probe, AJR 148:623, 1987.

69. Rusnak, B, et al: An improved dilator system for percutaneous nephrostomies, Radiology 144:174, 1982.

70. Sheffner, AL: The reduction *in vitro* in viscosity of mucoprotein solutions by a new mucogenic agent, N-acetylcysteine, Ann NY Acad Sci 1:298, 1963.

71. Solmi, L, et al: Echo guided fine needle biopsy of pancreatic masses, Am J Gastroenterol 82:744, 1987.

72. Sones, PJ: Percutaneous drainage of abdominal abscesses, AJR 142:35, 1984.

73. Sundaram, M, et al: Utility of CT guided abdominal aspiration procedures, AJR 139:1111, 1982.

74. van Sonnenberg, E, Mueller, PR, and Ferrucci, JT, Jr: Percutaneous drainage of 250 abdominal abscesses and fluid collections. I. Results, failures and complications, Radiology 151:337, 1984.

75. van Sonnenberg, E, Wittenberg, J, and Ferrucci, J: Triangulation method for percutaneous needle guidance: the angled approach to upper abdominal masses, AJR 137:757, 1981.

76. van Sonnenberg, E, et al: Temporizing effect of percutaneous drainage of complicated abscesses in critically ill patients, AJR 142:821, 1984.

77. van Waes, PFGM, et al: Management of loculated abscesses that are difficult to drain: a new approach, Radiology 147:57, 1983.

78. Wittenberg, J, et al: Percutaneous core biopsy of abdominal tumors using 22-gauge needles: further observations, AJR 139:75, 1982.

79. Wunschik, F, George, I, and Pastyr, O: Stereotaxic biopsy using computed tomography, J Comput Assist Tomogr 8:32, 1984.

80. Yamamoto, R, Tatsuta, CM, and Noguchi, S: Histologic diagnosis of pancreatic cancer by percutaneous aspiration biopsy under ultrasonic guidance, Am J Clin Pathol 83:409, 1985.

81. Zornoza, J, et al: Percutaneous needle biopsy of abdominal lymphoma, AJR 136:97, 1981.

82. Zornoza, J, et al: Fine needle aspiration biopsy of retroperitoneal lymph nodes and abdominal masses: an updated report, Radiology 125:87, 1987.

83 *Overview*

CHRISTOPH D. BECKER
H. JOACHIM BURHENNE

GENERAL CONSIDERATIONS

Interventional radiology began with manipulative procedures in the gastrointestinal (GI) tract. By 1955, 1838 treatments of intussusception in children had been reported from Scandinavia.[54] The term *interventional radiology* was coined by Margulis in 1967.[43] It defines the growing body of therapeutic procedures performed by the radiologist with the guidance of imaging techniques. In the 2 decades since, interventional radiology has expanded rapidly and now involves a wide range of indications for benign, malignant, and postoperative conditions in virtually every organ system in combination with almost all new imaging modalities. Significant developments in interventional radiology of the alimentary tract emerged concurrently in the early 1970s with the angiographic control of gastrointestinal bleeding[2] and nonoperative removal of bile duct calculi.[9] In the mid 1970s the simultaneous introduction of ultrasonography, computed tomography (CT), and the 22-gauge thin-wall Chiba needle provided the means for a safe, accurate pathologic diagnosis of intraabdominal mass lesions and fluid collections.[32] In the late 1970s drainage of abdominal abscesses under ultrasonic, fluoroscopic, and CT guidance was developed.[26] These procedures are now standard in many radiologic departments, and the search for new interventional techniques continues.

Radiologists performing interventional procedures undergo a substantive change from their traditional role of consultant and diagnostician to that of clinician and therapist. This requires not only close contact with the patient's referring physician, but also explanatory discussions with the patient before the procedure, obtaining informed consent, verification of drug or allergy history and bleeding parameters, familiarity with the options of pain control during interventional procedures, on-call availability, and follow-up visits after intervention. Some interventional radiologists have gone as far as to suggest that the radiology department should provide primary care services for inpatients and outpatients undergoing interventional procedures.[39,62] Others, however, believe that the disadvantages of such a system outweigh the advantages[11,22] and that most radiology departments are not prepared to provide the time, staff, and clinical skills necessary for quality patient care. Cooperation rather than adversity between medical specialties is required to keep interventional radiology growing. Furthermore, it should not be forgotten that it is the surgeon who has to take care of any complications of interventional radiologic procedures. We therefore believe that radiologists should not compete with their clinical colleagues as admitting physicians but rather seek close interdisciplinary cooperation.[11] Many nonoperative interventions require combinations of endoscopy, radiology, and surgery.

GASTROINTESTINAL TRACT

Percutaneous gastrostomy is an alternative to surgical gastrostomy, usually as a temporary or palliative procedure in patients with disorders of the central nervous system or intractable pharyngeal or esophageal obstruction.[72] Using guidewire techniques, a gastrostomy tube can be advanced under fluoroscopic control through the pylorus and duodenum into the jejunum, permitting small bowel decompression or jejunostomy feeding.[69] *Percutaneous cecostomy* has been used to decompress the massively distended cecum in impending cecal perforation caused by large bowel obstruction.[17] *Transesophageal intubation* of the stomach and small bowel under fluoroscopic control is widely used for diagnostic radiologic contrast examinations, enteric alimentation,[46] and radiologically guided *balloon dilatation* of esophagogastrointestinal strictures. Radiologic dilatation preceding surgical tube placement for esophageal cancer has resulted in significant reduction in procedural complications and mortality.[18] Favorable long-term results have also been reported with dilatation of strictures of inflammatory, anastomotic, and neoplastic origin throughout the GI tract.[47,48] The radial dilating force as opposed to the frictional component involved with the traditional bougienage technique is probably the reason for the low complication rate of the balloon technique. Fluoroscopically guided balloon dilatation now has a definite role, particularly in benign anastomotic strictures, as a noninvasive treatment.[21]

BILIARY TRACT

Percutaneous basket removal of retained bile duct stones through a T-tube tract initiated interventional radiology of the biliary tract in 1973.[9] The success of this procedure is based on a high efficacy (between 90% to 95%) in three major series published to date[10,23,25] and a complication rate that is clearly lower than that of surgical bile duct exploration[50] or endoscopic retrograde stone extraction with sphincterotomy.[64] Failures usually occur with very large calculi or those impacted in an anatomically inaccessible position, such as in a cystic duct remnant or distal to a biliary stricture. Extracorporeal shock-

wave lithotripsy has recently been found to be a valuable adjunct to radiologic intervention in such problem cases.[4,15] The interventional radiologist is ideally suited to conduct biliary lithotripsy because of the difficulty in targeting requiring several imaging technologies.[12]

Percutaneous transhepatic intervention may be indicated in certain cases of recurrent choledocholithiasis after previous cholecystectomy. Although endoscopic retrograde sphincterotomy with stone extraction is the standard treatment in this situation, retrograde bile duct cannulation can be quite difficult or even impossible because of special anatomic situations such as duodenal diverticula or distortion of the anatomy by surgical anastomoses. A transhepatic catheter can then provide guidance for the endoscopic sphincterotome into Vater's ampulla. Successful antegrade sphincterotomy has been performed successfully in some instances.[13,20] The transhepatic approach can also be used for fragmentation of bile duct calculi[19] or for bile duct opacification to facilitate extracorporeal lithotripsy.[3] Direct dissolution of bile duct calculi with agents such as monooctanoin[19] or more recently methyl tertiary butyl ether[8] (MTBE) has been performed by several investigators. The effect of the agents is limited to the cholesterol component of gallstones, whereas bile duct stones often have a major component of calcium bilirubinate. The side effects of the dissolving agents are also not negligible and include nausea, abdominal discomfort, diarrhea, and possibly inflammatory reaction (with monooctanoin) or sedation and burning pain (with MTBE). At present, dissolution of bile duct calculi must therefore still be considered investigational.

Percutaneous transhepatic biliary drainage (PTD) is now a well-established technique. However, with increasing clinical experience and the concurrent development of new endoscopic techniques, its indications need to be reappraised. Although initial investigations had also suggested that establishment of PTD before surgery for obstructive jaundice reduced complications during the postoperative course, prospective controlled studies have failed to confirm a significant beneficial effect from this approach.[49,59] Combined with antibiotic treatment, PTD can be recommended to stabilize patients with obstructive cholangitis and biliary sepsis before more definitive treatment.[42] Palliative PTD is indicated in patients with unresectable tumors obstructing the biliary system to relieve symptoms such as pruritus and fever and to improve coagulopathy and nutritional status by internal biliary drainage. Local radiotherapy by afterloading of internal biliary drainage catheters has been used for palliative treatment of hilar cholangiocarcinoma[35] and appears to be a sound alternative to palliative surgery or percutaneous drainage alone. Biliary endoprostheses[40] should be reserved for terminally ill patients with advanced tumors and an expected prognosis of less than 6 months' survival. Considerable technical advances have been made using endoscopic retrograde placement of biliary endoprosthesis that can be exchanged with less difficulty.[66] Particularly in distal strictures, such as those caused by pancreatic carcinoma, the endoscopic approach, although quite operator dependent, now appears preferable. Unfortunately, only very limited prospective control data are available comparing the outcome of palliative biliary drainage with palliative bypass surgery.[7] Poor surgical candidates with advanced disease are the most common candidates for palliative radiologic drainage procedures. Such patient selection bias is probably a major reason for the relatively poor results of palliative nonsurgical drainage compared with palliative bypass surgery.

Benign bile duct strictures constitute a difficult therapeutic problem and often require repeat surgical interventions. *Endoluminal balloon dilatation of biliary strictures* with or without additional postprocedural stenting has recently shown good results. The long-term patency rates after this procedure were somewhat better for strictures localized in the bile ducts than in anastomotic strictures. Strictures from sclerosing cholangitis have a less favorable prognosis.[52,71] Balloon dilatation of biliary strictures can be performed through a transhepatic approach, although access through a T-tube tract should be preferred if it is available. A surgically created cutaneous jejunostomy using the proximal limb of a Roux-en-Y choledochojejunostomy or hepaticojejunostomy can also be used effectively as an interventional access to the biliary tree in patients with a high likelihood of developing stricture recurrence.[33] Percutaneous transjejunal biliary intervention by direct puncture of a jejunostomy loop has been proved feasible in some instances.[44]

GALLBLADDER

Increasing interest is focused on nonsurgical intervention for cholecystolithiasis. Unlike the bile ducts, the gallbladder is poorly accessible by means of endoscopy, whereas radiologic gallbladder intervention can be performed through a subhepatic or transhepatic approach.

Surgical cholecystostomy is performed for external decompression of the acutely inflamed gallbladder in patients who are at high risk for formal cholecystectomy. The surgical cholecystostomy tract can be used as an access for gallstone extraction under fluoroscopic control. To minimize surgical trauma and the need for anesthetics in high-risk patients, the *minicholecystostomy approach* has been designed and used successfully at our institution.[14] With this method a short, straight, wide surgical gallbladder access permits early radiologic re-

moval of calculi from the gallbladder, the cystic duct, or even the common bile duct.[29]

Direct percutaneous gallbladder puncture under ultrasonic guidance through either a transhepatic or subhepatic route can be used for both diagnostic opacification of the biliary system and to establish gallbladder drainage.[41,45,58,67] Some investigators have also removed gallbladder calculi transhepatically,[38] but mechanical cholecystolithotomy requires considerable dilatation of the percutaneous tract and therefore appears quite invasive. More recently MTBE has been instilled into the gallbladder to dissolve cholesterol calculi. This method requires only a small catheter (for example, 5 French) but is quite time consuming and not without potential hazards. Passage of the MTBE through the patent cystic duct into the common bile duct and duodenum may lead to systemic absorption and subsequent heavy sedation.[1] *Extracorporeal shockwave lithotripsy* (ESWL) has been used to disintegrate gallbladder calculi to make them amenable to systemic dissolution therapy by orally administered bile acids.[63] The first follow-up results with this form of treatment have shown that even in ideally selected patients the disappearance of gallstone fragments produced by ESWL may take as long as 6 months or 1 year.[63] Possibly the combination of ESWL with direct MTBE dissolution will improve nonoperative gallstone treatment and, if so, the radiologist's role in the treatment of this common disease would likely increase considerably.

Present research in percutaneous gallbladder intervention is also focused on techniques to occlude the cystic duct permanently.[5] Successful cystic duct occlusion would not only prevent passage of MTBE into the duodenum but might also enable subsequent obliteration of the gallbladder mucosa by chemical sclerosing agents to prevent recurrent cholelithiasis after successful nonsurgical gallstone removal, thus offering a possible alternative to cholecystectomy.

DRAINAGE OF ABDOMINAL FLUID COLLECTIONS

Percutaneous abscess drainage was originally restricted to well-defined unilocular lesions, preferably with extraperitoneal access routes. More recently the radiologic drainage approach has also been applied to more complex, loculated, or multiple abscesses. Transperitoneal access routes, even traversing normal organs such as the liver or stomach, have been used successfully for percutaneous drainage. A trial of percutaneous drainage can now be recommended in virtually all simple abscesses and many complex abscesses with clinical response as the key determinant for the need of operative intervention.[28] It has also been suggested that certain patients be treated as outpatients with their percutaneous drainage catheters still in place to avoid the expense of prolonged hospitalization.[61] Although percutaneous abscess drainage is in most cases technically not very demanding, it is important to observe certain diagnostic and clinical criteria for successful treatment. *Liver abscesses,* for example, should be drained percutaneously if proved pyogenic by diagnostic fine needle aspiration,[34] but drainage is not indicated in most amebic abscesses, because these usually respond well to medical treatment.[60] Percutaneous drainage of *pancreatic pseudocysts* can be attempted in lesions that increase over 5 cm in size or persist longer than 4 to 6 weeks after the acute inflammatory period, because these carry an increased risk of complications, such as hemorrhage or rupture. The transgastric approach has been used without complications as an access route for drainage.[55] Some investigators have recently described new techniques to accomplish internal pseudocyst drainage using a percutaneous approach.[6,30] Loculated, infected pancreatic fluid collections—that is, infected pancreatic pseudocysts or well-loculated abscesses—are also often amenable to external catheter drainage, and a trial with this treatment appears to be indicated. *Pancreatic phlegmons,* on the other hand, whether infected or not, are usually impossible to drain with percutaneous catheters because of their widespread, semisolid nature and should therefore be treated by surgical debridement.[27]

Percutaneous catheter drainage of abscesses that arise as a complication of acute inflammatory bowel disease, such as appendicitis, Crohn's disease, or diverticulitis, has long been discouraged because standard surgical measures can provide abscess drainage and treatment of the underlying cause (usually bowel perforation) at the same time. Recently, however, it has been shown that percutaneous abscess drainage may be well suited as a temporizing measure in the acute inflammatory stage, thus simplifying surgical treatment, sometimes reducing two- or three-step bowel resections to single-step procedures or obviating surgery completely.[53,65,70]

INTRAVASCULAR INTERVENTION

Angiographic techniques for the localization and *control of severe GI tract hemorrhage* are among the most important and best established interventional radiologic procedures yet developed. Arterial hemorrhage may be treated by vasoconstrictive infusion therapy or selective embolization. Vasopressin, a potent vasoconstrictor, also causes muscular contraction of the gastrointestinal wall and is particularly well suited to control diffuse mucosal hemorrhage. Selective embolization with particulate material (for example, Gelfoam) is usually preferred to control bleeding from a more localized source, such as gas-

troduodenal ulcer, colonic diverticula, arteriovenous malformations, or hemobilia.[31,36,51] Permanent vessel occlusion with Ivalon, bucrylate, or Gianturco steel coils may be indicated in malignant bleeding sources, such as gastric carcinoma.

Interventional techniques also offer several options for the treatment of patients with portal hypertension. *Hemorrhage from gastroesophageal varices* may be treated by vasopressin infusion directly into the superior mesenteric artery. Direct embolization of bleeding varices can be performed by percutaneous transhepatic cannulation of the portal venous system with various substances, including particulate material and sclerosants such as ethanol and sotradecol. Recent experimental developments are aimed at creating intrahepatic portacaval shunts to treat chronic portal hypertension by expandible stents inserted through the transjugular route.[57] Existing surgical or spontaneous portosystemic shunts that lead to portal encephalopathy can be treated by embolization through the transarterial, transhepatic, or transvenous route.[68]

Transluminal angioplasty of the celiac and superior mesenteric artery has been used successfully for the treatment of intestinal angina from arteriosclerotic stenoses of these visceral arteries.[56] New techniques for the recanalization of arteries and veins include laser[24] and rotational tip catheters.[37] Selective embolization of hepatic neoplasms[16,31] and selective intraarterial perfusion therapy with cytotoxic agents are now performed in many centers; the effect of the latter approach is closely related to the efficacy of the administered drugs.

Continuing advances in interventional radiologic imaging techniques instrumentation offer a large potential of new interventional procedures to complement, obviate, or replace traditional surgical techniques. Some of these procedures are derived in principle from their surgical counterparts (for example, percutaneous abscess drainage), and others use entirely new approaches (for example, balloon dilatation, transcatheter embolization techniques, expandible stents, and laser techniques). Evaluation of these new interventional procedures requires intensive laboratory investigation and well-controlled clinical trials. Radiologists are well advised to initiate prospective, controlled studies to compare their interventional techniques with traditional surgical procedures to avoid patient selection bias. The goal is to improve patient care by providing less invasive and less expensive treatment modalities that equal or surpass surgery in efficacy and safety.

REFERENCES

1. Allen, MJ, et al: Rapid dissolution of gallstones by methyl tert-butyl ether: preliminary observations, N Engl J Med 312:217, 1985.

2. Baum, S, and Nusbaum, M: The control of gastrointestinal bleeding by selective mesenteric arterial infusion of vasopressin, Radiology 98:499, 1971.

3. Becker, CD, et al: Choledocholithiasis: treatment with extracorporeal shockwave lithotripsy, Radiology 165:407, 1987.

4. Becker, CD, et al: Treatment of retained cystic duct stones using extracorporeal shockwave lithotripsy, AJR 148:1121, 1987.

5. Becker, CD, Quenville, NF, and Burhenne, HJ: Long-term occlusion of the porcine cystic duct by means of endoluminal radiofrequency electrocoagulation, Radiology 167:63, 1988.

6. Bernardino, ME, and Amerson, JR: Percutaneous gastrocystostomy: a new approach to pancreatic pseudocyst drainage, AJR 143:1096, 1984.

7. Bornman, PC, et al: Prospective controlled trial of transhepatic biliary endoprosthesis versus bypass surgery for incurable carcinoma of head of pancreas, Lancet 1:69, 1986.

8. Brandon, JC, et al: Common bile duct calculi: updated experience with dissolution with methyl tertiary butyl ether, Radiology 166:665, 1988.

9. Burhenne, HJ: Nonoperative retained biliary tract stone extraction: a new roentgenologic technique, AJR 117:388, 1973.

10. Burhenne, HJ: Percutaneous extraction of retained biliary tract stones: 661 patients, AJR 134:888, 1980.

11. Burhenne, HJ: Open forum: interventional cholelithotomy as an alternative to cholecystecotmy with or without the surgeon? Invest Radiol 21:594, 1986.

12. Burhenne, HJ: Perspective: the promise of extracorporeal shockwave lithotripsy for the treatment of gallstones, AJR 149:233, 1987.

13. Burhenne, HJ, and Scudamore, CH: Antegrade transcholecystic sphincterotomy: canine study of a new interventional technique, Gastrointest Radiol 11:73, 1986.

14. Burhenne, HJ, and Stoller, JL: Minicholecystostomy and radiologic stone extraction in high-risk cholelithiasis patients: preliminary experience, Am J Surg 149:632, 1985.

15. Burhenne, HJ, et al: Biliary lithotripsy: an integrated approach of nonoperative intervention, AJR 150:1279, 1988.

16. Carrasco, et al: Transcatheter embolization of neoplasms, Semin Intervent Radiol 1:137, 1984.

17. Casola, G, et al: Percutaneous cecostomy for decompression of the massively distended cecum, Radiology 158:793, 1986.

18. Chisholm, RJ, et al: Radiologic dilatation preceding surgical tube placement for esophageal cancer, Am J Surg 151:397, 1986.

19. Clouse, ME, et al: Bile duct stones: percutaneous transhepatic removal, Radiology 160:525, 1986.

20. Cobourn, C, et al: Percutaneous transhepatic sphincterotomy in the management of biliary tract disease, Gastrointest Radiol 22:273, 1986.

21. deLange, EE, and Shaffer, HA: Anastomotic strictures of the upper gastrointestinal tract: results of balloon dilation, Radiology 167:45, 1988.

22. Evens, RG: The radiologist as an attending physician: routine or special procedure? Radiology 154:545, 1985.

23. Ferrucci, JT, Jr, Butch, RJ, and Mueller, PR: Biliary stone removal. In Ferrucci, JT, Jr, et al, editors: Interventional radiology of the abdomen, ed 2, Baltimore, 1984, Williams & Wilkins.

24. Furui, S, et al: Hepatic inferior vena cava obstructions: clinical results of treatment with percutaneous transluminal laser-associated angioplasty, Radiology 166:673, 1988.

25. Garrow, DG: The removal of retained biliary tract stones: report of 105 cases, Br J Radiol 50:777, 1977.

26. Gerzof, SG, et al: Percutaneous catheter drainage of abdominal abscesses guided by ultrasound and computed tomography, AJR 133:1, 1979.

27. Gerzof, SG, et al: Percutaneous drainage of infected pancreatic pseudocysts, Arch Surg 119:888, 1984.

28. Gerzof, SG, et al: Expanded criteria for percutanous abscess drainage, Arch Surg 120:227, 1985.

29. Gibney, RG, et al: Combined surgical and radiologic intervention for complicated cholelithiasis in high-risk patients, Radiology 165:715, 1987.

30. Hancke, S, and Henriksen, FW: Percutaneous pancreatic cystogastrostomy guided by ultrasound scanning and gastroscopy, Br J Surg 72:916, 1985.

31. Hemingway, AP, and Allison, DJ: Complications of embolization: analysis of 410 procedures, Radiology 166:669, 1988.

32. Holm, HH, et al: Ultrasonically guided percutaneous puncture, Radiol Clin North Am 14:493, 1975.

33. Hutson, DG, et al: Balloon dilatation of biliary strictures through a choledochojejuno-cutaneous fistula, Ann Surg 199:637, 1984.

34. Johnson, RD, et al: Percutaneous drainage of pyogenic liver abscesses, AJR 144:463, 1985.

35. Karam, J, et al: Internal biliary drainage and local radiotherapy with iridium-192 wire in treatment of hilar cholangiocarcinoma, Clin Radiol 36:603, 1985.

36. Keller, FS, editor: Nonoperative management of gastrointestinal hemorrhage, Semin Intervent Radiol 5:1, 1988.

37. Kensey, KR, et al: Recanalization of obstructed arteries with a flexible, rotating tip catheter, Radiology 165:387, 1987.

38. Kerlan, RK, Jr, La Berge, SM, and Ring, EJ: Percutaneous cholelithotomy: preliminary experience, Radiology 157:653, 1985.

39. Kinnison, ML, et al: Inpatient admissions for interventional radiology: philosophy of patient management, Radiology 154:349, 1985.

40. Lammer, J, and Neumayer, K: Biliary drainage endoprostheses: experience with 201 placements, Radiology 159:625, 1986.

41. Lohela, P, et al: Ultrasonic guidance for percutaneous puncture and drainage in acute cholecystitis, Acta Radiol [Diagn] 27:543, 1986.

42. Lois, JF, et al: Risks of percutaneous transhepatic drainage in patients with cholangitis, AJR 148:367, 1987.

43. Margulis, AR: Interventional diagnostic radiology: a new subspecialty, AJR 99:761, 1967.

44. Maroney, TP, and Ring, EJ: Percutaneous transjejunal catheterization of Roux-en-Y biliary-jejunal anastomoses, Radiology 164:151, 1987.

45. McGahan, JP: A new catheter design for percutaneous cholecystostomy, Radiology 166:49, 1988.

46. McLean, GK, et al: Enteric alimentation: radiologic approach, Radiology 160:155, 1986.

47. McLean, GK, et al: Radiologically guided balloon dilation of gastrointestinal strictures. I. Technique and factors influencing procedural success, Radiology 165:35, 1987.

48. McLean, GK, et al: Radiologically guided balloon dilation of gastrointestinal strictures. II. Results of long-term follow-up, Radiology 165:41, 1987.

49. McPherson GD, et al: Preoperative percutaneous transhepatic biliary drainage: the results of a controlled trial, Br J Surg 71:371, 1984.

50. McSherry, CK, and Glenn, F: The incidence and causes of death following surgery for nonmalignant biliary tract disease, Ann Surg 191:271, 1980.

51. Mitchell, SE, et al: Biliary catheter drainage complicated by hemobilia: treatment by balloon embolotherapy, Radiology 157:645, 1985.

52. Mueller, PR, et al: Biliary stricture dilatation: multicenter review of clinical management in 73 patients, Radiology 160:17, 1986.

53. Mueller, PR, et al: Sigmoid diverticular abscesses: percutaneous drainage as an adjunct to surgical resection in 24 cases, Radiology 164:321, 1987.

54. Nordentoft, JM, and Hansen, H: Treatment of intussusception in children: brief survey based on 1,838 Danish cases, Surgery 38:311, 1955.

55. Nuñez, D, Jr, et al: Transgastric drainage of pancreatic fluid collections, AJR 145:815, 1985.

56. Odurny, A, Sniderman, KW, and Colapinto, RF: Percutaneous transluminal angioplasty of the celiac and superior mesenteric arteries, Radiology 167:59, 1988.

57. Palmaz, JC, et al: Expandable intrahepatic portacaval shunt stents in dogs with chronic portal hypertension, AJR 147:1251, 1986.

58. Pearse, DM, et al: Percutaneous cholecystostomy in acute cholecystitis and common duct obstruction, Radiology 152:365, 1984.

59. Pitt, HA, et al: Does preoperative percutaneous biliary drainage reduce operative risk or increase hospital cost? Ann Surg 201:545, 1985.

60. Ralls, PW, et al: Medical treatment of hepatic amebic abscess: rare need for percutaneous drainage, Radiology 165:805, 1987.

61. Rifkin, MD, et al: Outpatient therapy of intraabdominal abscesses following early discharge from the hospital, Radiology 155:333, 1985.

62. Ring, EJ, and Kerlan, RK, Jr: Inpatient management: a new role for interventional radiologists, Radiology 154:543, 1985.

63. Sackmann, M, et al: Shockwave lithotripsy of gallbladder stones: the first 175 patients, N Engl J Med 318:383, 1988.

64. Safrany, L, and Cotton, PB: Endoscopic management of choledocholithiasis, Surg Clin North Am 62:825, 1982.

65. Safrit, HD, Mauro, MA, and Jaques, PF: Percutaneous abscess drainage in Crohn's disease, AJR 148:859, 1987.

66. Siegel, JH, and Snady, H: The significance of endoscopically placed endoprostheses in the management of biliary obstruction due to carcinoma of the pancreas: results of nonoperative decompression in 277 patients, Am J Gastroenterol 81:634, 1986.

67. Teplick, SK, Haskin, PH, and Sammon, JK: Common bile duct obstruction: assessment by transcholecystic cholangiography, Radiology 161:135, 1986.

68. Uflacker, R, et al: Chronic portosystemic encephalopathy: embolization of portosystemic shunts, Radiology 165:721, 1987.

69. vanSonnenberg, E, et al: Percutaneous gastrostomy and gastroenterostomy. II. Clinical experience, AJR 146:581, 1986.

70. vanSonnenberg, E, et al: Periappendiceal abscesses: percutaneous drainage, Radiology 163:23, 1987.

71. Williams, HJ, Jr, Bender, CE, and May, GR: Benign postoperative biliary strictures: dilation with fluoroscopic guidance, Radiology 163:629, 1987.

72. Wills, JS, and Oglesby, JT: Percutaneous gastrostomy: further experience, Radiology 154:71, 1985.

PART XVIII

CLINICAL OVERVIEW

84 *Oncology*

THEODORE L. PHILLIPS
VERNON SMITH
MICHAEL COLLIER

GENERAL CONSIDERATIONS

Gastrointestinal (GI) cancer represents approximately 35% of all cancers diagnosed in the United States. This range of diseases includes some of the most aggressive cancers with the poorest prognosis, but they also include those sites with some of the highest cure rates among major malignancies.

Special features

Special features of GI cancer include the involvement of a lumen with frequent bleeding and obstruction and often delayed diagnosis because of lack of symptoms and the deep-seated location of the tumor mass. Generally, early diagnosis and good prognosis is possible when bleeding or obstruction occur early before deep invasion or metastasis.

Incidence

Tumors of the GI tract vary widely in incidence, with carcinoma of the colon being the most common. Approximately 20% of all cancers occur in the colon, representing 100,000 cases per year in the United States. Next highest in frequency is carcinoma of the rectum at 5%, with approximately 25,000 cases per year. Both stomach and pancreatic cancers account for about 3% of tumors, with approximately 25,000 cases per year. Carcinomas of the esophagus, biliary tract, anus, and pharynx are less common, with between 1200 and 9000 cases per year at these sites.

Current overview of management

The treatment of GI cancers is extremely complex and involves a thorough integration of surgery, radiotherapy, and chemotherapy. In addition, a number of experimental treatments with immune system modulators are under investigation. At present diagnosis is generally made either radiographically or endoscopically. Histologic documentation is obtained either through a primary exploration and resection or biopsy, or more and more frequently, through endoscopic biopsy or fine-needle aspiration directed with computed tomography (CT).

After the diagnosis is made, optimal treatment is chosen. This chapter discusses specific treatments for each site. In general, however, surgical resection is the treatment of choice for all but early superficial lesions in the pharynx, esophagus, and anus. Radiotherapy can provide an alternative to surgery at these sites and in early rectal cancer. Radiotherapy also plays a role in the control of large, unresectable tumors and in their palliation. Chemotherapy is useful as an adjuvant, with several studies showing improved survival. Chemotherapy is also a useful enhancer of radiation response, leading to improved local regional response and control rates.

Cancers of the pharynx are generally treated by a combination of radiation and surgery, with no evidence yet that adjuvant chemotherapy improves survival. Esophageal cancers are generally treated either by radiation or by surgery, depending on stage and location. Simultaneous radiotherapy and chemotherapy in early studies appears to show improved local regional control. Gastric cancers are best treated surgically, with some benefit with adjuvant radiation and chemotherapy. Carcinomas of the pancreas are rarely resectable, but when they are, they can be controlled by surgical procedures. Radiotherapy for unresectable lesions is the only viable option in most patients, with radioactive implants and intraoperative irradiation playing a role. Adjuvant chemotherapy appears to improve survival.

Hepatic and biliary cancers are generally curable only if they are resectable. Recent studies with chemoembolization, isotopically labeled antibodies, and hepatic artery infusion are promising, at least in terms of increasing tumor response in the liver and prolonging disease-free survival. Carcinomas of the colon and rectum are generally treated by surgical resection, with recent evidence showing that adjuvant chemotherapy and radiotherapy improve local regional control and survival. Anal cancers, previously treated by surgical resection, are now highly curable by combined radiation therapy and simultaneous chemotherapy, which is the treatment of choice. Thus the management of each of these sites is an integrated one, and knowledge of the usefulness of surgery, radiotherapy, and chemotherapy is essential.

To diagnose these lesions properly and especially to plan adequate treatment, absolutely accurate information as to site, extent, and patterns of spread is required. This chapter concentrates on the role of imaging in oncology of the GI system; treatment planning for radiotherapy, in particular using imaging techniques; and a general outline of the oncologic factors at each specific site, including an overview, staging, pathologic classification, current treatment options, and some details of radiation oncology.

IMAGING NEEDS IN ONCOLOGY

The diagnosis of neoplasms of the alimentary tract is clearly a joint effort between the diagnostic imager and the endoscopist. Once the location and nature of the neoplasm is established with histologic proof, the needs for imaging switch to considerations of staging and treatment planning.

Staging of a neoplasm in the GI tract is extremely important in predicting prognosis. It is also important in delineating patterns of spread so that adequate resection or radiotherapy will be administered. Thus the needs of imaging procedures will often be more demanding for staging than for initial diagnosis and may require additional studies. Although a diagnosis of rectal cancer may be made simply by endoscopy, a magnetic resonance imaging (MRI) scan of the pelvis would be required to describe the exact extent of deep invasion. MRI or CT would also delineate enlarged lymph nodes for the design of a surgical procedure, the definition of operability, and the definition of irradiation treatment ports.

Accurate imaging, especially with CT and MRI, are required for modern treatment by radiotherapy. Definition of primary tumor extent and critical radiosensitive normal structures and localization of lymphatic metastases require a three-dimensional image or reconstruction to allow visualization of dose distribution in relationship to these structures. Thus a combination of contrast film examinations with CT and MRI will often generate the optimal three-dimensional image, which can then be reconstructed and displayed using several computer software and hardware systems. Superimposition of radiation dose distributions on these three-dimensional images then allows for optimization of the treatment plan.

Evaluation of response is another function of imaging in GI oncology. Often the tumors are not palpable and only can be superficially appreciated by endoscopy. Follow-up with films, particularly three-dimensional techniques such as MRI and CT, is essential to evaluate response. This is especially true with modalities such as radiotherapy and chemotherapy, where gross tumor is remaining. A number of algorithms exist in computer programs for the MRI and CT units that can calculate the volume of tumor and follow tumor response as a function of time.

Because of the necessity to make decisions about operability and placement of high-energy radiation ports, resolution of the imaging studies used for oncologic staging and treatment planning must be high. Both differentiation between tumor and normal tissue and spatial resolution with accuracy are essential. Fortunately the modern generations of CT and MRI units allow sufficient accuracy, quantification, and resolution.

RADIOTHERAPY TREATMENT PLANNING AND IMAGING

For initial planning in simple cases, current management entails standard radiologic methods and fluoroscopy. These tools are available in most modern radiotherapy departments on a radiation therapy simulator. This unit is an isocentric device fitted with a high-output x-ray tube with large and small focal spots and an opposing large-field image intensifier system. Field-defining wires are present and operate separately from the collimator leaves. A couch, which allows reproduction of all motions possible on the treatment accelerator, is an integral part of this unit. The isocenter of the unit and of the couch motions are aligned. Patients are immobilized as they will be for treatment, and films are taken at least in anterior, posterior, and lateral orthogonal positions. If a pre-determined plan of simple opposing portals or four portals is to be used, they are generally filmed at this time. Standard contrast agents may be employed, such as normal or thickened barium, intravenous iodinated contrast, small bowel contrast, or rectal contrast. Contours of the patients are made, and fiducial marks are placed to allow realignment with either the simulator or the treatment unit. Generally, laser marking systems are present, which allow anterior, posterior, lateral, and centerline fiducial marks relative to the treatment machine. This procedure may be aided by fluoroscopy for quickly determining port centers, checking for organ mobility, and setting up small portals.

CT and MR images play an increasing role in radiotherapy treatment planning and are essential for most curative treatments. Their adequate use requires a method of indexing the CT to films taken on the radiotherapy simulator, as well as to portal films taken on the treatment delivery machine. Although it is possible to use a CT or MRI for treatment planning alone, this is not generally done. Often their use is quite difficult because the images obtained do not correlate directly with those obtained on the treatment machine. Those taken on the simulator do correlate exactly with those on the treatment machine and generally are used for portal verification and checking.

To employ CT and MRI data, one must take the CT or MR images with the patient in the exact treatment position previously decided on at the simulation session. Immobilizing devices such as casts and plastic masks or jackets are often used and must be mountable on the CT or MRI unit. Fiducial marks should be placed on the patient's skin at the position marked during the simula-

tion session. Often it is best to put a long, vertical plastic rod at the center and edges of the portals in both the anteroposterior and the lateral position so that the rod will show in each MRI or CT slice. Plastic is ideal for CT, and catheters filled with oil are useful for MRI. Both anteroposterior and lateral scout views should be obtained so that the slice locations can be indexed to the simulator and to subsequent treatment machine verification films.

Slice thickness is important for CT scanning. If it is necessary later to reconstruct in sagittal and coronal planes for adequate treatment portal localization, slices of 3 to 5 mm thickness should be used.

Treatment planning is then conducted using a computer system. Several commercial systems and many research-type systems are available that allow display of the CT and MRI data on a high-resolution device, which allows overlays of radiation isodose curves. The most advanced systems allow display of this information not only in the transverse slices, but in all possible planes using reconstruction techniques. Some of these systems also allow tiling or wire frame–type outlining of various structures and tumors to allow true three-dimensional display. Superimposed on this is a three-dimensional image of the dose distribution.

When two-dimensional CT based planning is performed, the image is generally displayed, and superimposed on it are the isodose distributions calculated for the treatment device in use. An example of this is shown in Fig. 84-1. Correction for dose inhomogeneity caused by density differences is included in this charged particle plan using neon ions. Bowel gas has been eliminated as a factor through a computer adjustment.

A very useful technique in most of the advanced two-dimensional and all three-dimensional computerized treatment planning systems is the ability to display the results of contouring on simulated radiographs. In this technique the essential normal structures as well as the patient outline are created on each slice. This may be done for many organs by autocontouring and is generally done for the tumor through physician outlining. Some advanced systems can also autocontour certain organs such as kidney and liver. After these slices are outlined, they may be displayed in the anteroposterior and lateral positions or in an arbitrary angle on a reconstructed image of that angle.

The most useful reconstructed image is that of a simulated radiograph, or digitally reconstructed radiograph (DRR), which superimposes all pixels in that particular orientation. In the most advanced systems the DRR corrects for beam diversion, which would be expected in a true radiograph. This allows for direct comparison with simulator or machine portal films. Fig. 84-2 is an example of a DRR of a carcinoma of the pancreas showing

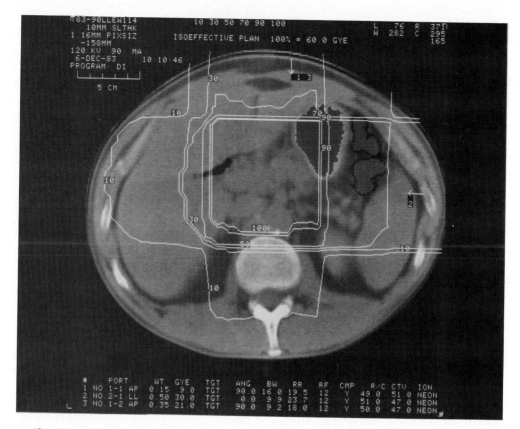

Fig. 84-1 CT-based treatment plan for carcinoma of pancreas using neon ions with three beams, or portals. Correction for density on pixel-by-pixel basis is included. Because of day-to-day changes, air density in bowel has been converted to water density.

the outlines of the pancreatic tumor in the center surrounded by a portal definition and the outlines of the kidneys.

Thus the computer has been used to define portal and, in particular, portals at angles other than the standard anteroposterior and lateral positions. The patient is returned to the simulator for verification films taken at the exact angle defined by the computer planning and often with the shaping blocks by the computer in place. Shaping is done by tracing the computer-generated portal shapes into a device that constructs cerabend (alloy with a low melting point) collimators for use on the blocking x-ray of the treatment machine. Thus multiple fields can be made from multiple angles to conform to the exact shape of the tumor, greatly reducing normal tissue exposure. In some systems the generation of these collimators is automated by a connection between the computer and a device that cuts molds for pouring the cerabend blocks.

The final step is to set up the patient in the position originally decided, align the fields determined by computer planning, and take portal films. These are then compared to the DRRs and the simulator verification films to ensure exact placement.

This complex system allows an order-of-magnitude enhancement of accuracy and a great reduction of normal tissue irradiation. It requires very close coordination between the radiation oncologist and the diagnostic radiologist so that the necessary immobilization, fiducial marks, slice thickness, and scout views are obtained.

Ideal tumor localization and treatment planning occur through the use of a combination of imaging studies. A few computer programs now have the ability to use both the MRI and the CT data. In some systems the two images are compared side by side, and reconstruction techniques ensure that the slice location and angle are identical. In other systems one can superimpose these two images and use, for example, the bony images from CT and soft tissue images from MRI. In three-dimensional displays one can, for example, show the CT data in one set of planes and the MR data in another. Through proper fiducial marks and image-correlated mathematic techniques, one can ensure accurate alignment of the two studies. Using similar techniques, film imaging tech-

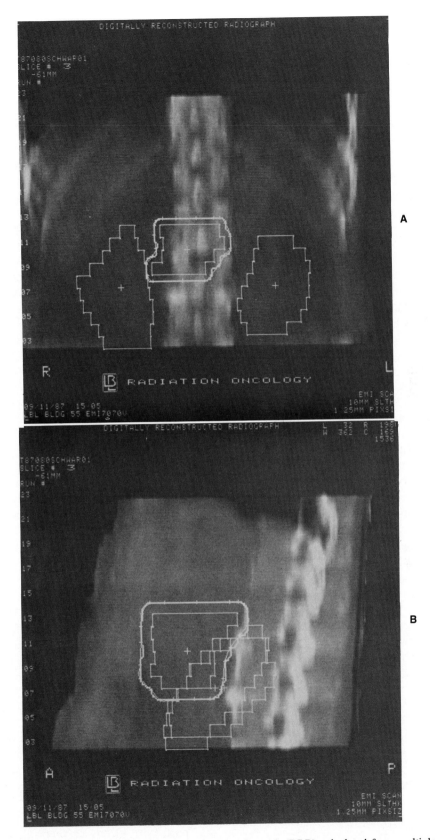

Fig. 84-2 A, Digitally reconstructed anteroposterior radiograph (DRR) calculated from multiple-slice CT data. Outlines of kidneys and tumor target volume are shown and are derived from outlines on each slice. Planned treatment portal for pancreatic cancer is shown around tumor outline. **B,** Lateral DRR from same case as **A.** Note position of kidneys and target volume.

niques such as arteriograms or portal films may also be aligned with three-dimensional CT and MRI images, although not directly incorporated in them because of their fixed two-plane nature.

ONCOLOGY OF SPECIFIC SITES
Pharynx
Overview

Management of patients with carcinoma of the head and neck, including the pharynx, requires careful evaluation of extent of disease and a multidisciplinary team approach, often using prospective patient management tumor conferences.

Besides imaging studies, mapping of the lesion under general endoscopy is essential. Esophagoscopy should be carried out in addition to laryngoscopy because of the high incidence of second tumors (10% to 15%).

A close relationship exists between prognosis and tumor size and between prognosis and tumor location, with tumors in the upper pharynx showing cure rates higher than those lower and adjacent to the esophagus.

Most treatment failures occur within 2 years, and patient follow-up must therefore be done frequently and carefully. Between 10% and 30% of head and neck cancer patients develop second primary tumors in either the upper aerodigestive tract or lungs, and long-term follow-up is important. Although distant metastases probably occur most frequently in a hypopharyngeal cancer, of all head and neck cancers, they still remain the minority compared to local regional failure.

Diagnosis of hypopharyngeal cancer is generally made by indirect mirror examination or by endoscopy and biopsy, generally using rigid laryngoscopes and endoscopes. CT and MRI are important in delineating the depth of invasion and in discovering clinically undetectable cervical adenopathy. Our experience with MRI has been that it is superior to CT in almost all locations for the hypopharynx, especially in delineating tumor from muscle density material and in separating a tumor from fibrosis following treatment.

The general approaches to treatment involve either surgery or radiotherapy for the early stages of disease. Because hypopharyngeal cancer is rarely seen at an early stage, almost all patients are managed by a combination of surgical resection and irradiation. Chemotherapy is under investigation and, although there are some interesting results, there is not yet a proven benefit of adjuvant chemotherapy in altering survival of hypopharyngeal cancer patients.

Staging and prognosis

The staging systems used for pharyngeal carcinomas are based on those devised by the American Joint Committee on Cancer Staging, such as the TNM (tumor, lymph node, metastasis) classification, as well as on clinical findings. The results of imaging examinations are used as well.

The extent of the primary tumor is defined by tumor location and extent, with T_1 a tumor confined to one site, T_2 a tumor with extension to adjacent regions or sites without fixation, and T_3 a tumor with extension and fixation of the larynx. T_4 describes a massive tumor invading the bone or soft tissues of the neck.

Lymph node staging is similar to that for other head and neck sites, with N_1 describing a clinically positive node 3 cm or less in diameter on the side of the lesion. N_2 denotes a condition with a positive node greater than 3 and less than 6 cm in diameter or multiple ipsilateral nodes. N_3 disease is massive ipsilateral nodes, greater than 6 cm in diameter, or bilateral or contralateral lymph node involvement.

Stage 1 disease is defined at T_1N_0 and has a 5-year survival in the 80% to 90% range. Stage 2 disease is indicated as T_2N_0 and has a 50% to 60% 5-year survival. Patients with T_3N_0 or T_1N_1, T_2N_1, or T_3N_1 fall into the stage 3 disease category and have a 30% to 50% 5-year survival rate. Stage 4 disease involves T_4 patients or any patients with a N_2 or N_3 condition. Five-year survival in this group is very low, 10% to 20%.

Pathologic classification

Most tumors of the pharynx are of squamous cell origin and can be preceded by precancerous in situ lesions. They are divided into keratinizing and nonkeratinizing. Less common but not rare are minor salivary gland tumors. Grading is carried out, but it has not generally been correlated with prognosis.

Current treatment options

The major lymphatic drainage from the hypopharynx is into jugulodigastric, juguloomohyoid and deep cervical lymph nodes, as well as into the retropharyngeal lymph node. Tumor can extend up into the high retropharyngeal nodes at the level of the nasopharynx even from a hypopharyngeal primary tumor.

The hypopharynx is divided into three regions: (1) pyriform fossa, (2) postcricoid region, and (3) posterior hypopharyngeal wall. The pyriform fossa is the most frequently involved site in the hypopharynx, accounting for more than two thirds of all patients. Cervical node metastasis occurs in 70% of patients in the pyriform fossa and approximately 45% in the other sites.

In defining the optimal treatment approach in the hypopharynx, clearly no single treatment offers improved survival over any other treatment. Recent reviews have indicated that the use of surgical resection with lymph node dissection and pre- or postoperative irradiation gives optimal local regional control. This approach is now standard.

Treatment of stage 1 hypopharyngeal cancer may be selected from radiotherapy and surgery options. Tumors in this stage are extremely rare, representing only a small percentage of patients seen. If the lesion is exophytic, radiotherapy alone is often the treatment of choice because of preservation of the larynx. The supraglottic laryngectomy may be performed for lesions near the superior part of the pyriform fossa. Otherwise, even for stage 1 disease, laryngopharyngectomy and neck dissection are indicated. In this stage postoperative irradiation would be indicated only for lesions with deep penetration or close or positive margins.

Stage 2 and stage 3 hypopharyngeal cancers are treated with combined radiotherapy and surgery. Total laryngectomy, radical neck dissection, and postoperative irradiation are most often performed and have yielded local regional control rates between 70% and 80%.

Stage 4 hypopharyngeal cancer, if resected, is managed in a way similar to that for stages 2 and 3, although more extensive resection of the pharynx with myocutaneous flap reconstruction may be required. This approach is generally followed by postoperative irradiation.

Patients with unresectable tumors are treated by radiotherapy and generally treated in an experimental mode. Approaches under investigation to improve the results of local irradiation in unresectable disease include hypoxic cell sensitizers and cytotoxic chemotherapy. Although neoadjuvant chemotherapy before irradiation has been explored, it does not appear to improve results in this stage of disease. Simultaneous administration of radiotherapy and chemotherapy with drugs such as 5-fluorouracil, bleomycin, cisplatin, and mitomycin-C have shown improved local and regional control. Adjuvant chemotherapy in conjunction with surgery and radiotherapy has been tested in a large national trial but has not been shown to improve survival rates over combined radiotherapy and surgery alone.

Radiation oncology

Carcinoma of the pharynx generally requires visualization at simulation with plain radiographs, sometimes accompanied by contrast. CT or preferably MRI is useful in delineating the stage of disease and unexpected lymph node involvement. CT or MRI is also useful when three-dimensional treatment planning is advisable because of the need to deliver a higher dose.

The patient is immobilized in the supine position. The head is generally fixed using either a molded plastic shell or a bite block fixed to an adjustable mechanism. Films are taken in the anteroposterior and lateral orthogonal positions. Additional films of the supraclavicular region are used.

Treatment of the pharynx does not always involve

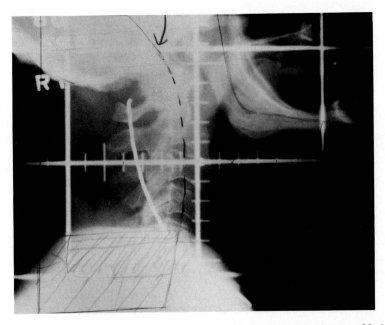

Fig. 84-3 Simulator film for treatment of patient with hypopharyngeal carcinoma with 4 meV x-rays. Note coverage of entire retropharyngeal node area in this postoperative patient. Incision is marked.

computerized or three-dimensional treatment planning, although for lesions in difficult locations, techniques involving three-dimensional images are employed.

Treatment of the pharynx generally involves the use of opposed lateral fields and an anterior supraclavicular field. Often it is necessary to treat the retropharyngeal nodes to the level of the nasopharynx, as well as the base of tongue beyond the surgical margin and the entire lymph node–bearing regions of the neck. To cover the supraclavicular region adequately, one must join a second portal here, taking great care to avoid overlapping on the spinal cord. This may be done by lateral field blocking or by using split fields in combination with table rotation. Compensating filters are generally used to prevent overdose in the anterior regions of the neck. An example of this lateral port technique is shown in Fig. 84-3.

Carcinoma of the hypopharynx is rarely treated by means of interstitial therapy. Occasionally the posterior pharyngeal wall may be implanted with catheters transfixing the neck in a single plane and loaded with iridium. The base of tongue following surgical resection may be implanted if margins are positive. Base of tongue implantation is often used for primary carcinomas in the base of tongue as well (Fig. 84-4). Unresectable carcinomas of the hypopharynx may be implanted by transfixing the larynx and hypopharyngeal wall with catheters afterloaded with temporary iridium-192 (^{192}Ir). Unre-

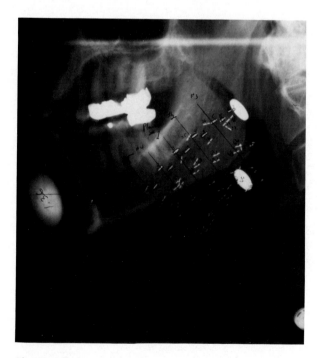

Fig. 84-4 Base of tongue implant loaded with ^{192}Ir seeds. Loops have been passed from skin surface through base of tongue and pharyngeal wall.

sectable cervical adenopathy may be implanted in a similar fashion. These advanced cases with such implants are often treated in conjunction with interstitial hyperthermia.

Esophagus
Overview

Carcinoma of the esophagus is generally treatable for palliation, but it is only rarely curable. The overall 5-year survival rate ranges from 5% to 20% in patients suitable for curative resection or definitive radiotherapy. The disease is usually diagnosed late in the United States, at a point where deep invasion and lymphatic permeation has occurred. Hepatic metastases are also a major problem.

The problem faced by the oncologist in approaching a patient with carcinoma of the esophagus is to delineate both the depth of invasion and the distal and proximal spread, as well as to rule out metastases to the liver and other organs. Most useful is an esophogram to delineate the linear spread of the lesion, then CT of the thorax and upper abdomen to delineate depth of invasion and localized enlarged lymph nodes and to evaluate the liver.

A carcinoma of the esophagus may be treated by surgical resection or by radiotherapy. Historically surgery has been used for lesions of the distal third and radiotherapy for those of the proximal and middle thirds. Combined radiotherapy and surgery have been employed with success in about 30% of patients tolerating the entire procedure. Recently chemotherapy in conjunction with radiotherapy appears to have improved local regional response rates.

Staging and prognosis

Carcinoma of the esophagus is staged clinically. T_1 disease is tumor involving 5 cm or less of the length of the esophagus without obstruction or extraesophageal spread. A T_2 tumor involves more than 5 cm of the length of the esophagus without extraesophageal spread or is any tumor that produces obstruction or involves the entire circumference. T_3 tumors are any tumors with evidence of spread through the esophageal wall to adjacent organs.

Imaging is essential in staging, since generally it is radiographic evidence of obstruction of the contrast material that denotes the T_2 nature of the tumor and evaluates extension beyond the esophagus. Although the latter may be obtained from contrast radiographs, today it is most often diagnosed by CT. Lymph node disease classification is confined to the cervical region and described simply as N_1, which is unilateral and palpable; N_2, which is bilateral and palpable; and N_3, which is fixed nodes. No clinical nodal staging system is in use for the middle and distal thirds.

Pathologic classification

More than 90% of esophageal tumors are squamous cell in origin and 10% are caused by adenocarcinomas. These either arise from a Barrett esophagus or from glands at the immediate gastroesophageal junction.

Current treatment options

Tumors of the cervical esophagus and mid-thoracic esophagus are generally treated by radiotherapy. In patients with a high performance status and lesions confined to the esophagus, resection with postoperative irradiation or preoperative irradiation and resection can be considered. In selected series these have shown improved survival (30% versus 5% to 10%), but one must realize that these series were selected. Because of the poor prognosis with both radiation or surgery alone, such combined approach is indicated in the favorably disposed patient.

Most patients, however, appear with more advanced stages of the disease, T_2 or T_3. The current approach to this problem is to use combined radiation and chemotherapy followed by reevaluation. It is unclear after such treatment whether surgical resection adds to survival,

since all patients found to have persistent tumor after combined modality treatment succumb to the disease in spite of surgical resection. The treatment generally chosen is simultaneous irradiation, with doses of 50 Gy or higher in combination with 5-fluorouracil chemotherapy. This is accompanied either by mitomycin-C or by cisplatin.

Postoperative irradiation may be used for tumors arising in any location and of either histology if there is a deep and extensive lymphatic invasion or positive margins. In small series of such patients survival has been in the 25% range.

Adjuvant chemotherapy has not proved to be valuable in carcinoma of the esophagus, either when used with surgery or with radiotherapy, except for the simultaneous administration program previously discussed.

Radiation oncology

Carcinoma of the esophagus is treated by radiotherapy strictly on the basis of imaging studies. Conventional esophagograms are necessary to define the length of esophagus, which must be irradiated. In general one attempts

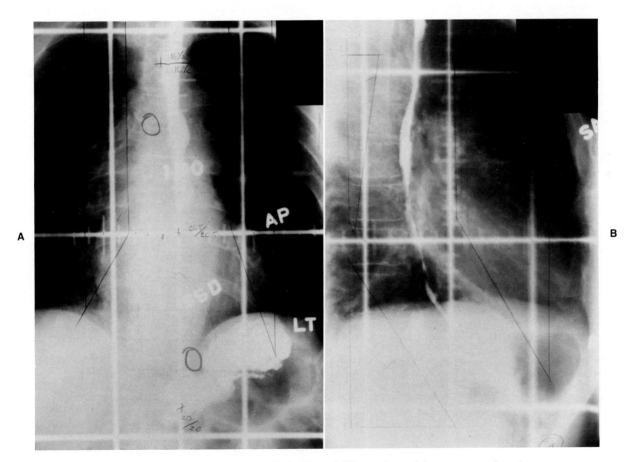

Fig. 84-5 Simulator films of anterior (**A**) and lateral (**B**) portals used for treatment of carcinoma of esophagus.

to irradiate almost the entire esophagus, and studies are needed to delineate the gastroesophageal junction and the cricoid. Reduced volumes and boost treatments require more specific delineation of the upper and lower margins of the lesions. CT is necessary to define the depth of invasion and localized enlarged lymph nodes.

Patients are immobilized in the supine position and anteroposterior and lateral orthogonal films are taken. Generally, esophageal contrast with barium is inserted, often with a thickened esophotrast-type barium. Patient contours are made so that transverse images may be associated with the location of the esophagus and the tumor, as well as other with thoracic structures. Two- and three-dimensional computerized treatment planning is often used in carcinoma of the esophagus. The use of multiple beams and reduced fields after 45 Gy limits the spinal cord dose to 45 Gy and limits the volume of lung and heart irradiated (Fig. 84-5).

Teletherapy techniques involve at least three and often four fields. Generally, anterior and posterior films, combined with reduced dose given by way of lateral portals, or posterior oblique films are used. More complex combinations and rotational techniques may be used for the final portion of the treatment. Total doses are generally in the range of 60 to 70 Gy.

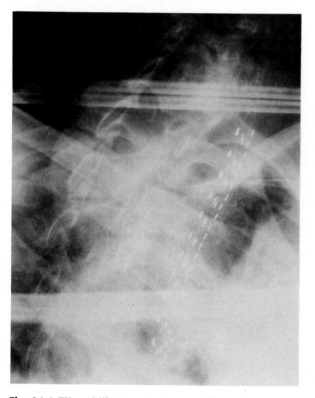

Fig. 84-6 Film of ^{192}Ir insertion into special esophageal tube containing six channels for seeds in surface. Tube was inserted over guidewire under fluoroscopic control.

Brachytherapy may be employed in the treatment of carcinoma of the esophagus for either an initial or current disease. An additional brachytherapy treatment may be given before teletherapy to shrink the lesion and allow rapid alimentation. It may be used as a boost at the end of external beam irradiation to increase the surface dose in the esophagus. It is also used at the time of recurrence to create more long-lasting relief of obstruction than can be obtained with dilatation or laser resection.

Brachytherapy is delivered using a specially designed esophageal tube that contains 6 channels for afterloading of ^{192}Ir seeds in ribbons. The catheter is generally inserted under fluoroscopic control over a guidewire into the stomach. The level of the lesion is then localized with contrast relative to the tube, and the radioactive sources are inserted into the channels to the appropriate depths (Fig. 84-6).

Stomach
Overview

Carcinoma of the stomach is often quite advanced when diagnosed. Early-stage disease accounts for only about 20% of all cases in the United States, and in this group more than 50% can be cured. Eighty percent have metastatic disease or advanced local disease, including extensive lymph node involvement.

Surgical resection is the standard treatment for gastric cancer for curative purpose. Radiotherapy in conjunction with chemotherapy remains experimental, although the combination can be very effective in achieving local regional response and palliation.

Imaging is the key to the diagnosis and staging of gastric cancer. Together with the findings of endoscopy, contrast films can delineate the location of esophageal gastric and duodenal lumen and the exact location of the primary tumor on the stomach wall. CT can define the extent of penetration and the presence of enlarged lymph nodes.

Staging and prognosis

Staging of carcinoma of the stomach is by the TNM classification and is generally obtained at surgery. T_1 disease is tumor limited to the mucosa or submucosa, regardless of extent or location. T_2 tumors involve the mucosa and the submucosa and may extend to but not penetrate the serosa. T_3 tumors penetrate the serosa but do not invade contiguous structures, whereas T_4 tumors do.

Nodal diseases are classified as N_1 when tumor involves the perigastric lymph nodes within 3 cm of the primary tumor; N_2 when it involves lymph nodes more than 3 cm from the primary tumor, which are, however, resected; and N_3 when it involves other intraabdominal lymph nodes, including the periaortic and mesenteric.

Stage 1 disease involves patients with T_1N_1 tumors,

which carry a 5-year survival of approximately 85%. Stage 2 disease includes T_2 and T_3 tumors. Survival is in the 50% range for T_2 but drops to below 20% for T_3 tumors. Stage 3 disease includes patients with T_1 through T_3 with nodal involvement in the N_1 and N_2 classification and those with early T_4 disease and less than N_3 nodal involvement. Five-year survival is approximately 15% to 20%.

Stage 4 tumors involve patients with T_3 or advanced T_4 disease or a distant metastasis. Their survival is less than 5% at 5 years.

Pathologic classification

The pathologic classification of stomach cancer involves adenocarcinomas, which can be subdivided into fungating, ulcerating, superficial spreading, and diffuse spreading, or linitis plastica types. Lymphomas and sarcomas also occur in the stomach but are not discussed here.

Current treatment options

Current treatment options for early-stage gastric cancer include a radical surgical procedure involving either a total distal gastrectomy, a total proximal gastrectomy, or a total gastrectomy for patients with diffuse tumor. Treatment of stage 2 tumors is similar. For patients with stage 3 disease resection is still the treatment of choice, but because of the high incidence of local and distant failure, investigational treatment should be considered. Such investigational treatment would include postoperative irradiation with or without chemotherapy. Patients with metastatic or unresectable stage 4 disease can receive palliative chemotherapy. Periods of such therapy often includes 5-fluorouracil in combination with other agents, such as doxorubicin, mitomycin-C, BCNU, as well as cisplatin.

Radiation oncology

As for carcinoma of the esophagus, localization of the stomach for radiotherapy requires diagnostic imaging techniques. Outlining the lumen with barium or other contrast is essential using radiographs. This helps delineate the upper and lower margins relative to the bowel lumen and identifies large masses as well as certain normal organs. Accurate treatment planning, however, requires CT, usually in addition with contrast in the bowel as well as intravenously.

Patients are simulated in a supine position and immobilized in that location. Left upper quadrant orthogonal films are obtained with barium contrast (Fig. 84-7). In addition, intravenous contrast is essential to delineate the kidneys.

CT taken through the delineated areas is extremely useful. Two-dimensional and three-dimensional com-

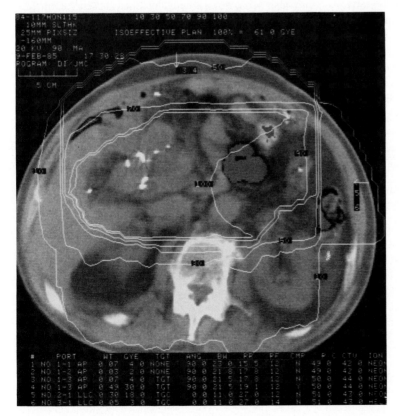

Fig. 84-7 Simulator anteroposterior field with oral barium contrast for carcinoma of stomach.

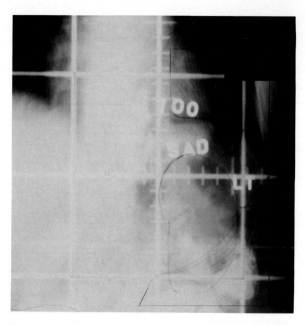

Fig. 84-8 Treatment plan on CT slice for carcinoma of stomach. Neon and helium ions have been used and arrangement spares kidneys and spinal cord.

puterized treatment plans are useful, as shown in Fig. 84-8. Such plans are essential if the irradiation of the kidneys and spinal cord, sparing as much liver as possible, is to be achieved.

Teletherapy techniques involve the use of high-energy machines in the 6 to 25 meV range and multiple portals. Often anteroposterior and lateral films, with wedge filters in the anteroposterior film, are used.

Brachytherapy is not generally employed for treatment of carcinoma of the stomach, although an occasional patient with residual tumor or very close surgical margins would be subjected to an intraoperative placement of catheters for afterloading with ^{192}Ir seeds. Intraoperative irradiation with electron beams has been widely explored, particularly for treating the periaortic and celiac lymph nodes following gastric resection. It can also be employed for unresectable residual masses.

Liver
Overview

Hepatocellular carcinoma is relatively rare in the United States. It is common, however, in China. Tumor is rarely curable by surgical resection, but this should always be considered because, if the lesion is localized to one lobe and can be resected, cure is possible. The hepatocellular carcinoma is associated with cirrhosis in more than half of the patients, and it is also frequently associated with hepatitis B infection. The presence or absence of elevated α-fetoprotein is an important prognostic indicator with patients exhibiting normal levels and having a better prognosis.

Imaging studies are essential in the evaluation, staging, and treatment planning for hepatocellular cancer. CT and more recently MRI delineate the location of the lesion and involvement of one or more lobes and are useful in positioning needles for fine-needle aspiration biopsy to establish the diagnosis. Angiography is often important in delineating the operability of the lesion. Spread to the peritoneal surface and other abdominal as well as thoracic organs is also delineated by CT.

There is no TNM classification for hepatic carcinomas, but generally they are defined as unresectable, localized, or metastatic. Resectable tumors are confined to a solitary mass in one portion of the liver, which allows complete resection with clean margins. Survival in these cases ranges from 10% to 30%. Patients with localized unresectable disease have tumor confined to the liver, which is unresectable because of extension across anatomic lines, thus not allowing complete en bloc surgery. These patients have 5-year survival rates less than 1%. The advanced tumor that has spread throughout the entire liver or to sites outside the liver carries essentially no 5-year survival.

Pathologic classification

The malignant tumors of the liver are primarily adenocarcinomas exhibiting 2 cellular types: hepatocellular carcinoma and cholangiocarcinoma. The hepatic types may be divided further into liver cell carcinoma and the fibrolamellar variant of hepatocellular carcinoma. One may also see a mix of hepatocellular and cholangiocarcinoma and undifferentiated tumors. Hepatoblastomas occur in children. The fibrolamellar variant is important because it is frequently diagnosed in young women and has a higher cure rate if resected.

Current treatment options

For a patient with resectable primary liver cancer, surgery is the treatment of choice. Surgery ranges from segmental to trisegmental resection. Hepatic carcinoma is often multifocal, however, and it involves multiple sites throughout the liver, preventing such curative resection. Adjuvants to surgery have been explored but remain experimental and include regional arterial infusion of chemotherapy postoperatively.

Patients with unresectable tumor still localized to the liver should generally be considered for investigational treatment. Such treatments include external beam irradiation with chemotherapy, followed by radiolabeled antiferritin; infusion of chemotherapy continuously using an implanted pump through catheters in the hepatic artery; and embolization of the hepatic artery with biodegradable microspheres, combined with chemotherapy. Surgery may be combined with chemotherapy or radiotherapy. Patients with advanced tumor really do not have many other options. Isotopic immunotherapy has been

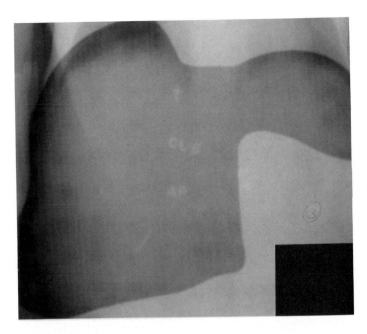

Fig. 84-9 Portal film for whole liver anterior field with block for left kidney.

explored in such patients, with occasional responses even in distant metastases.

Radiation oncology

To irradiate the liver properly, certain imaging studies are essential. Primary among these is a CT scan of the entire liver, which also involves the lower thorax and the abdomen adjacent to the liver. Use of contrast to delineate the kidneys and the bowel is also essential.

Patients are generally simulated in the supine position and anteroposterior films are taken with contrast administered to delineate the kidneys. In some situations portal films may be taken with isocentric localization so that oblique views can be employed (Fig. 84-9). In either situation it is necessary to evolve a plan that will spare at least one-third to one-half the total renal volume.

CT-based treatment planning is extremely useful in the treatment of the entire liver. After slices at 1 cm intervals are taken throughout the liver, planning is done in a two-dimensional mode on multiple slices. Anterior and posterior oblique views are often combined with a right-angle opposite oblique port.

Teletherapy techniques involve use of high energy, at least 6 meV, with 18 meV or higher if possible. Brachy therapy and intraoperative irradiation are rarely used for primary hepatic cancers.

Extrahepatic bile duct
Overview

Carcinomas arising in the extrahepatic bile duct occur infrequently and are curable in less than 10% of cases. The prognosis depends on the location of the tumor, which affects not only the stage in which it is diagnosed but also its resectability. Only about 25% of tumors are resectable. These represent primarily those in the distal bile duct.

In many situations the tumor is not completely resectable, and additional therapy with radiation or chemotherapy is indicated.

Imaging is very important in both diagnosis and staging of the tumor. Although some diagnoses may be made by endoscopy, this is extremely rare. Contrast studies carried out either through the percutaneous route or endoscopic route delineate the location of the lesion, whereas CT images define its dimensions and depth of invasion.

Staging and diagnosis

Tumors of the bile duct are generally classified as localized or unresectable. Patients with localized cancer can be completely resected and represent a small minority of patients with an overall 5-year survival rate of 10%. This can approach 25% for the distal duct.

Unresectable patients represent the remainder of the cases, with essentially no 5-year survival. Invasion of the adjacent liver and frequently seeding of the peritoneal surface usually occur, as well as regional lymph node disease.

Pathologic classification

There are two major types of extrahepathic bile duct tumor: the malignant epithelial tumors and the malignant mesenchymal tumors. Among the epithelial tumors are adenocarcinoma, squamous cell carcinoma, adenosquamous carcinoma, and cholangiocarcinoma. The rare mesenchymal tumors include include embryonal rhabdomyosarcoma, leiomyosarcoma, and malignant fibrosis histiocytoma.

Current treatment options

Patients with localized extrahepatic tumors are treated by means of surgical resection, which varies according to location. External beam irradiation may be added to the primary treatment if narrow or positive margins are present. Clips for localizing the areas of tumor placed at surgery can be useful but should be of a material that will not greatly interfere with CT scanning.

Patients with unresectable tumors may receive palliative irradiation. Again, this is improved if surgical localizing clips have been placed at the time of resection. Generally a bypass procedure has been performed, and often a tube is left in place that passes through the lesion, allowing brachytherapy.

Radiation oncology

Contrast films are needed of the entire intra- and extrahepatic bile duct system and adjacent to duodenum in order to localize the lesion. Contrast films of these organs are used in conjunction with CT scans. Ideally the CT scans will be with contrast. It is sometimes difficult to localize the exact dimensions of the tumor because of failure to contrast it with the substance of the liver. The role of MRI in assisting with such delineation is not yet clear.

Simulation is carried out with the patient in the supine position. Orthogonal isocentric films are taken centered at the portal hepatis (Fig. 84-10). Fiducial marks are placed and CT scans obtained.

Computerized treatment planning involves directing multiple high-energy beams at the site of residual tumor and adjacent liver. This is generally accomplished by three-dimensional treatment planning and often may include beams that are not coplanar with the usual transverse axis in order to decrease further the exposure to the adjacent normal liver and the kidneys.

Teletherapy techniques involve multiple high-energy beams in the 6 to 18 meV or higher range. Doses of 60 to 70 Gy are delivered and required for any level of local control. Whole liver irradiation has been attempted in conjunction with local irradiation to attempt to control micrometastases, but this has had little success and risks radiation hepatopathy. Intraoperative irradiation of the porta hepatis and involved ducts can be quite useful in conjunction with partial resection and in unresectable disease.

Brachytherapy has become quite popular in conjunction with the placement of bypass tubes, as long as the location of the tumor relative to the tube can be determined. Linear sources containing high-intensity ^{192}Ir or cesium seeds are then inserted and deliver a dose that can be in the 30 to 60 Gy range within 1 cm of the catheter. This will provide for palliation, but because of the limited depth of penetration, is generally not curative (Fig. 84-11).

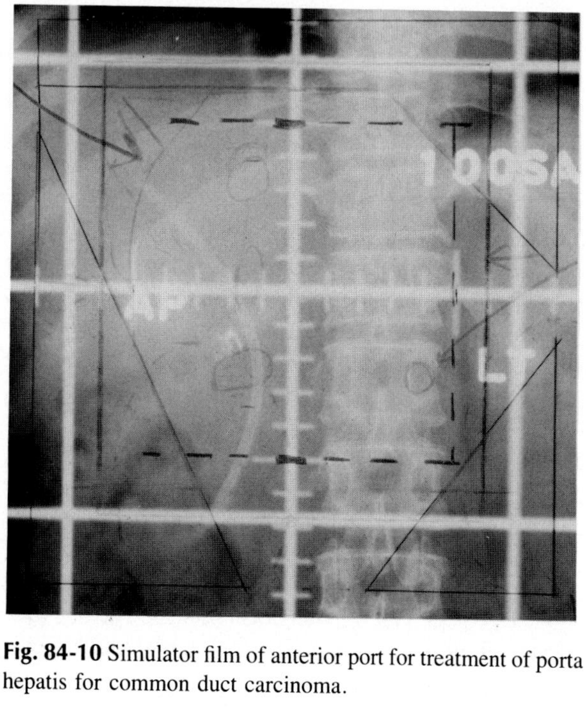

Fig. 84-10 Simulator film of anterior port for treatment of porta hepatis for common duct carcinoma.

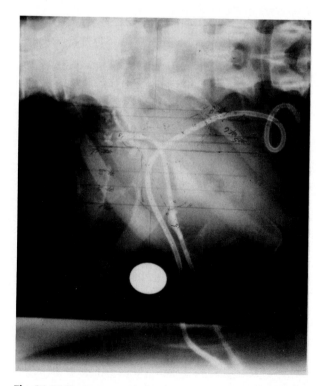

Fig. 84-11 Percutaneous drainage tubes in biliary tree with ^{192}Ir seeds in intrahepatic and extrahepatic bile ducts for bile duct carcinoma.

Pancreas
Overview

Pancreatic cancer is rarely curable because of its generally delayed diagnosis. In less than 20% of patients there is tumor localized to the pancreas, and even in this stage only approximately 5% are cured with surgical resection. The median survival range is from 8 to 12 months. Palliation of symptoms may be achieved with aggressive radiotherapy. Chemotherapy has been shown to improve median survival, but it does not cure. Surgical bypass is the most frequently used approach.

Imaging is essential in the diagnosis and staging of this lesion. Most pancreatic cancers are now detected through the use of CT scans and biopsies with fine-needle aspiration. Indications for superiority of MRI in this lesion are not clear. Contrast films may be useful in delineating the margins of the pancreas, but in general CT is the method of choice for localization and staging.

Staging and prognosis

The staging system for carcinoma of the pancreas is still under development but has progressed beyond the determination of resectable and unresectable. T_1 disease involves patients with no direct extension beyond the pancreas. In T_2 there is limited direct extension to duodenal bile ducts or stomach, but resection is possible. In T_3 direct extension occurs to adjacent organs, preventing resection. Nodal involvement is simply defined as present or absent.

Stage 1 is T_1 or T_2 without lymph node involvement and has a 3-year survival of about 15%. Stage 2 consists of patients with T_3N_0 disease, with a 3-year survival rate at 2%. Stage 3 patients have T_1 through T_3 with N_1 disease and a 3-year survival of 2%. Stage 4 is any disease more extensive than stage 2.

Pathologic classification

Approximately 90% of the patients exhibit duct cell carcinoma with other tumors, including acinar cell carcinoma and adenosquamous carcinoma. There are rare undifferentiated carcinomas, islet cell tumors, and cystadenocarcinomas.

Current treatment options

Because of the poor survival with any stage of pancreatic cancer, investigational treatment is often used. Curative resection is the primary modality, and adjuvant radiotherapy and/or chemotherapy may also be employed. Intraoperative irradiation and brachytherapy have been examined extensively, as has adjuvant radiation and chemotherapy after gross surgical resection.

Radiation oncology

To plan treatment for carcinoma of the pancreas, a high-quality CT scan is essential. This should preferably be done with 5 or even 3 mm slices so that reconstructions can be carried out.

Simulation is carried out with the patient supine, and generally anterior and lateral orthogonal films are taken and fiducial marks placed on the patient (Fig. 84-12).

Computerized treatment planning is essential, with at least a two-dimensional display of isodose curves on the tumor and surrounding normal tissue anatomy. Three-dimensional planes using other than coplanar portals are also useful.

Teletherapy techniques generally involve at least three portals with an anterior and two wedge laterals and energies in the 6 to 25 meV range. High-energy anterior electron portals are also useful, and charged particles such as helium have demonstrated improved dose distributions in the pancreas but have not improved median survival or cure rates (Fig. 84-13).

Intraoperative irradiation has been extensively tested both after surgical resection and for unresectable masses. In combination with external beam irradiation, it probably provides the longest survival time for patients exhibiting localized but unresectable tumor and may increase survival in patients who have resection. Implantation of the pancreas either at the time of surgery with permanent iodine seeds, or through transabdominal CT and stereotactic localization, also useful.

Colon
Overview

Cancer of the colon is generally treatable and often curable if discovered at a time when it is still localized to the bowel wall. It is second in incidence to carcinoma of the lung in the United States, and the second greatest cause of cancer death.

Screening tests for carcinoma of the colon include stool occult blood measurements, colonscopy, and barium enemas. The cost-effectiveness of all these is yet to be proved and probably should be confined to patients over age 50. Measurement of the carcinoembryonic antigen (CEA) often leads to earlier diagnosis of recurrence after initial treatment.

Surgical resection remains the treatment of choice, with removal of a significant portion of the bowel and reanastomosis. Adjuvant chemotherapy has recently been shown to give improved disease-free survival for Dukes' B and C tumor patients receiving postoperative chemotherapy consisting of 5-fluorouracil, methyl-CCNU, and vincristine.

Imaging is important in the diagnosis, staging, and treatment of colon cancer. Although fiberoptic colonscopy can yield the diagnosis in many patients, delineation of the exact extent and depth of invasion requires conventional and air contrast barium enemas and CT. MRI is useful in the low pelvis.

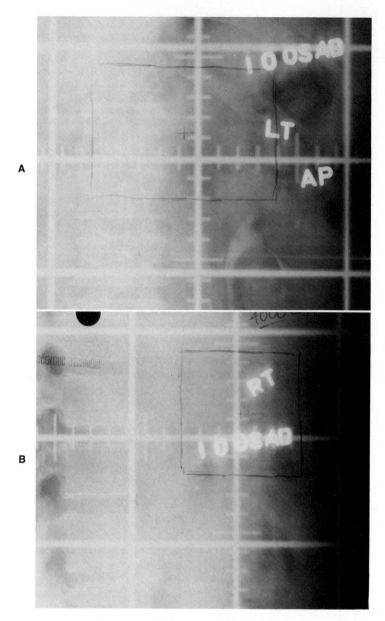

Fig. 84-12 Simulator films for anterior (**A**) and lateral (**B**) portals used in treatment of carcinoma of pancreas. Reduced volume cone down is also indicated.

Staging and prognosis

There is an available TNM staging system for colon carcinoma, but it is rarely employed. Staging is generally categorized by the traditional Dukes' system or by the Astler-Coller system. Stage 1 consists of patients with Dukes' A tumor limited to the bowel wall. In the Astler-Coller system stage A is tumor limited to the mucosa and B_1 is tumor extending into the muscularis. Stage 2 is defined as Dukes' B, with tumor spread through to the serosa, and is identical with Astler-Coller B_2. Stage 3 is defined as Dukes' C, with the exception that it also includes patients with tumor extension beyond the serosa

into contiguous tissues and/or organs. It also includes patients with any lymph node involvement. It is similar to Dukes' C, in which regional lymph nodes are involved, and Astler-Coller B_3, in which contiguous organs but no lymph nodes are involved. It also includes Astler-Coller C_1 for tumor limited to the bowel wall with involved nodes and Astler-Coller C_2, with tumor penetrating the bowel wall and with involved nodes. Survival is 75% to 100% in stage 1, 50% to 75% in stage 2, and 30% to 50% in Stage 3. Stage 4 disease includes any patients with distant metastases. These patients show survival at 5 years of less than 10%.

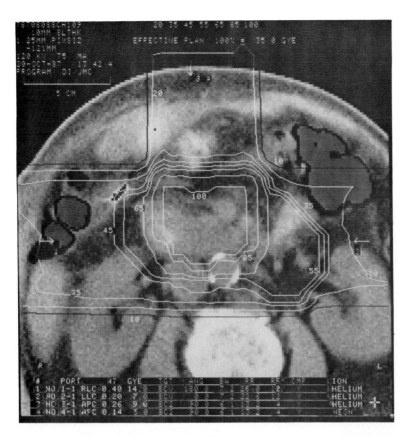

Fig. 84-13 Three-field treatment plan for carcinoma of pancreas using helium ions. Note excellent coverage of tumor and low doses to critical normal organs.

Pathologic classification

Tumors of the colon are classified as adenocarcinomas and subdivided according to mucinous, signet ring, or scirrhous patterns.

Current treatment options

The primary treatment of colon cancer is surgical resection of the primary and regional lymph nodes. In addition, solitary hepatic metastases can be cured with surgical resection in about 20% of patients. A recent study indicates that patients with stage B and C colon cancer also benefit from adjuvant chemotherapy with 5-fluorouracil, methyl-CCNU, and vincristine. This improvement is about 10% in survival and disease-free survival. This small gain was detected because of the large size of the study (1166 patients).

Radiotherapy has been used as an adjuvant to surgery for colon cancer in situations where there is complete penetration of the bowel wall and involvement of contiguous structures, but no peritoneal carcinomatosis or extensive lymph node disease.

Radiation oncology

The treatment of colon cancer is almost completely confined to postoperative irradiation of areas of microscopic or gross residual disease after resection. Therefore

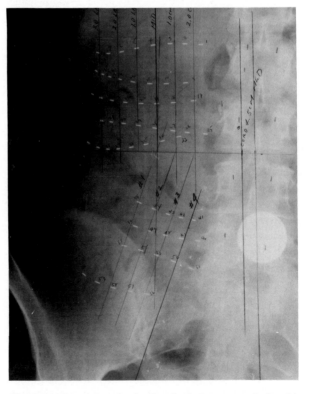

Fig. 84-14 Intra-operative implant loaded postoperatively with ^{192}Ir in retroperitoneal area. Region treated contained residual tumor after resection.

films imaging clips placed during surgery and CT scans are the major techniques employed.

Simulation is carried out with the patient in the supine position, and orthogonal radiographs are taken with contrast in the adjacent normal organs, including intravenous contrast for the kidneys and intraluminal contrast for small bowel and colon.

Computerized treatment planning is essential at least in the two-dimensional mode for localization of residual tumor together with adjacent organs. Reconstruction in other planes is often necessary.

Teletherapy techniques involve multiport irradiation of the region of residual tumor, designed in a way to minimize injury to small bowel and kidney. Whole abdomen irradiation in conjunction with this local treatment has been explored experimentally in an attempt to control liver and peritoneal recurrence, but as yet there has been no definitive study. Intraoperative electron beam irradiation has also been employed for positive margins or gross residual tumor.

Brachytherapy may be performed for areas of positive margin or gross residual tumor. In particular, retroperitoneal implants with removable catheters that are afterloaded with ^{192}Ir seeds have been used (Fig. 84-14).

Rectum
Overview

Carcinoma of the rectum is a highly curable tumor both in its localized form or with regional lymphatic involvement. Surgery is the primary treatment, with prognosis clearly related to depth of penetration and lymph node involvement. Recurrence in the pelvis is a major problem and outweighs both peritoneal seating and liver metastasis. For this reason post- or preoperative irradiation has been employed in a number of studies, as has the combination of radiation and chemotherapy. Because the incidence of this tumor is high, it is important to identify high-risk groups and attempt adjuvant treatment following surgery to reduce the problem of local and regional failure. Systemic chemotherapy has also been employed experimentally in an attempt to reduce metastases to the liver and peritoneum.

Imaging plays an important role in the staging and treatment planning. Diagnosis is generally made through endoscopy. Imaging can delineate the superior and lateral margins of extension, and both CT and MRI can assist in determination of resectability. CT and MRI are also important in radiotherapy treatment planning.

Staging and prognosis

As for the colon, there is an existing TMN staging classification system for rectal cancer as well as the Dukes' and Astler-Coller modification of the Dukes' system. Staging is the same for colon and rectal tumors and

will not be repeated. Five-year survival for stage 1 is generally 75% to 100%; for stage 2, 50% to 75%, for stage 3, 30% to 50%; and for stage 4, less than 5%.

Pathologic classification

Classification for rectal cancer is similar to that for colon cancer, with adenocarcinoma found in most cases. Subsets, including mucinous, signet ring, and scirrhous tumors, are recognized.

Current treatment options

The standard treatment for rectal cancer is surgical resection of the primary and regional lymph nodes for localized disease. Tumors in the early stage of disease, which are superficial and low lying, may be treated by fulguration or by a combination of intraluminal contact radiation therapy and radioactive implantation, carried out using a template on the perianal perineum.

Radiotherapy may be used alone for palliation and occasional control of patients with unresectable tumors. The combination of surgery, radiotherapy, and chemotherapy for more advanced B$_2$ and C lesions has improved local regional control and survival. Another study has shown improved survival for such patients treated with adjuvant chemotherapy alone using 5-fluorouracil and methyl-CCNU, as in the first study, and also vincristine. Disease-free survival was significantly improved, whereas overall survival was improved only marginally. Postoperative irradiation in this trial reduced local regional recurrence but did not affect survival when used alone. This study did not evaluate the combination, which may be more advantageous. It appears that chemotherapy, when combined with radiotherapy, not only improves its effectiveness in terms of local regional control, reducing failures by half, but also has an impact on distant metastases. Studies are underway that again are evaluating the combination of radiation and chemotherapy compared with chemotherapy alone. A trial in another group of patients has shown the advantage of the combination over radiation alone.

Radiation oncology

Proper treatment planning for either definitive or postoperative irradiation of rectal cancer requires localization of the position of the small intestine and the colon using barium contrast, with small bowel follow-through before simulation. Simulation is carried out with the patient in the prone position with a full bladder to minimize small bowel intrusion into the treatment volume. The prior administration of small bowel contrast allows localization of the small bowel and its shielding at least in the lateral portals. Orthogonal films are taken (Fig. 84-15). Generally a four-field isocentric technique is used with radiation energies from 6 to 25 meV. From 30% to 50%

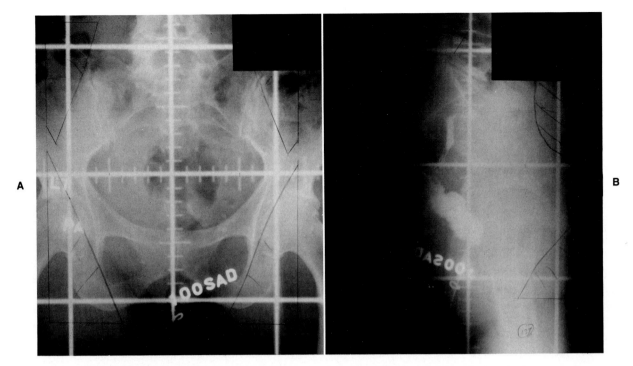

Fig. 84-15 Simulator films for postoperative treatment of carcinoma of rectum. **A,** Anterior port. **B,** Lateral port.

of the dose is delivered to the lateral portals, where shielding of the small bowel is possible.

Computerized treatment planning has not been widely used in rectal cancer because of the large volume, which is generally irradiated in the adjuvant or even definitive situation. Such planning could be useful for small-field boosts applied to gross residual tumor in the case of tumor unresectability.

Intraoperative irradiation has had widespread testing in rectal cancer and appears to be of benefit in the marginally resected patient.

Brachytherapy has been used extensively in the treatment of the very low-lying rectal lesions, particularly in the avoidance of abdominoperineal resection. It is useful for T_1 and T_2 tumors and may be combined with several films with intraluminal contrast materials with low-energy x-rays. It is almost always combined with external beam irradiation for half of the treatment and can yield control rates in the 90% range for T_1 lesions.

Anus
Overview

Anal cancer is often curable and recently has proved to be particularly amenable to a combination of radiation and chemotherapy. Abdominoperineal resection is the usual alternative but can be avoided in 75% or more of patients today. The major prognostic factors include the site (i.e., anal canal or perianal skin), the size, and the differentiation.

Although anal cancer has been an uncommon malignancy and appears mainly in elderly women, more recently it has occurred more frequently and has been identified as having increased in incidence in male homosexuals.

Imaging is important in anal cancer in delineating upward spread using both MRI and CT techniques and in delineating occult lymph node metastases. It is also essential in planning for radiotherapy treatment, with particular emphasis on multifield irradiation, perianal irradiation, and implantation.

Staging and prognosis

Stage 1 anal cancer involves only the anal mucosa without sphincter involvement and has a greater than 95% five-year survival. In stage 2 cancer there is involvement of the musculature of the wall of the anus but not of the lymph nodes. There may, however, be sphincter involvement. The 5-year survival rate is greater than 50%. Stage 3 carcinoma involves regional lymph nodes and has a prognosis in the 50% range if only perirectal nodes are involved and in the 10% range if higher pelvic nodes or inguinal nodes are involved. In stage 4 disease there is spread to the adjacent bony structures, distant nodes, or other organs, and 5-year survival is rare. It appears likely that the survival in stage 2 anal cancer has been improved by recent developments in the use of combined radiation and chemotherapy.

Pathologic classification

Carcinoma of the anus consist primarily of squamous cell or epidermoid carcinomas. There is an important subset of cloacogenic and basaloid tumors. It is unclear whether the histologic subtype influences survival.

Current treatment options

Surgical resection, often abdominoperineal, has been the mainstay of treatment of all but the earliest anal lesions, for which local excision or very local superficial irradiation has been used.

For larger stage 1 and stage 2 tumors immediate surgery has been replaced by the use of combined radiation and chemotherapy. Several administrations of combined 5-flurouracil and mitomycin-C in conjunction with radiotherapy doses between 40 and 55 Gy have yielded extremely high complete response rates. Even with lower doses complete response in the 70% range was observed and, with the doses described, this range extends to greater than 90%. Generally treatment is delivered to 40

to 50 Gy, and a biopsy is done at 6 weeks. If it is positive but tumor is limited, an additional 10 Gy dose may be given with another chemotherapy course. If tumor persists, abdominoperineal resection is performed. Between 75% and 90% of patients can avoid such surgery, however, and very high early local control and survival rates have been reported.

Radiotherapy alone has been used successfully for anal cancer with high control rates, but most experts now believe that the lower doses used in combination with chemotherapy yield somewhat better function and even higher control rates. Lymph nodal disease may be controlled by irradiation and chemotherapy or subsequent radical lymph node resection.

Radiation oncology

Treatment of anal cancer requires imaging of the location of the rectum in conjunction with portal definition and is generally carried out using films and barium contrast. For planning of implants, a CT scan or MRI with markers on the perineum is useful for determination of lesion depth and needle insertion depth.

Simulation is performed with the patient in the prone position. For perineal fields the supine lithotomy position

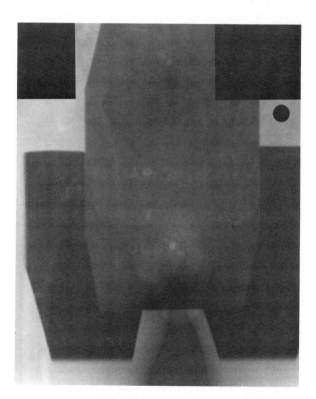

Fig. 84-16 Anterior port for treatment of stage 3 carcinoma of anus. Inguinal lymph nodes are treated from anterior port only, and partial thickness blocks are used to even the dose in region also treated posteriorly.

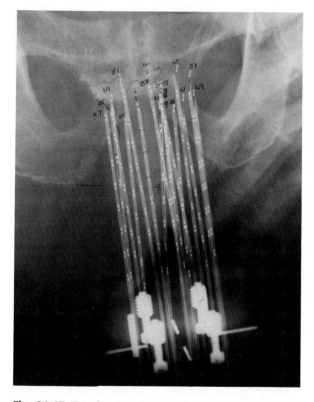

Fig. 84-17 Template-based perineal implant for anal carcinoma. Stainless steel needles are left in place and loaded with [192]Ir.

is used. The anus and rectum are localized with contrast in the rectum and a radiopaque marker in the anal canal and on the anus. Orthogonal films as well as contours are taken.

Computerized treatment planning based on CT or MRI is useful in delineating small-volume boost therapy, but it can be done on the basis of previously described simulator films.

Teletherapy techniques involve the use of a direct perineal field together with anterior and posterior wedged portals or use of a rotational technique in combination with a perineal field. Generally, small volumes limited to the rectum, anus, and perirectal tissue are sufficient for T_1 and limited T_2 tumors. The large T_2 and T_3 tumors require irradiation of the whole pelvis and the inguinal lymph nodes, as shown in Fig. 84-16.

In some patients a radioactive implant similar to that used for low rectal lesions can be useful to deliver a portion of the dose. It is important to avoid implantation of the entire circumference of the anal canal and sphincter to minimize complications. An example is shown in Fig. 84-17.

BIBLIOGRAPHY

Akine, Y, Hosoba, M, and Berardo, PA: Clinical merit of simulation images generated from CT, Radiology 145:528, 1982.

Al-Sarraf, M, et al: Concurrent radiotherapy and chemotherapy with cisplatin in inoperable squamous cell carcinoma of the head and neck: an RTOG study, Cancer 59:259, 1987.

American Joint Committee on Cancer: Manual for staging of cancer, ed 2, Philadelphia, 1983, JB Lippincott.

Badcock, PC: The role of CT scanning in the radiotherapy planning of pelvic tumors, Int J Radiat Oncol Biol Phys 9:905, 1983.

Campbell, WR, et al: Therapeutic alternatives in patients with esophageal cancer, Am J Surg 150:665, 1985.

Chang, AE, et al: A prospective randomized trial of regional versus systemic continuous 5-fluorodeoxyuridine chemotherapy in the treatment of colorectal liver metastases, Ann Surg 206(6):685, 1987.

Choi, Tk, Lee, NW, and Wong, J: Chemotherapy for advanced hepatocellular carcinoma, Cancer 53(3):401, 1984.

Coia, LR, Engstrom, PF, and Paul, AR: Nonsurgical management of esophageal cancer: report of a study of combined radiotherapy and chemotherapy, J Clin Oncol 5(11):1783, 1987.

Connolly, MM, et al: Survival in 1001 patients with carcinoma of the pancreas, Ann Surg 206(3):366, 1987.

Coppa, GF, et al: Hepatic resection for metastatic colon and rectal surgery, Ann Surg 202(2):203, 1985.

Cummings, B, et al: Results and toxicity of the treatment of anal canal carcinoma by radiation therapy or radiation therapy and chemotherapy, Cancer 54(10):2062, 1984.

Dahlin, H, et al: User requirements on CT-based computed dose planning systems in radiation therapy, Acta Radiol (Oncol) 22:397, 1983.

Daling, JR, et al: Correlates of homosexual behavior and the incidence of anal cancer, JAMA 247(14):1988, 1982.

Duttenhaver, JR, et al: Adjuvant postoperative therapy in the management of adenocarcinoma of the colon, Cancer 57(5):955, 1986.

Eisenberg, B, et al: Carcinoma of the colon and rectum: the natural history reviewed in 1704 patients, Cancer 49(6):1131, 1982.

Ellert, J, and Kreel, L: The value of CT in malignant colonic tumors, CT 4(3):225, 1980.

Ensminger, WD, et al: Totally implanted drug delivery system for hepatic arterial chemotherapy, Cancer Treat Rep 65(516):393, 1981.

Fisher, B, et al: Adjuvant chemotherapy or postoperative radiation for rectal cancer: 5 year results of NSABP protocol R-01, Proc Am Soc Clin Oncol 6A:359, 1987.

Fraass, BA, et al: Integration of magnetic resonance imaging into radiation therapy treatment planning. I. Technical considerations, Int J Radiat Oncol Biol Phys 13:1897, 1987.

Gastrointestinal Tumor Study Group: Therapy of locally unresectable pancreatic carcinoma: a randomized comparison of high-dose (6000 rads) radiation alone, moderate-dose radiation (4000 rads + 5-fluorouracil), and high-dose radiation + 5-fluorouracil, Cancer 48(8):1705, 1981.

Gastrointestinal Tumor Study Group: A comparison of combination chemotherapy and combined modality therapy for locally advanced gastric carcinoma, Cancer 49(9):1771, 1982.

Gastrointestinal Tumor Study Group: Controlled trial of adjuvant chemotherapy following curative resection for gastric cancer, Cancer 49(6):1116, 1982.

Gastrointestinal Tumor Study Group: Pancreatic cancer: adjuvant combined radiation and chemotherapy following curative resection, Arch Surg 120(8):899, 1985.

Gastrointestinal Tumor Study Group: Survival after postoperative combination treatment of rectal cancer, N Engl J Med 315(20):1294, 1986.

Gastrointestinal Tumor Study Group: Prolongation of the disease-free interval in surgically treated rectal carcinoma, N Engl J Med 312(23):1465, 1985.

Gastrointestinal Tumor Study Group: Further evidence of effective adjuvant combined radiation and chemotherapy following curative resection of pancreatic cancer, Cancer 59(12):2006, 1987.

Gerard, A, et al: Interim analysis of a phase II study on postoperative radiation therapy in resectable rectal carcinoma: trial of the Gastrointestinal Tract Cancer Cooperative Group of the European Organization for Research on the Treatment of Cancer (EORTC), Cancer 55(10):2372, 1985.

Glatstein, E, et al: The imaging revolution and radiation oncology: use of CT, ultrasound, and NMR for localization, treatment planning and treatment delivery, Int J Radiat Oncol Biol Phys 11:299, 1985.

Goitein, M: Future prospects in planning radiation therapy, Cancer 55:2234, 1985.

Goitein, M, and Abrams, M: Multi-dimensional treatment planning. I. Delineation of anatomy, Int J Radiat Oncol Biol Phys 9:777, 1983.

Goiten, M, et al: Prospective study of the value of CT in radiotherapy treatment planning, Int J Radiat Oncol Biol Phys 5:1787, 1979.

Goiten, M, et al: Multi-dimensional treatment planning. II. Beam's eye-view, back projection, and projection through CT sections, Int J Radiat Oncol Biol Phys 9:789, 1983.

Green, N, Mikkelsen, WP, and Kernen, JA: Cancer of the common hepatic bile ducts: palliative radiotherapy, Radiology 109:687, 1973.

Greenall, MJ, et al: Epidermoid cancer of the anal region: pathologic features, treatment and clinical results, Am J Surg 149(1):95, 1985.

Gunderson, LL, and Sosin, H: Areas of failure found at reoperation (second or symptomatic look) following "curative surgery" for adenocarcinoma of the rectum: clinicopathologic correlation and implications for adjuvant therapy, Cancer 34(4):1278, 1974.

Gunderson, LL, and Sosin, H: Adenocarcinoma of the stomach: areas of failure in a reoperation series (second or symptomatic looks): clinicopathologic correlation and implications for adjuvant therapy, Int J Radiat Oncol Biol Phys 8:1, 1982.

Gunderson, LL, et al: Intraoperative irradiation: a pilot study combining external beam irradiation with "boost" dose intraoperative electrons, Cancer 49:2259, 1982.

Hancock, SL, and Glatstein, E: Radiation therapy of esophageal cancer (review), Semin Oncol 11:144, 1984.

Harmer, MH, editor: TNM classifications of malignant tumors, ed 3, Geneva, 1978, UICC.

Heald, RJ, and Ryall, RD: Recurrence and survival after total mesorectal excision for rectal cancer, Lancet 1(8496):1479, 1986.

James, RD, Pointon, RS, and Martin, S: Local radiotherapy in the management of squamous carcinoma of the anus, Br J Surg 72(4):282, 1985.

Jose, B, et al: Computed tomography and radiotherapy in the treatment of cancer, J Surg Oncol 23:83, 1983.

Karlin, DA, Fisher, RS, and Krevsky, B: Prolonged survival and effective palliation in patients with squamous cell carcinoma of the esophagus following indoscopic laser therapy, Cancer 59(11):1969, 1987.

Kavanah, MT, et al: New surgical approach to minimize radiation-associate small bowel injury in patients with pelvic malignancies requiring surgery and high-dose irradiation, Cancer 56(6):1300, 1985.

Kemeny, N, et al: Intrahepatic or systemic infusion of fluorodeoxyuridine in patients with liver metastases from colorectal carcinoma, Ann Int Med 107(4):459, 1987.

Kligerman, MM, et al: Preoperative irradiation of rectosigmoid carcinoma including its regional lymph nodes, Am J Roentgenol 114:498, 1972.

Kopelson, G, et al: The role of radiation therapy in cancer of the extrahepatic biliary system: an analysis of thirteen patients and a review of the literature of the effectiveness of surgery, chemotherapy and radiotherapy, Int J Radiat Oncol Biol Phys 2(9/10):883, 1977.

Krook, J, et al: Radiation vs. sequential chemotherapy-radiation-chemotherapy: a study of the North Central Cancer Treatment Group, Duke University, and the Mayo Clinic, Proc Am Soc Clin Oncol 5:82, 1986.

Leichman, L, et al: Combined preoperative chemotherapy and radiation therapy for cancer of the esophagus: the Wayne State University, Southwest Oncology Group and Radiation Therapy Oncology Group Experience, Semin Oncol 11(12):178, 1984.

Leichman, L, et al: Cancer of the anal canal: model for postoperative adjuvant combined modality therapy, Am J Med 78(2):211, 1985.

Levi, JA, et al: Analysis of a prospectively randomized comparison of doxorubicin versus 5-fluorouracil, doxorubicin and BCNU in advanced gastric cancer: implications for future studies, J Clin Oncol 4(9):1348, 1986.

Martin, SA, et al: Carcinoma of the pyriform sinus: predictors of TNM relapse and survival, CA 46(9):1974, 1980.

Mendhall, WM, et al: Squamous cell carcinoma of the pyriform sinus treated with surgery and/or radiotherapy, Head Neck Surg 10(2):88, 1987.

Moertel, CG, et al: Combined 5-fluorouracil and supervoltage radiation therapy of locally unresectable gastrointestinal cancer, Lancet 2(7626):865, 1969.

Moertel, CG, et al: A phase II study of combined 7 fluorouracil, doxorubicin and cisplatin in the treatment of advanced upper gastrointestinal adenocarcinoma, J Clin Oncol 4(7):1053, 1986.

Munzenrider, JE, Verhey, L, and Doucett, J: A critical appraisal of the value of CT to the radiotherapist: the abdomen. In Husband, JE, and Hobday, PA, editors: Computerized axial tomography in oncology, Edinburgh, 1981, Churchill Livingstone.

Mustafa, AA, and Jackson, DF: The relation between X-ray CT numbers and charged particle stopping powers and its significance for radiotherapy treatment planning, Phys Med Biol 28:169, 1983.

O'Connell, MJ, Krook, JE, and Mayo Clinic North Central Cancer Treatment Group: Phase III randomized comparison of MeCCNU/5-FU vs. 5-FU alone followed by postoperative adjuvant radiotherapy and comparison of bolus vs. continuous 5-FU as a radioenhancer in patients with Stages B2/3 and C1-3 rectal carcinoma, MAYO-864751:NCCTG-9864751, active investigational protocol, last modified April 1988.

Order, SE, et al: Iodine 131 antiferritin, a new treatment modality in hepatoma: a Radiation Therapy Oncology Group study, J Clin Oncol 3(12):1573, 1985.

Papillon, J, et al: A new approach to the management of epidermoid carcinoma of the anal canal, Cancer 51(10):1830, 1983.

Paradis, P, Douglass, Ho, and Holyoke, ED: The clinical implications of a staging system for carcinoma of the anus, Surg Gynecol Obstet 141(3):411, 1975.

Purdy, JA: Computer applications in radiation therapy treatment planning, Radiat Med 1:161, 1983.

Schad, LR, et al: Three dimensional image correlation of CT, MR, and PET studies in radiotherapy treatment planning of brain tumors, J Comput Assist Tomogr 11:948, 1987.

Silverberg, E: Cancer Statistics: 1985, CA vol 19, 1985.

Steinberg, SM, et al: Prognostic indicators of colon tumors: the Gastrointestinal Tumor Study Group experience, Cancer 57(9):1866, 1986.

Thawley, SE, et al: Comprehensive management of Head and Neck Tumors, New York, 1986, WB Saunders.

Withers, HR, Romsdahl, MM, and Saxton, JP: Postoperative radiotherapy for cancer of the rectum and rectosigmoid, ASTRO Proc Int J Radiat Oncol Biol Phys 6(10):1380, 1980.

Wolmark, N, and Fisher, B: An analysis of survival and treatment failure following abdominoperineal and sphincter-saving resection in Dukes B and C rectal carcinoma: a report of the NSABP clinical trial, Ann Surg 204(4):480, 1986.

Wolmark, N, et al: Adjuvant therapy in carcinoma of the colon: five year results of the NSABP protocol C-01, Proc Am Soc Clin Oncol 6:A358, 1987.

Wong, JW, and Henkelman, RM: A new approach to CT pixel-based photon dose calculations in heterogeneous media, Med Phys 10:199, 1983.

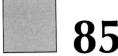

85 *Cost-Effectiveness*

HARVEY V. FINEBERG
JACK WITTENBERG

GENERAL CONSIDERATIONS

Cost-effectiveness analysis is an effort to measure and compare the costs, risks, and benefits of medical care. As strictly construed by economists, the aim of a cost-effectiveness assessment is to identify the most efficient use of limited economic resources. Cost-effectiveness analysis addresses such questions as what expenditure of resources can produce the greatest net benefit within a limited budget and what is the least costly way to achieve a particular level of benefit.* As used more loosely by a number of writers, the term *cost-effectiveness* also refers to any measurement of the costs and effects of medical services even if there are no explicit budget constraints or considerations of alternative ways of providing the services. The less constrained question in this sense involves the cost and service or benefit gained or lost if resources are deployed in a particular way.

This chapter describes an approach to conducting a cost-effectiveness analysis with reference to issues in the evaluation of imaging equipment and procedures. No standard methodology exists for conducting a cost-effectiveness analysis, but it is useful to remember certain principles and pitfalls. A cost-effective analysis should not be the sole determinant in any decision. Questionable assumptions and sometimes more serious shortcomings usually arise in an analysis. At its best, a cost-effectiveness analysis can array the gains and costs that attend different practices or strategies, but the physician, patient, or policy maker, collectively or individually, still has to judge whether the benefits are worth the costs. A later section discusses a cost-effective attitude toward radiologic practice as epitomized by an algorithmic approach to the choice of diagnostic tests.

IMPETUS FOR COST-EFFECTIVENESS

The interest in cost-effectiveness has grown along with the rise in expenditures for medical care. Between

---

*Economists distinguish cost-effectiveness from cost-benefit studies. The essential difference is that a cost-benefit study attempts to measure all effects, benefits as well as costs, in monetary terms, whereas a cost-effectiveness study considers benefits in terms of health (such as years of life gained) and does not convert benefits to dollar equivalents. Our emphasis here is on cost-effectiveness.

1965 and 1987 the costs of health care in the United States burgeoned from $43 billion to more than $500 billion, and expenditures are projected to exceed $750 billion in *1990*.[8] National health expenditures are expected to continue to grow faster than the gross national product (GNP), accounting for 9.5% of the GNP in 1980 and 11.5% in 1990.[8] As health costs have increased, it has become fashionable to question the value of many medical services, especially those, such as radiology, that rely on new technology. Physicians, economists, and other analysts have thus been motivated to assess both sides of the cost-effectiveness equation, clinical benefits as well as resource costs.

The number of published studies that assess the costs and benefits of a health program or medical practice increased more than sixfold during the first 7 years of the 1970s, from 16 studies in 1970 to 102 in 1977.[16] The growing interest of physicians in cost-effectiveness is evidenced by the especially rapid rise in publications in medical journals after 1975.[16] Studies have covered a full range of preventive, diagnostic, and therapeutic programs. The most frequently assessed medical intervention has been computed tomography (CT) scanning, with at least 18 published cost-effectiveness studies and numerous additional references to the implications of CT for cost-effectiveness.[16] Magnetic resonance imaging (MRI) has superseded CT as a major technologic breakthrough and is currently the focus of intense clinical evaluation. Accomplishing excellent multiplanar images in the absence of ionizing radiation and intravenous contrast material, MRI has proved to be comparable or superior in accuracy to CT scanning in many, but not all, anatomic areas.[14a] The experience gained with cost-effectiveness studies of CT will provide not only excellent methodologies to be used in evaluating MRI, but also will allow a more meaningful comparison of their cost-effectiveness.[16]

PRINCIPLES OF ANALYSIS

Several recent publications outline principles and steps in conducting a cost-effectiveness analysis in medical practices.[15,20,22,23] All exhort the analyst to be clear about the subject and purpose of an analysis, explicit about assumptions, and systematic in measuring costs and benefits. Although differing in details and emphasis, these methods are all consistent with one general approach, a version of which we present here. The following five steps are used in a formal cost-effectiveness analysis, with particular attention given to the requirements for assessing imaging procedures, equipment, and policies:

1. Define object and perspective.
2. Identify alternative approaches.
3. Measure benefits.
4. Measure costs.
5. Reach conclusions.

Define object and perspective

The object of a cost-effectiveness analysis can be a clinical procedure, a piece of equipment, a patient management strategy, or a health program. One analyst might want to assess the cost-effectiveness of alternative diagnostic strategies in patients with suspected colon cancer. Another might want to measure more narrowly the costs and yield of barium studies in patients with a suspected colon carcinoma. A third might be interested in the potential costs and effects of dietary changes that might alter the incidence of colon cancer. Each objective may be worthwhile; each requires examining a different range of medical interventions and potential consequences.

Many cost-effectiveness analyses in radiology focus on a particular procedure, (such as upper gastrointestinal series or arteriography), or a particular piece of equipment, such as CT or ultrasound scanner. In either case it is essential also to specify the range of patients to be included in the analysis. The pertinent population may be defined according to a demographic characteristic (women between the ages of 40 and 45), a presenting sign or symptom (guaiac-positive stool), or a clinical or pathologic diagnosis (colon carcinoma).

An important question is whether the objective of analysis is to encompass all patients examined with a specific procedure or equipment or just those with a single diagnosis. If the objective is to assess the overall cost-effectiveness of a diagnostic procedure or piece of equipment, this requires aggregating the full range of patients who may be examined. The comparative effectiveness and costs of the target procedure are likely to vary across these patient groups. One reason for this is the varying capability of the target equipment for different clinical problems; another is that applicability of alternative procedures varies among different patient groups. For example, if the target equipment for evaluation is computed body tomography, this procedure would encompass comprehensive examinations of the thorax and abdomen. Ultrasound is an alternative diagnostic procedure for the abdomen but not for the thorax.

In general, as the object of analysis encompasses a wider spectrum of patients, it becomes increasingly difficult to conduct a comprehensive cost-effectiveness analysis. On the other hand, a narrower analysis, focused on a restricted set of patients, may not address the question of prime concern, namely, what is the overall cost-effectiveness of the equipment?

The costs and benefits of any medical intervention must be calculated from a defined vantage point: costs and benefits to whom? In most cost-effectiveness studies the analyst takes a societal perspective, examining the aggregate net benefits to all patients and the social resource costs. The cost-effectiveness of a procedure to an individual patient differs from that to society if the patient has insurance that reduces or eliminates personal expenditures. A hospital's view of the cost-effectiveness of a new piece of machinery, a perspective in which units of service are the desired effect and revenues depend on someone else's costs, obviously differs from the patient's or society's perspective. Different vantage points serve distinct purposes, and no single vantage point is appropriate in all studies. In any one study it is essential to be consistent in terms of the perspective from which costs and benefits are calculated.

Identify alternative approaches

Every cost-effectiveness assessment is relative to some alternative use of available resources. A clinical procedure or piece of machinery is more or less cost-effective in comparison to specified alternatives. An existing piece of equipment may produce many new diagnoses at a relatively low cost and still be an unwise investment if an even more advanced device is available, more accurate, and equally or less expensive. In a different case, a more costly diagnostic procedure may be sufficiently cost-effective to be recommended if one is willing to pay the necessary price to achieve the possible benefit. The conclusions depend on the available alternatives.

Therefore any cost-effectiveness analysis is relative in two senses. First, for each available alternative, costs are measured relative to benefits. Second, costs and benefits of one device, procedure, or strategy are each relative to those of alternative approaches to reach the same objectives.

Measure benefits

Most discussions of cost-effectiveness analysis tend to describe health benefits in terms of ultimate health effects, usually measured in terms of mortality and morbidity. Several combined measures of mortality and morbidity have been used, such as the number of quality-adjusted life years[23] or the number of well years.[9] These measures of ultimate benefit reflect the aims of health care, but they are remote from the immediate product of an imaging test, an intelligible representation of anatomy and pathology. When analyzing the product and consequences of an imaging device, it is useful to consider it as a test system that includes the equipment, technician, patient, radiologist, and referring physician.[6]

The application of a diagnostic procedure engenders a hierarchy of efficacy, beginning with the technical performance of the test and extending through diagnostic information, therapeutic decision making, and finally the health outcome[7,12] (Fig. 85-1). This hierarchy stresses the value of the test to the patient undergoing examination and neglects possible research benefits for future patients and any larger effects on society. Some would argue that an imaging technique should be judged only on its ac-

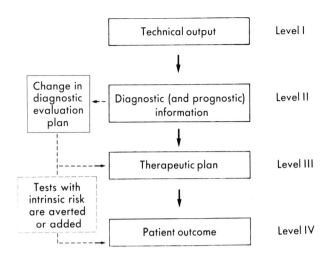

Fig. 85-1 Levels of clinical efficacy related to use of diagnostic test.

curacy in identifying normal and abnormal conditions. We think this view is too restrictive. The initial test may also prompt the performance or avoidance of additional tests. Alterations in the use of other tests as well as in treatment can change the net risks and expected benefits for the patient.

A useful, if still inconclusive, cost-effectiveness analysis could adopt a measure of effect, such as the impact on therapeutic decision making, more immediate than the ultimate health benefit, such as mortality. The advantage of such measures is their accessibility to be studied; the limitation is their tenuous connection with the ultimate benefits. For example, the discovery of an unresectable pancreatic carcinoma by CT may not alter the mortality but can avoid the need for exploratory laparotomy. The requirements for measures of benefit at any level are that it be attributable to the target equipment or procedures, that only incremental effects (effects beyond those of the alternatives) are included, and that negative as well as positive consequences are fully considered.

Each level of the efficacy hierarchy can provide indicators of a test's performance. At the level of technical performance, a measure of effect could be simply the number of studies performed or the number of interpretable examinations produced. In the evaluation of any imaging device, its day-to-day reliability and examination-to-examination reproducibility are also useful measures. More specific measures may apply to particular tests or devices; for example, different CT scanners can be compared according to contrast scale and noise, spatial resolution, radiation dose, scanning speed, and anatomic capacity.

A variety of measures can be used to represent the contribution of an imaging test to diagnostic understanding. In circumstances in which an independent confirmation of the presence or absence of disease is available, the test's sensitivity (frequency of positive results among patients with disease) and specificity (frequency of negative results among patients without disease) can be estimated. The sensitivity and specificity of a test depend on the quality of the image produced, the discriminating ability of the interpreter, and the criteria employed in defining a test result positive or negative. If more stringent decision criteria are used, there are fewer false-positive results but fewer true-positive results as well. Each test applied to a particular group of patient generates a set of possible combinations of true-positive and false-positive rates results; the actual performance among these possibilities depends on the stringency of the positivity criterion. The set of possible trade-offs among the true-positive rates for a given test is represented by the test's receiver operating characteristics (ROC) curve.[21]

The ability of a test to improve predictions of a disease depends not only on its sensitivity and specificity, but also on the prevalence or prior probability of the disease. The precise quantitative relation between posttest and pretest probability of disease is calculated with Bayes' formula (Fig. 85-2). One version of Bayes' formula states that the probability of disease following a positive test result is equal to a ratio. The numerator of the ratio is the product of the pretest probability of disease times the test's sensitivity. The denominator of the ratio is the sum of two products: (the pretest probability times the test's sensitivity) plus [(one minus the pretest probability) times (one minus the test's specificity)]. For example, suppose that the barium enema examination has a sensitivity of 0.90 in the detection of colon cancer (correctly diagnosed cancer in 9 of 10 patients with cancer) and a specificity of 0.95 (correctly ruled out cancer on 19 of 20 patients without the disease). If an 85-year-old patient with anemia has a pretest likelihood of colon cancer of 0.50 and a positive result on the barium enema examination, then the posttest likelihood of cancer is calculated as follows:

$$\frac{0.5 \times 0.90}{(0.5 \times 0.90) + [(1 - 0.5) \times (1 - 0.95)]}$$

The likelihood is almost 0.95. The same test would produce a much lower likelihood of cancer if it were applied to a population of women 40 to 45 years of age with anemia because the prior likelihood of cancer would be much smaller, perhaps 0.01. In this case a positive test result would increase the probability of disease only to 0.15.

Both normal and abnormal examinations of results are potentially valuable. What matters is not the diagnostic findings in themselves but the extent to which the findings alter prior beliefs about the patient's condition. Learning that a disease is absent in a patient previously thought to have the condition may be as important as or more im-

$$P(D/T^+) = \frac{P(D) \times P(T^+/D)}{P(D) \times P(T^+/D) + [1 - P(D)] \times [1 - P(T^-/\bar{D})]}$$

$P(D/T^+)$ = Probability of disease among patients with a positive test; that is, the posttest probability of disease given a positive test result

$P(D)$ = Pretest probability of disease

$P(T^+/D)$ = Test sensitivity; that is, the probability of a positive test result among patients with disease

$P(T^-/\bar{D})$ = Test specificity; that is, the probability of a negative test result among patients without disease

Fig. 85-2 Bayes' formula.

portant than confirming the presence of disease. Altering the probability of disease up or down affects the physician's confidence in the diagnosis and possibly provides better prognostic information for the patient. An imaging test can also serve as a critical adjunct to a definitive diagnosis, such as when used to guide a biopsy needle.

It is possible to assess diagnostic information provided by an imaging modality either in the context of clinical care or under conditions of controlled observation.[21] The latter approach offers a precise comparison of different diagnostic modalities and allows quantitative comparison of different observers. Studies in a clinical context can use the starting point of diagnostic knowledge before the test and measure its actual marginal contribution to the understanding of a patient's condition. Both types of studies can be useful and in fact complement each other.

The results of one diagnostic test can influence the choice of further tests, either prompting or avoiding the selection of them. This induced effect has the greatest impact on the net benefit when the potential tests are relatively risky or uncomfortable. The potential impacts on costs, also important, are discussed in the next section.

As to the level of effect on treatment, an analyst seeks to identify the changes in the treatment plan consequent to the test. These therapeutic changes may result from the confirmation or exclusion of a diagnosis or from a more exact definition of the extent of a suspected or known disease. Such a change may entail the addition of new treatments, the abandonment of a previously planned therapy, or improvements in the precision with which a previously planned treatment is administered. In addition, the increasing physician's and patient's confidence in a previously planned treatment can be of some value even when the treatment to be administered does not change. When the radiologist directly performs a therapeutic maneuver, as in percutaneous abscess drainage, its cost-effectiveness can be compared directly to

	Value rating
Diagnostic understanding (check one):	
-CT *confused* my understanding of this patient's disease and *led* to investiaations I would not otherwise have done	D1
-CT *confused* my understanding of this patient's disease but *did not* lead to any additional investigations.	D2
-CT had *no effect* or *little effect* on my understanding of this patient's disease.	D3
-CT provided information that *substantially* improved my understanding of this patient's disease.	D4
-My understanding of this patient's disease depended on diagnostic information provided *only* by CT (unavailable from any other nonsurgical procedure).	D5
Choice of therapy (check one):	
-CT led me to choose therapy that in retrospect was *not* in the best interests of the patient.	T1
-CT was of *no influence* in my choice of therapy.	T2
-CT did not alter my choice of therapy but did *increase my confidence* in the chosen treatment.	T3
-CT contributed to a change in my chosen therapy, but other factors (underline which: imaging tests, other diagnostic tests, changes in patient status) were *equally* or *more important.*	T4
-CT was *very important* compared with other factors in leading to a beneficial change in therapy.	T5
Did CT affect the precision with which you carried out therapy (for example, surgical approach, adjustment of medication dose)?	
Yes _____ No_____	

Fig. 85-3 Questionnaire on overall contribution of CT.

alternative treatments.[5] In selected categories of patients in which a particular level of confidence in a diagnosis leads to a specific therapy, the effect of a test on therapy plans might be inferred directly from the diagnostic information provided by the test.

The measurement of actual treatment effects can be conducted only in the clinical setting. In general, studies to measure effects on treatment require the collaboration of clinicians who are responsible for the care of patients. The radiologist's interpretation of a study establishes a potential benefit; the eventual gains depend on the credence given the radiologist's report and the range of therapeutic alternatives available.

An example of an evaluation of clinical efficacy is a study of computed body tomography that was conducted at Massachusetts General Hospital from 1976 to 1982.[26] Patients were prospectively classified into one of 12 protocols according to the principal clinical problem and anatomic region to be examined.

Before the CT examination, referring physicians completed questionnaires that prospectively indicated their diagnostic considerations and treatment plans. After performance of the CT examination, the radiologist provided the usual formal report, as well as a written estimate of the probabilities of each possible diagnosis, to facilitate later review of the examination's contribution. At the time of discharge or approximately 4 weeks after examination of outpatients, the physician completed a follow-up questionnaire on the overall contribution of CT (Fig. 85-3). These ratings of diagnostic and therapeutic contributions of CT were interviewed independently by the investigators and checked for consistency against the patient's record.

Tabulation of the responses of more than 300 physicians provided the data base of 2619 scanned patients. The study analysis was divided into three time phases that corresponded to the availability of each body CT unit (EMI CT 5005 prototype 18-second scanner, EMI 5005 production model 18-second scanner, EMI CT 7070 prototype 3-second scanner). The efficacy ratings for all protocols by time phase and over the entire study are summarized in Fig. 85-4. Overall, 53% of examinations produced a substantial or unique contribution to diagnostic understanding (D4 or D5). This proportion was significantly higher ($p < 0.05$) in phase 3 (57%) with the 3-second scanner than in phase 2 (51%) or phase 1 (49%) with the 18-second scanner. The proportion of patients in whom CT contributed to a change in treatment was 15% overall but did not significantly vary with technologic improvements. The 3-second scanner in phase 3 did produce a significantly higher ($p < 0.001$) proportion of patients with increased physician's confidence in

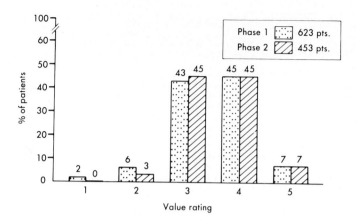

Fig. 85-4 Impact of CT on diagnostic decision making.

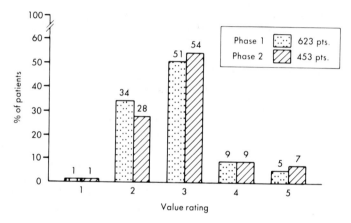

Fig. 85-5 Impact of CT on therapeutic decision making.

the previously chosen treatment (T3) than accomplished with the 18-second scanners in either phase 1 or 2.

Performance among the 12 different protocols varied considerably (Fig. 85-5). Lymphoma, pancreas, retroperitoneum, lung, and liver ranked in the top half for both diagnostic and therapeutic efficacy, whereas pelvis, urology, and colon fell in the bottom third. Updating by means of a survey during the last 4 months of 1987 revealed a frequency of protocol utilization very similar to these hierarchic results. The single exception was the addition in the top half of a new protocol, abscess search.

The effect of CT on proposed therapeutic measures such as surgery as well as utilization of alternative radiologic examinations was measured by comparing pre-CT proposals with post-CT actions. More surgery than planned was carried out on 15 patients rated T1 ($p < 0.01$) and considerably less surgery than planned was done on the 385 patients rated T4 or T5 ($p < 0.001$). Overall the 832 procedures actually performed represented a net reduction of 14% under the expected number.

Significant decreases in the frequency of angiographic, ultrasonic, and lymphangiographic examinations were also observed.

A test ultimately has its principal effect on the health outcome to the extent that appropriate treatment is chosen as a result of the test and that treatment can influence the course of disease. As the definition of health outcomes broadens to include such valued intangible qualities as peace of mind, the ultimate effects of an intervention become increasingly difficult to quantify. The measurement of effects on the health outcome typically requires the long-term follow-up of patient groups.

Measure costs

Providing a service such as a radiologic examination requires resources, and the economic cost of the service is equal to the value of the resources consumed. A product such as a radiologic examination may also engender an increase or decrease in the number of tests performed and changes in treatment that entail additional costs or savings. The net cost assigned to a test should reflect the overall effects of the test on the consumption of health resources. Uncertainty in predicting the magnitude of induced effects on other tests and the treatment broadens the possible range of the ultimate costs of a diagnostic procedure.

The production costs of a radiologic procedure have direct and indirect components (see following outline). Direct costs are those that are wholly attributable to the procedure itself. Indirect costs are those that are shared by many services concurrently; a portion of these costs is attributed to the procedure. Conventional methods of cost-accounting can be used to assign a value to each component of production costs.[4] Equipment can be valued most simply by straight-line depreciation, although some economists regard the amortized annual cost as a superior measure of societal cost because it includes both the purchase price and the foregone interest from investing in the equipment.[22] Labor is valued according to salary and materials according to purchase price. Overhead costs, such as rent, utilities, billing, and administrative services, may equal or even exceed the direct production costs and need to be taken into account.[4]

COMPONENTS OF HEALTH RESOURCE COSTS

I . Production costs
  A. Direct costs
    1. Equipment acquisition, maintenance, improvement
    2. Labor—professional and nonprofessional
    3. Materials
  B. Indirect costs (overhead)
    1. Rent and building depreciation
    2. Space preparation and upkeep
    3. Utilities
    4. Billing
    5. Insurance
    6. Other administrative and support services
II. Induced costs and savings
  A. Tests added or averted
  B. Treatments added or averted

Some components of production cost are *fixed*; that is, they do not change with the volume of service. This is true, for example, of equipment depreciation. Other components, such as materials, are *variable costs* because they increase directly with volume. There may be intermediate cost categories, such as some equipment maintenance, that are partly fixed (a function of time) and partly variable (a function of volume); these are called *semivariable costs.*

If radiologic procedures are performed, the average cost per procedure is the total of fixed, semivariable, and variable costs divided by n. If a service is intended just to pay for itself, charges would be set equal to the projected average cost plus an allowance for unpaid debts.

Because some costs are fixed, the average cost for a service declines as the volume increases, up to the capacity of the equipment.

In a cost-effectiveness analysis the focus should be on the incremental cost rather than on average cost. The incremental cost of the nth unit of service is the difference in the total costs required to produce n and those to produce $n - 1$ units of service. More generally the incremental costs or savings from any decision are the difference in net resource consumption before and after the decision. Decisions that lead to the purchase of new equipment entail incremental costs that include the fixed cost of acquisition. If the new service reduces the number of other procedures being performed with existing facilities, the short-term economic savings equal only the variable costs of the other procedures. Because a fair charge includes fixed as well as variable components, the savings are normally less than the sum of the fair charges for the volume of procedures reduced. This factor increases the difficulty of justifying the acquisition of new services purely on grounds of cost savings even when other tests will be used less.

Alternative investment decisions typically entail different streams of costs and benefits over time. Analysts prefer to compare the cost-effectiveness of alternative services in terms of their present values. Even after compensating for inflation, the present value of future costs is smaller than the same amount of immediate costs because dollars not spent today can be productively invested to produce a larger number of real dollars in the future. Analysts recommend discounting future costs at some social discount rate to make them comparable with present expenditures. The general formula for the present value of a future cost as follows:

$$P = \frac{C}{(1 + r)^n}$$

P is the present value, C is the future cost, r is the discount rate, and n is the number of years in the future that the cost in incurred. For example, with an 8% discount rate, a $1000 cost 5 years in the future would have the following present value:

$$\frac{\$1000}{(1 + 0.08)^5} = \$681$$

The rationale for discounting does not depend on inflation in the monetary price of goods and services; after adjusting for inflation, it is still appropriate to discount future costs. Many analysts recommend discounting future benefits as well as costs, but this method is more controversial.

An accurate and complete assessment of costs, therefore, requires an accounting approach toward resources consumed, including indirect production costs and induced effects; careful attention to incremental rather than average effects; and discounting of future costs to their present value.

Reach conclusions

Rarely, if ever, can a cost-effectiveness analysis produce unqualified conclusions. Almost every cost-effectiveness analysis rests on certain assumptions that may be inappropriate. It is generally advisable to perform a sensitivity analysis on baseline results and to vary key assumptions systematically to determine what effect these have on the conclusions. For example, if the risk of a procedure were to double, as it might at a different hospital, what impact would this have on the measured cost-effectiveness? Conclusions are strengthened when their general thrust holds up to this sort of systematic testing.

The results of any cost-effectiveness study must be qualified in terms of the institutional settings where it has been conducted. In general, evaluation studies tend to be carried out at teaching centers with experienced physicians and staff. Physicians practicing in less sophisticated settings may be unlikely to achieve equally good results. This discrepancy between ideal and average effectiveness may be especially noticeable with new and technically demanding procedures, such as percutaneous transluminal angioplasty.[2] On the other hand, it is possible that a typically definitive and relatively simple diagnostic test would make a greater contribution in a community hospital setting (where, before the addition of the test, the diagnosis would be less certain) than in a teaching hospital.

The applicability of any cost-effectiveness analysis to the future depends on possible changes in the objects of study over time. In assessments of imaging procedures, three of the most important changes are (1) technologic developments in equipment, (2) advances in scientific knowledge and clinical technique, and (3) shifts in the patterns of disease.

Any cost-effectiveness study applies to the *equipment* and *technique* of a particular technologic capability. As advances occur, for example, with successive generations of faster and more versatile CT scanners[18,19] or with improved interventional techniques,[5] the initial findings may no longer apply. Some technologic advances will possibly have a limited effect on efficacy or cost-effectiveness, but that possibility is an empiric question. Because cost-effectiveness is based on comparisons with alternative strategies, technologic advances in other areas can alter the apparent contribution of the imaging test being evaluated. For example, advances in CT alter the incremental contribution of invasive imaging techniques,[26] new diagnostic chemistry tests can change the

added value of an imaging,[17] and new biopsy techniques can enhance the contribution of an existing imaging procedure.[25]

Evolution in the *pattern of a disease* also affects the projected cost-effectiveness of a diagnostic test or clinical intervention. For example, the incidences of ulcer disease and carcinomas of the stomach have been declining. From a population point of view, the cost-effectiveness of tests designed to detect these diseases would also be declining, assuming a fixed sensitivity and specificity of the test. Pancreatic cancer, in contrast, has been increasing in incidence, and the cost-effectiveness of tests to detect this disease would be expected to improve even without any further technologic advances.

Above all, the conclusions of cost-effectiveness analysis rest on the correctness of each of the preceding steps: defining the object and perspective, identifying alternatives for the analysis, and measuring the benefits and costs. An accurate array of the net incremental benefits and costs attributable to a procedure, properly qualified with respect to anticipated future patterns, can serve as a useful guide to physicians, patients, and policy makers.

COST-EFFECTIVE RADIOLOGIC PRACTICE

In addition to undertaking and participating in formal cost-effectiveness studies, radiologists have an opportunity and responsibility to promote a more efficient and safe use of radiologic resources. This objective may be reached by eliminating or reducing radiation exposure of the patient, optimizing the number of films or slices per examination, and consulting with referring physicians on the selection of patients for examinations or particular procedures.

More broadly, a number of radiologists have advocated an orderly, integrated approach to diagnostic imaging through use of algorithms.[13,24] The many radiologic alternatives in both diagnostic and therapeutic procedures have created the potential for more expeditious and safer patient care. Without a systematic approach, the number of choices could present even the most astute clinician with an unending maze of possibilities.[24]

Clinical algorithms have been developed and tested for a variety of common ambulatory medical problems.[10] Some evaluations of widely used conventional imaging procedures have yielded more efficient selection criteria for patients.[3,14] In general the radiologic algorithm is a responsible attempt to foster more cost- and time-efficient solutions to diagnostic problems. The algorithm should represent an institution's consensus for a uniform diagnostic approach to common clinical problems. The strategy represented by the algorithm must take into account factors such as technologic availability, patient endurance, and risks as well as the accuracy and purpose of

☐ **TABLE 85-1**

Recommendations for CT examination: MGH Department of Radiology

Disease state	Preceding imaging examination*	Disease state	Proceding imaging examination*
Perirenal, renal, and retroperitoneal		Pancreas—cont'd	
Renal mass whose presence, cause, or extent is unresolved with other techniques	IVP, US	Adenocarcinoma in body or tail	—
		Cystadenoma or cystadenocarcinoma	—
Adrenal hyperfunction; primary tumor suspected	—	Epigastric mass	US
Adrenal insufficiency in patient with known primary malignancy	—	Hepatic or perihepatic	
		Metastasis	—
Biopsy-proven lymphoma	—	Fatty liver	—
Mass lesion documented by other noninvasive imaging techniques; cause or extent unresolved	—	Hemochromatosis	—
		Liver defects complicating cirrhosis: regenerating nodule	RN
Suspected retroperitoneal metastases	—	Perihepatic or portal mass	—
Suspected hematoma or abscess	—	Abscess or hematoma	US
		Perihepatic abscess	US
Jaundice		Hemangioma	—
Bilirubin level greater than 3 mg/dl; obstruction suspected but unresolved with other techniques	US	Abscess	US
		Vascular occlusion	US
Suspected and proven malignancy, preoperative evaluation	—	Aspiration biopsy	
		Mass smaller than 3 cm	—
Metastases	US	Mass; unsuccessful biopsy with ultrasound	—
		Mass; location of gastrointestinal tract necessary	—
Pancreas		Gastrointestinal malignancy	
Acute pancreatitis	—	Documented malignancy; evaluation of extraenteric extent	—
Chronic pancreatitis	—		
Pseudocyst	US	Recurrent malignancy	—
Abscess, phlegmon, or necrosis		Mesenteric malignancy	—
Adenocarcinoma in head, staging	US, ERCP		
Obstructive jaundice	US		

*The decision to proceed from preceding examinations to CT will be made in collaboration with primary physician. IVP, Intravenous pyelogram; US, ultrasound; RN, radionuclide scan; ERCP, endoscopic retrograde cholangiopancreatography

alternative tests in different patient populations. The set of algorithms incorporating CT currently used at the Massachusetts General Hospital (MGH) for abdominal imaging is summarized in Table 85-1.

The increasing frequency with which ultrasound has been successfully substituted for CT at a screening procedure is a consequence of the technologic improvement in ultrasound equipment. Consequently, CT availability for its more uniquely targeted applications thus has presumably increased.

To be clinically acceptable and effective, the algorithm must satisfy the needs of many participants, particularly the primary care physician. The radiologist should be prepared to modify the diagnostic strategy as indicated by the sound judgment of informed clinicians. This approach preserves the traditional role of the referring physician as the ultimate patient manager. An algorithm cannot be a rigid dictator; it merely generates guidelines for effective patient care that may be altered by either the clinician or radiologist.

Major deviations from the accepted conventions should be anticipated and accepted before their institution. For example, the radiologist should discuss in advance with the referring physician the advisability of performing a percutaneous aspiration biopsy of a suspected pancreatic carcinoma. If an unexpected lesion is discovered, a consultation on the spot with the physician is mandatory before attempting biopsy. The referring physician may also initiate an alteration in the conventional approach. For example, a surgeon may decide to forego the performance of percutaneous cholangiography with a jaundiced, febrile patient who demonstrates dilated ducts and gallstones by ultrasound. In addition, there are always patients whose diagnostic problems fit no previously prepared algorithm. In such circumstances it should be the prerogative of the referring physician to request a formal, comprehensive consultation with the radiologist before the initiation of any imaging tests.

The algorithmic approach certainly places new and growing demands on the role of the radiologist. Time is required for the preliminary preparation, recurrent discussion, modification, and effectiveness evaluation of acceptable algorithms. Any strategy requires an intimate familiarity with the performance characteristics of competing technologies, costs, and departmental availabilities. It is hardly persuasive to recommend CT as an effective, noninvasive alternative to lymphangiography for investigating retroperitoneal adenopathy when the next CT schedule opening is 4 days away. The enlarging role of radiologists in therapeutic intervention places further demands on their capacity for the clinical integration and mastery of technique.

These broadening responsibilities can effect a cost savings for the health care system. Most evaluations of test avoidance have been carried out with CT scanning because of the controversy that has surrounded this high-cost technology. Whalen[24] and Wittenberg et al.[26] have both documented a decreasing number of lymphangiograms that corresponds to the introduction of CT into clinical use. Interestingly, not only did the number of performed lymphangiograms decline, but there was also an upward trend in the percentage of positive examinations.[24] The cost savings attending the radiologic evaluation of the patient with a suspected lymphoma since the introduction of CT has been estimated by Margulis[13] to be $1667. CT has also led to an avoidance of pancreatic angiograms at a rate of 77% in a study of 185 patients scanned for pancreatic disease.[26] Similar reductions in pancreatic angiography as the result of CT or ultrasound have been documented by Whalen.[24] In 65 patients for whom endoscopic retrograde cholangiopancreatography (ERCP) was planned, CT resulted in 67% avoidance rate, and this effect was accompanied by an increased incidence of positive results in ERCP when CT has been performed.[26] Thus new technologies can also make other more invasive tests more effective on the average. The decreasing use of angiography for diagnostic testing undoubtedly has not resulted in the closing of many angiography suites, but it is likely that CT has slowed the demand for additional equipment and construction to satisfy the needs for the new important procedures of interventional angiography.[2,11]

Just as CT has substantially altered use of angiography, it is inevitable that MRI will similarly affect the further diffusion and clinical use of CT scanning. Avoiding the risks of ionizing radiation and intravenous contrast material while providing comparable accuracy, MRI is already being advocated as a substitute for CT in a number of common clinical problems. However, it is extremely unlikely that CT scanning equipment will become obsolete, since it has demonstrated its versatility and has an acknowledged predictable superiority to MRI in certain anatomic areas. The decade of the 1990s will witness an intense scrutiny of comparative clinical accuracy, the need for which will be heightened by progressive demands for cost containment.

The potential benefits of these societal savings to the radiologist are less easy to document and probably more controversial. Time saved in routine consultations because of established available imaging strategies undoubtedly is a major benefit. Similarly, invasive examinations such as pancreatic angiography are personnel-intense procedures that are not necessarily appropriately remunerated and certainly require more physician time than CT or ultrasound examinations. If the imaging role of radiologists requires frequent patient-specific comprehensive consultations, however, such a service may require the creation of a consultation fee. The personal and institutional benefits of imaging algorithms may hold future dividends as the health care reimbursement system changes. If cost reimbursement becomes predicated on the final diagnosis rather than on the numbers and types of diagnostic tests, the careful and prompt evaluation of patients will result in greater cost savings and benefits to all.

Every radiologist can introduce cost-effective principles into daily practice by establishing examination criteria and monitoring their implementation. These practices can complement more formal cost-effectiveness studies, and they can also directly and substantially improve the allocation of available resources. The success of these efforts depends on a shared attitude of all medical practitioners toward improving efficiency.

REFERENCES

1. Abrams, HL: The "overutilization" of x-rays, N Engl J Med 300:1213, 1979.
2. Athanasoulis, CA: Percutaneous transluminal angioplasty: general principles, AJR 135:893, 1980.
3. Cummins, RO, et al: High-yield referral criteria for post-traumatic skull roentgenography, JAMA 244:673, 1980.
4. Evens, RG: Cost accounting in radiology and nuclear medicine, CRC Crit Rev Clin Radiol Nucl Med 6:67, 1975.
5. Ferrucci, JT, Jr, and Wittenberg, J: Interventional radiology of the abdomen, Baltimore, 1981, Williams & Wilkins.
6. Fineberg, HV, and Sherman, H: Tutorial on the health and social value of computerized medical imaging, IEEE Trans Biomed Eng 28:50, 1979.

7. Fineberg, HV, Bauman, R, and Sosman, M: Computerized cranial tomography: effect on diagnostic and therapeutic plans, JAMA 238:224, 1977.

8. Freeland, M, Calat, G, and Schendler, CE: Projections of national health expenditures: 1980, 1985 and 1990, Health Care Fin Rev 1(3):1, 1980.

9. Kaplan, RM, Bush, SW, and Berry, CC: Health status: types of validity and the index of well-being, Health Serv Res 11:478, 1976.

10. Komaroff, AL, and Winickoff, RN, editors: Common acute illnesses: a problem-oriented textbook with protocols, Boston, 1977, Little, Brown & Co.

11. Levin, DC, et al: Impact of CT on cardiovascular radiology: implications for future manpower needs, AJR 135:200, 1980.

12. Lusted, LB: General problems in medical decision making with comments on ROC analysis, Semin Nucl Med 8:299, 1978.

13. Margulis, AR: Radiologic imaging, changing costs, greater benefits, AJR 136:657, 1981.

14. Marton, KI, et al: The clinical value of the upper gastrointestinal tract roentgenogram series, Arch Intern Med 140:191, 1980.

14a. National Institutes of Health Consensus Development Conference: Magnetic resonance imaging [statement], October 26-28, 1987.

15. Office of Technology Assessment, United States Congress: The implication of cost-effectiveness analysis of medical technology, Washington, DC, September 1980, US Government Printing Office.

16. Office of Technology Assessment, United States Congress: The implications of cost-effectiveness analysis of medical technology. Background paper No. 1; methodological issues and literature review, Washington, DC, September 1980, US Government Printing Office.

17. Podolsky, DK, et al: Galactosyltransferase isoenzyme II in the detection of pancreatic cancer, N Engl J Med 304:1313, 1981.

18. Robbins, AH, et al: Further observations on the medical efficacy of computed tomography of the chest and abdomen, Radiology 137:719, 1980.

19. Robbins, AH, et al: An assessment of the role of scan speed in perceived image quality of body computed tomography, Radiology 139:139, 1981.

20. Shepard, DS, and Thompson, MS: First principles of cost-effectiveness analysis in health, Public Health Rep 94:535, 1979.

21. Swets, JA, et al: Assessment of diagnostic technologies, Science 205:753, 1979.

22. Weinstein, MC, and Fineberg, HV: Clinical decision analysis, Philadelphia, 1980, WB Saunders.

23. Weinstein, MC, and Stason, WB: Foundations of cost-effectiveness analysis for health and medical practices, N Engl J Med 296:716, 1977.

24. Whalen, JP: Radiology of the abdomen: impact of new imaging methods, AJR 133:585, 1979.

25. Wittenberg, J, and Ferrucci, JT, Jr: Radiographically guided needle biopsy of abdominal neoplasms: who, how, where, why? J Clin Gastroenterol 1:273, 1979.

26. Wittenberg, J, et al: Clinical efficacy of computed body tomography, AJR 154:1111, 1980.

86 *Abdominal Imaging from the Clinician's Viewpoint*

DAVID C. CARTER

GENERAL CONSIDERATIONS

The last 20 years have seen a dramatic increase in the number and variety of techniques available for the diagnosis of alimentary tract disorders. As the list of available diagnostic methods has grown, constant readjustment of diagnostic algorithms has become essential. Furthermore, the development of nonoperative management by interventional radiology and endoscopic means now offers a real alternative to surgery in the treatment of a number of important alimentary disorders. More than ever before there is a pressing and continuing need for clinician and radiologist to work in close collaboration, to maintain detailed mutual feedback, and to be fully aware of the other's strengths and limitations. Only by these means can appropriate decisions be made about the optimal path to diagnosis and subsequent management of individual patients in a given institution. In this context it cannot be overemphasized that not all radiologists have equal diagnostic and interventional skills, and similarly, not all surgeons have equal operative ability. For example, surgeons learn quickly that a confident ultrasonic diagnosis of gallstones in a patient with acute pancreatitis may be a firm basis for operative intervention when made by one radiologist but a fragile and untrustworthy platform when made by another radiologist. Equally, radiologists soon appreciate that comprehensive and invasive investigation to establish that a pancreatic cancer is potentially resectable may be valueless (or even dangerous) if the surgeon concerned is unwilling or unable to undertake safe resection. We must bear in mind that the international gold standards for diagnostic and interventional radiology and for surgical management are rarely attainable (and are sometimes not even approached) in all areas of alimentary disease in a given institution. Radiologist and clinician must pool their resources effectively to offer the best local blend of diagnostic and therapeutic skills to the patients entrusted to their care.

This brief review cannot provide comprehensive coverage of the current interface between the radiologist and

2139

his or her clinical colleagues. Examples are drawn predominantly from my own area of special interest, namely pancreatic-biliary surgery. There is no doubt that the pace of introduction of advances in diagnosis and therapy will not slow. Only by continuing dialogue can we hope to continue to apply these advances wisely and to the full benefit of our patients.

APPROPRIATE USE OF DIAGNOSTIC METHODS

Obstructive jaundice is an excellent example of a diagnostic problem that can usually be resolved safely and efficiently by the careful selection of a small number of key investigations. On the other hand, it also provides an excellent example of a disorder that can be mismanaged if numerous unproductive, time-consuming, and potentially hazardous investigations are ordered.

Before even considering radiologic investigation, the clinician must confirm that the patient is indeed jaundiced and that the jaundice is likely to be obstructive. In the rush for sophisticated investigation it is all too easy to neglect the mainstays of clinical diagnosis, namely a full history and comprehensive physical examination. A dark urine, pale stool, and pruritus (caused by inability to excrete bile salts) all favor a diagnosis of obstructive jaundice, and the contention is strengthened if bilirubin is present in the urine and hyperbilirubinemia is associated with significant elevation in serum alkaline phosphatase levels. The duration, depth, and constancy of the jaundice are all valuable pointers. For example, a 1-month history of progressive unrelenting jaundice associated with weight loss in an elderly patient favors neoplastic obstruction, whereas a history of intermittent jaundice associated with rigors and pain is more suggestive of choledocholithiasis.

Given that the clinical and biochemical diagnosis of obstructive jaundice is secure, the following questions have to be addressed:

1. Is obstruction confined to the smaller biliary canaliculi, or does it affect the major branches of the biliary tree?
2. If the larger radicles are obstructed, is the site of obstruction intrahepatic or extrahepatic?
3. What is the nature of the obstruction?
4. What are the implications for treatment?

In the past a jaundiced patient thought clinically to have carcinoma of the head of the pancreas might have been subjected to some or all of the following investigations. A plain abdominal film might have been obtained, looking for radioopaque calculi as an alternative explanation for the obstruction. An intravenous cholangiogram or some form of infusion cholangiogram might have been attempted in those with minimal jaundice in the forlorn hope of outlining the biliary tree. A hypotonic

duodenogram might have been performed to look for abnormalities in the configuration of the duodenum and its mucosal lining. A ^{75}Se-seleno-methionine scan of the pancreas might have been obtained to try to distinguish between carcinoma of the pancreas and chronic pancreatitis. It is not my purpose to argue that these investigations are *never* helpful in defining the cause of obstructive jaundice; rather, I wish to point out that they are low-yield investigations now rendered virtually obsolete by investigations with higher specificities, sensitivities, and diagnostic accuracies. Furthermore, given the increased morbidity and mortality that accompany delayed resolution of jaundice, such low-yield tests carry the added danger of delaying appropriate treatment. Fortunately, investigation has now improved far beyond the point where laparotomy is needed as a diagnostic tool. Laparatomy is frequently a poor method of diagnosing the cause of obstructive jaundice. Indeed, given the availability of nonoperative methods of relieving obstruction, the very operation may well be inappropriate. Even when operation is appropriate, the process of obtaining a diagnosis may prolong the procedure and involve otherwise unnecessary maneuvers during surgery. For example, it may prove difficult to distinguish at laparotomy between a stone impacted at the lower end of the bile duct and a carcinoma of the head of the pancreas. Appropriate preoperative investigation is a much easier and more accurate means of resolving the dilemma, and given the presence of calculous obstruction, the patient may have been much better served by endoscopic papillotomy and stone retrieval to avoid potentially hazardous surgery in the presence of deep obstructive jaundice.

What then constitutes appropriate modern investigation of the patient with clinical and biochemical obstructive jaundice? In constructing an algorithm (Figure 86-1) all would now accept the claims that ultrasonography or computed tomography (CT) is the preliminary noninvasive investigation. These techniques appear to have equal sensitivities, but I suspect that in most hospitals logistics dictate the routine use of ultrasonography in this context. The first objective is to determine whether distention of the biliary tree is present, bearing in mind that intrahepatic bile ducts of normal caliber cannot usually be resolved by ultrasonography. It must also be stressed that a dilated biliary system does not necessarily contain a surgically remediable cause of obstruction, and conversely, obstruction to flow can be present despite a system that appears to be of normal caliber. Furthermore, an obstructive biochemical picture can be produced by medical rather than surgical causes, such as the drug-induced cholestasis associated with agents such as chlorpromazine. Ultrasonography offers a reliable means of defining the level of the obstructing lesion, as both the intrahepatic and extrahepatic parts of the biliary tree can

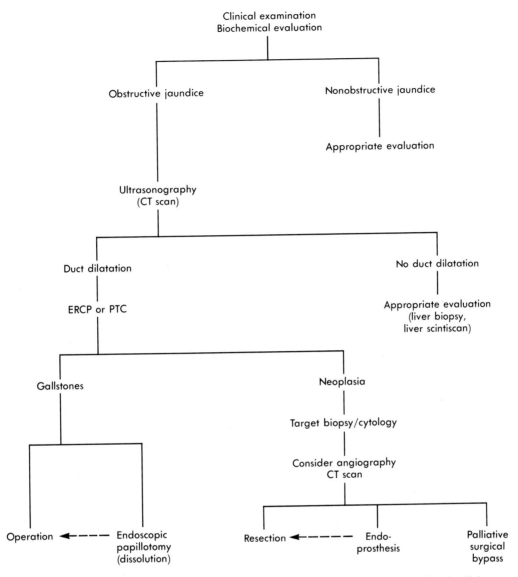

Fig. 86-1 One diagnostic algorithm that can be used to evaluate patients with jaundice. For simplicity attention has been concentrated on gallstones and neoplasia as common causes of obstructive jaundice.

be visualized. With definition of the site of blockage, much can be inferred about its nature. For example, obstruction at the confluence of the right and left hepatic duct is much more likely to be due to neoplasia than calculous obstruction. Conversely, blockage at the lower end of the common bile duct is due commonly to neoplasia or gallstones. It must be remembered that although ultrasonography is a reliable means of diagnosing the presence of stones in the gallbladder, it is much less reliable in the detection of stones in the lower reaches of the common bile duct.

Given that major duct obstruction is confirmed on ultrasonography, judgment must now be exercised in the choice of subsequent investigations. In the years following its introduction percutaneous transhepatic cholangiography (PTC) was used widely as the next procedure. In skilled hands a cholangiogram was virtually always obtained in patients with distended ducts, the use of slim flexible needles markedly reduced the risk of bleeding or bile leakage, and the avoidance of overdistention minimized the risk of precipitating bacteremia and septicemia. All of these risks were reduced further by careful patient preparation with particular attention to coagulation status and provision of antibiotic cover. Despite its accuracy and improved safety, PTC still has appreciable disadvantages. Although minimized, its risks do still pertain, and unless meticulous technique is employed, there is a small risk of introducing infection into a previously sterile biliary system. On occasions this can have far-reaching consequences. For example, in a patient with unresectable hilar cholangiocarcinoma or a high bile duct stricture, surgical decompression may be possible using part of the left hepatic duct system for a hepaticojejunal anastomosis.[8,31] In benign strictures the left hepatic duct can be made available by lowering the hilar plate, whereas in hilar cholangiocarcinoma it can be approached as it enters heaptic segment III, just to the left of the falciform ligament. Neither approach decompresses the right hepatic duct system, but both can allow jaundice to abate and liver function to return to normal. As long as infection has not been introduced into the right duct system, asymptomatic atrophy of the right liver then follows.

A further disadvantage of PTC is the relative lack of opportunity for therapeutic intervention if this is deemed appropriate. The technique of inserting an indwelling catheter for percutaneous transhepatic drainage has been used as a preparation for subsequent surgery, but most controlled studies indicate that eventual morbidity and mortality are not significantly improved[21,24,28]; indeed, introduction of sepsis by percutaneous drainage is a recognized and major hazard.[7,18] On the other hand, percutaneous transhepatic insertion of stents to allow bile to drain through an obstructing lesion may still prove useful, although as will be discussed, it has come under increasing challenge from transduodenal stent insertion after endoscopic papillotomy.[29]

Once cholangiography has defined the likely cause of obstruction, the diagnostic pathways diverge. For example, if gallstones are shown on ERCP, most endoscopists would relieve the obstruction there and then by endoscopic papillotomy and stone retrieval. The decision on the need for surgery can then be postponed until the patient's general condition has improved. If on the other hand the obstruction is due to neoplasia, the help of the radiologist is invaluable, first to facilitate target biopsy or fine-needle aspiration cytology under ultrasonographic or radiologic control, and then to assess resectability.

The diagnostic algorithm shown in Fig. 86-1 is by no means the only one that can be constructed for the evaluation of patients with obstructive jaundice. Nevertheless, it demonstrates the way in which diagnostic pathways can be defined to minimize delay and unnecessary investigation.

DEFINITION OF TUMOR RESECTABILITY

Once a neoplasm has been located and its nature confirmed by biopsy or fine-needle aspiration cytology, CT can provide useful information on tumor size, local invasion, and dissemination. Indeed, it can be argued that CT provides enough information to obviate the need for

cholangiography in many patients with neoplastic biliary obstruction. When contemplating the treatment of primary or secondary liver tumors, ultrasonography and CT are particulary helpful, but as will be discussed, the information provided can now be supplemented with that obtained by intraoperative ultrasonography.

The place of selective angiography in assessing the resectability of neoplasms of the pancreas and biliary tree remains controversial. In patients with pancreatic cancer, vascular encasement will be apparent in some two thirds of cases, while portal vein invasion or displacement by tumor may be detected in the late phase of angiography. Venous invasion is generally taken as a sign of inoperability, although some surgeons are still willing to undertake resection with reconstruction of the portal vein and/or major arteries if wider dissemination is not detected at laparotomy.[15,32] As Trede[32] has pointed out, the rare cystadenocarcinoma of the pancreas may show signs of portal vein obstruction and yet remain resectable and indeed curable. While the case for routine *diagnostic* angiography has now been dispelled by the availability of techniques such as ERCP, PTC, and CT scanning, a strong argument remains for angiography as a means of defining vascular invasion and displaying congenital anomalies of the arterial system when resection is contemplated. Origin of the right or common hepatic artery from the superior mesenteric artery may be particularly troublesome, as the anomalous vessel frequently runs in or near the line normally used for division of the pancreas in the operation of pancreaticoduodenectomy. An even stronger case can be made for selective angiography and indirect portal venography when cholangiography has revealed high bile duct cancer in patients thought to be candidates for resection. Tumor involvement of the main trunk of the portal vein or both of its branches is usually taken to indicate unresectability, but unilateral involvement of the hepatic artery and portal vein may not preclude resection with partial hepatectomy.[1]

It is interesting that the availability of modern diagnostic techniques may as yet have failed to reduce diagnostic delay or improve survival rates in patients with malignant obstruction.[16] However, there is encouraging evidence from some centers that in cancer of the head of the pancreas, tumor size at operation may be falling while resectability rates have risen.[23,32]

RADIOLOGY AND THE NEED FOR HISTOLOGIC CONFIRMATION

In many alimentary diseases the surgeon is willing to accept the radiologic detection of a lesion as sufficient basis for management. For example, the unequivocal demonstration of a duodenal ulcer by barium meal examination does not normally need endoscopic confirmation. On the other hand, the radiologic detection of a gastric ulcer can never be left unsupported. The difficulties of distinguishing radiologically between a benign peptic ulcer of the stomach and an ulcerating gastric cancer are well recognized, and endoscopy with multiple biopsy is mandatory if medical management is to be employed. Even when all biopsies show no evidence of malignancy, most clinicians routinely reendoscope and rebiopsy the area of the ulcer after 6 to 8 weeks of medical treatment. The risk of overlooking early ulcerating (and occasionally curable) gastric cancer cannot be overemphasized.

Although modern radiologic techniques have undoubtedly reduced the risk of misdiagnosing benign biliary obstruction as malignant, considerable care must still be exercised, and the need for cytologic or histologic confirmation remains paramount. Impaction of a gallstone masquerading at laparotomy as operable pancreatic cancer should now seldom cause confusion, but biliary obstruction from chronic pancreatitis remains a source of real diagnostic uncertainty (Fig. 86-2). Other benign conditions that can cause confusion include sclerosing cholangitis, benign inflammatory bile duct tumors, compression of the bile ducts by an inflamed gallbladder, and the Mirizzi syndrome, in which an impacted cystic duct stone is thought by some to trigger contraction of the common hepatic duct.[34] The problem is further complicated by

the fact that secondary deposits of cancer, notably from lymphoma, breast cancer, and bronchogenic carcinoma, can obstruct the biliary tree and simulate primary malignant obstruction (Fig. 86-3).

Of the primary malignant tumors that may obstruct the bile duct, periampullary cancer is the most accessible lesion, and multiple biopsies can be taken endoscopically under vision. Although a diagnosis of invasive carcinoma is secure, the pathologist is sometimes unable to give a confident diagnosis for a neoplastic lesion that shows suggestive but not definitive evidence of malignancy. In many ways the situation is analogous to some cases of colonic neoplasia, in which there is uncertainty about the presence of malignancy elsewhere in what appears to be a benign polyp. Under these circumstances excision of the entire neoplasm may be the only way to resolve diagnostic doubt.

A preoperative diagnosis of pancreatic cancer can now be obtained safely by percutaneous fine-needle aspiration cytology in lesions targeted by ultrasonography, CT, or ERCP. False positivity is extremely rare, but sampling error is a potential source of false negativity. The technique can confirm the diagnosis in about 80% of patients with pancreatic cancer,[20] although more recent reports indicate that diagnostic accuracy in some centers ap-

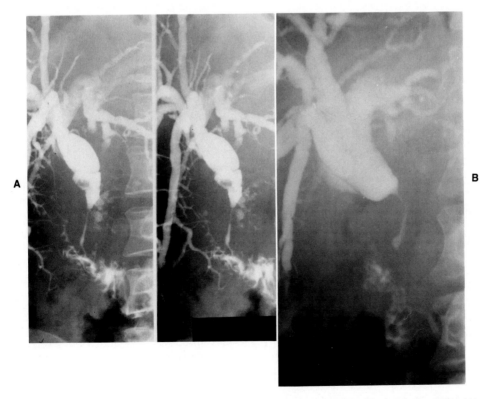

Fig. 86-2 PTC demonstrating obstruction of common bile duct caused by chronic pancreatitis (**A**) and pancreatic carcinoma (**B**). Although pancreatic calcification may help to differentiate between two lesions, configuration of stricture may pose major difficulties in diagnosis. Note elevation of distended bile duct from tumor mass in **B**.

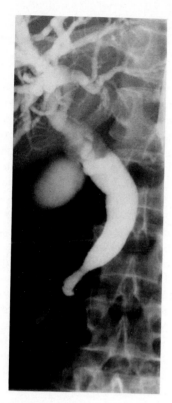

Fig. 86-3 PTC showing obstruction of lower common bile duct caused by deposits of lymphoma.

proaches 100%.[35] Cutaneous seeding of tumor has now been reported on at least three occasions,[25] suggesting that multiple passes may carry a small risk of dissemination. Laparoscopy also affords an opportunity to obtain histological or cytologic confirmation of diagnosis and may spare patients unnecessary surgery in the face of tumor spread to the liver, parietal peritoneum, or omentum.[33] If a tissue diagnosis has not been made before surgery, operative fine-needle aspiration cytology is worthwhile, although operative sampling is less accurate than needle aspiration targeted by ultrasonography or CT. Trucut biopsy, performed transduodenally if possible, may be more accurate but carries a slightly increased risk of bleeding, abscess, and fistula. The technique is also subject to sampling error, and the shortcomings of frozen-section pancreatic biopsy are demonstrated by a 30% failure rate in one recent study of patients with pancreatic cancer.[12] Multiple biopsies are best avoided, as evidence suggests that rapid serosal spread may be facilitated.

The greatest controversy surrounds the problem of confirmation of a radiologic diagnosis of cholangiocarcinoma. Cameron and co-workers[11] stress the difficulties of obtaining an adequate biopsy from small fibrotic tumors and believe that cholangiography taken in conjunction with the clinical presentation allows easy and ac-

curate differentiation in the great majority of patients. However, as has been mentioned, benign conditions not infrequently masquerade as cancer. It may be argued that resection is indicated regardless of whether the lesion is benign or malignant, but failure to define the true diagnosis assumes greater importance in patients treated by intubation or palliative bypass. The difficulties of biopsy should not be underestimated; many surgeons attempt to confirm the diagnosis cytologically by recovery of bile at the time of PTC, targeted percutaneous fine-needle aspiration, or biliary brush cytology at the time of surgery. Other methods described include curettage and cholangioscopically directed punch biopsy. The reported rates for confirmation of cholangiocarcinoma vary greatly, but by using a combination of preoperative and intraoperative methods, Blumgart and co-workers[9] were able to obtain a positive tissue diagnosis in no less that 91 of their 94 patients with hilar cholangiocarcinoma. An added factor in diagnosis is the recognition that polypoid and papillary neoplasms may carry a much better prognosis than nodular, scirrhous, constricting and diffusely infiltrating forms of cholangiocarcinoma.[30]

INTERVENTIONAL TECHNIQUES AS AN ALTERNATIVE TO SURGERY

The vast majority of patients coming to surgery with pancreatic or biliary cancer are elderly, have extensive disease, or are so ill that resection for attempted cure is seldom feasible. Jaundice is the main indication for palliation, and cholecystojejunostomy is the operation usually performed. Although the issue is debated, many surgeons add gastroenterostomy on the grounds that some 15% of patients will otherwise have trouble with duodenal obstruction. Collected reviews indicate that mean duration of survival following operative biliary bypass is only 5.4 months, and that the mean operative mortality is almost 20%.[27]

It is hardly surprising that these poor results have prompted the assessment of alternative methods of palliation. Although it is now generally agreed that external drainage by percutaneously inserted transhepatic catheters is undesirable, methods of internal drainage have provided encouraging results. In the prospective Cape Town trial in patients with pancreatic cancer, the 30-day mortality after percutaneous transhepatic placement of an endoprosthesis was 8% as opposed to 20% in patients randomized to surgical bypass.[10] The patients with endoprosthesis had a significantly shorter initial hospital stay, although this advantage was offset by the need to deal with prosthesis blockage in some cases. There was no significant difference in survival time.

In a recently reported randomized trial of endoscopically inserted as opposed to percutaneously placed stents in patients with malignant obstructive jaundice,[29] all of whom were deemed unfit for open operation, endoscopic insertion had a significantly lower 30-day mortality (15% versus 33%) and a significantly higher success rate in relieving jaundice (81% versus 61%). The higher mortality after percutaneous stenting was attributed to the complications of liver puncture, notably hemorrhage and bile leak. Therefore it seems reasonable to attempt endoscopic stenting in the first instance. If this fails, it may be worth using the percutaneous route to pass a guidewire through the obstructing lesion. An endoscope can then be used to retrieve the end of the guidewire from the duodenum and introduce a stent from below. In one recent report the success rate of endoscopic stenting was increased from 69% to 97% by this combined approach.[26]

It is worth stressing that some patients with malignant biliary obstruction may be too ill to undergo curative resection. This may be particularly problematic in patients with periampullary carcinoma and distal cholangiocarcinoma, in whom the prospects for cure following resection are greatly superior to those of patients with pancreatic cancer. Although external percutaneous transhepatic drainage is now seldom employed, there is a strong case for preliminary endoscopic papillotomy and stenting to allow jaundice to settle and so radically reduce the risks of resection.

In patients who with choledocholithiasis, and in whom T-tube access is no longer available, endoscopic papillotomy with stone retrieval now offers a valid alternative to surgery. Even if the stone cannot be retrieved, a nasobiliary catheter can be left in the duct to allow stone dissolution with agents suich as monooctanoin.[22] Endoscopic papillotomy can now be regarded as the emergency treatment of choice in patients with acute cholangitis.[17] In patients with choledocholithiasis collected reviews suggest that stones can be retrieved in some 80% to 90% of cases, with an estimated complication rate that approaches 10% and a mortality of approximately 1%. Duodenal perforation, biochemical (and occasionally clinical) pancreatitis, and bleeding from the papillotomy site are the major reported complications. Nevertheless, obtained as they are in groups of patients who are often elderly and ill, these results are undoubtedly superior to those of urgent surgical intervention. In one recent series of 80 elderly patients with choledocholithiasis[19] the ducts were cleared in 86% of cases, and only eight patients required subsequent surgery for duct clearance. Nine patients subsequently underwent cholecystectomy (but only four because of persistent symptoms), and most impressive of all, none of the patients died.

Even these impressive results may soon be of historic interest. Extracorporeal shock wave lithotripsy is beginning to be applied to the destruction of gallstones and laser lithotripsy at ERCP may offer an alternative approach to treatment. Further studies will soon be forthcoming to define the place of these novel approaches.

DEVELOPMENTS IN LIVER SURGERY

Recent years have seen a growing awareness of the importance of a thorough understanding of hepatic surgical anatomy.[13] In functional terms the right and left sides of the liver are separated by the main portal scissura (Cantlie's line), which runs from the middle of the gallbladder fossa to the left side of the vena cava. The right and left sides of the liver are independent in their portal and arterial blood supply, and the middle hepatic vein runs in the plane of Cantlie's line. Each side of the liver can be divided into two sectors, and further subdivision allows the description of eight segments[2] (Fig. 86-4). Resections may consist of hepatectomy (left or right), sectoriectomy, or segmentectomy, whereas right hepatectomy can be extended to include removal of segment IV (the line of resection being the umbilical fissure).

In classic surgical resection techniques preliminary vascular control is achieved by first dividing the portal pedicle and hepatic vein before transecting the liver parenchyma. Alternatively, resection can be commenced by dividing the liver parenchyma so that hilar vessels and hepatic veins are approached and ligated within the liver substance. A detailed prior knowledge of the patient's vascular anatomy is essential to facilitate the intrahepatic surgical approach, although blood loss may be minimized by prior hilar dissection so that the portal and arterial pedicles can be encircled and occluded temporarily without dividing them. When dealing with large vascular tumors, complete vascular occlusion of the liver can be achieved by simultaneously clamping the portal pedicle and occluding the inferior vena cava above and below the liver.

Intraoperative ultrasonography[3,5] is being used increasingly to supplement the information gained by preoperative ultrasonography, CT, and selective angiography. In one review of 77 patients with primary liver cancer, intraoperative ultrasonography gave additional information in one third of cases, modified the intended procedure in 21, and in 10 patients allowed subsegmental resection by facilitating guided cannulation and occlusion by balloon catheter of the branch of the portal vein supplying the part concerned[5] (Fig. 86-5). Intraoperative ultrasonography may be particularly useful in cirrhotic patients who develop hepatocellular carcinoma, as it may detect small tumors and minimize the amount of liver that must be resected to remove them. Clearly, such minimal resections may be critically important in cirrhotic patients with borderline hepatic reserve. In a recent review of 270 cirrhotic patients with hepatocellular cancer, 35 underwent resection ranging from subsegmentectomy to right hepatic lobectomy, the operative mor-

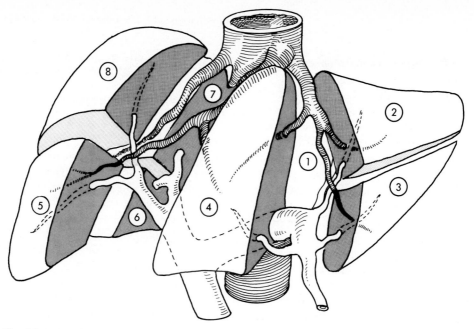

Fig. 86-4 Segmental anatomy of liver as described by Couinaud.[13] Eight segments are defined. Segment *1* is caudate lobe; segments *2* and *3* constitute left lobe; and segment *4*, also part of left hemiliver, contains quadrate lobe. Segments *5* to *8* comprise right side of liver, which can be divided into anterior and posterior portions.
(Redrawn from Bismuth, H, and Castaing, D: Operative ultrasound of the liver and biliary ducts, Berlin, 1987, Springer-Verlag.)

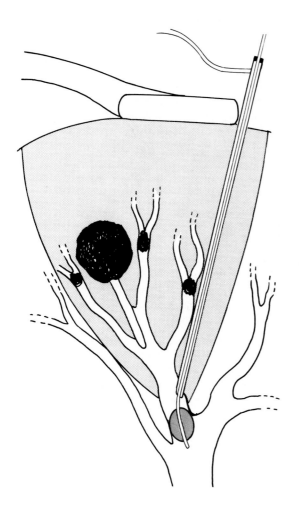

Fig. 86-5 Diagrammatic representation of intraoperative ultrasonography showing primary liver tumor surrounded by satellite metastases that have disseminated by portal propagation of tumor thrombosis. Balloon catheter has been guided ultrasonically into appropriate branch of portal vein. It can be used to delineate segment or sector to be resected and to occlude its blood supply during removal.
(Redrawn from Bismuth, H, and Castaing, D: Operative ultrasound of the liver and biliary ducts, Berlin, 1987, Springer-Verlag.)

tality being 14%.[6] Although experience of such resections in cirrhotic patients is growing, notably in Japan, it still remains to be seen whether favorable long-term results can be obtained in Western patients.

There is also growing interest in the use of liver resection for the treatment of hepatic metastases from colorectal cancer. It is now recognized that CT may detect occult hepatic metastases in approximately one quarter of patients thought not to have such metastases at the time of surgery.[14] Intraoperative ultrasonography may prove useful in this context as a means of detection of secondary liver tumors at operation. Given that liver involvement is detected and that subsequent CT scans and isotopic bone scans show no evidence of tumor elsewhere, controversy centers on the role of liver resection. In one series of 54 such patients hepatic resection was achieved without operative mortality, its extent ranging from right lobectomy to metastasectomy.[4] It is not yet known whether liver resection actually influences the natural history of the cancer in these selected patients, but 1- and 3-year survival rates of 81% and 41%, respectively, have been reported.[4]

It seems likely that liver surgery will be a growing specialty in the coming decade. The value of preoperative ultrasonography, CT, and selective angiography (including portal venography) in assessment is unquestioned. However, the technique of intraoperative ultrasonography also seems destined to grow in importance, as it provides a means of tumor detection and of defining vascular and biliary anatomy.

REFERENCES

1. Beazley, RM, et al: Clinicopathological aspects of high bile duct cancer: experience with resection and bypass surgical treatments, Ann Surg 199:623, 1984.
2. Bismuth, H: Surgical anatomy and anatomical surgery of the liver, World J Surg 6:3, 1982.
3. Bismuth, H, and Castaing, D: Operative ultrasound of the liver and biliary ducts, Berlin, 1987, Springer-Verlag.
4. Bismuth, H, Castaing, D, and Arrisueno Gomez do la Torre, C: Chirurgie d'exerese des metastases hepatique des cancers colorectaux, Chirurgie 112:45, 1986.
5. Bismuth, H, Castaing, D, and Garden, OJ: Operative ultrasound in surgery of primary liver tumours, World J Surg, 1988. (In press.)
6. Bismuth, H, et al: Liver resections in cirrhotic patients: a Western experience, World J Surg 10:311, 1986.
7. Blenkharn, JI, McPherson, GAD, and Blumgart, LH: Septic complications of percutaneous transhepatic biliary drainage: evaluation of a new dose drainage system, Am J Surg 147:318, 1984.
8. Blumgart, LH, and Kelley, CJ: Hepaticojejunostomy in benign and malignant high bile duct stricture: approaches to the left hepatic ducts, Br J Surg 71:257, 1984.
9. Blumgart, LH, et al: Surgical approaches to cholangiocarcinoma at confluence of hepatic ducts, Lancet 1:66, 1984.
10. Bornman, PC, et al: Prospective controlled trial of transhepatic biliary endoprosthesis versus bypass surgery for incurable carcinoma of head of pancreas, Lancet 1:69, 1986.
11. Cameron, JL, Broe, P, and Zuidema, GD: Proximal bile duct tumors: surgical management with silastic transhepatic biliary stents, Ann Surg 196:412, 1982.
12. Campanale, RP: Reliability and sensitivity of frozen-section pancreatic biopsy, Arch Surg 120:283, 1985.
13. Couinaud, C: Le Foie: etudes anatomiques et chirurgicales, Paris, 1957, Masson.
14. Finlay, IG, and McArdle, CS: Occult hepatic metastases in colorectal carcinoma, Br J Surg 73:732, 1986.
15. Fortner, JG: Regional pancreatectomy for cancer of the pancreas, ampulla and other related sites: tumor sampling and results, Ann Surg 199:418, 1984.
16. Kairaluoma, MI, et al: Impact of new imaging techniques on survival in cancer of the head of the pancreas and the periampullary region, Acta Chir Scand 151:69, 1985.
17. Leese, T, et al: Management of acute cholangitis and the impact of endoscopic sphincterotomy, Br J Surg 73:988, 1986.
18. Lewis, WD, et al: Avoidance of transhepatic drainage prior to hepatico-jejunostomy for obstruction of the biliary tract, Surg Gynecol Obstet 165:381, 1987.
19. Martin, DF, and Tweedle, DEF: Endoscopic management of common duct stones without cholecystectomy, Br J Surg 74:209, 1987.
20. McLoughlin, MJ, et al: Fine needle aspiration biopsy of malignant lesions in and around the pancreas, Cancer 41:2418, 1978.
21. McPherson, GAD, et al: Pre-operative percutaneous transhepatic biliary drainage: the results of a controlled trial, Br J Surg 71:371, 1984.
22. Neoptolemos, JP, Hofmann, AE, and Moossa, AR: Chemical treatment of stones in the biliary tree, Br J Surg 73:515, 1986.
23. Nix, GAJJ, et al: Carcinoma of the head of the pancreas: therapeutic implications of endoscopic retrograde cholangiopancreatography findings, Gastroenterology 87:37, 1984.
24. Pitt, HA, et al: Does preoperative percutaneous biliary drainage reduce operative risk or increase hospital cost? Ann Surg 201:545, 1985.
25. Rashleigh-Belcher, HJC, Russell, RCG, and Lees, WR: Cutaneous seeding of pancreatic carcinoma by fine-needle aspiration biopsy, Br J Radiol 59:182, 1986.
26. Robertson, DAF, et al: Experiences with a combined percutaneous and endoscopic approach to stent insertion in malignant obstructive jaundice, Lancet 2:1449, 1987.
27. Sarr, MG, and Cameron, JL: Surgical management of unresectable carcinoma of the pancreas, Surgery 91:123, 1982.
28. Smith, RC, et al: Preoperative percutaneous transhepatic internal drainage in obstructive jaundice: a randomised, controlled trial examining renal function, Surgery 97:641, 1985.
29. Speer, AG, et al: Randomised trial of endoscopic versus percutaneous stent insertion in malignant obstructive jaundice, Lancet 2:57, 1987.
30. Todoroki, T, et al: Gross appearance of carcinoma of the main hepatic duct and its prognosis, Surg Gynecol Obstet 150:33, 1980.
31. Traynor, O, Castaing, D, and Bismuth, H: Left intrahepatic cholangio-enteric anastomosis (round ligament approach): an effective palliative treatment for hilar cancers, Br J Surg 74:952, 1987.
32. Trede, M: The surgical treatment of pancreatic carcinoma, Surgery 97:28, 1985.
33. Warshaw, AL, Tepper, JE, and Shipley, WU: Laparoscopy in the staging and planning of therapy for pancreatic cancer, Am J Surg 151:76, 1986.
34. Weiss, SL, et al: Mirizzi syndrome simulating a tumor by ERC, Dig Dis Sci 31:100, 1986.
35. Yamamoto, R, et al: Histocytologic diagnosis of pancreatic cancer by percutaneous aspiration biopsy under ultrasonic guidance, Am J Clin Pathol 83:409, 1985.

INDEX

Electropapillotomy, percutaneous antegrade, 2050
Elimination of drugs, 121-122
Embolism, visceral, angiography and, 1889, 1891, 1892
Embolization
    angiographic, 1879, 1880-1881
        pancreas and, 1114
    barium, upper gastrointestinal studies and, 548
    hepatic metastases and, 1938
    lymphography and, 1705
    of pseudoaneurysms, 1939, 1943
Embryology, 215-230
    abnormal, 217-218
    diaphragm and, 228-229
    duodenum and, 223
    esophagus and, 221-222
    gallbladder and, 227-228
    ileum and, 224-226
    jejunum and, 224-226
    large intestine and, 226-227
    liver and, 227-228
    mouth and, 218-221
    normal, 215-217
    pancreas and, 228
    pharynx and, 218-221
    spleen and, 229
Emergency study, duodenal, 545-546
Emission tomography, 62-69
Emperonium, 467
Emphysema
    cholecystitis and, 304-305, 1213-1214
    gastritis and, 298, 299, 562, 563, 585
    interstitial gastric, 586
Empyema, gallbladder, 303-304, 1213
Endocrine cell tumors
    of colon, 883-884
    of pancreas, 1098
        and islet cell neoplasms, 1187
Endocrine cells in gut
    location of, 275
    tumor and, 883-884
Endocrine disorders, 1197-1198
    esophageal motility and, 446
    islet cell neoplasms and, 1187
    pediatric, 1767
Endocrine pancreas, 284
    tumors of, 1098
Endoluminal balloon dilatation of biliary stricture, 2101
Endometrial adenocarcinoma, 1400
Endometrioma, small bowel, 343
Endometriosis
    colon, 885, 886, 1033, 1034, 1077-1079
    double contrast enema and, 161, 164
    small bowel and, 343, 724
Endoprosthesis
    endoscopic retrograde placement of biliary, 2101
    fine-needle aspiration biopsy of pancreas and, 1120
Endoscopic papillotomy, common duct stones and, 2048-2050
Endoscopic retrograde cholangiopancreatography, 130, 1179-1180
    angiography of pancreas and, 1118
    biliary endoprosthesis placement in, 2101
    biliary tract disease and, 1142
    biliary tract imaging and, 1239-1241
    common duct stones and, 2048-2050
    complications of, 1369-1370
    contraindications to, 1367

Endoscopic retrograde cholangiopancreatography—cont'd
    correlation of, 1137, 1138
    development of, 1367
    diagnostic and therapeutic potential of, 1367
    differential diagnosis and, 1371
    duodenum and, 680
    functional signs and, 1386
    history of, 19
    indications for, 1367
    jaundice and, 1240, 1241, 1409
    nonvisualized gallbladder during, 1378-1380
    normal anatomy in, 1117, 1368-1369
    pancreas in
        chronic pancreatitis of, 1128, 1137, 1138, 1142
        diagnostic examination of, 1113
        interventional procedures for, 1114
        phlegmon and, 1150
        preoperative and postoperative radiologic evaluation of, 1155, 1156, 1157, 1158
    planning of percutaneous access routes for catheter drainage and, 1148, 1149, 1150
    primary sclerosing cholangitis and, 1257, 1258
    technique of, 1117, 1368-1369
        fine-needle aspiration biopsy of pancreas and, 1120
Endoscopic sclerotherapy, 1983
Endoscopic sonography; *see* Endoscopic ultrasonography
Endoscopic sphincterotomy
    choledochocele and, 1245
    common duct stone removal and, 2050, 2064
Endoscopic ultrasonography, 211, 595
    in gastric carcinoma, 599-600
    in pancreas, 1100-1101
Endoscopy; *see also* Liver and biliary tract endoscopy
    antral diaphragm and, 556, 557
    biliary tract interventional radiology and, 2048-2050
    colon carcinoma differential diagnosis and, 1053, 1076
    diagnostic value of in duodenum, 670
    erosive gastritis and, 557
    esophagus and, 427
        foreign bodies of, 454
        infectious esophagitis in, 463
        monilial esophagitis in, 464
        reflux esophagitis in, 462
        rings of, 470, 471
        strictures of, 474, 475
        varices of, 479-481
        viral esophagitis in, 465
    gastric carcinoma and, 211, 597-600
    gastric obstruction and, 326
    gastric pseudolymphoma and, 564
    gastroesophageal reflux and, 449
    of pancreas, 2078-2079
    upper gastrointestinal, 700
        bleeding and, 545-546
Endothelial mesothelioma, diaphragmatic, 493
End-to-end grafts, 1672
End-to-side grafts
    for aortic aneurysmectomy, 1672
    for aortoiliac stenosis, 1672
    dilatation of small bowel after, 1745
Enema
    air
        small bowel exam and, 177
        ultrasonography and, 201
    barium; *see* Barium examination